What Recent Students and Other NCLEX–RN Candidates Have Said About ADDISON-WESLEY'S NURSING EXAMINATION REVIEW

- "The sample test questions were wonderful! It helped to know what we would be facing in the RN licensure exam."
- "The format is very thorough! The combination of having a review section followed by sample questions and rationales is excellent."
- "The material was well organized, and the tests at the end of the units were an excellent gauge of my knowledge."
- "The concise outline format with many tables and charts makes it easy to read and understand."
- "Very well written and precise. The questions were tough, and that's good. It will make us more prepared for NCLEX-RN. *Keep* this book."
- "The very best—I have several kinds of review books, and this one is the best."

What Faculty Say About ADDISON-WESLEY'S NURSING EXAMINATION REVIEW

- "The test-taking technique section is essential and concise and provides information that is well tested and effective."
- "The Lagerquist text is close to being the ideal review text."
- "Its three major strengths are that it is comprehensive, provides rationales to questions, and is easy to use with the Lagerquist videotapes."
- "The authors have the ability to present complex theories and interventions in a clear, simple, concise nursing process format. The material is superior to all other review books."
- "The Orientation unit is an excellent introduction for the student. It is very easy to read and to comprehend. It sets the tone, gives specific directions for studying, and describes what students can expect in the testing process. The relaxation techniques are very effective."
- "The tables and figures are informative, straightforward, helpful, and clear. The coverage provides a comprehensive overview without burdening the reader with superfluous detail. The material is up-to-date and shows that contributors are active in their respective specialty areas."
- "The Pre, Post, and Prep tests are well written and reflect clinical situations that are reality-based. The clear and accurate rationale provided for each answer is a definite strength of this book and reflects sound test construction."
- "Most of our students have preferred Lagerquist's book over the others because they felt it was more comprehensive, accurate, easy to read, and more attuned to drill and practice if a weak area is identified for further review."

What [illegible] Say About ADDISON-WESLEY'S NURSING EXAMINATION REVIEW

- [illegible]
- [illegible]
- [illegible]
- [illegible]
- [illegible]
- [illegible]

What Faculty Say About ADDISON-WESLEY'S NURSING EXAMINATION REVIEW

- [illegible]
- [illegible]
- [illegible]
- [illegible]
- [illegible]
- [illegible]
- [illegible]
- [illegible]

FOURTH EDITION

Addison-Wesley's

NURSING EXAMINATION REVIEW

Sally Lambert Lagerquist, RN, MS, Editor

Contributing Authors

Geraldine C. Colombraro, RN, MA

Carol Howley, RN, MSN

Sally Lambert Lagerquist, RN, MS

Robyn M. Nelson, RN, DNSc

Janice Horman Stecchi, RN, EdD

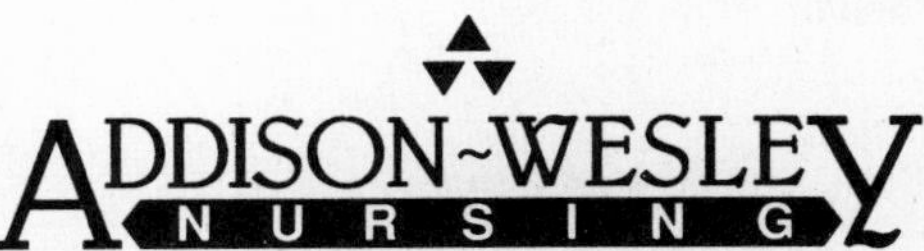

A Division of The Benjamin/Cummings Publishing Company, Inc.

Redwood City, California ▪ Menlo Park, California
Reading, Massachusetts ▪ New York ▪ Don Mills, Ontario ▪ Wokingham, U.K.
Amsterdam ▪ Bonn ▪ Sydney ▪ Singapore ▪ Tokyo ▪ Madrid ▪ San Juan

Sponsoring Editor: Mark McCormick
Editorial Assistant: Michèle Mangelli
Production Editor: Larry Olsen
Book and Cover Designer: Joe di Chiarro
Artist: Elizabeth Morales-Denney
Composition: Harrison Typesetting, Inc.

Library of Congress Cataloging in Publication Data

Addison-Wesley's nursing examination review / Sally Lambert Lagerquist, editor ; contributing authors, Geraldine C. Colombraro . . . [et al.]. — 4th ed.
p. cm.
Includes bibliographical references.
Includes index.
ISBN 0-8053-4002-5
1. Nursing—Outlines, syllabi, etc. 2. Nursing—Examinations, questions, etc. I. Lagerquist, Sally L. II. Colombraro, Geraldine C. III. Title: Nursing examination review.
[DNLM: 1. Nursing—examination questions. WY 18 A227]
RT52.A3 1991
610.73'076—dc20
DNLM/DLC
for Library of Congress 90-14475
CIP

ISBN 0-8053-4002-5
4 5 6 7 8 9 10-CRS-97 96 95 94 93

The authors and publishers have exerted every effort to ensure that drug selections and dosages set forth in this text are in accord with current recommendations and practice at the time of publication. However, in view of ongoing research, changes in government regulations, and the constant flow of information relating to drug therapy and drug reactions, the reader is urged to check the package insert for each drug for any change in indications of dosage and for added warnings and precautions. This is particularly important where the recommended agent is a new and/or infrequently employed drug.

Addison-Wesley Nursing
A Division of The Benjamin/Cummings Publishing Company, Inc.
390 Bridge Parkway
Redwood City, California 94065

Brief Contents

Contents

■ UNIT 2

Nursing Care of the Childbearing Family 116

Carol Howley

■ UNIT 3

Nursing Care of Children and Families 217

Geraldine C. Colombraro

Preface

With a conceptual framework based on *categories of human functions* and an emphasis on *nursing process, Addison-Wesley's Nursing Examination Review,* Fourth Edition, differs significantly from other nursing review books.

PROVEN RESULTS

This book has evolved from more than 20 years of experience in presenting nursing exam review courses throughout the United States. These courses emphasize a comprehensive review of commonalities in client care throughout the life span and in a variety of clinical settings. The content, the framework, the sequence of topics, the test-taking guidelines, and the practice exam questions and answers in this book have been tested during the past 15 years with *actual examination candidates* who have passed the RN licensure exam with highly successful results. This gives the material an authenticity and relevance that is difficult to attain in any other way.

CONCEPTUAL FRAMEWORK

The conceptual framework of the Fourth Edition concentrates on nursing concerns for *client needs* and the essential requirements for safe, effective, competent nursing care. The text emphasizes *practical application* of clinically relevant data. Each unit is organized in terms of the categories of human functions: (1) Protective, (2) Comfort, Rest, Mobility, and Activity; (3) Sensory-Perceptual, (4) Growth and Development, (5) Fluid-Gas Transport, (6) Elimination, and (7) Psycho-Social-Cultural functions. (See Appendix B for definitions of these key terms, and see Appendix C for an index of these key categories in the text.) Separate units emphasize the content areas of *nutrition, pharmacology, common treatments and nursing procedures,* and *ethical and legal aspects* of nursing.

Unlike other nursing review books, *Addison-Wesley's Nursing Examination Review* integrates the concepts of anatomy and physiology with the nursing concepts rather than presenting them as an introduction to disorders. Integrating these principles with the discussion of the steps of the nursing process promotes recall and understanding of their relevance and application in the clinical setting.

NEW AND SPECIAL FEATURES

The new and special features of the Fourth Edition include:

- Emphasis on the five steps of the nursing process, especially *health teaching* and specific outcome criteria for *evaluation* of the effectiveness of nursing care.
- 1990 NANDA-approved *nursing diagnoses* as a structure for presenting nursing interventions.
- Many easy-to-use and easy-to-find tables that summarize information for quick review and emphasize nursing responsibilities.
- New, easy-to-find content divisions marked with black page tabs at the outer margin of each page.
- New *boxed* lab data, and diagnostic tests indexed by a *triangle* symbol in the margin for quick reference.
- A special, thorough question-and-answer review at the end of each unit in a nursing process format reflecting diverse cultural influences.
- New *indexes* to *Detailed NCLEX-RN Test Plan on Client Needs:* Knowledge, Skills, and Abilities (Appendix I), Content Related to Categories of Human Functions (Appendix C), and *Nursing Process Questions* at ends of units (Appendix J) to facilitate review for repeat exam-takers.

This Fourth Edition has been revised and updated to incorporate the latest knowledge and current trends in nursing practice as well as to parallel the latest NCLEX-RN. All content has been submitted to outstanding educators and nursing practitioners for their review and critique. We would like to express our appreciation to this editorial review panel for their contributions, which make *Addison-Wesley's Nursing Examination Review* the best book to use for a *complete* nursing review.

In Unit 1, *Nursing Care of Behavioral and Emotional Problems Throughout the Life Span,* we have included coverage of midlife crises, alterations in self-concept, amphetamine abuse, panic disorders, posttraumatic disorders, dissociative disorders, sleep disturbances, and affective disorders. Psychiatric disorders have been reorganized under DSM-III-R guidelines. New content has been added on suicide precautions and culture assessment, and a chart has been added on reality orientation.

Unit 2, *Nursing Care of the Childbearing Family,* has been streamlined and updated to include the most exam-relevant content for both pregnancy and care of the neonate. The unit contains detailed information regarding many new diagnostic tests, such as chorionic villi sampling and biophysical profile testing, to identify the woman and fetus at risk. We include the latest information on perinatal acquired immune deficiency syndrome, sexually transmitted diseases, and preterm labor. We provide new information regarding drug therapies recommended during the perinatal period, such as hepatitis B vaccination for the at-risk infant. *Client teaching* and *nursing interventions* are delineated for each of these new areas of practice. The question and answer sections also address these advances in technology and care.

Unit 3, *Nursing Care of Children and Families,* includes much updated information concerning cardiac, respiratory, and orthopedic systems that has been synthesized into table format for easier reading, recall, and application to client care. New diagrams have been added showing tracheoesophageal fistulas and the dislocated hip in an infant. New coverage is provided for Reye's syndrome, Kawasaki disease, and Tylenol poisoning. Content includes normal developmental concerns and parental counseling as well as appreciation of cultural diversity in assessment and nursing interventions.

Unit 4, *Nursing Care of the Acutely Ill and the Chronically Ill Adult,* has been updated to present content under appropriate categories of human functions. *Risk factors* have been identified for all conditions, *goals of nursing* are clearly stated, and a brief description of *pathophysiology* has been incorporated with each condition. Tables on fluid and electrolyte imbalances, acid-base disorders, assessment differences with valvular defects, hazards of immobility, complications of diabetes, and malignant disorders supplement the condensed and consolidated content. New content includes acquired immune deficiency syndrome, Lyme disease, compartment syndrome, Crohn's disease, ulcers, external fixation devices for fractures, and lithotripsy. Assessment of the older adult now includes material on the normal changes of aging. The *many new tables, charts, and diagrams* include hip fractures, the Glasgow Coma Scale, breast and testicular self-exam, chest drainage, hepatitis non-A, non-B, preventing TPN complications, and TPN dressing changes. *Nursing interventions* are now grouped according to the goal of care and identify appropriate treatments and drug therapies. More detailed discussions follow in two *special* units on *nursing treatments* and *pharmacology* in Units 6 and 7.

Unit 5, *Review of Nutrition,* now contains new information regarding ethnic food patterns, nutritional needs of the elderly, religious food preferences, and cultural disease treatments involving food.

Unit 6, *Review of Pharmacology,* contains new classifications and drug treatments. Pediatric medication administration and obstetric analgesia are two topics that have been updated and cross-referenced to Unit 4.

In Unit 7, *Common Nursing Treatments,* content on gastrointestinal tubes has been clarified. Many other tests and procedures have been added.

Unit 8, *Ethical and Legal Aspects in Nursing,* contains a new section on bioethics and client rights.

New *Appendices* in this Fourth Edition are Appendix C, Index to Content Related to Categories of Human Functions; Appendix D, Community Resources; Appendix E, Communicating With Clients From Different Cultures; Appendix F, Family Assessment: Cultural Profile; and Appendix J, Index to Nursing Process Questions. Appendix I, Index to Detailed NCLEX-RN Test Plan: Knowledge, Skills, and Abilities, provides references to topics in the NCLEX-RN exam that are covered in the text.

FOUR UNIQUE SELF-EVALUATION TOOLS

This Fourth Edition of *Nursing Examination Review* contains three special integrated tests to help each of you assess your knowledge before taking the NCLEX-RN exam. The *Pre Test* is intended for students to take *before* reading this book. It is a preassessment tool to let you find your areas of strength and weakness before beginning focused study. The *Post Test* is intended to be taken *after* reviewing the material in this book. The *Prep Test* is a new *practice* exam tool designed to give computerized feedback to each student regarding performance compared with a normative sample of geographically distributed candidates who take this test and the NCLEX-RN exam. Students who wish to have this specific feedback should take the *Prep Test* using the answer sheet found inside the front cover of this book. By submitting the answer sheet with a scoring fee in the envelope provided, students will receive a detailed computerized evaluation of their answers, pinpointing areas that need further review. Appendices C, I, and J are designed to guide this review.

In addition to these tests, there are review questions and answers *following* each unit. Their purpose is to help students review each content area *separately* before taking the integrated tests. All questions at the end of units and in the integrated tests have been field-tested for several years with students from all over the United States, with a diverse group of candidates who have successfully passed the exam. These questions have also been reviewed by our editorial panel for appropriateness. The Answers/Rationale sections contain detailed explanations about why a particular answer is best or wrong. We expect that these special integrated tests and review question and answer sections will prove to be an invaluable review tool for each and every student.

In each of the end-of-unit review questions and the *Pre* and *Post Tests* you will find a three-part boldface code to help you understand exactly what is being tested by the question. The *first* code refers you to the part of the *nursing process* that applies to that question: AS, Assessment; AN, Analysis; PL, Plan; IMP, Implementation; EV, Evaluation. The *second* code refers to the relevant *category of human function:* 1, Protective; 2, Sensory-Perceptual; 3, Comfort, Rest, Activity, and Mobility; 4, Nutrition; 5, Growth and Development; 6, Fluid-Gas Transport; 7, Psycho-Social-Cultural Function; 8, Elimination. The *third* code refers to *client needs:* SECE, Safe, Effective Care Environment; PhI, Physiological Integrity; PsI, Psychosocial Integrity; HPM, Health Promotion/Maintenance. You may use these codes to help you answer the questions, or you may cover them up and use them as a guide for review when you find you did not select the right answer. These codes are unique to *Addison-Wesley's Nursing Examination Review.* They are an added study tool to help you assess your strengths and pinpoint problem areas as you prepare for the NCLEX-RN.

DOUBLE USE, DOUBLE VALUE

Many students find *Addison-Wesley's Nursing Examination Review* to be an ideal study tool for all undergraduate courses. Using this book in the last semester or two of your nursing program can help you study nursing content so that the material is familiar to you by the time you review for NCLEX-RN. The more questions you answer for practice, the better prepared you will be. This book can save you time—*now* when studying for nursing school exams and *later* when you are preparing for the licensure exam.

Now please turn to the Orientation section on page 1 for further information about the NCLEX-RN exam. My very best wishes on your successful exam results!

Sally L. Lagerquist

List of Figures

List of Tables

■ About the Authors

■ Sally Lambert Lagerquist, RN, MS

Sally Lambert Lagerquist is founder and president of Review for Nurses, Inc. and Review for Nurses Tapes Company of San Francisco. She is the author and editor of *Practice Questions and Answers for NCLEX-RN,* published by Review for Nurses Tapes Co., and *How To Pass Nursing Exams,* published by Review Press. She has coordinated RN licensure exam review courses on campuses nationwide since 1976. She is presently lecturer on test-taking techniques at workshops held nationwide for graduating senior nursing students. She has produced and developed The NCLEX-RN Board Game and audio and videotapes on Nursing Review and Successful Test-Taking Techniques for Nurses. She originated, developed, and has presented national satellite telecourses for NCLEX-RN review since June 1989. She is also a marriage, family, and child counselor and a member of Sigma Theta Tau. She has been a faculty member at the University of California at San Francisco School of Nursing for over ten years, where she also received her BS and MS degrees.

To Tom, my Aquarian lifemate
(23 years so far!)
. . . without whom there would
be no joyfulness.
"Plus qu'hier, moins que demain."
It's time for us to laugh more,
to dance to La Bamba again, to
pick more daisies all year.

To our daughter, Elana
. . . In celebration of your 21st
birthday.
It's time to hitch your wagon
to a star.
"May the road rise up to meet
you; may the wind be always
gentle at your back . . ."
Udu c Bogom, Dochinka!

To our Svensk pojke, Kalen
During this time of transition
for you, with accelerated self-
change, may you learn and accept
the challenge of the symbolic
language of the Viking Runes.
Let their meaningful names and
signifying sounds be "a mirror for
the magic of your Knowing Self"—
intuitively, spontaneously, and
lovingly.
May you always see inner choices.
You become a winner when you learn
from what takes place.

To my mother, Sonia
L'chaim! To life . . .
Take time to enjoy, to add
quality to your years.

To my father, in memoriam
Shalom! In Peace . . .
If only I could have made a
difference one more time, Petyinka.

To Larry Olsen:
We couldn't have done it without your
commitment to excellence and flexibility.

To all the nurses whose paths cross
with mine . . .
You have my best wishes for your
success. May you always take the time
to make a difference in someone
else's life.

Sally

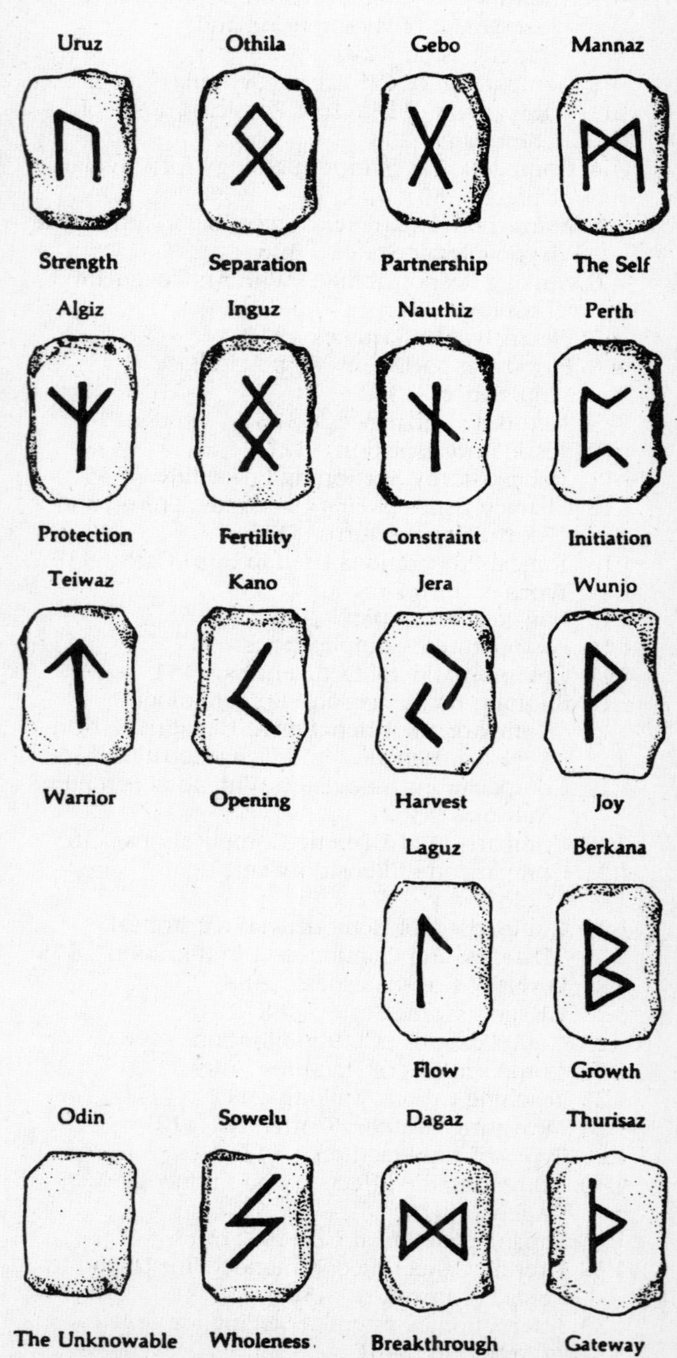

Source: Courtesy of Ralph Blum, *The Book of Runes.* New York: St. Martin's Press, 1987.

▪ Geraldine C. Colombraro, RN, MA

Geraldine Colombraro is presently the Assistant Dean for Continuing Education in Nursing at the Lienhard School of Nursing, Pace University, in New York. She received her BSN cum laude from Hunter College, Bellevue School of Nursing, in New York City, and she received her master's degree in nursing from New York University. She is currently completing her Ph.D. in nursing at New York University. Ms. Colombraro has had extensive clinical and educational experience in the nursing care of infants, children, and adolescents and their families. She has been a faculty member with *Review with Sally Lagerquist* since 1981, during which time she has presented NCLEX-RN reviews throughout the country. In addition, she has taught the first nationally broadcast, live-by-satellite NCLEX-RN reviews since 1989. She is a contributing author to *Practice Questions and Answers for NCLEX-RN* and authored the Pediatric Nursing videotape for Review for Nurses Tapes Company. She is a member of ANA/NYSNA, NLN, and Sigma Theta Tau.

I dedicate this edition to my husband of eighteen years, Bruce, who has given me so much love and support. This book would have never been written, and its contents would have never been taught, without you. Also, to our children, Jonathan and Jacqueline, who have given us so much joy and love. Thank you for helping us always remember what's really important in life.

Gerrie

▪ Carol Howley, RN, MSN

Carol Howley is presently a faculty member at Indiana University. She received her BSN and MSN from the University of Wisconsin and is currently completing her Ph.D. at Rush University in Chicago. She has authored several publications in nursing journals and textbooks. Previously she was a maternal-child nursing faculty member at the University of Illinois and Skidmore College. She has been a faculty member for *Review with Sally Lagerquist* for over eight years. She is a member of ANA, INA, and Sigma Theta Tau.

To my husband Joe, thank you for 18 years of love and laughter.

To my little daughters, Anne, Ruth, and Catherine. Always be happy, look to the future, laugh, and follow your dreams.

To my father in memoriam: I wish you could see what I have become.

Carol

▪ Robyn M. Nelson, RN, DNSc

Robyn M. Nelson is a professor of nursing and graduate coordinator at California State University, Sacramento. She received her BS in nursing from Loma Linda University, her MS from Boston University, and Doctor of Nursing Science degree from University of California at San Francisco. In addition to *Addison-Wesley's Nursing Examination Review,* she has developed a number of audio and visual aids for students and contributed to *Practice Questions and Answers for NCLEX-RN* published by Review for Nurses Tapes Company. Dr. Nelson has been a lecturer for *Review with Sally Lagerquist* for over eleven years. She was also one of the faculty for the first-ever satellite review offered nationally. She holds memberships in Sigma Theta Tau, International Honor Society, ANA, CNA, and NLN.

To my husband, Dean: There will never be a house big enough for my projects, but thanks for trying—I love you.

To my daughter, Kelly: Never lose your enthusiasm for life, fun, and friends, but clean your room first—you are loved.

To my parents, Gordon and Patty: Always interested, always generous, always supportive, and always there—love always.

To Tina, RN, and those students soon to be nurses: Feel proud, feel powerful, and with this book feel prepared—you are the future of health care.

Robyn

▪ Janice Horman Stecchi, RN, EdD

Janice Horman Stecchi is chairperson and a professor of nursing at University of Lowell, Massachusetts. Dr. Stecchi received her BS in nursing from Boston College, a master's degree in education from Salem State College, and her MS with a major in medical surgical nursing and a doctorate in education from Boston University. In addition to *Addison-Wesley's Nursing Examination Review,* she is contributor to *Practice Questions and Answers for NCLEX-RN* and several publications in nursing journals. Her most recent funded grants have been in identifying health status of the elderly post hospital discharge and the development of health promotion materials for minority populations. She has been a lecturer for *Review with Sally Lagerquist* for over a decade. She is a founder and charter member of Eta Omega chapter, Sigma Theta Tau, and holds membership in many organizations, including Who's Who in Nursing. She is a hospital trustee of St. John's Medical Center in Lowell. She has chaired the cabinet on education for the Massachusetts Nurses Association and is a past director of the Massachusetts division of the American Cancer Society.

To Dave, my husband and my best friend: I love you and I know I always will; we are indeed fortunate to have such a special marriage; words will never be enough to say thank you for your understanding and help as I have taken on new responsibilities; I could never do these things without you.

To my three sons, Dave, Bill, and Joe: You bring me so much joy; your sense of humor has always kept things in proper perspective; I hope that you find as much satisfaction in your chosen careers as I have enjoyed in nursing; you have my love.

To Pamela: Thank you for making Bill so happy; it is wonderful finally having a daughter; you are an important member of our family; Dave and I love you very much.

To my parents, Esther and Joe Horman: Thank you for always being there; your continual encouragement has helped me accomplish many things I never thought were possible.

To Helen and Dave Stecchi: Thanks for the greatest guy on Earth.

To all nurses reading this book: There are so many wonderful opportunities ahead of you; my wish for you is that nursing will be as exciting for you as it has been for me; good luck!

Janice

Orientation

HOW TO USE THIS REVIEW BOOK AS A STUDY GUIDE

Although nursing students may know that they are academically prepared to take the National Council Licensure Examination (NCLEX–RN), many find that reviewing nursing content for the licensure examination itself presents special concerns about *what* and *how* to study.

Some typical concerns about *what to study* are reflected in the following questions:

- Since there will be about 372 questions on the exam, how does one select what is the most important content for review? How does one narrow the focus of study and distinguish the relevant from the irrelevant material?
- What areas should be emphasized?
- How detailed should the review be?
- How does one know what areas to review first?
- Should basic sciences, such as anatomy, physiology, microbiology, and nutrition, be included in the study?

Concerns relating to *how to study* include:

- How does one make the best of limited review time to go over content that may be in lecture and clinical notes compiled during two to four years of schooling?
- Is it best to review from all the major textbooks used in nursing school?
- Should material be memorized, or should one study from broad principles and concepts?

We have written this nursing review book with the *general* intent of assisting nurses in identifying what they need to study in a format designed to use their study time effectively, productively, and efficiently while preparing for the examination.

Each contributing author has selected content and developed a style of presentation that has been tested by thousands of nursing students attending review courses coordinated by the editor in various cities throughout the United States. *Addison-Wesley's Nursing Examination Review* is the result of this study.

This review book can be used in a variety of ways: (a) as a *starting point* for review of essential content specifically aimed at NCLEX or Canadian exam preparation, (b) as an *end point* of studying for the examinations, (c) as an *anxiety-reduction tool,* (d) as a general guide and *refresher* for nurses not presently in practice, and (e) as a guide for graduates of *foreign* nursing schools.

As a Starting Point

This text can be used in early review when a longer study period is needed to *fill in gaps* of knowledge. One cannot remember something if one does not know or understand it. A lengthy review before the exam allows students time to rework and organize notes accumulated during two to four years of basic nursing education. In addition, an early review allows time for *self-evaluation.* We have provided questions and answers to help students identify areas requiring further study and to help them *integrate* unfamiliar material with what they already know.

As an End Point

This text can also be used for a *quick review* (a) to *promote retention and recall* and (b) to aid in determining *nursing actions* appropriate to specific health situations. During the time immediately preceding the examination, the main objective might be to *strengthen previous learning* by refreshing the memory. Or a brief overview may serve to *draw together* the isolated points under key concepts and principles in a way that shows their relationships and relative importance.

As an Anxiety-Reduction Tool

In some students, anxiety related to taking examinations in general may reach such levels that it causes students to be unproductive in study and to function at a lower level during the actual examination. Sections of this text are directed toward this problem and provide simple, *practical approaches to the reduction of general anxiety.* For anxiety specifically related to unknown aspects of the licensure examination itself, the section on the *structure, format, and mechanics of the RN examination* might bring relief through its focus on basic examination information.

For anxiety related to lack of confidence or skill in test-taking "know-how," the special section on *test-taking techniques* may be helpful.

As a General Study Guide and As a Refresher for Nurses Not Presently in Practice

Many nursing students will find this review book useful throughout their education as a general study guide as they prepare client care plans and study for midterm and final exams. It will help them put information into perspective as they learn it. And nurses who have not been in practice for several years will find it a useful reference tool and review device.

As a Guide for Graduates of Foreign Nursing Schools

Nurses who are foreign educated can use this book to serve their special needs.

1. To check their experiences, skills, and knowledge for *equivalency* to those of nursing candidates from U.S. programs, in terms of their ability to deliver effective and safe health care as determined by U.S. standards of practice.
2. To identify cultural differences in perception of client needs, nursing responses and actions.
3. To learn the necessary requirements in the various states for application to take the RN licensure exam.
4. To learn about the structure and format of the exam.
5. To learn how to prepare for the exam, including what books to read.
6. To practice taking tests made up of multiple choice questions.
7. To assess the level of language difficulty in reading the exam.

If you are a foreign-educated nurse and wish to compare your preparation with that of U.S.-educated nurses, you will find that the practice questions with detailed answers that are included at the end of each major content unit can serve as an effective self-assessment guide. If you find that you need further in-depth study after taking the practice test questions and reviewing the essential content presented in outline format throughout the book, you may wish to seek assistance from review courses or self-paced review on audiocassette tapes. A list of suggested references is provided at the end of the book to guide you in selecting textbooks frequently used in the United States. In addition, Unit 6 may help you review drugs used in the U.S. that may be called by other names outside the U.S.

Cultural differences may be one cause of incorrect answers stemming from your different perception of clients' needs or nursing action. In addition, Unit 8 contains the code of ethics and standards of nursing practice and legal aspects that pertain to nursing *in the U.S.* We suggest that the foreign-educated nurse become familiar with these sections in order to determine what is *emphasized* in this country. Appendix H addresses important client needs, and Appendices E and F address communicating with clients from different cultures.

To assist the nurse in making contact with Boards of Registered Nursing, Appendix A contains a directory of addresses to write for information about each state's specific requirements for application to take the RN licensing exam.

This Orientation unit is designed to help the foreign-educated nurse know what to expect during the two-day exam, what the exam structure and format will be like, what content will be covered, and how it will be scored. It will also help him or her learn how to study for the test, how to take a multiple choice test, and how to reduce test-taking anxiety.

If you are not familiar with or proficient in taking exams with multiple choice questions, the approximately 1000 sample test questions in this book will provide you with sufficient practice for taking such a test. In addition, if after reading this unit you feel that additional assistance in test-taking techniques or anxiety-reduction approaches might be useful, refer to the Bibliography and audiocassette tapes listed at the end of the book.

If you are concerned about your ability to read and comprehend English as it might be used in the exam, first check yourself by looking at the exam questions in this book. The terms used here are those used in the health care field and are considered to be those a nurse needs to know and use. If the vocabulary is different from yours or is difficult, consult local colleges for courses in *English as a second language (ESL courses).*

Where To Begin

In using this review book to prepare for the licensure examination, the nurse must:

1. Be prepared mentally.
   a. Know the purpose of the examination.
   b. Know the purpose of reviewing.
   c. Anticipate what is to come.
   d. Decide on a good study method—set a study goal before beginning a particular subject area (number of pages, for example); plan the length of the review period by the amount of material to be covered, not by the clock.
2. Plan the work to be done.
   a. Select one subject at a time for review, and establish and follow a sequence for review of each subject.
      (1) Using the answer circles provided beside each possible answer, answer the practice questions following the outline of the selected subject area. (Set a time limit, as pacing is important.)
      (2) Compare your answers with those provided following the questions as a means of evaluating areas of competence.

b. Identify those subjects that will require additional concentrated study in this review book as well as in basic textbooks.

c. Study the review text outlines, noting headings, subheadings, and *italics* and **boldface** type for emphasis of relative importance.

d. Study the content presented in chart format to facilitate memorization, understanding, and application.

e. Repeat the self-evaluation process by taking the test again.

f. Look up the answers for the correct response to the multiple choice questions. Do not memorize the answers. Read the rationale explaining *why* it was the correct response. (These explanations serve to correct as well as reinforce. Understanding the underlying principles also serves as an aid in applying the same principles to questions that may be based on the rationale and therefore phrased differently on the actual examination.)

g. If necessary, refer to the annotated bibliography for other basic textbooks to relearn any unclear aspects of anatomy, physiology, nutrition, or basic nursing procedures. Look up unfamiliar terminology in a medical dictionary.

While Reviewing

1. Scan the outline for main ideas and topics.
   a. Do not try to remember verbatim what is on each page.
   b. Paraphrase or explain this material to another person.
2. Refer to basic textbooks for details and illustrations as necessary to recall specific information related to basic sciences.
3. Integrate reading with experience.
   a. Think of examples that illustrate the key concepts and principles.
   b. Make meaningful associations.
   c. Look for implications for nursing actions as concepts are reviewed.
4. Take notes on the review outline—use stars and arrows, underscore, highlight with highlighter pens, and write comments in margins, such as "most important" and "memorize," to reinforce the relative importance of points of information.

After Reviewing

1. Repeat the self-evaluation process as often as necessary to gain mastery of content essential to safe nursing practice.
2. Continue to refer to major textbooks to fill in gaps where greater detail or in-depth comprehension is required.
3. Look for patterns in your selection of responses to the multiple choice practice questions—identify sources of difficulty in choosing the most appropriate answers.

KEY POINTS TO RECALL FOR BETTER STUDY

1. *Schedule*—study time should be scheduled so that review begins close to the time at which it will be used. Retention is much better following a well-spaced review. It may be helpful to group material into small learning segments. Study goals should be set before beginning each period of study (number of pages, for example).
2. *Overlearn*—many students have better retention of material after they have reorganized and relearned it.
3. *Rephrase and explain*—try to rephrase material in your own words or explain it to another person. Reinforce learning through repetition and usage.
4. *Decide on order of importance*—organize study time in terms of importance and familiarity.
5. *Use mechanical memory aids*—mnemonic (memory) devices simplify recall. For example, in "On Old Olympus's Towering Top a Finn and German Viewed Some Hops," the first letter of each word identifies the first letter of a cranial nerve.
6. *Association*—associate new material with related concepts and principles from past experience.
7. *Original learning*—if an unfamiliar topic is presented, do more than review. Seek out sources of additional information such as those given in the bibliographies.
8. *Make notes*—look for key words, phrases, and sentences in the outlined review material, and mark them for later reference.
9. *Definitions*—look up unfamiliar terms in a dictionary or the glossary of a basic text.
10. *Additional study*—refer to other textbook references for more detailed information.
11. *Distractors*—keep a pad of paper on hand to jot down extraneous thoughts; get them out of the mind and onto the paper.

THE MECHANICS OF THE NATIONAL COUNCIL LICENSURE EXAMINATIONS FOR REGISTERED NURSES (NCLEX—RN)

Frequently, candidates for the nursing licensing examination have many questions about the structure and format of the test itself and the rules and regulations concerning the examination procedure.

As an aid to reducing apprehension and time spent on speculation, this chapter is intended to provide information that candidates commonly seek. The information in this section was verified as correct at the time that it was compiled from a survey of responses by each state's board of nursing registration, as well as from literature distributed by the National Council of State Boards of Nursing, Inc., and the National League for Nursing. If you have further questions, contact the board of nursing in your state.

1. *What is required for admission to the examination center?* In some states a 2- by 2-inch or 3- by 3-inch head and shoulders photo of the candidate must be

attached to the admission card. The photo must be a recent likeness of the candidate for positive identification. In some states, only those holding these admission cards and photos will be admitted to the examination room.

2. *Can I bring any material into the examination room?* No, do *not* take any study materials, including books, notes, calculators, or cameras, into the examination building. You may be asked to place your personal belongings (purses, books, etc.) on tables provided.
3. *Is there assigned seating?* Yes, in some states. At the examination, each table will be identified with a number corresponding to the numbers assigned on admittance slips. The proctor will check your admittance slip and personal I.D. as you enter the examination room each time. You need to find your assigned seat.
4. *Can I bring my own pencil to blacken the circles?* Yes. In some states you must provide your own No. 2 pencil; plan to bring two to three *sharpened* No. 2 pencils with erasers. Blacken the circle corresponding to the answer you have chosen.
5. *What do I do when I finish the test?* You must turn in the test booklet to the proctor before leaving the exam room.
6. *Where do the exam questions come from?* The individual state boards nominate item writers who represent various regions and types of nursing programs to the National Council of State Boards of Nursing, which selects persons meeting the criteria for item-writing to write questions for the RN licensure examination. The state boards administer the exam under the control of the National Council of State Boards of Nursing, Inc. The test-writing service is the California Test Bureau, a division of McGraw-Hill.
7. *Are there any questions with which I may not have had previous experience in my basic nursing program?* Most of the questions are about clients with conditions familiar to you and are representative of common health problems on a national basis. Some questions may relate to nursing problems with which you may not have had prior experience. Their purpose is to test your ability to *apply* knowledge of specific principles from the physical, biologic, and social sciences to *new* situations.
8. *Will there be questions on nutrition and diet therapy, pharmacology, nursing fundamentals, and communicable diseases?* Yes. In addition to questions related to major health areas, the tests will include questions from such areas as nutrition and diet therapy, pharmacology, fundamentals of nursing, communicable disease nursing, psychosocial aspects of nursing, natural and behavioral sciences, legal aspects, and ethical responsibilities.
9. *How many questions does the total test contain?* 360–372 questions. The exam is divided into four 1½-hour parts, with approximately 90–93 questions in each part. As many as 70 questions may be "field test" questions that will not count in scoring.
10. *Are all the questions multiple choice?* Yes.
11. *How many choices are included?* Four.
12. *Do some questions have more than one answer?* No. Only *one* of the four suggested alternatives is the *best* answer. Mark only *one* answer to each question.
13. *What will happen if I mark more than one response to a question?* You will receive no credit for that question.
14. *When I do not know the answer, is it advisable to guess?* Answer those questions for which you *think* you know the right answer, even though you may not be sure. There is no penalty for guessing, which means that leaving many questions blank may adversely affect your score.
15. *Will I get partial credit for selecting the next-to-the-best answer?* No.
16. *May I make marks throughout the test booklets?* No, but you may make marks on the pages provided at the beginning or end of the test booklets.
17. *How is the exam scored?* It is scored by machine. Standardization and conversion tables are used to convert raw scores into standard scores. *Criterion referencing* is the method used in scoring. Please consult your State Board of Registered Nursing for further information.
18. *How much time is usually allowed for each part?* On the first day: two test booklets will be given out, with 1½ hours allowed for each booklet. On the second day: two additional test booklets will be given, with 1½ hours allowed for each.
19. *Is there time for lunch?* Yes, 1 to 2 hours.
20. *What if I need to leave my seat during a test?* You must get permission from the examiner or a designee. Without this permission, your papers will not be counted if you leave. You may be accompanied by a proctor.
21. *How often is the exam given?* Twice a year, on the same date in every state. The scheduled dates for NCLEX–RN are as follows:

1991	February 5–6	July 9–10
1992	February 5–6	July 8–9
1993	February 3–4	July 7–8
1994	February 2–3	July 13–14
1995	February 8–9	July 12–13
1996	February 6–7	July 9–10
1997	February 4–5	July 15–16
1998	February 3–4	July 14–15
1999	February 2–3	July 13–14

22. *Do I have to repeat the entire exam if I do not pass only one or two parts?* Yes. The exam is on a pass/fail basis.
23. *Can the exam be retaken before results from the previous exam are known?* No.
24. *How many times can the exam be repeated?* An unlimited number of times within two to three years in 16 states; other states have limits and may require remedial work. Currently, many states require an applicant to pass in no more than three writings within an 18-month period. However, each state can set its own limits. Please check with the individual State Board of Nursing for the most current information (see Appendix A for addresses and phone numbers).
25. *Does the exam fee have to be paid each time the test is repeated by an applicant?* It varies from state to state. In some states, if it is within one year from the first sitting, there is no additional fee. In most states, a new fee is required.

26. *Do diploma graduates take the same test as associate or baccalaureate degree graduates?* Yes.
27. *Do the different states have different exams?* All states as well as Guam and the Virgin Islands use the examination from the National Council Licensure Examination.
28. *When will the exam results be known?* It varies from six to eight weeks to two to four months, with an average time span of 50 days.
29. *Who grants the nursing license?* The State Board of Nursing for which you wrote the exam.
30. *Will every candidate have the same exam booklet at a given location?* Not necessarily. There may be as many as 30 different test forms distributed at a given time to the candidates.
31. *How is the current test different from the previous one?* Prior to 1982, the exam tested for nursing abilities in ten categories and was divided into five subject areas. The current test plan focuses on *nursing behaviors:* assessment, analysis, planning, implementation, and evaluation. It is *one comprehensive exam* divided into four booklets, with a pass or fail score. The questions test mainly for *application* of knowledge in a given situation and *analysis* of data, not merely recall of facts.
32. *Is the current exam supposed to be harder than the one prior to 1982?* No. The range of complexity level is the same.
33. *Why was the test changed rather than updated?* The implied framework of the former test, which utilized five headings (medical, surgical, obstetric, pediatric, and psychiatric nursing), was criticized as following the medical model rather than a nursing model.

    Also, new information became available from a project that was designed to provide a data base to study the validity of the licensing exam. Eleven thousand critical incidents in practice were collected and analyzed. These were events in which a nurse did or did not do something that influenced the client's well-being. The events reflected current nursing practice for providing safe and effective care and were used as a resource for the new exam.
34. *How is the exam constructed?* The Examination Committee of the National Council of State Boards of Nursing (12 members selected from 53 Boards of Registered Nursing, representing all regions of the U.S.) prepare the test *plan*. The plan is approved by delegates of the National Council (who represent the boards of nursing). States take turns submitting names of item writers (each state nominates every fourth year). Board of Directors of the National Council select item writers on the basis of their credentials and expertise in a particular area of nursing, types of nursing program, and region of the U.S. Item writers may be faculty, clinical nurse specialists, or beginning practitioners.

    For a week, item writers meet as a group, to be instructed by staff of the test service on how to write questions. At this time, no reference books are used to write common clinical situations and series of questions, to ensure that the language of any *particular* textbook is *not* used. *After* the questions are written, current nursing journals and textbooks are checked to validate correctness of the answers.

■ TABLE O.1 Exam Weight Given to Each Category of Health Needs of Clients Based on Job Analysis Study in 1986, 1988

Client Health Needs Tested	Percentage of Test Items
Safe, effective care environment	25–31%
Physiological integrity	42–48%
Psychosocial integrity	9–15%
Health promotion and maintenance	12–18%

After the exam questions are written, they are sent to the Boards of Nursing for suggestions for revision and their recommendation on whether to revise, accept, or reject questions and to rate priority. Up to this point, each question has been reviewed by item writers composed of faculty and clinical specialists, test service staff, members of the 12 participating State Boards of Nursing, and by members of the Executive Committee of the National Council of State Boards of Nursing.

These questions are then interspersed among the four booklets and field tested as experimental test questions at the actual licensure exam. The scores on these test items do *not* affect the passing score. Information attained by this nationwide field test serves to eliminate questions that may be unclear, vague, confusing, ambiguous, irrelevant, or not equally applicable to all regions of the United States.

35. *What is the purpose of the licensure exam?* To test for competencies needed by a newly licensed nurse to perform his or her work safely and effectively, as reported in a job analysis study that reflects nursing practice today.
36. *What does the current exam cover? Nursing behaviors* applied to client situations are selected from all stages in the *life cycle* as well as *common* health problems drawn from the major health areas and based on current morbidity studies.

    Most of the items on a given test (80%) will test for the ability to *apply* knowledge (principles, ideas, theories) and *analyze* data (break information down into elements or parts, set priorities, and see relationships between ideas); others will test for recall and comprehension.*
37. *What is the current test plan?* See Tables O.1 and O.2 for *samples* of how items *may* be selected for testing behaviors in accordance with the established test plan; the *client needs* and *nursing process* are the bases for this test plan.†
38. *What categories of nursing knowledge are included in this exam?* (Comments in parentheses indicate how and where this book covers this content.)*
    1. Normal growth and development (see Units 1 and 3).
    2. Basic human needs (see Unit 1).

---

* *Source:* A new licensing exam for nurses. 1980 (*American Journal of Nursing*, April), pp. 723–725.

† *Source:* National Council of the State Boards of Nursing.

3. Individual coping mechanisms (see Unit 1).
4. Actual or potential health problems (see Units 2, 3, and 4).
5. Effect of age, sex, culture, ethnicity, and/or religion on health needs (sociocultural components are integrated into all units. For special emphasis, see Unit 1, Tables 1.1 through 1.7, Table 1.10, Unit 5 on diet, and Appendices E and F.)
6. Ways by which nursing can assist individuals to maintain health and cope with health problems (see *nursing plan/implementation* sections in *each* unit of this book).

39. *What other concepts relevant to nursing practice are integrated throughout the exam?**
    1. Management
    2. Accountability (see Unit 8).
    3. Life cycle (consult the Contents to see how the conceptual framework of this book is organized by life cycle).
    4. Client environment. (There is continual reference throughout this book related to protection from harm against airborne irritants, cold, and heat; identification of environmental discomforts such as noise, odors, dust, and poor ventilation; elimination of potential *safety hazards;* maintenance of environmental order; and *cleanliness*.)

40. *What weight will be given to the questions?* Table O.1 lists the percentage of test items for each of the four categories of health needs covered on the exam.

    About half of the items will emphasize meeting the clients' physical needs in actual or potential life-threatening, chronic, recurring *physiological* conditions and the needs of clients who are at risk for complications or untoward effects of treatment. Subcategories include (1) physiological adaptation, (2) reduction of risk potential, (3) mobility, (4) comfort, (5) providing basic care.

    The second highest category in terms of emphasis *(Safe, effective care environment)* focuses on (1) coordinated care, (2) quality assurance, (3) goal-oriented care, (4) environmental safety, (5) preparation for treatment and procedures.

    The next highest category of emphasis *(Health promotion and maintenance)* covers (1) growth and development throughout the life cycle, (2) self care, (3) support systems, and (4) prevention and early treatment of disease.

    Finally, 9–15% of the items will be on *psychosocial coping and adaptation* in stress- and crisis-related situations throughout the life cycle.

    Table O.2 shows the weight given to various *nursing behaviors*. Each step is weighed equally (i.e., 15–25% of items will be on assessment; 15–25% on analysis; etc.).

    The test plan also calls for questions that test for levels of cognitive ability. Most items will be at the *application* and *analysis* level but will include *knowledge* and *comprehension*. Weighting (i.e., the number of items assigned to each level) is not specified for these levels.

Source: A new licensing exam for nurses. 1980 (*American Journal of Nursing,* April), pp. 723–725.

TABLE O.2 Exam Weight Given to Various Nursing Behaviors

Nursing Behavior Tested	Percentage of Test Items
Assessment	15–25%
Analysis	15–25%
Planning	15–25%
Implementation	15–25%
Evaluation	15–25%

HOW TO PREPARE FOR AND SCORE HIGHER ON EXAMS

The Psychology of Test Taking

Many nursing students know the nursing material they are being tested on and can demonstrate their nursing skills in practice but do not know how to prepare themselves for taking and passing the examination.

It is not just a matter of taking exams but of *knowing how* to take them, making educated guesses, and utilizing the allotted time in the most productive way. You must learn to use strategy and judgment in answering questions when you are not sure of the right answer. This section discusses practical strategies for eliminating wrong answers and for increasing your chances of selecting the best ones.

1. *Your first hunch is usually a good one.* Pay attention to your intuition, which may indicate which answer "feels" best.
2. *If you cannot decide between two choices, make a note of the numbers of the two choices about which you are not sure.* This will narrow down your focus when you come back to this question. Leave the question; do not spend much time on the ones in doubt. When you have completed the test, go back and spend more time on those with which you had trouble.
3. *Answer the easy questions first.* This is a basic rule of exam-taking. Too often examinees focus on one question for ten minutes, for example, instead of going on to answer 20 additional questions during this time. The main purpose is to answer correctly as many questions as possible.
4. *Be wise about the timing.* Divide your time. For example, if you have 93 questions and 1½ hours for the test, aim for an average of 1 question per minute. Keep working! Do not lose time looking back at your answers.
5. *Exercise care and caution when using electronically scored booklets.* You will receive an exam booklet containing the test questions that will be electronically scored. It is essential that you use the special No. 2 pencil required by the examiners. This pencil contains lead that the electrical grading scanner will pick up. If you need to erase, erase completely. A trace of lead in the wrong space might throw out the answer. Be especially careful to place your answers by the

correct question number. It might be helpful to say to yourself as you answer each question, "Choice No. 4 to question No. 3," to make sure that the right answer goes with each question.

6. *Stay the entire time allotted.* If you complete the section early, check your answers. On a second look (after you have completed the entire section), you may find something that you are *now sure* you marked in error the first time. Also, look for and erase stray marks. If you were undecided between two possible answers on any questions, use leftover time to reconsider those questions.
7. *On the morning of the exam, avoid excessive oral intake of products that act as diuretics for you.* If you know that coffee or cigarettes, for example, increase urgency and frequency, it is best to limit their intake. Undue physiologic discomforts can distract your focus from the exam at hand. Avoid carbohydrates such as doughnuts, which slow down thinking.
8. *Increase your oral intake of foods high in glucose and protein.* These foods reportedly have been helpful to some examinees for keeping up their blood-sugar level. This may enhance your concentration and problem-solving ability at the times when you most need to function at a high level.
9. *Prior to examination days, avoid eating exotic or highly seasoned foods to which your system may not be accustomed.* Avoid possible gastrointestinal distress when you least need it!
10. *Use hard candy or something similar* during the test to help relieve the discomfort of a dry mouth related to a state of anxiety. However, some states may not allow anything on the exam table except the exam booklet and pencils.
11. *Wear comfortable clothes that you have worn before.* The day of the exam is not a good time to wear new clothes or footwear that may prove to be constricting, binding, or uncomfortable, especially at the waistline and shoulder seams.
12. Anxiety states can bring about rapid increases and decreases in body temperature. *Wear clothing that can be shed or added on.* For example, you might bring a sweater that can be put on when you feel chilled or removed when your body temperature fluctuates again.
13. *Women need to be prepared for late, irregular, or unanticipated early onset of menses on exam day, a time of stress.*
14. Exam jitters can elicit anxietylike reactions, both physiologic and emotional. Since anxiety tends to be contagious, *try to limit your contacts with those who are also experiencing exam-related anxiety or who elicit those feelings in you.*
15. *The night before the exam is a good time to engage in a pleasurable activity* as a means of anxiety reduction. The exam involves many hours of endurance for sitting, thinking, and reacting. Give yourself a chance for restful, not energy- or emotion-draining, activities in the days before the exam.
16. *Get an early start* on the day you take the examination, to avoid raising your anxiety level before the actual exam starts. Allow yourself time for delays in traffic and in public transportation or for finding a parking place. Even allow for a dead battery, flooded engine, flat tire, or bus breakdown. If you are unfamiliar with the city in which you will take the exam, find the examination building the day before.
17. *Try a relaxation process* if anxiety reaches an uncomfortable level that cannot be channeled into the service of learning (see *How to Reduce Anxiety,* later in this chapter).
18. When you arrive home after the exam, *jot down content areas that were unfamiliar to you.* This may serve as a key focus for review.
19. If your anxiety level is high *after* the exam because you did not answer every question, remember that *you do not need to get all the answers right to pass.* The exam is not designed for obtaining a perfect passing score. Achieving scores on the high end of the continuum of a passing score on the NCLEX–RN will not earn you a gold star on your license or a differently designated license.
20. Aim to do as well as you can, but avoid the same competitive pressures and strivings to attain an "A" grade that you might have previously experienced in working for school or college grades. Good luck!

Purpose of Memorization

You'll need to memorize some items before you can rapidly assess or apply that knowledge to a particular situation; for example, you need to be able to recall the standard and lethal doses of a drug before deciding to administer it. Items you should memorize include, but are not limited to:

1. Names of common drugs.
2. Lethal and therapeutic doses.
3. Lab norms and values.
4. Growth and development norms.
5. Foods high or low in iron, protein, sodium, potassium, or carbohydrates.
6. Conversion formulas.
7. Anatomical names.
8. List of cranial nerves and their innervations.

How To Memorize: The Strategy of Memory Training

1. Before you work on training your mind to remember, you must *want* to remember the material.
2. You cannot memorize something that you do not understand; therefore *know* your material.
3. Visualize what you want to memorize; picture it; draw a picture.
4. Use the familiar to provide vivid mental pictures, to peg the unfamiliar.
   a. When needing to remember a *sequence,* use your body to turn material into a picture. Draw a person, then list the first item to be memorized on top of the head, the next item on the forehead, and so on for nose, mouth, neck, chest, abdomen, thighs, knees, and feet.
   b. Use what you already know to tie in with what you want to remember; make it memorable.
   c. Use as pegs the unexpected, the exaggerated. Weird imagery is easiest to recall.

5. Use the blank-paper technique:
   a. Place a large blank sheet on the wall.
   b. After you have studied, draw on the blank paper what you remember.
   c. When you have drawn all that you can recall, check with the book and study what you did correctly and incorrectly.
   d. Take another sheet and do it again. Purpose: to reinforce what you already know and work with what you want to remember.
6. Make up and use mnemonic devices to help you remember the important elements.
7. Repetitively explain to another person the material you want to memorize.
8. Saturate your environment with the material you want to memorize.
   a. Purpose: to overcome the mind's tendency to ignore.
   b. Tape facts, formulas, concepts on walls.
9. Above all, feel confident in your ability to memorize!

Strategies in Answering Questions

If you can intelligently eliminate false answers, you can reduce a four-answer question to a two-answer one and thereby make your chances as good as those in the true-false type of question; that is, odds will favor your guessing half of the answers correctly.

We think that the following pointers will assist you to narrow down your choices intelligently.

1. *Always, all, never, none.* Answers that include global words such as these should be viewed with caution because they imply that there are no exceptions. There are very few instances in which a correct answer is that absolute. Any suggested answer, such as:

   Nurses should exercise caution in interviewing alcoholics because:

   (1) Alcoholics *always* exaggerate.

   (2) Alcoholics are *never* consistent.

   should be looked at with care because any exception will make that a false response. A more reasonable answer to the preceding might be "Alcoholics may not be reliable historians."
2. *Broadest, most comprehensive answers.* Choose the answer that includes all the others, which is referred to here as the "umbrella effect." For example, in answering the question:

   A main nursing function in group therapy is to:

   (1) Help clients give and receive feedback in the group.

   (2) Encourage clients to bring up their concerns.

   (3) Facilitate group interaction among the members.

   (4) Remind clients to address their comments to the group.

   Number 3 is the best choice because all the other choices fall under it.
3. Test how *reasonable* the answer is by posing a specific situation to yourself. For example, the question might read, "The best approach when interviewing children who have irrational fears is to (1) help them analyze why they feel this way." Ask yourself if it is reasonable to use Freudian analysis with 2-year-old children.
4. *Focus on the client.* Usually the reason for doing something with a client is *not* to preserve the good reputation of the doctor, hospital, or nurse or to enforce rules. Wrong choices would focus on enlisting the client's cooperation for the purpose of fulfilling orders or because it is the rule. On seeing a client out of bed against orders, instead of just saying, "It's against doctor's orders for you to get up," you might better respond by focusing on how the client is reacting to the restriction on his mobility, by saying, for example, "I can see that you want to get up and that it is upsetting to you to be in bed now. Let me help you get back to bed safely and see what I can do for you."
5. *Eliminate any answer that takes for granted that anyone is unworthy or ignorant.* For example, in the question, "The client should not be told the full extent of her condition because . . . ," a poor response would be, "she would not understand."
6. *Look for the answer that may be different from the others.* For example, if all choices but one are stated in milligrams and that one reads, "1 g," that choice may be a distractor. In that case, you can narrow your selection to the other choices.
7. Read the question carefully to see if a *negative verb* is used. If the question asks, "Which of the following are *not* applicable," be sure to gear your thinking accordingly. You may want to underline a key word like *not* as you read the questions.
8. *Do not look for a pattern* in the answers shaded under a given numbered choice. If you have already shaded four successive answers under choice three for each of the four questions, do not be reluctant to shade choice three for the fifth question in a row if you think that it is the correct response.
9. *Look for the choices that you know are either correct or incorrect.* You can save time and narrow your selection by using this strategy.
10. In eliminating potentially wrong answers, remember to look for examples of what has been included in the *nontherapeutic response* list in Unit 1, Nursing Care of Behavioral and Emotional Problems Throughout the Life Span.
11. Wrong choices tend to be either *very brief* in response or *very long and involved.*
12. Better choices to select are those responses that (a) focus on *feelings:* "How did that make you feel?" (b) *reflect* the client's comments: "You say that made you angry," (c) communicate *acceptance* of the client by the nurse rather than criticism or a value judgment, (d) *acknowledge* the client: "I see that you are wincing," and (e) stay in the *here-and-now:* "What will help now?" Examples of better choices can be found in the *therapeutic responses* list in Unit 1, Nursing Care of Behavioral and Emotional Problems Throughout the Life Span.
13. Look for the *average, acceptable, safe, common, "garden variety"* responses, not the "exception to the rule," esoteric, or controversial responses.
14. Eliminate the response that may be the best for a *physician* to make. Look for an *RN role-appropriate* response; for example, *psychiatrists* analyze the *past,*

and *nurses* in general focus on *present* feelings and situations.

15. *Look for similarities and groupings* in responses and the one-of-a-kind key idea in multiple choice responses. For example:

    At which activity would it be important to protect the client who is on phenothiazines from the side effects of this drug?

    (1) Sunday church services.

    (2) A twilight concert.

    (3) A midday movie in the theater.

    (4) A luncheon picnic on the hospital grounds.

    Choices 1, 2, and 3 all involve indoor activities. Choice 4 involves outdoor exposure during the height of the sun's rays. Clients need to be protected against photosensitivity and burns when on phenothiazines.

16. Be sure to note whether the question asks for what is the *first* or *initial* response to be made or action to be taken by the nurse. The choices listed may all be correct, but in this situation selecting the response with the *highest priority* is important.

17. When you do not know the specific facts called for in a question, use your *skills of reasoning;* for example, when an answer involves amounts or time (mainly numbers) and you do not know the answer and cannot find any basis for reasoning (all else being equal), avoid the extreme responses (the highest or lowest numerical values).

18. *Give special attention to questions in which each word counts.* The purpose of this type of question may be not only to test your knowledge but also to see if you can read accurately and find the main point. In such questions, each answer may be a profusion of words, but there may be one or two words that make the critical difference.

19. All else being equal, select the response that you best *understand.* Long-winded statements are likely to be included as distractors and may be a lot of words signifying little or nothing, such as "criteria involved in implementing conceptual referents for standardizing protocol."

20. *Apply skim-reading techniques.* Read the descriptive case quickly. Pick out *key* words (write them down, if that is helpful to you). Translate, into *your own* words, the gist of what is asked in the question. You might close your eyes at this point and see if the answer "pops" into mind. *Then,* skim the answer choices, looking for the response that corresponds to what first came into your mind. Key ideas or themes to look for in responses have been covered in this section—look for a "feeling" response, acceptance, acknowledgment of the patient, and reflection, for example.

HOW TO REDUCE ANXIETY

Most people have untapped inner resources for achieving relaxation and tension-release in stressful situations (such as during an examination) when they need to function at their highest potential. The goal of this discussion is to help you experience a self-guided approach to reducing your anxiety level to one that is compatible with learning and high performance.

In anxiety-producing settings whenever you feel overwhelmed or blocked, a fantasy experience can be of help in mastering the rising anxiety by promoting a feeling of calm, detached awareness and a sense of deeper personal coping resources. Through the fantasy you can gain access to a zone of *tranquility* in the center of your being. Guided imagery often carries with it feelings of serenity, warmth, and comfort.

Fantasy experiences are, of course, highly individual. Techniques that help one person experience serenity may frustrate another. Try out the self-guided experiences suggested here, make up your own, and select ones that are best for you. There are endless possibilities for fantasy journeys. The best approach is to work with whatever fantasy occurs to you at the moment. The ideas for a journey presented here are meant to be a springboard for variations of your own.

A fantasy will be more effective if you take as comfortable a physical position as possible, with eyes closed and attention focused on the inner experience. Get in touch with physical sensations, your pattern and rate of breathing, your heart beat, and pressure points of your body as it comes in contact with the chair and floor.

When you take a fantasy journey by yourself, it is important for you to read over the instructions several times so that you will be able to recall the overall structure of the fantasy. *Then,* close your eyes and take your trip without concern for following the instructions in detail.

Progressive Relaxation

Relaxation approaches are used in a variety of anxiety states whenever stress interferes with the ability to function.

Progressive relaxation training was originated in 1929 by Dr. Edmund Jacobson. It is a technique for attaining self-control over skeletal muscles in order to induce low-level tonus in the major muscle groups. The approach involves learning systematically and sequentially to tense and relax various muscle groups throughout the body.

The *objectives* of this approach are to soothe nerves, combat hypertonus in muscles, and substitute relaxing activities for stressful ones in order to feel comfortable in and more alert to the internal and external environments.

The *theory* behind this method takes as its basis the idea that muscular relaxation and anxiety states produce directly opposite physiologic effects and thus cannot coexist. In other words, it is not possible to be tense in any body part that is completely relaxed.

The *physiologic changes* during relaxation include decreased oxygen consumption, decreased carbon dioxide elimination, and decreased respiratory rate.

The basic factors vital to eliciting a relaxation response include:

1. *Quiet setting*—eliminate unnecessary internal and external stimuli.
2. *Passive, "let-it-happen" attitude*—empty your mind of thoughts and distractions.
3. *Comfortable position*—sit or recline in one position for 20 minutes or so.
4. *Constant stimulus on which to focus*—a repetitive sound, constant gaze on an object or image, or attention to one's own breathing pattern.

Relaxation training is a procedure that can be defined, specified, and memorized until you can go through the exercises mechanically. If you regularly practice relaxation, you will be able to cope more effectively with difficult situations by reaping the physiologic and psychologic benefits of a balanced and relaxed state.

Instructions

- Sit comfortably in a chair. Shut your eyes and chase your thoughts for a minute; go where your thoughts go.
- Then, let the words go. Becomes aware of how you *feel*, here and now, not how you would like to feel.
- Shift your awareness to your feet. Do not move them. Become aware of what they are doing.
- Spend 20 to 30 seconds focusing progressively on different parts of your body. Relax each part in turn:

  Relax each of your toes; the tops of your feet; the arch of each foot; the insteps, balls, and heels; your ankles, calves, knees, thighs, and buttocks. Become aware of how your body is contacting the chair in which you are sitting. Let go of your abdominal and chest muscles; relax your back. Release the tension in your shoulders, arms, elbows, forearms, wrists, hands, and each finger in turn; relax the muscles in your throat, lips, and cheeks. Wrinkle your nose; relax your eyelids and eyebrows (first one and then the other); relax the muscles in your forehead and top and back of your head. Relax your whole body.

  Concentrate on your breathing: become aware of how you breathe. Allow yourself to inhale and exhale in your usual way. Become aware of the depth of your breathing. Are you expanding the lungs all the way? Or is your breathing shallow? Increase your depth of breathing. Now focus on the rate at which you are breathing. See if you can slow the rate down. When you breathe in, can you feel an inflow of energy that fills your entire body?

- Now concentrate on the sounds in the room.
- Focus on how you feel right now.
- Slowly open your eyes.

Suggestions for Additional Experiential Vignettes

- Imagine yourself leaving the room. In your mind's eye go through the city and over the fields. Come to a meadow covered with fresh, new grass and flowers. Look out on the meadow and focus on what you see, hear, smell, and feel. Walk through the meadow. See the length and greenness of the grass; see the brilliance and feel the warmth of the sunlight.
- For a more expansive feeling, visualize a mountain in the distance. Fantasize going to the country and slowly ascending a mountain. Walk through a forest. Climb to the top until at last you reach a height where you can see forever. Experience your awareness.
- Focus on a memory of a beautiful place you have been to, enjoyed, and would like to enjoy again. Be there; experience it.
- Imagine that you are floating on your back down a river. It may help at first to breathe deeply and feel yourself sinking. Visualize that you are coming out on a gentle river that is slowly winding its way through a beautiful forest. The sun is out and the rays feel warm on your skin. You pass trees and meadows of beautiful flowers. Smell the grass and flowers. Hear the birds. Look up in the blue sky; see the lazy tufts of clouds floating by. Leave the river and walk across the meadow. Enjoy the grass around your ankles. Come to a large tree . . .

Fill in the rest of the trip—what do you see now? Where do you want to go from here?

Sally L. Lagerquist

UNIT

1 Nursing Care of Behavioral and Emotional Problems Throughout the Life Span

The chief *objective* of this unit is to highlight the most commonly observed behavioral, emotional problems and disorders in the mental health field, as well as coping behaviors during the life span. The emphasis is on (a) main points for *assessment,* (b) *analysis* of data based on underlying *basic concepts and general principles* drawn from a psychodynamic and interpersonal theoretical framework, and (c) *nursing interventions* based on the therapeutic use of self as the cornerstone of a helping process. Nursing actions are listed in *priority* whenever possible. Hence the **nursing process framework** is followed throughout. Note that nursing interventions are divided into *planning* and *implementation* (covering long-term and short-term *goals* and stressing *priority* of actions) and *health teaching. Evaluation* of results is listed separately, although this step of the nursing process is circular and relates back to "assessment" and "goals."

I recognize that the categorization of psychiatric-emotional disorders can be complex and controversial. For purposes of clarity and simplicity, an attempt has been made here to capsulize many theoretical principles and component skills of the helping process that these disorders have *in common.* The term *client* has replaced *patient* to reflect the interpersonal rather than medical model of psychiatric nursing. The diagnostic categorization of disorders (based on a synthesis of NANDA and PND-I classification system for psychiatric nursing diagnoses)* is included here to update the reader in current terminology in the mental health field.

The underlying organizational framework for this unit is based on applicable **categories of human functions** (Growth and Development; Protective Functions; Comfort, Rest, Activity, and Mobility; Sensory-Perceptual Functions; and Psycho-Social-Cultural Functions; see Appendices B and C).

These categories have been incorporated into the diagnostic profile sent to the NCLEX–RN examinees as part of a report of their performance on the licensure exam. The categories reflect four **client needs** and are based on clusters of nursing activities designed to meet these needs; for example, protecting the clients, assisting clients with mobility needs.

■ GROWTH AND DEVELOPMENT

MAJOR THEORETICAL MODELS

I. Medical/biologic model (Kraepelin)

A. Assumptions: disturbances seen as diagnosable diseases with classifiable symptoms (or syndromes) that have a characteristic course, prognosis, and treatment.

B. Focus on diagnostic categories, e.g.:

1. Neurosis (anxiety, dissociative, phobias).
2. Psychosis (schizophrenia, affective).
3. Psychophysiologic.
4. Personality disorders.

C. Caused by organic conditions, such as:

1. Arrested mental development (Down syndrome).

* *Source:* ANA Classification of Individual Human Responses of Concern for Psychiatric Mental Health Nursing Practice (PND-I), 1986.

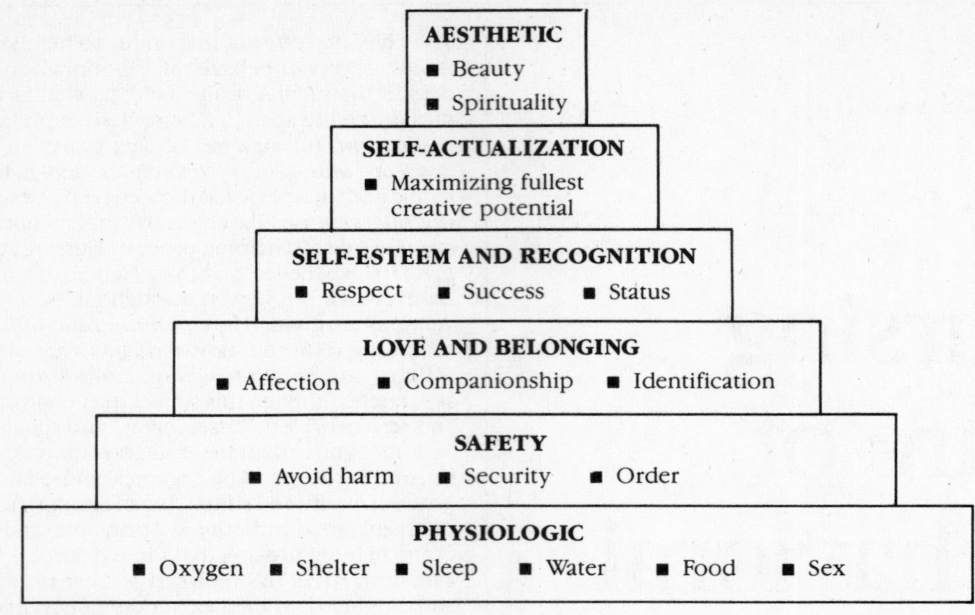

■ **FIGURE 1.1**
Maslow's hierarchy of needs.

3. Infectious (meningitis, tertiary syphilis).
4. Metabolic (hepatic and renal failure, COPD).
5. Drug-induced (alcoholism, LSD).
6. Neoplasm (cancer of the brain).
7. Traumatic (blow on the head).
8. Endocrine (thyroid disease).

II. Psychodynamic model (Freud)

A. Assumptions and key ideas

1. No human behavior is accidental; each psychic event is determined by preceding ones.
2. Unconscious mental processes occur with very great frequency and significance.
3. Psychoanalysis is used to uncover childhood trauma, which may involve conflict and repressed feelings.
4. Psychoanalytic methods are used: therapeutic alliance, transference, regression, dream association, catharsis.

B. *Freud*—shifted from classification of behavior to understanding and explaining in psychologic terms and changing behavior under structured conditions.

1. Structure of the mind: id, ego, superego; unconscious, preconscious, conscious.
2. Stages of psychosexual development (Table 1.1).
3. Coping mechanisms. (Refer to sections on coping mechanisms and glossary in this unit.)

III. Psychosocial development model (Erikson, Maslow, Piaget, Duvall)

A. *Erik Erikson—Eight Stages of Man* (1963)

1. Psychosocial development—interplay of biology with social factors, encompassing total life span, from birth to death, in progressive developmental tasks.
2. *Stages of life cycle*—life consists of a series of developmental phases (Table 1.2). (See also Table 1.4 for comparison summary.)
   a. Universal sequence of biologic, social, psychologic events.

■ **TABLE 1.1** **Freud's Stages of Psychosexual Development**

Stage	Age	Behaviors
Oral	Birth–1 year	Dependency and oral gratification.
Anal	1–3 years	Creativity, stinginess, cruelty, cleanliness, self-control, punctuality.
Phallic or Oedipal	3–6 years	Sexual, aggressive feelings; guilt.
Latency	6–12 years	Reactivation of pregenital impulses; intellectual and social growth.
Genital	12–18 years	Displacement of pregenital impulses; learns responsibility for self; establishes identity.

■ **TABLE 1.2** **Erikson's Stages of the Life Cycle**

Age and Stage of Development	Conflict Areas Needing Resolution	Evaluation: Result of Resolution/Nonresolution
Infancy (birth–18 months)	Trust	Shows affection, gratification, recognition; trusts self and others; begins to tolerate frustrations; develops *hope.*
	Mistrust	Withdrawn, alienated.
Early childhood (18 months–3 years)	Autonomy	Cooperative, self-controlled, self-expressive, can delay gratification; develops *will.*
	Shame and doubt	Exaggerated self-restraint; defiance; compulsive; overly compliant.
Late childhood (3–5 years)	Initiative	Realistic goals; can evaluate self; explorative; imitates adult, shows imagination; tests reality; anticipates roles; develops *purpose,* self-motivation.
	Guilt	Self-imposed restrictions relative to jealousy, guilt, and denial.
School age (5–12 years)	Industry	Sense of duty; acquires social and school *competencies;* persevering in real tasks.
	Inferiority	School and social drop-out; social loner; incompetent.
Adolescence (12–18 years)	Identity	Has ideologic commitments, self-actualizing; sense of self; experiments with roles; experiences sexual polarizations; develops *fidelity.*
	Role diffusion	Ambivalent, confused, indecisive; may act out (antisocial acts).
Young adulthood (18–25 years)	Intimacy, solidarity	Makes commitments to love and work relationships; able to sustain mutual *love* relationships.
	Isolation	Superficial, impersonal, biased.
Adulthood (25–60 years)	Generativity	Productive, creative, procreative, concerned for others; develops *care.*
	Self-absorption, stagnation	Self-indulgent.
Late adulthood (60 years–death)	Ego integrity	Appreciates past, present, and future; self-acceptance of own contribution to others, of own self-worth, and of changes in life-style and life cycle; can face "not being"; develops *wisdom.*
	Despair	Preoccupied with loss of hope, of purpose; contemptuous, fears death.

b. Each person experiences a series of normative conflicts and crises and thus needs to accomplish specific psychosocial tasks.

c. Two opposing energies (positive and negative forces) coexist and need to be synthesized.

d. How each age-specific task is accomplished influences the developmental progress of the next phase and the ability to deal with life.

B. *Abraham Maslow—Hierarchy of Needs* (1962)

1. Beliefs regarding emotional health based on a comprehensive, multidisciplinary approach to human problems, involving all aspects of functioning.
   a. *Premise:* mental illness cannot be understood without prior knowledge of mental health.
   b. *Focus:* positive aspects of human behavior (e.g., contentment, joy, happiness).
2. *Hierarchy of needs:* as each stage is mastered, the next stage becomes dominant (Figure 1.1).
3. *Characteristics of optimal mental health*—keep in mind that wellness is on a continuum with cultural variations.
   a. *Self-esteem:* entails self-confidence and self-acceptance.
   b. *Self-knowledge:* involves accurate self-perception of strengths and limitations.
   c. *Satisfying interpersonal relationships:* able to meet reciprocal emotional needs through collaboration rather than exploitation or power struggles or jealousy; able to make full commitments in close relationships.
   d. *Environmental mastery:* can adapt, change, and solve problems effectively; can make decisions, choose from alternatives, and predict consequences. Actions are conscious, not impulsive.
   e. *Stress management:* can delay seeking gratification and relief; does not blame or dwell on past; assumes self-responsibility; either modifies own expectations, seeks substitutes, or withdraws from stressful situation when cannot reduce stress.

C. *Jean Piaget—Cognitive and Intellectual Development* (1963)

1. **Assumptions**—child development is steered by interaction of environmental and genetic influences; therefore focus is on environmental and social forces (Table 1.3). (See also Table 1.4 for comparison with other theories.)
2. **Key concepts**
   a. *Assimilation*—process of acquiring new knowledge, skills, and insights by using what they already know and have.

TABLE 1.3 Piaget's Age-Specific Developmental Levels

Age	Stage	Abilities
Infancy–2 years	Sensorimotor	Preverbal; uses all senses; coordinates simple motor actions.
2–4 years	Preconceptual	Can use language; egocentric; imitation in play, parallel play.
4–7 years	Intuitive	Asks questions; can use symbols and associate subjects with concepts.
7–11 years	Concrete	Sees relationships, aware of viewpoints; understands cause and effect; can make conclusions; solves concrete problems.
11 years and on	Formal operational thought	Abstract and conceptual thinking; can check ideas, thoughts, and beliefs; lives in present and nonpresent; can use formal logic and scientific reasoning.

b. *Accommodation*—adjusts to change by solving previously unsolvable problems because of newly assimilated knowledge.

c. *Adaptation*—coping process to handle environmental demands.

D. *E. M. Duvall—Family Development* (1971)—developmental tasks are family-oriented, presented in eight stages throughout the life cycle:

1. *Married couple*
   a. Establishing relationship.
   b. Defining mutual goals.
   c. Developing intimacy: issues of dependence-independence–interdependence.
   d. Establishing mutually satisfying relationship.
   e. Negotiating boundaries of couple with families.
   f. Discussing issue of childbearing.
2. *Childbearing years*
   a. Working out authority, responsibility, and caretaker roles.
   b. Having children and forming new unit.
   c. Facilitating child's trust.
   d. Need for personal time and space while sharing with each other and child.
3. *Preschool-age years*
   a. Experiencing changes in energy.
   b. Continuing development as couple, parents, family.
   c. Establishing own family traditions without guilt related to breaks with tradition.
4. *School-age years*
   a. Establishing new roles in work.
   b. Children's school activities interfering with family activities.
5. *Teenage years*
   a. Parents continue to develop roles in community other than with children.
   b. Children experience freedom while accepting responsibility for actions.
   c. Struggle with parents in emancipation process.
   d. Family value system is challenged.
   e. Couple relationships may be strong or weak depending on responses to needs.
6. *Families as launching centers*
   a. Young adults launched with rites of passage.
   b. Changes in couple's relationship due to empty nest and increased leisure time.
   c. Changes in relationship with children away from home.
7. *Middle-aged parents:* Dealing with issues of aging of own parents.
8. *Aging family members*
   a. Sense of accomplishment and desire to continue to live fully.
   b. Coping with bereavement and living alone.

IV. Community mental health model (Gerald Kaplan)—levels of prevention

A. *Primary prevention*—lower the risk of mental illness and increase capacity to resist contributory influences by providing anticipatory guidance and maximizing strengths.

B. *Secondary prevention*—decrease disability by shortening its duration and reducing its severity through detection of early-warning signs and effective intervention following case-finding.

C. *Crisis intervention*—see pp. 51–53.

D. *Tertiary prevention*—avoid permanent disorder through rehabilitation.

V. Behavioral model (Pavlov, Watson, Wolpe, and Skinner)

A. Assumptions

1. Roots in neurophysiology.
2. Stimulus-response learning can be *conditioned* through *reinforcement.*
3. Behavior is what one does.
4. Behavior is observable, describable, predictable, and controllable.
5. Classification of mental disease is clinically useless, only provides legal labels.

B. Aim: change *observable* behavior. There is *no underlying* cause, *no internal* motive.

VI. Comparison of models—Table 1.4 compares four theories.

TABLE 1.4 Summary of Theories of Psychosocial Development Throughout the Life Cycle

Freud	Piaget	Sullivan	Erikson
Emphasis On			
Pathology (Intrapsychic).	*Normal* children.	Pathology (Interpersonal).	Both health and illness.
Anxiety.	*No* emphasis on ego, anxiety, identity, libido.	Anxiety.	
Unconscious, uncontrollable drives.	Cognitive development.	Unconscious, uncontrollable drives.	Problems are manageable and can be solved.
Ego needing defense.	Tasks can be accomplished through learning process.	Self-system needing defense.	Need to integrate individual and society.
Pathologic Development Influenced By			
Early feelings. Repressed experiences in unconscious mind.	Individual differences and social influences on the mind.	Unconscious mind *and* interpersonal relationships.	Ego, anxiety, identity, libido concepts *combined* with social forces.
Change Possible With			
Understanding content and meaning of unconscious.	Socialization process to facilitate cognitive development.	Improved interpersonal relationships (IPR) and understanding basic good-bad transformations.	Integration of attitudes, libido, and social roles for strong ego identity.
Age Group			
First five years of life.	Middle childhood years.	Adolescence.	Middle age, old age.
Focus On			
Emotional development.	Cognitive skills.	Emotional and interpersonal development.	Emotional, interpersonal, spiritual.
Psychosexual aspects.	Cognitive, interactive aspects.	Psychosocial aspects.	Psychosocial aspects.
Cause of Conflicts and Problems			
Oral, anal, genital stage problems (especially unresolved Oedipal/castration conflicts).	Faulty adaptation between individual and environment for intellectual development.	Threats to self-system. Disturbed communication process; 7 stages not complete.	Unresolved conflicts, crises in 8 successive life cycle stages.
Prognosis			
Few changes possible after age 5.	Little change in adult cognitive structure after middle adolescence.	Change usually possible with improved IPR.	Change not only possible but *expected* throughout life.
Sexual problems part of disturbed behavior.	Sex as a variable in learning (age, IQ).	Sexual problems are only one type of faulty IPR affecting behavior.	Sexual identity as one of many problems solved by interaction of desire and social process.

DEVELOPMENT OF BODY IMAGE THROUGHOUT THE LIFE CYCLE

I. Definition—"Mental picture of body's appearance; an interrelated phenomenon which includes the surface, depth, internal and postural picture of the body, as well as the attitudes, emotions, and personality reactions of the individual in relation to his body as an object in space, apart from all others."*

II. Operational definition†

A. Body image is created by social interaction.

1. Approval given for "normal" and "proper" appearance, gestures, posture, etc.
2. Behavioral and physical deviations from normality not given approval.
3. Body image formed by the person's response to the approval and disapproval of others.
4. Person's values, attitudes, and feelings about self continually evolving and unconsciously integrated.

B. Self-image, identity, personality, sense of self, and body image are interdependent.

C. Behavior is determined by body image.

III. Concepts related to persons with problems of body image

A. Image of self changes with *changing posture* (walking, sitting, gestures).

---

*From Kolb, L.: "Disturbances in body image," *American handbook of psychiatry,* S. Arieti, New York, 1959, Basic Books, pp. 749–769.
†From Norris, C.: "Body image," *Behavioral concepts and nursing intervention,* 2nd ed., C. Carlson and B. Blackwell, Philadelphia, 1978, J. B. Lippincott Co., p. 6.

TABLE 1.5 Four Phases of Body Image Crisis

Phase	Assessment	Nursing Plan/Implementation
Acute shock	Anxiety, numbness, helplessness.	Provide sustained support, be available to listen, express interest and concern. Allow time for silence and privacy.
Denial	Retreats from reality; fantasy about the wholeness and capability of the body; euphoria; rationalization; refusal to participate in self-care.	Accept denial without reinforcing it. Avoid arguing and overloading with reality. Gradually raise questions, reply with doubt to convey unrealistic ideas. Follow client's suggestions for personal-care routine to help increase feelings of adequacy and to decrease helplessness.
Acknowledgment of reality	Grief over loss of valued body part, function, or role; depression, apathy; agitation, bitterness; physical symptoms (insomnia, anorexia, nausea, crying) serve as outlet for feeling; redefinition of body structure and function, with implications for change in life-style; acceptance of and cooperation with realistic goals for care and treatment; preoccupation with body functions.	Expect and accept displacement onto nurse of anger, resentment, projection of client's inadequacy. Examine own behavior to see if client's remarks are justified. Simply listen if this is the only way the client can handle feelings at this time. Offer sustained, nonjudgmental listening without being defensive or taking remarks personally. Help dispel anger by encouraging its ventilation. Encourage self-care activities. Support family members as they cope with changes in client's health or body image, role changes, treatment plans.
Resolution and adaptation	Perceives crisis in new light; increased mastery leads to increased self-worth; can look at, feel, and ask questions regarding altered body part; tests others' reactions to changed body; repetitive talk on painful topic of changed self; concentration on *normal* functions in order to increase sense of control.	Teaching and counseling by same nurse in warm, supportive relationship. Assess level of knowledge; begin at that level. Consider motivational state. Provide gradual, nontechnical medical information and specific facts. Repeat instructions frequently, patiently, consistently. Support sense of mastery in self-care; draw on inner resources. Do not discourage dependence while gradually encouraging independence. Focus on necessary adaptations of life-style due to realistic limitations. Provide follow-up care via referral to community resources after client is discharged.

B. *Mental picture of self* may not correspond with the actual body; subject to continual but slow revision.

C. The degree to which people like themselves (good self-concept) is directly related to how well defined they perceive their body image to be.

1. *Vague, indefinite, or distorted body image* correlates with the following personality traits:
   a. Sad, empty, hollow feelings.
   b. Mistrustful of others; poor peer relations.
   c. Low motivation.
   d. Shame, doubt, sense of inferiority, poor self-concept.
   e. Inability to tolerate stress.
2. *Integrated body image* tends to correlate positively with the following personality traits:
   a. Happy, good self-concept.
   b. Good peer relations.
   c. Sense of initiative, industry, autonomy, identity.
   d. Able to complete tasks.
   e. Assertive.
   f. Academically competent; high achievement.
   g. Able to cope with stress.

D. Child's concept of body image can indicate degree of *ego strength* and personality integration; vague, distorted self-concept may indicate schizophrenic processes.

E. *Successful* completion of various developmental phases determines body concept and degree of *body boundary definiteness.* (See Table 1.6.)

F. *Physical changes* of height, weight, and body build lead to changes in perception of body appearance and of how body is used.

G. Success in *using* one's body (motor ability) influences the value one places upon self (self-evaluation).

H. *Secondary sex characteristics* are significant aspects of body image (too much, too little, too early, too late, in the wrong place, may lead to disturbed body image). Sexual differences in body image are in part related to differences in anatomical structure and body function, as well as to contrasts in life-styles and cultural roles.

I. Different *cultures and families* value bodily traits and bodily deviations differently.

J. Different *body parts* (for example, hair, nose, face, stature, shoulders) have varying personal significance; therefore there is variability in degree of threat, personality integrity, and coping behavior.

K. *Attitudes* concerning the self will influence and be influenced by person's physical appearance and ability. Society has developed stereotyped ideas regarding outer body structure (body physique) and inner personalities (temperament). Current stereotypes are:

1. *Endomorph*—talkative, sympathetic, good natured, trusting, dependent, lazy, fat.
2. *Mesomorph*—adventuresome, self-reliant, strong, tall.
3. *Ectomorph*—thin, tense and nervous, suspicious, stubborn, pessimistic, quiet.

L. Person with a *firm ego boundary or body image* is more likely to be independent, striving, goal oriented, influential. Under stress, may develop skin and muscle disease.

M. Person with *poorly integrated body image and weak ego boundary* is more likely to be passive, less goal oriented, less influential, more prone to external pressures. Under stress, may develop heart and GI diseases.

N. Any situation, *illness,* or *injury* that causes a change in body image is a crisis, and the person will go through the *phases of crisis* in an attempt to reintegrate the body image (see Table 1.5).

IV. Assessment—see Table 1.6.

V. Analysis—*body image development disturbance* may be related to:

A. *Obvious loss* of a major body part—amputation of an extremity, hair, teeth, eye, breast.

B. Surgical procedures in which the relationship of body parts is *visibly* disturbed—colostomy, ileostomy, gastrostomy, ureteroenterostomy.

C. Surgical procedures in which the loss of body parts is *not visible* to others—hysterectomy, lung, gallbladder, stomach.

D. Repair procedures (plastic surgery) that do *not* reconstruct body image as assumed—rhinoplasty, plastic surgery to correct large ears, breasts.

E. *Changes in body size and proportion*—obesity, emaciation, acromegaly, gigantism, pregnancy, pubertal changes (too early, too late, too big, too small, too tall).

F. Other changes in *external body* surface—hirsutism in women, mammary glands in men.

G. Skin *color* changes—chronic dermatitis, Addison's disease.

H. Skin *texture* changes—scars, thyroid disease, excoriative dermatitis, acne.

I. *Crippling* changes in bones, joints, muscles—arthritis, multiple sclerosis, Parkinson's.

J. Failure of a body part to *function*—quadriplegia, paraplegia, cerebrovascular accident (CVA).

K. Distorted ideas of structure, function, and significance stemming from *symbolism* of disease seen in terms of *life and death* when heart or lungs are afflicted—heart attacks, asthmatic attacks, pneumonia.

L. *Side effects* of drug therapy—moon face, hirsutism, striated skin, changes in body contours.

M. *Violent attacks* against the body—incest, rape, shooting, knifing, battering.

N. *Mental, emotional disorders*—schizophrenia with depersonalization, somatic delusions, and hallucinations about the body; anorexia nervosa, hypochondriasis; hysteria, malingering.

O. *Diseases requiring isolation* may convey attitude that body is undesirable, unacceptable—tuberculosis, malodorous conditions (for example, gangrene, cancer).

P. *Women's movement and sexual revolution*—use of body for pleasure, not just procreation, sexual freedom, wide range of normality in sex practices, legalized abortion.

Q. *Medical technology*—organ transplants, life-saving but scar-producing burn treatment, alive but hopeless, alive but debilitated with chronic illnesses.

VI. General nursing plan/implementation:

A. *Protect from psychologic threat* related to impaired *self-attitudes.*

1. Emphasize person's *normal* aspects.
2. Encourage self-performance.

B. *Maintain warm, communicating relationship.*

1. Encourage awareness of positive responses from others.
2. Encourage expression of feelings.

C. *Increase reality perception.*

1. Provide *reliable* information about health status.
2. Provide *kinesthetic* feedback to paralyzed part; e.g., "I am raising your leg."
3. Provide *perceptual* feedback; e.g., touch, describe, look at scar.
4. Support a realistic assessment of the situation.
5. Explore with the client his or her strengths and resources.

D. *Help achieve positive feelings about self, about adequacy.*

1. Support strengths *despite* presence of handicaps.
2. Assist client to look at self in *totality* rather than focus on limitations.

E. *Health teaching:*

1. Teach client and family about expected changes in functioning.

TABLE 1.6 Body Image Development and Disturbance Through the Life Cycle: Assessment

Age Group	Development of Body Image	Developmental Disturbances in Body Image
Infant and toddler	Becomes aware of body boundaries and separateness of own external body from others through sensory stimulation. Explores external body parts; handles and controls the environment and body through play, bathing, and eating. Experiences pain, shame, fear, and pleasure. Feels doubt or power in mastery of motor skills and strives for autonomy. Learns who one is in relation to the world.	*Infant* Inadequate somatosensory stimulation → impaired ego development, increased anxiety level, poor foundation for reality testing. Continues to see external objects as extension of self → unrealistic, *distorted* perceptions of significant persons, inability to form normal attachments to others (possessive, engulfing, autistic, withdrawn). *Toddler* If body fails to meet parental expectations → shameful, self-deprecating feelings. Failure to master environment and control own body → helplessness, inadequacy, and doubt.
Preschool and school-age	Experiences praise, blame, derogation, or criticism for body, its part or use (pleasure, pain, doubt, or guilt). Explores genitals—discovers anatomical differences between sexes with joy, pride, or shame. Begins awareness of sexual identity. Differentiates self as a body and self as a mind. Beginning of self-concept; of self as male or female. Learns mastery of the body (to *do*, to protect *self*, to protect *others*) and environment (run, skip, skate, swim); feels pleasure, competence, worth, or inadequacy.	*Preschool* Distortion of body image of genital area due to conflict over pleasure versus punishment. If body build does not conform to sex-typed expectations and sex role identification → body image confusion. *School-age* Physical impairments (speech, poor vision, poor hearing) → feelings of inadequacy and inferiority. Overly self-conscious about, and excessive focus on, body changes in puberty.
Adolescent	Physical self is of more concern than at any other time except old age. Forced body awareness due to physical changes (new senses, proportions, features); feelings of pleasure, power, confidence, or helplessness, pain, inadequacy, doubt, and guilt. Adult body proportions emerge. Anxiety over ideal self versus emerging/emerged physical self; body is compared competitively with same-sex peers. Use of body (adolescents' values and attitudes) to relate with opposite sex. Body image crucial for self-concept formation, status achievement, and adequate social relations. Physical changes need to be integrated into evolving body image (strong, competent, powerful, or weak and helpless).	Growth and changes may produce distorted view of self → overemphasis on defects with compensations; inflated ideas of body ability, beauty, perfection; preoccupation with body appearance or body processes, females more likely than males to see body fatter than it is; egocentrism.
Early adulthood	Learns to accept own body without undue preoccupation with its functions or control of these functions. Stability of body image.	
Middle Age	New challenges due to differential rates of aging in various body parts. Body not functioning as well; unresolved fears, misconceptions, and experiences in relation to body image persist and become recognized.	Less dependable, less likable body → regression to adolescent behavior and dress due to denial of aging, defeat, depression, self-pity, egocentrism due to fear of loss of sexual identity, withdrawal to early old age. Females more likely to judge themselves uglier than do males or younger and older females.

continued

TABLE 1.6 *(Continued)*

Age Group	Development of Body Image	Developmental Disturbances in Body Image
Old age	Accelerated physical decline with influence on self-concept and life-style.	
	Can accept self and personality as a whole; continued emphasis on physical self, with increased emphasis on inner, emotional self.	Ill health → fear of invalidism, hypochondriasis. Denial related to feelings of threatened incapacity and fear of declining functions.
		Despair over loss of beauty, strength, and youthfulness, with self-disgust about body → projection of criticism onto others.
		Regression.
		Isolation (separation of affect and thought) leads to less intense response to death, disease, aging.
		Compartmentalization (focus on one thing at a time) causes narrowing of consciousness, resistance, rigidity, repetitiveness.
		Resurgence of egocentrism.

2. Explain importance of maintaining a positive self-attitude.
3. Advise that negative responses from others be regarded with minimum significance.

VII. Evaluation:

A. Able to resume function in activities of daily living rather than prolonging illness.

B. Able to accept limits imposed by physical or mental conditions and not attempt unrealistic tasks.

C. Can shift focus from reminiscence about the healthy past to present and future.

D. Less verbalized discontent with present body; diminished display of self-displeasure, despair, weeping, and irritability.

BODY IMAGE DISTURBANCE—SELECTED EXAMPLES

I. Definition—a body image disturbance arises when a person is unable to accept the body as is and to adapt to it; a conflict develops between the body as it actually is and the body that is pictured mentally, that is, the ideal self.

II. Analysis/nursing diagnosis: *body image disturbance* may be related to:

A. Sensation of *size change* due to obesity, pregnancy, weight loss.

B. Feelings of being *dirty*—may be imaginary due to hallucinogenic drugs, psychoses.

C. Dual change of body *structure and function* due to trauma, amputation, stroke, etc.

D. Progressive *deformities* due to chronic illness, burns, arthritis.

E. Loss of body boundaries and *depersonalization* due to sensory deprivation, such as blindness, immobility, fatigue, stress, anesthesia. May also be due to psychoses or hallucinogenic drugs.

III. Assessment—see Table 1.6.

Body Image Disturbance Caused by Amputation

A. Assessment:

1. Loss of self-esteem; feelings of helplessness, worthlessness, shame, and guilt.
2. Fear of abandonment may lead to appeals for sympathy by exhibiting helplessness and vulnerability.
3. Feelings of castration (loss of self) and symbolic death; loss of wholeness.
4. Existence of phantom pain (most clients).
5. Passivity, lack of responsibility for use of disabled body parts.

B. Nursing plan/implementation:

1. Avoid stereotyping person as being less competent now than previously by not referring to client as the "amputee."
2. Foster independence; encourage self-care by assessing what client *can* do for himself or herself.
3. Help person set *realistic* short-term and long-term goals by exploring with the client his or her strengths and resources.
4. *Health teaching:*
   a. Encourage family members to work through their feelings, to accept person as he or she presents self.
   b. Teach how to set realistic goals and limitations.
   c. Explain what phantom pain is, that it is a normal experience.
   d. Explain role and function of prosthetic devices, where and how to obtain them, and how to find assistance in their use.

C. Evaluation:

1. Can acknowledge the loss and move through three stages of mourning (shock and disbelief, developing awareness, and resolution).

2. Can discuss fears and concerns about loss of body part, its meaning, the problem of compensating for the loss, and reaction of persons (repulsion, rejection, and sympathy).

Body Image Disturbance in CVA (Stroke)

A. Assessment:

1. Feelings of shame (personal, private, self-judgment of failure) due to loss of bowel and bladder control, speech function.
2. Body image boundaries disrupted; contact with environment is hindered by inability to ambulate or manipulate environment physically; may result in personality deterioration due to diminished number of sensory experiences. Loses orientation to body sphere; feels confused, trapped in own body.

B. Nursing plan/implementation:

1. Reduce frustration and infantilism due to communication problems by:
   a. Rewarding all speech efforts.
   b. Listening and observing for all nonverbal cues.
   c. Restating verbalizations to see if correct meaning is understood.
   d. Speaking slowly, using two- to three-word sentences.
2. Assist *reintegration* of body parts and function; help regain awareness of paralyzed side by:
   a. Tactile stimulation.
   b. Verbal reminders of existence of affected parts.
   c. Direct visual contact via mirrors and grooming.
   d. Use of safety features like the Posey belt.
3. *Health teaching:* control of bowel and bladder function; how to prevent problems of immobility.

C. Evaluation: dignity is maintained while relearning to control elimination.

Body Image Disturbance in Myocardial Infarction (MI)

Emotional problems (such as anxiety, depression, sleep disturbance, fear of another MI) during convalescence can seriously hamper rehabilitation. The adaptation and convalescence is influenced by the multiple symbolic meanings of the heart, for example:

1. Seat of emotions (love, pride, fear, sadness).
2. Center of the body (one-of-a-kind organ).
3. Life itself (can no longer rely on the heart; failure of the heart means failure of life).

A. Assessment:

1. *Attitude*—overly cautious and restrictive; may result in boredom, weakness, insomnia, exaggerated dependency.
2. *Acceptance* of illness—Use of denial may result in noncompliance.
3. *Behavior*—self-destructive.
4. *Family conflicts*—over activity, diet.
5. *Effects of MI on:*
   a. *Changes in life-style*—eating, smoking, drinking; activities, employment, sex.
   b. *Family members*—may be anxious, overprotective.
   c. *Role in family*—role reversal may result in loss of incentive for work.
   d. *Dependence–independence*—issues related to family conflicts (especially restrictive attitudes about desirable activity and dietary regimen).
   e. *Job*—social pressure to "slow down" may result in loss of job, reassignment, forced early retirement, "has-been" social status.

B. Nursing plan/implementation:

1. Prevent "cardiac cripple" by shaping person's and family's attitude toward damaged organ.
   a. Instill optimism.
   b. Encourage *productive* living rather than inactivity.
2. Set up a physical and mental activity program with client and mate.
3. Provide anticipatory guidance regarding expected weakness, fear, uncertainty.
4. *Health teaching:* nature of coronary disease, interpretation of medical regimen, effect on sexual behavior.

C. Evaluation:

1. Adheres to medical regimen.
2. Modifies life-style without becoming overly dependent on others.

Body Image and Obesity

A. Definition: body weight exceeding 20% above the norm for person's age, sex, and height constitutes obesity. Although a faulty adaptation, obesity may serve as a protection against more severe illness; it represents an effort to function better, be powerful, stay well, or be less sick. The *problem* may *not* be difficulty in losing weight; reducing may *not* be the appropriate *cure*.

B. Assessment—characteristics:

1. Age—one out of three under 30 years of age is more than 10% overweight.
2. Increased risks of CVA, MI.
3. Feelings: self-hate, self-derogation, failure, helplessness; tendency to avoid clothes shopping and mirror reflections.
4. Viewed by others as ugly, repulsive, lacking in will power, weak, unwilling to change, neurotic.
5. Discrepancy between actual body size (real self) and person's concept of it (ideal self).
6. Pattern of successful weight loss followed quickly and repetitively by failure, that is, weight gain.
7. Eating in response to outer environment (for example, food odor, time of day, food availability, degree of stress, anger), *not inner* environment (hunger, increased gastric motility).
8. Experiences less pleasure in physical activity; less active than others.
9. All obese people are *not* the same.
   a. In *obese newborns and infants,* there is an increased *number* of adipocytes via *hyperplastic* process.
   b. In *obese adults,* there may be increased body fat

deposits, resulting in increased *size* of adipocytes via *hypertrophic* process.

c. When an *obese infant becomes an obese adult,* the result may be an increased *number* of cells available for fat *storage.*

10. Loss of control of own body or eating behavior.

C. Analysis/nursing diagnosis: *Defensive coping* related to eating disorder. Contributing factors:

1. Genetic.
2. Thermodynamic.
3. Endocrine.
4. Neuroregulatory.
5. Biochemical factors in metabolism.
6. Ethnic and family practices.
7. *Psychologic:*
   a. Compensation for feelings of helplessness and inadequacy.
   b. Maternal overprotection; overfed and forcefed, especially formula-fed infants.
   c. Food offered and used to relieve anxiety, frustration, anger, and rage can lead to difficulty in differentiating between hunger and other needs.
   d. As a child, food offered instead of love.
8. *Social:*
   a. Food easily available.
   b. Use of motorized transportation and labor-saving devices.
   c. Refined carbohydrates.
   d. Social aspects of eating.
   e. Restaurant meals high in salt, sugar.

D. Nursing plan/implementation:

1. Encourage *prevention* of life-long body image problems.
   a. Support *breastfeeding,* where infant determines quantity consumed, not mother; work through her feelings against breastfeeding (fear of intimacy, dependence, feelings of repulsion, concern about confinement, and inability to produce enough milk).
   b. Help mothers to *not overfeed* the baby if formula-fed: suggest water between feedings; do not start solids until 6 months old or 14 pounds; do not enrich the prescribed formula.
   c. Help mothers *differentiate* between hunger and other infant cries; help her to try out different responses to the expressed needs other than offering food.
2. Use *case findings* of obese infants, young children, and adolescents.
3. Assess current eating patterns.
4. Identify need to eat, and relate need to preceding events, hopes, fears, or feelings.
5. Employ behavior-modification techniques.
6. Encourage outside interests not related to food or eating.
7. Alleviate guilt, reduce stigma of being obese.
8. *Health teaching:*
   a. Promote awareness of certain *stressful* periods that can produce maladaptive responses such as obesity—e.g., puberty, postnuptial, postpartum, menopause.
   b. Assist in drawing up a meal plan for slow, steady weight loss.
   c. Advise eating five small meals a day.

E. Evaluation: goal for desired weight is reached; weight-control plan is continued.

SCOPE OF HUMAN SEXUALITY THROUGHOUT THE LIFE CYCLE

Human sexuality refers to all the characteristics of an individual (social, personal, and emotional) that are manifest in his or her relationships with others and that reflect gender-genital orientation.

I. Components of sexual system

A. *Biological sexuality*—refers to chromosomes, hormones, primary and secondary sex characteristics, and anatomical structure.

B. *Sexual identity*—based on own feelings and perceptions of how well traits correspond with own feelings and concepts of maleness and femaleness; also includes gender identity.

C. *Gender identity*—a sense of masculinity and femininity shaped by biologic, environmental, and intrapsychic forces as well as cultural traditions and education.

D. *Sex role behavior*—includes components of both sexual identity and gender identity. Aim: sexual fulfillment through masturbation, heterosexual, and/or homosexual experiences. Selection of behavior is influenced by personal value system and sexual, gender, and biologic identity. Gender identity and roles are learned and constantly reinforced by input and feedback regarding social expectations and demands (Table 1.7).

II. Concepts and principles of human sexual response

A. Human sexual response involves not only the genitals but the total body.

B. Factors in early postnatal and childhood periods influence gender identity, gender role, sex typing, and sexual responses in later life.

C. Cultural and personally subjective variables influence ways of sexual expression and perception of what is satisfying.

D. Healthy sexual expressions vary widely.

E. Requirements for human sexual response:

1. Intact central and peripheral nervous system to provide *sensory* perception, *motor* reaction.
2. Intact circulatory system to produce *vasocongestive* response.
3. Desirable and interested partner, if sex outlet involves mutuality.
4. *Freedom* from guilt, anxiety, misconceptions, and interfering conditioned responses.
5. Acceptable physical *setting,* usually private.

TABLE 1.7 Sexual Behavior Throughout the Life Cycle

Age	Development of Sexual Behavior
First 18 months	Major source of pleasure from touch and oral exploration.
18 months–3 years	Pleasurable and sexual feelings are associated with genitals (acts of urination and defecation). Masturbation without fantasy or eroticism.
3–6 years	Beginning resolution of Oedipal and Electra complexes; foundation for heterosexual relationships; masturbation with curiosity about genitals of opposite sex.
6–12 years	Peer relations with same sex; onset of sex play; morality and sexual attitudes taught and learned; phase of sexual tranquility.
12– 18 years (adolescence)	Onset of puberty with biologic development of secondary sex characteristics; menstruation and ejaculation occur. Frequent masturbation. Intense anxiety and guilt may occur over heterosexual or homosexual behavior (petting, coitus, masturbation, VD, pregnancy, genital size).
18–23 years (early adulthood)	Maximum interpersonal and intrapsychic self-consciousness about sexuality. Issues: premarital coitus, sexual freedom. Anxiety about: sexual competency, genital size, impotence, fear of pregnancy, rejection.
23–30 years	Focus on sexual activity in coupling and parenthood; mutual masturbation.
30–45 years (middle adulthood)	For females—peak sexuality without new sexual experiences. Conflict regarding extramarital sex may increase.
	Purpose of Intercourse
	Need for body contact (and procreation until age 35 +)
	Physical expression of trust, love, and affection.
	Reaffirmation of self-concept as sexually desirable and sexually competent due to worry about effects of aging.
	Sexual Dysfunctions
	Men: impotence, premature ejaculation, decreasing libido.
	Women: intermittent lack of orgasmic response, vaginismus, dyspareunia.
	For either or both: changes or divergences in degree of sexual interest.
	Causes of Sexual Dysfunction (Men)
	Overindulgence in food or drink.
	Preoccupation with career and economic pursuits.
	Mental or physical fatigue.
	Boredom with monotony of relationship.
	Drug dependency: alcohol, tobacco, certain medications.
	Fear of failure.
	Chronic illness: diabetes, alcoholism → peripheral neuropathy → impotence; (smoking and drinking may result in decreased testosterone production) excessive smoking → vascular constriction → decreased libido; spinal-cord injuries.
	Self-devaluation due to accumulation of role function losses, sexual self-image, and body image.
	Past history of lack of sexual enjoyment in younger years.
	Causes of Sexual Dysfunction (Women)
	Belief in myths regarding "shoulds and should nots" of frequency, variations, and enjoyment.
	Widowhood: inhibition and loyalty to deceased.
45–60 years (later adulthood)	Menopause occurs.
	Little or no fear of pregnancy; evidence of sexual activity differences in male and female: women may have increased pleasure, men take longer to reach orgasm; may prefer less strenuous mutual masturbation.
Over 60 years (old age)	Activity depends on earlier sexual attitude.
	May suffer guilt and shame when engaging in sex.
	Can have active and enjoyable sex life with continuing sex needs.
	Age is not a barrier provided there is opportunity for sexual activity with a partner or for sublimated activities. Women in this age group outnumber men; single women outnumber single men by an even larger margin.

SEXUAL-HEALTH COUNSELING

General Issues

I. Issues in sexual practices with implications for counseling:

A. *Sex education*—need to provide accurate and complete information on all aspects of sexuality to all people.

B. *Sexual-health care*—should be part of total health care planning for all.

C. *Sexual orientation*—need to avoid discrimination based on sexual orientation (such as homosexuality); the right to satisfying, nonexploitative relationships with others, regardless of gender.

D. *Sex and the law*—sex between consenting adults not a legal concern.

E. *Explicit sexual material* (pornography)—can be useful in fulfilling various needs in life, as in quadriplegia.

F. *Masturbation*—a natural behavior at all ages; can fulfill a variety of needs. (See I. Masturbation, pp. 25–26.)

G. Availability of *contraception* for minors—the right of access to medical contraceptive care should be available to all ages.

H. *Abortion*—confidentiality for minors.

I. *Treatment for STD*—naming of partners as part of STD control.

J. *Sex and the elderly*—need opportunity for sexual expression; need privacy when in communal living setting.

K. *Sex and the disabled*—need to have possible means available for rewarding sexual expressions.

II. Sexual myths*

A. *Myth:* Ignorance is bliss.

Fact: What you don't know *can* hurt you (note the high frequency of STD and abortions); myths can perpetuate fears and such misinformation as:

1. *Masturbation causes mental illness.*
2. *Women don't or shouldn't have orgasms.*
3. *Tampons cause STD.*
4. *Plastic wrap works better than condoms.*
5. *Coca-Cola is an effective douche.*

Fact: Lack of knowledge during initial experiences may result in fear and set precedent for future sexual reactions.

B. *Myths:* The planned sex act is not O.K. and is somewhat immoral for "nice" girls. If a woman gets pregnant, it is her own fault. Contraceptives are solely a woman's responsibility.

Fact: Sex and contraception are the prerogative and responsibility of both partners.

C. *Myth:* A good relationship is harmonious, free of conflict and disagreement (which are signs of rejection and incompatibility).

Fact: Conflict can induce growth in self-understanding and in understanding of others.

D. *Myth:* Sexual deviance (such as homosexuality) is a sign of personality disturbance.

Fact: No single sexual behavior is the most desirable, effective, or satisfactory. Personal sexual choice is a fundamental right.

E. *Myth:* A woman's sexual needs and gratification should be secondary to her partner's; a woman's role is to satisfy others.

Fact: A woman has as much right to sexual freedom and experience as a man.

F. *Myth:* Menopause is an affliction signifying the end of sex.

Fact: Many women do not suffer through menopause, and many report renewed sexual interest.

G. *Myth:* Sexual activity past 60 years of age is not essential.

Fact: Sexual activity is therapeutic as it:

1. Affirms identity.
2. Provides communication.
3. Provides companionship.
4. Meets intimacy needs.

H. *Myth:* A woman's sex drive decreases in postmenopausal period.

Fact: The strength of the sex drive becomes greater as androgen overcomes the inhibitory action of estrogen.

I. *Myth:* Men over age 60 cannot achieve an erection.

Fact: According to Masters and Johnson, a major difference between the aging male and the younger man is the duration of each phase of the sexual cycle. The older male is slower in achieving an erection.

J. *Myth:* Regular sexual activity cannot help the aging person's loss of function.

Fact: Research is revealing that "disuse atrophy" may lead to loss of sexual capacity. Regular sexual activity helps preserve sexual function.

III. Basic principles of sexual-health counseling

A. There is no universal consensus about acceptable values in human sexuality. Each social group has very definite values regarding sex.

B. Counselors need to examine own feelings, attitudes, values, biases, knowledge base.

C. Help reduce fear, guilt, ignorance.

D. Offer guidance and education rather than indoctrination or pressure to conform.

E. Each person needs to be helped to make personal choices regarding sexual conduct.

IV. Counseling in sexual health

A. General considerations

1. Create atmosphere of *trust and acceptance* for objective, nonjudgmental dialogue.
2. Use *language* related to sexual behavior that is mutually comfortable and understood between client and nurse.
   a. Use alternative terms for definitions.
   b. Determine exact meaning of words and phrases since sexual words and expressions have different

*From Sedgwick, R.: "Myths in human sexuality: a social-psychological perspective," *Nurs Clin N Am,* 10(3):539–550, September 1975. W. B. Saunders 1975.

TABLE 1.8 Suggested Format for Assessment Interview

Interview Step	Rationale
1. Open the discussion of sexual matters subtly with an open-ended question: "People with your illness or stresses often experience other difficulties, sometimes with sexual functioning."	This gentle opening lets the client know that other people have difficulties, too. It gives the client permission to talk with the nurse about sexual matters without labeling these matters as problems.
2. Follow up with another open-ended question about the client's current status: "Has your illness or stresses made any difference in what it's like for you to be a wife or husband (lover, boy friend, girl friend, sexual partner)?"	The phrasing of this question enables the client to acknowledge a problem without admitting a shortcoming.
3. If the client speaks of having a dysfunction, ask about its effect: "How does this affect you?" or "How do you feel about it?"	This indicates that the nurse is willing to explore sexual matters more completely.
4. Ask about the severity and duration of the dysfunction: "Is it always difficult to control your ejaculation?" "Tell me when you first noticed this."	These questions are directed at identifying the specific problem.
5. Ask about the effects on the client's sexual partner: "Has this affected your relationship with your partner?"	This question is directed toward exploring the interactional aspects of the identified problem.
6. Ask what the client has already done to alleviate the situation: "Have you made any adjustments in your sexual activity?"	This question yields data that will help the nurse to formulate an intervention plan.
7. Ask the client if and how he or she would like the situation changed: "How would you like to change the situation to make it more satisfying?"	This question conveys the negotiated nature of the therapeutic relationship, in which the client's own goals play an important part.

Source: Adapted from Whitley MP, Willingham W: "Adding a Sexual Assessment to the Health Interview," *Journal of Psychiatric Nursing and Mental Health Services,* Vol. 16, No. 4, April 1978, pp. 17–27.

meanings to people with different backgrounds and experiences.

3. *Desensitize* own stress reaction to the emotional component of taboo topics.
   a. Increase awareness of own sexual values, biases, prejudices, stereotypes, and fears.
   b. Avoid overreacting, underreacting.
4. Become sensitively aware of *interrelationships* between sexual needs, fears, and behaviors and other aspects of living.
5. Begin with *commonly* discussed areas (such as menstruation) and progress to discussion of individual sexual experiences (such as masturbation). Move from areas where there is less voluntary control (nocturnal emissions) to more responsibility and voluntary behavior (premature ejaculation).
6. Offer *educational information* to dispel fears, myths; give tacit permission to explore sensitive areas.
7. Bring into awareness possibly *repressed* feelings of guilt, anger, denial, and suppressed sexual feelings.
8. Explore possible *alternatives* of sexual expression.
9. Determine *interrelationships* among mental, social, physical, and sexual well-being.

B. Assessment parameters

1. Self-awareness of body image, values, and attitudes toward human sexuality; comfort with own sexuality.
2. Ability to identify sex problems on basis of own satisfaction or dissatisfaction.
3. Developmental history, sex education, family relationships, cultural and ethnic values, and available support resources.
4. Type and frequency of sexual behavior.
5. Nature and quality of sex relations with others.
6. Attitude toward and satisfaction with sexual activity.
7. Expectations and goals. See Table 1.8 for a guideline in conducting an *assessment* interview.

C. Nursing plan/implementation:

1. *Long-term goals*
   a. Increase knowledge of reproductive system and types of sex behavior.
   b. Promote positive view of body and sex needs.
   c. Integrate sex needs into self-identity.
   d. Develop adaptive and satisfying patterns of sexual expression.
   e. Understand effects of physical illness on sexual performance.
2. *Primary sexual health interventions*
   a. Goals: minimize stress factors, strengthen sexual integrity.
   b. Provide education to uninformed or misinformed.
   c. Identify stress factors (myths, stereotypes, negative parental attitudes).
3. *Secondary sexual health interventions:* identify sexual problems early and refer for treatment.

D. Evaluation:

1. Reduced impairment or dysfunction from acute sex problem or chronic, unresolved sex problem.
2. Evaluate how client's goals were achieved in terms of *positive* thoughts, feelings, and *satisfying* sexual behaviors.

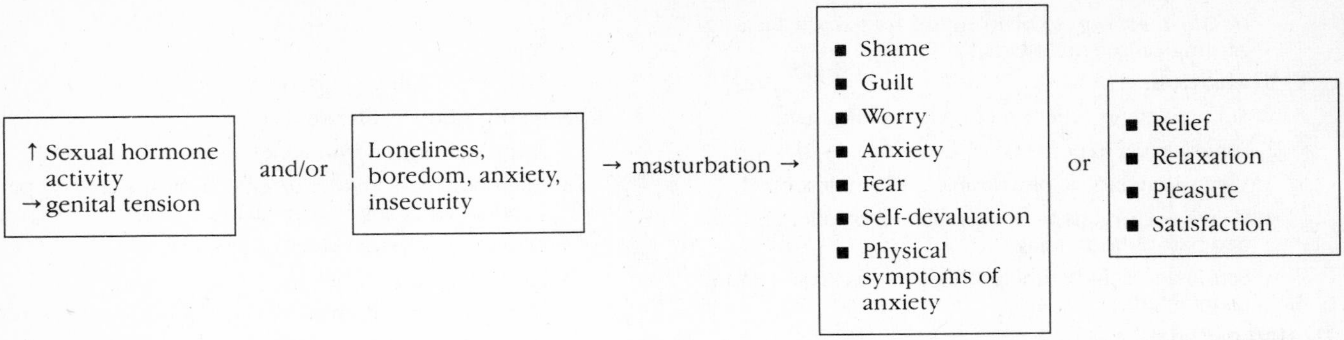

↑ Sexual hormone activity → genital tension	and/or	Loneliness, boredom, anxiety, insecurity	→ masturbation →	■ Shame ■ Guilt ■ Worry ■ Anxiety ■ Fear ■ Self-devaluation ■ Physical symptoms of anxiety	or	■ Relief ■ Relaxation ■ Pleasure ■ Satisfaction

■ **FIGURE 1.2**
Operationalization of the behavioral concept of masturbation.

Specific Situations

I. Masturbation

A. Definition—act of achieving sexual arousal and orgasm through manual or mechanical stimulation of the sex organs.

B. Characteristics

1. Can be an interpersonal as well as a solitary activity.
2. "It is a healthy and appropriate sexual activity, playing an important role in ultimate consolidation of one's sexual identity."*
3. Accompanied by fantasies that are important for:
   a. Physically disabled.
   b. Fatigued.
   c. Compensation for unreachable goals and unfulfilled wishes.
   d. Rehearsal for future sexual relations.
   e. Absence or impersonal action of partner.
4. Can help release tension harmlessly.

C. Concepts and principles related to masturbation

1. Staff's feelings and reactions influence their responses to client and affect continuation of masturbation (that is, negative staff actions increase client's frustration, which increases masturbation).
2. Masturbation is normal and universal, *not* physically or psychologically harmful in itself.
3. Pleasurable genital sensations important for increasing *self-pride,* finding *gratification* in *own* body, increasing sense of *personal value* of being lovable, helping to *prepare for adult* sexual role.
4. Excessive masturbation—some needs not being met through interpersonal relations; may use behavior to *avoid* interpersonal relations.
5. Activity may be related to:
   a. Curiosity, experimentation.
   b. Tension reduction, pleasure.
   c. Enhanced interest in sexual development.
   d. Fear and avoidance of social relationships.

D. Nursing plan:

1. *Long-term goals*
   a. Gain insight into *preference* for masturbation.
   b. Relieve accompanying guilt, worry, self-devaluation (Figure 1.2).
2. *Short-term goals*
   a. Clarify myths regarding masturbation.
   b. Help client see masturbation as an acceptable sexual activity for individuals of all ages.
   c. Set limits on masturbation in inappropriate settings.

E. Nursing implementation:

1. Examine, control nurse's own negative feelings; show respect.
2. *Avoid* reinforcement of guilt and self-devaluation; scorn; threats, punishment, anger, alarm reaction; use of masturbation for rebellion in power struggle between staff and client.
3. *Identify* patient's or client's unmet needs; consider purpose served by masturbation (may be useful behavior).
4. *Examine* pattern in which behavior occurs.
5. Intervene when degree of functioning in other daily life activities is *impaired.*
   a. Remain calm, accepting, but nonsanctioning.
   b. Promptly help clarify client's or patient's feelings, thoughts, at stressful time.
   c. Review precipitating events.
   d. Be a neutral "sounding board"; avoid evasiveness.
   e. If unable to handle situation, find someone who can.
6. For clients who masturbate at *inappropriate* times or in inappropriate places:
   a. Give special attention when they are not masturbating.
   b. Encourage new interests and activities, but not immediately after observing masturbation.
   c. Keep clients distracted, occupied with interesting activities.

---

*Marcus, I. M., and Francis, J. J.: *Masturbation from infancy to senescence,* New York, 1975, International Universities Press.

7. *Health teaching:* explain myths and teach facts regarding cause and effects.

F. Evaluation:

1. Acknowledges function of own sexual organs.
2. States sexual experience is satisfying.
3. Views sexuality as pleasurable and wholesome.
4. Views sex organs as acceptable, enjoyable, and valued part of body image.
5. Self-image as fully functioning person is restored and maintained.

II. Homosexuality

A. Definition—alternative sexual behavior; applied to sexual relations between persons of the same sex.

B. Theories regarding causes

1. Hereditary tendencies.
2. Imbalance of sex hormones.
3. Environmental influences and conditioning factors, related to learning and psychodynamic theories.
   a. Defense against unsatisfying relationship with father.
   b. Unsatisfactory and threatening early relationships with opposite sex.
   c. Oedipal attachment to parent.
   d. Seductive parent (incest).
   e. Castration fear.
   f. Labeling and guilt leading to sexual acting out.
   g. Faulty sex education.
4. Preferred choice as a life-style.

C. Nursing plan/implementation:

1. Nurse needs to be aware of and work through own attitudes that may interfere with providing care.
2. Accept and respect life-style of gay (male homosexual) or lesbian (female homosexual) client.
3. Assess and treat for possible sexually transmitted diseases and hepatitis.
4. *Health teaching:* assess and add to knowledge base alternatives in sexual behavior. Teach specific assessment measures related to sexual activities.

D. Evaluation: expresses self-confidence and positive self-image; able to sustain satisfying sexual behavior with chosen partner.

III. Sex and the disabled person

A. Assessment parameters

1. Previous level of sex functioning and conflict.
2. Client's view of sex activity (self and mutual pleasure, tension release, procreation, control).
3. Cultural environment (influence on body image).
4. Degree of acceptance of illness.
5. Support system (partner, family, support group).
6. Body image and self-esteem.
7. Outlook on future.

B. Analysis/nursing diagnosis: *Sexual dysfunction* associated with physical illness related to:

1. Disinterest in sexual activity.
2. Fear of precipitating or aggravating physical illness through sexual activity.
3. Use of illness as excuse to avoid feared or undesired sex.
4. Physical inability or discomfort during sexual activity.

C. Nursing plan/implementation:

1. Approach with nonjudgmental attitude.
2. Elicit concerns about current physical state and perceptions of changes in sexuality.
3. Observe nonverbal clues of concern.
4. Identify genital assets.
5. Support client and partner during adjustment to current state.
6. Explore culturally acceptable sublimation activities.
7. Promote adjustment to body image change.
8. *Health teaching:*
   a. Teach self-help skills.
   b. Teach partner to care for client's physical needs.
   c. Teach alternate sex behaviors and acceptable sublimation (touching, for example).

D. Evaluation: attains satisfaction with adaptive alternatives of sexual expressions; has a positive attitude toward self, body, and sexual activity.

IV. Inappropriate sexual behavior

A. Assessment: public exhibitions of sexual behaviors that are offensive to others; making sexual advances to other clients or staff.

B. Analysis/nursing diagnosis: *Conflict with social order* related to:

1. Acting out angry and hostile feelings.
2. Lack of awareness of hospital and agency rules regarding acceptable public behavior.
3. Variation in cultural interpretations of what is acceptable public behavior.
4. Reaction to unintended seductiveness of nurse's attire, posture, tone, or choice of terminology.

C. Nursing plan/implementation:

1. Maintain calm, nonjudgmental attitude.
2. Set firm limits on unacceptable behavior.
3. Encourage verbalization of feelings rather than unacceptable physical expression.
4. Reinforce appropriate behavior.
5. Provide constructive diversional activity for clients or patients.
6. *Health teaching:* explain rules regarding public behavior; teach acceptable ways to express anger.

D. Evaluation: verbalizes anger rather than acting out; accepts rules regarding behavior in public.

CONCEPT OF DEATH THROUGHOUT THE LIFE CYCLE

I. Ages 1 to 3

A. No concept per se, but experiences *separation anxiety and abandonment* any time significant other disappears from view over a period of time.

B. *Coping* means: fear, resentment, anger, aggression, regression, withdrawal.

C. **Nursing plan/implementation**—help the family:
1. Facilitate transfer of affectional ties to another nurturing adult.
2. Decrease separation anxiety of hospitalized child by encouraging family visits and by reassuring child that she or he will not be alone.
3. Provide stable environment through consistent staff assignment.

II. Ages 3 to 5

A. Least anxious about death.
B. Denial of death as inevitable and final process.
C. Death is separation, being alone.
D. Death is *sleep* and sleep is death.
E. "Death" is part of vocabulary; seen as real, gradual, *temporary,* not permanent.
F. Dead person is seen as alive, but in altered form, that is, lacks movement.
G. There are *degrees* of death.
H. Death means not being here anymore.
I. "Living" and "lifeless" are not yet distinguished.
J. Illness and death seen as *punishment* for "badness"; fear and guilt about sexual and aggressive impulses.
K. Death happens, but only to others.
L. **Nursing plan/implementation** (in addition to above):
1. Encourage play for expression of feelings; use clay, dolls, etc.
2. Encourage verbal expression of feelings using children's books.
3. Model appropriate grieving behavior.
4. Protect child from the overstimulation of hysterical adult reactions by limiting contact.
5. Clearly state what death is—death is final, no breathing, eating, awakening—and that death is *not* sleep.
6. Check child at night and provide support through holding and staying with child.
7. Allow a choice of attending the funeral and, if child decides to attend, describe what will take place.
8. If parents are grieving, have other family or friends attend to child's needs.

III. Ages 5 to 10

A. Death is cessation of life; question of what happens after death.
B. Death seen as definitive, *universal,* inevitable, *irreversible.*
C. Death occurs to all living things, including self; may express, "It isn't fair."
D. Death is distant from self (an eventuality).
E. Believe death occurs by accident, happens only to the very *old* or very sick.
F. Death is personified (as a separate person) in fantasies and magical thinking.
G. Death anxiety handled by *nightmares, rituals,* and *superstitions* (related to fear of darkness and sleeping alone because death is an external person, like a skeleton, who comes and takes people away at night).
H. Dissolution of bodily life seen as a perceptible result.
I. Fear of body mutilation.
J. **Nursing plan/implementation** (in addition to above):
1. Allow child to experience the loss of pets, friends, and family members.
2. Help child talk it out and experience the appropriate emotional reactions.
3. Understand need for increase in play, especially competitive play.
4. Involve child in funeral preparation and rituals.
5. Understand and accept regressive or protest behaviors.
6. Rechannel protest behaviors into constructive outlets.

IV. Adolescence

A. Death seen as inevitable, *personal,* universal, and *permanent;* corporal life stops; body decomposes.
B. Does not fear death, but concerned with how to *live now,* what death feels like, *body changes.*
C. Experiences *anger, frustration, and despair* over lack of future, lack of fulfillment of adult roles.
D. Openly asks *difficult,* honest, *direct* questions.
E. Anger at healthy peers.
F. Conflict between *developing* body versus *deteriorating* body, *independent* identity versus *dependency.*
G. **Nursing plan/implementation** (in addition to above):
1. Facilitate full expression of grief by answering direct questions.
2. Help let out feelings, especially through creative and esthetic pursuits.
3. Encourage participation in funeral ritual.
4. Encourage full use of peer group support system, by providing opportunities for group talks.

V. Young adulthood

A. Death seen as *unwelcome* intrusion, *interruption* of what might have been.
B. Reaction: *rage, frustration, disappointment.*
C. **Nursing plan/implementation:** all of above, especially peer group support.

VI. Middle age

A. Concerned with *consequences* of own death and that of significant others.
B. Death seen as disruption of involvement, responsibility, and *obligations.*
C. End of plans, projects, experiences.
D. Death is *pain.*
E. **Nursing plan/implementation** (in addition to above): assess need for counseling when also in midlife crisis.

VII. Old age

A. *Philosophic* rationalizations: death as inevitable, final process of life, when "time runs out."
B. *Religious* view: death represents only the dissolution of life and is a doorway to a new life (a preparatory stage for another life).
C. Time of rest and peace, supreme refuge from turmoil of life.
D. **Nursing plan/implementation** (in addition to above):
1. Help person prepare for own death by helping with

funeral prearrangements, wills, and sharing of mo-mentos.

2. Facilitate life review and reinforce positive aspects.
3. Provide care and comfort.
4. Be present at death.

DEATH AND DYING

Too often the process of death has had such frightening aspects that people have suffered alone. Today there has been a vast change in attitudes; death and dying are no longer taboo topics. There is a growing realization that we need to accept death as a natural process. Elisabeth Kübler-Ross has written extensively on the process of dying, describing the stages of *denial* ("not me!"), *anger* ("why me?"), *bargaining* ("yes me—but"), *depression* ("yes, me"), and *acceptance* ("my time is close now, it's all right"), with implications for the helping person.

I. Concepts and principles related to death and dying

A. Persons may know or *suspect* they are dying and may want to talk about it; often they look for someone to share their fears and the process of dying.

B. Fear of death can be reduced by helping clients feel that they are *not alone.*

C. The dying need the opportunity to live their final expe-riences to the fullest, in their *own* way.

D. People who are dying remain more or less the *same* as they were during life; their approaches to death are consistent with their approaches to life.

E. Dying persons' need to review their lives may be a purposeful attempt to reconcile themselves to what "was" and "what could have been."

F. *Three ways* of facing death are (a) quiet acceptance with inner strength and peace of mind, (b) restlessness, impa-tience, anger, and hostility, and (c) depression, with-drawal, and fearfulness.

G. *Four tasks* facing a dying person are (a) reviewing life, (b) coping with physical symptoms in the end-stage of life, (c) making a transition from known to unknown state, (d) reaction to separation from loved ones.

H. Crying and tears are an important aspect of the grief process.

I. There are many *blocks* to providing a helping relation-ship with the dying and bereaved:

1. Nurses' unwillingness to share the process of dying—minimizing their contacts and blocking out their own feelings.
2. Forgetting that a dying person may be feeling lonely, abandoned, and afraid of dying.
3. Reacting with irritation and hostility to the person's frequent calls.
4. Nurses' failure to seek help and support from team members when feeling afraid, uneasy, and frustrated in caring for a dying person.
5. Not allowing client to talk about death and dying.
6. Nurses' use of technical language or social chit-chat as a defense against their own anxieties.

II. Assessment of death and dying:

A. *Physical*

1. Observable deterioration of physical and mental capacities—person is unable to fulfill physiologic needs, such as eating and elimination.
2. Circulatory collapse (blood pressure and pulse).
3. Renal or hepatic failure.
4. Respiratory decline.

B. *Psychosocial*

1. Fear of death is signaled by agitation, restlessness, and sleep disturbances at night.
2. Anger, agitation, blaming.
3. Morbid self-pity with feelings of defeat and failure.
4. Depression and withdrawal.
5. Introspectiveness and calm acceptance of the inevita-ble.

III. Analysis/nursing diagnosis:

A. *Altered feeling patterns* related to fear of being alone.

B. *Altered comfort patterns* related to pain.

C. *Altered meaningfulness* related to depression, hope-lessness, helplessness, powerlessness.

D. *Altered social interaction* related to withdrawal.

IV. Nursing plan/implementation:

A. *Long-term goal:* foster environment where person and family can experience dying with dignity.

B. *Short-term goals*

1. Express feelings (person and family).
2. Support person and family.
3. Minimize physical discomfort.

C. Explore your own feelings about death and dying with team members; form support groups.

D. Be aware of the *normal grief* process.

1. Allow person and family to do the work of grieving and mourning.
2. Allow crying and mood swings, anger, demands.
3. Permit yourself to cry.

E. Allow person to *express* feelings, fears, and concerns.

1. Avoid pat answers to questions about "why."
2. Pick up symbolic communication.

F. Provide care and comfort with *relief from pain;* do not isolate person.

G. Stay *physically close.*

1. Use touch.
2. Be available to form a consistent relationship.

H. *Reduce isolation and abandonment* by assigning per-son to room in which it is less likely to occur and by allowing flexible visiting hours.

I. Keep activities in room as *near normal* and *constant* as possible.

J. Speak in *audible* tones, not whispers.

K. Be alert to cues when person needs to be alone *(disen-gagement process).*

L. Leave room for *hope.*

M. Help person die with peace of mind by lending support and providing opportunities to express anger, pain, and fears to someone who will accept her or him and not censor verbalization.

N. *Health teaching:* teach grief process to family and friends; teach methods to relieve pain.

V. Evaluation:

A. Remains comfortable and free of pain as long as possible.

B. Dies with dignity.

GRIEF

Grief is a typical reaction to the loss of a source of psychologic gratification. It is a syndrome with somatic and psychologic symptoms that diminish when grief is resolved. Grief processes have been extensively described by Erich Lindemann and George Engle.*

I. Concepts and principles related to grief:

A. Cause of grief: reaction to loss (real or imaginary, actual or pending).

B. Healing process can be interrupted.

C. Grief is universal.

D. Uncomplicated grief is a self-limiting process.

E. Grief responses may vary in degree and kind (for example, absence of grief, delayed grief, and unresolved grief).

F. People go through stages similar to stages of death described by Elisabeth Kübler-Ross.

G. Many factors influence successful outcome of grieving process:

1. The more *dependent* the person on the lost relationship, the greater the difficulty in resolving the loss.
2. A *child* has greater difficulty resolving loss.
3. A person with *few meaningful relationships* also has greater difficulty.
4. The *more losses* the person has had in the past, the more affected that person will be, as losses tend to be cumulative.
5. The more *sudden* the loss, the greater the difficulty in resolving it.
6. The more *ambivalence* (love–hate feelings, with guilt) there was toward the dead, the more difficult the resolution.
7. *Loss of a child* is harder to resolve than loss of an older person.

II. Assessment—characteristic stages of grief responses:

A. *Shock and disbelief* (initial and recurrent stage)

1. *Denial* of reality. ("No, it can't be.")
2. Stunned, *numb* feeling.
3. Feelings of loss, *helplessness,* impotence.
4. Intellectual acceptance.

B. *Developing awareness*

1. Anguish about loss.
   a. *Somatic* distress.
   b. Feelings of emptiness.
2. *Anger* and hostility toward person or circumstances held responsible.
3. Guilt feelings—may lead to self-destructive actions.
4. Tears (inwardly, alone; or inability to cry).

C. *Restitution*

1. Funeral *rituals* are an aid to grief resolution by emphasizing the reality of death.
2. Expression and sharing of feelings by gathered family and friends are a source of acknowledgment of grief and support for the bereaved.

D. *Resolving the loss*

1. Increase *dependency* on others as an attempt to deal with painful void.
2. More aware of own *bodily sensations*—may be identical with symptoms of the deceased.
3. Complete *preoccupation* with thoughts and memories of the dead person.

E. *Idealization*

1. All hostile and negative feelings about the dead are *repressed.*
2. Mourner may *assume* qualities and attributes of the dead.
3. Gradual lessening of preoccupation with the dead; *reinvesting* in others.

III. Analysis—see Table 1.9.

IV. Nursing plan/implementation in grief states:

A. *Apply crisis theory and interventions.*

B. *Demonstrate unconditional respect* for cultural, religious, and social mourning customs.

C. *Utilize knowledge of the stages of grief* to anticipate reactions and facilitate the grief process.

1. Anticipate and permit expression of different manifestations of shock, disbelief, and denial.
   a. News of impending death is best communicated to a family group (rather than an individual) in a private setting.
   b. Let mourners see the dead or dying, to help them accept reality.
   c. Encourage description of circumstances and nature of loss.
2. Accept guilt, anger, and rage as a common response to coping with guilt and helplessness.
   a. Be aware of potential suicide by the bereaved.
   b. Permit crying; stay with the bereaved.
3. Mobilize social support system; promote hospital policy that allows gathering of friends and family in a private setting.
4. Allow dependency on staff for initial decision making while person is attempting to resolve loss.
5. Respond to somatic complaints.
6. Permit reminiscence.
7. Encourage mourner to relate accounts connected with the lost relationship that reflect positive and negative feelings and remembrances; *place loss in perspective.*
8. Begin to encourage and reinforce new interests and social relations with others by the end of the idealization stage, loosen bonds of attachment.

---

*Engle, G.: Grief and grieving, *Am J Nurs* 9(64):93–98, September 1964.

TABLE 1.9 Analysis/Nursing Diagnosis: *Altered Feeling Patterns* Related to Grief

Problem Classification	Characteristics
1. Somatic distress	Occurs in waves lasting from 20 minutes to 1 hour.
	Deep, sighing respirations most common when discussing grief.
	Lack of strength.
	Loss of appetite and sense of taste.
	Tightness in throat.
	Choking sensation accompanied by shortness of breath.
2. Preoccupation with image of deceased.	Similar to daydreaming.
	May mistake others for deceased person.
	May be oblivious to surroundings.
	Slight sense of unreality.
	Fear that he or she is becoming "insane."
3. Feelings of guilt	Accuses self of negligence.
	Exaggerates existence and importance of negative thoughts, feelings, and actions toward deceased.
	Views self as having failed deceased—"If I had only . . ."
4. Feelings of hostility	Irritability, anger, and loss of warmth toward others.
	May attempt to handle feelings of hostility in formalized and stiff manner of social interaction.
5. Loss of patterns of conduct	Inability to initiate or maintain organized patterns of activity.
	Restlessness, with aimless movements.
	Loss of zest—tasks and activities are carried on as though with great effort.
	Activities formerly carried on in company of deceased have lost their significance.
	May become strongly dependent on whoever stimulates him or her to activity.

Source: Wilson HS, Kneisl CR, *Psychiatric Nursing,* 3rd ed. (Redwood City, CA: Addison-Wesley, 1988).

9. Identify high-risk persons for maladaptive responses. (See I.G. Many factors influence successful outcome of grieving process, p. 29.)
10. *Health teaching:*
    a. Explain that emotional response is appropriate and common.
    b. Explain and offer hope that emotional pain will diminish with time.
    c. Describe normal grief stages.

V. Evaluation: outcome may take one year or more—can remember comfortably and realistically both pleasurable and disappointing aspects of the lost relationship.

A. Can express feelings of sorrow caused by loss.

B. Can describe ambivalence (love, anger) toward lost person, relationship.

C. Able to review relationship, including pleasures, regrets, etc.

D. Bonds of attachment are loosened and new object relationships are established.

MENTAL AND EMOTIONAL DISORDERS IN CHILDREN AND ADOLESCENTS

Children have certain developmental tasks to master in the various stages of development (for example, learning to trust, control primary instincts, and resolve basic social roles; see Unit 3, Nursing Care of Children and Families).

I. Concepts and principles related to mental and emotional disorders in children and adolescents

A. Most emotional disorders of children are related to family dynamics and the place the child occupies in the family group.

B. Children must be understood and treated within the context of their *families.*

C. Many disorders are related to the phases of development through which the children are passing. (Erik Erikson's developmental tasks for children are: trust, autonomy, initiative, industry, identity, and intimacy.)

D. Table 1.10 summarizes key age-related disturbances, lists main *symptoms and analyses of causes,* and highlights medical interventions and *nursing plan/implementation.*

E. Children are not miniature adults; they have special needs.

F. Play and food are important media to make contact with children and help them release emotions in socially acceptable forms, prepare them for traumatic events, and develop skills.

G. Children who are physically or emotionally ill regress, giving up previously useful habits.

H. Adolescents have special problems relating to need for *control* versus need to *rebel, dependency* versus *interdependency,* and search for *identity* and *self-realization.*

I. Adolescents often *act out* their underlying feelings of insecurity, rejection, deprivation, and low self-esteem.

J. Strong feelings may be evoked in nurses working with children; these feelings should be expressed, and each nurse should be supported by team members.

II. Assessment of selected disorders:

A. *Autistic disorders* (previously called childhood schizophrenia):

1. Disturbance in how perceptual information is processed; normal abilities present.
   a. Behave as though they cannot hear, see, etc.
   b. Do not react to external stimulus.
   c. Mute or echolalic.
2. Lack of self-awareness as a unified whole—may not relate bodily needs or parts as extension of themselves.
3. Severe difficulty in communicating with others—may be mute and isolated.
4. Bizarre postures and gestures (head-banging, rocking back and forth).
5. Disturbances in learning.
6. Etiology is unknown.
7. Prognosis depends on severity of symptoms and age of onset.

B. *Developmental disorders* (brain injury) characteristics:

1. Hyperactivity.
2. Explosive outbursts.
3. Distractibility.
4. Impulsiveness.
5. Perceptual difficulties (visual distortions, such as figure–ground distortion and mirror-reading; body-image problems; difficulty in telling left from right).
6. Receptive or expressive language problems.

C. *Elimination disorders* (Functional enuresis)—related to feelings of insecurity due to unmet needs of attention and affection; important to preserve their self-esteem.

D. *Anxiety disorders of childhood* (School phobias)—anxiety about school is accompanied by physical distress. Usually observed with fear of leaving home, rejection by mother, fear of loss of mother, or history of separation from mother in early years.

E. *Disruptive behavior disorders*—include lying, stealing, running away, truancy, substance abuse, sexual delinquency, vandalism, and fire-setting; chief motivating force is either overt or covert hostility; history of disturbed parent–child relations.

III. Analysis/nursing diagnosis:

A. *Altered feeling patterns:* anxiety, fear, hostility related to personal vulnerability and poorly developed or inappropriate use of defense mechanisms.

B. *Altered interpersonal processes:*

1. *Impaired verbal communication* related to cerebral deficits and psychological barriers.
2. *Altered conduct/impulse processes:* aggressive, violent behaviors toward self, others, environment related to feelings of distrust and altered judgment.
3. *Dysfunctional behaviors:* age-inappropriate behaviors, bizarre behaviors; disorganized and unpredictable behaviors related to inability to discharge emotions verbally.
4. *Impaired social interaction:* social isolation/withdrawal related to feelings of suspicion and mistrust.
5. *Altered values:* inability to internalize values associated with refusing limits, related to unresolved emotions and altered judgment.
6. *Altered parenting* related to ambivalent family relationships and failure of child to meet role expectations.

C. *Sensory/perceptual alterations:* altered attention related to disturbed mental activities.

D. *Altered cognition process:* altered decision making, judgment, knowledge and learning processes; altered thought content and processes related to perceptual or cognitive impairment and emotional dysfunctioning.

IV. Nursing plan/implementation in mental and emotional disorders in children and adolescents:

A. *General goals:* corrective behavior—behavior modification.

B. Help children gain self-awareness.

C. Provide *structured* environment to orient children to reality.

D. Impose *limits* on destructive behavior toward themselves or others without rejecting the children.

1. *Prevent* destructive behavior.
2. *Stop* destructive behavior.
3. *Redirect* nongrowth behavior into constructive channels.

E. Be *consistent.*

F. Meet *developmental and dependency* needs.

G. Recognize and encourage each child's strengths, growth behavior, and reverse regression.

H. Help these children reach the next step in social growth and development scale.

I. Use play and projective media to aid working out feelings and conflicts and in making contact.

J. Offer support to parents and strengthen the parent-child relationship.

K. *Health teaching:* teach parents methods of behavior modification.

TABLE 1.10 Emotional Disturbances in Children

Stage	Disturbance	Assessment: Symptoms or Characteristics	Analysis: Behavior Related To	Plan/Implementation
Oral (Birth–1 year)	Feeding disturbances	Refusal of food.	1. Rigid feeding schedule. 2. *Psychologic* stress. 3. Incompatible formula. 4. *Physiologic:* pyloric stenosis.	Pediatric evaluation, especially if infant is not gaining weight or is losing weight. Rule out physiologic etiology or incompatible formula. Evaluate *feeding style* of caretaker. Is baby on demand feeding? Is caretaker sensitive to infant's needs or communications about holding, hunger, or satiation?
		Colic. Crying is usually confined to one part of day and starts after a feeding. Commonly lasts from first to third month.	Periodic tension in infant's immature nervous system, causing gas and sharp intestinal pains.	Reassure parents and teach about condition and how to relieve it with *hot water bottle, rocking, rubbing back, pacifier,* which may soothe infant.
	Sleeping disturbances	Infant resists being put down for sleep or going to sleep.	1. Need for parental attention. 2. A pattern formed during period of colic or other illness. 3. Emotional disturbance related to *anxiety.*	If it is attention-getting strategy, suggest parental lack of response for few nights to break pattern. If emotional disturbance is suspected, evaluate *infant–caretaker interaction* and refer for pyschotherapeutic intervention.
	Failure to thrive	Infant does not grow or develop over a period of time.	1. *Psychologic:* inadequate caretaking. 2. *Physicologic:* heart, kidneys, central nervous system (CNS) malfunction.	*Hospitalization* is essential. Assist in evaluation of physiologic functioning, especially heart, kidneys, and CNS. *Nurturing plan* for infant, using specifically assigned personnel and the caretaker parent. If the infant grows and develops with nurturing, thus confirming problems of parenting as causative factor, psychotherapeutic and child protective interventions are necessary.
	Severe disturbances	*Autistic psychosis:* Very early onset; lack of response to others; bizarre, repetitive behavior; normal to above normal intelligence; failure to develop language or use communicative speech. Autism is one of the most severe and debilitating psychiatric disturbances.	1. Etiology is uncertain; *regression* or *fixation* at earlier developmental stage, before child differentiates "me" from "not me." 2. A "*nature versus nurture*" controversy that exists over the causative factors. These are variously thought to be: a. *Environment only:* Infant is tabula rasa and all disturbance is directly attributable to the environment (primarily the parenting). b. *Heredity only:* For genetic, biochemical, or other predetermined reasons, some infants will be psychotic regardless of the environment. c. *Combination of environment and heredity* plus *the interaction between them:* A *susceptible* infant, *less* than optimal parenting, and *negative* interaction between parent and infant will combine to produce disturbance.	The severely disturbed child requires intensive psychotherapy and often milieu therapy available in residential or day care programs. Therapy is usually indicated for parents also. Nurses can work on a *primary level* of prevention by assessing parenting skills of prospective parents and *teaching* them these skills. On a *secondary level* of *prevention,* nurses can be knowledgeable about and *teach* others the early signs of childhood psychosis, making appropriate referrals. The earlier the intervention, the better the prognosis. On a *tertiary level of prevention,* nurses work with severely disturbed children and their families in child guidance clinics and residential and day care settings. *Health teaching would include:* play activities that foster support, acceptance, and a nonthreatening mode of communication and interaction with a significant other.

■ **TABLE 1.10 *(Continued)***

Stage	Disturbance	Assessment: Symptoms or Characteristics	Analysis: Behavior Related To	Plan/Implementation
Oral (cont.)		*Symbiotic psychosis:* Identified later than autistic type, usually between 2 and 5 years of age. These children seem to be unable to function independently of the caregiving parent. A situational stress, such as hospitalization of parent or child or entry into school, may precipitate a psychotic break in the child.	The same *"nature versus nurture"* controversy exists with respect to the origin of symbiotic psychosis. The child progresses beyond the self-absorbed autistic stage to form an object relationship with another (usually the mother). Having progressed to this stage, the child then *fails to differentiate his or her own identity* from that of the mother.	
Anal (1–3 years)	Disturbances related to toilet training	*Constipation*	1. *Diet.* 2. Child withholding due to history of one or two painful, *hard bowel movements.* 3. *Psychologic* causation: child withholds from parents to *express anger, opposition,* or passage through a very *independent* development stage.	Evaluate *diet* and consistency of stools. Fecal softener may be prescribed if necessary. In all cases, *help parent* avoid making an issue of constipation with the child. Enemas are contraindicated. If child is withholding, *work with parents* around not forcing rigid toilet training on child. Most children are more cooperative about *toilet training* at 18–24 months.
		Encopresis (soiling)	Child's expression of anger or hostility. It is usually directed toward the parent with whom the child is experiencing conflict and is rarely physiologic.	Medical evaluation, then assessment and intervention in the child–parent relationship. Therapy for child (and possibly for parent) may be indicated.
	Excessive rebelliousness	Frequent temper tantrums, fighting, destruction of toys and other objects, consistent oppositional behavior.	1. Fear caused by inconsistency in handling the child, the setting of rigid limits, or the parents' refusal or inability to set limits, which can all create insecurity and fear in the child. 2. Excessive rebelliousness usually indicates a *frightened* child and should not be confused with expression of negativism normal at around age 2, which is a necessary (though trying) developmental stage.	The nurse should offer parent counseling if necessary. When working with the child, the nurse needs to be receptive and sympathetic while establishing and maintaining firm limits.
	Excessive conformity	Lack of spontaneity, anxious desire always to please all adult authority figures, timidity, refusal to assert own needs, passivity.	*These children have:* 1. Established very rigid control in an attempt to handle fears. 2. Harsh *toilet training,* resulting in an overcompliant child. These children need help as much as over-rebellious children, but they get it less frequently because their behavior is not a "problem"—that is, it is not difficult for parents to tolerate.	Excessive conformity can lead to compulsive, ritualistic, or obsessive behavior later. The nurse needs to be able to identify such a child, then work with the child and parents to encourage *self-expression* in the child. Referral for psychotherapy may be necessary to help the child deal with repressed anger.
		Enuresis. Ordinarily refers to wetting while asleep (nocturnal enuresis), though some enuretic children wet themselves during the day also. Enuresis is a *symptom,* not a diagnosis or disease entity.	1. *Faulty toilet training* (especially if child wets during the day also) or 2. *Psychologic stress.* 3. *Physiologic* etiology, such as genitourinary (GU) tract infections or CNS disease, is	Many approaches have been tried with varying degress of success. These include Trofand, *fluid restriction, behavioral intervention* (in which a buzzer wakes the child when the child starts to wet), and psycho-

continued

TABLE 1.10 *(Continued)* **Emotional Disturbances in Children**

Stage	Disturbance	Assessment: Symptoms or Characteristics	Analysis: Behavior Related To	Plan/Implementation
Anal (cont.)			rare. The child under 4 years old is usually not considered enuretic but is included in this section because bladder training is part of toilet training. Etiology is uncertain.	therapy. *Educating parents in bladder training* techniques and attitudes can help solve the problem on a *primary* level. It is important when working with enuretic children or their parents to *suggest* ways to help the child *overcome feelings of shame and guilt.* These feelings are often exacerbated by well-meaning but misguided parents.
Oedipal (3–6 years)	Excessive fears	Child will be frightened even in nonthreatening situations. *Nightmares and other sleep disturbances* occur. Usually, child will be very "clingy" with parents in an attempt to gain reassurance.	*Anxiety* as the causative factor. Anxiety can be induced by many things, such as: 1. Parental *failure to set appropriate limits.* 2. *Physical or psychologic abuse.* 3. *Illness.* 4. Fear of *mutilation.* 5. *Imaginary* worries are common at this age, so a 4-year-old who is suddenly afraid of the dark, or dogs, or fire engines is not necessarily suffering from excessive fears.	If possible, identify and deal with the factors that are producing the anxiety. Offer child calm reassurance. *Night-light and open doors* can help allay night fears, but *counsel parents* that it is unwise to allow the child to sleep with the parents, which may make the child feel that the Oedipal retaliation has succeeded. With the hospitalized child, the nurse needs to be aware of and work with the mutilation fears common at this age. Fears around certain procedures (like injections) can often be resolved by helping the child *play out fears.*
	Excessive masturbation	Touching and fondling of genitals excessively, sometimes in a preoccupied or absentminded manner.	1. *Insecurity.* 2. Exploration and stimulation of the genital area is *normal* and common in this age group. However, if it is compulsive, the behavior is a signal that the child is *insecure.* 3. Occasionally, a *specific fear.* For example, a boy viewing a baby sister's genitals may have castration fears. These can be dealt with directly.	*Assess* the child's masturbating activity. When does it occur and why? Then help the child develop other *strategies* for coping with anxiety. *Answer questions about sexuality* in an open manner. *Counsel parents* that *threats and shaming are contraindicated,* and help parents deal with *their* feelings about masturbation.
	Regression	Resumption of activities (such as *thumb sucking, soiling and wetting, baby talk*) characteristic of earlier developmental levels.	1. Child's attempt to regain a more comfortable, previous level of development in response to a *threatening* situation (such as a new baby), or 2. A response to difficulty resolving Oedipal *conflicts.*	*Counsel parents* not to make an issue of behavior. Offer child emotional support and acceptance, though not approval of regressive behavior.
	Stuttering	Articulation difficulty characterized by many stops and repetitions in speech pattern.	1. Anxiety. 2. Frustration. 3. Insecurity. 4. Excitement. Stuttering usually occurs when the affected child feels *anxious, frustrated, insecure,* or *excited.* Parental concerns and attention to stuttering focuses attention on it and increases anxiety. The origins of stuttering are not understood. It is *common around 2–3 years of age* and is not a cause for concern at that time.	Speech therapy is usually indicated. Psychotherapy may also be indicated, if stuttering is an expression of anxiety and conflict, persisting beyond age 6.

■ **TABLE 1.10 *(Continued)***

Stage	Disturbance	Assessment: Symptoms or Characteristics	Analysis: Behavior Related To	Plan/Implementation
Latency (6–12 years)	Hyperactivity and hyperkinesis	Both hyperactivity and hyperkinesis are occasionally observed in school children; characterized by a *short attention span,* restlessness, distractibility, and *impulsivity.*	1. An *organic disturbance* of the *CNS,* of uncertain origin, is the basis of *hyperkinesis.* Because the primary symptom—difficulty with attention span—is the same as that presented by the hyperactive child, the hyperactive child is frequently and incorrectly labeled hyperkinetic. 2. *Hyperactive child*—attempts to *control* anxiety through *reducement* and *can* attend when interested or relaxed. Does not fit smoothly into environment, but problem may be with the environment rather than the child. In other words, the school situation requires a high degree of conformity. The child who does not fit the mold is *not* necessarily emotionally disturbed.	For the *hyperkinetic* child, psychopharmaceutical intervention—usually *Ritalin*—is most often employed. Psychotherapy and special education classes may also be indicated. Ritalin is also frequently prescribed for the *hyperactive* child—which raises the issue of whether an individual should be medicated to fit more smoothly into the environment. Therapy can help the hyperactive child *decrease anxiety* and *increase self-esteem,* thus reducing the symptoms.
	Withdrawal	Reduced body movement and verbalization, lack of close relationships, *detachment,* timidity, and seclusiveness.	1. Need to withdraw as a defensive behavior, through which the child controls anxiety by *reducing contact* with the outer world. Like the overcompliant child, the withdrawn child is frequently not identified as needing help because this behavior is not a "problem."	Offer *positive reinforcement* when child is more active. Help child *assert* self and *experience success* at certain tasks. The nurse needs to work with the parents who are overprotective. Therapy may be useful to work through anxiety and provide child with a chance to form a *trusting* relationship with another.
	Psychophysiologic symptoms	The child experiences physical symbtoms (such as *vomiting, headaches, eczema, asthma, colitis*) with no apparent physiologic cause.	*Conversion* of anxiety into physical symptoms	After medical evaluation has established lack of physiologic etiology, psychotherapy is usually indicated. Family therapy may be treatment of choice since *dysfunctional interpersonal family dynamics* are common in these cases. The nurse can also provide the child with a healthy interpersonal relationship. Nurses are frequently in a position to talk to parents and teachers about the importance of mental health counseling for children with physical symptoms.
	School "phobia"	Sudden and seemingly inexplicable fear of going to school. These children often don't know what it is they fear at school. Frequently occurs *after an illness* and absence from school or birth of sibling.	Not actually a phobia but an *acute anxiety reaction related to separation* from home.	If the child is allowed to stay home, the dread of returning to school usually increases. The child and parent should have psychiatric intervention quickly (before the problem becomes worse) to help the child separate from the parent.
	Learning disabilities	Failure or difficulty in learning at school	1. Emotional disorders can cause school failure. 2. Feelings of *inferiority, discouragement,* and loss of	A comprehensive evaluation is essential. Ideally, this would include assessments by a pediatric neurologist, a mental health

continued

■ TABLE 1.10 *(Continued)* **Emotional Disturbances in Children**

Stage	Disturbance	Assessment: Symptoms or Characteristics	Analysis: Behavior Related To	Plan/Implementation
Latency (cont.)			confidence from school failure. Learning disabilities may be caused by many factors or combinations of factors, including *anxiety, poor sensory or sensorimotor integration, dyslexia, receptive aphasia.*	worker such as a psychiatric nurse or psychiatrist, a learning disabilities teacher specialist, and possibly an occupational therapist trained to work with sensory integration. Treatment is then based on the specific problem or problems.
	Behavior problems	Behavior that is nonproductive; that is repeated in spite of threats, punishments, or rational argument; and that usually leads to punishment. Persistent *stealing a ıd truancy* are examples.	*Conflicts* that are expressed and communicated through behavior rather than verbally. Child knows what he or she is doing but is unaware of the underlying motivations for the problem behavior.	Counseling or therapy for the child by a child psychiatric nurse or other mental health worker can allow the child to resolve the basic conflict, thus making the problem behavior unnecessary.

Source: Adapted from Wilson HS, Kneisl CR, *Psychiatric Nursing,* 3rd ed. (Redwood City, CA: Addison-Wesley 1988).

V. Evaluation:

A. Destructive behavior is inhibited.

B. Demonstrates age-appropriate behavior on developmental scale.

MIDLIFE CRISIS: PHASE OF LIFE PROBLEMS

Midlife crisis is a time period that marks the passage between early maturity and middle age.

I. Assessment:

A. Commonly occurs between ages 35 and 45.

B. Preoccupied with *visible* signs of aging, own mortality.

C. *Feelings: urgency* that time is running out ("last chance") for career achievement and unmet goals; *boredom* with present, *ambivalence, frustration, uncertainty* about the future.

D. Time of *reevaluation:*

1. Reassess: meaning of time and parental role (omnipotence as a parent is challenged).
2. Reexamine and contemplate change in career, marriage, family life.

E. *Personality changes* may occur. *Women:* traditional definitions of femininity may be challenged as become more assertive. *Males:* may be more introspective, sensitive to emotions, make external changes (younger mate, improve looks, new sports activity), mood swings.

F. Presence of *helpful elements* necessary to turn life's obstacles into opportunities.

1. Willingness to take risks.
2. Strong support system.
3. Sense of purpose.
4. Accumulated wisdom.

II. Analysis/nursing diagnosis:

A. *Self-esteem disturbance (low self-esteem)* related to: loss of youth, faltering physical powers, and facing discrepancy between youthful ambitions and actual achievement (no longer a promising person with potential).

B. *Altered role performance (role reversal):* related to parents who previously provided security and comfort but now need care.

C. *Altered emotional processes (depression):* related to disappointments and diminished optimism as life is reconsidered in light of the reality of aging and death.

III. Nursing plan/implementation—*long-term goal:* help individual to rebuild life structure.

A. Help client reappraise meaning of his life in terms of past, present, and future, and integrate aspects of time. Encourage introspection and reflection with questions.

1. What have I done with my life?
2. What do I really get from and give to my spouse, children, friends, work, community, and self?
3. What are my strengths and liabilities?
4. What have I done with my early dream, and do I want it now?

B. Assist client to complete *four major tasks:*

1. Terminate era of early adulthood by *reappraising* life goals identified and achieved during this era.
2. Initiate movement into middle adulthood by beginning to make *necessary changes* in *unsuccessful* aspects of the current life while trying out new choices.
3. Cope with *polarities* that divide life.
4. Directly confront *death of own parents.*

C. *Health teaching:* stress management techniques; how to do self-assessment of aptitudes, interests; how to plan for retirement, aloneness, and use of increased leisure time; dietary modification and exercise program.

IV. Evaluation:

A. Gives up *idealized* self of early 20s for more *realistically* attainable self.

1. Talks less of early hopes of eminence and more on modest goal of *competence.*
2. Shifts values from sexuality to platonic relationships: replaces romantic dreams with *satisfying* friendships and companionships.
3. Modifies early illusions about own capacities.
4. Shifts values away from physical attractiveness and strength to *intellectual* abilities.

B. Comes to accept that life is finite and reconciles what *is* with what *might have been;* appreciates everyday human experience rather than glamor or power.

C. Through self-confrontation, self-discovery, and change, experiences time of restabilization; is reinvigorated, adventuresome.

D. Develops *alternative* abilities that release new energies.

E. Tries *less* to please everyone; others' opinions less important.

F. Makes more efficient and well-seasoned decisions from well-developed sense of judgment.

MENTAL HEALTH PROBLEMS OF THE AGED

In general, problems affecting the elderly are *similar* to those affecting persons of *any* age. This section will highlight the *differences* from the viewpoint of etiology, frequency, and prognosis.

I. Concepts and principles related to mental health problems of the aged.

A. The elderly *do* have capacity for growth and change.

B. Human beings, regardless of age, need sense of future and *hope* for things to come.

C. An inalienable right of all individuals should be to make or participate in all decisions concerning themselves and their possessions as long as they can.

D. Physical disability due to the aging process may enforce dependency, which may be unacceptable to elderly patients and may evoke feelings of anger and ambivalence.

E. In an attempt to reduce feelings of loss, elderly patients may cling to concrete things that most represent, in a *symbolic* sense, all that has been significant to them.

F. As memory diminishes, *familiar objects* in environment and *familiar routines* are important in helping to keep clients oriented and in contact with reality.

G. *Familiarity of environment brings security;* routines bring a sense of security about what is to happen.

H. If individuals feel unwanted, they may tell *stories* about their *earlier* achievements.

I. Many of the traits in the elderly result from *cumulative* effect of *past* experiences of frustrations and *present* awareness of limitations rather than from any primary consequences of physiologic deficit.

II. Assessment:

A. *Psychologic characteristics of the aged:*

1. Increasingly *dependent* on others, not only for physical needs but also for emotional security.
2. Concerns focus more and more *inward,* with narrowed outside interests.
   a. Decreased emotional energy for concern with social problems unless these issues affect them.
   b. Tendency to *reminisce.*
   c. May appear selfish and unsympathetic.
3. Sources of pleasure and gratification are more childlike: *food, warmth, and affection,* for example.
   a. Tangible and frequent evidence of affection is important (letters, cards, and visits, for example).
   b. May hoard articles.
4. *Attention span and memory are short;* may be forgetful and accuse others of stealing.
5. Deprivation of any kind is *not* tolerated:
   a. Easily frustrated.
   b. Change is poorly tolerated; need to have favorite chairs and established daily routine, for example.
6. Main *fears* in the aged include: fear of *dependency,* chronic *illness, loneliness, boredom,* fear of being unloved, forgotten, *deserted* by those close to them, fear of *death;* fear of *loss of control* of one's own life; a failing *cognition;* loss of *purpose* and *productivity.*
7. *Nocturnal delirium* may be due to problems with night vision and inability to perceive *spatial* location.

B. *Psychiatric problems in aging*

1. *Loneliness*—related to *loss* of mate, diminishing circle of friends and family through death and geographical separation, *decline* in physical energy, loss of work (retirement), sharp loss of income, and loss of a life-long life-style.
2. *Insomnia*—pattern of sleep changes in significant ways: disappearance of *deep* sleep, frequent *awakening, daytime* sleeping.
3. *Hypochondriasis*—anxiety may shift from concern with finances, job, or social prestige to concern about own bodily function.
4. *Depression*—common problem in the aging, with a *high suicide rate;* partly because of bodily changes that influence the *self-concept,* the older person may direct hostility toward self and therefore may be subject to feelings of depression and loneliness.
5. *Senility*—four early symptoms:
   a. Change in attention span.
   b. Memory loss for *recent* events and *names.*
   c. Altered intellectual capacity.
   d. Diminished ability to respond to others.

C. *Successful aging*

1. Being able to *perceive* signs of aging and limitations resulting from the aging process.
2. *Redefining* life in terms of effects on social and physical aspects of living.
3. Seeking *alternatives* for meeting needs and finding sources of pleasure.
4. Adopting a *different outlook* about self-worth.
5. *Reintegrating* values with goals of life.

D. *Causative factors* of mental disorder in the aged related to:

1. *Nutritional* problems and *physical ill health* related to *acute and chronic illness:*

a. Cardiovascular diseases (heart failure, stroke, hypertension).
b. Respiratory infection.
c. Cancer.
d. Alcohol dependence and abuse.
e. Dentition problems.

2. Faulty adaptation related to *physical* changes of aging; e.g., depression, hypochondriases.
3. Problems related to *loss, grief, and bereavement.*
4. *Retirement* shock related to lose of status and financial security.
5. Social isolation and loneliness related to *inadequate sensory stimulation.*
6. *Environmental change* (relocation within a community or from home to institution): loss of family, privacy.
7. *Hopelessness, helplessness* related to condition and circumstances.
8. *Altered body image* (negative) related to aging process.
9. Depression related to *helplessness,* inability to express anger.

III. Analysis/nursing diagnosis:

A. *Altered self-concept* related to disturbance in self-esteem and body image and altered family role.

B. *Impaired social interaction* related to social isolation and environmental changes.

C. *Dysfunctional grieving* related to loss and bereavement.

D. *Altered emotional and valuation processes* related to hopelessness, anxiety, fear, powerlessness.

E. *Altered physiologic processes* related to physical ill health.

F. *Sleep pattern disturbance* related to insomnia and altered sleep/arousal patterns.

IV. Nursing plan/implementation:

A. *Long-term goal:* to help reduce hopelessness and helplessness.

B. *Short-term goal:* to focus on ego assets.

C. Help elderly *preserve* what facet of life they can and *regain* that which has already been lost.

1. Help minimize regression as much as possible.
2. Help retain their *adult* status.
3. Help preserve their *self-image* as useful individuals.
4. Identify and preserve their *abilities* to perform, emphasizing what they *can* do.

D. Attempt to *prevent* loss of dignity and loss of worth—address them by titles, not "Gramps."

E. *Reduce* feelings of *alienation* and loneliness. Provide *sensory* experiences for those with visual problems:

1. Let them touch objects of various textures and consistencies.
2. Encourage heightened use of remaining senses to make up for those that are diminished or lost.

F. *Reduce* depression and feelings of isolation.

1. Allow time to *reminisce.*
2. *Avoid changes* in surroundings or routine.

G. *Protect* from rush and excitement.

1. Use simple, unhurried conversation.
2. Allow *extra* time to organize thoughts.

H. Be sensitive to *concrete* things they may want to *keep.*

I. *Health teaching:*

1. How to keep track of time (for example, by marking off days on a calendar), to promote orientation.
2. How to keep track of medications.
3. Exercises to promote blood flow.
4. *Retirement counseling:*
   a. Obtaining satisfaction from leisure time.
   b. Nurturing relationships with younger generations.
   c. Adjusting to changes: physical health, retirement, loss of loved ones.
   d. Developing connections with own age group.
   e. Taking on new social roles.
   f. Maintaining a satisfactory and appropriate living situation.
   g. Coping with dependence on others, especially one's children.

V. Evaluation:

A. Less confusion and fewer mood swings.

B. Increased interest in activities of daily living and interaction with others.

C. Lessened preoccupation with death, dying, physical symptoms, feelings of sadness.

D. Reduced insomnia and anorexia.

E. Expresses feelings of belonging and being needed.

■ PROTECTIVE FUNCTIONS

COMMON BEHAVIORAL PROBLEMS

I. Anger

A. Definition: feelings of resentment in response to anxiety when threat is perceived; need to discharge tension of anger.

B. Assessment:

1. *Degree of anger and frequency:* Scope of anger ranges on a continuum from everyday mild annoyance → frustration from interference with goal accomplishment → assertiveness (behavior used to deal with anger effectively) → anger related to helplessness and powerlessness that may interfere with functioning → rage and fury, when coping means are depleted or not developed.
2. *Mode of expression of anger*
   a. *Covert,* passive expression of anger: being overly nice; body language with little or no eye contact, arms close to body, soft voice, little gesturing; sarcasm through humor; sublimation through art and music; projection onto others; denying and pushing anger out of awareness; psychosomatic illness in response to internalized anger, e.g., headache.

b. *Overt,* active expression of anger: physical activity to work off excess physical energy associated with biologic response (e.g., hitting punching bag, taking a walk); aggression, assertiveness.

3. *Physiologic behaviors*—result of secretion of epinephrine and sympathetic nervous system stimulation preparing for fight–flight.
   a. *Cardiovascular* response: increased blood pressure and pulse, increased free fatty acid in blood.
   b. *Gastrointestinal* response: increased nausea, salivation, decreased peristalsis.
   c. *Genitourinary* response: urinary frequency.
   d. *Neuromuscular* response: increased alertness, increased muscle tension and deep tendon reflexes, ECG changes.
4. *Positive functions of anger*
   a. Energizes behavior.
   b. Protects positive image.
   c. Provides ego defense during high anxiety.
   d. Gives greater control over situation.
   e. Alerts to need for coping.
   f. A sign of a healthy relationship.

C. Analysis/nursing diagnosis: *Defensive coping* related to source of stress (stressors):

1. *Biologic stressors*—instinctual drives (Lorenz, on aggressive instincts, and Freud), endocrine imbalances, seizures, tumors, hunger, fatigue.
2. *Psychologic stressors*—inability to resolve frustration that leads to aggression; real or imagined threatened loss of self-esteem; conflict, lack of control; anger as a learned expression and a reinforced response. Prolonged stress; an attempt to protect self; a desire for retaliation; a normal part of grief process.
3. *Sociocultural stressors*—lack of early training in self-discipline and social skills; crowding, personal space intrusion; role-modeling of abusive behavior by significant others and by media personalities.

D. Nursing plan/implementation—*long-term goals:* constructive use of angry energy to accomplish tasks and motivate growth.

1. *Prevent* and *control* violence.
   a. Approach unhurriedly.
   b. Provide atmosphere of acceptance; listen attentively, refrain from arguing and criticizing.
   c. Encourage expression of feelings.
   d. Offer feedback of client's expressed feelings.
   e. Encourage mutual problem solving.
   f. Encourage realistic perception of others and situation and respect for the rights of others.
2. *Limit-setting:*
   a. Clearly state expectations and consequences of acts.
   b. Enforce consequences.
   c. Encourage client to assume responsibility for behavior.
   d. Explore reasons and meaning of negative behavior.
3. Promote *self-awareness* and *problem-solving* abilities. Encourage and assist client to:
   a. Accept self as a person with a right to experience angry feelings.
   b. Explore reasons for anger.
   c. Describe situations where anger was experienced.
   d. Discuss appropriate alternatives for expressing anger (including assertiveness training).
   e. Decide on one feasible solution.
   f. Act on solution.
   g. Evaluate effectiveness.
4. *Health teaching:*
   a. Explore other ways to express feelings, and provide activities that allow appropriate expression of anger.
   b. Recommend that behavior limits be set (by the family).
   c. Explain how to set behavioral limits.
   d. Advise against causing defensive patterns in others.

E. Evaluation:

1. Demonstrates insight (awareness of factors that precipitate anger; identifies disturbing topics, events, and inappropriate use of coping mechanisms).
2. Uses appropriate coping mechanisms.
3. Reaches out for emotional support before stress level becomes excessive.
4. Evidence of increased reality perception and problem-solving ability.

II. Combative-aggressive behavior

A. Definition: acting out feelings of frustration, anger, anxiety, etc. through physical or verbal behavior.

B. Assessment—recognize precombative behavior:

1. Demanding, fist-clenching.
2. Boisterous, loud.
3. Vulgar, profane.
4. Limited attention span.
5. Sarcastic, taunting, verbal threats.
6. Restless, agitated, elated.
7. Frowning.

C. Analysis/nursing diagnosis: *Potential for violence* related to:

1. Frustration as response to breakdown of self-control coping mechanisms.
2. Acting out as customary response to anger *(Defensive coping).*
3. Confusion *(Sensory/perceptual alterations).*
4. Physical restraints, such as when postoperative patient discovers wrist restraints.
5. Fear of intimacy, intrusion on emotional and physical space *(Altered thought processes).*
6. Feelings of helplessness, inadequacy *(Situational or chronic low self-esteem).*

D. Nursing plan/implementation:

1. *Long-term goal*—channel aggression—help person express feelings rather than act them out.
2. *Immediate goal*—prevent injury to self and others.

a. Calmly call for assistance; do *not* try to handle *alone*.

b. Approach cautiously. Keep client within *eye contact*, observing client's personal space.

c. *Protect* against self-injury and injury to others; be aware of your position in relation to the weapon, door, escape route.

d. *Minimize* stimuli, to control the environment—clear the area, close doors, turn off TV so person can hear you.

e. *Divert* attention from the act; engage in talk and lead away from others.

f. Assess triggering cause.

g. Identify immediate problem.

h. Focus on remedy for immediate problem.

i. Choose one calm, quieting individual to interact with person; nonauthoritarian, nonthreatening.

j. Maintain *verbal contact* to keep communication open; offer empathetic ear, but be firm and consistent in setting *limits* on dangerous behavior.

k. Negotiate, but don't make false promises or argue.

l. Restraints may be necessary as a *last* resort.

m. Place person in quiet room so he or she can calm down.

3. *Health teaching:*

a. Explain how to obtain release from stress and how to rechannel emotional energy into acceptable activity.

b. Advise against causing defensive responses in others.

c. Explain what is justifiable aggression.

d. Emphasize importance of how to recognize tension in self.

e. Explain why self-control is important.

f. Explain to family, staff, how to set behavioral limits.

g. Explain causes of maladaptive coping related to anger.

h. Teach how to use problem-solving method.

E. Evaluation:

1. Is aware of causes of anger; can recognize the feeling of anger and utilize alternative methods of expressing anger.
2. Expression of anger is appropriate, congruent with the situation.
3. Replaces aggression and acting-out with assertiveness.

III. Confusion/disorientation

A. Definition: loss of reality orientation as to person, time, place, events, ideas.

B. Assessment—note unusual behavior:

1. Picking, stroking movements in the air or on clothing and linens.
2. Frequent crying or laughing.
3. Alternating periods of confusion and lucidity (for example, confused at night, when alone in the dark).
4. Fluctuating mood, actions, rationality (argumentative, combative, withdrawn).
5. Increasingly restless, fearful, leading to insomnia, nightmares.
6. Acts bewildered; has trouble identifying familiar people.
7. Preoccupied; irritable when interrupted.
8. Unresponsive to questions; problem with concentration and setting realistic priorities.
9. Sensitive to noise and light.
10. Has unrealistic perception of time, place, and situation.
11. Nurse no longer seen as supportive but as threatening.

C. Analysis/nursing diagnosis: *Altered thought processes and sensory/perceptual alterations* related to:

1. *Physical and physiologic disturbances*—metabolic (uremia, diabetes, hepatic dysfunction), fluid and electrolyte imbalances, cardiac arrhythmias, congestive heart failure; anemia, massive blood loss with low hemoglobin; organic brain disease; nutritional deficiency; pain; sleep disturbance; drugs (antidepressants, tranquilizers, sedatives, antihypertensives, diuretics, alcohol, PCP, street drugs).
2. *Unfamiliar environment*—unfamiliar routine and people; procedures that threaten body image; noisy equipment.
3. *Loss of sensory acuity* from partial or incomplete reception of orienting stimuli or information.
4. *Disability in screening out* irrelevant and excessive sensory input.
5. *Memory impairment.*

D. Nursing plan/implementation:

1. Check *physical signs;* for example, vital signs, neurologic status, fluid and electrolyte balance, and blood urea nitrogen.
2. Be calm; make contact to *reorient to reality:*

a. Avoid startling if person is alone, in the dark, sedated.

b. Make sure person can see, hear, and talk to you—turn off TV; turn on light, put on client's glasses, hearing aids, dentures.

c. Call by name, clearly and distinctly.

d. Approach cautiously, close to *eye* level.

e. Keep your hands visible; for example, on bed.

3. *Take care of immediate problem;* for example, disconnected IV tube or catheter.

a. Give instructions slowly and distinctly; avoid threatening tone and comments.

b. *Stay* with person until reoriented.

c. Put *siderails* up.

4. Use conversation to *reduce* confusion:

a. Use simple, concrete phrases; language the person can understand; repeat as needed.

b. Avoid shouting, arguing, false promises, use of medical abbreviations (for example, NPO).

c. Give more time to concentrate on what you said.

d. Focus on reality-oriented topics or objects in the environment.

5. *Prevent confusion by establishing a reality-oriented relationship.*

a. Introduce self by name.

b. Jointly establish routines to prevent confusion from unpredictable changes and variations. Determine client's usual routine; attempt to incorporate this to lessen disruption in life-style.

c. Explain what to expect in understandable words—where client is and why, what will happen, noises and activities client will hear and see, people client will meet, tests and procedures client will have.

d. Find out what meaning hospitalization has to client; reduce anxiety related to feelings of apprehension and helplessness.

e. Spend as much time as possible with client.

6. *Maintain orientation by providing nonthreatening environment*

a. Assign to room near nurse's station.

b. Surround with familiar objects from home (for example, photos).

c. Provide clock, calendar, and radio.

d. Have flexible visiting hours.

e. Open curtain for natural light.

f. Keep glasses, dentures, hearing aids nearby.

g. Check client often, especially at night.

h. Avoid using intercom to answer calls.

i. Avoid low-pitched conversation.

7. *Take care of other needs*

a. Promote sleep according to usual habits and patterns in order to *prevent sleep deprivation.*

b. Avoid sedatives, which may lead to or increase confusion.

c. Promote independent functions, self-help activities, to *maintain dignity.*

d. Encourage *nutritional* adequacy; incorporate familiar foods, ethnic preferences.

e. Maintain *routine;* avoid being late with meals, medication, or procedures.

f. Have *realistic expectations.*

g. *Discover hidden fears.*

(1) Do not assume confused behavior is unrelated to reality.

(2) Look for clues to meaning from client's background, occupation.

h. *Provide support to family.*

(1) Encourage expression of feelings; avoid being judgmental.

(2) Check what worked in previous situations.

8. *Health teaching:* explain possible causes of confusion. Reassure that it is common. Teach family, friends how to react to confused behavior.

E. Evaluation:

1. Less restlessness, fearfulness, mood lability.
2. More frequent periods of lucidity; oriented to time, place, and person; responds to questions.

IV. Demanding behavior

A. Definition: a strong and persistent struggle to obtain satisfaction of self-oriented needs (such as control, self-esteem) or relief from anxiety.

B. Assessment:

1. Attention-seeking behavior.
2. Multiple requests.
3. Frequency of questions.
4. Lack of reasonableness; irrationality of request.

C. Analysis/nursing diagnosis: *Defensive coping and impaired social interaction* related to:

1. Feelings of helplessness and hopelessness.
2. Feelings of powerlessness and fear.
3. A way of coping with anxiety.

D. Nursing plan/implementation:

1. *Control* own irritation; assess reasons for own annoyance.
2. *Confront* with behavior; discuss reasons for behavior.
3. *Anticipate* and meet client's needs; set time to discuss requests.
4. *Ignore* negative attention-seeking and reinforce appropriate requests for attention.
5. Make plans with *entire staff* to set *limits.*
6. Set up *contractual* arrangement for brief, frequent, regular, uninterrupted attention.
7. *Health teaching:* teach appropriate methods for gaining attention.

E. Evaluation: fewer requests for attention; assumes more responsibility for self-care.

V. Denial of illness

A. Definition: an attempt or refusal to acknowledge some anxiety-provoking aspect of oneself or external reality. Denial may be an acceptable first phase of coping as an attempt to allow time for adaptation.

B. Assessment:

1. Observe for coping mechanisms such as dissociation, repression, selective inattention, suppression, displacement of concern to another person.

2. Note behaviors that may indicate denial of diagnosis:

a. Failure to follow treatment plan.

b. Missed appointment.

c. Refusal of medication.

d. Inappropriate cheerfulness.

e. Ignoring symptoms.

f. Use of flippant humor.

g. Use of second or third person in reference to illness.

h. Flight into wellness, overactivity.

3. Use of earliest and most primitive defense by closing eyes, turning head away to separate from what is unpleasant and anxiety-provoking.

4. Note *range* of denial: *explicit* verbal denial of obvious facts, disowning or *ignoring* aspects or *minimizing* by understatement.

5. Be aware of situations such as long-term physical disability that make people more prone to denial of anger. Denial of illness protects the ego from overwhelming anxiety.

C. Analysis/nursing diagnosis: *Ineffective denial* related to:

1. Untenable wishes, needs, ideas, deeds, or reality factors.
2. Inability: to adapt to full realization of painful experience or to accept changes in body image or role perception.
3. Intense stress and anxiety.

D. Nursing plan/implementation:

1. *Long-term goal*—understand needs met by denial.
2. *Short-term goal*—avoid reinforcing denial patterns.
   a. Recognize behavioral cues of denial of some reality aspect; be aware of level of awareness and degree to which reality is excluded.
   b. Determine if denial interferes with treatment.
   c. Support moves toward greater reality orientation.
   d. Determine person's stress tolerance.
   e. Supportively help person discuss events leading to, and feelings about, hospitalization.
3. *Health teaching:*
   a. Explain that emotional response is appropriate and common.
   b. Explain to family and staff that emotional adjustment to painful reality is done at own pace.

E. Evaluation: indicates desire to discuss painful experience.

VI. Dependence

A. Definition: reliance on other people to meet basic needs, usually for love and affection, security and protection, and support and guidance; acceptable in early phases of coping.

B. Assessment:

1. Excessive need for advice and answers to problems.
2. Lack of confidence in own decision-making ability and lack of confidence in self-sufficiency.
3. Clinging, too-trusting behavior.
4. Gestures, facial expressions, body posture, recurrent themes conveying "I'm helpless."

C. Analysis/nursing diagnosis:

1. *Low self-esteem* related to inability to meet basic needs or role expectations.
2. *Helplessness* and *hopelessness* related to inadvertent reinforcement by staff's expectations.
3. *Powerlessness* related to holding a belief that one's own actions cannot affect life situations.

D. Nursing plan/implementation:

1. *Long-term goal*—increase self-esteem, confidence in own abilities.
2. *Short-term goals*—provide activities that promote independence.
   a. *Limit-setting*—clear, firm, consistent; acknowledge when demands are made; accept client but refuse to respond to demands.
   b. *Break cycle* of: nurse avoids client when he or she is clinging and demanding → client's anxiety increases → demands for attention increase → frustration and avoidance on nurse's part increase.
   c. *Give attention before* demand exists.
   d. Use behavior modification approaches—
      (1) *Reward* appropriate behavior (such as making decisions, helping others, caring for own needs) with attention and praise.
      (2) Give *no response* to attention-seeking, dependent, infantile behavior; goal is to increase incidence of mature behavior as client realizes little gratification from dependent behavior.
   e. *Avoid secondary gains* of being cared for, which impede progress toward above goals.
   f. Assist in developing *ability to control* panic by responding less to client's high anxiety level.
   g. Help client develop ways to seek gratification other than excessive turning to others.
   h. *Resist* urge to act like a parent when client becomes helpless, demanding, and attention-seeking.
   i. *Promote decision making* by not giving advice.
   j. *Encourage accountability* for own feelings, thoughts, and behaviors.
      (1) Help identify feelings through nonverbal cues, thoughts, recurrent themes.
      (2) Convey expectations that client does have opinions and feelings to share.
      (3) Role model how to express feelings.
   k. *Reinforce self-esteem* and ability to work out problems independently. (Consistently ask: "How to you feel about . . ." "What do you think?")
   l. *Health teaching:*
      (1) Teach family ways of interacting to enforce less dependency.
      (2) Teach problem-solving skills, assertiveness.

E. Evaluation:

1. Performs self-care.
2. Asks less for approval and praise.
3. Seeks less attention, proximity, physical contact.

VII. Hostility

A. Definition: a feeling of intense anger or an attitude of antagonism or animosity, with the destructive component of intent to inflict harm and pain to another or to self; may involve hate, anger, rage, aggression, regression.

B. Operational definition:

1. Past experience of frustration, loss of self-esteem, unmet needs for status, prestige, or love.
2. Present expectations of self and others not met.
3. Feelings of humiliation, inadequacy, emotional pain, and conflict.
4. Anxiety experienced and converted into hostility, which can be:
   a. Repressed, with result of becoming withdrawn.
   b. Disowned to the point of overreaction and extreme compliance.
   c. Overtly exhibited: verbal, nonverbal.

C. Concepts and principles:

1. Aggression and violence are two *outward* expressions of hostility.
2. Hostility is often unconscious, automatic response.
3. Hostile wishes and impulses may be underlying motives for many actions.
4. Perceptions may be distorted by hostile outlook.
5. Continuum: from extreme politeness to *externalization* as murderous rage or homicide or *internalization* as depression or suicide.
6. Hostility seen as a defense *against* depression as well as a *cause* of it.
7. Hostility may be repressed, dissociated, or expressed covertly or overtly.
8. *Normal* hostility may come from justifiable fear of *real* danger; *irrational* hostility stems from *anxiety*.
9. Developmental roots of hostility—
   a. *Infants* look away, push away, physically move away from threat; give defiant look. Role modeling by parents.
   b. *Three-year-olds* replace overt hostility with protective shyness, retreat, and withdrawal. Feel weak, inadequate in face of powerful person against whom cannot openly ventilate hostility.
   c. Frustrated or unmet needs for status, prestige, or power serve as a basis for *adult* hostility.

D. Assessment:

1. Fault-finding, scapegoating, sarcasm, derision.
2. Arguing, swearing, abusiveness, verbal threatening.
3. Deceptive sweetness, joking at others' expense, gossiping.
4. Physical abusiveness, violence, murder, vindictiveness.

E. Analysis/nursing diagnosis:

1. *Causes*
   a. *Anxiety* related to a learned means of dealing with an interpersonal threat.
   b. *Potential for violence* related to a reaction to *loss of self-esteem* and *powerlessness*.
   c. *Defensive coping* related to intense frustration, insecurity, and/or apprehension.
   d. *Impaired social interaction* related to low anxiety tolerance.
2. *Situations with high potential for hostility:*
   a. *Enforced illness and hospitalization* cause anxiety, which may be expressed as hostility.
   b. Dependency feelings related to acceptance of illness may result in hostility as a coping mechanism.
   c. Certain illnesses or physical disabilities may be conducive to hostility:
      (1) *Preoperative cancer* client may displace hostility onto staff and family.
      (2) Postoperatively, if diagnosis is *terminal,* the family may displace hostility onto nurse.
      (3) Anger, hostility is a *stage of dying* the person may experience.
      (4) *Amputee* may focus frustration on others due to dependency and jealousy.
      (5) Patients on *hemodialysis* are prone to helplessness, which may be displaced as hostility.

F. Nursing plan/implementation:

1. *Long-term goal:* help alter response to fear, inadequacy, frustration, threat.
2. *Short-term goal:* express and explore feelings of hostility without injury to self or others.
   a. Remain calm, nonthreatening; endure verbal abuse in impartial manner, within limits; speak quietly.
   b. *Protect from self-harm,* acting out.
   c. Discourage hostile behavior while showing acceptance of client.
   d. Offer support to *express* feelings of frustration, anger, and fear *constructively, safely,* and *appropriately.*
   e. Explore hostile feelings *without* fear of retaliation, disapproval.
   f. *Avoid* arguing, advice-giving, reacting with hostility, punitiveness, fault-finding.
   g. *Avoid* joking, teasing, which can be misinterpreted.
   h. *Avoid* words like *anger, hostility;* use client's words (*upset, irritated*).
   i. Do not minimize problem or give client reassurance or hasty, general conclusions.
   j. *Do not stop verbal* expression of anger unless detrimental.
   k. Respond *matter-of-factly* to attention-seeking behavior, not defensively.
   l. *Avoid* physical contact; allow client to set pace in "closeness."
   m. Look for clues to antecedent events and focus *directly* on those areas; *do not evade* or ignore.
   n. Constantly focus on *here and now* and affective component of message rather than on content.
   o. Reconstruct what happened and why, discuss client's reactions; seek observations, *not* inferences.
   p. Learn how client would like to be treated.
   q. Look for ways to help client relate better without defensiveness, *when ready.*
   r. Plan to channel feelings into *motor* outlets (occupational and recreational therapy, physical activity, games, debates).
   s. Explain procedures beforehand; approach frequently.
   t. Withdraw attention, *set limits,* when acting out.
3. *Health teaching:* teach acceptable motor outlets for tension.

G. Evaluation: identifies sources of threat and experiences success in dealing with threat.

VIII. Manipulation

A. Definition: process of playing upon and using others by unfair, insidious means to serve own purpose without regard for others' needs; may take many forms; occurs consciously, unconsciously to some extent, in all interpersonal relations.

B. Operational definition (Figure 1.3):

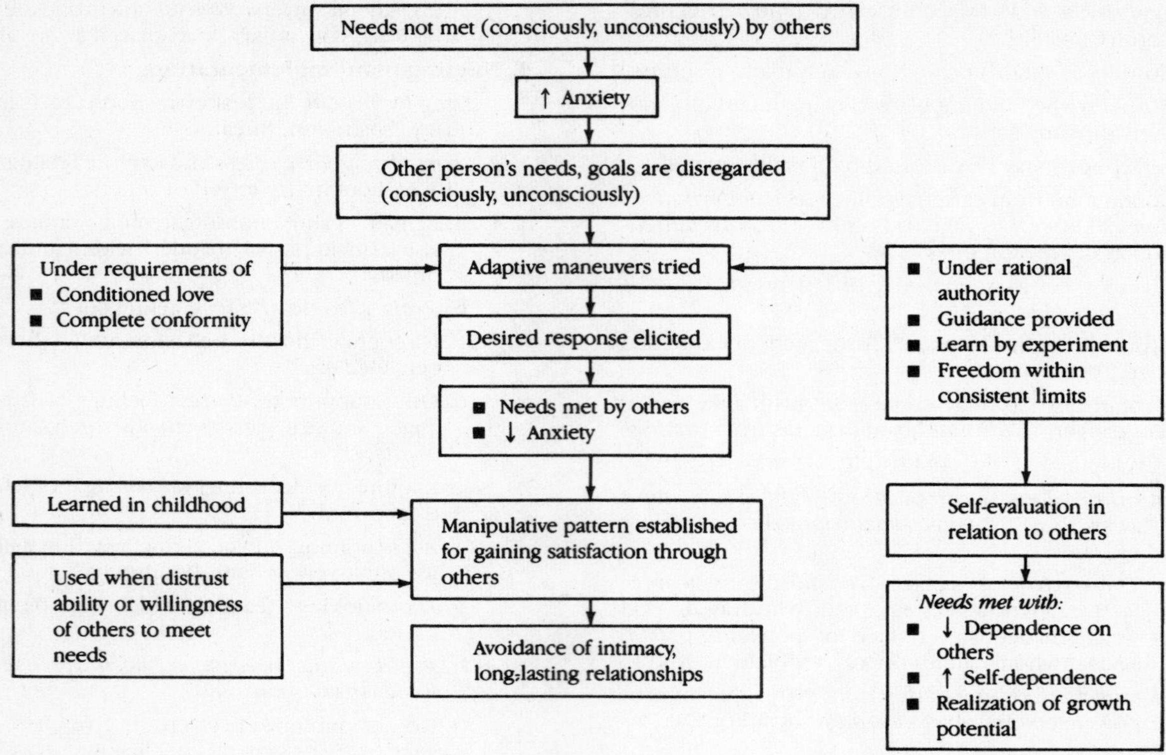

FIGURE 1.3
Operationalization of the behavioral concept of manipulation.

1. Conflicting needs, goals exist between client and other person (e.g., nurse).
2. Other person perceives need as unacceptable, unreasonable.
3. Other person refuses to accept client's need.
4. Client's tension increases, and he begins to relate to others as objects.
5. Client increases attempts to influence others to fulfill his need.
   a. Appears unaware of others' needs.
   b. Exhibits excessive dependency, helplessness, demands.
   c. Sets others at odds (especially staff).
   d. Rationalizes, gives logical reasons.
   e. Uses deception, false promises, insincerity.
   f. Questions and defies nurse's authority and competence.
6. Nurse feels powerless and angry at having been used.

C. Assessment:

1. Acts out sexually, physically.
2. Dawdles, always last minute.
3. Uses insincere flattery; expects special favors, privileges.
4. Exploits generosity and fears of others.
5. Feels no guilt.
6. Plays one staff member against another.
7. Tests limits.
8. Finds weaknesses in others.
9. Makes excessive, unreasonable, unnecessary demands for staff time.
10. Pretends to be helpless, lonely, distraught, tearful.
11. Can't distinguish between truth and falsehood.
12. Plays on sympathy or guilt.
13. Offers many excuses, lacks insight.
14. Pursues unpleasant issues without genuine regard for or feelings of individuals involved.
15. Intimidates, derogates, threatens, bargains, cajoles, violates rules to obtain reactions or privileges.
16. Betrays information.
17. Uses communication as a medium for manipulation, as verbal, nonverbal means to get others to cooperate, to behave in certain way, to get something from another for own use.
18. May be coercive, illogical or skillfully deceptive.
19. Unable to learn from experience; i.e., repeats unacceptable behaviors despite negative consequences.

D. Analysis/nursing diagnosis: *Impaired adjustment* related to:

1. Mistrust and contemptuous view of others' motivations.
2. Life experience of rejection, deception.
3. Low anxiety tolerance.
4. Inability to cope with tension.
5. Unmet dependency needs.

6. Need to avoid anxiety when cannot obtain gratification.
7. Need to obtain something that is forbidden, or need for instant gratification.
8. Attempt to put something over on another when no real advantage exists.
9. Intolerance of intimacy, maneuvering effectively to keep others at a safe distance in order to dilute the relationship by withdrawing and frustrating others or distracting attention away from self.
10. Attempt to demand attention, approval, disapproval.

E. Nursing plan/implementation:

1. *Long-term goal*—define relationship as a mutual experience in learning and trust rather than a struggle for power and control.
2. *Short-term goal*—increase awareness of self and others; increase self-control; learn to accept limitations.
3. Promote use of cooperation, compromise, collaboration rather than exploitation or deception.
4. *Decrease level and extent of manipulation.*
   a. Set *firm, realistic goals,* with clear, consistent expectations and limits.
   b. *Confront* client regarding exploitation attempts; examine, discuss behavior.
   c. Give *positive reinforcement* with concrete reinforcers for nonmanipulation, to lessen need for exploitative, deceptive, and self-destructive behaviors.
   d. *Ignore* "wooden-leg" behavior (feigning illness to evoke sympathy).
   e. *Allow verbal* anger; don't be intimidated; avoid giving desired response to obvious attempts to irritate.
   f. Set *consistent, firm, enforceable limits* on *destructive,* aggressive behavior that impinges on others' health, rights, and interests, and on excessive dependency; *give reasons* when you can't meet requests.
   g. Keep staff informed of rules and reasons; obtain staff *consensus.*
   h. Enforce *direct* communication; encourage openness about *real* needs, feelings.
   i. Do *not* accept gifts, favors, flattery, or other guises of manipulation.
5. Increase responsibility for *self-control* of actions.
   a. Decide who (client, nurse) is responsible for what.
   b. Provide opportunities for *success* to increase self-esteem, experiencing acceptance by others.
   c. Evaluate actions, *not* verbal behavior; point out the difference between talk and action.
   d. Support efforts to be responsible.
   e. Assist client to increase emotional repertoire; explore *alternative* ways of relating interpersonally.
   f. *Avoid submission* to control based on fear of punishment, retaliation, loss of affection.
6. Facilitate awareness of, and *responsibility* for, manipulative behavior and its *effects on others.*
   a. Reflect back client's behavior.
   b. Discourage distortion and misuse of information.
   c. *Increase tolerance* for differences and *delayed gratification* through behavior modification.
   d. Insist on clear, consistent staff communication.
7. Avoid:
   a. Labeling client as a "problem."
   b. Hostile, negative attitude.
   c. Making a public issue of client's behavior.
   d. Being excessively rigid or permissive, inconsistent or ambiguous, argumentative or accusatory.
8. *Health teaching:* act as a role model; demonstrate how to deal with mistakes, human imperfections, by admitting mistakes in nonshameful, nonvirtuous ways.

F. Evaluation: accepts limits; able to compromise, cooperate rather than deceive and exploit; acts responsible, self-dependent.

IX. Noncompliance and uncooperative behavior

A. Definition: consistently failing to meet the requirements of the prescribed treatment regimen; for example, refusing to adhere to dietary restrictions or take required medications.

B. Assessment:

1. Refuses to participate in routine or planned activities.
2. Refuses medication.
3. Violates rules, ignores limits, and abuses privileges; acts out anger and frustration.

C. Analysis/nursing diagnosis: *Noncompliance* related to:

1. *Psychologic factors:* lack of knowledge; attitudes, beliefs, and values; denial of illness; rigid, defensive personality type; anxiety level (very high or very low); can't accept limits or dependency (rebellious counterdependency).
2. *Environmental factors:* finances, transportation, lack of support system.
3. *Health care agent–client relationship:* client feels discounted and like an "object"; sees staff as uncaring, authoritative, controlling.
4. *Health care regimen:* too complicated; not enough benefit from following regimen; results in social stigma or social isolation; unpleasant side effects.

D. Nursing plan/implementation:

1. *General goal:* reduce need to act out by nonadherence.
   a. Take *preventive* action—be alert to signs of noncompliance, such as intent to leave against medical advice.
   b. *Explore* feelings and reasons for lack of cooperation.
   c. Assess and *allay fears* in client in reassuring manner.
   d. Provide *adequate* information about, and reasons for, rules and procedures.
   e. *Avoid* threats or physical restraints; maintain calm composure.
   f. Demonstrate *tact and firmness* when confronting violations.

g. Offer *alternatives.*

h. Firmly insist on cooperation in selected important activities but not all activities.

2. *Health teaching:* increase knowledge base regarding health-related problem, procedures, or treatments, consequences.

E. Evaluation: follows prescribed regimen.

PSYCHIATRIC EMERGENCIES*

I. Definition—sudden onset (days or weeks, not years) of unusual (for that individual), disordered (without pattern or purpose), or socially inappropriate behavior caused by emotional or physiologic situation. For example: suicidal feelings or attempts, overdose, acute psychotic reaction, acute alcohol withdrawal, acute anxiety.

II. General characteristics:

A. Assessment: the presence of great distress without reasonable explanation; *extreme* behavior in comparison with antecedent event.

1. *Fear*—related to a particular person, activity, or place.
2. *Anxiety*—fearful feeling without any obvious reason, not specifically related to a particular person, activity, or place (for example, adolescent turmoil).
3. *Depression*—continual pessimism, easily moved to tears, hopelessness, and isolation (for example, student despondency around exam time, middle-aged crisis, elderly hopelessness).
4. *Mania*—unrealistic optimism.
5. *Anger*—many events seen as deliberate insults.
6. *Confusion*—diminished awareness of who and where one is; memory loss.
7. *Loss of reality contact*—hallucinations or delusion (as in acute psychosis).
8. *Withdrawal*—neglect or giving away of belongings and neglect of appearance; loss of interest in activities; apathy.

B. Analysis/nursing diagnosis: *Ineffective individual coping* related to degree of seriousness:

1. *Life-threatening emergencies*—violence toward self or others (for example, suicide, homicide).
2. *Serious emergencies*—confused and unable to care for or protect self from dangerous situations (as in substance abuse).
3. *Potentially serious emergencies*—anxious and in pain; disorganized behavior; can become worse or better (as in grief reaction).

C. General nursing plan/implementation:

1. *Remove* from stressful situation and persons.
2. Engage in *dialogue* at a nonthreatening distance, to offer help.
3. Use *calm, slow, deliberate* approach to relieve stress and disorganization.
4. *Explain* what will be done about the problem and the likely outcome.
5. *Avoid* using force, threat, or counterthreat.
6. Use *confident, firm, reasonable* approach.
7. Encourage client to relate.
8. Elicit *details.*
9. Encourage *ventilation* of feelings without interruption.
10. Accept distortions of reality *without arguing.*
11. Give form and *structure* to the conversation.
12. Contact significant others to gain information and to be with client, including previous therapist.
13. Treat emergency as *temporary* and *readily resolved.*
14. Check every half hour if cannot remain with client.

III. Categories of psychiatric emergencies:

A. *Acute nonpsychotic reactions,* such as acute anxiety attack or panic reaction (for symptoms, see Anxiety and Anxiety Disorders, pp. 71, 72, and 74).

1. **Assessment** includes differentiating hyperventilation that is anxiety-connected from asthma, angina, and heart disease.
2. **Nursing plan/implementation** in hyperventilation syndrome—*Goal:* prevent paresthesia, tetanic contractions, disturbance in awareness; reassure client that vital organs are not impaired.
   a. Increase CO_2 in lungs by rebreathing from paper bag.
   b. Minimize secondary gains; avoid reinforcing behavior.
   c. *Health teaching:* demonstrate how to slow down breathing rate.
3. **Evaluation:** respirations slowed down; no evidence of effect of hyperventilation.

B. *Delirium or acute organic mental disorders*—conditions produced by changes in the cerebral chemistry or tissue by metabolic toxins, direct trauma to the brain, drug effects, and/or withdrawal.

1. *Acute alcohol intoxication* (see also Alcohol Abuse and Dependence, pp. 57–59).
   a. **Assessment:** signs of head or other injury (past and recent), emotional lability, memory defects, loss of judgment, disorientation.
   b. **Nursing plan/implementation:**
      (1) Observe, monitor *vital signs.*
      (2) *Prevent aspiration* of vomitus by positioning.
      (3) *Decrease* environmental stimuli:
         (a) Place in quiet area of emergency room.
         (b) Speak and handle calmly.
      (4) Give medication (Valium) to control agitation.
   c. **Evaluation:** oriented to time, place, person; appears calmer.
2. *Hallucinogenic drug intoxication*—LSD, mescaline, amphetamines, cocaine, scopolamine, and belladonna.
   a. **Assessment:**
      (1) Perceptual and cognitive distortions (for example, feels heart stopped beating).

---

*Adapted from Aguilera, Donna, and Messick, J., *Crisis Intervention: Therapy for Psychological Emergencies,* Mosby Medical Library, 1982.

(2) Anxiety (apprehension → panic).

(3) Subjective feelings (omnipotence → worthlessness).

(4) Interrelationship of dose, potency, setting, expectations, and experiences of user.

(5) Eyes: red—marijuana; *dilated*—LSD, mescaline, belladonna; *constricted*—heroin and derivatives.

b. **Nursing plan/implementation:**

(1) "Talk down."

(a) Establish *verbal* contact, attempt to have client verbally express what is being experienced.

(b) *Environment*—few people, normal lights, calm, supportive.

(c) Allay fears.

(d) Encourage to keep eyes *open.*

(e) Have client focus on *inanimate* objects in room as a bridge to reality contact.

(f) Use simple, *concrete, repetitive* statements.

(g) *Repetitively* orient to time, place, and temporary nature.

(h) Do *not* moralize, challenge beliefs, or probe into life-style.

(i) Emphasize confidentiality.

(2) *Medication (minor tranquilizer—Valium, Librium):*

(a) Allay anxiety.

(b) Reduce aggressive behavior.

(c) Reduce suicidal potential; check client every 5–15 minutes.

(d) Avoid anticholinergic crisis (precipitated by use of phenothiazines, belladonna, and scopolamine ingestion) with 2–4 mg IM or PO of physostigmine salicylate.

(3) *Hospitalization:* if hallucinations, delusions last more than 12–18 hours; if client has been injecting amphetamines for extended time; if client is paranoid and depressed.

c. **Evaluation:** less frightened; oriented to time, place, person.

3. *Acute delirium*—seen in postoperative electrolyte imbalance, systemic infections, renal and hepatic failure, oversedation, metastatic cancer.

a. **Assessment:**

(1) Disorientation regarding time, at night.

(2) Hallucinations, delusions, illusions.

(3) Alterations in mood.

(4) Increased emotional lability.

(5) Agitation.

(6) Lack of cooperation.

(7) Withdrawal.

(8) Sleep pattern reversal.

(9) Alterations in food intake.

b. **Nursing plan/implementation:**

(1) Identify and remove *toxic* substance.

(2) Reality orientation—well-lit room; constant attendance to inform *repetitively* of place and time and to *protect* from injury to self and others.

(3) Simplify environment.

(4) *Avoid* excessive medication and restraints; use low-dose phenothiazines; do not give barbiturates or sedatives (these increase agitation, confusion, disorientation).

c. **Evaluation:** oriented to time, place, person; cooperative; less agitated.

C. *Acute psychotic reactions*—disorders of mood or thinking characterized by hallucinations, delusions, excessive euphoria (mania), or depression.

1. *Acute schizophrenic reaction* (see also Schizophrenic Disorders, pp. 78–81).

a. **Assessment:**

(1) History of previous hospitalization, no illicit drug ingestion; use of major tranquilizers and recent withdrawal from them or alcohol.

(2) Auditory hallucinations and delusions.

(3) Violent, assaultive, suicidal behavior directed by auditory hallucinations.

(4) Assault, withdrawal, and panic related to paranoid delusions of persecution; fear of harm.

(5) Disturbance in mental status (associative thought disorder).

b. **Nursing plan/implementation** (see also II. C. Hallucinations, pp. 79–80).

(1) Hospitalization.

(2) Medication—phenothiazines.

(3) *Avoid* physical restraints or touch when fears and delusions of sexual attack exist.

(4) Allow client to *diffuse* anger and intensity of panic through talk.

(5) Use simple, *concrete* terms, avoid figures of speech or content subject to multiple interpretations.

(6) Do *not* agree with reality distortions; point out that client's thoughts are difficult to understand but you are willing to listen.

c. **Evaluation:** doesn't hear frightening voices; less fearful and combative behavior.

2. *Manic reaction* (see also Bipolar Disorders, pp. 85–87).

a. **Assessment:**

(1) History of depression requiring antidepressants.

(2) Thought disorder (flight of ideas, delusions of grandeur).

(3) Affect (elated, irritable, irrational anger).

(4) Speech (loud, pressured).

(5) Behavior (rapid, erratic, chaotic).

b. **Nursing plan/implementation:**

(1) Hospitalization to protect from injury to self and others.

(2) Medication: lithium carbonate.

(3) Same as for acute schizophrenic reaction, *ex-*

cept do not encourage talk, as need to decrease stimulation.

(4) Provide food and fluids that can be consumed while on-the-go.

c. **Evaluation:** speech and activity slowed down; thoughts less disordered.

D. *Homicidal or assaultive reaction*—seen in acutely drug-intoxicated, delirious, paranoid, acutely excited manic, or acute anxiety-panic conditions.

1. **Assessment**—history of obvious antisocial behavior, paranoid psychosis, previous violence, sexual conflict, rivalry, substance abuse, recent moodiness, and withdrawal.

2. **Nursing plan/implementation:**

a. Physically restrain if client has a weapon; use group of trained people to help.

b. Allow person to "save face" in giving up weapon.

c. *Separate* from intended victims.

d. Approach: calm, unhurried; *one person* to offer support and reassurance; use clear, unambiguous statements.

e. Immediate and rapid admission procedures.

f. Observe for *suicidal* behavior that may follow homicidal attempt.

3. **Evaluation:** client regains impulse control.

E. *Suicidal reaction*—seen in anxiety attacks, substance intoxication, toxic delirium, schizophrenic auditory hallucinations, and depressive reactions.

1. **Concepts and principles related to suicide:**

a. *Based on social theory:* Suicidal tendency is a result of collective social forces rather than isolated individual motives (Durkheim's *Le Suicide*).

(1) Common factor: increased *alienation* between person and social group; psychologic isolation, called "anomie," when links between groups are weakened.

(2) "Egoistic" suicide: results from lack of integration of individual with others.

(3) "Altruistic" suicide: results from insufficient individualization.

(4) *Implication:* increase group cohesiveness and mutual interdependence, making group more coherent and consistent in fulfilling needs of each member.

b. *Based on symbolic interaction theory:*

(1) Person evaluates self according to *others' assessment.*

(2) Thus, suicide stems from *social rejection* and disrupted social relations.

(3) Perceived failure in relationships with others may be inaccurate but seen as real by the individual.

(4) *Implication:* need to recognize difference in perception of alienation between own viewpoint and others'.

c. *Based on psychoanalytic theory:*

(1) Suicide stems mainly from the individual, with external events only as precipitants.

(2) There is a strong life urge in people.

(3) *Universal death instinct* is always present (Freud).

(4) Person may be balancing life wishes and death wishes. When self-preservation instincts are diminished, death instincts may find direct outlet via suicide.

(5) When *love instinct* is frustrated, *hate* impulse takes over (Menninger).

(a) Desire to kill → desire to be killed → desire to kill oneself.

(b) Suicide may be an act of extreme hostility, manipulation, and revenge to elicit guilt and remorse in significant others.

(c) Suicide may also be act of self-punishment to handle own guilt or to control fate.

d. *Based on synthesis of social and psychoanalytic theories:*

(1) Suicide is seen as *running away* from an intolerable situation in order to interrupt it rather than *running to* something more desirable.

(2) Process *defined in operational terms* involves:

(a) Despair over inability to cope.

(b) Inability to feel hope or adequacy.

(c) Frustration with others when others cannot fill needs.

(d) Rage and aggression experienced toward significant other is turned inward.

(e) Psychic blow acts as precipitant.

(f) Life seen as harder to cope with, with no chance of improvement in life situation.

(g) *Implication:* persons who experience suicidal impulses can gain a certain amount of control over these impulses through the support they gain from meaningful relationships with others.

e. *Based on crisis theory (Dublin):* concept of emotional disequilibrium:

(1) Everyone at some point in life is in a crisis, with temporary inability to solve problems or to master the crisis.

(2) Usual coping mechanisms do not function.

(3) Person unable to relate to others.

(4) Person searches consciously and unconsciously for useful coping techniques, with suicide as one of various solutions.

(5) With inadequate communication of needs and isolation, suicide is possible.

f. *Based on the view that suicide is an individual's personal reaction and decision, a final response to own situation:*

(1) *Process* of anger turned inward → self-inflicted, destructive action.

(2) *Definition* of concept in operational steps:

(a) Frustration of individual needs → anger.

(b) Anger turned inward → feelings of guilt, despair, depression, incompetence, hopelessness, and exhaustion.

(c) Stress felt and perceived as unbearable and overwhelming.

(d) Attempt to communicate hopelessness and defeat to others.

(e) Others do not provide hope.

(f) Sudden change in behavior, as noted when depression appears to lift, may indicate *danger,* as person has more energy to act on suicidal thoughts and feelings.

(g) Decision to end life → plan of action → self-induced, self-destructive behavior.

(3) May be *pseudo-suicide* attempts, where there is no actual or realistic desire to achieve finality of death. Intentions or causes may be:

(a) "Cry for help," where nonlethal attempt notifies others of deeper intentions.

(b) Desire to manipulate others.

(c) Need for attention and pity.

(d) Self-punishment.

(e) Symbol of utter frustration.

(f) Wish to punish others.

(g) Misuse of alcohol and other drugs.

(4) Other reasons for self-destruction, where the individual *gives his life* rather than takes it, include:

(a) Strong parental love that can overcome fear and instinct of self-preservation to save child's life.

(b) "Sacrificial death" during war, such as kamikaze pilots in WWII.

(c) Submission to death for religious beliefs (martyrdom).

2. **Assessment of suicide:**

a. *Assessment of risk regarding statistical probability of suicide—composite picture:* over-45-year-old male, unemployed, divorced, living alone, depressed (weight loss, somatic delusions, sleep disturbance, preoccupied with suicide), history of substance abuse and suicide within family.

b. *Ten factors* to predict potential suicide and assess risk:

(1) *Age, sex, and race*—teenage, older age; more women make attempts; more men complete suicide act. Highest risk: older women rather than young boys; older men rather than young girls. Suicide occurs in all races and socioeconomic groups.

(2) *Recent stress*—family problems: death, divorce, separation, alienation; financial pressures; loss of job; loss of status; failing grades.

(3) *Clues to suicide:* suicidal thoughts are usually time-limited and do not last forever. Early assessment of behavioral and verbal clues is important.*

(a) *Verbal clues—Direct:* "I am going to shoot myself." *Indirect:* "It's more than I can bear." *Coded:* "This is the last time you'll ever see me." "I want you to have my coin collection."

(b) *Behavioral clues—Direct:* trial run with pills or razor, for example. *Indirect:* sudden lifting of depression, buying a casket, giving away cherished belongings, putting affairs in order, writing a will.

(c) *Syndromes—Dependent-dissatisfied:* emotionally dependent but dislikes dependent state, irritable, helpless. *Depressed:* detachment from life; feels life is a burden; hopelessness, futility. *Disoriented:* delusions or hallucinations, confusion, delirium tremens, organic brain syndromes. *Willful-defiant:* active need to direct and control environment and life situation, with low frustration tolerance and rigid set, rage, shame.

(4) *Suicidal plan*—the more details about method, timing, and place, the higher the risk.

(5) *Previous suicidal behavior*—history of prior attempt increases risk. Eight out of ten suicide attempts give verbal and behavioral warnings as listed above.

(6) *Medical status*—chronic ailments, terminal illness, and pain increase suicidal risk.

(7) *Communication*—the more withdrawn and apathetic, the greater potential for suicide, unless extreme psychomotor retardation is present.

(8) *Style of life*—high risks include substance abusers, those with sexual-identity conflicts, unstable relationships (personal and job-related). Suicidal tendencies are not inherited but learned from family and other interpersonal relationships.

(9) *Alcohol*—can reinforce helpless and hopeless feelings; may be lethal if used with barbiturates; can decrease inhibitions, result in impulsive behavior.

(10) *Resources*—the fewer the resources, the higher the suicide potential. Examples of resources: family, friends, colleagues, religion, pets, meaningful recreational outlets, satisfying employment.

c. Assess *needs* commonly communicated by individuals who are suicidal:

(1) To trust.

(2) To be accepted.

(3) To bolster self-esteem.

(4) To "fit in" with groups.

(5) To experience success and interrupt the failure syndrome.

(6) To expand capacity for pleasure.

(7) To increase autonomy and sense of self-mastery.

(8) To work out an acceptable sexual identity.

3. **Analysis/nursing diagnosis:** *Potential for self-directed violence* related to:

a. Feelings of alienation.

b. Feelings of rejection.

c. Feelings of hopelessness, despair.

d. Feelings of frustration and rage.

4. **Nursing plan/implementation:**

a. *Long-term goals*

(1) Increase client's self-reliance.

(2) Help client achieve more realistic and positive feelings of self-esteem, self-respect, acceptance by others, and sense of belonging.

(3) Help client experience success, interrupt failure pattern, and expand views about pleasure.

b. *Short-term goals*

(1) Medical: assist as necessary with gastric lavage; provide respiratory and vascular support; assist in repair of inflicted wounds.

(2) Provide protection from self-destruction until client is able to assume this responsibility.

(3) Allow outward and constructive expression of hostile and aggressive feelings.

(4) Provide for physical needs.

c. *Suicide precautions* to institute under emergency conditions:

(1) One-to-one supervision at *all* times for maximum precautions; check whereabouts every 15 minutes, if on basic suicide precautions.

(2) Prior to instituting these measures, explain to client what you will be doing and why; MD must also explain; document this explanation.

(3) Do not allow client to leave the unit for tests, procedures.

(4) Look through client's belongings *with* the client and remove any potentially harmful objects, e.g., pills, matches, belts, razors, glass, tweezers.

(5) Allow visitors and phone calls, but maintain one-to-one supervision during visits.

(6) Check that visitors do not leave potentially harmful objects in the client's room.

(7) Serve meals in an isolation meal tray that contains no glass or metal silverware.

(8) Do not discontinue these measures without an order.

d. *General approaches*

(1) *Observe* closely at all times to assess suicide potential.

(2) Be *available.*

(a) Demonstrate concern for client as a person.

(b) Be sensitive, warm, and consistent.

(c) Listen with empathy.

(d) Avoid imposing your own feelings of reality on client.

(e) Avoid extremes in your own mood when with client (especially exaggerated cheerfulness).

(3) *Focus directly* on client's self-destructive ideas.

(a) Reduce alienation and immobilization by discussing this "taboo" topic.

(b) Acknowledge suicidal threats with calmness and without reproach—do not ignore or minimize threat.

(c) Find out details about suicide plan and reduce environmental hazards.

(d) Help client verbalize aggressive, hostile, and hopeless feelings.

(e) Explore death fantasies—try to take "romance" out of death.

(4) Acknowledge that suicide is one of several options.

(5) *Make a contract* with the client, and structure a plan of alternatives for coping when next confronted with the need to commit suicide (for example, the client could call someone, express feeling of anger outwardly, or ask for help).

(6) Point out client's *self-responsibility* for suicidal act.

(a) Avoid manipulation by client who says, "You are responsible for stopping me from killing myself."

(b) Emphasize protection against self-destruction *rather than* punishment.

(7) *Support* the part of the client that wants to live.

(a) Focus on ambivalence.

(b) Emphasize meaningful past relationships and events.

(c) Look for reasons left for wanting to live. Elicit what is meaningful to the client at the moment.

(d) Point out effect of client's death on others.

(8) *Remove sources of stress.*

(a) Decrease uncomfortable feelings of *alienation* by initiating one-to-one interactions.

(b) Make all *decisions* when client is in severe depression.

(c) Progressively let client make simple decisions: what to eat, what to watch on TV, etc.

(9) *Provide hope.*

(a) Let client know that problems can be solved with help.

(b) Bring in new resources for help.

(c) Talk about likely changes in client's life.

(d) Review past effective coping behaviors.

(10) *Provide with opportunity to be useful.* Reduce self-centeredness and brooding by planning diversional activities within the client's capabilities.

(11) *Involve as many people as possible.*

(a) Gradually bring in others, for instance, other therapists, friends, staff, clergy, family, co-workers.

(b) Prevent staff "burn-out," found when only one nurse is working with suicidal client.

(12) *Health teaching:* teach client and staff principles of crisis intervention and resolution. Teach new coping skills.

5. **Evaluation:** physical condition is stabilized; client able to verbalize feelings rather than acting them out.

CRISIS INTERVENTION

Crisis intervention is a type of brief psychiatric treatment in which individuals and/or their families are helped in their efforts to forestall the process of mental decompensation in reaction to severe emotional stress by direct and immediate supportive approaches.

I. Definition of crisis—sudden event in one's life that disturbs homeostasis, during which usual coping mechanisms cannot resolve the problem. Types of crisis:

A. *Maturational* (internal): see Erik Erikson's eight stages of developmental crises anticipated in the development of the infant, child, adolescent, and adult (Unit 3).

B. *Situational* (external): occurs at any time; for example, loss of job, loss of income, death of significant person, illness, hospitalization.

II. Concepts and principles related to crisis intervention:

A. Crises are turning points where changes in behavior patterns and life-styles can occur; individuals in crisis are most amenable to altering old and unsuccessful coping mechanisms and are most likely to learn new and more functional behaviors.

B. Social milieu and its structure are contributing factors in both the development of psychiatric symptoms and eventual recovery from them.

C. If crisis is handled effectively, the person's mental stability will be maintained; individual may return to a precrisis state or better.

D. If crisis is not handled effectively, individual may progress to a worse state with exacerbations of earlier conflicts; future crises may not be handled well.

E. There are a number of universal developmental crisis periods (maturational crises) in every individual's life.

F. Each person tries to maintain equilibrium through use of adaptive behaviors.

G. When individuals face a problem they cannot solve, tension, anxiety, narrowed perception, and disorganized functioning occur.

H. *Immediate relief* of symptoms produced by crisis is more urgent than *exploring* their cause.

III. Characteristics of crisis intervention:

A. Acute, sudden onset related to a stressful precipitating event of which individual is aware but which immobilizes previous coping abilities.

B. Responsive to brief therapy with focus on immediate problem.

C. Focus shifted from the psyche in the individual to the *individual in the environment;* deemphasis on intrapsychic aspects.

D. Crisis period is *time-limited* (usually up to six weeks).

IV. Nursing plan/implementation in crises:

A. General goals:

1. Avoid hospitalization if possible.
2. Return to precrisis level and preserve ability to function.
3. Assist in problem solving, with *here-and-now* focus.

B. *Assess* the crisis:

1. Identify stressful *precipitating* events: duration, problems created, and degree of significance.
2. Assess *suicidal and homicidal risk.*
3. Assess amount of *disruption* in individual's life and effect on significant others.
4. Assess *current coping skills,* strengths, and general level of functioning.

C. *Plan* the intervention:

1. Consider *past coping* mechanisms.
2. Propose *alternatives* and untried coping methods.

D. *Implementation:*

1. Help client relate the crisis event to current feelings.
2. Encourage expression of all feelings related to disruption.
3. Explore past coping skills and *reinforce adaptive* ones.
4. Use all means available in *social network* to take care of client's *immediate needs* (significant others, law enforcement agencies, housing, welfare, employment, medical, and school, for example).
5. Set limits.
6. *Health teaching:* teach additional problem-solving approaches.

V. Evaluation:

A. Client returns to precrisis level of functioning.

B. Client learns new, more effective coping skills.

C. Client can describe realistic plans for future in terms of own perception of progress, support system, and coping mechanisms.

Selected Specific Crisis Situations

I. Rape-trauma syndrome

A. Definition: forcible perpetration of an act of sexual intercourse on the body of an unwilling person.

B. Assessment:

1. *Signs of physical trauma*—physical findings of entry.
2. *Symptoms of physical trauma*—verbatim statements regarding type of sexual attack.
3. *Signs of emotional trauma*—tears, hyperventilation, extreme anxiety, withdrawal, self-blame, anger, embarrassment, fears, sleeping and eating disturbances, desire for revenge.
4. *Symptoms of emotional trauma*—statements regarding method of force used and threats made.

C. Analysis/nursing diagnosis: *Rape-trauma syndrome* related to phases of response to rape:

1. *Acute response:* volatility, disorganization, disbelief, shock, incoherence, agitated motor activity, nightmares, guilt (should have been able to protect self), phobias (crowds, being alone, sex).
2. *Outward coping:* denial and suppression of anxiety and fear (silent rape syndrome), feelings appear controlled.
3. *Integration and resolution:* confronts anger with attacker; realistic perspective.

D. Nursing plan/implementation in counseling rape victims. Figure 1.4 is a summary of self-care decisions a victim faces the first night following a sexual assault.

1. Overall goals:

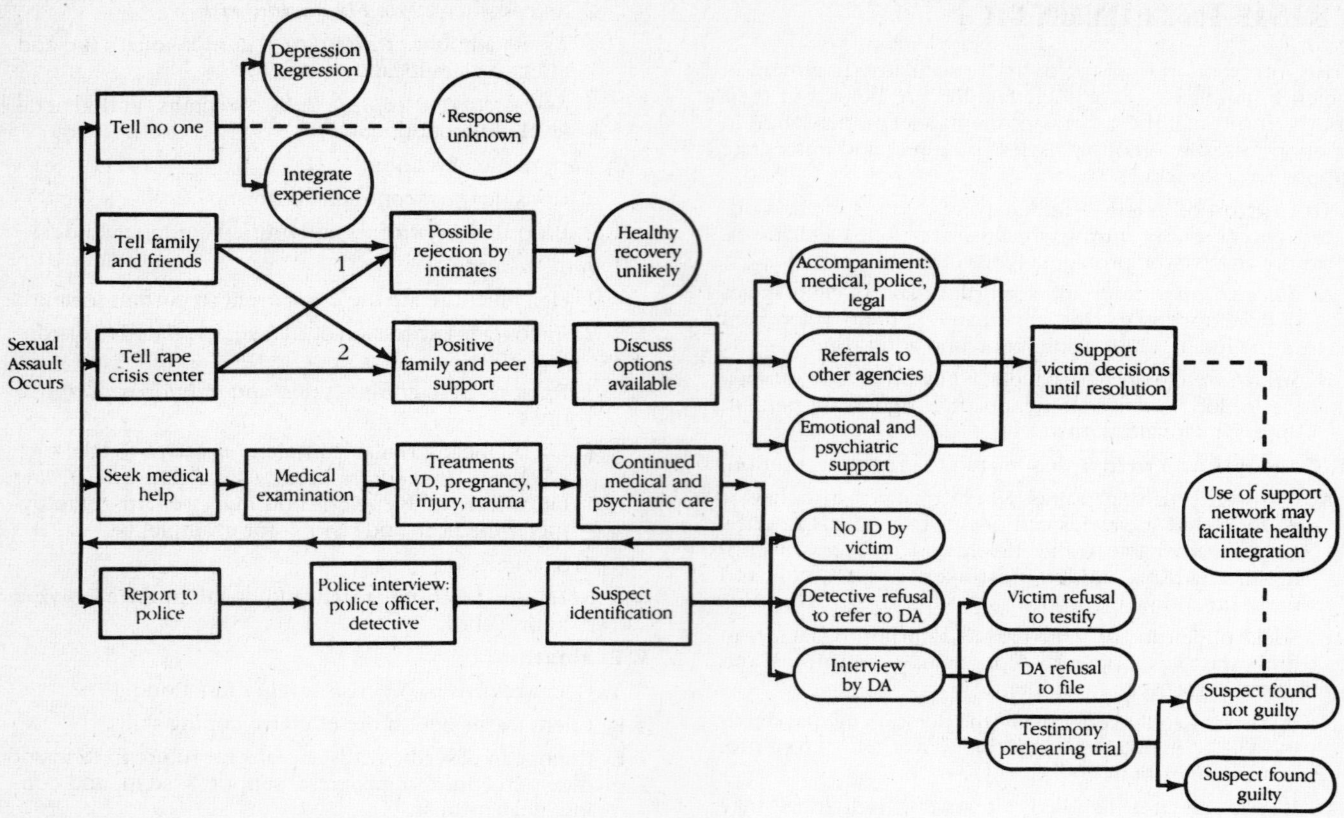

■ **FIGURE 1.4**
Victim decisions following a sexual assault. (From the Rape Crisis Services of the YWCA, Greater Harrisburg, PA.)

a. Acknowledge feelings.
b. Face feelings.
c. Resolve feelings.
d. Maintain and restore self-respect, dignity, integrity, and self-determination.

2. Work through issues:
   a. Handle legal matters and police contacts.
   b. Clarify facts.
   c. Get medical attention if needed.
   d. Notify family and friends.
   e. Understand emotional reaction.
   f. Attend to practical concerns.
   g. Evaluate need for psychiatric consultations.
3. Acute phase:
   a. Decrease victim's stress, anxiety, fear.
   b. Seek medical care.
   c. Increase self-confidence and self-esteem.
   d. Identify and accept feelings and needs (to be in control, cared about, to achieve).
   e. Reorient perceptions, feelings, and statements about self.
   f. Help resume normal life-style.
4. Outward coping phase:
   a. Remain available and supportive.
   b. Reflect words, feelings, and thoughts.
   c. Explore real problems.
   d. Explore alternatives regarding contraception, legal issues.
   e. Evaluate response of family and friends to victim and rape.
5. Integration and resolution phase:
   a. Assist exploration of feelings (anger) regarding attacker.
   b. Explore feelings (guilt and shame) regarding self.
   c. Assist in making own decisions regarding health care.
6. Maintain confidentiality and neutrality—facilitate person's own decision.
7. Search for alternatives to advice-giving.
8. *Health teaching:*
   a. Explain procedures and services to victim.
   b. Counsel to avoid isolated areas and being helpful to strangers.
   c. Counsel where and how to resist attack (scream, run unless assailant has weapon).
   d. Teach what to do if pregnancy or STD are outcome.

E. Evaluation: little or no evidence of possible long-term effects of rape (guilt, shame, phobias, denial).

II. Sexual abuse of children

A. Assessment—characteristic behaviors:

1. *Relationship* of offender to victim: many filling paternal role (uncle, grandfather, cousin) with repeated, unquestioned access to the child.
2. Methods of *pressuring* victim into sexual activity: offering material goods, misrepresenting moral standards ("it's O.K."), exploiting need for human contact and warmth.
3. Method of pressuring victim to *secrecy* (in order to conceal the act) is inducing fear of: punishment, not being believed, rejection, being blamed for the activity, abandonment.
4. Disclosure of sexual activity via:
   a. Direct visual or verbal confrontation and *observation* by others.
   b. *Verbalization* of act by victim.
   c. *Visible clues:* excess money and candy, new clothes, pictures, notes.
   d. *Signs and symptoms:* bed-wetting, excessive bathing, tears, avoiding school, somatic distress (GI and urinary tract pains).

B. Analysis/nursing diagnosis:

1. *Altered protection* related to inflicted pain.
2. *Potential for injury* related to neglect, abuse.
3. *Personality identity disturbance* related to abuse as child and feeling guilty and responsible for being a victim.
4. *Ineffective individual coping* related to high stress level.
5. *Sleep pattern disturbance* related to traumatic sexual experiences.
6. *Ineffective family coping.*
7. *Altered family processes* related to use of violence.
8. *Altered parenting* related to violence.
9. *Powerlessness* related to feelings of being dependent on abuser.
10. *Social isolation/withdrawal* related to shame about family violence.

C. Nursing plan/implementation:

1. Establish safe environment and the termination of trauma.
2. Encourage child to verbalize feelings about incident to dispel tension built up by secrecy.
3. Ask child to draw a picture or use dolls and toys to show what happened.
4. Observe for symptoms over a period of time.
   a. *Phobic* reactions when seeing or hearing offender's name.
   b. *Sleep pattern* changes, recurrent dreams, nightmares.
5. Look for *silent reaction* to being an accessory to sex (that is, child keeping burden of the secret activity within self); help deal with unresolved issues.
6. Establish therapeutic alliance with abusive parent.
7. *Health teaching:*
   a. Teach child that his (her) body is private and to inform a responsible adult when someone violates privacy without consent.
   b. Teach adults in family to respond to victim with sensitivity, support, and concern.

D. Evaluation:

1. Child's needs for affection, attention, personal recognition, or love met without sexual exploitation.
2. Perpetrator accepts therapy.
3. Conspiracy of silence is broken.

■ COMFORT, REST, ACTIVITY, AND MOBILITY FUNCTIONS

SLEEP DISTURBANCE

I. Types of sleep:

A. *Rapid eye movement (REM) sleep:* Colorful, dramatic, emotional, implausible dreams.

B. *Non-REM sleep—stages:*

1. Stage 1: lasts 30 seconds to 7 minutes—falls asleep, drowsy; easily awakened; fleeting thoughts.
2. Stage 2: more relaxed; no eye movements, clearly asleep but readily awakens; 45% of total sleep time spent in this stage.
3. Stage 3: (Delta sleep) deep muscle relaxation; ↓ TPR.
4. Stage 4: (Delta sleep) very relaxed; rarely moves.

C. *Sleep cycle*—common progression of sleep stages:

1. Stages 1, 2, 3, 4, 3, 2, REM, 2, 3, 4, etc.
2. *Delta* sleep most common during first third of night, with *REM* sleep periods increasing in duration during night from 1–2 minutes at start to 20–30 minutes by early morning.
3. REM sleep varies.
   a. Adolescents spend 30% of total sleep time in REM sleep.
   b. Adults spend 15% of total sleep time in REM sleep.

II. Sleep deprivation (Dyssomnias):

A. Assessment:

1. *Non-REM sleep loss:* physical fatigue due to less time spent in normal deep sleep.
2. *REM sleep loss:* psychologic effects—irritability, confusion, anxiety, short-term memory loss, paranoia, hallucinations.
3. *Desynchronized sleep:* occurs when sleep shifts more than 2 hours from normal sleep period. Irritability, anoxia, decreased stress tolerance.

B. Analysis/nursing diagnosis: *Sleep pattern disturbance* may be related to:

1. Interrupted sleep cycles before 90-minute sleep cycle is completed.
2. Unfamiliar sleeping environment.
3. Alterations in normal sleep/activity cycles (e.g., jet lag).
4. Preexisting sleep deficits prior to hospital admission.

5. Medications, e.g., alcohol withdrawal or abruptly discontinuing the use of hypnotic or antidepressant medications.
6. Pain.

C. Nursing plan/implementation:

1. Obtain sleep history as part of nursing assessment. Determine: normal sleep hours, bedtime rituals, factors that promote or interrupt sleep.
2. Duplicate normal bedtime rituals when possible.
3. Make *environment* conducive to sleep: lighting, noise, temperature.
   a. Close door, dim lights, turn off unneeded machinery.
   b. Encourage staff to muffle conversation at night.
4. Encourage *daytime* exercise periods.
5. Allow *uninterrupted periods of 90 minutes of sleep*. Group nighttime treatments and observations that require touching the client.
6. *Minimize* use of hypnotic medications.
   a. Substitute backrubs, warm milk, relaxation exercises.
   b. Encourage physician to consider prescribing hypnotics that minimize sleep disruption (e.g., chloral hydrate and Dalmane).
   c. *Taper* off hypnotics rather than abruptly discontinuing.
7. Observe client while asleep.
   a. Evaluate quality of sleep.
   b. It may be sleep apnea if client is extremely restless and snoring heavily.
8. *Health teaching:* avoid caffeine and hyperstimulation at bedtime; teach how to promote sleep-inducing environment, relaxation techniques.

D. Evaluation: verbalizes satisfaction with amount, quality of sleep.

■ SENSORY-PERCEPTUAL FUNCTIONS

SENSORY DISTURBANCE

I. Types of sensory disturbance:

A. *Sensory deprivation*—amount of stimuli *less* than required, such as isolation in bed or room, deafness, stroke victim.

B. *Sensory overload*—receives *more* stimuli than can be tolerated; for example, bright lights, noise, strange machinery, barrage of visitors.

C. *Sensory deficit*—impairment in functioning of sensory or perceptual processes; for example, blindness, changes in tactile perceptions.

II. Assessment—based on awareness of behavioral changes:

A. *Sensory deprivation*—boredom, daydreaming, increasing sleep, thought slowness, inactivity, thought disorganization, hallucinations.

B. *Sensory overload*—same as above, plus restlessness and agitation, confusion.

C. *Sensory deficit*—may not be able to distinguish sounds, odors, and tastes or differentiate tactile sensations.

III. Analysis/nursing diagnosis: problems related to sensory disturbance:

A. *Altered thought processes.*

B. *Confusion.*

C. *Anger, aggression.*

D. *Body image disturbance.*

E. *Sleep pattern disturbance.*

IV. Nursing plan/implementation:

A. *Management of existing* sensory disturbances in:

1. *Acute sensory deprivation*
   a. Increase interaction with staff.
   b. Use TV.
   c. Provide touch.
   d. Help clients choose menus that have aromas, varied tastes, temperatures, colors, textures.
   e. Use light cologne or after-shave lotion, bath powder.
2. *Sensory overload*
   a. Restrict number of visitors and length of stay.
   b. Reduce noise and lights.
   c. Reduce newness by establishing and following routine.
   d. Organize care to provide for extended rest periods with minimal input.
3. *Sensory deficits*
   a. Report observations about hearing, vision.
   b. May imply need for new glasses, medical diagnosis, or therapy.

B. *Health teaching: prevention* of sensory disturbance involves *education* of parents during child's growth and development regarding tactile, auditory, and visual stimulation.

1. Hold, talk, and play with infant when awake.
2. Provide bright toys with different designs for children to hold.
3. Change environment.
4. Provide music and auditory stimuli.
5. Give foods with variety of textures, tastes, colors.

V. Evaluation:

A. Client is oriented to time, place, person.

B. Little or no evidence of mood or sleep disturbance.

ANOREXIA NERVOSA/BULIMIA

Anorexia nervosa is an eating disorder, usually seen in adolescence, when a person is underweight and emaciated and refuses to eat. It can result in death due to irreversible metabolic processes.

Bulimia nervosa is another type of eating disorder, also encountered among older women and younger men as well. It is characterized by at least two binge-eating episodes of large quantities of high calorie food over a couple of hours followed by disparaging self-criticism and depression. Self-induced vomiting is commonly associated since it decreases physical pain of abdominal distention, may reduce post-binge anguish, and may provide a method of self-control. Bulimic episodes may occur as part of anorexia nervosa, but these clients rarely become emaciated, and not all have a body image disturbance.

I. Concepts and principles related to anorexia nervosa:

A. *Not* due to lack of appetite or problem with appetite center in hypothalamus.

B. Normal stomach hunger is *repressed, denied, depersonalized;* no conscious awareness of hunger sensation.

II. Assessment of anorexia nervosa:

A. *Body image disturbance*—delusional, obsessive (for example, doesn't see self as thin and is bewildered by others' concern).

B. Usually *preoccupied* with food, yet dreads gaining too much weight. *Ambivalence:* avoids food, hoards food.

C. Feels ineffectual, with low sex drive. *Repudiation of sexuality.*

D. *Pregnancy* fears, including misconceptions of oral impregnation through food.

E. *Self-punitive* behavior leading to starvation.

F. *Physical signs and symptoms*

1. Weight loss (20% of previous "normal" body weight).
2. Amenorrhea and secondary sex organ atrophy.
3. Hyperactivity; compulsiveness.
4. Constipation.
5. Hypotension, bradycardia, hypothermia.
6. Hyperkeratosis of skin.
7. Blood: leukopenia, anemia, hypoglycemia, hypoproteinemia, hypercholesterolemia, hypokalemia.

III. Analysis/nursing diagnosis:

A. *Potential for self-inflicted injury* related to starvation from refusal to eat or ambivalence about food.

B. *Altered physiological processes:* amenorrhea related to starvation; hypotension, bradycardia.

C. *Altered nutrition, less than body requirements,* related to attempts to vomit food after eating and refusal to eat, related to need to demonstrate control.

D. *Body image disturbance* related to anxiety over assuming an adult role and concern with sexual identity.

E. *Compulsive physical activity* related to need to maintain control of self, represented by losing weight.

IV. Nursing plan/implementation:

A. Help reestablish connections between body sensations (hunger) and responses (eating). Use *stimulus-response conditioning* methods to set up eating regimen (see Behavior Modification, pp. 87–88).

B. *Monitor* physiologic signs and symptoms (amenorrhea, constipation, hypoproteinemia, hypoglycemia, anemia, secondary sexual organ atrophy, hypothermia, hypotension, leg cramps and other signs of hypokalemia).

1. *Weigh* regularly, at same time and with same amount of clothing.
2. Make sure water drinking is avoided before weighing.
3. Give one-to-one supervision during and 30 minutes after mealtimes to *prevent* attempts to vomit food.

C. *Health teaching:*

1. Explain normal sexual growth and development to improve knowledge deficit.
2. Use behavior modification to reestablish awareness of hunger sensation and to relate it to the clock and regular meal times.
3. Teach parents skills in communication related to dependence/independence needs of adolescent.

V. Evaluation:

A. Attains and maintains minimal normal weight for age and height.

B. Eats regular meal (standard nutritional diet).

C. No incidence of self-induced vomiting, bulimia, or compulsive physical activity.

D. Acts on increased internal emotional awareness and recognition of body sensation of hunger (i.e., talks about being hungry and feeling hunger pangs).

E. Relates increased sense of effectiveness with less need to control food intake.

ORGANIC MENTAL DISORDERS

Organic mental disorders include etiology associated with: (1) the *aging process* (Dementias arising in the senium or presenium, includes primary degenerative dementia of the Alzheimer type and multiinfarct dementia); (2) *psychoactive substance-induced organic mental disorder* (e.g., alcohol, barbiturates, opioids, cocaine, amphetamines, PCP, hallucinogens, *cannabis,* nicotine, and caffeine). The organic mental disorders are further classified under ten syndromes, as listed in I.D., below.

Dementias Arising in the Senium and Presenium

I. Concepts and principles:

A. Course may be progressive, with steady deterioration.

B. Alternative pathways and compensatory mechanisms may develop to show a clinical picture of remissions and exacerbations.

C. Etiologic factors:

1. Aging.
2. Substance-induced.

D. DSM IIIR lists *ten different syndromes:*

1. Intoxication.
2. Withdrawal.
3. Delirium.
4. Dementia.
5. Amnestic disorder *(Alzheimer's disease):* progressive, irreversible loss of cerebral function due to cortical atrophy; exists in 10–20% of people over 80 years old; may begin at ages 40–60; may lead to death within two years.
   a. Progressive decline in intellectual capacity: memory, judgment, affect, motor coordination and loss of social sense, apathy or restlessness.
   b. *Problems with* speech, recognition of familiar objects (even parts of own body).
6. Delusional disorder.

7. Hallucinosis.
8. Mood disorder.
9. Anxiety disorder.
10. Personality disorder.

II. Assessment:

A. *Most common areas of difficulty* for the person with an organic brain syndrome can be grouped under the mnemonic term *JOCAM: J*—judgment, *O*—orientation, *C*—confabulation, *A*—affect, and *M*—memory.

1. *Judgment:* impaired, resulting in socially inappropriate behavior (such as hypersexuality toward inappropriate objects) and inability to carry out activities of daily living.
2. *Orientation:* confused, disoriented; perceptual disturbances (for example, illusions, misidentification of other persons and objects; misperception to make unfamiliar more familiar; *visual, tactile, and auditory* hallucinations may appear as images and voices or disorganized light and sound patterns). *Paranoid delusions* of persecution.
3. *Confabulation:* common use of this defense mechanisms in order to fill in memory gaps with invented stories.
4. *Affect:* mood changes and unstable emotions; quarrelsome, with outbursts of morbid anger (as in cerebral arteriosclerosis); tearful; withdrawn from social contact; *depression* is a frequent reaction to loss of physical and social function.
5. *Memory:* impaired, especially for names and *recent* events; may compensate by confabulating and by using *circumstantiality* and *tangential* speaking patterns.

B. *Other areas of difficulty*

1. *Seizures* (in Alzheimer's disease and cerebral arteriosclerosis, for example).
2. *Intellectual capacities diminished.*
   a. Difficulty with abstract thought.
   b. Compensatory mechanism is to stay with familiar topics; repetition.
   c. Short concentration periods.
3. *Personality changes*
   a. Loss of ego flexibility; adoption of more rigid attitudes.
   b. Ritualism in daily activities.
   c. Hoarding.
   d. Somatic preoccupations (hypochondriases).
   e. Restlessness.

III. Analysis/nursing diagnosis:

A. *Potential for injury* related to cognitive deficits and altered motor behavior (restlessness, hyperactivity).

B. *Altered conduct/impulse processes* (irritability and aggressiveness) related to neurologic impairment.

C. *Sensory/perceptual alterations:* visual, auditory, kinesthetic, gustatory, tactile, olfactory.

D. *Altered attention and memory* related to progressive neurological losses.

E. *Total incontinence* related to sensory/perceptual alterations.

F. *Altered nutrition, more or less than body requirements,* related to confusion.

G. *Self-care deficit* (feeding, bathing/hygiene, dressing, toileting) related to physical impairments (poor vision, uncoordination, forgetfulness).

H. *Altered sleep/arousal patterns* resulting in disorientation at night, related to confusion.

I. *Altered abstract thinking and agnosia* related to destruction of cerebral tissue and inability to utilize information to make judgments and transmit messages.

J. *Impaired communication* related to poverty of speech and withdrawal behavior, progressive neurological losses, and cerebral impairment.

K. *Altered role performance* related to decreases in intellectual competence.

IV. Nursing plan/implementation in organic brain syndrome. Also see interventions in III. Confusion/disorientation, p. 40.

A. *Long-term goal:* minimize regression related to memory impairment.

B. *Short-term goal:* provide structure and consistency to increase security.

C. Make *brief, frequent* contacts, as attention span is short.

D. Allow clients *time* to talk and to complete projects.

E. Stimulate *associative* patterns to improve recall (by repeating, summarizing, and focusing).

F. Allow clients to *review* their lives and focus on the past.

G. Utilize *concrete* questions in interviewing.

H. *Reinforce* reality-oriented comments.

I. Keep environment the *same* as much as possible (same room and placement of furniture, for example); *routine* is important to diminish stress.

J. Recognize the importance of *compensatory* mechanisms (confabulation, for example) to increase self-esteem; build psychologic reserve.

K. Give recognition for each accomplishment.

L. Use *recreational* and physical therapy.

M. *Health teaching:* give *specific* instructions for diet, medication, and treatment; how to use many sensory approaches to learn new information; how to use existing knowledge, old learning, and habitual approaches to deal with new situations.

V. Evaluation:

A. Symptoms occur *less* frequently and are less severe in areas of emotional lability and appropriateness; false perceptions; self-care ability; disorientation, memory, and judgment; and decision making.

B. Client is able to preserve optimum level of functioning and independence while allowing basic needs to be met.

C. Stays relatively calm and noncombative when upset or fearful.

D. Accepts own irritability and frustrations as part of illness.

E. Asks for assistance with self-care activities.

F. Knows and adheres to daily routine; knows own nurse, location of room, bathroom, clocks, calendars.

G. Uses supportive community services.

Psychoactive Substance Use Disorders

I. Definition: ingesting in any manner a chemical that has an effect on the body.

II. General assessment:

A. *Behavioral* changes exist while under the influence of substance.

B. Engages in regular *use* of substance.

1. *Substance abuse:*
   a. Pattern of *pathologic* use (i.e., day-long intoxication; inability to stop use, even when contraindicated by serious physical disorder (overpowering need or desire to take the drug despite legal, social, or medical problems); daily need of substance for functioning; repeated medical complications from use.
   b. *Interference* with social, occupational functioning.
   c. Willingness to obtain substance by any means, including illegal.
   d. Pathologic use for more than one month.
2. *Substance dependence:*
   a. More severe than substance abuse; body *requires* substance to continue functioning.
   b. Physiologic dependence (i.e., either develops a *tolerance*—must increase dose to obtain desired effect—or has *physical withdrawal symptoms* when substance intake is reduced or stopped).
   c. Person feels it's impossible to get along without drug.

C. Effects of substance on *central nervous system.*

III. General analysis: only in recent years has substance abuse been viewed as an illness rather than moral delinquency or criminal behavior. The disorders are very complex and little understood. There are physiologic, psychologic, and social aspects to their causality, dynamics, symptoms, and treatment, where personality disorder has a major part.

A. *Physiologic aspects*—current unproven theories include "allergic" reaction to alcohol, disturbance in metabolism, genetic susceptibility to dependency, and hypofunction of adrenal cortex. There are *organic effects* of chronic excessive use.

B. *Psychologic aspects*—disrupted parent–child relationship and family dynamics; deleterious effect on ego function.

C. *Social and cultural aspects*—local customs and attitudes vary about what is excessive.

D. *Maladaptive behavior related to:*

1. Low self-esteem.
2. Anger.
3. Denial.
4. Rationalization.
5. Social isolation.
6. A rigid pattern of coping.
7. Poorly defined philosophy of life, values, mores.

E. *Nursing diagnosis* in acute phase of abuse, intoxication:

1. *Potential for injury* related to impaired coordination, disorientation, and altered judgment (worse at night).
2. *Potential for violence:* self-directed or directed at others, related to misinterpretation of stimuli and feelings of suspicion or distrust of others.
3. *Sensory/perceptual alterations:* visual, kinesthetic, tactile, related to intake of mind-altering substances.
4. *Altered thought processes* (delusions, incoherence) related to misinterpretation of stimuli.
5. *Sleep pattern disturbance* related to mind-altering substance.
6. *Ineffective individual coping* related to inability to tolerate frustration and to meet basic needs or role expectations, resulting in unpredictable behaviors.
7. *Noncompliance* with abstinence and supportive therapy, related to inability to stop using substance because of dependence and refusal to alter life-style.
8. *Impaired communication* related to mental confusion or CNS depression related to substance use.
9. *Altered health maintenance* related to failure to recognize that a problem exists and inability to take responsibility for health needs.

Alcohol Abuse and Dependence

Alcohol dependence is a chronic disorder in which the individual is unable, for physical or psychologic reasons or both, to refrain from frequent consumption of alcohol in quantities that produce intoxication and disrupt health and ability to perform daily functions.

I. Concepts and principles related to alcohol abuse and dependence:

A. Alcohol affects cerebral cortical functions:

1. Memory.
2. Judgment.
3. Reasoning.

B. Alcohol as a *depressant:*

1. Relaxes the individual.
2. Lessens use of repression of unconscious conflict.
3. Releases inhibitions, hostility, and primitive drives.

C. Drinking represents a tension-reducing device and a relief from feelings of insecurity. Strength of drinking habit equals degree of anxiety and frustration intolerance.

D. Alcohol abuse and dependence is a *symptom* rather than a disease.

E. Underlying fear and anxiety, associated with inner conflict, motivate the alcoholic to drink.

F. Alcoholics can never be cured to drink normally; cure is to be a "sober alcoholic," with total abstinence.

G. The spouse of the alcoholic often unconsciously contributes to the drinking behavior because of own emotional needs *(co-alcoholic* or *co-dependent).*

H. Intoxication occurs with a blood alcohol level of *0.15%* or above. *Signs of intoxication* are:

1. Incoordination.
2. Slurred speech.
3. Dulled perception.

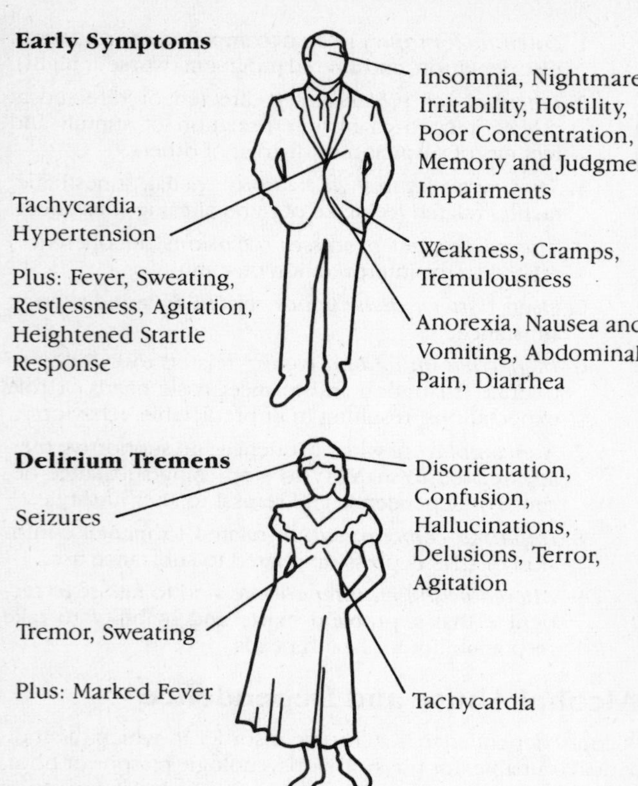

■ **FIGURE 1.5**
Symptoms associated with alcohol withdrawal. (From Wilson HS, Kneisl CR: *Psychiatric Nursing,* 2nd ed., Addison-Wesley, Menlo Park, CA, 1983, p. 388.)

I. Tolerance occurs with alcohol dependence. Increasing amounts of alcohol must be consumed in order to obtain the desired effect.

II. Assessment:

A. *Vicious cycle*—(a) low tolerance for coping with frustration, tension, guilt, resentment, (b) uses alcohol for relief, (c) new problems created by drinking, (d) new anxieties, and (e) more drinking.

B. Coping mechanisms used: *denial, rationalization, projection.*

C. *Complications of abuse and dependence.*

1. *Alcohol withdrawal delirium (delirium tremens—DTs)* (see Figure 1.5)—result of nutritional deficiencies and toxins; requires sedation and constant watchfulness against unintentional suicide and convulsions.
   a. *Impending* signs relate to *central nervous system*—marked nervousness and restlessness, increased irritability; gross tremors of hands, face, lips; weakness; also *cardiovascular*—increased blood pressure, tachycardia, diaphoresis; *depression; gastrointestinal*—nausea, vomiting, anorexia.
   b. *Actual—serious* symptoms of mental confusion, convulsions, hallucinations (visual, auditory, tactile). Without cure, *15–20%* may die.
2. *Wernicke's syndrome*—a neurologic disturbance manifested by confusion, ataxia, eye movement abnormalities, and memory impairment. Other problems include:
   a. Disturbed vision.
   b. Mind-wandering.
   c. Stupor and coma.
3. *Alcohol amnestic syndrome (Korsakoff's syndrome)*—degenerative neuritis due to *thiamine* deficiency.
   a. Impaired thoughts.
   b. Confusion, loss of sense of time and place.
   c. Use of confabulation to fill in severe memory loss.
   d. Follows episode of Wernicke's encephalopathy.
4. *Polyneuropathy*—sensory and motor nerve endings are involved, causing pain, itching, and loss of limb control.
5. Others—*gastritis, esophageal varices, cirrhosis, pancreatitis, diabetes,* pneumonia, REM sleep deprivation, *malnutrition.*

III. Analysis/nursing diagnosis:

A. *Potential for self-directed violence:* tendency for *self-destructive* acts related to intake of mind-altering substances.

B. *Altered nutrition, less than body requirements,* related to a lack of interest in food.

C. *Defensive coping* related to tendency to be domineering and critical, with difficulties in *interpersonal* relationships.

D. *Conflict with social order* related to extreme dependence coupled with resentment *of authority.*

E. *Spiritual distress* or general dissatisfaction with life related to *low frustration* tolerance and demand for immediate need satisfaction.

F. *Dysfunctional behaviors* related to tendency for *excess* in work, sex, recreation, marked *narcissistic* behavior.

G. *Social isolation* related to use of coping mechanisms that are primarily *escapist.*

IV. Nursing plan/implementation:

A. *Detoxification phase*

1. *Administer adequate sedation* to control anxiety, insomnia, agitation, tremors.
2. *Administer anticonvulsants* to prevent *withdrawal seizures.*
3. *Control nausea and vomiting* to avoid massive GI bleeding or rupture of esophageal varices.
4. *Assess fluid and electrolyte balance* for dehydration (may need IV fluids) or overhydration (may need a diuretic).
5. *Reestablish proper nutrition:* high protein (as long as no severe liver damage), carbohydrate, vitamins C and B complex.
6. *Provide calm, safe environment:* bedrest with rails, well-lit room to reduce illusions; constant supervision and reassurance about fears and hallucinations, assess depression for suicide potential.

B. *Recovery-rehabilitation phase:* encourage participation in *group* activities; *avoid sympathy* when client tends to rationalize behavior and seeks special privileges—use acceptance and a *nonjudgmental,* consistent, firm, but kind approach; *avoid* scorn, contempt, and moralizing or punitive and rejecting behaviors; do *not* reinforce feelings of worthlessness, self-contempt, hopelessness, or low self-esteem.

C. *Problem behaviors*

1. *Manipulative*—be firm and consistent; avoid "bid for sympathy."
2. *Demanding*—set limits.
3. *Acting out*—set limits, enforce rules and regulations, strengthen impulse control and ability to delay gratification.
4. *Dependency*—place responsibility on client; avoid advice-giving.
5. *Superficiality*—help client make realistic self-appraisals and expectations in lieu of grandiose promises and trite verbalizations; encourage formation of lasting interpersonal relationships.

D. *Common reactions among staff*

1. Disappointment—instead, set realistic goals, take one step at a time.
2. Moral judgment—instead, support each other.
3. Hostility—instead, offer support to each other when feeling frustrated from lack of results.

E. Refer client from hospital to *community resources* for follow-up treatment with social, economic, and psychologic problems, as well as to self-help groups, in order to reduce "revolving door" situation in which client comes in, is treated, goes out, and comes in again the next night.

1. *Alcoholics Anonymous (AA)*—a self-help group of addicted drinkers who confront, instruct, and support fellow drinkers in their efforts to stay sober one day at a time through fellowship and acceptance.
2. *Alanon*—support group for *families* of alcoholics. *Alateen*—support group for *teenagers* when parent is alcoholic.
3. *Antabuse* (Disulfiram)—drug that produces intense headache, severe flushing, extreme nausea, vomiting, palpitations, hypotension, dyspnea, and blurred vision when alcohol is consumed while person is taking this drug.
4. *Aversion therapy*—client is subjected to revulsion-producing or pain-inducing stimuli at the same time he takes a drink, to establish alcohol rejection behavior.
5. *Group psychotherapy*—the goals of group psychotherapy are for the client to give up alcohol as a tension reliever, identify cause of stress, build different means for coping with stress, and accept drinking as a serious symptom.

F. *Health teaching:* teach improved coping patterns to tolerate increased stress; teach substitute tension-reducing strategies; prepare in advance for difficult, painful events; teach how to reduce irritating or frustrating environmental stress.

V. Evaluation: everyday living patterns are restructured for a satisfactory life without alcohol; demonstrates feelings of increased self-worth, confidence, and reliance.

Other Psychoactive Substance Use Disorders

I. Concepts and principles:

A. *Three* interacting key factors give rise to dependence—*psychopathology* of the individual; frustrating *environment;* and *availability* of powerful, addicting, and temporarily satisfying drug.

B. According to conditioning principles, substance abuse and dependence proceed in *several phases:*

1. *Use* of sedatives-hypnotics, CNS stimulants, hallucinogens and narcotics, for relief from daily tensions and discomforts or anticipated withdrawal symptoms.
2. Habit is *reinforced* with each relief by drug use.
3. Development of *dependency*—drug has less and less efficiency in reducing tensions.
4. Dependency is further reinforced as addict *fails* to maintain adequate drug intake—increase in frequency and duration of periods of tension and discomfort.

II. Assessment:

A. Abuse

1. *Hallucinogens* (LSD, marijuana, STP, PCP, peyote): euphoria and rapid mood swings, flight of ideas; perceptual impairment, feelings of omnipotence, "bad trip" (panic, loss of control, paranoia), flashbacks, suicide.
2. *CNS stimulants* (amphetamines and cocaine abuse): euphoria, hyperactivity, hyperalertness, irritability, persecutory delusions; insomnia, anorexia → weight loss; tachycardia; tremulousness; hypertension; hyperthermia → convulsions.
3. *Narcotics* (opium and its derivatives, e.g., morphine, heroin, codeine, Demerol): used by "snorting," "skin popping," and "mainlining." May lead to abscesses and hepatitis. Decreased pain response, respiratory depression; apathy, detachment from reality; impaired judgment; loss of sexual activity; pinpoint pupils.
4. *Sedatives-hypnotics (barbiturate abuse):* like alcohol-induced behavior, e.g., euphoria followed by depression, hostility; decreased inhibitions; impaired judgment; staggering gait; slurred speech; drowsiness; poor concentration; progressive respiratory depression.

B. *Withdrawal symptoms*

1. *Narcotics:* begins within 12 hours of last dose, peaks in 24–36 hours, subsides in 72 hours, and disappears in 5–6 days.
   a. Pupil dilation.
   b. Muscle: twitches, tremors, aches, pains.
   c. Goose flesh (piloerection).
   d. Lacrimation, rhinorrhea, sneezing, yawning.
   e. Diaphoresis, chills.
   f. Potential for fever.
   g. Vomiting, abdominal distress.
   h. Dehydration.
   i. Rapid weight loss.
   j. Sleep disturbance.

2. *Barbiturates:* may be gradual or abrupt ("cold turkey"); latter is dangerous or *life-threatening;* should be hospitalized.
   a. *Gradual* withdrawal reaction from barbiturates:
      (1) Postural hypotension.
      (2) Tachycardia.
      (3) Elevated temperature.
      (4) Insomnia.
      (5) Tremors.
      (6) Agitation, restlessness.
   b. *Abrupt* withdrawal from barbiturates:
      (1) Apprehension.
      (2) Muscular weakness.
      (3) Tremors.
      (4) Postural hypotension.
      (5) Twitching.
      (6) Anorexia.
      (7) *Grand mal seizures.*
      (8) *Psychosis-delirium.*
3. *Amphetamines:* depression, lack of energy, somnolence.

C. *Difference* between alcohol and other abused substances (e.g., opioid).
1. Above drugs may need to be obtained by illegal means, making it a legal and criminal problem as well as a medical and social problem; *not* so with alcohol abuse and dependency.
2. Opium and its derivatives inhibit aggression, whereas alcohol *releases* aggression.
3. As long as she or he is on large enough doses to avoid withdrawal symptoms, abuser of narcotics, sedatives, or hypnotics is comfortable and functions well, whereas chronically intoxicated alcoholic *cannot* function normally.
4. Direct physiologic effects of long-term opioid abuse and dependence on above drugs are much *less critical* than those with chronic alcohol dependence.

III. Analysis/nursing diagnosis:

A. *Altered physiological processes* (cardiac, circulation, gastrointestinal, sleep pattern disturbance) related to use of mind-altering drugs.

B. *Altered conduct/impulse processes* related to rebellious attitudes toward authority.

C. *Altered social interaction* (manipulation, dependency) related to hostility and personal insecurity.

D. *Altered judgment* related to misinterpretation of sensory stimuli and low frustration tolerance.

E. *Altered feeling patterns* (denial) related to underlying self-doubt and personal insecurity.

IV. Nursing plan/implementation: generally the same as in treating antisocial personality and alcohol abuse and dependence.

A. Maintain *safety* and optimum level of *physical* comfort. Supportive physical care: vital signs, nutrition, hydration, seizure precautions.

B. *Assist with medical treatment* and offer support and *reality orientation* to reduce feelings of panic.
1. *Detoxification (or dechemicalization)*—give medications according to detoxification schedule.
2. *Withdrawal*—may be gradual (barbiturates, hypnotics, tranquilizers) or abrupt ("cold turkey" for heroin). Observe for symptoms and report immediately.
3. *Methadone*—person must have been dependent on narcotics at least two years and have failed at other methods of withdrawal before admission to program of readdiction by methadone.
   a. *Characteristics*
      (1) Synthetic.
      (2) Appeases desire for narcotics without producing euphoria of narcotics.
      (3) Given by mouth.
      (4) Distributed under federal control (*N*arcotic *A*ddict *R*ehabilitation *A*ct).
      (5) Given with urinary surveillance.
   b. *Advantages*
      (1) Prevents narcotic withdrawal reaction.
      (2) Tolerance not built up.
      (3) Person remains out of prison.
      (4) Lessens perceived need for heroin or morphine.

C. *Participation in group therapy—goals:* peer pressure, support, and identification.

D. *Rehabilitation phase:*
1. Refer to halfway house and group living (e.g., Daytop).
2. Support *employment* as therapy (work training).
3. Expand client's *range of interests* to relieve characteristic boredom and stimulus hunger.
   a. Provide *structured* environment and planned routine.
   b. Provide educational therapy (academic and vocational).
   c. Arrange activities to include current events discussion groups, lectures, drama, music, and art appreciation.

E. Achieve role of *stabilizer and supportive* authoritative figure; this can be achieved through frequent, regular contacts with the same client.

F. *Health teaching:* how to cope with pain, fatigue, and anxiety without drugs.

V. Evaluation: replaces addictive life-style with self-reliant behavior.

■ PSYCHO-SOCIAL-CULTURAL FUNCTIONS

MENTAL STATUS ASSESSMENT

I. Components of mental status exam

A. *Appearance*—appropriate dress, grooming, facial expression, stereotyped movements, mannerisms, rigidity.

B. *Behavior*—anxiety level, congruence with situation, co-

Physical and intellectual

1. Presence of physical illness and/or disability.
2. Appearance and energy level.
3. Current and potential levels of intellectual functioning.
4. How client sees personal world, translates events around self; client's perceptual abilities.
5. Cause and effect reasoning, ability to focus.

Socioeconomic factors

1. Economic factors—level of income, adequacy of subsistence; how this affects life-style, sense of adequacy, self-worth.
2. Employment and attitudes about it.
3. Racial, cultural, and ethnic identification; sense of identity and belonging.
4. Religious identification and link to significant value systems, norms, and practices.

Personal values and goals

1. Presence or absence of congruence between values and their expression in action; meaning of values to individual.
2. Congruence between individual's values and goals and the immediate systems with which client interacts.
3. Congruence between individual's values and assessor's values; meaning of this for intervention process.

Adaptive functioning and response to present involvement

1. Manner in which individual presents self to others—grooming, appearance, posture.
2. Emotional tone and change or constancy of levels.
3. Style of communication—verbal and nonverbal; ability to express appropriate emotion, follow train of thought; factors of dissonance, confusion, uncertainty.
4. Symptoms or symptomatic behavior.
5. Quality of relationship individual seeks to establish—direction, purposes, and uses of such relationships for individual.
6. Perception of self.
7. Social roles that are assumed or ascribed; competence in fulfilling these roles.
8. Relational behavior:
   a. Capacity for intimacy.
   b. Dependence-independence balance.
   c. Power and control conflicts.
   d. Exploitiveness.
   e. Openness.

Developmental factors

1. Role performance equated with life stage.
2. How developmental experiences have been interpreted and used.
3. How individual has dealt with past conflicts, tasks, and problems.
4. Uniqueness of present problem in life experience.

■ **FIGURE 1.6**
Individual assessment. (From Wilson HS, Kneisl CR: *Psychiatric Nursing,* 2nd ed., Addison-Wesley, Menlo Park, CA, 1983, pp. 204–205.)

operativeness, openness, hostility, reaction to interview, consistency.

C. *Speech characteristics*—relevance, coherence, meaning, repetitiveness, qualitative (*what* is said), quantitative (*how much* is said), abnormalities, inflections, affectations, congruence with level of education, impediments, tone quality.

D. *Mood*—appropriateness, intensity, hostility turned inwards or toward others, duration, swings.

E. *Thought content*—delusions, hallucinations, obsessive ideas, phobic ideas, themes, areas of concern, self-concept.

F. *Thought processes*—organization and association of ideas, coherence, ability to abstract and understand symbols.

G. *Sensorium*

1. *Orientation* to person, time and place, situation.
2. *Memory*—immediate, rote, remote, and recent.
3. *Attention and concentration*—susceptibility to distraction.
4. *Information and intelligence*—account of general knowledge, history, and reasoning powers.
5. *Comprehension*—concrete and abstract.
6. *Stage of consciousness*—alert/awake, somnolent, lethargic, delirious, stuporous, comatose.

H. *Insight and judgment*

1. Extent to which client sees self as having problems, needing treatment.
2. Client awareness of intrapsychic nature of own difficulties.
3. Soundness of judgment.

II. Individual assessment—consider the following (see Figure 1.6):

A. Physical and intellectual factors.

B. Socioeconomic factors.

C. Personal values and goals.

D. Adaptive functioning and response to present involvement.

E. Developmental factors.

III. Cultural assessment*

A. Knowledge of ethnic beliefs and cultural practices can

* *Source:* Ross B, Cobb KL: *Family Nursing.* Redwood City, CA: Addison-Wesley, 1990.

assist the nurse in the planning and implementation of holistic care.

B. Consider the following:

1. *Demographic data:* is this an "ethnic neighborhood"?
2. *Socioeconomic status:* occupation, education (formal and informal), income level; who is employed?
3. *Ethnic/racial orientation:* ethnic identity, value orientation.
4. *Country of immigration:* date of immigration; where were the family members born? Where has the family lived?
5. *Languages spoken:* does family speak English? Language and dialect preferences.
6. *Family relationships:* what are the formal roles? Who makes the decisions within the family? What is the family life-style and living arrangements?
7. *Degree of acculturation* of family members: how are the family customs and beliefs similar to or different from the dominant culture?
8. *Communication patterns:* social customs, nonverbal behaviors.
9. *Religious preferences:* what role do beliefs, rituals, and taboos play in health and illness? Is there a significant religious person? Are there any dietary symbolisms or preferences or restrictions due to religious beliefs?
10. *Cultural practices related to health and illness:* does the family use folk medicine practices or a folk healer? Are there specific dietary practices related to health and illness?
11. *Support Systems:* do extended family members provide support?
12. *Health beliefs:* response to pain and hospitalization; disease predisposition and resistance.
13. Other significant factors related to ethnic identity: what health care facilities does the family use?
14. Communication barriers:
    a. Differences in language.
    b. Technical languages.
    c. Inappropriate place for discussion.
    d. Personality or gender of the nurse.
    e. Distrust of the nurse.
    f. Time-orientation differences.
    g. Differences in pain perception and expression.
    h. Variable attitudes toward death and dying.

IV. Interviewing

A. Definition: a goal-directed method of communicating facts, feelings, and meanings. For interviewing to be successful, interaction between two persons involved must be effective.

B. Nine principles for verbal interaction

1. *Client's initiative* begins the discussion.
2. *Indirect approach,* moving from the periphery to the core.
3. *Open-ended* statements, using incomplete forms of statements such as "You were saying . . ." to prompt rather than close off an exchange.
4. *Minimal verbal activity* in order not to obstruct thought process and client's responses.
5. *Spontaneity,* rather than fixed interview topics, may bring out much more relevant data.
6. *Facilitate expression of feelings* to help assess events and reactions by asking, for example, "What was that like for you?"
7. *Focus on emotional areas* about which client may be in conflict, as noted by repetitive themes.
8. *Pick up cues, clues, and signals from client,* such as facial expressions and gestures, behavior, emphatic tones, and flushed face.
9. *Introduce material related to content* already brought up by client; do not bring in a tangential focus from "left field."

C. Purpose and goals of interviewing

1. *Initiate and maintain a positive nurse–client relationship,* which can decrease symptoms, lessen demands, and move client toward optimum health when nurse demonstrates understanding and sharing of client's concerns.
2. *Determine client's view of nurse's role* in order to utilize it or change it.
3. *Collect information on emotional crisis* to plan goals and approaches in order to increase effectiveness of nursing interventions.
4. *Identify and resolve crisis;* the act of eliciting cause or antecedent event may in itself be therapeutic.
5. *Channel feelings directly* by exploring interrelated events, feelings, and behaviors in order to discourage displacement of feelings onto somatic and behavioral symptoms.
6. *Channel communication* and transfer significant information to the physician and other team members.
7. *Prepare for health teaching* in order to help the client function as effectively as possible.

GENERAL PRINCIPLES OF HEALTH TEACHING

One key nursing function is to promote and restore health. This involves teaching patients or clients new psychomotor skills, general knowledge, coping attitudes, and social skills related to health and illness (such as proper diet, exercises, colostomy care, wound care, insulin injections, urine testing). The teaching function of the nurse is vital in assisting normal development and helping patients and clients meet health-related needs.

I. Purpose of health teaching

A. *General goal:* motivate health-oriented behavior.

B. *Nursing interventions*

1. Fill in *gaps* in information.
2. *Clarify* misinformation.
3. Teach necessary *skills.*
4. *Modify* attitudes.

II. Educational theories on which effective health teaching is based:

A. *Motivation theory*

1. Health-oriented behavior is determined by the degree to which person sees health problem as *threatening*, with *serious consequences, high probability of occurrence,* and *belief in availability of effective course of action.*
2. Non–health-related motives may *supersede* health-related motives.
3. Health-related motives may not always give rise to health-related behavior, and vice versa.
4. Motivation may be influenced by:
   a. *Phases of adaptation* to crisis (poor motivation in early phase).
   b. *Anxiety and awareness of need* to learn. (Mild anxiety is highly motivating.)
   c. *Mutual* versus externally imposed goal setting.
   d. Perceived *meaningfulness* of information and material. (If within client's frame of reference, both meaningfulness and motivation increase.)

B. *Theory of planned change*

1. *Unfreeze* present level of behavior—develop awareness of problem.
2. Establish *need* for change and relationship of trust and respect.
3. *Move* toward change—examine alternatives, develop intentions into real efforts.
4. *Freeze* on a new level—generalize behavior, stabilize change.

C. Elements of *learning theory*

1. *Drive* must be present based on experiencing uncertainty, frustration, concern, or curiosity; hierarchy of needs exists.
2. *Response* is a learned behavior that is elicited when associated stimulus is present.
3. *Reward and reinforcement* are necessary for response (behavior) to occur and remain.
4. *Extinction of response,* that is, elimination of undesirable behavior, can be attained through conditioning.
5. Memorization is the easiest level of learning, but least effective in changing behavior.
6. Understanding involves the incorporation of generalizations and specific facts.
7. After introduction of new material, there is a period of floundering when assimilation and insight occur.
8. Learning is a two-way process between learner and teacher; defensive behavior in either makes both activities difficult, if not impossible.
9. Learning flourishes when client feels respected, accepted by enthusiastic nurse; learning occurs best when differing value systems are accepted.
10. Feedback increases learning.
11. Successful learning leads to more successes in learning.
12. Teaching and learning should take place in the area where *targeted activity* normally occurs.
13. Priorities for learning are dependent on client's *physical and psychologic status.*
14. Decreased visual and auditory perception leads to decreased readiness to learn.
15. Content, terminology, pacing, and spacing of learning needs to correspond to client's *capabilities, maturity level, feelings, attitudes, and experiences.*

III. Assessment of the client-learner:

A. *Characteristics:* age, sex, race, medical diagnosis, prognosis.

B. *Sociocultural-economic:* ethnic, religious group beliefs and practices; family situation (roles, support); job (type, history, options, stress); financial situation, living situation (facilities).

C. *Psychologic:* own and family's response to illness; premorbid personality; current self-image.

D. *Educational:*

1. Client's *perception* of current situation: What is wrong? Cause? How will life-style be affected?
2. *Past experience:* previous hospitalization and treatment; past compliance.
3. *Level of knowledge:* What has he been told? From what source? How accurate? Known others with the same illness?
4. *Goals:* what he *wants* to know.
5. *Needs:* what nurse thinks he *should* know for self-care.
6. Readiness for learning.
7. *Educational* background; ability to read and learn.

IV. Analysis of factors influencing learning:

A. *Internal*

1. Physical condition.
2. Senses (sight, hearing, touch).
3. Age.
4. Anxiety.
5. Motivation.
6. Experience.
7. Values (cultural, religious, personal).
8. Comprehension.
9. Education and language deficiency.

B. *External*

1. Physical environment (heat, light, noise, comfort).
2. Timing, duration, interval.
3. Teaching methods and aids.
4. Content, vocabulary.

V. Teaching plan needs to be:

A. Compatible with the *three* domains of learning—

1. *Cognitive* (knowledge, concepts): use written and audiovisual materials, discussion.
2. *Psychomotor* (skills): use demonstrations, illustrations, role models.
3. *Affective* (attitudes): use discussions, maintain atmosphere conducive to change; use role models.

B. Appropriate to educational material.

C. Related to client's abilities and perceptions.

D. Related to objectives of teaching.

VI. Implementation—*teaching guidelines* to use with clients:

■ TABLE 1.11 Summary of Beginning (Orientation) Phase of the Therapeutic Nursing Process

Objective	Therapeutic Tasks/Plans	Approaches/Implementation
Establishment of contact in the form of a working relationship with the client.	Clarification of purpose of relationship, role of nurse, and responsibilities of client.	*Educative:* 1. Provide information regarding purpose, roles, and responsibilities. 2. Address misconceptions, fantasies, and fears regarding relationship and/or nurse.
	Addressing client's suffering.	Use facilitative characteristics, especially empathic understanding. Avoid premature reassurance (allow trust to evolve). Be explicit about who has access to client's revelations (degree of confidentiality).
	Negotiation of therapeutic contract (client's definition of personal goals for treatment and nurse's professional responsibilities).	Encourage delineation of goals that: 1. Are specific. 2. Address behavioral patterns. 3. Designate degree of change necessary for client self-satisfaction. Determine place, duration, and time of meeting. Consider optional referral sources.

Source: Wilson HS, Kneisl CR: *Psychiatric Nursing,* 3rd ed. (Redwood City, CA: Addison-Wesley, 1988).

- **A.** Select conducive *environment* and best *timing* for activity.
- **B.** Assess the client's *needs,* interests, *perceptions,* motivations, and *readiness* for learning.
- **C.** State purpose and *realistic goals* of planned teaching/learning activity.
- **D.** Actually involve the client by giving him or her the opportunity to *do, react, experience,* and *ask questions.*
- **E.** Make sure that the client views the activity as useful and worthwhile and that it is within the client's grasp.
- **F.** Use comprehensible terminology.
- **G.** Proceed from the *known to the unknown,* from *specific to general* information.
- **H.** Provide opportunity for client to *see results* and progress.
- **I.** Give *feedback* and *positive reinforcement.*
- **J.** Provide opportunities to achieve *success.*
- **K.** Offer repeated practice in *real-life* situations.
- **L.** *Space and distribute* learning sessions over a period of time.

VII. Evaluation:

- **A.** Client's deficit of knowledge is lessened.
- **B.** Increased compliance to treatment.
- **C.** Length of hospital stay is reduced.
- **D.** Rate of readmission to hospital is reduced.

THE THERAPEUTIC NURSING PROCESS

A *therapeutic nursing process* involves an interaction between the nurse and client in which the nurse offers a series of planned, goal-directed activities that are useful to a particular client in relieving discomfort, promoting growth, and satisfying interpersonal relationships.

I. Characteristics of therapeutic nursing:

- **A.** Movement from first contact through final outcome:
  1. *Eight general phases* occur in a typical unfolding of a natural process of problem solving.
  2. Stages are not always in the same sequence.
  3. Not all stages are present in a relationship.
- **B. Phases***
  1. *Beginning* the relationship. *Goal:* build trust (Table 1.11).
  2. *Formulating* and clarifying a problem and concern. *Goal:* clarify client's statements.
  3. *Setting a contract* or working agreement. *Goal:* decide on terms of the relationship.

*Lawrence M. Brammer, *The Helping Relationship: Process and Skills,* p. 55. Copyright © 1973, Prentice-Hall, Inc., Englewood Cliffs, N.J.

■ **TABLE 1.12 Summary of Middle (Working) Phase of the Therapeutic Nursing Process**

Objective	Therapeutic Tasks/Plans	Approaches/Implementation
Mutual determination of dynamics of client's behavior patterns, especially those considered dysfunctional.	Identify and explore important behavior patterns.	Explore behavior pattern in depth, including origin, causes, operation, and effect of pattern (intrapersonally and interpersonally).
		Separate environmental factors (familial, political, economic, cultural) from intrapersonal factors.
		Link elements of one behavior pattern to other patterns as appropriate, for a gradual unfolding of central life patterns.
	Analyze client's mode of conflict resolution.	Encourage detailed exploration of how client reacts to reduce anxiety associated with conflict.
		Increase awareness of defenses employed to ward off anxiety awakened by such exploration.
	Facilitate client self-assessment of growth-producing and growth-inhibiting behavior patterns.	Encourage client to assert own needs when external environmental conditions (group, agency, institution) are an inhibiting force.
Institution of behavioral change, especially in dysfunctional behavior patterns.	Address forces that inhibit desired change (problematic thoughts, feelings, and behaviors).	Assist client in challenging client's personal resistance to change.
		Use problem-solving strategies, active decision making, and personal accountability.
		Encourage client to assert own needs when external environmental conditions (group, agency, institution) are an inhibiting force.
	Create an atmosphere that offers permission for active experimentation to test and assess effectiveness of new behaviors.	Allow freedom to make and assess mistakes and blunders.
		Avoid parental judgment of any behavioral experimentation—encourage client self-assessment instead.
	Facilitate the development of coping skills to deal with anxiety associated with behavioral change.	Address, rather than avoid, anxiety and its manifestations.
		Strengthen existing growth-promoting coping skills, especially regarding unalterable conditions (e.g., terminal illness, physical deformity, loss of significant other by death).
		Encourage development of new coping skills and their application to actual life experiences.

Source: Wilson HS, Kneisl CR: *Psychiatric Nursing,* 3rd ed. (Redwood City, CA: Addison-Wesley, 1988).

4. *Building* the relationship. *Goal:* increase depth of relationship and degree of commitment.
5. *Exploring goals* and solutions, gathering data, expressing feelings. *Goals:* (a) maintain and enhance relationship (trust and safety), (b) explore blocks to goal, (c) expand self-awareness, and (d) learn skills necessary to reach goal.
6. *Developing action plan. Goals:* (a) clarify feelings, (b) focus on and choose between alternate courses of action, and (c) practice new skills.
7. *Working through* conflicts or disturbing feelings. *Goals:* (a) channel earlier discussions into specific course of action and (b) work through unresolved feelings (Table 1.12).
8. *Ending* the relationship. *Goals:* (a) evaluation of goal attainment and (b) leave-taking (Table 1.13).

II. Therapeutic nurse–client interactions

A. Plans/goals:

1. Demonstrate unconditional *acceptance,* interest, concern, and respect.
2. Develop trust—be *consistent and congruent.*

TABLE 1.13 Summary of End (Resolution) Phase of the Therapeutic Nursing Process

Objective	Therapeutic Tasks/Plans	Approaches/Implementation
Termination of contact in a mutually planned, satisfying manner.	Assist client evaluation of therapeutic contract and of psychotherapeutic experience in general.	Encourage client's appraisal of personal therapeutic goals (motivation, effort, progress, outcome).
		Provide appropriate feedback regarding appraisal of goals.
		Underline client's assets and therapeutic gains.
		Underline areas for further therapeutic work.
	Encourage transference of dependence to other support systems.	Encourage client to develop reliance on others in client's immediate environment (spouse, relative, employer, neighbor, friend) for empathic emotional support.
	Participate in explicit therapeutic good-bye with client.	Be alert to surfacing of any behavior arising on termination (repression, regression, acting out, anger, withdrawal, acceptance, etc.).
		Assist client in working through feelings associated with these behaviors.
		Anticipate own reaction to separation and share in a manner that does not burden client.
		Allow "time" and "space" for termination; the longer the duration of the one-to-one relationship, the more time is needed for the resolution phase.

Source: Wilson HS, Kneisl CR: *Psychiatric Nursing,* 3rd ed. (Redwood City, CA: Addison-Wesley, 1988).

3. Make *frequent* contacts with the client.
4. Be *honest* and *direct, authentic* and spontaneous.
5. Offer support, security, and empathy, *not* sympathy.
6. Focus comments on concerns of client *(client-centered),* not self (social responses). *Refocus* when client changes subject.
7. Encourage expression of *feelings;* focus on feelings and *here-and-now* behavior.
8. Give attention to a client who complains.
9. Give information at client's level of understanding, at appropriate time and place.
10. Use open-ended questions; ask *how, what, where, who,* and *when* questions; avoid *why* questions; avoid questions that can be answered by *yes* or *no*.
11. Use feedback or reflective listening.
12. Maintain hope, but *avoid* false reassurances, clichés, and pat responses.
13. *Avoid* verbalizing value judgments, giving personal opinions, or moralizing.
14. Do not change the subject *unless* the client is redundant or focusing on physical illness.
15. Point out *reality;* help the client leave "inner world."
16. Set *limits* on behavior when client is acting out unacceptable behavior that is self-destructive or harmful to others.
17. Assist clients in arriving at their own decisions by demonstrating problem solving or involving them in the process.
18. Do not talk if it is not indicated.
19. Approach, sit, or walk with agitated clients; stay with the person who is upset, if he or she can tolerate it.
20. Focus on nonverbal communication.
21. Remember the *psyche has a soma!* Do not neglect appropriate physical symptoms.

B. Examples of **therapeutic** responses as interventions:

1. Being *silent*—being able to sit in silence with a person can connote acceptance and acknowledgment that the person has the right to silence. (Dangers: the nurse may wrongly give the client the impression that there is a lack of interest, or the nurse may discourage verbalization if acceptance of this behavior is prolonged; it is not necessarily helpful with acutely psychotic behavior.)
2. Using *nonverbal communication*—nodding head, moving closer to the client, and leaning forward, for example; use as a way to encourage client to speak.
3. Give encouragement to continue with *open-ended leads*—nurse's responses: "Then what?" "Go on," "For instance," "Tell me more," "Talk about that."
4. *Accepting, acknowledging*—nurse's responses: "I hear your anger," or "I see that you are sitting in the corner."

5. *Commenting on nonverbal behavior* of client—nurse's responses: "I notice that you are swinging your leg," "I see that you are tapping your foot," or "I notice that you are wetting your lips." Client may respond with, "So what?" If she does, the nurse needs to reply why the comment was made—for example, "It is distracting," "I am giving the nonverbal behavior meaning," "Swinging your leg makes it difficult for me to concentrate on what you are saying," or "I think when people tap their feet it means they are impatient. Are you impatient?"
6. Encouraging clients to *notice with their senses* what is going on—nurse's response: "What did you see (or hear)?" or "What did you notice?"
7. Encouraging *recall and description* of details of a particular experience—nurse's response: "Give me an example," "Please describe the experience further," "Tell me more," or "What did you say then?"
8. *Giving feedback by reflecting, restating, and paraphrasing* feelings and content:

   Client: I cried when he didn't come to see me.

   Nurse: You cried. You were expecting him to come and he didn't?
9. *Picking up on latent content* (what is implied)—nurse's response: "You were disappointed. I think it may have hurt when he didn't come."
10. *Focusing, pinpointing,* asking "what" questions:

    Client: They didn't come.

    Nurse: Who are 'they'?

    Client: [Rambling.]

    Nurse: Tell it to me in a sentence or two. What is your main point? What would you say is your main concern?
11. *Clarifying*—nurse's response: "What do you mean by 'they'?" "What caused this?" or "I didn't understand. Please say it again."
12. *Focusing on reality* by expressing doubt on "unreal" perceptions:

    Client: Run! There are giant ants flying around after us.

    Nurse: That is unusual. I don't see giant ants flying.
13. *Focusing on feelings,* encouraging client to be aware of and describe personal feelings:

    Client: Worms are in my head.

    Nurse: That must be a frightening feeling. What did you feel at that time? Tell me about that feeling.
14. Helping client to *sort and classify impressions, make speculations, abstract* and *generalize* by making connections, seeing common elements and similarities, making comparisons, and placing events in logical sequence—nurse's responses: "What are the common elements in what you just told me?" "How is this similar to . . ." "What happened just before?" or "What is the connection between this and . . ."
15. *Pointing out discrepancies* between thoughts, feelings, and actions—nurse's response: "You say you were feeling sad when she yelled at you; yet you laughed. Your feelings and actions do not seem to fit together."
16. *Checking perceptions* and *seeking agreement* on how the issue is seen, *checking* with the client to see if the message sent is the same one that was received—nurse's response: "Let me restate what I heard you say," "Are you saying that . . ." "Did I hear you correctly?" "Is this what you mean?" or "It seems that you were saying . . ."
17. *Encouraging client to consider alternatives*—nurse's response: "What else could you say?" or "Instead of hitting him, what else might you do?"
18. *Planning a course of action*—nurse's response: "Now that we have talked about your on-the-job activities and you have thought of several choices, which are you going to try out?" or "What would you do next time?"
19. *Imparting information*—give additional data as new input to help client; for example, state facts and reality-based data that client may lack.
20. *Summing up*—nurse's response: "Today we have talked about your feelings toward your boss, how you express your anger, and about your fear of being rejected by your family."
21. *Encouraging client to appraise and evaluate* the experience or outcome—nurse's response: "How did it turn out?" "What was it like?" "What was your part in it?" "What difference did it make?" or "How will this help you later?"

C. Examples of **nontherapeutic** responses:

1. *Changing the subject, tangential response,* moves away from problem and/or focuses on incidental, superficial content:

   Client: I hate you.

   Nurse: Would you like to take your shower now?

   Suggested responses reflect, "You hate me; tell me about this," or "You hate me; what does hate mean to you?"

   Client: I want to kill myself today.

   Nurse: Isn't today the day your mother is supposed to come?

   Suggested responses: (a) give open-ended lead, (b) give feedback: "I hear you saying today that you want to kill yourself," or (c) clarifying: "Tell me more about this feeling of wanting to kill yourself."
2. *Moralizing:* saying with approval or disapproval that the person's behavior is good or bad, right or wrong; *arguing* with stated belief of person; directly opposing the person:

   Nurse: That's good. It's wrong to shoot yourself.

   Client: I have nothing to live for.

   Nurse: You certainly do have a lot!

   Suggested response: similar to those in 1. (See above.)
3. *Agreeing with client's autistic inventions:*

   Client: The eggs are flying saucers.

   Nurse: Yes, I see. Go on.

   Suggested response: use clarifying response first: "I don't understand," and then, depending on client's response, use either *accepting and ac-*

knowledging, focusing on reality, or *focusing on feelings.*

4. *Agreeing with client's negative view of self:*

   Client: I have made a mess of my life.

   Nurse: Yes, you have.

   Suggested response: use clarifying response about "mess of my life"—"Give me an example of one time where you feel you messed up in your life."

5. *Complimenting, flattering:*

   Client: I have made a mess of my life.

   Nurse: How could you? You are such an attractive, intelligent, generous person.

   Suggested response: same as in 4. (See above.)

6. *Giving opinions and advice* concerning client's life situation—examples of poor responses include: "In my opinion . . ." "I think you should . . ." or "Why not?"

   Suggested response: (a) encourage the client to consider alternatives ("What else do you think you could try?"); (b) encourage the client to appraise and evaluate for himself or herself ("What is it like for you?").

7. *Seeking agreement* from client with nurse's personal opinion—examples of poor responses include: "I think. . . Don't you?" and "Isn't that right?"

   Suggested responses: (a) it is best to keep personal opinion to oneself and only to give information that would aid the client's orientation to reality; (b) if you give an opinion as a *model* of orienting to reality, ask client to *state his or her* opinion ("My opinion is. . . What is your opinion?").

8. *Probing* and/or *offering premature solutions and interpretations;* jumping to conclusions:

   Client: I can't find a job.

   Nurse: You could go to an employment agency.

   Client: I'd rather not talk about it.

   Nurse: What are you unconsciously doing when you say that? What you really mean is . . .

   Client: I don't want to live alone.

   Nurse: Are you afraid of starting to drink again?

   Suggested responses: use responses that seek clarification and elicit more data.

9. *Changing client's words* without prior validation:

   Client: I am *not feeling well* today.

   Nurse: What makes you feel so *depressed?*

   Suggested response: "In what way are you not feeling well?" Use the same language as the client.

10. *Following vague content* as if understood or *using vague global* pronouns, adverbs, and adjectives:

    Client: People are so *unfair.*

    Nurse: I know what you mean.

    Suggested response: clarify vague referents such as "people" and "unfair."

    Client: I feel sad.

    Nurse: Everyone feels that way at one time or another.

    Suggested response: "What are you sad about?"

11. *Questioning on different topics without waiting for a reply:*

    Client: [Remains silent.]

    Nurse: What makes you so silent? Are you angry? Would you like to be alone?

    Suggested response: choose one of the above and wait for a response before asking the next question.

12. *Ignoring client's questions or comments:*

    Client: Am I crazy, nurse?

    Nurse: [Walking away as if he did not hear her.]

    Suggested responses: "I can't understand what makes you bring this up at this time," or "Tell me what makes you bring this up at this time." Ignoring questions or comments usually implies that the nurse is feeling uncomfortable. It is important not to "run away" from the client.

13. *Closing off exploration* with questions that can be answered by *yes* or *no:*

    Client: I'll never get better.

    Nurse: Is something making you feel that way?

    Suggested response: "What makes you feel that way?" Use open-ended questions that start with *what, who, when, where,* etc.

14. *Using clichés* or stereotyped expressions:

    Client: The doctor took away my weekend pass.

    Nurse: The doctor is only doing what's best for you. Doctor knows best. [Comment: also an example of moralizing.]

    Suggested response: "Tell me what happened when the doctor took away your weekend pass."

15. *Overloading:* giving too much information at one time:

    Nurse: Hello, I'm Mr. Brown. I'm a nurse here. I'll be here today, but I'm off tomorrow. Ms. Anderson will assign you another nurse tomorrow. This unit has five RNs, three LVNs, and students from three nursing schools who will all be taking care of you at some time.

    Suggested response: "Hello, I'm Mr. Brown, your nurse today." Keep your initial orienting information simple and brief.

16. *Underloading:* not giving enough information, so that meaning is not clear; withholding information:

    Client: What are visiting hours like here?

    Nurse: They are flexible and liberal.

    Suggested response: "They are flexible and liberal, from 10 A.M. to 12 noon and from 6 to 8 P.M." Use specific terms and give specific information.

17. *Saying no without saying no:*

    Client: Can we go for a walk soon?

    Nurse: We'll see. Perhaps. Maybe. Later.

    Suggested response: "I will check the schedule in the nursing office and let you know within an hour." Vague, ambiguous responses can be seen as "putting the client off." It is best to be clear, specific, and direct.

18. *Using double-bind communication:* sending con-

flicting messages that do not have "mutual fit," or are incongruent:

Nurse: [continuing to stay and talk with the client] It's time for you to rest.

Suggested response: "It's time for you to rest and for me to leave [proceeding to leave]."

19. *Protecting:* defending someone else while talking with client; implying client has no right to personal opinions and feelings:

Client: This hospital is no good. No one cares here.

Nurse: This is an excellent hospital. All the staff were chosen for their warmth and concern for people.

Suggested response: focus on feeling tone or on clarifying information.

20. *Asking "why" questions* implies that the person has immediate conscious awareness of the reasons for his or her feelings and behaviors. Examples of this include: "Why don't you?" "Why did you do that?" or "Why do you feel this way?"

Suggested response: ask clarifying questions using *how, what,* etc.

21. *Coercion;* using the interaction between people to force someone to do *your* will, with the implication that if they don't "do it for your sake," you won't love them or stay with them:

Client: I refuse to talk with him.

Nurse: Do it for my sake, before it's too late.

Suggested response: "Something keeps you from wanting to talk with him?"

22. Focusing on *negative* feelings, thoughts, actions:

Client: I can't sleep; I can't eat; I can't think; I can't do anything.

Nurse: How long have you not been sleeping, eating, or thinking well?

Suggested response: "What *do* you do?"

23. *Rejecting* client's behavior or ideas:

Client: Let's talk about incest.

Nurse: Incest is a bad thing to talk about; I don't want to.

Suggested response: "What do you want to say about incest?"

24. *Accusing, belittling:*

Client: I've had to wait five minutes for you to change my dressing.

Nurse: Don't be so demanding. Don't you see that I have several people who need me?

Suggested response: "It must have been hard to wait for me to come when you wanted it to be right away."

25. *Evading a response* by asking a question in return:

Client: I want to know your opinion, nurse. Am I crazy?

Nurse: Do you think you are crazy?

Suggested response: "I don't know. What do you mean by 'crazy'?"

26. *Circumstantiality:* communicating in such a way that the main point is reached only after many side comments, details, and additions:

Client: Will you go out on a date with me?

Nurse: I work every evening. On my day off I usually go out of town. I have a steady boyfriend. Besides that, I am a nurse and you are a client. Thank you for asking me, but no, I will not date you.

Suggested response: abbreviate your response to: "Thank you for asking me, but no, I will not date you."

27. *Making assumptions* without checking them:

Client: [Standing in the kitchen by the sink, peeling onions, with tears in her eyes.]

Nurse: What's making you so sad?

Client: I'm not sad. Peeling onions always makes my eyes water.

Suggested response: use simple acknowledgment and acceptance initially, such as "I notice you have tears in your eyes."

28. *Giving false, premature reassurance:*

Client: I'm scared.

Nurse: Don't worry; everything will be all right. There's nothing to be afraid of.

Suggested response: "I'd like to hear about what you're afraid of, so that together we can see what could be done to help you." Open the way for clarification and exploration, and offer yourself as a helping person—not someone with magic answers.

ALTERATIONS IN SELF-CONCEPT

I. Assessment:

A. Self-derisive; self-diminution; and criticism.

B. Denies own pleasure due to need to punish self; doomed to failure.

C. Disturbed interpersonal relationships (cruel, demeaning, exploitive of others; passive-dependent).

D. Exaggerated self-worth or rejects personal capabilities.

E. Feels guilty, worries (nightmares, phobias, obsessions).

F. Sets unrealistic goals.

G. Withdraws from reality with intense self-rejection (delusional, suspicious, jealous).

H. Views life as either-or, worst-or-best, wrong-or-right.

I. Postpones decisions due to ambivalence (procrastination).

J. Physical complaints (psychosomatic).

K. Self-destructive (substance abuse or other destructiveness).

II. Analysis/nursing diagnosis: *Altered self-concept* may be related to:

A. *Low self-esteem* related to parental rejection, unrealistic parental expectations, repeated failures.

B. *Altered personal identity (negative):* self-rejection and self-hate related to unrealistic self-ideals.

C. *Identity confusion* related to role conflict, role overload, and role ambiguity.

D. *Feelings of helplessness, hopelessness,* worthlessness, fear, vulnerability, inadequacy related to extreme *dependency* on others and *lack of personal responsibility.*

E. *Disturbed body image.*

F. Depersonalization.

G. Physiologic factors that produce self-concept distortions (e.g., fatigue, oxygen and sensory deprivation, toxic drugs, isolation, biochemical imbalance).

III. Nursing plan/implementation:

A. *Long-term goal:* Facilitate client's self-actualization by helping him or her to grow, develop, and realize potential while compensating for impairments.

B. *Short-term goals:*

1. Expand client's *self-awareness:*
   a. Establish open, trusting relationship to *reduce fear* of interpersonal relationships.
      (1) Offer unconditional acceptance.
      (2) Nonjudgmental response.
      (3) Listen and encourage discussion of thoughts, feelings.
      (4) Convey that client is valued as a person, is responsible for self *and* able to help self.
   b. Strengthen client's capacity for *reality-testing, self-control,* and *ego integration.*
      (1) Identify ego strengths.
      (2) Confirm identity.
      (3) Reduce panic level of anxiety.
      (4) Use undemanding approach.
      (5) Accept and clarify communication.
      (6) Prevent isolation.
      (7) Establish simple routine.
      (8) Set limits on inappropriate behavior.
      (9) Orient to reality.
      (10) Activities: gradual increase; provide positive experiences.
      (11) Encourage self-care; assist in grooming.
   c. Maximize *participation in decision making* related to self.
      (1) Gradually increase participation in own care.
      (2) Convey expectation of ultimate self-responsibility.
2. Encourage client's *self-exploration.*
   a. Accept client's feelings and assist *self-acceptance* of emotions, beliefs, behaviors, and thoughts.
   b. Help *clarify* self-concept and relationship to others.
      (1) Elicit client's perception of own strengths and weaknesses.
      (2) Ask client to describe: ideal self, how client believes he or she relates to other people and events.
   c. Nurse needs to be aware of *own* feelings as a model of behavior and to limit countertransference.
      (1) Accept own positive and negative feelings.
      (2) Share own perception of client's feelings.
   d. Respond with *empathy,* not sympathy, with the belief that client is subject to own control.
      (1) Monitor sympathy and self-pity by client.
      (2) Reaffirm that client is *not* helpless or powerless but is responsible for own choice of maladaptive or adaptive coping responses.
      (3) Discuss: alternatives, areas of ego *strength,* available coping resources.
      (4) Utilize family and group-support system for self-exploration of client's conflicts and maladaptive coping responses.
3. Assist client in *self-evaluation.*
   a. Help to clearly *define* problem.
      (1) Identify relevant stressors.
      (2) Mutually identify: faulty beliefs, misperceptions, distortions, unrealistic goals, areas of strength.
   b. Explore use of adaptive *and* maladaptive coping responses and their positive and negative *consequences.*
4. Assist client to formulate a *realistic action plan.*
   a. Identify alternative solutions to client's *inconsistent perceptions* by helping him or her to change:
      (1) Own beliefs, ideals, to bring closer to reality.
      (2) Environment, to make consistent with beliefs.
   b. Identify alternative solutions to client's *self-concept not consistent with his or her behavior* by helping him or her to change:
      (1) Own behavior to conform to self-concept.
      (2) Underlying beliefs.
      (3) Self-ideal.
   c. Help client set and clearly define *goals* with *expected concrete* changes. Use role rehearsal, role modeling, and role playing to see practical, reality-based, emotional consequences of each goal.
5. Assist client to become committed to decision to *take necessary action* to replace maladaptive coping responses and maintain adaptive responses.
   a. Provide opportunity for success and give assistance (vocational, financial, and social support).
   b. Provide positive reinforcement; strengths, skills, healthy aspects of client's personality.
   c. Allow enough time for change.
6. *Health teaching:* how to focus on strengths rather than limitations; how to apply reality-oriented approach.

IV. Evaluation:

A. Client able to discuss perception of self and accept aspects of own personality.

B. Client assumes increased responsibility for own behavior.

C. Client able to transfer new perceptions into possible solutions, alternative behavior.

ANXIETY

Anxiety is a subjective warning of danger in which the specific nature of the danger is usually not known. It occurs when a person faces a new, unknown, or untried situation. Anxiety is also felt when a person perceives threat in terms of past experiences. It is a general concept underlying most disease states. In its milder form, anxiety can contribute to learning and is necessary for problem solving. In its severe form, anxiety can impede a client's treatment and recovery. The general feelings elicited on all levels of anxiety are nervousness, tension, and apprehension.

It is essential that nurses recognize their own sources of anxiety and behavior in response to anxiety as well as help client recognize the manifestations of anxiety in themselves.

I. Assessment:

A. *Physiologic* manifestations:

1. Increased heart rate and palpitations.
2. Increased rate and depth of respiration.
3. Increased urinary frequency and diarrhea.
4. Dry mouth.
5. Decreased appetite.
6. Cold sweat and pale appearance.
7. Increased menstrual flow.
8. Increased or decreased body temperature.
9. Increased or decreased blood pressure.
10. Dilated pupils.

B. *Behavioral* manifestations—stages of anxiety:

1. *Mild anxiety:*
   a. Increased perception (visual and auditory).
   b. Increased awareness of meanings and relationships.
   c. Increased alertness (notice more).
   d. Ability to utilize problem-solving process.
2. *Moderate anxiety:*
   a. Selective inattention (for example, may not hear someone talking).
   b. Decreased perceptual field.
   c. Concentration on relevant data; "tunnel vision."
   d. Muscular tension, perspiration, GI discomfort.
3. *Severe anxiety:*
   a. Focus on many fragmented details.
   b. Physical and emotional discomfort (headache, nausea, dizziness, dread, horror, trembling).
   c. Not aware of total environment.
   d. Automatic behavior aimed at getting immediate relief instead of problem solving.
   e. Poor recall.
   f. Inability to see connections between details.
   g. Drastically reduced awareness.
4. *Panic state of anxiety:*
   a. Increased speed of scatter; does not notice what goes on.
   b. Increased distortion and exaggeration of details.
   c. Feeling of terror.
   d. Dissociation (hallucinations, loss of reality, and little memory).
   e. Inability to cope with any problems; no self-control.

C. *Reactions in response to anxiety:*

1. *Fight:*
   a. Aggression.
   b. Hostility, derogation, belittling.
   c. Anger.
2. *Flight:*
   a. Withdrawal.
   b. Depression.
3. *Somatization* (psychosomatic disorder).
4. *Impaired cognition:* blocking, forgetfulness, poor concentration, errors in judgment.
5. *Learning* about or searching for causes of anxiety, and identifying behavior.

II. Analysis/nursing diagnosis: *Anxiety* related to:

A. *Physical causes:* threats to biologic well-being (e.g., sleep disturbances, interference with sexual functioning, food, drink, pain, fever).

B. *Psychologic causes: Disturbance in self-esteem* related to:

1. Unmet wishes or expectations.
2. Unmet needs for prestige and status.
3. *Impaired adjustment:* inability to cope with environment.
4. *Altered role performance:* not utilizing own full potential.
5. *Altered meaningfulness:* alienation.
6. *Conflict with social order:* value conflicts.
7. Anticipated disapproval from a significant other.
8. *Altered feeling patterns: guilt.*

III. Nursing plan/implementation:

A. *Moderate to severe anxiety*

1. Provide *motor outlet* for tension energy, such as working at a simple, concrete task, walking, crying, or talking.
2. Help clients *recognize* their anxieties by talking about how they are behaving and by exploring their underlying feelings.
3. Help the clients *gain insight* into their anxieties by helping them to understand how their behavior has been an expression of anxiety and to recognize the threat that lies behind this anxiety.
4. Help the clients *cope* with the threat behind their anxieties by reevaluating the threats and learning new ways to deal with them.
5. *Health teaching:*
   a. Explain and offer hope that emotional pain will decrease with time.
   b. Explain that some tension is normal.
   c. Explain how to channel emotional energy into activity.

d. Explain need to recognize highly stressful situations and to recognize tension within oneself.

B. *Panic state*

1. Give simple, clear, *concise* directions.
2. *Avoid* decision making by client. Do not try to reason with client, for he or she is irrational and cannot cooperate.
3. *Stay* with client.
   a. Do not isolate.
   b. *Avoid* touching.
4. Allow client to seek *motor* outlets (walking, pacing).
5. *Health teaching:* advise activity that requires no thought.

IV. Evaluation:

A. Uses more positive thinking and problem-solving activities and is less preoccupied with worrying.

B. Uses values-clarification to resolve conflicts and establish realistic goals.

C. Demonstrates regained perspective, self-esteem, and morale; expresses feeling more in control, more hopeful.

D. Fewer or absent physical symptoms of anxiety.

Patterns of Adjustment (Coping Mechanisms)

Coping mechanisms (ego defense mechanisms or mental mechanisms) consist of all the *coping* means used by individuals to seek relief from emotional conflict and to ward off excessive anxiety.

I. Definitions*

blocking a disturbance in the rate of speech when a person's thoughts and speech are proceeding at an average rate but are very suddenly and completely interrupted, perhaps even in the middle of a sentence. The gap may last from several seconds up to a minute. Blocking is often a part of the thought disorder found in schizophrenic disorders.

compensation making up for real or imagined handicap, limitation, or lack of gratification in one area of personality by overemphasis in another area to counter the effects of failure, frustration, and limitation; e.g., the blind compensate by increased sensitivity in hearing; the unpopular student compensates by becoming an outstanding scholar; small men compensate for short stature by demanding a great deal of attention and respect; a nurse who does not have manual dexterity chooses to go into psychiatric nursing.

confabulating filling in gaps of memory by inventing what appear to be suitable memories as replacements. This symptom may occur in various organic psychoses but is most often seen in Korsakoff's syndrome (deterioration due to alcohol) and in organic mental disorders.

conversion psychologic difficulties are translated into physical symptoms *without conscious* will or knowledge; e.g., pain and immobility on moving your writing arm the day of the exam.

denial an intolerable thought, wish, need, or reality factor is disowned automatically; e.g., a student, when told of a failing grade, acts as if he never heard of such a possibility.

displacement transferring the emotional component from one idea, object, or situation to another, more acceptable one. Displacement occurs because these are painful or dangerous feelings that cannot be expressed toward the original object; e.g., kicking the dog after a bad day at school or work; anger with clinical instructor gets transferred to classmate who was late to meet you for lunch.

dissociation splitting off or separation of differing elements of the mind from each other. There can be separation of ideas, concepts, emotions, or experiences from the rest of the mind. Dissociated material is deeply repressed and becomes encapsulated and inaccessible to the rest of the mind. This usually occurs as a result of some very painful experience, for example, split of affect from idea in anxiety disorders and schizophrenia.

fixation a state in which personality development is arrested in one or more aspects at a level short of maturity; e.g., "She is anally fixated" (controlling, stingy, holding onto things and memories).

idealization overestimation of some admired aspect or attribute of another person; e.g., "She was a perfect human being."

ideas of reference fixed, false ideas and interpretations of external events as though they had direct reference to self; e.g., client thinks that TV news announcer is reporting a story about client.

identification the wish to be like another person; situation in which qualities of another are unconsciously transferred to oneself; e.g., boy identifies with his father and learns to become a man; a woman may fear she will die in childbirth because her mother did; a student adopts attitudes and behavior of her favorite teacher.

introjection incorporation into the personality, without assimilation, of emotionally charged impulses or objects; a quality or an attribute of another person is taken into and made part of self; e.g., a girl in love introjects the personality of her lover into herself—his ideas become hers, his tastes and wishes are hers; this is also seen in severe depression following death of someone close—patient may assume many of deceased's characteristics; similarly, working in a psychiatric unit with a suicidal person brings out depression in the nurse.

isolation temporary or long-term splitting off of certain feelings or ideas from others; separating emotional and intellectual content; e.g., talking emotionlessly about a traumatic accident.

projection attributes and transfers own feelings, attitudes, impulses, wishes, or thoughts to another person or object in the environment, especially when ideas or impulses are too painful to be acknowledged as belonging to oneself; e.g., in hallucinations and delusions by alcoholics; or, "I flunked the course because the teacher doesn't know how to teach"; "I hate him" reversed into "He hates me"; or a student impatiently accusing an instructor of being intolerant.

rationalization justification of behavior by formulating a logical, socially approved reason for past, present, or proposed behavior. Commonly used, conscious or unconscious, with false or real reason; e.g., upon losing a class election, a student states she really did not want all the extra work and is glad she lost.

* From Kalkman, M.: *Psychiatric Nursing,* 3rd ed., New York, 1967, © McGraw-Hill Book Company, pp. 83–93. Copyrighted by the C. V. Mosby Co., St. Louis.

reaction formation going to the opposite extreme from what one wishes to do or is afraid one might do; e.g., being overly concerned with cleanliness when one wishes to be messy, being an overly protective mother through fear of own hostility to child, or showing great concern for a person whom you dislike, going out of your way to do special favors.

regression when individuals fail to solve a problem with the usual methods at their command they may resort to modes of behavior that they have outgrown but that proved successful at an earlier stage of development; retracing developmental steps; going back to earlier interests or modes of gratification; e.g., a senior nursing student about to graduate becomes dependent on a clinical instructor for directions.

repression involuntary exclusion of painful and unacceptable thoughts and impulses from awareness. *Forgetting* these things solves the situation by not solving it; e.g., by not remembering what was on the difficult exam after it was over.

sublimation channeling a destructive or instinctual impulse that cannot be realized into a *socially acceptable,* practical, and less dangerous outlet, with some relation to the original impulse for emotional satisfaction to be obtained; e.g., sublimation of sexual energy into other creative activities (art, music, literature) or hostility and aggression into sports or business competition; or an infertile person putting all energies into pediatric nursing.

substitution when individuals cannot have what they wish and accept something else in its place for symbolic satisfaction; e.g., pin-up pictures in absence of sexual object, or a person who failed an RN exam signs up for an LVN (LPN) exam.

suppression a deliberate process of blocking from the conscious mind thoughts, feelings, acts, or impulses that are undesirable; e.g., "I don't want to talk about it," "Don't mention his name to me," or "I'll think about it some other time"; or willfully refusing to think about or discuss disappointments with exam results.

symbolism sign language that stands for related ideas and feelings, conscious and unconscious. Used extensively by children, primitive peoples, and psychotic patients. There is meaning attached to this sign language that makes it very important to the individual; e.g., a student wears dark, somber clothing to the exam site.

undoing a coping mechanism against anxiety, usually unconscious, designed to negate or neutralize a previous act; e.g., Lady Macbeth's attempt to wash her hands (of guilt) after the murder. A repetitious, symbolic acting out, in reverse of an unacceptable act already completed. Responsible for compulsions and magical thinking.

II. Characteristics of coping mechanisms:

- **A.** Coping mechanisms are utilized to some degree by everyone occasionally; they are normal processes by which the ego reestablishes equilibrium—unless they are used to an extreme degree, in which case they interfere with maintenance of self-integrity.
- **B.** Much overlapping:
    1. Same behavior can be explained by more than one mechanism.
    2. May be used in combination—e.g., isolation and repression, denial and projection.
- **C.** Common defense mechanisms compatible with mental well-being.
    1. Compensation.
    2. Compromise.
    3. Identification.
    4. Rationalization.
    5. Sublimation.
    6. Substitution.
- **D.** Typical coping mechanisms in:
    1. *Paranoid disorders*—denial, projection.
    2. *Dissociative disorders*—denial, repression, dissociation.
    3. *Obsessive-compulsive behaviors*—displacement, reaction-formation, isolation, denial, repression, undoing.
    4. *Phobic disorders*—displacement, rationalization, repression.
    5. *Conversion disorders*—symbolization, dissociation, repression, isolation, denial.
    6. *Major depression*—displacement.
    7. *Bipolar disorder, manic episode*—reaction-formation, denial, projection, introjection.
    8. *Schizophrenic disorders*—symbolization, repression, dissociation, denial, fantasy, regression, projection, insulation.
    9. *Organic mental disorders*—regression.

III. Concepts and principles related to coping mechanisms:

- **A.** Unconscious process—coping mechanisms are used as a substitute for more effective problem-solving behavior.
- **B.** *Main functions*—increase *self-esteem; decrease,* inhibit, minimize, alleviate, avoid, or eliminate *anxiety;* maintain feelings of personal worth and adequacy and soften failures; *protect the ego; increase security.*
- **C.** *Drawbacks*—involve high degree of self-deception and reality distortion; may be maladaptive because they superficially eliminate or disguise conflicts, leaving conflicts unresolved but still influencing behavior.

IV. Nursing plan/implementation with coping mechanisms:

- **A.** Accept coping mechanisms as normal, but not when overused.
- **B.** Look beyond the behavior to the need that is expressed by the use of the coping mechanism.
- **C.** Discuss alternative coping mechanisms that may be more compatible with mental health.
- **D.** Assist the person to translate defensive thinking into nondefensive, direct thinking; a problem-solving approach to conflicts minimizes the need to use coping mechanisms.

ANXIETY DISORDERS (ANXIETY AND PHOBIC NEUROSES)

I. Definition: emotional illnesses characterized by *fear* and *autonomic nervous system symptoms* (palpitations, tachycardia, dizziness, tremor); related to *intrapsychic conflict* and psychogenic origin where instinctual impulse (related to sexuality, aggression, or dependence) may be in conflict with the ego, superego, or sociocultural environment; related to sudden object loss.

An *anxiety disorder* is a mild to moderately severe functional disorder of personality in which *repressed* inner conflicts between drives and fears are manifested in behavior patterns, including *generalized anxiety* and *phobic, obsessive-compulsive disorders.* (Other related disorders are *dissociative, conversion,* and *hypochondriasis*.)

II. General concepts and principles related to anxiety disorders:

- **A.** Behavior may be an attempt to "bind" anxiety: to *fix* it in some particular area (hypochondriasis) or to *displace* it from the rest of personality (phobic, conversion, and dissociative disorders—amnesia, fugue, multiple personalities; obsessive-compulsive disorders).
- **B.** *Purpose of symptoms:*
  1. To intensify *repression* as a defense.
  2. To exhibit some repressed content in *symbolic* form.

III. General assessment of anxiety disorders:

- **A.** Uses behavior to *avoid* tense situations.
- **B.** Frightened, suggestible.
- **C.** Prone to *minor* physical complaints (for example, fatigue, headaches, and indigestion) and reluctance to admit recovery from physical illnesses.
- **D.** Attitude of martyrdom.
- **E.** Often feels helpless, insecure, inferior, inadequate.
- **F.** Uses *repression, displacement, and symbolism* as key coping mechanisms.

Anxiety States

I. *Generalized anxiety disorder:*

A. Assessment:

1. Persistent, diffuse, free-floating, painful anxiety for at least one month.
2. Motor tension, autonomic hyperactivity.
3. Hyperattentiveness expressed through vigilance and scanning.

B. Analysis/nursing diagnosis:

1. *Anxiety: excessive worry* related to threat to security.
2. *Alteration in concentration* related to overwhelming anxiety.
3. *Fear* related to sudden object loss.
4. *Guilt* related to inability to meet role expectations.
5. *Disturbance in self-concept* related to feelings of inadequacy.
6. *Altered role performance* related to inadequate support system.
7. *Impaired social interaction* related to use of avoidance in tense situations.
8. *Distractibility* related to pervasive anxiety.
9. *Hopelessness* related to feelings of inadequacy.

C. Nursing plan/implementation:

1. Fulfill needs as promptly as possible.
2. Listen attentively.
3. Stay with client.
4. Avoid decision making and competitive situations.
5. Promote rest; decrease environmental stimuli.
6. *Health teaching:* teach steps of anxiety reduction.

D. Evaluation: symptoms are diminished.

II. *Panic disorder:*

A. Assessment:

1. Three acute, terrifying panic attacks within 3-week period, *unrelated* to marked physical exertion, life-threatening situation, presence of organic illness, or exposure to specific phobic stimulus.
2. Discrete periods of apprehension, fearfulness (lasting from few moments to an hour).
3. *Mimics cardiac* disease: dyspnea, chest pain, smothering or choking sensations, palpitations, tachycardia, dizziness, fainting, sweating.
4. Feelings of unreality, paresthesias.
5. Hot, cold flashes and dilated pupils.
6. Trembling, sense of impending death, fear of becoming insane.

B. Analysis/nursing diagnosis:

1. *Ineffective individual coping* related to undeveloped interpersonal processes.
2. *Altered comfort pattern:* distress, anxiety, fear related to threat to security.
3. *Decisional conflict* related to apprehension.
4. *Altered thought processes* related to impaired concentration.

C. Nursing plan/implementation:

1. *Reduce immediate anxiety* to more moderate and manageable levels.
   - a. Stay *physically close* to reduce feelings of alienation and terror.
   - b. *Communication approach:* calm, serene manner; short, simple sentences; firm voice to convey that nurse will provide external controls.
   - c. *Physical environment:* remove to smaller room to minimize stimuli.
2. Provide *motor outlet* for diffuse energy generated at high anxiety levels; e.g., moving furniture, scrubbing floors.
3. Administer *antianxiety medications* as ordered.
4. *Health teaching:* recommend more effective methods of coping.

D. Evaluation: can endure anxiety while searching out its causes.

III. *Obsessive-compulsive disorder:*

A. Assessment—chief characteristic: fear that client can harm someone or something.

1. *Obsessions*—recurrent, persistent, involuntary, senseless *thoughts, images, ideas, or desires* that may be trivial or morbid; e.g., fear of germs, doubts as to performance of an act, thoughts of hurting family member, death, suicide.
2. *Compulsions*—uncontrollable, persistent urge to perform repetitive, stereotyped *behaviors* that provide relief from unbearable anxiety; e.g., handwashing, counting, touching, checking and rechecking

doors to see if locked, elaborate dressing and undressing rituals.

B. Analysis/nursing diagnosis:

1. *Ineffective individual coping* related to:
   a. *Intellectualization* and *avoidance* of awareness of feelings.
   b. Limited ability to express emotions (may be disguised or delayed).
   c. Exaggerated feelings of *dependence and helplessness*.
   d. High need to *control* self, others, and environment.
   e. Rigidity in thinking and behavior.
   f. Poor ability to tolerate anxiety and depression.
2. *Social isolation* related to:
   a. Resentment.
   b. Self-doubt.
   c. Exclusion of pleasure.

C. Nursing plan/implementation:

1. *Accept* rituals permissively (excessive handwashing, for example); stopping ritual will increase anxiety.
2. *Avoid* criticism or "punishment," making demands, or showing impatience with client.
3. *Allow* extra time for slowness and client's need for precision.
4. *Protect* from rejection by *others*.
5. *Protect* from *self-inflicted* harmful acts.
6. Engage in nursing therapy *after* the ritual is over, when client is most comfortable.
7. *Redirect* client's actions into substitute outlets.
8. *Health teaching:* teach how to prevent health problems related to rituals; i.e., use rubber gloves, hand lotion.

D. Evaluation: avoids situations that increase tension and thus reduces need for ritualistic behavior as outlet for tension.

IV. *Phobic disorders*—Intense, *irrational, persistent* fear in response to *external* object, activity, or situation; e.g., *agoraphobia*—fear of being alone or in public places; *claustrophobia*—fear of closed places; *acrophobia*—fear of heights; *simple phobias* such as *mysophobia*—fear of germs. *Social phobias:* fear of situations that may be humiliating or embarrassing. *Dynamics: displacement* of anxiety from original source onto avoidable, *symbolic,* external, and specific object (or activity or situation); i.e., phobias help person control intensity of anxiety by providing specific object to attach it to, which he or she can then avoid.

A. Assessment: same as for anxiety symptoms; fear that someone or something will harm them.

B. Analysis/nursing diagnosis: *social isolation;* avoidance; irrational *fear* out of proportion to actual danger; *defensive coping* with high need to control self, others, environment.

C. Nursing plan/implementation—promote psychologic and physical calm:

1. *Use systematic desensitization*—never force contact with feared object or situation.
2. *Health teaching:* progressive relaxation, meditation, biofeedback training, or other behavioral conditioning techniques.

D. Evaluation: phobia is eliminated (i.e., able to come into contact with feared object with lessened degree of anxiety).

V. *Posttraumatic stress disorder:*

A. Assessment:

1. Precipitant: severe traumatic event (natural or man-made disaster) that is not an ordinary occurrence; e.g., rape, fire, flood, earthquake, tornado, bombing, torture, kidnapping.
2. Self-report of reexperiencing incident; intrusive memories.
3. Numb, unresponsive, detached, estranged reaction to external world (unable to feel tenderness, intimacy).
4. Change in sleep pattern (insomnia, recurrent dreams, nightmares), memory loss, hyperalertness (startle response).
5. Guilt rumination about survival.
6. Avoids activities reminiscent of trauma; phobic responses.
7. Difficulty with task-completion and concentration.
8. Depression.
9. Increased irritability may result in unpredictable, explosive outbursts.
10. Impulsive behavior, sudden life-style changes.

B. Analysis/nursing diagnosis:

1. *Victim-abuse syndrome* related to overwhelming traumatic event.
2. *Fear* related to environmental stressor.
3. *Sleep pattern disturbance* related to fear and rumination.
4. *Decisional conflict (impaired decision making)* related to perceived threat to personal values and beliefs.
5. *Guilt* related to lack of social support system.
6. *Altered emotional processes:* emotional lability related to diminished sense of control over self and environment.

C. Nursing plan/implementation:

1. Crisis counseling: (listen with concern and sympathy).
   a. Ease way for client to talk out the experience and express fear.
   b. Help client to become aware and accepting of what happened.
2. *Health teaching:* suggest how to resume concrete activity and reconstruct life with available social, physical, and emotional resources. Help make contact with friends, relatives, and other resources.

D. Evaluation: can cry and express anger, loss, frustration, and despair; begins process of social and physical reconstruction.

DISSOCIATIVE DISORDERS (HYSTERICAL NEUROSES, DISSOCIATIVE TYPE)

I. Assessment:

A. *Psychogenic amnesia:* partial or total inability to recall the past; occurs during highly stressful events; client may have conscious desire to escape but be unable to accept escape as a solution; uses *repression.*

B. *Psychogenic fugue:* client not only forgets but also *flees* from stress.

C. *Multiple personality:* client exhibits two or more complete personality systems, each very different from the other; alternates from one personality to the other without awareness of change (*one* personality *may* be aware of others); each personality has well-developed emotions and thought processes that are in conflict; uses *repression.*

D. *Depersonalization:* loss of sense of self; feeling of self estrangement (as if in a dream); fear of going insane.

II. Analysis/nursing diagnosis:

A. Sudden *alteration in:*

1. *Consciousness* (*short- and long-term memory loss:* can't recall important personal events) related to repression.
2. *Personal and social identity* (amnesia: forgets own identity; becomes another identity) related to intense anxiety.

B. *Confusion* related to use of repression.

C. *Spiritual distress* related to conversion of conflict into physical or mental flights.

D. *Sensory/perceptual alteration* of external environment related to repression and escapism.

E. *Altered meaningfulness* (hopelessness, helplessness, powerlessness) related to lack of control over situation.

III. Nursing plan/implementation:

A. *Remove* client from immediate environment to reduce pressure.

B. *Alleviate* symptoms using behavior-modification strategies.

C. *Divert* attention to topics other than symptoms (not remembering names, addresses, and events).

D. Encourage *socialization* rather than isolation.

E. *Avoid* sympathy, pity, and oversolicitous approach.

F. *Health teaching:* teach families to avoid reinforcing dissociative behavior; teach client problem solving, with goal of minimizing stressful aspects of environment.

IV. Evaluation: recall returns to conscious awareness; anxiety kept within manageable limits.

SOMATOFORM DISORDERS

I. Main characteristic: involuntary, physical symptoms *without* demonstrable organic findings or identifiable physiologic bases; involve psychologic factors or nonspecific conflicts.

II. General assessment:

A. Precipitant: major emotional, interpersonal stress.

B. Occurrence of secondary gain from illness.

III. General analysis/nursing diagnosis:

A. *Fear* related to loss of dependent relationships.

B. *Powerlessness* related to chronic resentment over frustration of dependency needs.

C. *Altered feeling patterns:* inhibition of anger, which is discharged physiologically and is related to control of anxiety.

D. *Impaired judgment* related to denial of existence of any conflicts or relationship to physical symptoms.

E. *Altered role performance:* regression related to not having dependency needs met.

Somatization Disorder

Repeated, multiple, vague or exaggerated physical complaints of several years' duration *without* identifiable physical cause; clients constantly seek medical attention, undergo numerous tests; at risk for unnecessary surgery or drug abuse.

A. Assessment:

1. Onset and occurrence—teen years, more common in women.
2. Reports illness most of life.
   a. *Neuromuscular* symptoms—fainting, seizures, dysphagia, difficulty walking, back pain, urinary retention.
   b. *Gastrointestinal* symptoms—nausea, vomiting, flatus, food intolerance, constipation or diarrhea.
   c. *Female reproductive* symptoms—dysmenorrhea, hyperemesis gravidarum, dyspareunia.
   d. *Psychosexual* symptoms—sexual indifference, dyspareunia.
   e. *Cardiopulmonary* symptoms—palpitations, shortness of breath, chest pain.
   f. *Rule out:* Multiple sclerosis, systemic lupus erythematosus, porphyria, hyperparathyroidism.
3. Appears anxious and depressed.

B. Analysis/nursing diagnosis:

1. *Anxiety* related to threat to security and inability to meet role expectations.
2. *Self-care deficit* related to development of physical symptoms to escape stressful situations.
3. *Dysfunctional behaviors* related to inability to accept that physical symptoms lack a physiologic basis.
4. *Body image disturbance* and *altered role performance* related to passive acceptance of disabling symptoms.

Conversion Disorder (Hysterical Neuroses, Conversion Type)

Sudden symptoms of *symbolic* nature developed under *extreme* psychologic stress (e.g., war, loss, natural disaster) that *disappear* through hypnosis.

A. Assessment:

1. *Neurologic* symptoms—paralysis, aphonia, tunnel vision, seizures, blindness, paresthesias, anesthesias.
2. *Endocrinologic* symptoms—pseudocyesis.
3. Hysterical, dependent *personality profile:* exhibi-

tionistic dress and language; self-indulgent; suggestible; impulsive and global impressions and hunches; little capacity to concentrate, integrate, and organize thoughts or plan action or outcomes; little concern for symptoms, despite severe impairment ("La Belle Indifference").

B. Analysis/nursing diagnosis:

1. Prolonged *loss or alteration of physiological processes* related to severe psychologic stress and conflict that results in disuse, atrophy, contractures. *Primary gain*—internal conflict or need is kept out of awareness; there is a close relationship in time between stressor and occurrence of symbolic symptoms.
2. *Impaired social interaction:* chronic sick role related to attention-seeking.
3. *Noncompliance* with expected routines related to *secondary gain*—avoidance of upsetting situation, with support obtained from others.
4. *Impaired adjustment* related to *repression* of feelings through somatic symptoms, *regression, denial* and *isolation,* and *externalization.*
5. *Ineffective individual coping;* e.g., daydreaming, fantasizing, superficial warmth and seductiveness related to inability to control symptoms voluntarily or to explain them by known physical disorder.

Hypochondriasis (Hypochondriacal Neurosis)

Exaggerated concern for one's physical health; *unrealistic* interpretation of signs or sensations as abnormal; *preoccupation with fear* of having serious disease, *despite* medical reassurance of no diagnosis of physical disorder.

A. Assessment:

1. Preoccupation with symptoms; sweating, peristalsis, heartbeat, coughing, muscular soreness, skin eruptions.
2. Occurs in both men and women in adolescence, 30s, or 40s.
3. History of long, complicated shopping for doctors and refusal of mental health care.
4. Organ neurosis may occur (e.g., cardiac neurosis).
5. Personality trait: compulsive.
6. Prevalence of anxiety and depression.
7. Controls relationships through physical complaints.

B. Analysis/nursing diagnosis:

1. *Personal identity disturbance* related to perception of self as ill in order to meet needs for dependency, attention, affection.
2. Displaced *anxiety* related to inability to verbalize feelings.
3. *Fear* related to not being believed.
4. *Powerlessness* related to feelings of insecurity.
5. *Altered role performance:* disruption in work and interpersonal relations related to regression and need gratification through preoccupation with fantasized illness; and related to control over others through physical complaints.

IV. General nursing plans/implementation for somatoform disorders:

A. *Long-term goals:*

1. Develop interests *outside* of self. Introduce to new activities and people.
2. Facilitate experiences of increased feelings of *independence.*
3. Increase *reality perception* and *problem-solving ability.*
4. Emphasize *positive* outlook and promote positive thinking. Reassure that symptoms are anxiety-related, not a result of physical disease.
5. Develop mature ways for meeting *affection* needs.

B. *Short-term goals:*

1. *Prevent* anxiety from mounting and becoming uncontrollable by recognizing symptoms, for early intervention.
2. *Environment:* warm, caring, supportive interactions; instill hope that anxiety can be mastered.
3. Encourage client to *express* somatic concerns verbally. Encourage awareness of body processes.
4. Provide *diversional* activities.
5. Develop ability to relax rather than ruminate or worry. Help find palliative relief through anxiety reduction (slower breathing, exercise).
6. *Health teaching:*
   a. Relaxation training as self-help measures.
   b. Increase knowledge of appropriate and correct information on physiologic responses that accompany anxiety.

V. General evaluation:

A. Does not isolate self.
B. Discusses fears, concerns, conflicts that are self-originated and not likely to be serious.
C. Decides which aspects of situation can be overcome and ways to meet conflicting obligations.
D. Looks for things of importance and value.
E. Deliberately engages in new activities other than ruminating or worrying.
F. Talks self out of fears.
G. Decrease in physical symptoms; is able to sleep, feels less restless.
H. Makes fewer statements of feeling helpless.
I. Can freely express angry feelings in *overt* way and not through symptoms.

OTHER DISORDERS IN WHICH PSYCHOLOGIC FACTORS AFFECT PHYSICAL CONDITIONS (PSYCHOPHYSIOLOGIC DISORDERS)

This group of disorders occurs in various organs and systems, whereby emotions are expressed by affecting body organs.

I. Concepts and principles related to psychologic factors affecting physical conditions:

A. Majority of organs involved are usually under control of *autonomic* nervous system.

B. Coping mechanisms

1. *Repression or suppression* of unpleasant emotional experiences.
2. *Introjection*—illness seen as punishment.
3. *Projection*—others blamed for illness.
4. *Conversion*—physical symptoms rather than underlying emotional stresses are emphasized.

C. Clients often exhibit the following underlying *needs in excess:*

1. Dependency.
2. Attention.
3. Love.
4. Success.
5. Recognition.
6. Security.

D. Need to distinguish between:

1. Factitious disorders—deliberate, *conscious* exhibit of physical or psychological illness to avoid an uncomfortable situation.
2. *Conversion disorder*—affecting *sensory* systems that are usually under *voluntary* control; generally *non-life-threatening;* symptoms are symbolic solution to anxiety; *no* demonstrable *organic* pathology.
3. *Psychologic factors affecting physical condition*—e.g., psychophysiologic disorders; under *autonomic* nervous system control; structural *organic* changes; may be life-threatening.

E. A *decrease in emotional security* tends to produce an *increase in symptoms.*

F. When treatment is confined to physical symptoms, emotional problems are *not* usually relieved.

II. Assessment of physiologic factors:

A. Persistent psychologic factors may produce structural *organic* changes resulting in *chronic diseases,* which may be *life-threatening* if untreated.

B. *All* body systems are affected:

1. Skin (pruritus and dermatitis, for example).
2. Musculoskeletal (*backache,* muscle cramps, and rheumatism, for example).
3. Respiratory (*asthma,* hiccups, and hay fever, for example).
4. Gastrointestinal (*ulcers,* ulcerative colitis, irritable colon, heartburn, constipation, and diarrhea, for example).
5. Cardiovascular (paroxysmal tachycardia, *migraines,* palpitations, and hypertension, for example).
6. Genitourinary (dysuria and *dysmenorrhea,* for example).
7. Endocrine (hyperthyroidism, for example).
8. Nervous system (general fatigue, anorexia, and exhaustion, for example).

III. Analysis/nursing diagnosis: *Ineffective individual coping* related to inappropriate need-gratification through illness (actual illness used as means of meeting needs for attention and affection). Absence of life experiences that gratify needs for attention and affection.

IV. Nursing plan/implementation in disorders in which psychologic factors affect physical conditions:

A. *Long-term goal: release* of feelings through verbalization.

B. *Short-term goals:*

1. Take care of *physical* problems during acute phase.
2. *Remove* client from anxiety-producing stimuli.

C. Prompt attention in meeting clients' *basic needs,* to gratify appropriate needs for dependency, attention, and security.

D. Maintain an attitude of *respect and concern;* clients' pains and worries are very real and upsetting to them; do not belittle the symptoms. Do not say, "There is nothing wrong with you" because emotions do in fact cause somatic disabilities.

E. *Treat organic* problems as necessary, but without undue emphasis (that is, do not reinforce preoccupation with bodily complaints).

F. Help clients *express their feelings,* especially anger, hostility, guilt, resentment, or humiliation, which may be related to such issues as sexual difficulties, family problems, religious conflicts, and job difficulties. Help clients recognize that, when stress and anxiety are not released through some channel such as verbal expression, the body will release the tension through *"organ language."*

G. Provide *outlets* for release of tensions and diversions from preoccupation with physical complaints.

1. Provide social and recreational activities to decrease time for preoccupation with illness.
2. Encourage clients to use physical and intellectual capabilities in constructive ways.

H. *Protect* clients from any disturbing stimuli; help the healing process in the acute phase of illnesses (myocardial infarct, for example).

I. Help clients feel *in control* of situations and be as independent as possible.

J. Be *supportive;* assist clients to bear painful feelings through a helping relationship.

K. *Health teaching:*

1. Teach how to express feelings.
2. Teach more effective ways of responding to stressful life situations.
3. Teach the family supportive relationships.

V. Evaluation: can verbalize feelings more fully.

SCHIZOPHRENIC DISORDERS

Schizophrenia is a group of interrelated symptoms with a number of common features involving disorders of *mood, thought content, feelings, perception,* and *behavior.* The term means "splitting of the mind," alluding to the discrepancy between the content of *thought processes* and their emotional expression; this should *not* be confused with "multiple personality" (dissociative reaction).

Half of the clients in mental hospitals are diagnosed as schizophrenic; many more schizophrenics live in the community. The onset of symptoms for this disorder generally occurs between 15 and 27 years of age. Causes, psychodynamics, and psychopathology are still a matter of controversy.

I. Common subtypes of schizophrenia (without clear-cut differentiation):

disorganized type disordered, thinking ("word salad"), inappropriate effect (blunted, silly), regressive behavior, incoherent speech, preoccupied and withdrawn.

catatonic type disorder of muscle tension, with rigidity, waxy flexibility, posturing, mutism, violent rage outbursts, negativism, and frenzied activity. Marked decrease in involvement with environment and in spontaneous movement.

paranoid type disturbed perceptions leading to disturbance in thought content of *persecutory, grandiose,* or hostile nature; projection is key mechanism, with religion a common preoccupation.

residual continued difficulty in thinking, mood, perception, and behavior after schizophrenic episode.

undifferentiated type unclassifiable schizophreniclike disturbance with mixed symptoms of delusions, hallucinations, incoherence, gross disorganization.

II. Concepts and principles related to schizophrenic disorders:

A. *General:*

1. *Symbolic* language used expresses schizophrenic's life, pain, and progress toward health; all symbols used have meaning.
2. *Physical care* provides media for relationship; nurturance may be initial focus.
3. *Consistency, reliability,* and *empathic* understanding build trust.
4. *Denial, regression,* and *projection* are key defense mechanisms.
5. Felt anxiety gives rise to distorted thinking.
6. Attempts to engage in verbal communication may result in tension, apprehensiveness, and defensiveness.
7. Person rejects real world of painful experiences and creates fantasy world through illness.

B. *Withdrawal:*

1. Withdrawal from and resistance to forming relationships are attempts to reduce anxiety related to:
   a. Loss of ability to experience satisfying human relationships.
   b. Fear of rejection.
   c. Lack of self-confidence.
   d. Need for protection and restraint against potential destructiveness of *hostile* impulses (toward self and others).
2. *Ambivalence* results from need to approach a relationship and need to avoid it.
   a. Cannot tolerate swift emotional or physical closeness.
   b. Needs more time than usual to establish a relationship; time to test sincerity and interest of nurse.
3. Avoidance of client by others, especially staff, will reinforce withdrawal, thereby creating problem of mutual withdrawal and fear.

C. *Hallucinations:*

1. It is possible to replace hallucinations with satisfying interactions.
2. Person can relearn to focus attention on real things and people.
3. Hallucinations originate during *extreme* emotional stress when unable to cope.
4. Hallucinations are very real to client.
5. Client will react as the situation is perceived, *regardless* of reality or consensus.
6. Concrete experiences, *not* argument or confrontation, will correct sensory distortion.
7. Hallucinations are *substitutes* for human relations.
8. Purposes served by or expressed in falsification of reality:
   a. Reflection of problem in inner life.
   b. Statement of criticism, censure, self-punishment.
   c. Promotion of self-esteem.
   d. Satisfaction of instinctual strivings.
   e. Projection of unacceptable unconscious content in disguised form.
9. Perceptions *not* as *totally* disturbed as they seem.
10. Client attempts to restructure reality through hallucinations to protect remaining ego integrity.
11. Hallucinations may result from a variety of psychologic and biologic conditions (extreme fatigue, drugs, pyrexia, and organic brain disease, for example).
12. Hallucinating person needs to feel free to describe his perceptions if he is to be understood by the nurse.

III. Assessment of schizophrenic disorders:

A. Eugene Bleuler described four classic and *primary symptoms as the "four A's":*

1. *Associative looseness*—impairment of logical thought progression, resulting in confused, bizarre, and abrupt thinking. *Neologisms*—making up new words or condensing words into one.
2. *Affect*—exaggerated, apathetic, blunt, flat, inappropriate, inconsistent feeling tone that is communicated through face and body posture.
3. *Ambivalence*—simultaneous, conflicting feelings or attitudes toward person or object.
   a. Stormy outbursts.
   b. Poor, weak interpersonal relations.
4. *Autism—withdrawal* from external world; preoccupation with fantasies and idiosyncratic thoughts.
   a. *Delusions*—false, fixed beliefs, not corrected by logic; a defense against intolerable feeling. The two most common delusions are:
      (1) *Delusions of grandeur*—conviction in a belief related to being famous, important, or wealthy.
      (2) *Delusions of persecution*—belief that one's thoughts, moods, or actions are controlled or influenced by strange forces or by others.
   b. *Hallucinations*—false sensory impressions without observable external stimuli.
      (1) Auditory—affecting hearing (e.g., hears voices).

(2) Visual—affecting vision (e.g., sees snakes).

(3) Tactile—affecting touch (e.g., feels electric charges in body).

(4) Olfactory—affecting smell (e.g., smells rotting flesh).

(5) Gustatory—affecting taste (e.g., food tastes like poison).

c. *Ideas of reference*—clients interpret cues in the environment as having reference to them. Ideas *symbolize guilt, insecurity, and alienation;* may become delusions, if severe.

d. *Depersonalization*—feelings of strangeness and unreality about self or environment or both; difficulty in differentiating boundaries between self and environment.

B. *Regression*—extreme *withdrawal* and social isolation.

C. *Prodromal or residual symptoms:*

1. Social isolation, *withdrawal.*
2. Marked impairment in *role* functioning (e.g., as student, employee).
3. Markedly *peculiar* behavior (e.g., collecting garbage).
4. Marked impairment in personal *hygiene.*
5. *Affect:* blunt, inappropriate.
6. *Speech:* vague, overelaborate, circumstantial, metaphorical.
7. *Thinking:* bizarre ideation or magical thinking, e.g., ideas of reference, "others can feel my feelings."
8. Unusual *perceptual* experiences, e.g., sensing the presence of a force or person not physically there.

IV. Analysis/nursing diagnosis:

A. *Sensory/perceptual alterations* related to inability to define reality and distinguish the real from the unreal (hallucinations, illusions) and misinterpretation of stimuli.

B. *Altered communication process* with inability to *verbally* express needs and wishes related to difficulty with processing information and unique patterns of speech.

C. *Altered thought processes* related to intense anxiety and blocking (delusions).

D. *Altered emotional processes* related to anxiety about others (*inappropriate emotions*).

E. *Self-care deficit* with *inappropriate* dress and poor physical hygiene related to perceptual or cognitive impairment.

F. *Altered judgment* related to lack of trust, fear of rejection, and doubts regarding competence of others.

G. *Altered self-concept* related to *feelings of inadequacy* in coping with the real world.

H. *Body image disturbance* related to inappropriate use of defense mechanisms.

I. *Disorganized behaviors:* impaired relatedness to others, related to withdrawal, distortions of reality, and lack of trust.

J. *Diversional activity deficit* related to personal ambivalence.

V. Nursing plan/implementation in schizophrenic disorders:

A. *General:*

1. Set *short-range* goals, realistic to client's levels of functioning.
2. Use *nonverbal* level of communication to demonstrate concern, caring, and warmth, as client often distrusts words.
3. Set climate for free expression of *feelings* in whatever mode, without fear of retaliation, ridicule, or rejection.
4. Seek client out in his or her own fantasy world.
5. Try to understand meaning of symbolic language; help him or her communicate less symbolically.
6. Provide *distance,* as client needs to feel safe and to observe nurses for sources of threat or promises of security.
7. Help client tolerate nurses' presence and learn to *trust* nurses enough to move out of isolation and share painful and often unacceptable (to client) feelings and thoughts.
8. Anticipate and accept negativism; do *not* personalize.
9. *Avoid* joking, abstract terms, and figures of speech when client's thinking is literal.
10. Give antipsychotic medications.

B. *Withdrawn behavior:*

1. *Long-term goal:* develop satisfying interpersonal relationships.
2. *Short-term goal:* help client feel safe in one-to-one relationship.
3. Seek client out at every chance, and establish some bond.
   a. Stay with client, in silence.
   b. Initiate talk when he or she is ready.
   c. Draw out, but do not demand, response.
   d. Do *not* avoid the client.
4. Use simple language, specific words.
5. Use an *object or activity* as medium for relationship; initiate activity.
6. Focus on everyday experiences.
7. Delay decision making.
8. Accept one-sided conversation, with silence from the client; *avoid* pressuring to respond.
9. Accept the client's outward attempts to respond and inappropriate social behavior, without remarks or disdain; teach social skills.
10. Avoid making demands on client or exposing client to failure.
11. *Protect* from aggressive persons and from impulsive attacks on self and others.
12. Attend to *nutrition, elimination, exercise,* hygiene, and signs of physical illness.
13. Add structure to the day; tell him or her, "This is your 9 A.M. medication."
14. *Health teaching:* assist family to understand client's needs, to see small sign of progress; teach client to perform simple tasks of self-care in order to meet own biologic needs.

C. *Hallucinatory behavior:*

1. *Long-term goal:* establish satisfying relationships with *real* persons.

2. *Short-term goal:* interrupt *pattern* of hallucinations.
3. Provide a *structured* environment with routine activities. Use *real* objects to keep client's interest or to stimulate new interest (in painting or crafts, for example).
4. *Protect* against injury to self and others resulting from "voices" he thinks he hears.
5. *Short, frequent* contacts initially, increasing social interaction gradually (one person → small groups).
6. Ask person to describe experiences as hallucinations occur.
7. Respond to anything real the client says, for example, with acknowledgment or reflection. Focus more on *feelings,* not on delusional, hallucinatory content.
8. *Distract* client's attention to something real when he hallucinates.
9. *Avoid* direct confrontation that voices are coming from client himself; do not argue, but listen.
10. *Clarify* who "they" are:
    a. Use personal pronouns, avoid universal and global pronouns.
    b. Nurse's own language needs to be clear and unambiguous.
11. Use one sentence, ask only one question, at a time.
12. Encourage *consensual validation.* Point out that experience is not shared by you; voice doubt.
13. *Health teaching:*
    a. Recommend more effective ways of coping (e.g., consensual validation).
    b. Advise that highly emotional situations be avoided.
    c. Explain the causes of misperceptions.
    d. Recommend methods for reducing sensory stimulation.

D. *Delusions* (see *Nursing plan/implementation in paranoid disorders,* in following section).

VI. Evaluation:

A. Small behavioral changes occur (e.g., eye contact, better grooming).

B. Evidence of beginning trust in nurse (keeping appointments).

C. Initiates conversation with others; participates in activities.

D. Decreases amount of time spent alone.

E. Demonstrates appropriate behavior in public places.

F. Articulates relationship between feelings of discomfort and autistic behavior.

G. Makes positive statements.

DELUSIONAL (PARANOID) DISORDER

Paranoid disorders have a concrete and pervasive delusional system, usually *persecutory. Projection* is a chief coping mechanism of this disorder.

I. Concepts and principles related to paranoid disorders:

A. Delusions are attempts to cope with stresses and problems.

B. May be a means of allegorical or symbolic communication and of testing others for their trustworthiness.

C. Interactions with others and activities interrupt delusional thinking.

D. To establish a rational therapeutic relationship, gross distortions, misorientation, misinterpretation, and misidentification need to be overcome.

E. Delusional people have extreme need to maintain self-esteem.

F. False beliefs cannot be changed without first changing experiences.

G. A delusion is held because it *performs a function.*

H. When people who are experiencing delusions become at ease and comfortable with people, delusions will not be needed.

I. Delusions are misjudgments of reality based on a series of mental mechanisms: (a) *denial,* followed by (b) *projection* and (c) *rationalization.*

J. There is a *kernel of truth* in delusions.

K. Behind the anger and suspicion in a paranoid, there is a *lonely, terrified* person who *feels vulnerable* and *inadequate.*

II. Assessment of paranoid disorders:

A. Chronically *suspicious,* distrustful (thinks "people are out to get me.").

B. Distant, but *not* withdrawn.

C. Poor insight; blames others (*projects).*

D. Misinterprets and *distorts reality.*

E. Difficulty in admitting own errors; takes pride in intelligence and in being correct (superiority).

F. Maintains false persecutory belief despite evidence or proof (may refuse food and medicine, insisting they are poisoned).

G. Literal thinking *(rigid).*

H. Dominating and provocative.

I. Hypercritical and intolerant of others; *hostile,* quarrelsome, and aggressive.

J. *Very sensitive* in perceiving minor injustices, errors, and contradictions.

K. Evasive.

III. Analysis/nursing diagnosis:

A. *Severe anxiety* related to projection of threatening, aggressive impulses and misinterpretation of stimuli.

B. *Ineffective individual coping* related to lack of trust, fear of close human contact.

C. *Impaired cognitive functioning* related to rigidity of thought.

D. *Chronic low self-esteem* related to feelings of inadequacy.

E. *Impaired social interaction* related to lack of tender, kind feelings, feelings of grandiosity and/or persecution.

F. *Altered thought processes* related to lack of insight.

IV. Nursing plan/implementation in paranoid disorders:

A. *Long-term goals:* gain clear, correct perceptions and interpretations through corrective experiences.

B. *Short-term goals:*

1. Help client recognize distortions, misinterpretations.
2. Help client feel safe in exploring reality.

C. Help client learn to *trust self;* help to develop self-confidence and ego assets through positive reinforcement.

D. Help to *trust others.*

1. Be consistent and honest at all times.
2. Do not whisper, act secretive, or laugh with others in client's presence when he or she cannot hear what is said.
3. Do not mix medicines with food.
4. Keep promises.
5. Let client know ahead of time what he or she can expect from others.
6. Give reasons and careful, complete, and repetitive explanations.
7. Ask permission to contact others.
8. Consult client first about all decisions concerning him or her.

E. Help to *test reality.*

1. Present and repeat reality of the situation.
2. Do not confirm or approve distortions.
3. Help accept responsibility for own behavior rather than project.
4. Divert from delusions to reality-centered focus.
5. Let client know when behavior does not seem appropriate.
6. Assume nothing and leave no room for assumptions.
7. Structure time and activities to limit delusional thought, behavior.
8. Set limit for *not* discussing delusional content.
9. Look for underlying needs expressed in delusional content.

F. Provide *outlets* for anger and aggressive drives.

1. Listen matter of factly to angry outbursts.
2. Accept rebuffs and abusive talk as symptoms.
3. Do not argue, disagree, or debate.
4. Allow expression of negative feelings without fear of punishment.

G. Provide *successful group experience.*

1. Avoid competitive sports involving close physical contact.
2. Give recognition to skills and work well done.
3. Utilize managerial talents.
4. Respect client's intellect and engage him or her in activities with others requiring intellect (chess, puzzles, and Scrabble, for example).

H. Limit physical contact.

I. *Health teaching:* teach a more rational basis for deciding whom to trust by identifying behaviors characteristic of trusting and trustworthy people.

V. Evaluation: able to differentiate trustworthy from untrustworthy people; growing self-awareness, and able to share this awareness with others; accepting of others without need to criticize or change them; is open to new experiences; able to delay gratification.

PERSONALITY DISORDERS

Subtypes of personality disorders include: antisocial, histrionic, narcissistic, avoidant, and dependent personalities. A *personality disorder* is a syndrome in which the person's inner difficulties are revealed through general behaviors and by a pattern of living that seeks *immediate gratification of impulses* and instinctual needs without regard to society's laws, mores, and customs and *without censorship* of personal conscience.

Borderline personality disorder is subtype in which client is unstable in many areas: she or he has unstable but intense interpersonal relationships, impulsive and unpredictable behavior, wide mood swings; chronic feelings of boredom or emptiness; intolerance of being alone; uncertainty about identity; and is physically self-damaging.

Passive-aggressive subtype displays indirect resistance to demand for performance: procrastinates, forgets, and is inefficient.

I. Concepts and principles related to *antisocial personality disorders:*

A. One defense against severe anxiety is "acting out," or dealing with distressful feelings or issues through action.

B. Faulty or arrested emotional development in preoedipal period has interfered with development of adequate social control or superego.

C. Since there is a malfunctioning or *weakened superego,* there is little internal demand and therefore no tension between ego and superego to evoke guilt feelings.

D. The defect is *not* intellectual; person shows *lack of moral responsibility, inability to control emotions* and impulses, and *deficiency in normal feeling* responses.

E. "Pleasure principle" is dominant.

F. Initial stage of treatment is most crucial; treatment situation is very threatening because it mobilizes client's anxiety, and client ends treatment abruptly. Key underlying emotion: fear of closeness, with threat of exploitation, control, and abandonment.

II. Assessment—antisocial personality disorders:

A. Onset *before* age 15.

B. History of behavior that *conflicts with society:* truancy, expulsion or suspension from school for misconduct; delinquency, thefts, vandalism, running away from home; persistent lying; repeated substance abuse; initiating fights; chronic violation of rules at home or school; school grades below IQ level.

C. Inability to sustain consistent *work* behavior (e.g., frequent job changes or absenteeism).

D. Lack of ability to function as *responsible* parent (evidence of child's malnutrition or illness due to lack of minimal hygiene standards; failure to obtain medical care for seriously ill child; failure to arrange for caretaker when parent is away from home).

E. Failure to accept *social norms* with respect to *lawful* behavior (e.g., thefts, multiple arrests).

F. Inability to maintain enduring *intimate* relationship (e.g., multiple relations, desertion, multiple divorces); lack of respect or loyalty.

G. *Irritability* and *aggressiveness* (spouse, child abuse; repeated physical fights).

H. Failure to honor *financial* obligations.

I. Failure to *plan ahead.*

J. *Disregard for truth* (lying, "conning" others for personal gain).

K. *Recklessness* (driving while intoxicated, recurrent speeding).

L. *Violating* rights of others.

M. Does not appear to profit from experience; *repeats* same punishable or antisocial behavior; usually does not feel guilt or depression.

N. Exhibits *poor judgment;* may have intellectual, but not emotional, insight to guide judgments. Inadequate problem solving and reality testing.

O. Uses *manipulative* behavior patterns in treatment setting (see VIII. Manipulation, pp. 43–45).

1. Demands and controls.
2. Pressures and coerces, threatens.
3. Violates rules, routines, procedures.
4. Requests special privileges.
5. Betrays confidences and lies.
6. Ingratiates.
7. Monopolizes conversation.

III. Analysis/nursing diagnosis:

A. *Ineffective individual coping* related to:

1. Inability to tolerate frustration.
2. Verbal, nonverbal manipulation (lying).
3. Destructive behavior toward self or others.
4. Overuse of: denial, projection, rationalization, intellectualization.
5. Inability to learn from experience.

B. *Personal identity disturbance* related to:

1. *Self-esteem disturbance* as evidenced by grandiosity, depression.
2. Lack of responsibility, accountability, commitment.
3. Distancing relationships.

C. *Impulsive behavior* related to fear of real or potential loss.

D. *Noncompliance* related to excess need for independence.

IV. Nursing plan/implementation in personality disorders:

A. *Long-term goal:* help person accept responsibility and consequences of own actions.

B. *Short-term goal:* minimize manipulation and acting-out.

C. Set *fair, firm, consistent limits and follow through on consequences* of behavior; let client know what she or he can expect from staff and what the unit's regulations are, as well as the consequences of violations. Be explicit.

D. *Avoid* letting staff be played against one another by a particular client; staff should present a unified approach.

E. Nurses should *control* their *own* feelings of anger and defensiveness aroused by any person's manipulative behavior.

F. Change focus when client persists in raising inappropriate subjects (such as personal life of a nurse).

G. Encourage expression of *feelings* as an alternative to acting-out.

H. Aid client in realizing and accepting responsibility for own actions and *social responsibility* to others.

I. Use group therapy as a means of *peer control* and multiple feedback about behavior.

J. *Health teaching:* teach family how to use behavior-modification techniques to reward client's acceptable behavior (i.e., when he or she accepts responsibility for own behavior, is responsive to rights of others, adheres to social and legal norms).

V. Evaluation: less use of lying, blaming others for own behavior; more evidence of following rules; less impulsive, explosive behavior.

MOOD DISORDERS

Mood disorders include: (1) *Depressive disorders* and (2) *Bipolar disorders.* Bipolar disorders are further divided into (a) *manic,* (b) *depressed,* (c) *mixed* or (d) *cyclothemia.* The mood disturbance may occur in a number of patterns of severity and duration, alone or in combination, where client feels extreme sadness and guilt, withdraws socially, expresses self-deprecatory thoughts *(major depression), or* experiences an elevated, expansive mood with hyperactivity, pressured speech, inflated self-esteem, decreased need for sleep *(manic episode or disorder).*

Another specific mood disorder is *dysthymic* disorder (depressive neuroses), in which there is a chronic mood disturbance involving a depressed mood or loss of interest and pleasure in all usual activities, but not of sufficient severity or duration to be classified as a *major depressive episode.* Table 1.14 *summarizes* the main points of *difference between the two types of depression.*

These affective disorders should be distinguished from grief. Grief is *realistic* and proportionate to what has been *specifically* lost and involves *no loss of self-esteem.* There is a *constant* feeling of sadness over a period of 3–12 months or longer, with good reality contact (no delusions).

Major Depression

I. Concepts and principles

A. Self-limiting factors—most depressions are self-limiting disturbances, making it important to look for a change in functioning and behavior.

B. *Theories of cause of depression*

1. Aggression turned inward—*self-anger.*
2. Response to separation or object *loss.*
3. *Genetic* and/or *neurochemical* basis (Table 1.15).
4. *Cognitive*—negative mind-set of hopelessness.
5. *Personality*—negative self-concept, low self-esteem affect belief system and appraisal of stressors.
6. *Learned helplessness:* environment can't be controlled.
7. *Behavioral*—loss of positive reinforcement.
8. *Integrated*—interaction of chemical, experiential, and behavioral variables acting on diencephalon.

II. General assessment

A. *Physical*—early-morning awakening, *insomnia* at night, increased need for sleep during the day, fatigue, constipation, *anorexia* with weight loss, loss of sexual

TABLE 1.14 Comparison of the Two Different Types of Depression

Dimension	Major Depression	Dysthymic Depression
Cause	Primary disturbance in structure and function of brain and nervous sytem.	Severe, prolonged stress, unresolved conflicts; chronic anxiety, fears, anger.
Onset	Rapid and without apparent cause.	Gradual.
Form of depression	Restlessness and agitation, *or* psychomotor retardation; severe; tends to be worse in morning and better in evening.	Mixed; mild to severe; unpredictable mood; usually optimistic in morning and depressed in evening.
Sleep	Insomnia after being awakened.	Easily awakened, but goes back to deep sleep in morning.
Appetite	Anorexia leading to weight loss.	Varied (anorexia leading to compulsive eating).
Activity	Chronically tired; needs structure at all times.	Occasional energy bursts (feels embarrassed at lack of energy).
Self-esteem	Very low.	Fluctuates from high to low.
Fears	Intense fear of being alone.	Multiple fears about present and future.
Decision making	Totally indecisive.	O.K. on minor decisions; indecisive on important decisions.
Memory	Poor.	Unreliable.
Contact with reality	Poor; paranoid, self-deprecatory delusions, distorted judgment.	Varies.

interest, *psychomotor retardation,* physical complaints, amenorrhea.

B. *Psychologic*—inability to remember, decreased *concentration,* slowing or blocking of thought, all-or-nothing thinking, *less interest* and involvement with external world and own appearance, feeling worse at certain times of day or after any sleep, difficulty in enjoying activities, monotonous voice, *repetitive* discussions, *inability to make decisions* due to ambivalence, impaired coping with "practical problems."

C. *Emotional*—loss of self-esteem, feelings of *hopelessness* and *worthlessness,* shame and self-derogation due to *guilt, irritability,* despair and *futility* (leading to *suicidal* thoughts), alienation, *helplessness,* passivity, avoidance, *inertia,* powerlessness, denied anger; uncooperative, tense, crying, demanding, and *dependent* behavior.

III. Analysis/nursing diagnosis:

A. *Altered nutrition* (anorexia) related to lack of interest in food.

B. *Potential for violence* toward self (suicide) related to inability to verbalize emotions.

C. *Sleep pattern disturbance* (insomnia or excessive sleep) related to emotional dysfunctioning.

D. *Self-care deficit* related to disinterest in activities of daily living.

E. *Chronic low self-esteem* with self-reproaches and blame related to feelings of inadequacy.

F. *Altered feeling and meaning patterns* (sadness, loneliness, apathy) related to overwhelming feeling of unworthiness and dysfunctional grieving.

G. *Impaired social interaction* related to social isolation.

IV. Nursing plan/implementation:

A. Promote sleep and food intake—take nursing measures to ensure the *physical* well-being of the client.

B. Provide steady company to assess *suicidal* tendencies and to diminish feelings of loneliness and alienation.

1. Build trust in a one-to-one relationship.
2. Interact with client on a nonverbal level if that is his or her immediate mode of communication; this will promote feelings of being recognized, accepted, and understood.
3. Focus on *today,* not the past or far into the future.
4. Reassure that present state is temporary and that he or she will be protected and helped.

C. Make the *environment* nonchallenging and nonthreatening.

1. Use a kind, firm attitude, with warmth.
2. See that client has favorite foods; respond to other wishes and likes.
3. Protect from overstimulation and coercion.

D. Postpone client's *decision making* and resumption of duties.

1. Allow *more time* than usual to complete activity (dressing, eating) or thought process and speech.
2. Structure the environment for client to help reestablish a set schedule and predictable *routine* during ambivalence and problems with decisions.

E. *Provide nonintellectual activities* (for instance, sanding wood)—avoid chess and crossword puzzles, for example, as thinking capacity at this time tends to be circular.

F. Encourage expression of emotions, denial, hopelessness, helplessness, guilt, regret; provide *outlets for anger* that may be underlying the depression; as client

■ **TABLE 1.15 Theories of Causative Factors Related to the Development of Depression**

Biologic (Genetic, Biochemical)	Psychologic	Cognitive	Sociocultural
Possible genetic influence. Hormonal influence (drop in estrogen and progesterone). *Biochemical activities:* impaired neurotransmission of monoamine oxidase (MAO); high levels of catecholamines (dopamine and norepinephrine). Toxic reactions.	Dependency. Low self-esteem. Powerlessness. Ambivalence. Guilt. Lack of support system. Severe stress. Lack of clear goals. Feelings of failure. Inability to fulfill expectations.	Narrow, negative perspective called "cognitive triad": view of self, world, and the future. Draws conclusions on inadequate or contradictory evidence. Overgeneralizes from one instance. Focuses on a single detail rather than on the whole. Distortion of long-range consequences, hence bad judgment.	Social situations that contribute to feelings of powerlessness and low self-esteem: 1. Status of minority groups. 2. Status of women in male-oriented professional and business culture. 3. Role loss, such as loss of mother role in empty nest phase. 4. Being the object of cultural stereotypes (e.g., blacks, aged, Jews).

Source: Wilson HS, Kneisl CR: *Psychiatric Nursing,* 3rd ed. (Redwood City, CA: Addison-Wesley, 1988).

becomes more verbal with anger and recognizes the origin and results of anger, help client resolve feelings—allow client to complain and be *demanding* in initial phases of depression.

G. Discourage *redundancy in speech and thought*—redirect focus from a monologue of painful recounts to an appraisal of more neutral or positive attributes and aspects of situations.

H. Encourage client to *assess own* goals, unrealistic expectations, and perfectionist tendencies.

1. May need to change goals or give up some goals that are incompatible with abilities and external situations.
2. Assist client to recapture what was lost through substitution of goals, sublimation, or relinquishment of unrealistic goals—reanchor client's self-respect to other aspects of his or her existence; help him or her free self from *dependency* on one person or single event or idea.

I. Indicate that success is possible and not hopeless.

1. Explore what steps client has taken to achieve goals and suggest new or alternate ones.
2. Set *small, immediate goals* to help attain mastery.
3. Recognize client's efforts to mobilize self.
4. Provide positive reinforcement for client through exposure to activities in which client can experience a sense of *success, achievement, and completion* to build *self-esteem* and self-confidence.
5. Help client experience *pleasure;* help client start good relationships in social setting.

J. *Long-term goal:* to encourage interest in external surroundings, outside of self, to increase and strengthen social relationships.

1. Encourage purposeful activities.
2. Let client advance to activities at own pace (graded task assignments).
3. Gradually encourage activities with others.

K. *Health teaching:* explain need to recognize highly stressful situation and fatigue as stress factor; advise that negative responses from others be regarded with minimum significance; explain need to maintain positive self-attitude; advise occasional respite from responsibilities; emphasize need for realistic expectation of others.

V. Evaluation: performs self-care; expresses increased self-confidence; engages in activities with others; accepts positive statements from others; identifies positive attributes and skills in self.

Bipolar Disorders

Bipolar disorders are major emotional illnesses characterized by mood swings, alternating from depression to elation, with periods of relative normality between episodes. Most persons experience a single episode of manic or depressed type; some have recurrent depression or recurrent mania or mixed. There is increasing evidence that a biochemical disturbance may exist and that most individuals with manic episodes eventually develop depressive episodes.

I. Concepts and principles related to bipolar disorders:

A. The psychodynamics of manic and depressive episodes are related to hostility and guilt.

B. The struggle between unconscious impulses and moral conscience produces feelings of *hostility, guilt,* and *anxiety.*

C. To relieve the internal discomfort of these reactions, the person *projects* long-retained hostile feelings onto others or onto objects in the environment during *manic* phase; during *depressive* phase, hostility and guilt are *introjected* toward self.

D. Demands, irritability, sarcasm, profanity, destructiveness, and threats are signs of the *projection* of *hostility;* guilt is handled through *persecutory delusions and accusations.*

■ TABLE 1.16 Behaviors Associated With Mania and Depression

Mania (periods of predominantly and persistently elevated, expansive, or irritable mood)	**Depression (loss of interest or pleasure in usual activities)**
Affect	
Lack of shame or guilt; inflated self-esteem; euphoria; intolerance of criticism.	Anger, anxiety, apathy, denial, delusions of guilt, helplessness, feelings of doom, hopelessness, loneliness, low self-esteem (self-degradation).
Physiology	
Insomnia; inadequate nutrition, weight loss.	Insomnia; anorexia, constipation, indigestion, nausea, vomiting→weight loss.
Cognition	
Denial of realistic danger. *Thoughts:* flight of ideas, loose associations; illusions, delusions of grandeur; lack of judgment; distractibility.	Ambivalence, confusion, inability to concentrate, self-blame; loss of interest and motivation; self-destructive (preoccupied with suicide).
Behavior	
Hyperactivity (social, sexual, work)→irrationality, aggressiveness, sarcasm, exhibitionism, and acting-out in behavior and dress. Hostile, arrogant, argumentative, demanding, and controlling. *Speech:* rapid, rhyming, punning, witty, pressured.	Altered activity level, social isolation, substance abuse, overdependency, underachievement, inability to care for self, *psychomotor retardation.*

E. Feelings of inferiority and fear of rejection are handled by being light and amusing.

F. Both phases, though appearing distinctly different, have the *same objective: to gain attention, approval, and emotional support.* These objectives and behaviors are unconsciously determined by the client; this behavior may be either biochemically determined or *both* biochemically and unconsciously determined.

II. Assessment of bipolar disorders:

A. Manic and depressed types are *opposite* sides of the *same* disorder.

1. Both are disturbances of mood and self-esteem.
2. Both have underlying aggression and hostility.
3. Both are intense.
4. Both are self-limited in duration.

B. Comparison of behaviors associated with mania and depression: see Table 1.16.

III. Analysis/nursing diagnosis:

A. *Potential for injury* related to poor judgment.

B. *Altered nutrition, less than body requirements,* related to inability to sit down long enough to eat.

C. *Sleep pattern disturbance:* lack of sleep and rest related to restlessness, hyperactivity, emotional dysfunctioning.

D. *Self-care deficits* related to altered motor behavior due to anxiety.

E. *Altered feeling state* (anger), *judgment, thought content* (magical thinking), *thought processes* (altered concentration and problem solving) related to disturbance in self-concept.

F. *Impaired social interaction* related to internal and external stimuli (overload, underload).

IV. Nursing plan/implementation:

A. *Manic:*

1. Prevent *physical* dangers stemming from suicide and exhaustion—promote rest, sleep, and intake of nourishment.
   a. Use *suicide* precautions.
   b. Reduce outside stimuli or remove to quieter area.
   c. Diet: provide *high-calorie beverages, finger foods* within sight and reach.
2. Attend to client's personal care.
3. Absorb with understanding and without reproach behaviors such as talkativeness, provocativeness, criticism, sarcasm, dominance, profanity, and dramatic actions.
   a. Allow, postpone, or partially fulfill demands and freedom of expression *within limits* of ordinary social rules, comfort, and safety of client and others.
   b. Do not cut off manic stream of talk, as this increases anxiety and need for release of hostility.
4. Constructively utilize excessive energies with *activities* that do *not* call for concentration or follow-through.
   a. Outdoor walks, gardening, putting, and ball-tossing are therapeutic.
   b. Exciting, disturbing, and highly *competitive* activities should be *avoided.*
   c. Creative occupational therapy activities promote release of hostile impulses, as does creative writing.
5. Give tranquilizers as ordered until lithium affects symptoms (3 weeks); then give lithium carbonate as ordered.
6. Help client to recognize and express *feelings* (denial, hopelessness, anger, guilt, blame, helplessness).
7. Encourage realistic self-concept.
8. *Health teaching:* how to monitor effects of lithium; instructions regarding salt intake.

B. *Depressed:*

1. Take routine *suicide* precautions.
2. Give attention to *physical* needs for food and sleep and to hygiene needs. Prepare warm baths and hot beverages to aid sleep.
3. Initiate *frequent* contacts:
   a. Do not allow long periods of silence to develop or client to remain withdrawn.
   b. Use a kind, understanding, but emotionally neutral approach.
4. Allow dependency in severe depressive phase. Since dependency is one of the underlying concerns with depressive persons, if nurse allows dependency to occur as an initial response, he or she must plan for resolution of the dependency toward himself or herself as an example for the client's other dependent relationships.
5. Slowly repeat simple, direct information.
6. Assist in daily decision making until client regains self-confidence.
7. Select *mild* exercise and diversionary *activities* instead of stimulating exercise and competitive games, as they may overtax physical and emotional endurance and lead to feelings of inadequacy and frustration.
8. Give antidepressive drugs.
9. *Health teaching:* how to make simple decisions related to health care.

V. Evaluation:

A. *Manic:* speech and activity are slowed down; affect is less hostile; able to sleep; able to eat with others at the table.

B. *Depressed:* takes prescribed medications regularly. Does not engage in self-destructive activities. Able to express feelings of anger, helplessness, hopelessness.

■ TREATMENT MODES

MILIEU THERAPY

Milieu therapy consists of treatment by means of controlled modification of the client's environment to promote positive living experiences.

I. Concepts and principles related to milieu therapy:

A. Everything that happens to clients from the time they are admitted to the hospital or treatment setting has a potential that is either therapeutic or antitherapeutic.
1. Not only the therapists but all who come in contact with the clients in the treatment setting are important to the clients' recovery.
2. Emphasis is on the social, economic, and cultural dimension, the interpersonal climate, as well as the physical environment.

B. Clients have the right, privilege, and responsibility to make decisions about daily living activities in the treatment setting.

II. Characteristics of milieu therapy:

A. Friendly, warm, trusting, secure, supportive, comforting atmosphere throughout the unit.

B. An optimistic attitude about prognosis of illness.

C. Attention to comfort, food, and daily living needs; help with resolving difficulties related to tasks of daily living.

D. Opportunity for clients to take responsibility for themselves and for the welfare of the unit in gradual steps.
1. Client government.
2. Client-planned and client-directed social activities.

E. Maximum individualization in dealing with clients, especially regarding treatment and privileges in accordance with clients' needs.

F. Opportunity to live through and test out situations in a realistic way by providing a setting that is a microcosm of the larger world outside.

G. Opportunity to discuss interpersonal relationships in the unit among clients and between clients and staff (decreased social distance between staff and clients).

H. Program of carefully selected resocialization activities to prevent regression.

III. Nursing plan/implementation in milieu therapy:

A. *New structured relationships*—allow clients to develop new abilities and use past skills; support them through new experiences as needed; help build liaisons with others; set limits; help clients modify destructive behavior; encourage group solutions to daily living problems.

B. *Managerial*—inform clients about expectations; preserve orderliness of events.

C. *Environmental manipulation*—regulate the outside environment to alter daily surroundings.
1. Geographically move clients to units more conducive to their needs.
2. Work with families, clergy, employers, etc.
3. Control visitors for the benefit of the client.

D. *Team approach* uses the milieu to meet each client's needs.

IV. Evaluation:

A. *Physical dimension:* order, organization.

B. *Social dimension:* clarity of expectations, practical orientation

C. *Emotional dimension:* involvement, support, responsibility, openness, valuing, accepting.

BEHAVIOR MODIFICATION

Behavior modification is a therapeutic approach involving the application of learning principles so as to change maladaptive behavior.

I. Definitions:

conditioned avoidance (also *aversion therapy*) a technique whereby there is a purposeful and systematic production of strongly unpleasant responses in situations to which the client has been previously attracted but now wishes to avoid.

desensitization frequent exposure in small but gradually increasing doses of anxiety-evoking stimuli until undesirable behavior disappears or is lessened (as in phobias).

token economy desired behavior is reinforced by rewards, such as candy, money, and verbal approval, used as tokens.

operant conditioning a method designed to elicit and reinforce desirable behavior (especially useful in mental retardation).

positive reinforcement giving rewards to elicit or strengthen selected behavior or behaviors.

II. Objectives and process of treatment in behavior modification:

A. Emphasis is on changing unacceptable, overt, and observable behavior to that which is acceptable; emphasis is on changed way of *acting* first, not of thinking.

B. Mental health team determines behavior to change and treatment plan to use.

C. Therapy is based on the knowledge and application of *learning* principles, that is, *stimulus-response;* the unlearning, or *extinction,* of undesirable behavior; and the *reinforcement* of desirable behavior.

D. Therapist identifies what events are important in the life history of the client and arranges situations in which the client is therapeutically confronted with them.

E. Two primary aspects of behavior modification:

1. *Eliminate* unwanted behavior by *negative reinforcement* (removal of an aversive stimulus, which acts to reinforce the behavior that results in removal of the aversive stimulus) and *ignoring* (withholding positive reinforcement).
2. *Create* acceptable new responses to an environmental stimulus by *positive* reinforcement.

F. Useful with: disturbed children, rape victims, dependent and manipulative behaviors, eating disorders, obsessive-compulsive disorders, sexual dysfunction.

III. Assumptions of behavioral therapy:

A. Behavior is what an organism does.

B. Behavior can be observed, described, and recorded.

C. It is possible to predict the conditions under which the same behavior may recur.

D. Undesirable social behavior is not a symptom of mental illness but is behavior that can be modified.

E. Undesirable behaviors are learned disorders that relate to acute anxiety in a given situation.

F. Maladaptive behavior is learned in the same way as adaptive behavior.

G. People tend to behave in ways that "pay off."

H. *Three ways* in which behavior can be reinforced:

1. *Positive* reinforcer (adding something pleasurable).
2. *Negative* reinforcer (removing something unpleasant).
3. *Adverse* stimuli (punishing).

I. If an undesired behavior is ignored, it will be extinguished.

J. Learning process is the same for all; therefore, all conditions (except organic) are accepted for treatment.

IV. Nursing plan/implementation in behavior modification:

A. Find out what is a "reward" for the person.

B. Break the goal down into small, successive *steps.*

C. Maintain *close* and continual observation of the selected behavior or behaviors.

D. Be *consistent* with on-the-spot, immediate intervention and correction of undesirable behavior.

E. Record focused observations of behavior frequently.

F. Participate in close teamwork with the *entire* staff.

G. Evaluate procedures and results continually.

H. *Health teaching:* teach above steps to colleagues and family.

V. Evaluation: acceptable behavior is increased and maintained; undesirable behavior is decreased or eliminated.

ACTIVITY THERAPY

Activity therapy consists of a variety of recreational and vocational activities (RT, recreational therapy; OT, occupational therapy; and music, art, and dance therapy) designed to test and examine social skills and serve as adjunctive therapies.

I. Concepts and principles related to activity therapy:

A. Socialization counters the regressive aspects of illness.

B. Activities need to be selected for specific psychosocial reasons to achieve specific effects.

C. Nonverbal means of expression as an additional behavioral outlet add a new dimension to treatment.

D. Sublimation of sexual drives is possible through activities.

E. Indications for activity therapy; clients with low self-esteem who are socially unresponsive.

II. Characteristics of activity therapy:

A. Usually planned and coordinated by other team members, the recreational therapists or music therapists, for example.

B. Goals:

1. Encourage socialization in community and social activities.
2. Provide pleasurable activities.
3. Help client release tensions and express feelings.
4. Teach new skills, help client find new hobbies.
5. Offer graded series of experiences, from passive spectator role and vicarious experiences to more direct and active experiences.
6. Free and/or strengthen physical and creative abilities.
7. Increase self-esteem.

III. Nursing plan/implementation in activity therapy:

A. Encourage, support, and cooperate in client's participation in activities planned by the adjunct therapists.

B. Share knowledge of client's illness, talents, interests, and abilities with others on the team.

C. *Health teaching:* teach client necessary skills for each activity (e.g., sports, games, crafts).

IV. Evaluation: client develops occupational and leisure-time skills that will help provide a smoother transition back to the community.

GROUP THERAPY

Group therapy is a treatment modality in which two or more clients and one or more therapists interact in a helping process to relieve emotional difficulties, increase self-esteem and insight, and improve behavior in relations with others.

I. Concepts and principles related to group therapy:

A. People's problems usually occur in a social setting; thus they can best be evaluated and corrected in a social

TABLE 1.17 Curative Factors of Group Therapy

Factor	Definition
Instilling of hope	Imbuing the client with optimism for the success of the group therapy experience.
Universality	Disconfirming the client's sense of aloneness or uniqueness in misery or hurt.
Imparting of information	Giving didactic instruction, advice, or suggestions.
Altruism	Finding that the client can be of importance to others; having something of value to give.
Corrective recapitulation of the primary family group	Reviewing and correctively reliving early familial conflicts and growth-inhibiting relationships.
Development of socializing techniques	Acquiring sophisticated social skills, such as being attuned to process, resolving conflicts, and being facilitative toward others.
Imitative behavior	Trying out bits and pieces of th- behavior of others and experimenting with those that fit well.
Interpersonal learning	Learning that the client is the author of his or her interpersonal world and moving to alter it.
Group cohesiveness	Being attracted to the group and the other members with a sense of "we"-ness rather than "I"-ness.
Catharsis	Being able to express feelings.
Existential factors	Being able to "be" with others; to be a part of a group.

Source: Wilson HS, Kneisl CR: *Psychiatric Nursing,* 3rd ed. (Redwood City, CA: Addison-Wesley, 1988).

setting (see Table 1.17 for summary of curative factors).

B. *Not* all are amenable to group therapies. For example:

1. Brain-damaged.
2. Acutely suicidal.
3. Acutely psychotic.
4. Persons with very passive-dependent behavior patterns.
5. Acutely manic.

C. It is best to match group members for *complementarity in behaviors* (verbal with nonverbal, withdrawn with outgoing) but for *similarity in problems* (obesity, predischarge group, cancer patients, prenatal group) to facilitate empathy in the sharing of experiences and to heighten group identification and cohesiveness.

D. Feelings of *acceptance,* belonging, respect, and comfort develop in the group and facilitate change and health.

E. In a group, members can *test reality* by giving and receiving *feedback.*

F. Clients have a chance to experience in the group that they are not alone (concept of *universality*).

G. Expression and *ventilation* of strong emotional feelings (anger, anxiety, fear, and guilt) in the safe setting of a group is an important aspect of the group process aimed at health and change.

H. The group setting and the *interactions* of its members may provide *corrective emotional experiences* for its members. A key mechanism operating in groups is *transference* (strong emotional attachment of one member to another member, to the therapist, and/or to the entire group).

I. To the degree that people modify their behavior through corrective experiences and identification with others rather than through personal-insight analysis, group therapy may be of special advantage over individual therapy, in that the possible number of interactions is greater in the group and the patterns of behavior are more readily observable.

J. There is a higher client-to-staff ratio, and it is thus less expensive.

II. General group goals:

A. Provide opportunity for self-expression of ideas and feelings.

B. Provide a setting for a variety of relationships through group interaction.

C. Explore current behavioral patterns with others and observe dynamics.

D. Provide peer and therapist support and source of strength for the individuals to modify present behavior and try out new behaviors; made possible through development of identity and group identification.

E. Provide on-the-spot, multiple feedback (that is, incorporate others' reactions to behavior), as well as give feedback to others.

F. Resolve dynamics and provide insight.

III. Nursing plan/implementation in group setting:

A. Nurses need to fill different roles and functions in the group, depending on the type of group, its size, its aims, and the stage in the group's life cycle. The multifaceted roles may include:

1. Catalyst.
2. Transference object.
3. Clarifier.
4. Interpreter of "here and now."
5. Role model and resource person.
6. Supporter.

B. During the *first sessions,* explain the purpose of the group, go over the "contract" (structure, format, and goals of sessions), and facilitate introductions of group members.

C. In *subsequent sessions,* promote greater group cohesiveness.

1. Focus on *group concerns* and group process rather

TABLE 1.18 Differences Between Reality Orientation and Resocialization

Reality Orientation	Resocialization
1. Maximum use of assets.	1. Reality living situation in a community.
2. Structured.	2. Unstructured.
3. Refreshments *may* be served.	3. Refreshments served.
4. Constant reminders of who the clients are, where they are, and why and what is expected of them.	4. Reliving happy experiences; encouragement to participate in home activities.
5. Group size: 3–5, depending on degree and level of confusion or disorientation.	5. Group size: 5–17, depending on mental and physical capabilities.
6. Meetings: one-half hour daily, same time and place.	6. Meetings: 3 times per week for one-half to one hour.
7. Planned topics: reality-centered objects.	7. No planned topic; group-centered feelings.
8. Role of leader: eliciting response of participants.	8. Role of leader: clarification and interpretation.
9. Periodic reality-orientation test of participants' level of confusion.	9. Periodic progress note of participants' enjoyment and improvements.
10. Emphasis: time, place, person orientation.	10. Any topic freely discussed.
11. Use of mind function still intact.	11. Rely on memories and experiences.
12. Participant is greeted *by name*, thanked for coming, extended a handshake and/or physical contact.	12. Participant greeted on arrival, thanked, extended a handshake on leaving.
13. Conducted by trained aides and activity assistants.	13. Conducted by RN, LPN/LVN, aides, program assistants.

Source: Adapted by permission from Barns, E., Sack, A., Shore, H., *The Gerontologist* 1973: 13:513.

than on intrapsychic dynamics of individuals.

2. Demonstrate nonjudgmental acceptance of behaviors within the limits of the group contract.
3. Help group members handle their anxiety, especially during the initial phase.
4. Encourage silent members to interact at their level of comfort.
5. Encourage members to interact verbally without dominating the group discussion.
6. Keep the focus of discussion on related themes; *set limits and interpret group rules.*
7. Facilitate sharing and *communication* among members.
8. Provide *support* to members as they attempt to work through anxiety-provoking ideas and feelings.
9. Set the expectation that the members are to take responsibility for carrying the group discussion and exploring issues on their own.

D. *Termination phase:*

1. Make early preparation for group termination (end point should be announced at the first meeting).
2. Anticipate common reactions from group members to separation anxiety and help each member to work through these reactions:
   a. Anger.
   b. Acting-out.
   c. Regressive behavior.
   d. Repression.
   e. Feelings of abandonment.
   f. Sadness.

IV. Evaluation:

A. *Physical:* shows improvement in daily life activities (eating, rest, work, exercise, recreation).

B. *Emotional:* asks for and accepts feedback; states feels good about self and others.

C. *Intellectual:* is reality-oriented; greater awareness of self, others, environment.

D. *Social:* willing to take a risk in trusting others; sharing self; reaching out to others.

REALITY ORIENTATION AND RESOCIALIZATION

See Table 1.18 for differences between these two modes of therapy.

FAMILY THERAPY

Family therapy is a process, method, and technique of psychotherapy in which the focus is not on an individual but on the total family as an interactional system.

I. Developmental tasks of North American family (Duvall, 1971):

A. *Physical maintenance*—provide food, shelter, clothing, health care.

B. *Resource allocation*—(physical and emotional) allocate material goods, space, and facilities; give affection, respect, and authority.

C. *Division of labor*—decide who earns money, manages household, cares for family.

D. *Socialization*—guidelines to control food intake, elimination, sleep, sexual drives, and aggression.

E. *Reproduction, recruitment, release of family members*—give birth to, or adopt, children; rear children; incorporate in-laws, friends, etc.

F. *Maintenance of order*—ensure conformity to norms.

G. *Placement of members in larger society*—interaction in school, community, etc.

H. *Maintenance of motivation and morale*—reward achievements, develop philosophy for living; create rituals and celebrations to develop family loyalty. Show acceptance, encouragement, affection; meet crises of individuals and family.

II. Basic theoretical concepts related to family therapy:

A. The ill family member (called the *identified patient,* or *IP*), by symptoms, sends a message about the "illness" of the family as a *unit*.

B. *Family homeostasis* is the means by which families attempt to maintain the status quo.

C. *Scapegoating* is found in disturbed families and is usually focused on one family member at a time, with the intent to keep the family in line.

D. Communication and behavior by some family members bring out communication and behavior in other family members.

1. Mental illness in the IP is almost always accompanied by emotional illness and disturbance in other family members.
2. Changes occurring in one member will produce changes in another; that is, if the IP improves, another IP may emerge, or family may try to place original person back into IP role.

E. Human communication is a key to emotional stability and instability—to normal and abnormal health. *Conjoint* family therapy is a communication-centered approach that looks at interactions between family members.

F. *Double bind* is a "damned-if-you-do, damned-if-you-don't" situation; it results in helplessness, insecurity, anxiety, fear, frustration, and rage.

G. *Symbiotic tie* usually occurs between one parent and a child, hampering individual ego development and fostering strong dependence and identification with the parent (usually the mother).

H. *Three basic premises* of communication:*

1. One cannot *not* communicate; that is, silence is a form of communication.
2. Communication is a *multilevel* phenomenon.
3. The message sent is *not* necessarily the *same* message that is received.

I. Indications for family therapy.

1. Marital conflicts.
2. Severe sibling conflicts.
3. Cross-generational conflicts.
4. Difficulties related to a transitional stage of family life cycle (e.g., retirement, new baby, death).
5. *Dysfunctional family patterns:* overprotective mother and distant father, with timid child or destructive, acting-out teenager; overfunctioning "super wife" or "super husband" and the underfunctioning, passive, dependent, and compliant spouse; child with poor peer relationships or academic difficulties.

* From Watzlawick, P.: *An anthology of human communication*. Palo Alto, California, 1964, Science and Behavior Books, Inc.

III. Family assessment should consider the following factors:

A. *Family as a social system:*

1. Family as responsive and contributing unit within network of other social units.
   a. Family boundaries—permeability or rigidity.
   b. Nature of input from other social units.
   c. Extent to which family fits into cultural mold and expectations of larger system.
   d. Degree to which family is considered deviant.
2. Roles of family members:
   a. Formal roles and role performance (father, child, etc.).
   b. Informal roles and role performance (scapegoat, controller, follower, decision maker).
   c. Degree of family agreement on assignment of roles and their performance.
   d. Interrelationship of various roles—degree of "fit" within total family.
3. Family rules:
   a. Family rules that foster stability and maintenance.
   b. Family rules that foster maladaptation.
   c. Conformity of rules to family's life-style.
   d. How rules are modified; respect for difference.
4. Communication network:
   a. How family communicates and provides information to members.
   b. Channels of communication—who speaks to whom.
   c. Quality of messages—clarity or ambiguity.

B. *Developmental stage of family:*

1. Chronologic stage of family.
2. Problems and adaptations of transition.
3. Shifts in role responsibility over time.
4. Ways and means of solving problems at earlier stages.

C. *Subsystems operating within family:*

1. Function of family alliances in family stability.
2. Conflict or support of other family subsystems and family as a whole.

D. *Physical and emotional needs:*

1. Level at which family meets essential physical needs.
2. Level at which family meets social and emotional needs.
3. Resources within family to meet physical and emotional needs.
4. Disparities between individual needs and family's willingness or ability to meet them.

E. *Goals, values, and aspirations:*

1. Extent to which family members' goals and values are articulated and understood by all members.
2. Extent to which family values reflect resignation or compromise.
3. Extent to which family will permit pursuit of individual goals and values.

F. *Socioeconomic factors* (see list in Figure 1.6).

IV. Nursing plan/implementation in family therapy:

A. Establish a family *contract* (who attends, when, duration of sessions, length of therapy, fee, and other expectations).

B. Encourage family members to identify and clarify own *goals.*

C. *Set ground rules:*

1. Focus is on the family as a whole unit, not on the IP.
2. No scapegoating or punishment of members who "reveal all" should be allowed.
3. Therapists should not align themselves with issues or individual family members.

D. *Use self* to empathetically respond to family's problems; share own emotions openly and directly; function as a role model of interaction.

E. Point out and encourage the family to *clarify* unclear, inefficient, and ambiguous family communication patterns.

F. Identify family *strengths.*

G. Listen for repetitive interpersonal *themes, patterns,* and attitudes.

H. *Attempt to reduce guilt and blame* (important to neutralize the scapegoat phenomenon).

I. Present possibility of *alternate* roles and rules in family interaction styles.

J. *Health teaching:* teach clear communication to all family members.

V. Evaluation: each person clearly speaks for self; asks for and receives feedback; communication patterns are clarified; family problems are delineated; members more aware of each other's needs.

ELECTROCONVULSIVE THERAPY

Electroconvulsive therapy (ECT) is a physical treatment that induces grand mal convulsions by applying electric current to the head. It is also called electric shock therapy (EST).

I. Characteristics of electroconvulsive therapy:

A. Usually used in treating major depression, with severe suicide risk, extreme hyperactivity, severe catatonic stupor, or those with bipolar affective disorders not responsive to psychotropic medication.

B. Consists of a series of treatments (6–25) over a period of time (three times a week, for example).

C. Person is asleep through the procedure and for 20–30 minutes afterwards.

D. Convulsion may be seen as a series of minor, jerking motions in extremities (e.g., toes). Spasms are reduced by use of muscle-paralyzing drugs.

E. Confusion is present for 30 minutes after treatment.

F. Induces loss of memory for *recent* events.

II. Views concerning success of electroconvulsive therapy:

A. Posttreatment sleep is the "curative" factor.

B. Shock treatment is seen as punishment, with an accompanying feeling of absolution from guilt.

C. Chemical alteration of thought patterns results in memory loss, with decrease in redundancy and awareness of painful memories.

III. Nursing plan/implementation in electroconvulsive therapy:

A. Always tell the client of the treatment.

B. Inform client about temporary memory loss for recent events after the treatment.

C. *Pretreatment care:*

1. Take vital signs.
2. See to client's toileting.
3. Remove client's dentures, eyeglasses or contact lenses, and jewelry.
4. NPO for 8 hours beforehand.
5. Atropine sulfate subcutaneously 30 minutes before treatment to decrease bronchial and tracheal secretions.
6. Anesthetist gives anesthetic and muscle relaxant IV (succinylcholine chloride, or Anectine) and oxygen for 2–3 minutes and inserts airway. Often all three are given close together—anesthetic first, followed by another syringe with Anectine and atropine sulfate. Electrodes and treatment must be given within 2 minutes of injections, as Anectine is very short-acting (2 minutes).

D. *During the convulsion* the nurse needs to make sure the person is in a safe position, to avoid dislocation and compression fractures (although Anectine is given to prevent this).

E. *Care during recovery stage:*

1. Put up side rails while client is confused; side position.
2. Take blood pressure and respirations.
3. Stay until person awakens, responds to questions, and can care for self.
4. Orient client to time and place and inform that treatment is over.
5. Offer support to help client feel more secure and relaxed as the confusion and anxiety decrease.
6. Medication for nausea and headache.

F. *Health teaching:* teach family members what to expect of client after ECT (confusion, headache, nausea); how to reorient the client.

IV. Evaluation: feelings of worthlessness, helplessness, and hopelessness seem diminished.

GLOSSARY

affect *feeling* or *mood* communicated through the face and body posture. Can be blunted, blocked, flat, inappropriate, or displaced.

ambivalence coexisting *contradictory* (positive and negative) emotions, desires, or attitudes toward an object or person (e.g., love-hate relationship).

amnesia loss of memory due to physical or emotional trauma.

anxiety state of uneasiness or response to a *vague*, unspecific danger cued by a threat to some value that the individual holds essential to existence (or by a threat of loss of control); the danger may be *real or imagined. Physiologic* manifestations are increased pulse, respiration, and perspiration, with feeling of "butterflies."

autism self-preoccupation and absorption in fantasy, as found with schizophrenia, with a complete *exclusion* of *reality* and loss of interest in and appreciation of others.

catatonia type of schizophrenia characterized by muscular rigidity; alternates with periods of excitability.

compulsion an insistent, repetitive, intrusive, and unwanted urge to perform an *act* that is contrary to ordinary conscious wishes or standards.

conflict emotional struggle resulting from *opposing* demands and drives of the id, ego, and superego.

coping mechanism device used to ward off anxiety or uncomfortable thoughts and feelings; an activity of the ego that operates outside of awareness to hold impulses in check that might cause conflict (repression and regression, for example).

cyclothymia alterations in moods of elation and sadness, with mood swings out of proportion to apparent stimuli.

delusion a false fixed *belief*, idea, or group of ideas that are contrary to what is thought of as real and that cannot be changed by logic; arise out of the individual's needs and are maintained in spite of evidence or facts (e.g., grandeur and persecution).

depression morbid sadness or dejection accompanied by feelings of hopelessness, inadequacy, and unworthiness. *Distinguished from grief,* which is realistic and in proportion to loss.

disorientation loss of awareness of the position of self in relation to time, place, or person.

echolalia automatic repetition of heard *phrases or words.*

echopraxia automatic repetition of observed *movements.*

ego the "I," "self," and "person" as distinguished from "others"; that part of the personality, according to Freudian theory, that *mediates* between the primitive, pleasure-seeking, instinctual drives of the id and the self-critical, prohibitive, restraining forces of the superego; that aspect of the psyche that is *conscious* and most in touch with external reality and is directed by the *reality principle.* The part of the personality that has to make the *decision.* Most of the ego is conscious and represents the *thinking-feeling* part of a person. The *compromises* worked out on an unconscious level help to resolve intrapsychic conflict by keeping thoughts, interpretations, judgments, and behavior practical and efficient.

electroshock electroshock treatment (EST) or electroconvulsive treatment (ECT) is the treatment of certain psychiatric disorders (best suited for depression) by therapeutic administration of regulated electrical impulses to the brain to produce convulsions.

empathy an objective awareness of another's thoughts, feelings, or behavior and their meaning and significance; intellectual identification *versus* emotional identification (sympathy).

euphoria exaggerated feeling of physical and emotional well-being *not* related to external events or stimuli.

flight of ideas a *thought disorder* where one thought moves rapidly to another without reaching a main idea or point, as in manic behavior. The next sentence may be triggered by a word in the previous sentence or by something in the environment.

fugue dissociative state involving amnesia and actual *physical flight.*

hallucination *false sensory* perception in the absence of an actual external stimulus. May be due to chemicals or inner needs and may occur in any of the five senses. Seen in psychosis and acute and chronic brain disorder.

hypochondriasis state of morbid preoccupation about one's health (somatic concerns).

id psychoanalytic term for that division of the psyche that is unconscious, contains instinctual primitive drives that lead to immediate gratification, and is dominated by the *pleasure principle.* The id wants what it wants when it wants it.

illusion misinterpretation of a real, external sensory stimulus (e.g., a person may see a shadow on the floor and think it is a hole).

insanity *legal* term for mental defect or disease that is of sufficient gravity to bring person under special legal restrictions and immunities.

labile unstable and rapidly shifting (referring to emotions).

manipulation process of influencing another to meet one's own needs, *regardless* of the other's needs.

mental retardation term for mental deficiency or deficit in normal development of intelligence that makes intellectual abilities lower than normal for chronologic age. May result from a condition present at birth, from injury during or after birth, or from disease after birth.

narcissism *exaggerated self-love* with all attention focused on own comfort, pleasure, abilities, appearance, etc.

neologism a newly coined word or condensed combination of several words not readily understood by others; found in schizophrenia.

neurosis *an older* term for mild to moderately severe illness in which there is a disorder of feeling or behavior but no gross mental disorganization, delusions, or hallucinations, as in serious psychoses. Typical reactions include disproportionate anxiety, phobias, and obsessive-compulsive behavior.

obsession persistent, unwanted, and uncontrollable *urge* or *idea* that *cannot* be banished by logic or will.

organic psychosis mental disease resulting from defect, damage, infection, tumor, or other *physical cause* that can be *observed* in the body tissues.

paranoid adjective indicating feelings of suspicion and persecution; one type of schizophrenia.

personality disorder broad category of illnesses in which inner difficulties are revealed not by specific symptoms but by *antisocial* behavior.

phobia *irrational, persistent,* abnormal, *morbid,* and unrealistic dread of external object or situation displaced from unconscious conflict.

premorbid personality state of an individual's personality *before* the onset of an illness.

psyche synonymous with mind or the *mental and emotional* "self."

psychoanalysis theory of human development and behavior, method of research, and form of treatment described by Freud that attributes abnormal behavior to repressions in the unconscious mind. Treatment involves dream interpretation and free association to bring into awareness the origin and effects of unconscious conflicts in order to eliminate or diminish them.

psychodrama a therapeutic approach that involves a structured, dramatized, and directed *acting-out* of emotional problems and troubled interactions by the client in order to gain insight into individual's own difficulties.

psychogenic symptoms or physical disorders caused by emotional or mental factors, as opposed to organic.

psychopath *older,* inexact term for one of a variety of *personality disorders* in which person has poor impulse control, releasing tension through immediate action, without social or moral conscience.

psychosis severe emotional illness characterized by a disorder of *thinking, feeling, and action* with the following symptoms: loss of contact, denial of reality, bizarre thinking and behavior, perceptual distortion, delusions, hallucinations, and regression.

schizoid form of personality disorder characterized by shyness, introspection, introversion, withdrawal, and aloofness.

schizophrenia severe functional mental illness characterized in general by a disorder in perception, thinking, feeling, behavior, and interpersonal relationships.

sociopathic pertaining to a disorder of behavior in which a person's feelings and behavior are asocial, with impaired judgment and inability to profit from experience; the intellect remains intact. This term is often used interchangeably with "antisocial personality."

soma term meaning the body or *physical* aspects.

superego in psychoanalysis, that part of the mind that incorporated the parental or societal values, ethics, and standards. It guides, restrains, criticizes, and punishes. It is unconscious and learned and is sometimes equated with the term *conscience.*

transference unconscious projections of feelings, attitudes, and wishes that were originally associated with early significant others onto persons or events in the present; may be positive or negative transference.

waxy flexibility psychomotor underactivity in which the individual maintains the posture in which he or she is placed.

word salad meaningless mixture of phrases and words often seen in schizophrenic behavior, e.g., "the ridjams frast wolmix."

■ QUESTIONS

Select the one best answer for each question, and fill in the answer circle beside the answer number.

Mrs. Allen, a 28-year-old woman, is admitted to a psychiatric hospital with symptoms of severe depression. Fourteen months ago, her 9-month-old boy died of crib death. Since then, Mrs. Allen has lost weight, will not eat, spends most of her time immobile, and speaks only in monosyllabic responses. She pays little attention to her appearance. Questions 1 through 6 refer to this case.

1. Which one of the following nursing approaches would be best for Mrs. Allen while her symptoms are severe?
- ○ 1. Allow her time for quiet thought; remain silent. **IMP 7**
- ○ 2. Ask her to join you and the other clients in the TV lounge. **PsI**
- ○ 3. State that you would like to go with her for a short walk around the outside grounds, and assist her with her coat.
- ○ 4. Give her a choice of recreational activities.

2. One afternoon, Mrs. Allen comes to lunch with her hair combed and traces of lipstick. What could a nurse say to reinforce this change of behavior?
- ○ 1. "What happened? You combed your hair!" **IMP**
- ○ 2. "This is the first time I've seen you look so good." **7 PsI**
- ○ 3. "You must be feeling better. You look much better."
- ○ 4. "I see that your hair is combed and you have lipstick on."

3. Which of the following are important nursing approaches in depression?
- ○ 1. Providing motor outlets for aggressive, hostile feelings. **PL 7**
- ○ 2. Protecting against harm to others. **PsI**
- ○ 3. Reducing interpersonal contacts.
- ○ 4. Deemphasizing preoccupation with elimination, nourishment, and sleep.

4. When Mrs. Allen says to the nurse, "I can't talk; I have nothing to say," and continues being silent, what should the nurse do?
- ○ 1. Say, "All right. You don't have to talk. Let's play cards, instead." **IMP 7**
- ○ 2. Explain that talking is an important sign of getting well and that she is expected to do so. **PsI**
- ○ 3. Be silent until Mrs. Allen speaks again.
- ○ 4. Say, "It may be difficult for you to speak at this time; perhaps you can do so at another time."

5. In working with clients who are depressed, it is essential that the nurse know that depression may stem from:
- ○ 1. A sense of loss—actual, imaginary, or impending. **AN 7**
- ○ 2. Revived memories of a painful childhood. **PsI**
- ○ 3. A confused sexual identity.
- ○ 4. An unresolved Oedipal conflict.

6. Which of the following activities would be best for the nurse to suggest to a client who is depressed?
- ○ 1. Folding laundry or stapling paper sheets for charts. **IMP 3**
- ○ 2. Playing checkers. **PsI**
- ○ 3. Doing a crossword puzzle.
- ○ 4. Ice skating.

Mr. Short, a 35-year-old man, is brought to a psychiatric hospital by his wife. His history includes periodic episodes of manic behavior, alternating with depression. Questions 7 through 11 refer to this case.

7. When assessing clients who are in the depressed phase and those who are in the manic phrase of bipolar affec-

Key to codes following questions Nursing process: **AS**, Assessment; **AN**, Analysis; **PL**, Plan; **IMP**, Implementation; **EV**, Evaluation. Category of human function: **1**, Protective; **2**, Sensory-perceptual; **3**, Comfort, Rest, Activity, and Mobility; **4**, Nutrition; **5**, Growth and Development; **6**, Fluid-Gas Transport; **7**, Psycho-Social-Cultural; **8**, Elimination. Client needs: **SECE**, Safe, Effective Care Environment; **PhI**, Physiological Integrity; **PsI**, Psychosocial Integrity; **HPM**, Health Promotion/Maintenance. See frontmatter for full explanation.

tive disorders, which characteristic is the nurse likely to note that is common to both phases of the disorder?
- ○ 1. Suicidal tendency. **AS**
- ○ 2. Underlying hostility. **2**
- ○ 3. Delusions. **PsI**
- ○ 4. Flight of ideas.

8. A nursing care plan for a hospitalized hyperactive client in manic reaction needs to include:
- ○ 1. Involvement in a group activity and encouragement to talk. **PL** **2**
- ○ 2. Attention to adequate food and fluid intake. **PsI**
- ○ 3. Protection against suicide.
- ○ 4. Permissive acceptance of bizarre behavior.

9. One evening the nurse sees Mr. Short in the dayroom without any clothes. He is shouting vulgarities and dancing wildly about the room while other clients are watching TV. The best initial response by the nurse at this time would be:
- ○ 1. "Let's sit down with the others and watch TV; I'll put this blanket over you to keep you warm." **IMP** **2** **PsI**
- ○ 2. "We do not allow this behavior in the hospital. It is embarrassing the other clients."
- ○ 3. "Please put your clothes on."
- ○ 4. "Come put your clothes on, Mr. Short. I will help you."

10. When talking with a client who is in the acute manic phase with flight of ideas, the nurse primarily needs to:
- ○ 1. Speak loudly and rapidly to keep the client's attention, as the client is easily distracted. **PL** **2**
- ○ 2. Focus on the feelings conveyed rather than the thoughts expressed. **PsI**
- ○ 3. Encourage the client to complete one thought at a time.
- ○ 4. Allow the client to talk freely.

11. Which of the following activities could a nurse suggest that would be best for a client with manic behavior?
- ○ 1. Solitary activity, such as reading. **IMP**
- ○ 2. Hammering on metal in a jewelry-making class. **3** **PsI**
- ○ 3. Playing chess.
- ○ 4. Competitive games.

A nurse discovers John, a 19-year-old man, crouched in a corner of the psychiatric unit corridor. There is blood on the floor. He is holding on to a gushing wound on his right wrist and looks pale and frightened. A razor is nearby on the floor. Questions 12 through 15 refer to this case.

12. What should the nurse do first?
- ○ 1. Sit down on the floor, next to the client, and in a quiet, reassuring tone, say, "You seem frightened. Can I help?" **AN** **7** **PsI**
- ○ 2. Ask the aide to watch the client and run to get the doctor.
- ○ 3. Apply pressure on the wrist, saying to the client, "You are hurt. I will help you."
- ○ 4. Go back down the hall to get the emergency cart.

13. The next morning, John relates to the nurse, "I was going to kill myself." What is the best initial response by the nurse?
- ○ 1. Say nothing. Wait for his next comment. **IMP**
- ○ 2. "What were you going to do this time?" **7**
- ○ 3. "Have you felt this way before?" **PsI**
- ○ 4. "You seem upset. I am going to be here with you; perhaps you will want to talk about it."

14. The nurse must assess for high-risk suicide behavior when the behavior is related to:
- ○ 1. Depression with melancholia. **AN**
- ○ 2. Schizophrenic disorders. **7**
- ○ 3. Bipolar affective disorder, manic. **PsI**
- ○ 4. Psychologic factors affecting physical condition.

15. In caring for John, who is a suicide risk, the most important nursing consideration is:
- ○ 1. Maintain constant awareness of John's whereabouts. **PL** **7**
- ○ 2. Ignore John as long as he is talking about suicide, because a suicide attempt is unlikely. **PsI**
- ○ 3. Relax vigilance when John seems to be recovering from depression.
- ○ 4. Administer medication.

Jane Green is a 23-year-old who stands 5 feet high and weighs 180 pounds. She has, since the beginning of her teenage years, become more overweight. Ms. Green has a busy social life with other women in the office where she works as a consultant. However, she does not date and has had few social contacts with males. She went for a physical, and the physician suggested therapy, as there was no physical reason for her obesity problem. Questions 16 through 22 refer to this case.

16. Ms. Green was referred by the physician to the nurse for diet counseling. What action would the nurse take?
- ○ 1. Develop a weight control plan, together with her, that will allow gradual weight loss. **IMP** **4**
- ○ 2. Ask Ms. Green to describe her eating patterns. **PsI**
- ○ 3. Support her interests in other activities.
- ○ 4. Put Ms. Green on a diet with very limited number of calories so she will have an immediate weight loss.

17. Ms. Green says to the nurse, "My therapist told me I eat because I didn't get enough love from my mother. What does he mean?" What is the best response for the nurse to offer?
- ○ 1. "Tell me what you think the therapist means." **IMP**
- ○ 2. "We are here to deal with your diet, not with your psychological problems." **7** **PsI**
- ○ 3. "You need to ask your therapist."
- ○ 4. "What do you think is the connection between your not getting enough love and your overeating?"

18. Which of the following characteristics does the nurse need to be aware of that apply to a person engaged in other forms of gradual self-destructive behavior (such as in obesity, drug addiction, and smoking)?
- ○ 1. Acceptance of the death wish. **AN**
- ○ 2. Denial of possibility of death. **7**
- ○ 3. Ability to control own behavior. **PsI**
- ○ 4. Ignorance of the consequences of own behavior.

19. The nurse bases her plan of care on the knowledge that persons engaged in gradual self-destructive behavior:
- ○ 1. Believe they can stop this behavior at any time. **AN**
- ○ 2. Have decreased anxiety when they stop the behavior. **7** **PsI**
- ○ 3. Believe the behavior controls them.
- ○ 4. Believe the behavior, in some manner, is "good" for them.

20. Which of the following feelings is the nurse likely to identify as antecedent of self-destructive behavior?
- ○ 1. Omnipotence. **AN**

○ 2. Grandiosity. 7
○ 3. Low self-esteem. **PsI**
○ 4. Self-satisfaction.

21. One view about self-destructive behavior that a nurse needs to know about in planning patient care is that self-destructive behavior may be interpreted as the:
○ 1. Directing of hostile feelings toward self. **AN**
○ 2. Directing of hostile feelings toward others. 7
○ 3. Directing of hostile feelings toward an internalized love object. **PsI**
○ 4. Internalization of the fear of death.

22. In conducting an assessment interview, the nurse needs to be aware that self-destructive behavior is determined by:
○ 1. A variety of factors, with the same factors present in each individual. **AS** 7
○ 2. Genetic disturbances. **PsI**
○ 3. Interpersonal disturbances.
○ 4. A variety of factors, different for each individual.

Mrs. Betty Barnes, mother of a 5-year-old girl and an 11-year-old boy and long estranged from her husband, received a letter informing her that her husband had suddenly died. Her immediate reaction was stunned silence related to shock and grief, followed by expression of anger: "I suppose he didn't have any insurance benefits to leave to the children." Questions 23 through 25 refer to this case.

23. Which of the following indicates that the nurse best understands Mrs. Barnes' reaction?
○ 1. She is experiencing a normal grief reaction. **AN**
○ 2. Her reaction can best be understood if more was known about the marital relationship and breakup. 7 **PsI**
○ 3. The children and the injustice done to them by the father's death are her main concern.
○ 4. She is not reacting normally to the news.

24. Mrs. Barnes' resolution of grief would likely be complicated if:
○ 1. There are ambivalent feelings for the deceased. **AN** 7
○ 2. Mr. Barnes' death was due to a chronic illness. **PsI**
○ 3. It is the first loss to be experienced.
○ 4. There was little emotional dependency on the deceased.

25. Mrs. Barnes' mother-in-law comes to stay with them. Betty notices that her mother-in-law is acting more and more like her deceased son, even complaining of similar physical symptoms that her son had before he died. She is preoccupied solely with thoughts about his positive attributes. The nurse will see signs of grief resolution in Mrs. Barnes when she:
○ 1. Encourages Betty to remarry. **EV**
○ 2. Is able to talk about both the pleasurable and the painful aspects connected with her son. 7 **PsI**
○ 3. Tries to make up for his deficiencies, saying, "He would have wanted me to do this for you."
○ 4. Is finally able to feel anger toward her son and agree with Betty that he had failed them all.

26. *A 10-year-old boy diagnosed with acute leukemia, terminal stage, asks the nurse one morning while she is fixing his bed: "I am going to die, aren't I?" What would be the most appropriate response by the nurse?*
○ 1. "No, you're not. You are getting the latest treatment available and you have a very good doctor. Your white count was better yesterday." **IMP** 7 **HPM**
○ 2. "We are all going to die sometime."
○ 3. "What did the doctor tell you?"
○ 4. "I don't know. You have a serious illness. Do you have feelings that you want to talk about now?"

27. *Ruth, an acutely ill 40-year-old wife and mother hospitalized for treatment of metastatic lung carcinoma, begs the nurse to ask the doctor to give her a pass to attend her son's high school graduation in a city 100 miles from the hospital. "If only I could be free of pain to do just this one thing, then I'll be ready to die," she says. The nurse identifies Ruth's behavior as an example of:*
○ 1. Being unrealistic and denying the degree of her illness. **EV** 7
○ 2. Using bargaining as a reaction to death and dying. **HPM**
○ 3. Being manipulative to get her way.
○ 4. Being unaware of her diagnosis.

While Marshall Brown was driving the car with his wife in a blizzard one evening, the car slid on some ice and hit the edge of a bridge. His wife was killed instantly, and he was admitted to the hospital with severe chest injuries. His wife's family made and carried out the funeral arrangements for his wife. Before the accident, the couple appeared to be happily married. Because Marshall cannot attend the viewing of the body, the funeral, or the burial, you expect that he may later have difficulty with resolution of his grief. Questions 28 and 29 refer to this case.

28. Which of the following data regarding the present situation could help the nurse forecast Marshall's future difficulties?
○ 1. Feelings of anger toward the hospital staff for keeping him hospitalized during the funeral. **AN** 7
○ 2. Feelings of anger toward himself for having been injured but not killed in the accident. **PsI**
○ 3. His inability to participate in the cultural rituals of grief, wherein the reality of his wife's death is emphasized.
○ 4. His preoccupation with his own physical distress at this time.

29. As the nurse is giving morning care to Marshall, the nurse is aware that he is in the grief stage of developing awareness of his loss. What behavior might the nurse see him display at this stage in reaction to his wife's death?
○ 1. Crying and/or anger. **AS**
○ 2. Appearing dazed and repeatedly saying, "No, it can't be." 7 **PsI**
○ 3. Preoccupation with thoughts of how ideal the marriage had been.
○ 4. Responding with a brief complaint about his own physical pain.

Mr. Gonzalez is a 60-year-old, highly successful businessman who, in the last year, has refused to attend to his business, is now refusing to eat because he is too "bad" to eat, and has sat quietly in a chair mumbling to himself. Mr. Gonzalez is diagnosed as having major depression with psychotic features. Questions 30 through 33 refer to this case.

30. Mr. Gonzalez says, "I don't cry because my wife can't bear it." The nurse needs to be aware that this is an example of:
○ 1. Suppression. **AN**
○ 2. Undoing. 7

○ 3. Repression. PsI
○ 4. Rationalization.

31. What feeling tone is the nurse most likely to see the client demonstrate during major depression with psychotic features?
○ 1. Suspicion. AN
○ 2. Agitation. 7
○ 3. Loneliness. PsI
○ 4. Worthlessness.

32. After Mr. Gonzalez makes a home visit, his wife reports that it was a stressful time. In an interview, Mr. Gonzalez says, "We had a marvelous visit." The nurse is aware that this is an example of:
○ 1. Compensation. AN
○ 2. Denial. 7
○ 3. Symbolism. PsI
○ 4. Identification.

33. It would be important for the nurse to implement definite suicide precautions for Mr. Gonzalez if his mood changed suddenly to one of:
○ 1. Cheerfulness. EV
○ 2. Psychomotor retardation. 7
○ 3. Agitation. PsI
○ 4. Hostility.

A 23-year-old premedical student, Georgia, is admitted to a psychiatric hospital in a withdrawn catatonic state. She was an honor student and very active in student government and had become progressively withdrawn, silent, and mute. For two days prior to admission, she remained seated in one position without moving or speaking. On the ward, she continues to exhibit waxy flexibility as she sits all day. Questions 34 through 43 refer to this case.

34. During the initial phase of hospitalization, the nurse's first priority is to:
○ 1. Watch for edema and cyanosis of the extremities. PL 3
○ 2. Encourage Georgia to discuss her concerns leading to the catatonic state. PhI
○ 3. Provide a warm, nurturing relationship, with therapeutic use of touch.
○ 4. Identify the predisposing factors in her illness.

35. Georgia began having auditory hallucinations. When the nurse approaches her, Georgia whispers, "Did you hear that terrible man? He is scary!" Which would be the best response for the nurse to make initially?
○ 1. "What is he saying?" IMP
○ 2. "I didn't hear anything. What scary things is he saying?" 2 PsI
○ 3. "Who is he? Do you know him?"
○ 4. "I didn't hear a man's voice, but you look scared."

36. One day, Georgia looks at a mirror and cries out, "I look like a bird. My face is no longer me." Which would be the best response by the nurse?
○ 1. "Which bird?" IMP
○ 2. "That must be a distressing experience; your face doesn't look different to me." 2 PsI
○ 3. "Maybe it was the light at that particular time. Would you like to use another mirror?"
○ 4. "What makes you think that your face looks like a bird?"

The nurses on the unit are having a difficult time with Georgia, who continually talks about the "nofas are coming."

37. In responding to Georgia's neologism, it would be best for the nurse to:
○ 1. Divert the client's attention to an aspect of reality. PL 2
○ 2. State that what the client is saying has not been understood and then divert attention to something that is reality-bound. PsI
○ 3. Acknowledge that the word has some special meaning for the client.
○ 4. Try to interpret what the client means.

38. When interacting with clients who have autistic thinking and speaking patterns, which of the following is likely to pose the *greatest difficulty* for the nurse?
○ 1. Showing acceptance for their incomprehensible acts and verbalizations. IMP 7
○ 2. Ignoring their bizarre behavior. PsI
○ 3. Speaking in a way that clients can understand.
○ 4. Determining which of the clients' needs are being met by their autistic expressions.

39. The doctor asked you to activate this client when she is hallucinating, withdrawn, and negativistic. What might be your best approach with Georgia?
○ 1. Give her a long explanation of the benefits of activity. IMP 7
○ 2. Let her know that you need a partner for an activity. PsI
○ 3. Demand that she join a group activity.
○ 4. Mention that the "voices" would want her to participate.,

40. While communicating with Georgia when she is withdrawn, what would be important for the nurse to do at first?
○ 1. Remain silent and not encourage her to talk. PL
○ 2. Talk with her as you would to a normal person. 7
○ 3. Allow her to do all the talking. PsI
○ 4. Use simple, concrete language in speaking to her.

41. When a client's behavior is considered abnormal, the nurse first needs to:
○ 1. Ignore the client. PL
○ 2. Serve as a role model. 7
○ 3. Point out the client's disturbed behavior. PsI
○ 4. Focus on the feelings communicated by the client's behavior.

42. At times, Georgia seems preoccupied with her own thoughts as she grins, giggles, grimaces, and frowns. Although she is 23 years old, her behavior seems childish and regressed. She is unkempt, voids on the floor, disrobes, and openly masturbates. The main nursing care for Georgia at this time should be directed toward:
○ 1. Improving her social conduct to meet hospital standards. PL 7
○ 2. Controlling her narcissistic impulses. PsI
○ 3. Finding out why she is behaving this way.
○ 4. Showing acceptance of her.

43. The main nursing goal with clients with schizophrenic disorders is to:
○ 1. Set limits on their bizarre behavior. PL
○ 2. Establish a trusting, nonthreatening, reality-based relationship. 7 PsI
○ 3. Quickly establish a warm, close relationship to counteract their aloofness.
○ 4. Protect them from self-destructive impulses.

Mr. Carlson refuses to eat his meals in the hospital, stating that the food is poisoned. Questions 44 through 46 refer to this case.

44. The nurse is aware that Mr. Carlson is expressing an example of:
- ○ 1. Hallucination. **AN**
- ○ 2. Illusion. **7**
- ○ 3. Delusion. **PsI**
- ○ 4. Negativism.

45. Mr. Carlson cannot find his slippers. During the community meeting, he accuses clients and staff of stealing them during the night. The most therapeutic approach is to:
- ○ 1. Listen without reinforcing his belief. **PL**
- ○ 2. Logically point out that he is jumping to conclusions. **7** **PsI**
- ○ 3. Inject humor to defuse the intensity.
- ○ 4. Divert his attention.

46. Clients with symptoms such as Mr. Carlson's use projection. The nurse is aware that this mechanism is chiefly a way to:
- ○ 1. Provoke anger in others. **AN**
- ○ 2. Control delusional thought. **7**
- ○ 3. Handle their own unacceptable feelings. **PsI**
- ○ 4. Manipulate others.

Alice, an attractive, intelligent 15-year-old, has a history of truancy from school, running away from home, and "borrowing" other people's things without their permission. She denies that she steals, rationalizing instead that as long as no one was using the items, she thought it was all right to borrow them. She has been referred by the juvenile court to the local mental health center. Questions 47 through 50 refer to this case.

47. It is important for the nurse to understand that, psychodynamically, Alice's behavior may be largely attributed to a developmental defect related to the:
- ○ 1. Id. **AN**
- ○ 2. Ego. **5**
- ○ 3. Superego. **PsI**
- ○ 4. Oedipal complex.

48. In interacting with Alice, what would be the most therapeutic approach consistent with question 47?
- ○ 1. Reinforce her self-concept as a young woman. **PL**
- ○ 2. Gratify her inner needs. **7**
- ○ 3. Give her opportunities to test reality. **PsI**
- ○ 4. Provide external controls.

49. A new nursing student reports to the unit. He is assigned to take clients for an outing. Alice approaches him and says, "I like you. I'm glad you'll be the one to take us out. My doctor told me that I can go too." Which initial response by the nurse is best?
- ○ 1. "Since I am new here and not familiar with unit routine, I will go check with the staff and be back." **IMP** **7** **PsI**
- ○ 2. "It's a beautiful day, and I'm glad that you have ground privileges now."
- ○ 3. "When did the doctor tell you that?"
- ○ 4. "You seem pleased."

50. Alice arouses anxiety and frustration in the staff and tends to intimidate by her manipulative patterns. One morning Alice shouts at the nurse, "Since you won't give me a pass, go away, you fat pig, or I'll hit you." What is the most effective response by the nurse to a client who threatens or derogates?
- ○ 1. "You are rude and I don't like it. It makes me not want to talk with you." **IMP** **7**
- ○ 2. "That kind of talk will keep you here longer." **PsI**
- ○ 3. "What did I do wrong?"
- ○ 4. "I don't like to hear insults and threats. What is important about getting the pass today?"

Reva Jones, age 38 and mother of two children, ages 12 and 14, was brought to the emergency ward at a hospital by her husband, Paul. Her diagnosis was alcohol withdrawal. Questions 51 through 54 refer to this case.

51. On admission, the nurse is likely to note that Reva is exhibiting signs of:
- ○ 1. Perceptual disorders. **AS**
- ○ 2. Impending coma. **7**
- ○ 3. Recent alcohol intake. **PsI**
- ○ 4. Depression with mutism.

52. To relate therapeutically with Mrs. Jones, it is important that the nurse base his or her care on the understanding that alcohol dependence:
- ○ 1. Is hereditary. **AN**
- ○ 2. Is due to lack of willpower and true remorse. **7**
- ○ 3. Results in always breaking promises. **PsI**
- ○ 4. Cannot be cured.

53. The nursing care plan will need to incorporate a characteristic physiologic consequence of alcohol abuse and dependence, which is:
- ○ 1. Cardiac arrhythmia. **AN**
- ○ 2. Convulsive disorder. **7**
- ○ 3. Psychomotor hyperactivity. **PhI**
- ○ 4. Cirrhosis of the liver.

54. In establishing a therapeutic nursing approach with a client who abuses and is dependent on substances, the nurse primarily needs to:
- ○ 1. Promote a permissive, accepting environment. **PL** **7**
- ○ 2. Use a straightforward and confronting approach. **PsI**
- ○ 3. Meet the client's need for a chemical substitute for the drug.
- ○ 4. Prevent the client's use of the addictive drug.

Mr. David's behavior has been a source of concern to the staff. He refuses to attend group therapy sessions at 9:00 A.M. because he says he has to wash his hands for at least 45 minutes, from 9:00 A.M. until 9:45 A.M. At the team meeting, staff members discuss the problem. They feel it is important for Mr. David to participate in group therapy sessions to learn more successful methods of interaction with others. Questions 55 through 58 refer to this case.

55. Which concept does the staff need to keep in mind in planning nursing interventions for this client?
- ○ 1. Fears and tensions are often expressed in disguised form through symbolic processes. **AN** **7**
- ○ 2. Unmet needs are discharged through ritualistic behavior. **PsI**
- ○ 3. Ritualistic behavior makes others uncomfortable.
- ○ 4. Depression underlies ritualistic behavior.

56. To help reduce stress and to aid this client in using less maladaptive means of handling stress, the nurse could:
- ○ 1. Provide varied activities on the unit, as change in routine can break a ritualistic pattern. **IMP** **7**
- ○ 2. Give him ward assignments that do not require perfection. **PsI**
- ○ 3. Tell him of changes in routine at the last minute to avoid build-up of anxiety.
- ○ 4. Provide an activity in which positive accom-

plishment can occur so he can gain recognition.

57. Which of the following is an example of *limit-setting* as an effective nursing intervention in ritualistic behavior patterns?
- ○ 1. "I don't want you to wash your hands so often anymore." **IMP 7**
- ○ 2. "If you continue to wash your hands so frequently, the skin on your hands will break down." **PsI**
- ○ 3. "You may wash your hands before the group therapy meeting if you wish, but not during group therapy."
- ○ 4. "The doctor wrote an order that you are to stop washing your hands so often."

58. It is important that the nurse understand that Mr. David's repetitive handwashing is probably an attempt to:
- ○ 1. Punish himself for guilt feelings. **AN**
- ○ 2. Control unacceptable impulses or feelings. **7**
- ○ 3. Do what the voices tell him to do. **PsI**
- ○ 4. Seek attention from the staff.

In the last five years, Alice Adam has gone to a number of different doctors for nonspecific complaints of chest pains without any conclusive findings of an organic disease process. She has collected all the medical literature on the subject of coronary diseases. Most of her time is spent recounting details of her symptoms. Her latest internist has referred her to the local mental health center's day-treatment facility. Questions 59 through 64 refer to this case.

59. When meeting Alice for the first time at the day-treatment center, which approach by the nurse would be best initially?
- ○ 1. Allow the client to describe her physical problems to become familiar with them. **IMP 7**
- ○ 2. Comment on a neutral topic instead of using the usual conversation opener of "How are you today?" **PsI**
- ○ 3. Give the client a simple but direct explanation of the physiologic basis for her symptoms.
- ○ 4. Let the client know that you are familiar with her psychogenic problems and guide the discussion to other areas.

60. All of the following goals are important for Alice, who has the diagnosis of a somatoform disorder. Which would be appropriate for an *initial* nursing goal?
- ○ 1. Help Alice learn how to live with her functional organic disturbance without using her symptoms to control others. **PL 7 PsI**
- ○ 2. Assist Alice in developing new and varied interests outside of herself at which she can be successful.
- ○ 3. Accept Alice as a person who is sick and *needs* help.
- ○ 4. Help Alice see how she uses her illness to avoid looking at or dealing with her problems.

61. To formulate an effective care plan for this client, the nurse *needs* to have an understanding of which of the following psychodynamic principles related to somatoform disorder?
- ○ 1. The major fundamental mechanism is regression. **AN 7**
- ○ 2. An extensive, prolonged study of her symptoms will be reassuring to the client, as she seeks sympathy, attention, and love. **PsI**
- ○ 3. The symptoms of a somatoform disorder are an attempt to adjust to painful life situations or to cope with conflicting sexual, aggressive, or dependent feelings.
- ○ 4. The client's symptoms are imaginary and her suffering is faked.

62. In order to divert the client's focus from her physical state, it would *not* be helpful for the nurse to use logic and reason to assist the client with a somatoform disorder with conversion symptoms (such as paralysis of the arm) because:
- ○ 1. The client is not in contact with reality and thus is unable to "hear" or understand the nurse. **AN 7 PsI**
- ○ 2. The client may need the symptoms to handle feelings of guilt or aggression.
- ○ 3. The nature of the client's particular illness makes her suspicious of all medical personnel.
- ○ 4. Paralysis of the arm has become a habitual response to stress.

63. The most common coping mechanisms utilized in somatoform disorders are:
- ○ 1. Repression and symbolism. **AN**
- ○ 2. Sublimation and regression. **7**
- ○ 3. Substitution and displacement. **PsI**
- ○ 4. Reaction formation and rationalization.

64. Which adaptive behavior by a client with somatoform disorders might indicate to the nurse that she is showing the greatest improvement in her condition?
- ○ 1. She recognizes that her behavior is unreasonable. **EV 7**
- ○ 2. She agrees to go to occupational therapy and recreational therapy every day. **PsI**
- ○ 3. Her symptoms are replaced by expressions of hostility.
- ○ 4. She is verbalizing how she feels instead of demonstrating it by pathologic body languages.

Mr. Simon, a 35-year-old married clerk, had surgery for ulcerative colitis ten days ago. The physical symptoms have abated, but he continues to complain angrily and to be demanding of the nursing staff. He makes numerous requests, such as to open or close the windows, to bring him fresh water, and so on. Questions 65 through 70 refer to this case.

65. The nurse needs to understand that Mr. Simon's behavior might be saying:
- ○ 1. "You aren't doing your job." **AN**
- ○ 2. "I am alone and helpless and need to depend on you to take care of me when I need you." **7 PsI**
- ○ 3. "Everyone needs attention."
- ○ 4. "I'm going to get even with you for thinking I'm a crank by making you work."

66. Mr. Simon's family is ready to make discharge plans jointly with him and the staff. The nurse will need to determine that the greatest bearing on his rehabilitation course will be:
- ○ 1. The amount of emotional support his family gives him. **AS 7**
- ○ 2. His wife's interest in, and ability to take care of his postoperative dietary needs. **HPM**
- ○ 3. The family expectations of him to resume his role in the home.
- ○ 4. Mrs. Simon's understanding that the course of

his illness may have exacerbations and remissions.

67. In evaluating his progress, the nurse is aware that Mr. Simon's somatoform symptoms will probably show the most improvement when he:
- ○ 1. Accepts the fact that his physical symptoms have an emotional component. **EV 7 PsI**
- ○ 2. Finds more satisfying ways of expressing feelings through verbalization.
- ○ 3. Becomes involved in group activities and focuses less on his symptoms.
- ○ 4. Understands that his current way of reacting to stress is not healthy.

68. One day Mr. Simon became angry with a client who was monopolizing the group therapy meeting. What interpretation by the nurse regarding this noted change in Mr. Simon's behavior would indicate the nurse's understanding of the dynamics of his somatoform disorder?
- ○ 1. He is intolerant of others. **AN 7 PsI**
- ○ 2. He has strong competitive drives.
- ○ 3. He has his own ideas of how the group members should act.
- ○ 4. He is repressing fewer of his feelings.

69. When Mr. Simon asks his doctor about his prognosis, he becomes alternately depressed and agitated about his impending discharge. Which nursing approach would be best at this time?
- ○ 1. "You *are* much better than when you first were hospitalized. You have to decide whether you need to be hospitalized longer or whether you are ready to go home." **IMP 7 PsI**
- ○ 2. "You seem to have concerns about going home."
- ○ 3. "What is it about going home that bothers you?"
- ○ 4. "You seem sad about going home. Would you like to talk about it?"

70. What would be the most realistic statement a nurse could make about Mr. Simon's prognosis after a course of necessary treatment?
- ○ 1. His symptoms will recur. **EV 7 PsI**
- ○ 2. His ulcerative lesions will heal, but under stress the same symptoms will reappear.
- ○ 3. It is not possible to prognosticate the future course.
- ○ 4. Ongoing psychotherapy is essential for him to be free of symptoms.

One morning Mr. Allen, an 80-year-old client with organic mental disorder related to cerebral arteriosclerosis, said to the nurse, "I'm going to the university today to be their guest lecturer on aerodynamics." Questions 71 through 79 refer to this case.

71. Which response by the nurse would be most therapeutic for Mr. Allen?
- ○ 1. "Do you know that you are in the hospital now?" **IMP 5 PsI**
- ○ 2. "Are you saying that you would like to be asked to give a lecture at the university?"
- ○ 3. "How about watching a movie on television instead?"
- ○ 4. "It's more important that you don't tire yourself out."

72. The nurse is aware that the main function confabulation serves in clients, especially those with organic mental disorders (organic brain syndrome), is to:
- ○ 1. Impress others. **AN 2 PsI**
- ○ 2. Protect their self-esteem.
- ○ 3. Control others by distance maneuvers.
- ○ 4. Maintain a sense of humor.

73. Another key consideration in planning the general care of clients with organic mental disorders (organic brain syndrome) is that:
- ○ 1. They be protected from suicide attempts. **PL 2 SECE**
- ○ 2. Their capacity for physical activity is diminished.
- ○ 3. Team effort be aimed at increasing their independence.
- ○ 4. The staff be sympathetic when clients mention their failing abilities.

74. Which of the following will the nurse most commonly note in the clinical picture of organic mental disorders (organic brain syndrome)?
- ○ 1. Memory loss for events in the distant past. **AS 2 PsI**
- ○ 2. Quarrelsome behavior directly related to the extent of cerebral arteriosclerosis.
- ○ 3. Increased resistance to change.
- ○ 4. Insight into one's situation, its probable causes, and its logical consequences.

75. An important part of the nursing care for a client with chronic arteriosclerotic brain syndrome would be:
- ○ 1. Minimizing regression. **PL 2 SECE**
- ○ 2. Correcting memory loss.
- ○ 3. Rehabilitating toward independent functioning.
- ○ 4. Preventing further deterioration.

76. Due to his condition, in planning Mr. Allen's schedule, it is most important that the daily activities:
- ○ 1. Be highly structured. **PL 5 SECE**
- ○ 2. Be changed by the nurse each day to meet the client's needs for variety.
- ○ 3. Be simplified as much as possible to avoid problems with decision making.
- ○ 4. Provide many opportunities for making choices to stimulate the client's involvement and interest.

77. It is important for the nurse to be aware that the mental health of an aged client such as Mr. Allen is most directly influenced by:
- ○ 1. The attitude of relatives in providing for the client's needs. **AN 7 PsI**
- ○ 2. Societal factors such as role change, loss of loved ones, and loss of physical energy.
- ○ 3. The client's level of education and economic situation.
- ○ 4. The attitudes the client has toward life circumstances.

78. In preparing the nursing care plan for Mr. Allen, which of the following is the *most* common basic need of the aged that must be met?
- ○ 1. Sexual outlets and security. **PL 5 PsI**
- ○ 2. Unconditional acceptance by others of their impairments and deficits.
- ○ 3. Preservation of self-esteem.
- ○ 4. Socialization.

79. Based on knowledge of Erikson's stages of growth and development, the nurse determines that the task of old age is primarily concerned with:
- ○ 1. Ego integrity versus despair. **AN**

○ 2. Autonomy versus shame and doubt. 5
○ 3. Trust versus mistrust. HPM
○ 4. Industry versus inferiority.

80. *Mrs. Jacobson, a 90-year-old client who is hard of hearing, tells the same story over and over again to all personnel who come to take care of her in a convalescent home—about the exciting time when her family came out West in a covered wagon. Which of the following interpretations offered by the nurse would* not *demonstrate any understanding of this behavior?*
○ 1. Mrs. Jacobson has better recall for past events than for recent ones. AN 5
○ 2. She enjoys reliving pleasurable aspects of her life, since the present and future are bleak. PsI
○ 3. Repeating her stories is one way of interacting, to compensate for a two-way conversation that is difficult for her to sustain.
○ 4. She wants to impress others.

81. *Mr. Bell has Alzheimer's disease. One night, at 4 A.M., the nurse finds 88-year-old Mr. Bell in the hallway trying to open the door to the fire escape. Which response by the nurse would probably indicate the most accurate assessment of the situation?*
○ 1. "Mr. Bell, you look confused. Would you like to sit down and talk with me.?" IMP 7
○ 2. "That door leads to the fire escape. Why do you want to go outside now?" SECE
○ 3. "This is the fire escape door. Are you looking for the bathroom?"
○ 4. "Something seems to be bothering you. Let's go back to your room and talk about it."

Jenny, age 19, is brought to the emergency room because she slashed her wrists. Jenny is in the middle of her first year of college. She has always had many friends and has been popular with both sexes. She has, in the past, done well in school. Two weeks ago her boyfriend "dropped" her. Since then Jenny has had trouble concentrating on her studies and has refused to date other boys. Questions 82 through 88 refer to this case.

82. What is the nurse's first concern?
○ 1. Stabilization of physical condition. PL
○ 2. Determination of antecedent, causal factors relevant to Jenny's wrist-slashing. 7 PhI
○ 3. Reduction of anxiety.
○ 4. Obtaining a detailed nursing history.

83. Three days after her admission, Jenny meets with a crisis intervention nurse. The initial goal at this time is to:
○ 1. Determine the precipitating event, determine how many people are involved in the incident, and determine how angry Jenny is. PL 7 PsI
○ 2. Determine if Jenny has an immediate support system, determine what the people in the support system think of Jenny's cutting her wrists, and determine how angry Jenny is.
○ 3. Determine the precipitating event, determine if Jenny has an immediate support system, and assess the likelihood of immediate recurrence of the suicidal act.
○ 4. Assess the likelihood of immediate recurrence of the suicidal act.

84. In explaining the goal of therapy in crisis intervention to a new colleague, the nurse states that the goal is to:
○ 1. Restructure the personality. IMP
○ 2. Remove specific symptoms. 7
○ 3. Remove anxiety. SECE
○ 4. Resolve immediate problems.

85. The crisis nurse also explains to her colleague that the focus of treatment in crisis intervention is on the:
○ 1. Present and on restoration to the usual level of functioning. IMP 7
○ 2. Past and on freeing the unconscious. SECE
○ 3. Past in relation to the present.
○ 4. Present and on the repression of unconscious drives.

86. The nurse plans her or his goals based on a principle of crisis intervention therapy that crises:
○ 1. May go on indefinitely. PL
○ 2. Seldom occur in normal people's lives. 7
○ 3. Usually are resolved in 4–6 weeks. SECE
○ 4. Are related to deep, underlying problems.

87. At the first therapy session with Jenny, what does the crisis nurse need to do?
○ 1. Discourage discussion of Jenny's suicide attempt. PL 7
○ 2. Encourage Jenny to dwell on her feelings about how badly she was treated as a child. PsI
○ 3. Encourage Jenny to discuss the suicide attempt in detail.
○ 4. Help Jenny see how her suicide attempt hurt others.

88. The crisis intervention nurse and physician agree hospitalization is not necessary for Jenny; therefore, the nurse needs to:
○ 1. Wish Jenny luck and terminate the session. IMP
○ 2. Make an appointment for Jenny for tomorrow and give Jenny a telephone number where the nurse can be reached tonight. 7 SECE
○ 3. Make an appointment for Jenny in two weeks, when her wrists might be healed.
○ 4. Tell Jenny to make an appointment when she wants to, at her local mental health clinic.

Mr. Rains is a 47-year-old client who has been in a mental hospital for 10 years. His table manners are crude, and this upsets other clients. Questions 89 through 91 refer to this case.

89. Which of the following will probably be most therapeutic for Mr. Rains, a client on a behavior modification ward?
○ 1. Accept his table manners without comment. PL
○ 2. Urge him to eat like the other clients do. 2
○ 3. Offer him a reward for each improvement in his table manners. PsI
○ 4. Point out to him that his eating habits distress the other clients.

90. It is likely that the above approach will be most helpful because its main goal is to:
○ 1. Protect Mr. Rains from embarrassment about his table manners. PL 7
○ 2. Offer Mr. Rains an incentive for improving his behavior. SECE
○ 3. Help Mr. Rains achieve socially acceptable behavior.
○ 4. Permit Mr. Rains to examine his own behavior without further loss of self-esteem.

91. In their role in a behavior therapy program, it is essential that nurses:
○ 1. Ask clients about the content of their dreams. IMP

○ 2. Interact only with clients who are verbal. **7**
○ 3. Continually observe clients' behavior and immediately intervene if necessary. **SECE**
○ 4. Obtain a detailed account of each client's growth and development.

Betty, a client on the psychiatric unit, becomes increasingly agitated, in spite of the nurses' verbal attempts to stop her aggressive actions. Betty begins to throw furniture around, shouting insults and threats at the other clients and nursing staff. Questions 92 through 96 refer to this case.

92. When Betty starts demolishing the recreation room, what is the best response and action by the nurse?
○ 1. Firmly set limits on her behavior. **IMP**
○ 2. Allow her to continue, since she is seeking to express herself. **1** **SECE**
○ 3. Tell her she is trying to intimidate other clients.
○ 4. Let her know that she doesn't need to express her anger at the nurse by demolishing the recreation room.

93. Of the following nursing interventions with a person who is expressing anger, which is inappropriate?
○ 1. Stating your observations of the expressed anger. **IMP** **1**
○ 2. Assisting the person to describe the feelings. **PsI**
○ 3. Helping the person find out what preceded the anger.
○ 4. Helping the person refrain from expressing anger verbally.

94. The steps in therapeutic nursing intervention with an angry client would be to describe the situation, then:
○ 1. Discuss alternative solutions, decide on several, try them out, and evaluate their effectiveness. **IMP** **7** **SECE**
○ 2. Focus on one solution, try it out, and evaluate its effectiveness.
○ 3. Outline to the client exactly what to do about the anger.
○ 4. Discuss alternative solutions, decide on one, use it, evaluate its effectiveness, and continue repeating the process until the client is satisfied.

95. The nurse can determine that the expression of hostility is appropriate and useful when the:
○ 1. Energy from anger is utilized to accomplish what needs to be done. **EV** **7**
○ 2. Expression intimidates others. **PsI**
○ 3. Degree of hostility is less than the provocation.
○ 4. Expression of anger dissipates the energy.

96. Betty is placed in isolation for seclusion due to agitated behavior. The nurse knows that it is essential that:
○ 1. Restraints be applied. **PL**
○ 2. All the furniture be removed from the isolation room. **1** **SECE**
○ 3. A staff member have frequent contacts with Betty.
○ 4. Betty be allowed to come out after 4 hours.

Mrs. Dawn, age 28, has been married for three years and has one child. A year ago, while nursing the child, she discovered a lump in her breast. She refused to see a physician or have a biopsy, stating that the lump was cystic thickening as a result of nursing the infant. Questions 97 through 101 refer to this case.

97. Mrs. Dawn's refusal to see a physician about the lump in her breast can be interpreted by a nurse as:
○ 1. Rationalization. **AN**
○ 2. Projection. **2**
○ 3. Sublimation. **PsI**
○ 4. Denial.

98. The nurse bases her nursing care plan on the knowledge that body image is the:
○ 1. Conscious attitude the individual has toward his or her body. **AN** **2**
○ 2. Attitude others have about an individual's body. **HPM**
○ 3. Image the person sees of himself or herself in the mirror.
○ 4. Sum of the conscious and unconscious attitudes the person has toward his or her body.

Mrs. Dawn went to a physician for a routine physical. The physician discovered several lumps and suggested a biopsy and possible mastectomy. On biopsy, the tissue was discovered to be malignant, so a modified mastectomy was performed.

99. Immediately following surgery, what behaviors could the nurse expect Mrs. Dawn to display?
○ 1. Signs of grief reaction. **AS**
○ 2. Signs of deep depression. **7**
○ 3. Relief that the operation is over. **PsI**
○ 4. Denial of the possibility of carcinoma.

100. Two days after the operation, Mrs. Dawn was crying and saying, "My husband won't love me anymore." The nurse is aware that this statement might stem from:
○ 1. Mrs. Dawn's deep insecurity about her marriage. **AN** **7**
○ 2. Preexisting marital disharmony. **PsI**
○ 3. Mrs. Dawn's concerns about her body and a resultant change in her beliefs about her own self-worth.
○ 4. A momentary fear about her husband's fidelity.

101. Following Mrs. Dawn's statement in the preceding question, what would be most therapeutic for the nurse to respond at this time?
○ 1. "Of course your husband loves you." **IMP**
○ 2. "Tell me what has happened that makes you think your husband won't love you anymore." **7** **PsI**
○ 3. "If you stop crying and fix yourself up, you will look good to your husband."
○ 4. "Do you think your husband won't love you because you have lost a breast?"

Frank Gregg, a 19-year-old male, was an excellent student, president of the freshman class in college, on the freshman football team, and active in his church. Two months ago, while home from college on a visit, he got up one morning and started screaming at his mother, "I am not me. You are controlling me." He grabbed a knife and started chasing his mother. However, before he hurt her, he suddenly stopped chasing her and went to his room. For two days he did not talk or eat. After two days, his parents had him see a psychiatrist, who had him admitted to the psychiatric hospital. Questions 102 through 104 refer to this case.

102. From the above history, you could infer overcompliance with his parents' expectations for his behavior. The nurse knows that acceptance of the role Frank perceives his parents require could result in:
○ 1. Lack of development of a separate identity. **AN**

○ 2. Confusion of his sex role. 7
○ 3. Successful development of a separate identity. **HPM**
○ 4. Identification of a weak superego.

103. The nurse establishes a nurse–client relationship with Frank. One of the goals is to help him develop a separate self-identity. One way to do this is to:
○ 1. Call him by a "pet" name frequently. **IMP**
○ 2. Use "you" and "I" rather than "we." **7**
○ 3. Correct his opinions. **PsI**
○ 4. Encourage "should" responses.

104. Frank's parents asked the nurse what she thought Frank meant when he said to the mother, "You are controlling me." What would be the best response by the nurse?
○ 1. "He is upset and thinks you are taking charge of him." **IMP** **7**
○ 2. "He resents always having to be good." **PsI**
○ 3. "I can't tell you. You will have to ask Frank."
○ 4. "I think you can ask Frank that question. Do you want me to stay with you while you ask him?"

Maria Galvez, age 38, is a brilliant research chemist who came into the hospital with a diagnosis of paranoid disorder. Questions 105 through 111 refer to this case.

105. The nurse determines that the part of Maria's personality that is weak is called the:
○ 1. Id. **AN**
○ 2. Ego. **5**
○ 3. Superego. **PsI**
○ 4. "Not me."

When Maria was in the second grade, she had difficulty with the teacher. She began to misbehave in class. She was taken from the public school and placed in a private school where others in the neighborhood were going. Her grades were not good because she was attempting to make an adjustment to her new peers. Her father severely reprimanded her and forced her to study after school rather than play with other children.

106. At this point, what normal phase of development would the above data indicate to the nurse that Maria was deprived of forming?
○ 1. A love relationship with her father. **AN**
○ 2. Close relationships with her peers. **5**
○ 3. Heterosexual relationships. **HPM**
○ 4. A dependency relationship with her father.

107. In college Maria did exceptionally well. Her chemistry professor complimented her and arranged for her to be a lab assistant and to do advanced research. She was very thorough in her work. However, when given constructive criticism she became angry and stalked out of the lab for a few hours. The most plausible theoretical explanation the nurse could give to her bewildered colleague is that Maria:
○ 1. Knew she was right. **IMP**
○ 2. Thought the professor was jealous of her. **7**
○ 3. Needed to feel and know that she was perfect. **PsI**
○ 4. Felt anxiety as a result of a threat to her security and self-image.

108. Recently, when an experiment in the laboratory went wrong, Maria complained of a plot against her and accused the lab assistants of sending signals about her to each other. The nurse determines that this behavior is related to:
○ 1. Delusions of grandeur. **AN**
○ 2. Illusion. **7**
○ 3. Ideas of reference. **PsI**
○ 4. Echolalia.

109. Maria began to refuse to eat her husband's cooking because she thought he was poisoning her. The nurse is aware that this behavior is related to:
○ 1. Delusion of persecution. **AN**
○ 2. Ideas of reference. **7**
○ 3. Illusion. **PsI**
○ 4. Hallucination.

110. Maria is diagnosed as having a paranoid disorder. What implication might this have for the nurse?
○ 1. Let Maria talk about her suspicions without correcting misinformation. **IMP** **7**
○ 2. Avoid talking to other nurses when Maria can see them but can't hear what is being said. **PsI**
○ 3. Placate her by agreeing with what she says.
○ 4. Argue with her about her ideas.

111. One day Maria said to the nurse, "That woman over there is a lesbian." What is the best response by the nurse?
○ 1. "Are you afraid she will attack you?" **IMP**
○ 2. "That woman is not a lesbian." **7**
○ 3. "What did the woman do that makes you think she is a lesbian?" **PsI**
○ 4. "Then stay away from her."

The nurse has been asked to see John Sorenson, age 15, because he is disruptive in the school room. She knows that he has, on occasion, used alcohol and engaged in sexual activities with both males and females. His complaints are that no one will let him "do his own thing." Questions 112 through 116 refer to this case.

112. John comes to the first session and sits glaring at the nurse. What is the best response by the nurse?
○ 1. "I know you are angry, but how does being angry help?" **IMP** **7**
○ 2. "Stop being angry and tell me what is wrong." **PsI**
○ 3. "I think you are angry because you feel you don't need any help."
○ 4. "We have to meet because your parents are concerned about you."

113. During the session John says, "I suppose you have to tell my parents everything." What would be the best response by the nurse?
○ 1. "What are you going to tell me that is so secret that I can't tell your parents?" **IMP** **7**
○ 2. "If you tell me you are going to do something to hurt yourself I will have to tell your parents, but I will tell you first before I tell them." **SECE**
○ 3. "Everything you tell me is confidential. I will not tell your parents anything."
○ 4. "Everything you tell me I will need to tell your parents. They have a right to know."

114. During one session John says, "I want you to go tell the teacher I am sick and I am to be allowed to do what I want." The nurse determines that this statement best represents:
○ 1. Insight. **AN**
○ 2. Manipulation. **7**
○ 3. Dependency. **PsI**
○ 4. Trust.

115. To the statement, "I want you to go tell the teacher I am sick and I am to be allowed to do what I want," the best response by the nurse would be:
○ 1. "Certainly. You are sick and need some relaxation of rules in the classroom." **IMP** **7**

○ 2. "I am glad you recognize you are sick." **PsI**
○ 3. "No, John, you are expected to follow the rules of the classroom."
○ 4. "All teachers are too strict. I agree some rules need to be relaxed."

116. In discussions between parents and adolescents about their relationship, a desired outcome is that the adolescents will benefit because they will be able to:
○ 1. See themselves as the victims. **EV**
○ 2. View their parents and themselves realistically. **7**
○ 3. Enlist the therapist's aid as an ally against their parents. **HPM**
○ 4. See their parents as victims.

Mr. Sundowner is a 52-year-old man who has just been admitted to a general hospital for possible acute appendicitis. The nurse who admits him notices that he is wearing very thick glasses and a hearing aid. He does not seem to be having any trouble understanding what is being said. The nurse, in her orientation of Mr. Sundowner, tells him that if he goes to surgery, he will wake up in the postoperative recovery room, not in his hospital room. Mr. Sundowner immediately says, "Oh, I will need to have either my glasses or my hearing aid or preferably both with me in the recovery room or I will be confused and upset when I wake up." Questions 117 through 118 refer to this case.

117. The nurse determines that Mr. Sundowner is trying to tell her that he:
○ 1. Has periods of confusion and may have a psychiatric problem. **AN** **2**
○ 2. Is psychologically dependent on his hearing aid and glasses. **PhI**
○ 3. Needs his hearing aid and/or glasses in order to correctly perceive what is going on around him, and misperception will cause confusion.
○ 4. Needs his hearing aid and/or glasses because he wants to be sure people are taking proper care of him.

118. Which of the following statements by the nurse is the best response to the above situation?
○ 1. "You won't need your glasses or hearing aid. The nurses will take care of you." **IMP** **2**
○ 2. "I understand. You will be able to cooperate best if you know what is going on, so I will find out how I can arrange to have your glasses and hearing aid available to you in the recovery room." **PsI**
○ 3. "I understand you might be more cooperative if you have your aid and glasses, but that is just not possible. Rules, you know."
○ 4. "Do you get upset and confused often?"

Questions 119–166 are individual items.

119. One therapeutic nursing attitude is to be accepting and permissive. To convey this attitude most therapeutically, the nurse might:
○ 1. Wait for a client to initiate contact. **IMP**
○ 2. Let the client make decisions. **7**
○ 3. Ignore undesirable behavior. **PsI**
○ 4. Meet the client at his or her level of functioning.

120. The basic goal of nursing in a mental health setting is to:
○ 1. Plan activity programs for clients. **PL**
○ 2. Maintain a therapeutic environment. **7**
○ 3. Understand various types of family therapy and psychologic tests and how to interpret them. **SECE**
○ 4. Advance the science of psychiatry by initiating research and gathering data for current statistics on emotional illness.

121. The client was telling the nurse about her parent's impending divorce. She said, "I couldn't believe that he was going to leave us for someone else." Which would be best for the nurse to reply?
○ 1. "Was your mother expecting this to happen?" **IMP**
○ 2. "Yes, go on." **7**
○ 3. "Did you cry?" **HPM**
○ 4. "I can understand how you must feel."

122. Arnold related angrily to the nurse that his wife says he is selfish. Which would be the most helpful response by the nurse?
○ 1. "That's just her opinion." **IMP**
○ 2. "I don't think you're that selfish." **7**
○ 3. "Everybody is a little bit selfish." **HPM**
○ 4. "You sound angry—tell me more about what went on."

123. Lynn talks about her daughter who is mentally retarded: "She's really an inspiration to me, do you know what I mean?" Which would be the most appropriate initial comment by the nurse?
○ 1. "What makes her an inspiration?" **IMP**
○ 2. "It seems to be important to you to find something positive about her." **7** **HPM**
○ 3. "No, explain more about what you mean."
○ 4. "Tell me more about her."

124. The mother relates to the nurse, "When my baby had asthma five years ago, I thought he was going to die." What could the nurse say that would be the most appropriate?
○ 1. "What made you think that he was going to die?" **IMP** **7**
○ 2. "What did you do?" **HPM**
○ 3. "You thought he was dying?"
○ 4. "What were some of your feelings at that time?"

125. One effective way for a nurse to start an interaction with a client who is silent is to:
○ 1. Tell the client something about himself/herself and hope that the client does the same. **PL** **7**
○ 2. Remain silent, waiting for the client to bring up a topic. **PsI**
○ 3. Bring up a controversial topic to elicit the client's response.
○ 4. Introduce a neutral topic, giving the client a broad opening.

126. What might be the most therapeutic response the nurse could make to a student who begins crying on hearing that he or she failed an exam?
○ 1. "You'll make it next time." **IMP**
○ 2. "Failing an exam is an upsetting thing to happen." **7** **PsI**
○ 3. "How close were you to passing?"
○ 4. "It won't seem so important five years from now."

127. A client tells the nurse that he has something he wants to say to her but does not want her to tell anyone else. As the nurse, you:
○ 1. Agree not to "tell." **IMP**
○ 2. Refuse to agree to this. **7**
○ 3. Say nothing, allowing him to go on. **SECE**
○ 4. Let him know that you cannot promise this.

128. Which nursing intervention is effective when clients are severely anxious?
- ○ 1. Encourage group participation. **PL**
- ○ 2. Give detailed instructions before treatment procedure. **7** **SECE**
- ○ 3. Impart information succinctly and concretely.
- ○ 4. Increase opportunities for decision making.

129. When a client tells the nurse that she cannot sleep at night because of fear of dying, what would be the best initial response?
- ○ 1. "Don't worry, you won't die. You're just here for some tests." **IMP** **3**
- ○ 2. "Why are you afraid of dying?" **PsI**
- ○ 3. "Try to sleep. You need the rest before tomorrow's test."
- ○ 4. "It must be frightening for you to feel that way. Tell me more about it."

130. Which of the following common physiologic reactions occurring in response to anxiety is the nurse likely to note?
- ○ 1. Clammy hands and increased perspiration. **AS**
- ○ 2. Palpitations and pupillary constriction. **7**
- ○ 3. Diarrhea and vomiting. **PhI**
- ○ 4. Pupillary dilation, retention of feces and urine.

131. Which most characteristic behavior of a panic response is the nurse likely to note?
- ○ 1. Goal-directed behavior aimed at a "flight" from apparent threat. **AN** **7**
- ○ 2. Automatic behavior with poor judgment. **PsI**
- ○ 3. A severity of reaction that is not related to the severity of the threat to self-esteem.
- ○ 4. A delayed reaction in perceiving the danger.

132. The nurse is aware that the two major types of precipitating factors in anxiety are:
- ○ 1. Fear of disapproval and shame. **AN**
- ○ 2. Conflicts involving avoidance and pain. **7**
- ○ 3. Threats to one's biologic integrity and threats to one's self-system. **PsI**
- ○ 4. A person's poor health and poor financial condition.

133. Psychomotor manifestations of anxiety that a nurse may observe include:
- ○ 1. Decreased activity. **AS**
- ○ 2. Increased activity. **7**
- ○ 3. Increased lability of emotions. **PhI**
- ○ 4. Decreased lability of emotions.

134. The nurse needs to know that anxiety may increase intellectual functioning because anxiety may:
- ○ 1. Increase the perceptual field. **AN**
- ○ 2. Increase ability to concentrate. **7**
- ○ 3. Decrease the perceptual field. **PsI**
- ○ 4. Decrease random activity.

135. When working with a person who is anxious, what is the *overall* goal of nursing intervention?
- ○ 1. Remove anxiety. **PL**
- ○ 2. Develop the person's awareness of anxiety. **7**
- ○ 3. Protect the person from anxiety. **PsI**
- ○ 4. Develop the person's capacity to tolerate mild anxiety and to use it constructively.

136. Clients who are suspicious tend to use projection. The nurse is aware that the main purpose of this action is to:
- ○ 1. Control and manipulate others. **AN**
- ○ 2. Deny reality. **7**
- ○ 3. Handle feelings and thoughts not acceptable to the ego. **PsI**
- ○ 4. Express resentment toward others.

137. The nurse is aware that clients who exhibit reaction formation can be described as:
- ○ 1. Using a socially acceptable outlet for impulses from the id. **AN** **7**
- ○ 2. Adopting the feelings and attitudes of a hero. **PsI**
- ○ 3. Keeping unacceptable ideas or feelings from awareness.
- ○ 4. Adopting a feeling or attitude that is the opposite of the original attitude.

138. When the nurse is aware that the client is exhibiting regressive behavior, she or he knows that regression is common in physical and emotional illness. Which of the following best explains this mechanism?
- ○ 1. When faced with frustration, conflict, and/or anxiety, people may need to return to a previous level of functioning where they felt secure and comfortable. **AN** **7** **PsI**
- ○ 2. Immature behavior has secondary benefits.
- ○ 3. Childlike behavior is a way of getting away with expressing hostility.
- ○ 4. Individuals enjoy the sympathy and attention they received as children when they were ill.

139. When a client is described as exhibiting "fixation," the nurse is aware that this mode of coping is related to:
- ○ 1. Reversion to an earlier developmental phase. **AN**
- ○ 2. Behavior persisting into later life that was appropriate in an earlier developmental phase. **7** **PsI**
- ○ 3. A disturbance in the rate of speech.
- ○ 4. A wish to be like another and to assume attributes of the other.

140. An angry man may channel his hostilities into competitive sports in which there are many opportunities for combat. The nurse knows that this is:
- ○ 1. Sublimation. **AN**
- ○ 2. Repression. **7**
- ○ 3. Rationalization. **PsI**
- ○ 4. Reaction formation.

141. When the client exhibits signs of amnesia, the nurse knows that this behavior is probably related to:
- ○ 1. Selective forgetting and storing unacceptable thoughts, wishes, and impulses in the unconscious mind. **AN** **7** **PsI**
- ○ 2. Conscious, deliberate forgetting.
- ○ 3. Transferring to another situation an emotion felt in a previous situation where its expression would not have been acceptable.
- ○ 4. Unconscious imitating of the manners, behavior, and feelings of another.

142. Mary, a client who attempted suicide recently, remarks to the nurse the next morning, "Let's not think about that now. Maybe I'll feel like thinking about it later." The nurse identifies this as:
- ○ 1. Blocking. **AN**
- ○ 2. Denial. **7**
- ○ 3. Suppression. **PsI**
- ○ 4. Repression.

143. Repetitive handwashing is often seen when a client is experiencing guilt feelings. This ritualistic behavior can be described as a mechanism whereby the client attaches significance to the act of washing. The nurse would identify this behavior as:

○ 1. Symbolism. **AN**
○ 2. Fantasy. **7**
○ 3. Isolation. **PsI**
○ 4. Conversion.

144. The client shouts at the nurse one morning, "Why do you waste your time on me? I'm not sick; I don't need you. Go talk to Mr. Gomez. He's really sick!" The nurse identifies this as:
○ 1. Reaction formation. **AN**
○ 2. Denial. **7**
○ 3. Intellectualization. **PsI**
○ 4. Rationalization.

145. Which of the following terms would the nurse use to describe the experience of an individual who thought he heard a machine gun when his neighbor's lawnmower backfired as she was mowing the lawn?
○ 1. Delusion. **AN**
○ 2. Hallucination. **7**
○ 3. Identification. **PsI**
○ 4. Illusion.

146. The nurse knows that the most characteristic task of puberty and adolescence, according to Erikson's stages of psychosexual development, is:
○ 1. Identity versus role confusion. **AN**
○ 2. Initiative versus guilt. **5**
○ 3. Ego integrity versus despair. **HPM**
○ 4. Intimacy versus isolation.

147. Johnny, age 10 years, was admitted to the hospital for a tonsillectomy. In the morning, the nurse notes that the bedding is wet. There are several boys his age in the room. Which initial approach would best demonstrate a nurse's understanding of enuresis and Johnny's stage of growth and development?
○ 1. While proceeding to change the wet linens, ask Johnny what sports he likes best, purposely ignoring the wet bed by staying on impersonal topics. **IMP** **5** **HPM**
○ 2. Draw the curtains around his bed while changing the linen, saying, "I know that this must be embarrassing to you."
○ 3. Say nothing while changing the bed; return at another time, when the other boys are not in the room, and explain to Johnny the medical-emotional reasons for enuresis.
○ 4. Sit down on the bed and convey acceptance of him as a person rather than focusing on the wet bed.

148. In assessing the behavior of an autistic child, the nurse notes that a symptom that characteristically differentiates an autistic child from one with Down syndrome is:
○ 1. Retardation of activity. **AS**
○ 2. Short attention span. **5**
○ 3. Difficulty in responding to a nurturing relationship. **PsI**
○ 4. Poor academic performance.

149. What is a main goal (purpose) of milieu therapy?
○ 1. Inclusion of the family in the treatment process. **PL** **7**
○ 2. Permissiveness with rules or structure. **SECE**
○ 3. Client-planned, client-led activities.
○ 4. Staff's nonparticipation in decision making.

150. When a colleague is confused about the purpose of a therapeutic environment, the nurse explains to the colleague that in a therapeutic environment, rules and regulations:
○ 1. Need to be kept to a minimum. **IMP**
○ 2. Serve as solutions for commonly occurring problems. **7** **SECE**
○ 3. Teach clients self-control.
○ 4. Should be rigidly enforced.

151. A client in a therapeutic community setting approached the nurse one weekend evening, complained of being bored, and requested that some activity be provided. Which response by the nurse would be consistent with a milieu-therapy approach?
○ 1. "All right, I'm not busy. How about playing cards with me?" **IMP** **7**
○ 2. "I'll go ask the head nurse and see if we can come up with something." **PsI**
○ 3. "Why don't you ask Mr. Anderson to play cards with you?"
○ 4. "Let's get the clients and staff together and discuss this."

152. The nurse explains to a colleague that the major goal of group therapy is to:
○ 1. Give the therapist a chance to supply authoritative answers common to group problems. **PL** **7**
○ 2. Give the client an opportunity for feedback from several people regarding problems discussed in group. **SECE**
○ 3. Give the client an opportunity to hear other people's problems.
○ 4. Give the therapist the chance to interact with many clients.

153. The nursing role in group therapy may include all except:
○ 1. Role model and catalyst. **PL**
○ 2. Transference object. **7**
○ 3. Participant, observer, and facilitator. **SECE**
○ 4. Directive.

154. In family therapy sessions, the nurse should:
○ 1. Serve as an arbitrator during disputes. **PL**
○ 2. Focus on the person with the presenting problem. **7** **SECE**
○ 3. Neutralize the scapegoating phenomenon.
○ 4. Use paradoxical communication.

155. Electroconvulsive therapy is ordered as treatment for a client who is depressed. What is the most important point for the nurse to know to plan immediate posttreatment care?
○ 1. The client will not be as depressed as before and therefore will be a high suicide risk. **AN** **7**
○ 2. The client needs to be left alone and needs to sleep. **SECE**
○ 3. The client may look bewildered, be confused, and experience memory loss.
○ 4. The client will be hungry after being NPO and will need nourishment on awakening.

156. At 2:30 A.M., a client walked out to the nurse's station complaining that he was choking, suffocating, weakening, and dying. He demanded a cigarette. What is the best response by the nurse?
○ 1. Refuse and tell him it is against the rules. **IMP**
○ 2. Call the doctor and inform him of the client's request and behavior. **7** **PsI**
○ 3. Refuse and tell him the cigarettes are locked.
○ 4. Give him a cigarette and stay with him while he smokes.

157. What approach can the nurse use to best handle a client's disturbed behavior?

○ 1. Approve his behavior. PL 7 SECE
○ 2. Maintain consistency of approach.
○ 3. Encourage him not to express negative opinions.
○ 4. Interpret for him the reasons for his behavior.

158. In primary sex health intervention, what is the nurse's major task?
○ 1. Identifying sexual problems. PL 7 HPM
○ 2. Referring clients to other health care providers.
○ 3. Providing follow-up therapy after initial treatment for sexual dysfunction.
○ 4. Providing education to individuals who are uninformed or misinformed about the nature of human sexuality.

159. In response to a colleague's concern, which of the following statements can the nurse make that is most accurate about masturbation?
○ 1. It is unhealthy because it prevents a person from acknowledging the function of his or her sexual organs. IMP 7 HPM
○ 2. It is a healthy and appropriate sexual activity that enables a person to consolidate his or her own sexual identity.
○ 3. It prevents a person from enjoying heterosexual sexual activity.
○ 4. It is an unhealthy and inappropriate sexual activity that confuses a person's sexual identity.

160. The overall client goal in rape counseling is to help the victim:
○ 1. Forget the incident and repress her feelings in order to be able to carry on with her life. PL 1 HPM
○ 2. Identify the rapist in a court of law.
○ 3. Accept her part in the rape.
○ 4. Acknowledge, face and resolve the reaction she is experiencing.

161. Which of the following is the most appropriate in response to a client who states emphatically, "I hate them"?
○ 1. "I will stay with you as long as you feel this way." IMP 2 PsI
○ 2. "Tell me about your hate."
○ 3. "I understand how you can feel this way."
○ 4. "For whom do you have these feelings?"

162. The nurse observes for signs of heroin withdrawal, which may include:
○ 1. Rhinorrhea, sneezing, and high fever. AS 7 PhI
○ 2. Pupillary dilation, diaphoresis, and weight loss.
○ 3. Pupillary constriction, vomiting, and pruritus.
○ 4. Choreiform movements and frequent lip wetting.

163. The nurse will look for what likely outcome of methadone treatment for heroin abuse and dependence?
○ 1. Sedation. EV 7 PhI
○ 2. Euphoria.
○ 3. Neuritis.
○ 4. Blocking of the euphoric effect of heroin and elimination of craving.

164. An acutely agitated female client becomes increasingly aggressive. The staff's verbal attempts to stop her aggressive behavior are not effective. The client begins to shout threats at the staff and other clients, throws furniture, breaks windows, hits and kicks and bites other clients and staff. The client has a p.r.n. order for medication when she is agitated. Which of the following actions should the nurse take initially?
○ 1. Orient the client to reality and place her in a well-lit, quiet room. IMP 1 SECE
○ 2. Give the ordered tranquilizer and put the client in bed with the siderails up.
○ 3. Lock the client in her room and call the doctor.
○ 4. Have at least two staff members restrain the client physically and take her to a quiet room.

165. Heather Jackson, an 18-year-old former art student, is admitted to the mental health unit. She has a history of involvement in car thefts as well as traffic violations; she has been sexually active since age 10 and has frequently experimented with a variety of drugs. Her home environment has been permissive, with few controls. On the unit, she frequently calls nurses by their first name, offers to help them with their work, and tells them they are the nicest people she has ever known. Ms. Jackson is on a locked unit. A new nurse, about to leave, is holding the key as Ms. Jackson approaches her and eagerly offers to unlock the door for the nurse, saying, "The other nurses let me." Which first response by the nurse would be most appropriate?
○ 1. Let Ms. Jackson turn the key in the lock, but stay close to her while she does it. IMP 7 SECE
○ 2. Ask Ms. Jackson why she wants to unlock the door.
○ 3. Tell Ms. Jackson, in a nice way, that this is not allowed.
○ 4. Go to the head nurse and ask if it is all right for Ms. Jackson to unlock the door.

166. During a nursing-care conference, several staff members voice their frustrations about Mrs. Rawley's constant questions, such as "Should I go to the dayroom or should I stay in my room?" and "Should I have a cup of tea or a cup of coffee?" Which of the following interpretations about Mrs. Rawley's behavior will help the nursing staff deal effectively with this behavior?
○ 1. Her inability to make decisions reflects a basic anxiety about making a mistake and being a failure. AN 7 SECE
○ 2. Her indecisiveness is aimed at testing the staff's reaction and acceptance of her.
○ 3. Her dependence on others (staff) is a symptom that needs to be interrupted by firm limit-setting.
○ 4. Her need to ask questions is a bid for attention.

■ ANSWERS/RATIONALE

1. (3) This will reduce the isolation and withdrawal while at the same time not putting the burden of decision making on her. She needs a structured routine that is simple. She may not be able to handle close proximity to more than one person at this point, as in No. 2. No. 1 incorrectly allows her to *remain* isolated; No. 4 is incorrect because she needs a *structured* routine until she can make decisions for herself.

2. (4) A simple acknowledgment of what the nurse sees is the best response. No. 3 makes an assumption that she feels better if she looks better. Nos. 1 and 2 can be taken as a put-down.

3. (1) It is important to externalize the anger away from self. No. 2 is incorrect because usually the client is turning anger *inward,* toward the self. No. 3 increases her sense of isolation. The needs in No. 4 should be taken care of but *not* emphasized, as the depressed client often has somatic delusions.

4. (4) Meet the client at her level of functioning, and provide support and encouragement for a higher level in the near future. No. 1 implies that the nurse agrees that the client has nothing to say. No. 2 conveys no empathy or understanding. No. 3 is incorrect because silence reinforces silence and a sense of isolation.

5. (1) "Loss" is *most basic* to the development of depression. Nos. 2, 3, and 4 are *not essential* to development of depression.

6. (1) An undemanding task that the client could finish would allow a feeling of successful accomplishment. Nos. 2 and 3 require intellectual activity that is usually slowed down during a depressive phase. No. 4 requires a skill that the client may not have and that might frustrate the client to learn; also, the client may not have the psychomotor energy for ice skating.

7. (2) In the depressed phase, anger is turned inward; in the manic, it is noted in sarcasm, demanding behavior, and angry outbursts. Nos. 3 and 4 occur in the manic phase. No. 1 is a particular problem in the depressed phase.

8. (2) During the manic phase, the client may be too busy to eat and sleep. Nos. 1 and 3 are more appropriate for the depressed phase; No. 4 is more appropriate for schizophrenia with bizarre behavior. Clients in the manic phase exhibit hyperactive behavior.

9. (4) It is a matter-of-fact statement that is direct, while offering assistance and setting limits on inappropriate behavior. The following are not useful because: No. 1 reinforces inappropriate social behavior; No. 2 sets limits but does not state a positive expectation for the client to follow; No. 3 neither offers assistance nor sets limits, which he needs.

10. (2) Often the verbalized ideas are jumbled, but the underlying feelings are discernible and need to be acknowledged. Flight of ideas should be *curtailed;* thus, No. 4 is incorrect. The client may not be able to control the internal stimuli to focus on one idea at a time as in No. 3. A louder and more rapid tone by the nurse may only increase the external stimuli for the client, making No. 1 incorrect.

11. (2) It will provide energy release without the external stimuli and pressure of *competitive games* (Nos. 3 and 4). Reading usually requires sitting, which a manic client cannot readily do, as in No. 1.

12. (3) In Nos. 1 and 2 the client could suffer extensive blood loss if the nurse focuses on feelings at this point or leaves him without first attempting to control the bleeding. In No. 4, the client is left alone, bleeding, frightened, and with a razor still next to him.

13. (4) The client needs to have his feelings acknowledged, with encouragement to discuss feelings, and be reassured about the nurse's presence. The client may interpret the nurse's silence as discomfort in talking about his suicidal feeling and thoughts (No. 1). No. 2 focuses on facts too swiftly without providing an opportunity for the client to express his feelings. Also, No. 2 would be most appropriate in *crisis* intervention when client is *first* admitted, *not* the next morning. No. 3 moves away from focus on here-and-now to focus on the past.

14. (1) Another name for depression with melancholia is depression with psychotic features. Suicide risk is a part of all depressions. Nos. 2, 3, and 4 are incorrect because the diagnosis alone does not indicate suicide risk like the diagnosis of depression.

15. (1) The client needs to be constantly observed. No. 2 is incorrect because all suicidal talk and gestures are to be taken seriously. If the client *talks* about suicide, there *may* be an attempt. No. 3 is incorrect because suicide risk is greater when depression is lifting, requiring greater vigilance. No. 4 is incorrect because medication for depression may take up two weeks to decrease symptoms, and the client needs vigilant surveillance *now.*

16. (1) The nurse should formulate a weight control plan, in *cooperation* with the client, that allows for a *gradual* weight loss, *not immediate* loss as in No. 4. Nos. 2 and 3 *are incorporated* into No. 1.

17. (1) This reply asks for information that the nurse can use. If the client understands the statement, the nurse can support the therapist when focusing on connections between food, love, and mother. If the client does not understand the statement, the nurse can help her get clarification from the therapist. No. 2 alienates the client, and the nurse loses the chance for collaboration with the therapist. No. 3 shuts the client off. No. 4 is incorrect because it is asked before the nurse is sure the client understands the therapist's statement.

18. (2) Persons engaged in self-destructive behavior other than active suicide behavior fantasize *they can control* their behavior and deny the likelihood of death as a result. Thus Nos. 1, 3, and 4 are incorrect.

19. (1) These persons have not faced up to the idea that they are controlled by their behavior, and this relieves their anxiety. Contrary to No. 2, persons have *increased* anxiety if they stop the behavior. No. 3 is also incorrect (see question 18). No. 4 is incorrect because these persons *know* the behavior is bad for them.

20. (3) When feelings of low self-esteem are prevalent, self-destructive behavior reaches its peak. Hence, Nos. 1, 2, and 4 are incorrect.

21. (3) Correct by Freudian theory. Nos. 1, 2, and 4 are incorrect because they are incomplete.

22. (4) A variety of factors can cause self-destructive behavior, and these differ for each individual. Hence, Nos. 1, 2, and 3 are not the best choices because, although correct, they are *examples* of a *variety* of factors; No. 4 is more inclusive.

23. (1) Shock and anger are commonly the primary initial reactions. No. 2 is irrelevant; and No. 3 is a literal, concrete interpretation of Mrs. Barnes's reaction, not aimed at the possible latent feelings. No. 4 is incorrect because it contradicts correct answer No. 1.

24. (1) Love-hate feelings take longer to resolve. Reactions to loss tend to be cumulative in effect, in that the more loss experienced in the past, the greater the reaction the next time; thus, No. 3 is wrong. Reactivation of feelings connected with previous losses by the current loss accounts for the increased intensity of the reaction. Sudden, unexpected death, *rather* than death due to a chronic illness, as in No. 2, is harder to resolve, and strong, *not little,* emotional dependency (as in No. 4) also complicates grief resolution.

25. (2) When the mourner can pass through the idealization stage and be more realistic about the positive and negative aspects of the loss, resolution of grief is beginning. Nos. 3 and 4 occur in *earlier* stages of grief. No. 1 could be a sign of denial of grieving, an initial grief reaction.

26. (4) An honest, direct answer that focuses on feelings is the best approach. Nos. 1, 2, and 3 stop any further exploration of the client's feelings.

27. (2) Refer to Elisabeth Kübler-Ross's emotional stages of death and dying. She is being neither unrealistic (No. 1), manipulative (No. 3), nor unaware of her diagnosis (No. 4).

28. (3) One way to enhance the development of unresolved grief is *not* to participate in activities that demonstrate death. Nos. 1, 2, and 4 may occur, but they are *not* the best predictors of grief resolution difficulties.

29. (1) Correct according to Lindemann's and Engle's grief stages. Hence, incorrect are No. 2 ("shock" stage), No. 3 ("idealization" stage), and No. 4 ("resolving the loss" stage).

30. (4) *Rationalization* is the process of constructing plausible reasons for one's responses. No. 1, *suppression,* is the intentional exclusion of material from consciousness. No. 2, *undoing,* is an act that partially negates a previous one. No. 3, *repression,* is the involuntary exclusion of painful or conflicting thoughts or feelings from awareness.

31. (4) Feelings of worthlessness or low self-esteem are the underlying problem in depression. Nos. 1, 2, and 3 may occur but are *not most* apt.

32. (2) *Denial* is the act of avoiding disagreeable realities by ignoring them. No. 1 is incorrect because *compensation* is the process by which a person makes up for a deficiency in self-image by emphasizing an asset. No. 3, *symbolism,* is the use of one mental image to represent another. No. 4, *identification,* is also incorrect (see answer to question 145, No. 3).

33. (1) A person who has settled on a plan for suicide will become more cheerful. No. 2 is incorrect because a person who is severely retarded in the psychomotor area cannot carry out a suicide act. Nos. 3 and 4 are incorrect because Mr. Gonzalez is more likely to be hostile and agitated if he does not have a suicide plan. Agitated behavior can also represent the need to "repent" for sins thought to be committed.

34. (1) Circulation may be severely impaired in a client with waxy flexibility who tends to remain motionless for hours unless moved. No. 2 is *not the first* priority. "Touch" is *not* used in this stage, as in choice No. 3. And No. 4 is incorrect because she is *mute* and also because intellectual discussion of predisposing factors *ignores* the *feelings* of the client.

35. (4) This is a reality-based response, as well as one that acknowledges the client's nonverbal reaction. The following are *not* the best choices because: Nos. 1 and 3 focus on "voice," which reinforce the hallucination, and no doubt is placed; in No. 2 doubt is placed but focus is on "voice" and *not* on client's *feelings.*

36. (2) This acknowledges the experience and points out reality as the nurse sees it. Nos. 1, 4, and 3 do not focus on the client or attempt to explore feelings.

37. (3) It is important to acknowledge a statement, even if it is not understood. No. 1 is not a *direct* response; No. 2 leaves out the importance of the meaning of the neologism to the client; and No. 4 is less valid and important than *acknowledgment* of the meaning to the client.

38. (4) Decoding symbolic, autistic expressions calls for skill and sensitivity in understanding latent messages. No. 1 is not a good choice, since showing "acceptance" is a basic, initial nursing goal that does not require a complexity of skills. No. 2 points out a non-therapeutic nursing action, which is best not to use at all. No. 3 implies that the nurse use short sentences with clear, concise, unambiguous meaning; this *can* be accomplished with practice. Nos. 1 and 3 need to be accomplished before No. 4 is possible.

39. (2) You help do things by doing something with her. No. 1 is incorrect because the client won't hear a long explanation. No. 3 is incorrect because demanding won't work. She can't join in unless you are with her (as in No. 2). No. 4 is incorrect because you should not produce psychosis in order to motivate a person.

40. (4) Clients with withdrawn behavior in schizophrenic disorders tend to think in concrete terms. Therefore, use of simple language enables them to grasp meaning. No. 1 is incorrect because if you remain silent the client will remain silent. No. 2 is incorrect because if you are not concrete the client might have trouble understanding some terms in normal conversation. No. 3 is incorrect, as client has difficulty talking.

41. (4) Focusing on feelings is usually the best choice. Ignoring the client is rarely an acceptable intervention (No. 1). Pointing out disturbed behavior and role modeling by the nurse are valid, but *not* as first interventions (Nos. 2 and 3).

42. (4) The primary initial focus of the nurse–client relationship is in showing the client, through acceptance, that it is *the client* one is concerned about, *not* the *symptoms.* Nos. 1 and 2 are incorrect because the focus of *initial* nursing care is on the client, not on meeting hospital standards or controlling impulses. No. 3 is incorrect because it is an attempt to analyze the *whys* of behavior, which is not an appropriate *basic* nursing intervention and certainly *not* an initial aspect of care.

43. (2) A permissive atmosphere is the key, as well as a *slowly* evolving relationship (not quickly evolving, as in No. 3) with room for *distance.* Self-destruction is *not a persistent* problem requiring *major* focus for concern, as in No. 4. No. 1 is not the best response because "acceptance" of *bizarre* behavior is more important than setting limits.

44. (3) This is a false belief developed in response to an emotional need. In No. 1, the situation is *not* a perceptual disorder. In No. 2, the situation is *not* a misperception. In No. 4, although the client refuses meals, the reason for this is a false belief (delusion).

45. (1) Listening is probably the most effective response of the four choices. A key consideration in interacting with clients who are suspicious is to *avoid* the use of logic and argument; thus No. 2 is incorrect. Humor usually intensifies the anger and suspicion; thus No. 3 is incorrect. Changing the topic, as in No. 4, may serve to reinforce the client's belief in the guilt of others.

46. (3) Definition of *projection* as a coping mechanism. Nos. 1, 2, and 4 are incorrect because they have nothing to do with the coping mechanism of projection. Coping mechanisms in general function in the service of "self"—that is, they protect the ego and preserve self-esteem in an effort to cope with anxiety; the focus is *not* on *others,* as in Nos. 1 and 4. Mr. Carlson's symptoms of projection do in fact *express* delusional thought rather than *control* it, contrary to No. 2.

47. (3) This shows a weak sense of moral consciousness. According to Freudian theory, personality disorders stem from a *weak* superego. No. 1 is incorrect, as the id is *strong.* These disorders are *not* characterized by a weak ego, as in No. 2, whereas schizophrenia is. No. 4 is of relevance in sexual-identity difficulties rather than in personality disorders.

48. (4) A weak superego implies a lack of adequate controls. No. 1 is not relevant, as her *self-identity* as a woman is *not* a focus here. No. 2 is incorrect because Alice typically gratifies her own inner needs, which is part of the difficulty with a strong id and which requires external controls, such as that in No. 4. No. 3 is incorrect because she is *not* psychotic but has a personality disorder, for which reality testing is *not* impaired. She *is* aware of reality.

49. (1) This response aims to prevent use of manipulative patterns. In Nos. 2, 3, and 4, the nurse needs to seek validation, and these responses indicate acceptance without validation.

50. (4) Let the client know without anger how you feel and that you are not intimidated, then help her examine what she is doing and why. No. 1 is incorrect because it points the finger in an angry, accusatory way and labels the client in turn ("*You* are rude"). No. 2 makes the client sound like "Big Nurse"—authoritarian and punitive. No. 3 may place the nurse in a position to be intimidated and "kicked" by the client.

51. (1) Frightening visual hallucinations are especially common. No. 2, coma, is usually *not* an immediate consequence of alcohol withdrawal. No. 3 is incorrect because her diagnosis is *withdrawal* from alcohol, not alcohol intoxication (intake). No. 4 is incorrect because the client will be *agitated* and *rambling* in conversation, not mute and depressed.

52. (4) Arrest of the disease is possible through abstinence, not through change in psychophysiologic response to alcohol. Nos. 1, 2, and 3 are stereotyped statements, not generally or universally accepted.

53. (4) The liver is affected by both the direct effect of alcohol and nutritional deficiencies associated with alcohol abuse and dependence. Nos. 1, 2, and 3 are areas not usually affected by alcohol abuse and dependence.

54. (2) It is important to provide external support in helping develop the superego. No. 1 may promote manipulative behavior in the client. No. 3 may foster additional dependence. And preventing the client's use of drugs (No. 4) is *not* the primary step in building a nurse–client relationship based on therapeutic communication.

55. (1) Anxiety is generated by group therapy at 9 A.M. The ritualistic behavioral defense of handwashing decreases anxiety by avoiding group therapy. No. 2 is incorrect because *tension,* not unmet needs, is discharged through ritualistic behavior. No. 3 may be true, but it is not essential to planning care. No. 4 is incorrect, as depression is *not* characteristic of ritualism.

56. (4) The *opposite* of what is stated in the first three choices is true. The client seems to do best when (1) *routine* activities are set up and anxiety-provoking changes are avoided; (2) *perfection-type* activities bring satisfaction (cleaning and straightening a linen closet, for example); and (3) he knows *ahead of time* about changes in routine.

57. (3) This is the best example of setting limits on the behavior. Nos. 1 and 4 may be closely linked to non-therapeutic use of power. No. 2 is more of an example of a punishment approach.

58. (2) A ritual, such as compulsive handwashing, is an attempt to allay anxiety caused by unconscious impulses that are frightening. No. 1 is incorrect because it is the opposite of what the handwashing ritual is intended to do—the ritual is aimed at *absolving* guilt, not *punishing.* No. 3 is related to *psychotic* symptoms and not at all relevant to symptoms of ritualism. No. 4 is incorrect because handwashing is aimed at relief of guilt and self-help to reduce anxiety, *not* at seeking attention from staff.

59. (1) It shows acceptance by listening to the client's initial account of her physical problems. Neither a superficial focus nor a technical explanation of physical problems (Nos. 2 and 3) conveys acceptance of the client as a person; No. 4 is too abrupt for an initial response.

60. (3) Showing *acceptance* and gaining trust and confidence are usually the key initial nursing goals. You need to show acceptance before *helping* (Nos. 1 and 4) or *assisting* (No. 2). Note the lead verb: *accept* before *help* or *assist.*

61. (3) No. 1 is incorrect because conversion, *not regression,* is the major coping mechanism. And No. 2 is incorrect because, if a possible cause is identified and treatment relieves the discomfort, the client often develops another symptom. Frequently, clients do not want to be cured of their symptoms because they *need* the symptoms to control the behavior of others or because they do not know how else to get attention. In No. 4, the converse is true: the symptoms *are* real, not imagined or faked.

62. (2) This is a better choice than No. 4, which may be true but is a tangential and irrelevant reason. No. 1 is not correct because the client *is* aware of reality but may not understand the *cause* for her conversion disorder. No. 3 is more relevant in a *paranoid* reaction.

63. (1) The original source of conflict, pain, and/or guilt is repressed (pushed out of awareness), only to surface in a symbolic way. Nos. 2, 3, and 4 are only partially correct: in somatoform disorders, regression is common, *not sublimation;* displacement is common, *not substitution;* reaction formation is common, *not rationalization.*

64. (4) This answer also incorporates No. 3. Agreement to attend activities (No. 2) does not indicate the *greatest* improvement. The client *already* recognizes that her behavior is irrational but cannot understand the cause or banish the behavior by will, as in No. 1.

65. (2) Characteristic underlying needs in somatoform disorders are dependency, attention, and the need for security through trust. Nos. 1 and 4 are incorrect because the client's complaints are not aimed at blaming others or at seeking vengeance but at expressing dependency needs and seeking security. No. 3 is inappropriate because Mr. Simon is expressing his *own* need for attention; he is not speaking for everyone.

66. (1) Emotional support is a key need. No. 2 does *not* focus on emotional support. No. 3, role expectation, in itself has *no* bearing; emotional support of role would. No. 4 would help Mrs. Simon and her own emotional reaction but would *not* help Mr. Simon.

67. (2) All the other choices are correct but can be dovetailed into No. 2.

68. (4) One coping mechanism often seen in somatoform disorders is repression. As the client is better able to handle the anxiety connected with underlying feelings, the *need for repression lessens*. Nos. 1, 2, and 3 may be the content of his feelings, but they do not explain the dynamics, the *reason* he is expressing more feelings.

69. (2) It reflects the client's underlying concerns in the *most* open-ended manner. No. 1 is incorrect because the *nurse* cannot say how the client is feeling; she is *assuming* here that he *is* better, which is inappropriate. No. 4 only focuses on *one* aspect: *sadness*. What about the *agitation* he *also* expresses? No. 3 is not incorrect, but it is also not the *best* choice because it asks a direct question when a simple acknowledgment (as in No. 2) would be better *initially*.

70. (3) This answer is the best choice because the other choices seem *too certain* for a disorder that, although it has a pattern, can be altered *if* and *when* the client adopts different outlets for expressing his emotions.

71. (2) The other choices are *not* helpful, for the following reasons: Nos. 3 and 4 *switch* the focus and *ignore* the client's statement; No. 1 is too brusque an attempt to bring client back to reality.

72. (2) Since confabulation is a coping mechanism, the best choice is the one that defines one of the main functions of coping mechanisms—to protect self-esteem. Nos. 1 and 3 are incorrect because they focus on *others,* not on self. No. 4 is completely *irrelevant*.

73. (2) An important principle to remember here is that a program of care should not increase physiologic losses by overtaxing the client's physical capacities. It is important to remember that suicide is the *main* concern of *depression* and *not* a key concern of organic mental disorder, as in No. 1. Empathy *rather than* sympathy (No. 4) is a helpful behavior. No. 3, increasing independence, is *not realistic; maintaining* it *is*.

74. (3) One of the main needs experienced by most elderly clients with organic mental disorders is the need for most things to be the same. The other choices are wrong for the following reasons: There has been no demonstrable evidence of relationship between any behavior symptom and the extent or severity of pathophysiologic condition (No. 2); intellectual *blunting* usually occurs, which interferes with ability to deal with insight and abstract thoughts (No. 4); and memory loss is for *recent* events and names, *not* those in the distant past, as in No. 1.

75. (1) Memory loss is usually permanent, not corrective; thus, No. 2 is wrong. However, disorientation attributed to loss of memory can be minimized. Clients usually become *more* dependent in the course of illness *and* deteriorate progressively. Thus, Nos. 3 and 4 are incorrect. Use of regression as a coping response (No. 1) *can* be minimized.

76. (1) Elderly clients feel more secure when they can count on their environment being the same, predictable, and consistent in detail from day to day (hence, structured) to compensate for feelings of loss of the familiar in terms of body functions, social environment, and so on. Nos. 2 and 4 imply change, not routine. No. 3, while correct, is not the *most* important.

77. (4) Although all the other choices *are* valid and important, the fourth answer encompasses them all and is therefore the most *comprehensive* answer.

78. (3) Self-esteem is *the most basic* psychologic need at *any* age, especially so for the elderly. Nos. 1, 2, and 4, although also important, are not the most basic needs.

79. (1) No. 2 relates to toddler; No. 3 to infancy; No. 4 to latency period in childhood.

80. (4) Redundancy is *not* meant to impress others but is aimed at *pleasure* gained through focus on the *past* and need to *control* the conversation when memory or hearing deficit is present. Nos. 1, 2, and 3 *would* demonstrate understanding of this behavior.

81. (3) Nocturnal urination is a most common need, complicated by disorientation related to the client's age, disorder, and unfamiliar environment by night. To sit down (No. 1) or to go back to his room and talk (No. 4) does not take care of the possible problem, the need to urinate. Asking a person "why" questions (No. 2) is not helpful and is too literal a response to his behavior.

82. (1) Deal first with the *life-saving* situation. Nos. 2 and 3 are incorrect because they are done *following* stabilization of physical condition. No. 4 is incorrect because it is *not* a necessary life-saving concern.

83. (3) It incorporates all information a crisis intervention nurse needs immediately. Nos. 1 and 2 are incorrect because the nurse does not need to know about other people's involvement at this time. No. 4 is incorrect because it is *not as complete* an answer as No. 3.

84. (4) The major goal of crisis intervention is to resolve immediate problems. No. 1 is incorrect because restructuring personality is the goal of *psychoanalytic* therapy. Nos. 2 and 3 are incorrect because they are goals of *brief* psychotherapy, and, although they may occur in the resolution of immediate problems, they are *not the* goal.

85. (1) To resolve immediate problems, you focus on a person's ability to cope and usual level of functioning. No. 2 is incorrect because it is a *psychoanalytic* focus. Nos. 3 and 4 are incorrect because they are the focus of *brief* psychotherapy.

86. (3) Part of the definition of a crisis is a time span of 4–6 weeks. No. 1 is incorrect because, by definition, crises do *not* continue indefinitely. No. 2 is incorrect because *all* people have crises, and having crises does not determine normality. No. 4 is incorrect because, although crises may be related to deep, underlying problems, one of the principles of crisis intervention therapy is to deal with the immediate situation, not the underlying problem.

87. (3) Jenny needs to be aware of her actions and the possible ramifications of her actions. No. 1 is incorrect because she *needs to discuss* her actions. No. 2 is incorrect because the purpose of crisis intervention is to deal with the *present* problem and situation, *not* the past. No. 4 is incorrect because the focus needs to be on the client, *not* on others.

88. (2) On principle, the crisis intervention nurse needs to be *immediately* available to Jenny. No. 1 is incorrect because it abandons her. No. 3 is incorrect because Jenny needs to deal with the situation *immediately*. No.

4 is incorrect because Jenny might decide that the crisis intervention nurse is not interested in helping her, and she needs *immediate* assistance.

89. (3) A principle of behavior modification is to reward behavior. No. 1 is incorrect because this allows him to continue with unacceptable behavior. Nos. 2 and 4 are incorrect because they are not suitable reinforcers. If he could eat like others, he would, and it is doubtful that he is concerned about others' distress.

90. (2) A principle of behavior modification is to reward behavior. Nos. 1, 3, and 4 are not suitable reinforcers for a regressed client. See question 89.

91. (3) On-the-spot observation and intervention are key. Focus on dreams is part of Freudian analysis; thus, No. 1 is incorrect. Behavior modification is used in the treatment of *mute* clients also; thus, No. 2 is incorrect. The emphasis of behavioral therapy is the present (No. 3) and *not* the past developmental history, as in No. 4.

92. (1) The nurse needs to set limits to assure the safety of the client and others. No. 2 is incorrect because she may hurt herself or others. Nos. 3 and 4 are incorrect because they are interpretations that may or may not be correct, and they do *not control* her *unsafe* behavior.

93. (4) A person needs to be allowed to express anger appropriately. Nos. 1, 2, and 3 are *incorrect* choices here because they *are* things you assist a person to do when intervening in anger.

94. (4) It provides the complete steps. No. 1 is incorrect because of the phrase "decide on *several*"; it should be *one* solution at a time. No. 2 is incorrect because it *doesn't include* "discuss alternative solutions." No. 3 is incorrect because it does not describe a requested *series* of steps and because *giving* a person one answer is untherapeutic.

95. (1) This is the proper use of anger. No. 2 is incorrect because, although anger can be used to intimidate others, that use creates interpersonal problems. No. 3 is incorrect because, in order for hostility to be a good communication mechanism, the degree of hostility must be *appropriate* to the provocation. No. 4 is incorrect because this expression of anger does not produce positive accomplishment.

96. (3) Frequent contacts at times of stress are important, especially when a client is isolated. The following are not useful because: No. 1, isolation does not automatically imply the use of restraints; No. 2, *all* furniture need not be removed, depending on the institution and the type of behavior exhibited by the client; No. 4, there is *no specific* time limit, as time depends on individual behavior and the client's individual needs.

97. (4) Denial is defined as the avoidance of disagreeable realities by ignoring or refusing to recognize them; avoidance implies refusing to take action. No. 1 is incorrect because rationalization involves offering a socially acceptable or logical explanation to justify feelings or behavior. In rationalization, one does not need to take action; one merely offers an explanation. No. 2 is incorrect because projection involves attributing one's thoughts or impulses to others. No. 3 is incorrect because sublimation is the acceptance of a socially approved substitute for a drive that is blocked.

98. (4) This is the *most complete* description of body image. Nos. 1, 2 and 3 are *partial* answers and therefore incorrect.

99. (1) It is most likely that grief would be expressed because of object loss. No. 2 is incorrect because deep depression, if it occurs, would be the result of *lack* of resolution of grief over object loss. No. 3 is incorrect because relief is *not part* of the grief process. No. 4 is incorrect because the question asks for the client's *immediate* response. Denial of carcinoma, if it occurs, would probably occur *later.*

100. (3) A change in body image has made Mrs. Dawn feel unloved and unworthy of love. Nos. 1, 2, and 4 are incorrect because there are *no supporting data.*

101. (2) This question attempts to get a specific description of what has happened and will allow client to describe grief and feelings of low self-worth because of loss of breast. No. 1 is incorrect because it offers *false* reassurance. No. 3 is incorrect because it is a *stereotyped* response to a female and denies the client's actual loss. No. 4 is incorrect because it is an *interpretation* that, although possibly true, the client may reject. Resolution of grief, etc., is better achieved if the client can state connection.

102. (1) Overcompliance leads to lack of development of self-identity, one of the major problems in schizophrenic disorders. No. 2 is incorrect because there are *no substantiating data.* No. 3 is incorrect because it *contradicts* the correct statement in No. 1. No. 4 is incorrect because he probably has a *strong* superego due to an implied "should" system (overcompliance with his parents' expectations of behavior).

103. (2) Use of "you" and "I" forces him to acknowledge separate identities. No. 1 is incorrect because "pet names" are usually not a person's choice. Frank needs to be called by his real name. No. 3 is incorrect because he has no identity if he can't have his own opinions. No. 4 is incorrect because "should" responses imply others' ideas, not his.

104. (4) The parents need to ask Frank, not the nurse, but the nurse should also support the parents and encourage them to interact with Frank. Nos. 1 and 2 are incorrect because they are *interpretations* that state opinions about Frank without Frank's participation. No. 3 is incorrect because *no support is given* to the parents.

105. (2) A diagnosis of a paranoid disorder implies weak *ego* development. Nos. 1, 3, and 4 are incorrect because a client with a paranoid disorder might have *strong* id, superego, and "not me" components.

106. (2) In second grade a person needs to form close relationships with *peers.* No. 1 needs to occur *earlier* than second grade *or later* in early teen years. No. 3 occurs *later.* No. 4 is incorrect because her father's actions *make* her dependent on him rather than on her peers.

107. (4) This is the all-inclusive answer. Nos. 1, 2, and 3 may be part of No. 4.

108. (3) The meaning of "ideas of reference" is that all that goes on is somehow connected to a person. No. 1 is incorrect because delusions of grandeur mean a person has an *exalted* opinion of self. No. 2 is incorrect because illusion is a false perceptual experience occurring in response to a stimulus. No. 4 is incorrect because echolalia is a person's automatic *repetition* of what is said.

109. (1) Maria has ideas that someone (her husband) is out to kill her. No. 2 is incorrect because the problem is *beyond* just an "idea of reference" (she fears bodily harm).

No. 3 is incorrect because illusion is a false perceptual experience occurring in response to a stimulus. No. 4 is incorrect because a hallucination is a sensory experience triggered by a person's inner needs, functioning independently of stimulation from the environment.

110. (2) A client with paranoid disorder is suspicious, so a nurse must make every effort not to engage in behavior Maria can misinterpret. Nos. 1 and 3 are incorrect because a nurse *should* give her correct information about what she says and *not* placate her (she will sense the falseness). No. 4 is incorrect because arguing just solidifies her ideas. In a neutral voice, the nurse should give correct information.

111. (3) The nurse should encourage Maria to *explain* her statement in order to understand the experience Maria is having. No. 1 is incorrect because it offers an *interpretation* that may or may not be true. No. 2 is incorrect because it denies Maria's perception without clarification. No. 4 is incorrect because the nurse agrees with an unsupported statement.

112. (3) The nurse tells him she heard his statement about "not doing his own thing" and states she *thinks* he is angry. No. 1 is incorrect because the nurse states she *knows* he is angry. No. 2 is incorrect because an angry person *can't stop* being angry on command. No. 4 is incorrect because focusing on the parents puts the nurse on their side.

113. (2) Confidentiality cannot be guaranteed if there is a danger to the client or to others. No. 1 is incorrect because it is a *sarcastic* response and *denies* that the client has serious problems. No. 3 *contradicts* No. 2. No. 4 is incorrect because parents *do not* have the right to know the content of therapy sessions except in the circumstances described in No. 2.

114. (2) Manipulation is the attempt to control the behavior of others to achieve one's own goals. No. 1, insight, is understanding and using understanding to correct one's behavior. Nos. 3 and 4 are incorrect because, although the client may be trying to con the nurse into believing he *needs* her to do something for him and he *trusts* her, the *real* purpose of the request is manipulation.

115. (3) This response *stops* the manipulation and suggests John is responsible for his own behaviors. Nos. 1, 2, and 4 are incorrect because they indicate the nurse has been conned and manipulated.

116. (2) Part of maturing is learning to view one's parents *and* oneself realistically. Nos. 1, 3, and 4 are incorrect because they represent the *misinformation* that creates problems between individuals.

117. (3) A person with limited hearing and sight becomes confused and disturbed. Nos. 1 and 4 are *unwarranted* assumptions. No. 2 is incorrect because Mr. Sundowner's situation is *not psychologic* dependency but actual *sensory* need.

118. (2) Mr. Sundowner will be easier to care for if he has his hearing aid and glasses. In No. 1, the nurse is *denying* the client his right to the full information of his senses. No. 3 is incorrect because the nurse has the responsibility to change rules for clearly therapeutic reasons. No. 4 does *not* respond to the client's needs.

119. (4) If a particular client is nonverbal, for example, the nurse should not expect that client to function at a verbal level until ready. In No. 1, if the nurse waits for a withdrawn client, for example, to make contact, it may not be helpful. In No. 2, an ambivalent client may need assistance in making decisions. In No. 3, the client's undesirable behavior may be adversely affecting others.

120. (2) This is the most neutral answer by process of elimination. No. 1 is *mainly* the function of a *recreational-occupational* therapist, although nurses participate. No. 3 is *usually* filled by *psychologists* and social workers, and No. 4 is carried out *primarily by psychologists* or *statisticians,* although nurses are involved. "Maintenance of a therapeutic environment" fits more readily into a nursing role by virtue of the number of hours per day a nurse spends with the clients on a unit, in comparison with the number spent by other professionals.

121. (2) Offering a broad opening by giving a general lead is most therapeutic to elicit further description of the client's reaction and to clarify her feelings, which were vaguely stated. No. 1 is a *switch of focus* from the client to the mother. No. 3 is nontherapeutic because a question that can be *answered by a yes or no* often closes off further exploration. No. 4 could be a helpful intervention but is *premature* acknowledgment before feelings have been elaborated.

122. (4) It is important to pick up on a feeling tone and encourage exploration of the feelings and the situation. No. 1 *stops* exploration of the client's feeling. Nos. 2 and 3 *shift* the focus away from feelings to content of selfishness.

123. (3) An appropriate direct response to a "you know what I mean" comment is to say you do *not* automatically know what is meant. Nos. 1, 2, and 4 are not the best response because they *shift the focus* from the client's experience to the characteristics of the *other* person.

124. (4) Attempts to focus on encouraging the client to describe feelings are important. Nos. 1 and 2 ask for facts rather than focusing on feelings, and No. 3 is an example of reflecting—a therapeutic response, but in this case it only reflects a *thought,* not a feeling.

125. (4) This is the least threatening. No. 2 is not good because the nurse *needs* to intervene into a pattern of silence. It is not therapeutic for the focus to be on the *nurse,* as in Nos. 1 and 3, and bringing up a *controversial* topic (such as religion or politics) usually results in an exchange of opinions and arguments.

126. (2) Nos. 1 and 4 focus on *"there-and-then"* rather than "here-and-now" feelings and events, and No. 3 is *irrelevant* because the focus is on a *fact* rather than a feeling.

127. (4) Information that is given to the nurse that may interfere with the client's recovery needs to be related to other team members. The following are not the best response because: No. 1 is withholding information from other staff who are also responsible for care and may interfere with recovery needs; No. 2 is a refusal that may stop the interaction—a negotiation is needed; No. 3 does not provide a client with the clear feedback needed in order to work through conflict.

128. (3) Brief and specific information *can* be processed during severe anxiety. In severe anxiety, the person cannot respond to the social environment (as in No. 1); giving detailed information results in overload, as the client cannot retain and recall data (as in No. 2). Only directive information that is brief and specific is effective when the client cannot focus on what is happening. Decision making needs to be postponed until the person is less anxious; hence, No. 4 is wrong.

129. (4) Acknowledging a feeling tone is the most therapeutic response and provides a broad opening for the client to elaborate feelings. The following are not the best response because: No. 1 is false *reassurance* that does not allay feelings; No. 2 is asking a "*why*" question, which is confrontive and may increase anxiety; No. 3 gives *advice,* which stops exploration of underlying feelings.

130. (1) No. 1 is the best choice. Common reactions: pupilary dilation, *not* constriction (No. 2); diarrhea, *not* constipation (No. 4). Vomiting is not typical of an anxiety response (No. 3 is incorrect).

131. (2) In panic, a person is highly suggestible and follows "herd instinct" rather than exercising independent judgment and problem solving (No. 1). No. 3 is incorrect because the severity of the reaction *is* related to the severity of the threat. The more severe the perceived threat (actual or imaginary), the more intense the reaction to the danger, and *not* delayed as in No. 4.

132. (3) This is the most inclusive answer. Nos. 1, 2, and 4 are all *incorporated* into No. 3.

133. (2) Research shows *increased* activity is a psychomotor manifestation of anxiety; No. 1 is therefore wrong. Nos. 3 and 4 are incorrect because emotion is *not* a psychomotor manifestation.

134. (3) Research shows that anxiety *decreases* the perceptual field—No. 1 therefore is incorrect. Research also shows that anxiety *decreases* the ability to concentrate and *increases* random activity; therefore, Nos. 2 and 4 are incorrect.

135. (4) Some anxiety is necessary in order to learn. No. 2 is incorrect because it is *incomplete.* Nos. 1 and 3 are incorrect because anxiety *is necessary* for learning and growth.

136. (3) Projection is a coping mechanism. Most coping mechanisms are aimed at either reducing anxiety to the *self*-system or maintaining self-esteem. Although answer No. 2 may be correct at times, it is *not* so in *all* instances of projection. Denial may operate in *some* cases of projection. Nos. 1 and 4 are *not* good answers because the main focus of coping mechanisms is on *self, not on others.*

137. (4) By definition: No. 1 describes sublimation; No. 2, introjection; and No. 3, repression.

138. (1) It is the most comprehensive, inclusive choice, which may also *encompass* Nos. 2 and 4. Since regression is a coping mechanism, we know that the key purpose is to increase self-esteem and/or decrease anxiety; therefore, No. 3 does not fit, as expressing hostility does not necessarily increase esteem and/or decrease anxiety.

139. (2) No. 1 describes regression; No. 3, blocking; and No. 4, identification.

140. (1) By definition, this is the release of energy or impulses into socially acceptable outlets.

141. (1) By definition, No. 2 is suppression; No. 3, displacement; and No. 4, identification.

142. (3) By definition, this is the conscious, deliberate effort to avoid talking or thinking about painful, anxiety-producing experiences.

143. (1) Symbolism is the most clearly descriptive mechanism. No. 2, fantasy, is a mental activity; No. 3, isolation, is the exclusion from awareness of a feeling; and No. 4, conversion, is a disruption of motor or sensory functioning.

144. (2) Denial is the mind's way of protecting the self-system from a disturbing reality. No. 1, reaction formation, is an expression of an attitude opposite to unconscious feelings; No. 3, intellectualization, is giving rational reasons without expression of underlying feelings; No. 4, rationalization, is the attempt to make one's behavior look like the result of logical thinking.

145. (4) Correct by definition. No. 1 is incorrect because delusion is a fixed *idea* arising out of a person's inner needs and contrary to observed facts. No. 2 is incorrect because a hallucination is a misperception that is unrelated to an external stimulus. No. 3 is incorrect because identification is the process of taking on another person's attribute.

146. (1) No. 2 refers to preschool age; No. 3 is characteristic of "maturity" in later years of life; and No. 4 refers to young adulthood.

147. (4) The goal is to preserve ego strength through acceptance and respect of him as a person. No. 1 focuses on the tangential and irrelevant; No. 2 makes the problem more obvious to others in the room and makes an assumption without validation about how Johnny must feel; No. 3 is incorrect because it is usually not helpful to give a rational explanation for an emotional difficulty related to enuresis.

148. (3) Most children with Down are affectionate and enjoy being held and cuddled, whereas the *opposite* is usually the case with an autistic child. All other responses may apply to *both* Down and autism.

149. (3) Clients plan and lead activities rather than staff. Although families and significant others are brought in when needed, *family therapy* is neither a key feature nor an emphasis in milieu therapy. Thus, No. 1 is incorrect. Structured activities based on members' needs, rather than permissiveness (No. 2) is the keynote. Staff do participate *with* (not dominate) clients in discussing plans for activities; thus, No. 4 is wrong.

150. (1) If rules and regulations are at a minimum, clients can work out their own solutions. No. 2 is incorrect because imposed solutions do not allow for personal growth. No. 3 is incorrect because adults do not learn self-control from imposed rules but from working out their own rules. No. 4 is incorrect because it is important to teach people to reason and problem-solve about rules rather than to respond rigidly.

151. (4) This calls for *joint* client-staff planning and decision making. The other responses are typical of a high degree of direction by the staff, with clients in the passive-dependent role.

152. (2) One of the purposes of group therapy is to discover a universality of problems and a diversity of solutions. No. 1 is incorrect because people do not use authoritative answers, and to give authoritative answers lessens learning. No. 3 is incorrect because it is *not as complete* as No. 2. No. 4 is incorrect because the goal of therapy is to assist *clients,* not the therapist.

153. (4) The directive role decreases responsibility and independence in the client. All the other options are true.

154. (3) A contract early in therapy is essential to make expectations clear, which includes no scapegoating or blaming of one family member by another. The opposites of Nos. 2 and 4 are important to practice. It is crucial that nurses not take sides or try to referee a family fight, as suggested in No. 1.

155. (3) The client will be in a confused state after treatment and will require siderails and the reassuring presence of a nurse. Nos. 1 and 4 are incorrect because hunger and suicide are *not* immediate posttreatment concerns. No. 2 is incorrect because the client needs *someone* there to help orient him, as he is likely to wake up and be somewhat disoriented.

156. (4) The client is anxious and needs someone with him. No. 1 is incorrect because it *ignores* the client's anxiety and needs. No. 2 is incorrect because it also *ignores* the client's anxiety and uses the doctor as an excuse to ignore his needs. No. 3 is incorrect because it also *ignores* the client's anxiety and needs and gives a poor reason for refusal.

157. (2) Consistency lets clients know consequences of behavior and develops trust. No. 1 is incorrect because you *cannot approve all* behavior (e.g., destructive behavior). No. 3 is incorrect because it can be therapeutic *to express* negative opinions. No. 4 is incorrect because interpretation of behavior is *not* always advisable. Clients may use interpretations of behavior to avoid consequences of behavior or may see them as an excuse not to change behavior.

158. (4) Providing information is the *primary* sex health intervention. Nos. 1 and 2 are *secondary* health interventions. No. 3 is a *tertiary* intervention.

159. (2) Masturbation can provide appropriate sexual activity that enables a person to become comfortable with his or her sexual identity. No. 1 is incorrect because masturbation *can* be healthy. No. 3 is incorrect because masturbation *can* enhance heterosexual activity. No. 4 is the *opposite* of correct answer No. 2.

160. (4) The victim needs to engage in expression of the experience, which will assist her to work through her feelings so that the experience may not interfere in future interpersonal relations. To repress the incident, as in No. 1, would make it continually interfere in her relationship. No. 2 is only done *after* No. 4 has been accomplished. No. 3 is incorrect because the rape victim has *no* "part" in the rape.

161. (2) You are asking the client to clarify and further discuss feelings. No. 1 is incorrect because, while staying with the client *might* convey acceptance, it does *not help* him clarify or deal with feelings. No. 3 is incorrect because it cuts off any further response from the client and because it is *doubtful* that you can understand another person's feelings. No. 4 is incorrect because it is *more* important to *clarify* the client's *feelings* than it is to understand the *object* of hate.

162. (2) Note the eyes: when a person is *on* heroin, the pupils are constricted; during *withdrawal,* they are dilated. Withdrawal does *not* usually include high fever, pupil constriction, or choreiform movements, as in Nos. 1, 3, and 4.

163. (4) Methadone is a synthetic narcotic and has no euphoric effect. Methadone does not produce sedation (No. 1), euphoria (No. 2), or neuritis (No. 3).

164. (4) With concern for danger to the other clients, staff and the environment, it is essential for the client to be restrained at this time. The other choices are incorrect because: No. 1—orientation and a quiet environment *alone* do *not* provide for safety when the client's agitation is out of control; No. 2—the initial *delay* in onset of effectiveness of the tranquilizer does not *immediately* provide for the safety needs of other clients, staff, and the environment; No. 3—locking the client in her room eliminates only the danger to others, and additional measures would be needed to provide for the safety of this *client.*

165. (4) Based on the client's history of antisocial behavior, she is probably attempting to use the nurse for her own purpose and is not truthful. Therefore, it is best that the new nurse on the unit go directly to the head nurse to check on what is permissible and not accept the client's word that it is permissible. No. 1 is not helpful because allowing the client to unlock the door may feed into the manipulative attempt by the client to get off the unit. No. 2 is incorrect because asking a "why" question is not a therapeutic communication. No. 3 is incorrect because this option places the new nurse in an argumentative position with the client, who is likely to become defensive and say, "Oh, yes. I *am* allowed to open doors."

166. (3) Limit-setting is an important intervention with a client who exhibits excessive, constant dependence on others for simple, seemingly inconsequential decisions in everyday life. The other choices are wrong because the situation presented provides insufficient data on which to base interpretations related to fear of failure (No. 1), a need to test for staff acceptance of her (No. 2), or a bid for attention (No. 4).

MATERNAL-INFANT NURSING

■ UNIT

2

Nursing Care of the Childbearing Family

■ GROWTH AND DEVELOPMENT

BIOLOGIC FOUNDATIONS OF REPRODUCTION

General overview: This review of the structures, functions, and important assessment characteristics of the reproductive system provides essential components of the database required for accurate nursing judgments. Comparing normal characteristics and established patterns with nursing assessment findings assists in identifying client needs and in planning, implementing, and evaluating appropriate goal-directed nursing interventions.

Female Reproductive Anatomy and Physiology

I. Structure of pelvis (see Figure 2.1)

A. Two hip bones (right and left innominate: sacrum, coccyx).

B. False pelvis—upper portion above brim; supportive structure for uterus during last half of pregnancy.

C. True pelvis—below brim; pelvic inlet, midcavity, pelvic outlet comprise this structure. Fetus passes through during birth.

II. Pelvic measurements

A. Diagonal conjugate—12.5 cm or greater is adequate size; measured by examiner.

B. Conjugate vera—11 cm is adequate size; measured by X ray.

C. Obstetric conjugate—measured by X ray.

D. Tuber-ischial diameter—9 to 11 cm indicates adequate size; measured by examiner.

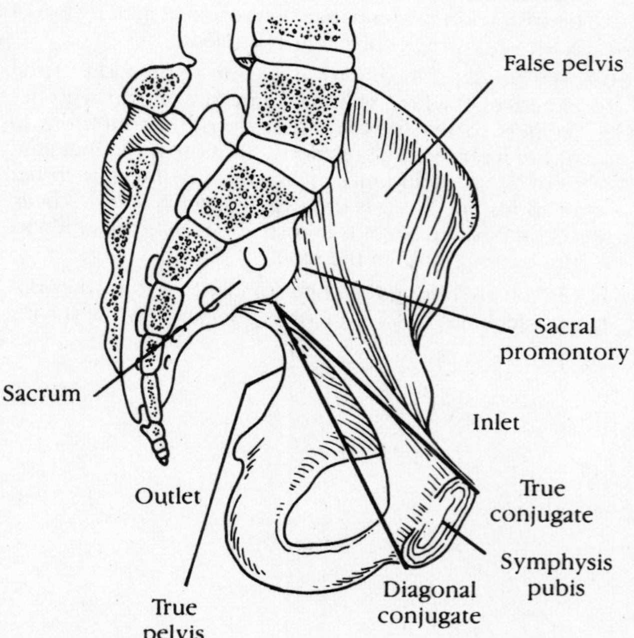

■ **FIGURE 2.1**
The female pelvis.

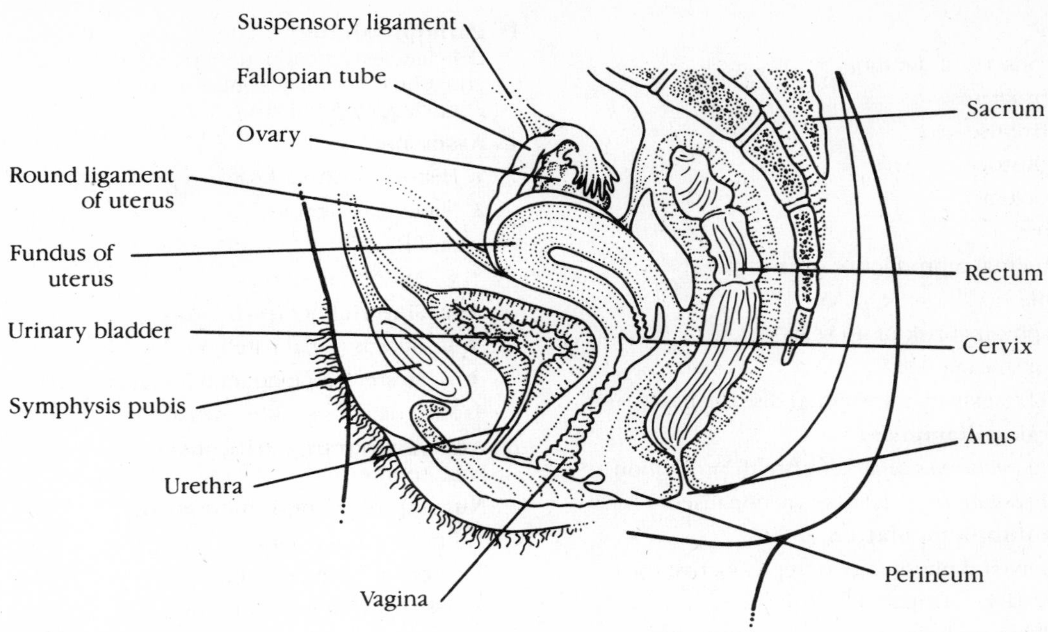

■ **FIGURE 2.2**
Female internal reproductive organs.

III. Female external organs

A. Mons veneris—protects symphysis.

B. Labia majora—covers, protects labia minora.

C. Labia minora—2 located within labia majora.

D. Clitoris—small erectile tissue.

E. Hymen—thin membrane at opening of vagina.

F. Urinary meatus—opening of urethra.

G. Bartholin glands—producer of alkaline secretions that enhance sperm motility, viability.

IV. Internal structures (see Figure 2.2)

A. Vagina—outlet for menstrual flow, depository of semen, lower birth canal.

B. Cervix—uterine outlet.

C. Uterus—muscular organ that houses fetus during gestation.

D. Fallopian tubes—2 tubes stretching from cornua of uterus to ovaries; transports ovum.

E. Ovaries—2 oval-shaped structures that produce ovum and hormones (estrogen and progesterone).

F. Breasts—2 mammary glands capable of secreting milk for infant nourishment.

V. Menstrual cycle

A. Reproductive hormones

1. *FSH* (Follicle Stimulating Hormone)—secreted during the first half of cycle; stimulates development of graafian follicle; secreted by anterior pituitary.
2. *ICSH or LH* (Interstitial Cell Stimulating Hormone, Luteinizing Hormone)—stimulates ovulation and development of corpus luteum; secreted by pituitary.
3. *Estrogen*—assists in ovarian follicle maturation; stimulates endometrial thickening; responsible for development of secondary sex characteristics; maintains endometrium during pregnancy. Secreted by ovaries and adrenal cortex during cycle and by placenta during pregnancy.
4. *Progesterone*—aids in endometrial thickening; facilitates secretory changes; relaxes smooth muscle; causes cervical secretions to become hostile to sperm once conception occurs. Secreted by corpus luteum and placenta.
5. *Prostaglandins*—substances produced by various body organs that act hormonally on the endometrium to influence the onset and continuation of labor. A medication that may be used to facilitate onset of second trimester abortion; also used to efface the cervix prior to induction of labor in term pregnancies.

B. Ovulation—growth and release of nonfertilized egg from ovary; generally occurs midcycle 14 days before beginning of next menses.

C. Menstruation—vaginal discharge of blood and fragments of the endometrium; cyclic; occurs in response to dropping levels of estrogen and progesterone.

D. Fertilization—impregnation of ovum by sperm.

E. Implantation—fertilized ovum attaches to uterine wall for growth.

F. Menopause—normally occurring cessation of menses with gradual decrease in amount of flow and increase in the time between periods at end of fertility cycle; average age, 53. Early menopause rare but may be influenced by hypothyroidism, surgical ovarian removal, overexposure to radiation. Treatments during menopause for symptom relief: hormonal replacement therapy, vitamins B and E for hot flashes, vaginal creams for dyspareunia (painful intercourse), and calcium for osteoporosis.

G. Spinnbarkheit—stretchable, thin cervical mucus present at ovulation.

VI. Assessment of reproductive tract/reproductive health

A. Health history
   1. Menarche: onset and duration.
   2. Menstrual problems.
   3. Contraceptive use.
   4. Pregnancy history.
   5. Fertility problems.

B. Physical exam
   1. External, internal reproductive organs.
   2. Breast exam.
   3. Mammography, if at risk or 40 years old.
   4. Periodic Pap smears.
   5. Tests for STD (sexually transmitted diseases).

VII. Analysis/nursing diagnosis:

A. *Health-seeking behaviors* related to health promotion.

B. *Health-seeking behaviors* related to menopause.

VIII. Nursing plan/implementation:

A. Discuss anatomy and physiology of reproductive tract.

B. Review menstruation, ovulation, fertilization.

C. Explain need for periodic Pap smears, annual gynecologic exams, including mammography.

IX. Evaluation: client displays basic understanding of anatomy and physiology; understands cycle and contraception; regularly seeks preventive care and performs monthly breast self-exams.

DECISION MAKING REGARDING REPRODUCTION

General overview: During the reproductive years, the sexually active client often faces the decision to postpone, prevent, or terminate a pregnancy. The nursing role focuses on assisting the client to make an informed decision consistent with individual needs.

I. Family planning

A. Assessment:
   1. Determine interest in and present knowledge of methods of family planning.
   2. Identify factors affecting choice of method: cultural and religious objections, contraindications for individual methods, motivation/ability to follow chosen method successfully, financial considerations.

B. Analysis/nursing diagnosis: *Knowledge deficit* regarding family planning methods/options.

C. Nursing plan/implementation—Goal: *health teaching*—to facilitate informed decision making, selection of option appropriate to individual needs, desires.
   1. Describe, explain, discuss options available and appropriate to individual client. Include information on advantages and hazards of each option (Tables 2.1, 2.2).
   2. Demonstrate, as necessary, method selected.

D. Evaluation:
   1. Avoids or achieves a pregnancy as desired.
   2. Expresses comfort and satisfaction with method selected.

II. Infertility

A. Definition: inability to conceive after 1 year of unprotected intercourse.

B. Pathophysiology: contributing factors—hormonal deficiencies, reproductive system mechanical disorders, congenital anomalies, male impotence, sexual knowledge deficit, debilitating disease.

C. Assessment:
   1. History—general health, reproduction, social history.
   2. Maternal diagnosis
      a. BBT.
      b. Endocrine studies.
      ▶ c. Sims-Huhner (postcoital).
      ▶ d. Rubins (tubal patency).
      ▶ e. Hysterosalpingogram (tubal patency).
   3. Male diagnosis—semen analysis.

D. Analysis/nursing diagnosis: *Altered sexuality* related to infertility.

E. Nursing plan/implementation:
   1. Emotional support.
   2. Explain testing procedures for diagnosis.
   3. Assist with referral process.

■ CHILDBEARING: PREGNANCY BY TRIMESTER

General overview: This review of the normal physiologic and psychosocial changes occurring during each trimester of pregnancy provides essential components of the data base for accurate nursing judgments and anticipatory guidance during the prenatal period. Complications of pregnancy are correlated with the trimester of common occurrence; relationships with other NCLEX categories of human function are described.

I. General aspects of nursing care

A. Assessment—based on nursing knowledge of:
   1. Biophysical and psychosocial aspects of conception and gestation.
   2. Parameters of normal pregnancy.
   3. Risk factors, signs, symptoms, and implications of deviations from normal patterns of maternal and fetal health.

B. Analysis/nursing diagnosis:
   1. *Knowledge deficit* re: normal pregnancy-related alterations (physiologic and emotional alterations/trimester).
   2. *Pain* related to normal physiologic alterations in pregnancy.
   3. *Altered urinary elimination* related to normal physiologic changes during pregnancy (polyuria, constipation).
   4. *Altered nutrition* related to increased metabolic needs due to pregnancy.
   5. *Impaired adjustment* related to altered self-image; anticipated role change; resurgence of old, unresolved conflicts.

C. Nursing plan/implementation:
   1. Goal: *emotional support.*
      a. Encourage verbalization of feelings, fears, concerns.

TABLE 2.1 Contraception

Method	Action	Advantages	Disadvantages and Side Effects	Effectiveness
Oral Contraceptives				
Combination of estrogen and progesterone.	Suppresses ovulation by suppressing production of FSH and LH.	Convenient. Easy to take. Menstrual cycles are predictable.	*Hazards*—thrombus formation, thrombophlebitis, pulmonary embolus, and hypertension in women over 35. *Contraindicated* in obesity, hypertension, sickle cell or liver disease, heavy smokers, diabetes, migraine headaches, and over 35 years of age.	Most efficient form of contraception (99.7%) if used consistently.
Minipill—progesterone (norethindrone 0.35 mg daily).	Antifertility effect. Makes cervical mucus impervious to sperm and alters endometrium. Ovulation does occur most of the time.	May reduce side effects found with other oral preparations.	Menstrual irregularity. Lumps in breast. Affects cholesterol.	Undetermined. Can reach 98% reliability if used exactly as prescribed.
Intrauterine Devices (IUDs)				
Made of soft plastic Medicated: • progesterone • copper	• Exerts progesterone effect on endometrium and cervical mucus. • Spermicidal effect.	No interference with hormonal regulation of menstrual cycle.	*Hazards*—unnoticed expulsion, uterine perforation, and/or intrauterine or fallopian infection. ↑risk of spontaneous abortion, preterm labor. *Side effects*—heavy flow, spotting between periods, and cramping.	Effectiveness rate, 90–99%.
Mechanical Barriers				
Diaphragm—shallow rubber device that fits over cervix.	Barrier preventing sperm from entering cervix if it is correct size and correctly placed.	Safety—no side effects.	Add spermicide before using. Must insert prior to intercourse and leave for 6 hours after last intercourse. Requires careful cleansing, checking for tears, and storage away from heat; powder with cornstarch. Recheck size after each baby, every 2 years, or after weight loss/gain of 10 lbs. or more.	Effectiveness improved if a spermicidal foam, jelly, or cream is also used. Effectiveness rate, 80–85%.
Condom—thin, stretchable latex sheath to cover penis.	Barrier preventing sperm from entering vagina. Is applied over erect penis.	Safety—no side effects. Protective measure against spread of sexually transmitted infections.	Preejaculatory drops also contain sperm; conception possible even when drops fall around *external* vaginal opening. Sheath may tear during intercourse.	Spermicidal foam, jelly, or cream is also used and sheath is held in place as penis is withdrawn. Effectiveness rate, 64–98% when used with spermicide.
Chemical Barriers				
Spermicide—foam, jelly, cream, or vaginal suppository, C-film.	Kills sperm. Decreases sperm motility.	Increases effectiveness of mechanical barriers. Ease of application. Aids lubrication of vagina. Requires no medical examination or prescription.	If it is only method being used, each intercourse should be preceded (by 30 minutes) by a fresh application. May be allergenic.	Effectiveness rate 70–98% when used with diaphragm or condoms.

continued

TABLE 2.1 (Continued)

Method	Action	Advantages	Disadvantages and Side Effects	Effectiveness
Other Methods				
Natural family planning—BBT each morning before any physical activity. Symptothermal variation—BBT plus cervical mucus changes.	Requires sexual abstinence during woman's fertile period (3 days before ovulation plus 1 day after).	Physically safe to use—no drugs or appliances are used. Meets requirements of most religions.	Effectiveness depends on high level of motivation and diligence. Requires fairly predictable menstrual cycle.	Effectiveness may be increased by accuracy of assessment. Effectiveness rate, 75–98%.

b. Validate normalcy of behavioral response to pregnancy.

2. Goal: *anticipatory guidance.*
   a. Facilitate achievement of developmental tasks.
   b. Strengthen coping techniques for pregnancy, labor, delivery. Suggest appropriate resources (preparation for childbirth classes).
3. Goal: *health teaching.* Describe, explain, discuss:
   a. Normal physiologic alterations during pregnancy.
   b. Common discomforts of pregnancy, management.

D. Evaluation:

1. Takes an active, informed part in own pregnancy-related care.
2. Copes effectively with common alterations associated with pregnancy (physiologic, psychologic, role-change).
3. Successfully carries an uneventful pregnancy to term.

II. Biologic foundations of pregnancy

A. Conception

1. *Egg*—life span, approximately 24 hours after ovulation.
2. *Sperm*—life span, approximately 72 hours after ejaculation into female reproductive tract.
3. *Conception* (fertilization)—usually occurs 12–24 hours after ovulation, within fallopian tube.
4. *Implantation* (nidation)—usually occurs within 7 days of conception, or about day 21 of a 28-day menstrual cycle.
5. *Ovum*—period of conception until primary villi have appeared; usually about 12–14 days.
6. *Embryo*—period from end of ovum stage until measurement reaches approximately 3 cm; 54–56 days (see Figure 2.3).
7. *Fetus*—period from end of embryo stage until the pregnancy is terminated.

B. Anatomic and physiologic modifications

1. *Bases of functional alterations*
   a. *Hormonal*—see Table 2.3 for discussion of the effects of estrogen and progesterone during pregnancy. Nursing implications provide the knowledge base for:
      (1) Anticipatory guidance regarding normal maternal adaptations.

TABLE 2.2 Sterilization

Method	Action	Advantages	Disadvantages and Side Effects	Effectiveness
Men				
Vasectomy	Vas deferens is ligated and severed, interrupting passage of sperm.	Relatively simple surgical procedure. Does not affect endocrine function, production of testosterone. Does not alter volume of ejaculate.	Some men become impotent due to psychologic response to procedure. Reversible in 20–40% of cases.	100% effective after ejaculate is free of sperm that was in vas deferens (about 3 months or ten ejaculations).
Women				
Tubal ligation	Both fallopian tubes are ligated and severed, preventing passage of eggs; fulguration of the tubes at the cornu is most effective.	Abdominal surgery utilizing 1-inch incision and laparoscopy.	Major surgery (if done by laparotomy) with possible complications of anesthesia, infection, hemorrhage, and trauma to other organs. Psychologic trauma in some.	Greater than 99.5% effective.

Source: Bobak I et al.: *Sterilization and Gynecologic Care*, St. Louis, 1989, Mosby.

First Trimester

- Great danger to teratogens.
- Heart functions at 3–4 weeks.
- Eye formation at 4–5 weeks.
- Arm and leg buds at 4–5 weeks.
- Recognizable face at 8 weeks.
- Brain: rapid growth.
- External genitalia at 8 weeks.
- Placenta formed at 12 weeks.
- Bone ossification at 12 weeks.

Second Trimester

- Less danger from teratogens after 12 weeks.
- Facial features formed at 16 weeks.
- Fetal heart beat heard at 20 weeks.
- Quickening at 18–20 weeks.
- Length: 10 in., weight: 8–10 oz.
- Vernix: present.

Third Trimester

- Iron stored.
- Surfactant production begins in increasing amounts.
- Size: 15 in., 2–3 lb.
- Calcium stored at 28–32 weeks.
- Reflexes present at 28–32 weeks.
- Subcutaneous fat deposits at 36 weeks.
- Lanugo shedding at 38–40 weeks.
- Average size: 18–22 in., 7.5–8.5 lb at 38–40 weeks.

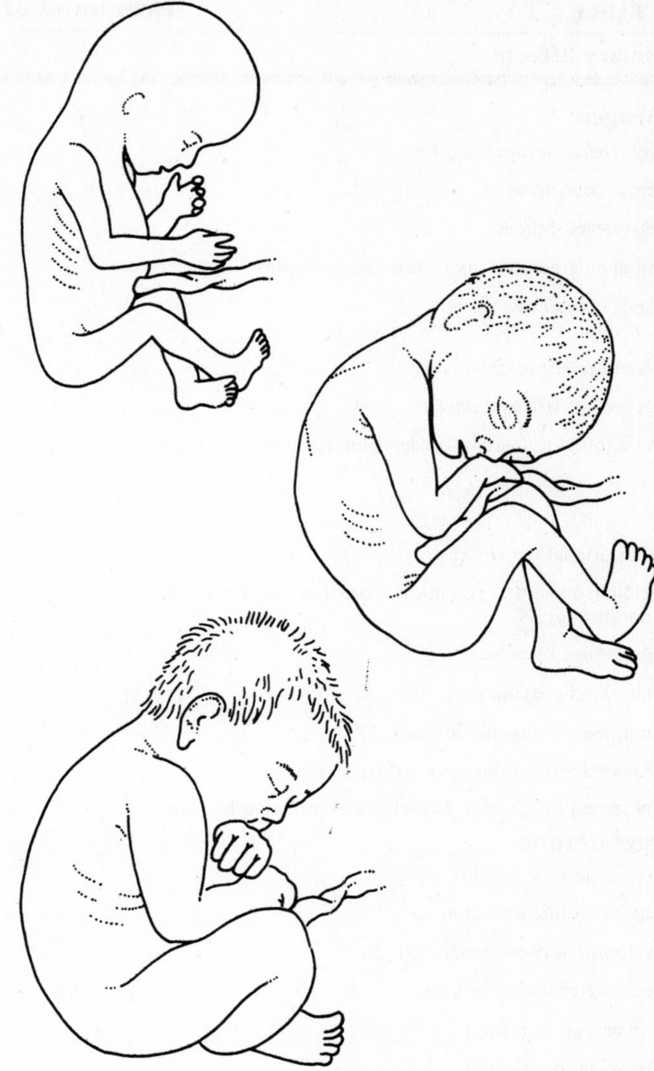

FIGURE 2.3
Milestones of embryonic development.

(2) Early identification of deviations from normal patterns.

b. *Mechanical*—enlarging uterus → displacement and pressure; increased weight of uterus and breasts → changes in posture and pressure.

2. *Breasts*—enlarged darkened areola; secrete colostrum.

3. *Reproductive organs*

a. *Uterus*

(1) Amenorrhea. Occasional spotting common, especially at time of first missed menstrual period.

(2) Increased vascularity adds to increase in size and softening of the lower uterine segment (*Hegar's sign*).

(3) Growth is due to hypertrophy and hyperplasia of existing muscle cells and connective tissue.

b. *Cervix*

(1) Increased vascularity → softening (*Goodell's sign*) and deepened blue-purple coloration (*Chadwick's sign*).

(2) Edema, hyperplasia, thickening of mucous lining, and increased mucus production; formation of mucous plug by end of second month.

(3) Becomes shorter, thicker, and more elastic.

c. *Vagina*

(1) Hyperemia deepens color (*Chadwick's sign*).

(2) Hypertrophy and hyperplasia thicken vaginal mucosa.

(3) Relaxation of connective tissue.

(4) pH acidic (4.0–6.0).

(5) Leukorrhea—nonirritating.

■ **TABLE 2.3** **Hormones of Pregnancy**

Primary Effects	Clinical Implications for Nursing Actions
Estrogen	
Level rises in serum and urine.	Basis of test for maternal/placental/fetal well-being.
Uterine development.	Probable sign of pregnancy.
Breast development.	Probable sign of pregnancy; increased tingling, tenderness.
Genital enlargement: increased vascularization, hyperplasia.	Vaginal growth facilitates vaginal birth.
Softens connective tissue.	Results in back- and leg ache; relaxes joints to increase size of birth canal and rib cage.
Alters nutrient metabolism:	*GI and metabolic changes:*
Decreases HCl and pepsin.	Digestive upsets.
Antagonist to insulin—makes glucose available to fetus.	Antiinsulin effect challenges maternal pancreas to produce more insulin; failure of β-cells to respond leads to "gestational" diabetes. For the insulin-dependent woman, insulin requirements increase by an average of 67% during the second half of pregnancy.
Supports fat deposition.	Protect source of energy for fetus.
Sodium and water retention; edema of lower extremities (nonpitting).	Meet increased plasma volume needs and maintain fluid reserve.
Hematologic changes:	
Increased coagulability.	Increased tendency to thrombosis.
Increased sedimentation rate (SR).	SR loses diagnostic value for heart disease.
Vasodilation: spider nevi; palmar erythema.	Resolves spontaneously after delivery.
Increased production of melanin-stimulating hormone.	Resolves spontaneously after delivery.
Progesterone	
Development of decidua.	High levels result in tiredness, listlessness, and sleepiness.
Reduces uterine excitability.	Protection against abortion/early delivery.
Development of mammary glands.	Prepares breasts for lactation.
Alters nutrient metabolism:	*Nutritional significance:*
Antagonist to insulin.	Diabetogenic.
Favors fat deposition.	Energy reserve.
Decreases gastric motility and relaxes sphincters.	Favors heartburn and constipation.
Increased sensitivity of respiratory center to CO_2.	Increased depth, some dyspnea, increased sighing.
Decreased smooth muscle tone:	*Decreased tone can lead to:*
Colon.	Constipation.
Bladder, ureters.	Stasis of urine with infection.
Veins.	Dependent edema; varicosities.
Gallbladder.	Gallbladder disease.
Increased basal body temperature (BBT) by 0.5° C.	Discomfort from hot flashes and perspiration.
Human Chorionic Gonadotropin	
Maintains corpus luteum during early pregnancy.	Placenta must "take over" after a few weeks.
Stimulates male testes.	Increased testosterone in male fetuses.
May suppress immune response.	May inhibit response to foreign protein, for example, fetal portion of placenta.
	Diagnostic value:
	Basis for pregnancy test.
	Hydatidiform mole.
	Decreased level with threatened abortion.
	Increased level with multiple pregnancy.

TABLE 2.3 *(Continued)*

Primary Effects	Clinical Implications for Nursing Actions
Human Placental Lactogen (Human Chorionic Somatotropin)	
Antagonizes insulin.	Diabetogenic; may→gestational diabetes or complicate management of existing diabetes.
Mobilizes maternal free fatty acids.	Increased tendency to ketoacidosis in pregnant diabetic.
Prolactin	
Suppressed by estrogen and progesterone.	No milk produced before delivery.
Increased level after placenta is delivered.	Milk production 2–3 days after birth.
Follicle Stimulating Hormone	
Production suppressed during pregnancy; level returns to prepregnant levels within 3 weeks after birth.	No ovulation during pregnancy. Ovulation usually returns: within 6 weeks for 15%, within 12 weeks for 30%.
Oxytocin	
Causes uterus to contract when the oxytocin levels exceed those of estrogen and progesterone.	Labor induction or augmentation. Treatment for postpartum uterine atony.

d. *Perineum*
   (1) Increases in size—hypertrophy of muscle cells, edema, and relaxation of elastic tissue.
   (2) Deepened color—increased vascularization/hyperemia.

e. *Ovaries*
   (1) Ovum production ceases.
   (2) Corpus luteum persists; produces hormones to week 10–12 until placenta "takes over."

C. Alterations affecting fluid-gas transport

1. *Cardiovascular system* (see Table 2.4)
   a. **Physiologic changes**
      (1) Heart displaced upward and to the left.
      (2) Circulation:
         (a) Cardiac volume increases by 20 to 30%.
         (b) Labor—cardiac output increases by 20 to 30%.
      (3) Hemoglobin and hematocrit values remain between 10–14 gm and 35–42%; normal drop is 10% during second trimester.
      (4) Hypercoagulability—increased levels of blood factors VII, IX, and X.
      (5) Nonpathologic increased sedimentation rate—due to 50% increase in fibrinogen level.
      (6) Blood pressure should remain stable with drop in second trimester.
      (7) Heart rate often increases 10–15 beats/min at term.
      (8) Compression of pelvic veins → stasis of blood in lower extremities.
      (9) Compression of inferior vena cava when supine → bradycardia → *reduced* cardiac output, faintness, sweating, nausea. *Fetal response:* marked bradycardia due to hypoxia secondary to decreased placental perfusion.
   b. **Assessment**
      (1) Apical systolic murmur.
      (2) Exaggerated splitting of first heart sound.
      (3) Physiologic anemia.
      (4) Dependent edema in third trimester.

TABLE 2.4 Blood Values

Component	Prepregnant	Pregnant	Postpartum*
WBC	4–11,000	9–16,000 (25,000–labor)	20,000–25,000 within 10–12 days of delivery, then returns to normal.
RBC volume	1600 mL	1900 mL	Prepregnant level of 1600 mL.
Plasma volume	2400 mL	3700 mL	Prepregnant level of 2400 mL.
Hct (PCV)	37–47%	32–42%	At 72°, returns to prepregnant level of 37–42%.
Hgb (at sea level)	12–16 g/dL	10–14 g/dL	At 72°, returns to prepregnant level of 12–16 g/dL.
Fibrinogen	250 mg/dL	400 mg/dL	At 72°, returns to prepregnant level of 250 mg/dL.

*Postpartum values depend on factors of amount of blood loss, mobilization and physiologic edema (excretion of extravascular water). Normal blood loss for vaginal delivery is 300–400 cc.

(5) Vena cava syndrome (supine hypotension)—drop in systolic blood pressure may occur due to compression of descending aorta and inferior vena cava when supine.

(6) Varicosities (vulvar, anal, leg).

c. **Nursing care plan/implementation:** Goal: *health teaching*

(1) Elevate lower extremities frequently.

(2) Apply support hose.

(3) Avoid excess intake of sodium.

(4) Assume left-side lying position at rest.

(5) Teach woman signs and symptoms of pregnancy-induced hypertension.

2. *Respiratory system*

a. **Physiologic changes**

(1) Increased tidal volume, vital capacity, respiratory reserve, oxygen consumption, production of CO_2.

(2) Diaphragm elevated, increased substernal angle → flaring of rib cage.

(3) Uterine enlargement prevents maximum lung expansion in third trimester.

b. **Assessment**

(1) Dyspnea on exertion and when lying flat in third trimester.

(2) Nasal stuffiness due to estrogen-induced edema.

(3) Deeper respiratory excursion.

c. **Nursing care plan/implementation:** Goal: *health teaching*

(1) Sit and stand with good posture.

(2) When resting assume semi-Fowler's position.

(3) Avoid overdistention of stomach.

D. Alterations affecting elimination

1. *Urinary system*

a. **Physiologic changes**

(1) Relaxation of smooth muscle results in conditions that can persist 4–6 weeks after delivery:

(a) Dilatation of ureters.

(b) *Decreased* bladder tone.

(c) Increased potential for urinary stasis and *infection* (UTI).

(2) *Increased* glomerular filtration rate (50%) during last two trimesters.

(3) *Increased* renal plasma flow (25–50%) during first two trimesters; returns to near normal levels by end of last trimester.

(4) *Increased* renal-tubular reabsorption rate—compensates for increased glomerular activity.

(5) Glycosuria common—reflects kidney's inability to reabsorb all glucose filtered by glomeruli (urine glucose not reliable index of diabetic status during pregnancy).

(6) *Increased* renal clearance of urea and creatinine (creatinine clearance used as test of renal function during pregnancy).

(7) Hormone-induced turgescence of bladder and pressure on bladder from gravid uterus.

b. **Assessment**

(1) Urinary frequency, first and third trimesters.

(2) Nocturia.

(3) Stress incontinence in third trimester.

c. **Nursing plan/implementation:** Goal: *health teaching*

(1) Void with urge to prevent bladder distention.

(2) Teach signs and symptoms of UTI.

(3) Decrease fluid intake in late evening.

(4) Teach Kegel exercises to reduce incontinence.

2. *Gastrointestinal system*

a. **Physiologic changes**

(1) General decrease in smooth muscle tone and motility due to actions of progesterone.

(2) *Intestines:* slowed peristalsis, increased water reabsorption in bowel.

(3) *Stomach*

(a) Gastric emptying time is delayed (e.g., 3 hours vs. 1½ hours).

(b) Gastric secretion of HCl and pepsin decreases.

(c) Decreased motility delays emptying; increased acidity.

(4) *Cardiac sphincter* relaxes.

(5) Increasing size of *uterus* and displacement of *intra-abdominal organs.*

(6) *Gallbladder:* decreased emptying.

b. **Assessment**

(1) Nausea and vomiting in first trimester.

(2) Constipation and flatulence.

(3) Hemorrhoids.

(4) Heartburn, reflux esophagitis, indigestion.

(5) Hiatal hernia.

(6) Epulis—edema and bleeding of gums.

(7) Ptyalism—excessive salivation.

(8) Jaundice.

(9) Gall stones.

(10) Pruritus due to increased retention of bile salts.

c. **Nursing care plan/implementation:** Goal: *health teaching*

(1) Nausea and vomiting

(a) Avoid fatty food; increase carbohydrates.

(b) Eat small, frequent meals.

(c) Eat dry crackers in A.M.

(d) Decrease liquids with meals.

(e) Avoid odors that predispose to nausea.

(2) Constipation and flatulence

(a) Increase fluids (6–8 glasses/day).

(b) Maintain exercise regimen.

(c) Add fiber to diet.

(d) Avoid mineral oil laxatives.

(e) Avoid gas-producing foods (i.e., beans, cabbage).

(3) Heartburn and indigestion

(a) Eliminate fatty or spicy foods.

(b) Eat small, frequent meals (6/day).

(c) Eat slowly.

(d) Avoid gastric irritants (i.e., alcohol, coffee).

(e) Perform "flying exercises."

(f) Avoid lying flat.

(g) Take antacids without sodium or phosphorus.

(h) Sip milk or eat yogurt with heartburn.

(i) Avoid sodium bicarbonate.

(4) Hemorrhoids

(a) Increase fluid and fiber intake.

(b) Maintain exercise regimen.

(c) Avoid constipation and straining to defecate.

(d) Take warm sitz baths.

(e) Apply witch hazel pads.

(f) Elevate hips and legs frequently.

(g) Use hemorrhoidal ointments only with advice of health care provider.

E. Alterations affecting nutrition:

1. **Physiologic changes**

a. *Gastrointestinal system*

(1) Gingivae soften and enlarge due to increased vascularity.

(2) Increased saliva production.

b. *Endocrine system*

(1) *Increased* size and activity of pituitary, parathyroids, adrenals.

(2) *Increased* vascularity and hyperplasia of thyroid.

(3) Pancreas—*increased* insulin production during second half of pregnancy, needed to meet rising maternal needs; placental HPL and insulinase deactivate maternal insulin; may precipitate *gestational diabetes* in susceptible women.

c. *Metabolism*

(1) Basal metabolic rate (BMR)—*increases* 25% as pregnancy progresses, due to increasing oxygen consumption; protein-bound iodine (PBI) *increases* to 7–10 μg/dL; metabolism returns to normal by sixth postpartal week.

(2) Protein—need *increased* for fetal and uterine growth, maternal blood formation.

(3) Water retention—*increased.*

(4) Carbohydrates—need *increases* in order to spare protein stores.

(a) *First half of pregnancy*—glucose rapidly and continuously siphoned across placenta to meet fetal growth needs; may lead to hypoglycemia and faintness.

(b) *Second half of pregnancy*—placental production of antiinsulin hormones; normal maternal hyperglycemia; affects coexisting diabetes.

(5) Fat—*increased* plasma-lipid levels.

(6) Iron—supplements recommended to meet *increased* need for red blood cells by maternal/placental/fetal unit.

2. **Assessment**

a. Weight gain: 20–30 lb (Average gain, 24 lb).

b. Normal pattern: first trimester, 1 lb/mo; remainder of gestation, 0.9–1 lb/wk.

3. **Nursing care plan/implementation:** Goal: *health teaching*

a. Evaluate diet for adequacy of nutrient and caloric intake.

b. Evaluate cultural, religious, and economic influences on diet.

c. Review dietary recommendation for pregnancy with woman.

d. Avoid dieting in pregnancy (even if obese).

e. Supplement diet with vitamins, iron, or folic acid on advice of health provider.

f. Ptyalism:

(1) Suck hard candies.

(2) Perform frequent oral hygiene.

(3) Maintain adequate oral intake (6–8 glasses/day).

(4) Use lip balm to prevent chapping.

g. Epulis:

(1) Frequent oral hygiene.

(2) Use soft toothbrush.

(3) Floss gently.

(4) See dentist regularly.

F. Alterations affecting protective functions—*integumentary system*

1. **Physiologic changes**—Estrogen-induced vascular and pigment changes.

2. **Assessment**

a. Increased pigmentation.

b. Striae gravidarum (stretch marks).

c. Increased sebaceous and sweat gland activity.

d. Palmar erythema.

e. Angiomas—vascular "spiders."

3. **Nursing care plan/implementation:** Goal: *health teaching*

a. Bathe or shower daily.

b. Reassure woman that skin changes decrease after pregnancy.

G. Alterations affecting comfort, rest, mobility—*musculoskeletal system*

1. Progesterone, estrogen, and relaxin-induced relaxation of joints, cartilage, and ligaments.

2. Function in childbearing—increases anteroposterior diameter of rib cage and enlarges birth canal.

3. **Assessment:**

a. Complaint of pelvic "looseness."

b. Duck-waddle walk.

c. Tenderness of symphysis pubis.

d. Lordosis (exaggerated lumbar curve)—*increased* weight of pelvis tilts pelvis forward; to compensate, woman throws head and shoulders backward; complaint of leg and back strain and fatigue.

4. **Nursing plan/implementation:** Goal: *health teaching*

■ TABLE 2.5 Common Discomforts During Pregnancy

Discomfort and Cause	Health Teaching
Morning sickness—first 3 months; nausea and vomiting; may occur anytime, day or night; *cause*: hormonal, psychologic, and empty stomach.	Alternate dry carbohydrate and fluids hourly; take dry carbohydrate before rising, stay in bed 15 more minutes; avoid empty stomach, offending odors, and food difficult to digest (food high in fat, for example).
Fatigue (sleep hunger)—first 3 months; *cause:* possibly hormones. Often returns in late pregnancy when physical load is great.	Iron supplement if anemic—foods high in iron, folic acid, and protein. Adequate rest.
Fainting (syncope)—early pregnancy; due to slightly decreased arterial blood pressure; late pregnancy, due to venous stasis in lower extremities.	Elevate feet; sit down when necessary. When standing, do not lock knees; avoid prolonged standing; prolonged fasting.
Urinary frequency—enlarging uterus presses on bladder, turgescence of structures from hormone stimulation; relieved somewhat as uterus rises from pelvis; recurs with lightening.	Kegel's exercises; limit fluids just before bedtime to ensure rest. Rule out urinary tract infection.
Vaginal discharge—months 2–9, mucus, acid, and increases in amount.	Cleanliness important. Treat only if infection sets in; douche contraindicated in pregnancy.
Hot flashes—heat intolerance, due to increased metabolism → diaphoresis.	Alter clothing, bathing, and environmental temperature p.r.n.
Headache—cause unknown; possibly blood pressure change, nutritional, tension (unless associated with preeclampsia).	If pain relief needed, consult physician (avoid aspirin without prescription). Reduce tension.
Nasal stuffiness—due to increased vascularization; allergic rhinitis of pregnancy.	Antihistamines and nasal sprays by *prescription only*.
Heartburn—enlarging uterus and hormones slow digestion; progesterone → reverse peristaltic waves → reflux of stomach contents into esophagus.	Physician may prescribe an antacid; "flying exercise"; avoid use of antacids containing sodium. Instead of leaning over, bend at the knees, keeping torso straight; sit on firm chairs; limit fatty and fried foods in diet; small, frequent meals.
Flatulence—altered digestion from enlarging uterus and hormones.	Maintain regular bowel habits, avoid gas-forming foods. Antiflatulent may be prescribed.
Insomnia—fetal movements, fears or concerns, and general body discomfort from heavy uterus.	Medication by prescription only. Exercise; side-lying positions with pillow supports; change position often; backrubs, ventilate feelings.
Shortness of breath—enlarging uterus limits expansion of diaphragm.	Good posture; cut down/stop smoking; position—supine and upright.
Backache—increased elasticity of connective tissue, increased weight of uterus, and increased lumbar curvature.	Correct posture, low-heeled, wide-base shoes, and diet; do pelvic rock often; avoid fatigue.
Pelvic joint pain—hormones relax connective tissue and joints and allow movement within joints.	Rest; good posture; will go away after delivery, in 6–8 weeks.
Leg cramps—pressure of enlarging uterus on nerve supplying legs; possible causes: lack of calcium, fatigue, chilling, and tension.	Stretch affected muscle and hold until it subsides; *do not rub* (may release a blood clot, if present).
Constipation—decreased motility (hormones, enlarging uterus) and increased reabsorption of water; iron therapy (oral).	Diet—prunes, fruits, vegetables, roughage, and fluids; regular habits; exercise; sit on toilet with knees up. Avoid enemas, mineral oil, laxatives.
Hemorrhoids—varicosities around anus; aggravated by pushing with stool and by uterus pressing on blood vessels supplying lower body.	As above, avoid constipation. Pure Vaseline or Desitin are mild and sometimes soothing; use any other preparation with prescription only.
Ankle edema—normal and nonpitting; gravity.	Rest legs often during day with legs and hips raised.
Varicose veins—lower legs, vulva, pelvis; pressure of heavy uterus; relaxation of connective tissue in vein walls; hereditary.	Progressively worse with subsequent pregnancies and obesity; elevate legs above level of heart; support hose may help.
Cramp in side or groin—round ligament pain; stretching of round ligament with cramping.	To get out of bed, turn to side, use arm and upper body and push up to sitting position.

TABLE 2.6 Behavioral Changes in Pregnancy

Assessment/Characteristics	Nursing Plan/Implementation
First Trimester	
Emotional lability (mood swings).	Encourage verbalization of feelings, concerns.
Displeasure with subjective symptoms of early pregnancy (nausea, fatigue, etc.).	Validate normalcy of feelings, behaviors.
Feelings of ambivalence.	*Health teaching:* diet, rest, relaxation, diversion.
Second Trimester	
Accepts pregnancy (usually coincides with awareness of fetal movement, i.e., "quickening").	Encourage exploration of feelings of dependency, introspection, mood swings.
Becomes introspective: Resolves old conflicts (feelings toward mother, sexual intimacy, masturbation).	Discuss childbirth preparation classes; refer, as necessary.
Reevaluates self, life-style, marriage.	
Daydreams, fantasizes self as "mother."	
Seeks out other pregnant women and new mothers.	
Third Trimester	
Altered body image.	Encourage verbalization of concerns, discomforts of late pregnancy.
Fears body mutilation (stretching of body tissues, episiotomy, cesarean delivery).	Help meet dependency needs. Reassurance, as possible.
Distress over loss of control over body functions (ptyalism, colostrum leakage, leukorrhea, urinary frequency, constipation, stress incontinence).	*Health teaching:* Kegel's exercises; preparation for labor. Anticipatory guidance and planning for needs of self, baby, and family in early postpartum.
Anxiety for baby (deformity, death).	
Fears pain, loss of control in labor.	
Acceptance of impending labor during last two weeks (ready to "move on").	

a. Good body alignment—tuck pelvis under; tighten abdominal muscles.

b. Pelvic-rock exercises.

c. Squat; bend at knees, *not* at waist.

d. Wear low-heeled, sturdy shoes.

e. Advise against tight-fitting clothing interfering with circulatory return in legs.

III. Psycho-social-cultural alterations

A. *Emotional changes*—affected by age, maturity, support system, amount of current stresses, coping abilities, physical and mental health status. *Developmental tasks of pregnancy:*

1. Accept the pregnancy as real: "I am pregnant"; progress from symbiotic relationship with the fetus to perception of the child as an individual.
2. Seek and ensure acceptance of child by others.
3. Seek protection for self and fetus through pregnancy and labor.
4. Prepare realistically for the coming child and for necessary role change: "I am going to be a parent."

B. *Physical bases of changes*

1. *Increased* metabolic demands may result in anemia and fatigue.
2. *Increased* hormone levels (steroids, estrogen, progesterone)—affect mood as well as physiology.

C. *Characteristic behaviors*—Table 2.6 describes behaviors commonly exhibited in each trimester.

D. *Sexuality and sexual expression*—feelings and expressions of sexuality may vary during pregnancy due to maternal adaptations.

E. *Intrafamily relationships*

1. Pregnancy a maturational crisis for the family.
2. Requires changes in life-style and interactions:
   a. Increased financial demands.
   b. Changing family and social relationships.
   c. Adapting communication patterns.
   d. Adapting sexual patterns.
   e. Anticipating new responsibilities and needs.
   f. Responding to reactions of others.

PRENATAL MANAGEMENT

I. Initial assessment goal: establish baseline for health supervision, teaching, emotional support, and/or referral.

II. Objectives:

A. Determine client's present health status and validate pregnancy.

B. Identify factors affecting and/or affected by pregnancy.

C. Describe current gravidity and parity.

D. Identify present length of gestation.

E. Establish an estimated date of delivery (EDD). Nagele's determination of EDD—Subtract 3 months, add 7 days to LMP.

F. Determine relevant knowledge deficit.

III. Assessment: history

A. *Family*—inheritable diseases, reproductive problems.

B. *Personal*—medical, surgical, gynecologic, past obstetric, average nonpregnant weight.

1. *Gravida*—a pregnant woman.
   a. *Nulligravida*—woman who has *never* been pregnant.
   b. *Primigravida*—woman with a *first* pregnancy.
   c. *Multigravida*—woman with a *second or later* pregnancy.
2. *Para*—refers to *past pregnancies* (not number of babies) that reached viability (whether or not born alive).
   a. *Nullipara*—woman who has *not* carried a pregnancy to viability; e.g., may have had one or more abortions.
   b. *Primipara*—woman who has carried *one* pregnancy to viability.
   c. *Multipara*—woman who has delivered *two or more* pregnancies that reached viability (24 weeks or more).
   d. *Grandmultipara*—woman who has delivered *six or more* viable pregnancies.
3. Examples of gravidity/parity. Several methods of describing gravidity and parity are in common use. One method describes number of pregnancies, term (or full-term infants), preterm infants, abortions, and number of living children (GTPAL).
   a. A woman who is pregnant for the *first* time and is currently *undelivered* is designated as 1-0-0-0-0. *After* delivering a full-term living neonate, she becomes 1-1-0-0-1.
   b. If a woman's second pregnancy ends in abortion and she has a living child from a previous pregnancy, delivered at term, she is designated as 2-1-0-1-1.
   c. A woman who is pregnant for the fourth time and whose previous pregnancies yielded one full-term neonate, premature twins, and one abortion (spontaneous or induced), and who now has three living children, may be designated as 4-1-1-1-3.
   d. Others record as follows: number gravida/number para. Applying this system to the examples given above, those mothers would be designated as follows: a—G1P1; b—G2P1; c—G4P2.
   e. Others include recording of abortions:
      G1P1 Ab0
      G2P1 Ab1
      G4P2 Ab1

IV. Assessment: initial physical aspects:

A. Height and weight.

B. Vital signs.

C. Blood work—hematocrit and hemoglobin for anemia; type and Rh factor; tests for sickle cell trait, syphilis, and rubella antibody titer (see also Table 2.4, p. 123).

D. Urinalysis—glucose, protein, acetone, signs of infection, and pregnancy test (HCG).

▶ **E.** Breast exam.

▶ **F.** Pelvic exam.

1. Signs of pregnancy.
2. Adequacy of pelvis and pelvic structures.
3. Size and position of uterus.
4. Papanicolau smear.
5. Smears for monilial and trichomonal infections.
6. Signs of pelvic inflammatory disease.
7. Tests for STD: GC, chlamydia.

G. *Validation of pregnancy*—physician or midwife makes differential diagnosis between presumptive/probable signs/symptoms of early pregnancy and other signs.

1. *Presumptive symptoms*—subjective experiences.
   a. Amenorrhea—more than 10 days past missed menstrual period.
   b. Breast tenderness, enlargement.
   c. Nausea and vomiting.
   d. Quickening (week 16–18).
   e. Urinary frequency.
   f. Fatigue.
   g. Constipation (50% of women).
   h. Vaginal changes (*Chadwick's sign*): purple hue in vulvar/vaginal area.
2. *Probable signs*—examiner's objective findings.
   a. Positive pregnancy test.
   b. Enlargement of abdomen/uterus.
   c. Striae gravidarum, linea nigra, chloasma (after week 16).
   d. Reproductive organ changes (after sixth week):
      (1) *Goodell's sign*—cervical softening.
      (2) *Hegar's sign*—softening of lower uterine segment.
   e. Ballottement (after 16–20 weeks).
   f. Braxton-Hicks contractions.
3. *Positive signs of pregnancy:*
   a. Fetal heart tones.
      (1) Doptone: week 10–12.
      (2) Fetoscope: week 20.
   b. Examiner feels fetal movements (usually after week 24).
   c. Sonographic examination (after week 14) when fetal head is sufficiently developed for accurate diagnosis.

V. Assessment: nutritional status:

A. Physical findings suggesting poor nutritional status:

1. Skin: rough, dry, scaly.
2. Lips: lesions in corners.
3. Hair: dull, brittle.
4. Mucous membranes: pale.
5. Dental caries.

B. Height, weight, age—average weight gain approximately 24 lb. Range from 24 to 32 lb is best for mother and neonate.

C. Laboratory values—Hemoglobin: <10.5/100 mg. Hct: <32% indicates anemia.

D. Nutrition history.

E. Analysis/nursing diagnosis:

1. *Altered nutrition: less than body requirements* related to anemia, vitamin/mineral deficit.
2. *Altered nutrition: more than body requirements* related to obesity.

F. Nursing plan/implementation: Goal: *health teaching.* Nutritional counseling for diet in pregnancy and/or lactation.

G. Evaluation:

1. If *underweight* at conception: should gain more than 24 pounds.
2. If *obese* at conception: should gain approximately 24 pounds; dieting contraindicated.

VI. Assessment: psychosocial aspects:

A. Pregnancy: planned or not; desired or not.

B. Present plans:

1. Carry pregnancy, keep baby.
2. Carry pregnancy, adoption.
3. Abortion.

C. Cultural, ethnic influences on decisions: will influence range of activities, types of safeguarding actions, diet, and health-promotion behaviors.

D. Parenting potential: actively seeking medical care and information about pregnancy, childbirth, parenthood.

E. Family readiness for childbearing/childrearing:

1. Physical maintenance.
2. Allocation of resources: identify support system.
3. Division of labor.
4. Socialization of family members.
5. Reproduction, recruitment, launching of family members into society.
6. Maintenance of order (relationships within family).

F. Perceptions of present and projected family relationships.

G. Review life-style for smoking, drugs, ETOH, attitudes to pregnancy, and health care practices.

VII. Analysis/nursing diagnosis:

A. *Altered role performance* related to stress imposed by developmental tasks.

B. *Ineffective coping: individual, family* related to stress caused by developmental tasks/crises.

C. *Altered family process* related to developmental tasks. First baby may precipitate individual or family developmental crisis.

VIII. Nursing plan/implementation:

A. Goal: *anticipatory guidance/support.*

1. Discuss mood swings, ambivalent feelings, negative feelings.
2. Reinforce "normalcy" of such feelings.

B. Goal: *increase individual/family coping skills, reduce intrafamily stress.*

1. Reinforce family strengths (both partners), sense of family identity.
   a. Encourage open communication between partners; share feelings and concerns.
   b. Increase understanding of mutual needs, encourage mutuality of support.
   c. Increase tendency of mother to turn to partner as most significant person (as opposed to physician).
   d. Enhance bond, success of childbirth preparation classes.
2. Promote understanding/acceptance of role change.
   a. Facilitate/support achievement of developmental tasks.
   b. Reduce probability of postpartal psychologic problems.
   c. Promote family bonding.

C. Goal: *health teaching.*

1. *Siblings:*
   a. Alert parents to sibling needs for security, love.
   b. Include sibling in pregnancy experience.
   c. Provide clear, simple explanations of happenings.
   d. Continue demonstrations of love.
   e. Describe increased status ("big sister/brother").
   f. Discuss possible misbehavior to gain attention.
2. *Relatives:* alert parents to possible negative feelings of in-laws.
3. Referral to childbirth preparation/parenting classes.
4. Appropriate community referrals for financial relief to decrease stress and provide aid.

IX. Evaluation:

A. Actively participates in pregnancy-related decision making.

B. Expresses satisfaction with decisions made.

C. Demonstrates growth and development in parenting role.

D. Prepared for the birth and for early parenthood.

ANTEPARTUM

I. Nursing care and obstetric support

A. General aspects of prenatal management

1. *Scheduled visits:*
   a. Once monthly—until week 32.
   b. Every 2 weeks—weeks 32–36.
   c. Weekly—week 36 until labor.
2. **Assessment:**
   a. General well-being, signs of deviations, concerns, questions.
   b. Weight gain pattern.
   c. Blood pressure (right arm, sitting).
   d. Abdominal palpation:
      (1) Fundal height; tenderness, masses, hernia.
      (2) Fetal heart rate (FHR).
      (3) Leopold's maneuvers for presentation (after week 32).
   e. Laboratory tests:
      (1) Urinalysis—for protein, sugar, signs of asymptomatic infection.

(2) Venous blood—for Hgb, Hct (done initially: VDRL, anti-Rh titer, sickle cell). HIV recommended for high-risk groups.

▶ (3) Cultures (vaginal discharge; cervical scrapings, for *Chlamydia trachomatis*) p.r.n.

(4) Tuberculosis screening in high-risk areas.

(5) Maternal alpha-fetoprotein screen, 16–18 wks optimum time.

(6) Serum glucose screen, 24–28 wks.

f. Follow-up on medications (vitamins, iron) and nutrition.

B. Common minor discomforts during pregnancy (For **Assessment,** see Table 2.5, p. 126.)

1. **Etiology:** normal maternal physiologic/psychologic alterations in pregnancy.

2. **Nursing plan/implementation:**

a. Goal: *anticipatory guidance.* Discuss the importance of adequate rest, exercise, diet, and hydration in minimizing symptoms.

b. Goal: *health teaching* (see Table. 2.5).

3. **Evaluation:** avoids, minimizes, and/or copes effectively with minor usual discomforts of pregnancy.

C. Danger signs:

1. **Etiology:** Specific disease processes are discussed under Complications, below.

2. **Nursing plan/implementation:** Goal: *health teaching*—to safeguard status. Signs to report *immediately:*

a. Persistent vomiting beyond first trimester or severe vomiting at any time.

b. Fluid discharge from vagina—bleeding or amniotic fluid (anything other than leukorrhea).

c. Severe or unusual pain: abdominal.

d. Chills or fever.

e. Burning on urination.

f. Absence of fetal movements after quickening.

g. Visual disturbances—blurring, double vision, "spots before eyes."

h. Swelling of fingers or face.

i. Severe, frequent, or continual headache.

j. Muscle irritability or convulsions.

3. **Evaluation:**

a. Actively participates in own health maintenance/pregnancy management.

b. Identifies early signs of potentially serious complications during the antepartal period.

c. Promptly reports and seeks medical attention.

II. Complications during the antepartum

A. General aspects:

1. **Etiology:**

a. Normal alterations and increasing physiologic stress of pregnancy affect status of coexisting medical disorders.

b. Conditions affecting mother's general health also affect ability to adapt successfully to normal physiologic stress of pregnancy.

c. Aberrations of normal pregnancy.

2. Goal: *reduce incidence of health problems affecting maternal/fetal health and pregnancy outcome.*

a. Identify presence of risk factors and signs and symptoms of complications early.

b. Treat emerging complications promptly and effectively.

c. Minimize effects of complications on pregnancy outcome.

3. **Assessment:** risk factors.

a. Age:

(1) Adolescent.

(2) Primigravida, age 35 or older.

(3) Multigravida, age 40 or older.

b. Socioeconomic level: lower.

c. Ethnic group: black, Latin.

d. Previous pregnancy history:

(1) Habitual abortion.

(2) Multiparity greater than 5.

(3) Previous stillbirths.

(4) Previous cesarean delivery.

(5) Preterm labor.

e. Multiple pregnancy.

f. Prenatal care:

(1) Enters health care system late in pregnancy.

(2) Irregular/episodic care visits.

(3) Noncompliance with medical/nursing recommendations.

g. Pre- or coexisting medical disorders:

(1) Cardiovascular: hypertension, heart disease.

(2) Diabetes.

(3) Other: renal, respiratory, infections, AIDS.

h. Substance abuse.

4. **Nursing plan/implementation:**

a. Goal: *health teaching* (discussed under specific health problem).

b. Goal: *early identification/treatment of emerging health problems* (if any).

(1) Monitor status and progress of pregnancy.

(2) Refer for medical management, as necessary.

c. Goal: *emotional support.*

5. **Evaluation:**

a. Understands present health status, interactions of coexisting disorder and pregnancy.

b. Accepts responsibility for own health maintenance.

c. Makes informed decisions regarding pregnancy.

d. Minimizes potential for complications of coexisting disorder/pregnancy.

(1) Avoids factors predisposing to health problems.

(2) Understands and implements therapeutic management of coexisting disorder/pregnancy.

(3) Increases compliance with medical/nursing recommendations.

e. Carries uneventful pregnancy to successful termination.

B. Disorders affecting fluid-gas transport: *cardiac disease*

1. **Pathophysiology:** cardiac overload → cardiac decompensation → right-sided failure → pulmonary edema.
2. **Etiology:**
   a. Congenital heart defects.
   b. Valvular damage—due to rheumatic fever (↓ incidence due to early identification and treatment).
   c. Increased circulating-blood volume and cardiac output—exceeds cardiac reserve. Greatest risk: *after 28 weeks gestation*—reaches maximum (30–50%) volume increase; *postpartum*—due to diuresis.
   d. Secondary to tx (e.g., tocolysis and B methasone)
3. Normal physiologic alterations during pregnancy that mimic cardiac disorders:
   a. Systolic murmurs, palpitations, tachycardia, and hyperventilation with some dyspnea on normal moderate exertion.
   b. Edema of lower extremities.
   c. Cardiac enlargement.
   d. Elevated sedimentation rate near term.
4. **Assessment:**
   a. Medical evaluation of cardiac status. Classification of severity of cardiac involvement.
      (1) *Class I*—least affected; asymptomatic with ordinary activity.
      (2) *Class II*—activities somewhat limited; ordinary activities cause fatigue, dyspnea, angina.
      (3) *Class III*—moderate/marked limitation of activity; common activities result in severe symptoms of fatigue, etc.
      (4) *Class IV*—most affected; symptomatic (dyspnea, angina) at rest; should avoid pregnancy.
   b. Signs of cardiac decompensation:
      (1) Pedal edema.
      (2) Moist, frequent cough; rales at base p̄ 2 inspirations.
      (3) Dyspnea on minimal physical activity.
      (4) Cyanosis of lips and nail bed.
      (5) Pulse: rapid, weak ($\geq$ 100/min), irregular.
      (6) Fatigue increased.
5. **Analysis/nursing diagnosis:**
   a. *Fluid volume excess* related to inability of compromised heart to handle increased workload (decreased cardiac reserve → congestive heart failure).
   b. *Impaired gas exchange* related to pulmonary edema secondary to congestive heart failure.
6. **Nursing plan/implementation:**
   a. *Medical management:* drug therapy.
      (1) Diuretics, electrolyte supplements.
      (2) Digitalis.
      (3) Antibiotics—prophylaxis against rheumatic fever; treatment of bacterial infections during pregnancy.
      (4) Oxygen, as needed.
   b. Goal: *health teaching.*
      (1) Need for compliance with therapeutic regimen, medical/nursing recommendations.
      (2) Drug actions, dosage, necessary client actions (how to take own pulse, reportable signs/symptoms).
      (3) Methods for *decreasing work of heart:*
         (a) Adequate *rest*—minimum 10 hours sleep each night; half-hour nap after each meal.
         (b) Avoid heavy physical *activity* (including housework), fatigue, excessive weight gain, emotional stress, infection.
         (c) Avoid *situations* of reduced ambient O_2, such as smoking, exposure to pollutants, flight in unpressurized small planes.
   c. Goal: *nutritional counseling.*
      (1) Well-balanced diet; adequate protein, fresh fruits and vegetables, water.
      (2) *Avoid* "junk food," stimulants (caffeine), excessive salt intake.
   d. *Anticipatory planning:* management of labor.
      (1) Goal: *minimize physiologic and psychologic stress.*
      (2) Medical management:
         (a) Reevaluation of cardiac status prior to EDD and labor.
         (b) Regional anesthesia for labor/delivery.
         (c) Low-outlet forceps delivery; episiotomy.
      (3) **Assessment:** continuous.
         (a) Physiologic response to labor stimuli—*frequent vital signs* (pulse rate most sensitive and reliable indicator of impending congestive heart failure).
         (b) Color, respiratory effort, diaphoresis.
         (c) Contractions, etc.—same as for any laboring mother.
   e. **Nursing plan/implementation:** *labor.*
      (1) Goal: *safeguard status.*
         (a) Report *promptly:* pulse rate over 100; respirations more than 24 between contractions.
         (b) Oxygen at 6 liters, as needed.
      (2) Goal: *emotional support*—to reduce anxiety, facilitate cooperation.
         (a) Encourage verbalization of feelings, fears, concerns.
         (b) Explain all procedures.
      (3) Goal: *promote cardiac function.* Position—semirecumbent; support arms and legs.
      (4) Goal: *promote relaxation/control over labor discomfort.* Encourage Lamaze (or other) breathing/relaxation techniques.
      (5) Goal: *reduce stress on cardiopulmonary system.* Discourage bearing-down efforts.
      (6) Goal: *relieve stress of pain, eliminate bearing-down.* Prepare for regional anesthesia.

(7) Goal: *maintain effective cardiac function.* Administer medications, as ordered (e.g., digitalis, diuretics, antibiotics).

7. *Anticipatory planning:* postpartal management.
   a. Factors increasing risk of cardiac decompensation.
      (1) Delivery → rapid, decreased intraabdominal pressure → vasocongestion and rapid rise in cardiac output.
      (2) Loss of placental circulation.
      (3) Normal diuresis increases circulating blood volume.
   b. **Assessment:**
      (1) Observe for tachycardia and/or respiratory distress.
      (2) Monitor blood loss, I&O—potential hypovolemic shock, cardiac overload due to diuresis.
      (3) Pain level—potential neurogenic shock.
      (4) Same as for any postpartum mother (fundus, signs of infection, etc.).
   c. **Nursing plan/implementation:** *postpartum.*
      (1) Goal: *minimize stress on cardiopulmonary system.*
         (a) Rest, dangle, ambulate with aid.
         (b) Gradual increase in activity—as tolerated without symptoms.
         (c) Position, semi-Fowler's if needed.
         (d) Extra help with newborn care.
   d. **Evaluation:**
      (1) Successfully carries uneventful pregnancy to term.
      (2) Experiences no cardiopulmonary embarrassment during labor, delivery, or postpartum.

C. Disorders affecting fluid-gas transport: *Rh incompatibility*

1. **Pathophysiology**—in an Rh-negative mother: Rh-positive fetal red blood cells enter the maternal circulation → maternal antibody formation → antibodies cross placenta and enter fetal bloodstream → attack fetal red blood cells → hemolysis → anemia, hypoxia.
   a. The pregnant Rh-positive mother carries her infant (Rh negative *or* positive) without incident.
   b. The pregnant Rh-negative mother carries an Rh-negative infant without incident.
   c. The pregnant Rh-negative mother *usually* carries her first Rh-positive child without problems *unless* she has been sensitized by inadvertent transfusion with Rh-positive blood. **Note:** Fetal cells do not usually enter the maternal bloodstream until placental separation (at abortion, abruptio placenta, or delivery).
2. **Etiology**
   a. The Rh factor is an antigen on the red blood cells of some people (these people are Rh positive); the Rh factor is dominant; a person may be homozygous or heterozygous for Rh factor.
   b. An Rh-negative person is homozygous for this recessive trait—does *not* carry the antigen; develops antibodies when exposed to Rh-positive red blood cells (isoimmunization) via transplacental (or other) transfusion.
   c. Following delivery of an Rh-positive infant, if fetal cells enter the mother's bloodstream, maternal antibody formation begins; antibodies remain in the maternal circulation.
   d. At time of next pregnancy with Rh-positive fetus, antibodies cross placenta → hemolysis. *Note: Degree* of hemolysis depends on *number* of maternal antibodies present.
3. Possible serious complication (fetal)—rare today. Hydrops fetalis—most severe hemolytic reaction: severe anemia, cardiac decompensation, hypoxia, edema, ascites, hydrothorax; may be stillborn.
4. **Assessment:**
   a. *Prenatal*—diagnostic procedures:
      (1) Maternal blood type and Rh factor.
      (2) Indirect Coombs test—to determine presence of Rh sensitization (titer indicates number of maternal antibodies).
      ▶ (3) Amniocentesis—as early as 26 weeks gestation—amount of bilirubin by-products indicates severity of hemolytic activity.
      (4) RhoGAM between 28–32 weeks to prevent antibody formation.
   b. *Intrapartal* observation of amniotic fluid (on membrane rupture).
      (1) Straw-colored fluid—mild disease.
      (2) Golden fluid—severe fetal disease.
   c. *Postnatal*—see III.A. Rh Incompatability, p. 199.
5. **Nursing plan/implementation:**
   a. Goal: *prevent isoimmunization.*
      (1) *Postabortion*—if no evidence of Rh sensitization (antibody formation) in the Rh-negative mother, administer RhoGAM.
      (2) *Prenatal*—if no evidence of sensitization, administer RhoGAM at 28 weeks gestation, as ordered, to all Rh− women.
      (3) *Postpartum*—if no evidence of sensitization, administer RhoGAM to mother within 72 hours of delivery to Rh− women who have delivered Rh+ baby.

Give RhoGAM to:
1. Rh− mother who delivers Rh+ neonate.
2. Rh− mother after spontaneous abortion.
3. Rh− mother after induced abortion (>8 wks).
4. Rh− mother after amniocentesis.
5. Rh− mother between 28 and 32 weeks gestation.

   b. Goal: *health teaching.*
      (1) Explain, discuss that RhoGAM suppresses antibody formation in susceptible Rh-negative women carrying Rh-positive fetus. *Note:* Cannot reverse sensitization if already present.
      (2) Required during and after each pregnancy, with Rh+ fetus.
6. **Evaluation:**
   a. Successfully carries pregnancy to term.

b. No evidence of Rh isoimmunization.

c. Delivery of viable infant.

D. Disorders affecting nutrition: *diabetes* (D.M.)

1. **Pathophysiology**—increased demand for insulin exceeds pancreative reserve → inadequate insulin production; enzyme (insulinase) activity breaks down circulating insulin → further reduction in available insulin; increased tissue resistance to insulin; glycogenolysis/gluconeogenesis → ketosis.

2. **Etiology**—increased metabolic rate; action of placental hormones (see below), enzyme (insulinase) activity.

3. Normal physiologic alterations during pregnancy that may affect management of the diabetic client, or precipitate gestational diabetes in susceptible women:

a. Hormone production:

(1) Human Placental Lactogen (HPL); Human Chorionic Somatotropin (HCS).

(2) Cortisol.

(3) Estrogen.

(4) Progesterone.

b. *Effects of hormones:*

(1) Decreased glucose tolerance.

(2) Increased metabolic rate.

(3) Increased production of adrenocortical and pituitary hormones.

(4) Decreased effectiveness of insulin (increased resistance to insulin by peripheral tissues).

(5) Increased gluconeogenesis.

(6) Increased size and number of islets of Langerhans to meet increased maternal needs.

(7) Increased mobilization of free fatty acids.

(8) Decreased renal threshold, increased glomerular filtration rate; glycosuria common.

(9) Decreased CO_2 combining power of blood; higher metabolic rate increases tendency to acidosis.

c. *Effect of pregnancy on diabetes:*

(1) Nausea and vomiting—predispose to ketoacidosis.

(2) Insulin requirements—relatively stable or may decrease in first trimester; rapid *increase* during second and third trimesters; rapid *decrease* in post-partum to prepregnant level.

(3) Pathophysiologic progression (nephropathy, retinopathy, and arteriosclerotic changes) may appear; existing pathology may worsen.

4. *Effect of diabetes on pregnancy*—increased incidence of:

a. Infertility.

b. Urinary tract infection (UTI).

c. Vaginal infections (moniliasis).

d. Spontaneous abortion.

e. Congenital anomalies (three times as prevalent).

f. Preeclampsia/eclampsia.

g. Hydramnios.

h. Premature labor and delivery.

i. Fetal macrosomia—cephalopelvic disproportion (CPD).

j. Stillbirth.

5. **Assessment:** gestational diabetes (D.M.)

a. History:

(1) Family history.

(2) Previous infant 4200 g or more.

(3) Unexplained fetal wastage—abortion, stillbirth.

(4) Obesity with very rapid weight gain.

(5) Hydramnios (excessive amniotic fluid).

(6) Previous infant with congenital anomalies.

(7) Increased tendency for intense vaginal and/ or urinary tract infections.

b. Symptoms: 3 "P's"—polydipsia, polyphagia, polyuria—and weight loss.

c. *Abdominal assessment:*

(1) Fetal heart rate.

(2) Excessive fundal height.

(a) Hydramnios.

(b) Large-for-gestational-age (LGA) fetus. *Note:* With vascular pathology, small-for-gestational-age (SGA) fetus.

d. *Medical diagnosis*—procedures:

▶ (1) Abnormal glucose tolerance test (GTT) (two or more of the following findings are not within normal limits; normal values follow).

(a) Fasting blood sugar (FBS)—60–80 mg/dL (90 mg/dL may be normal during first trimester).

(b) One hour—under 200 mg/dL.

(c) Two hours—under 150 mg/dL (~120).

(d) Three hours—under 150 mg/dL (~120).

(2) *Diabetic classification criteria*

(a) Class A—gestational or chemical diabetes (abnormal GTT).

(b) Class B—overt diabetes, onset after age 20, duration less than 10 years, no vascular involvement.

(c) Class C—overt diabetes, onset prior to age 20, duration 10–20 years, no vascular involvement.

(d) Class D—overt diabetes, onset prior to age 10, duration longer than 20 years, vascular involvement, benign retinopathy, leg calcification.

(e) Class F—renal impairment.

e. Known diabetic client—all classes.

(1) Knowledge and acceptance of disease and its management:

(a) Signs and symptoms of hyperglycemia/ hypoglycemia.

(b) Appropriate behaviors (e.g., skim milk for symptoms of hypoglycemia).

(2) Skill and accuracy in monitoring serum glucose (dextrometer use).

(3) Skill and accuracy in preparing and administering insulin dosage; site rotation; subcutaneous injection.

(4) Close monitoring—prenatal status assessment every 2 weeks until 30 weeks, then weekly until delivery. Alert to signs of emerging problems (need for insulin adjustment, hydramnios, macrosomia).

(5) Other—as for any pregnant woman.

6. **Analysis/nursing diagnosis:**

a. *Knowledge deficit* re: pathophysiology, interactions with pregnancy, management (e.g., insulin administration).

b. *Altered nutrition, more or less than body requirements,* related to weight gain.

c. High-risk pregnancy: potential for infection, ketosis, perinatal wastage, fetal macrosomia, cephalopelvic disproportion, hydramnios, preterm labor and delivery, congenital anomalies.

7. **Nursing plan/implementation:**

a. Goal: *health teaching.*

(1) Pathophysiology of diabetes, as necessary; effect of pregnancy on management.

(2) Signs and symptoms of hyperglycemia, hypoglycemia; appropriate management of symptoms.

(3) Hygiene—to reduce probability of infection.

(4) Exercise—needed to control serum-glucose levels, regulate weight gain, and for feeling of well-being.

(5) Need for close monitoring during pregnancy.

(6) Insulin regulation:

(a) Requirements vary through pregnancy: *first trimester*—may decrease with some periods of hypoglycemia due to fetal drain; *second trimester*—increased need for insulin; *third trimester*—needs may be triple prepregnant dose; acidosis more common in late pregnancy (precipitated by emotional stress, infection).

▶ (b) Serum-glucose testing—dextrometer, acucheck, or other.

(c) Preparation and self-administration of insulin injection, as necessary.

(d) Prompt reporting of fluctuating serum-glucose levels.

(7) Diagnostic testing/hospitalization:

(a) Nonstress test.

(b) Sonography.

(c) Amniocentesis.

b. Goal: *dietary counseling.*

(1) Optimal weight gain—about 24 lb.

(2) Needs 35 calories/kg of ideal body weight.

(3) Protein—20% (2 g/kg, or about 70 g daily).

(4) Carbohydrates: 30–45% in complex form (milk, bread).

(5) Fats—unsaturated.

(6) Appropriate exchanges.

c. *Medical management:* hospitalize client for:

(1) Regulation of insulin (oral hypoglycemics *contraindicated* in pregnancy, due to teratogenicity).

(2) Control of infection.

(3) Determination of fetal jeopardy and/or indications for early termination of pregnancy.

8. **Evaluation:**

a. Understands and accepts diagnosis of diabetes.

b. Actively participates in effective management of diabetes and pregnancy.

c. Maintains serum-glucose levels within acceptable parameters (e.g., 60–90 mg/dL after fasting; 2 hours postprandial, less than 120 mg/dL).

(1) Monitors serum-glucose levels accurately (dextrometer, acucheck, urine testing).

(2) Prepares and self-administers insulin appropriately.

(3) Demonstrates compliance with dietary regimen.

9. *Antepartal hospitalization*

a. **Assessment:**

(1) *Medical evaluation—procedures:*

(a) Serum-glucose levels (↓ 120 mg).

▶ (b) Sonography for fetal growth: biophysical profile (BPP) evaluates fetal physical well-being and volume of amniotic fluid.

▶ (c) Nonstress testing/contraction stress testing.

▶ (d) Amniocentesis for fetal maturity (*Note:* L/S ratio may be elevated in diabetic women); phosphatidylglycerol (PG) more accurate for diabetic clients.

(2) **Nursing assessment:**

(a) Daily weight, vital signs, FHR q4h, I&O.

(b) Fundal height on admission.

b. **Nursing plan/implementation.** Goal: *emotional support*—to reduce anxiety and tension, which contribute to insulin imbalance.

(1) Explain all procedures.

(2) Assist with tests for fetal status.

(3) Prepare for possibility of caesarean delivery.

10. *Anticipatory planning*—management of labor

a. **Assessment:** continuous.

(1) Signs and symptoms of hyperglycemia, hypoglycemia.

(2) Electronic fetal monitoring—to identify signs of fetal distress.

(3) Other—as for any laboring woman.

b. **Nursing plan/implementation:** Goal: *safeguard maternal/fetal status.* Position: left Sims—to reduce compression of inferior vena cava due to hydramnios or large for gestational age (LGA) baby. (Supine hypotensive syndrome results from compression; reduced placental perfusion increases incidence of fetal hypoxia/anoxia.)

c. *Medical management*—varies widely.

(1) Timing—amniocentesis to determine PG (phosphotidyglycerol and phosphotidilynosital) levels (estimate fetal pulmonary surfactant).

(2) Insulin added to intravenous infusion of 5–10% D/W, and titrated to maintain serum glucose between 100 and 150 mg/dL. D/W needed to prevent hypoglycemia that may lead to maternal ketoacidosis; hyperglycemia may result in newborn hypoglycemia.

(3) Ultrasound or X-ray pelvimetry to identify CPD.

11. *Anticipatory planning*—management of postpartum

a. Factors influencing serum-glucose levels:

(1) Loss of placental hormones that degrade insulin.

(2) Lower metabolic rate. Woman requiring large doses of insulin may need to triple caloric intake and decrease insulin by one-half.

b. **Assessment:**

(1) Observe for:

(a) Hypoglycemia.

(b) Infection.

(c) Preeclampsia/eclampsia (higher incidence in diabetic women).

(d) Hemorrhage (associated with hydramnios, macrosomia, induction of labor, forceps delivery, or caesarean delivery).

(2) Monitor healing of episiotomy/abdominal incision.

c. **Nursing plan/implementation:**

(1) *Medical management:* insulin calibration—requirement may drop to one-half or two-thirds pregnant dosage on first postpartum day if client is on full diet (due to loss of human placental lactogen and conversion of serum glucose to lactose).

(2) *Nursing management*

(a) Goal: *euglycemia.* Acucheck, insulin as ordered.

(b) Goal: *avoid trauma, reduce risk of UTI.* Avoid catheterization, where possible.

(c) Goal: *health teaching.* Nipple care—to prevent fissures and possible mastitis.

(d) Goal: *reduce serum-glucose and insulin needs.* Encourage/support breastfeeding → antidiabetogenic effect. **Note:** If *acetonuria* occurs, stop breastfeeding while physician readjusts diet/insulin balance; may pump breasts to maintain lactation. If *hypoglycemic,* adrenaline level rises → decreased milk supply and let-down reflex.

12. *Anticipatory guidance*—discharge planning

a. Goal: *counseling.* Reinforce recommendations of physicians/genetic counselors.

(1) Risk of infant inheriting gene for diabetes is greater if mother has early-onset disease.

(2) Increased risk of congenital disorders.

b. Goal: *family planning*

(1) Oral contraceptives **contraindicated** since they decrease carbohydrate tolerance; IUD contraindicated—due to impaired response to infection. Barrier contraceptives (diaphragm or condoms) recommended.

(2) Tubal ligation: if mother has vascular involvement, i.e., retinopathy or nephropathy, increased risk with later pregnancies (see Table 2.2).

c. Goal: *health teaching.*

(1) Self-care measures.

(2) Importance of eating on time, even if infant must wait to nurse.

(3) Importance of adequate rest and exercise to maintain insulin/glucose balance.

(4) Organize schedule to care for infant, other children, and her diabetes. Allow time for self.

13. **Evaluation:**

a. Successfully completes an uneventful pregnancy, labor, and delivery of a normal, healthy newborn.

b. Makes informed judgments regarding parenting, family planning, management of her diabetes.

E. Disorders affecting psycho-socio-cultural behaviors: *substance abuse*

1. **Assessment:** pregnant substance abuser

a. *Medical history*

(1) AIDS.

(2) Hepatitis.

(3) Cirrhosis of liver.

(4) Cellulitis.

(5) Endocarditis.

(6) Pancreatitis.

(7) Pneumonia.

(8) Psychiatric illness (depression, paranoia, violence).

b. *Obstetrical history*

(1) Spontaneous abortions.

(2) History of abruptio placentae.

(3) Preterm labor.

(4) Premature rupture of membranes.

(5) Fetal death.

(6) Low-birth-weight infants.

(7) Sexually transmitted diseases.

c. *Current pregnancy*

(1) Premature labor contractions.

(2) Hypoactivity—hyperactivity in fetus.

(3) Poor or decreased weight gain.

(4) Sexually transmitted disease.

(5) Vaginal bleeding.

(6) Drugs being used.

d. *Psychosocial history*

(1) Attitudes re: pregnancy.

(2) Current support system: lacking.

(3) Current living arrangements; lifestyle.

(4) History of psychiatric illness.

(5) History of physical, sexual abuse.

(6) Involvement with legal system.

e. *Physical exam*

f. *Commonly abused substances*

(1) Nicotine.

(2) Alcohol (F.A.S.).

(3) Marijuana.

(4) Stimulants—cocaine, crack, ice.

(5) Opiates—heroin, methadone, Darvon, Tylenol.

(6) Sedatives, hypnotics.

(7) Caffeine.

g. *Neonatal outcomes*

(1) LBW, small heads.

(2) Irritable, difficult to console.

(3) Disorganized suck-swallow reflex.

(4) Impaired motor development.

(5) Congenital anomalies: genitourinary, gastrointestinal, limb anomalies.

(6) Cerebral infarctions.

(7) Breastfeeding contraindicated unless mother is drug-free for 3 months.

(8) Poor, slow weight gain.

2. **Analysis/nursing diagnosis:**

a. *Altered nutrition: more than body requirements*—weight gain related to poor nutrition.

b. *Altered nutrition: less than body requirements*—slow fetal growth related to slow gain in weight.

c. *Altered placental function* related to potential for abruptio placentae.

d. *Noncompliance* with health care protocols related to persistent drug use.

e. *Altered parenting* related to psychologic illness (dependence).

3. **Nursing plan/implementation:**

a. Early identification of substance abuser.

b. Stabilize physiological status.

c. Fetal surveillance

d. Urge consistent obstetrical care.

e. Refer for social services.

4. **Evaluation:**

a. Seeks out and utilizes social services and drug treatment program.

b. Abstains from illicit substances during pregnancy.

c. Successfully completes an uneventful pregnancy, labor, and delivery of normal healthy infant.

III. Other high-risk clients

A. The pregnant adolescent

1. *General aspects:*

a. Pregnancy in female between 12 and 17 years old.

b. Incidence increasing dramatically; approximately one-third of all births are in adolescents.

c. *Predisposing factors:* early menarche, early experimentation with sex, poor family relationships, poverty, late or no prenatal care.

d. *Associated health problems:* Pregnancy Induced Hypertension (PIH), preterm labor, SGA (small for gestational age) infants, anemia, bleeding disorders, infections, cephalopelvic disproportion (CPD).

e. *Social problems:* poorly educated mothers, child abuse, single-parent families, mothers unemployed or working at minimum wage.

2. **Assessment:**

a. Present physical/health status.

b. Feelings toward pregnancy.

c. Plans for the future.

d. Factors influencing decisions related to self, pregnancy, baby.

e. Signs and symptoms of complications of pregnancy (see A.1.d. Associated health problems, above).

f. Potential for gestational diabetes.

g. Need/desire for health maintenance information (family planning).

3. **Analysis/nursing diagnosis:**

a. *Ineffective coping, individual/family,* related to need to alter life-style, plans, expectations.

b. *Altered family processes,* related to unexpected/unwanted pregnancy.

c. *Altered parenting* related to intrafamily stress secondary to unexpected pregnancy, developmental tasks.

d. *Self-esteem disturbance* related to altered self-concept, body image, role performance, personal identity.

e. *Knowledge deficit* related to family planning, health maintenance, risk factors, pregnancy options.

f. *Altered nutrition* related to anemia

4. **Nursing plan/implementation:**

a. Goal: *emotional support.*

(1) Establish acceptant, supportive environment.

(2) Encourage verbalization of feelings, concerns, fears, desires, etc.

(3) Maintain continuity of care—consistency of nursing approach, to establish trust, confidentiality.

b. Goal: *facilitate informed decision making.* Discuss available options; aid in exploration of implications of possible decisions.

c. Goal: *nutritional counseling* (anemia).

(1) Needs for own growth and that of fetus.

(2) High-quality diet—value for character of skin, return to prepregnant figure.

(3) Include pizza, hamburgers, milkshakes as ac-

ceptable—to minimize anger at being "different."

d. Goal: *health teaching.*

(1) Rest, exercise, hygiene—as for other women.

(2) Prevention of infection—STD, UTI, etc.

(3) Breast self-exam; Pap smear.

(4) Future family planning options (see Table 2.1, pp. 119–120).

e. Goal: *assist in achievement of normal developmental tasks.* Encourage exploration of new role and responsibilities.

f. Goal: *referral to appropriate resources.*

(1) Abortion.

(2) Preparation for childbirth and parenting classes.

(3) Family counseling.

(4) Social services.

g. Goal: *assist in facilitating continuing/completing basic education.*

(1) Communicate with school nurse.

(2) Explore other options available in community.

5. **Evaluation:**

a. Makes informed decisions appropriate to individual and family needs, desires.

b. Actively participates in own health maintenance.

(1) Complies with medical/nursing recommendations.

(2) Minimizes potential for complications of pregnancy.

c. Copes effectively with normal physiologic and psychosocial alterations of pregnancy.

d. Both woman and baby's father express satisfaction with decision and management of this pregnancy. If parenthood is chosen and pregnancy is successful, accepts parenting role.

B. Older parents: primigravida over age 35

1. *General aspects*—higher incidence of congenital anomalies (e.g., Down syndrome), increased possibility of complications of pregnancy, however generally it is a conscious decision to have postponed decision making. Individuals are usually used to making own decisions regarding career and health care.

2. **Assessment:**

a. Same as for other prenatal clients.

b. Reaction to reality of pregnancy.

c. Family response to pregnancy.

3. **Analysis/nursing diagnosis:**

a. *Fear* related to threat to pregnancy.

b. *Knowledge deficit* related to aspects of pregnancy care.

4. **Nursing plan/implementation:**

a. Goal: *anticipatory guidance.* Preparation for parenthood, altered life-style, potential change of career. Assist with realistic expectations. Refer to "over 30" parents' support group.

b. Goal: *health teaching.* Explain, discuss special diagnostic procedures. See Amniocentesis, p. 150.

c. Other—same as for other prenatal clients.

5. **Evaluation:**

a. Experiences normal, uncomplicated pregnancy, labor, and delivery of normal, healthy newborn.

b. Expresses satisfaction with decision and outcome of this pregnancy.

C. Older parents: multipara over age 40

1. *General aspects*

a. Increased incidence of pre- and coexisting medical disorders (hypertension, diabetes, arthritis).

b. Increased incidence of complications of pregnancy (preeclampsia/eclampsia, hemorrhage).

c. Smoking is major risk factor.

2. **Assessment:**

a. Same as for other prenatal clients.

b. Reaction to pregnancy (varies from pleasure at still being "young enough," to despair, if facing decision to abort).

c. History, signs and symptoms of coexisting disorders.

d. Indications of reduced physical ability to cope with normal physiologic alterations of pregnancy.

e. Family constellation: stage of family developmental cycle, responses to this pregnancy (especially adolescents' reaction to parents' pregnancy).

3. **Analysis/nursing diagnosis:** same as for over-35 age group.

4. **Nursing plan/implementation:**

a. Goal: *emotional support.* Encourage verbalization of feelings, fears, concerns.

b. Goal: *referral to appropriate resource.*

(1) Genetic counseling.

(2) Abortion/support groups.

(3) Preparation for childbirth classes.

c. Goal: *facilitate/support effective family process.* Involve family in preparation for birth and integration of newborn into family unit.

d. Other—same as for other prenatal clients.

5. **Evaluation:**

a. Makes informed decisions related to pregnancy.

b. Expresses satisfaction with decision and outcome of this pregnancy.

c. Experiences uncomplicated pregnancy, labor, and birth of normal, healthy newborn.

D. AIDS

1. *General aspects*—AIDS is a serious condition affecting the immune system. Heterosexual females are considered at risk if they or their sexual partners:

a. Are HIV positive.

b. Are IV drug users (50%).

c. Received blood between 1977 and 1985 (9%).

d. Are homosexual or bisexual males (39%).

e. Are hemophiliacs.

2. **Assessment**—general symptoms:

a. Malaise.

b. Chronic cough.

TABLE 2.7 Emergency Conditions

First Trimester

Assessment/Observations	Possible Problem	Nursing Plan/Implementation
Fluid-Gas Transport		
a. *Cramping*—with or without bleeding or passage of tissue.	Abortion (prior to 24 weeks). Threatened. Imminent, incomplete, septic.	Bedrest, sedation, avoid coitus—if threatened; bedrest, start IV fluids and draw blood for laboratory work; CBC, type/cross-match, electrolytes, platelets, HCG levels.
b. *Passage of tissue* (products of conception; grapelike vesicles) or *brown spotting;* fundus too high for gestational age; *blood pressure* elevated. Often associated with hyperemesis gravidarum and preeclampsia.	Hydatidiform mole (trophoblastic disease).	Vital signs q 5–15 minutes, p.r.n.
c. Severe *pain, shock* out of proportion to amount of overt blood; shoulder-strap pain (Kehr's sign), a "referred pain" that indicates intraabdominal bleeding (or rupture of ovarian cyst); amenorrhea of 6–12 weeks.	Ectopic pregnancy.	Save all pads or tissue passed through vagina for physician evaluation. No rectal or vaginal examination until physician is present.
d. Malodorous *discharge; hyperthermia and chills;* tender abdomen.	Septic abortion (self-induced or "criminal").	Take complete history, if possible. Convulsion precautions if hypertensive.
e. *Ecchymosis or bleeding*—with a history that includes any or all of the following: had symptoms of pregnancy, but they subsided; pregnancy test negative; uterine size diminishing; no FHT.	Missed abortion with possible DIC.	Emotional support for loss of pregnancy (through nurse's manner, tone of voice, touch, use of her name, keep her informed of what is happening). Oxygen, p.r.n.

Second Trimester

Assessment/Observations	Possible Problem	Nursing Plan/Implementation
Fluid-Gas Transport		
a. Cramping; passage of products of conception.	Late abortion.	Same as for first trimester.
b. Labor—cervical changes, "show."	Incompetent cervical os.	See MD immediately for possible cerclage.
c. *Prolonged* nausea and vomiting; unexplained *hypertension* or *preeclampsia;* passage of dark blood or grapelike vesicles; *absent FHTs;* excessive fundal height for gestation.	Hydatidiform mole.	Maintain hydration. Assess for dehydration. Refer to MD.
Sensory-Perceptual		
a. *Preeclampsia/eclampsia* *Assessment:* hypertension first noted after 24 weeks; followed by increased proteinuria. *Symptoms:* blurred or double vision; pain: headache, epigastric (late sign) *Signs:* BP 160/110; 3+ proteinuria. Edema: facial, digital; pulmonary. Oliguria. Hyperreflexia.	With increased severity: renal failure, circulatory collapse, CVA, coagulation defects (DIC); abruptio placentae.	Pharmacologic management of gravida with hypertension (see Unit 4). *Convulsion precautions:* 1. Emergency tray at bedside. 2. Oxygen/suction. 3. Start IV. 4. Padded siderails. 5. Indwelling catheter. 6. Constant observation. 7. Deep tendon reflexes. 8. Daily weight. 9. I&O. 10. Note any complaints and changes. 11. Prepare for lab work (type and cross-match, CBC, platelets, BUN, and creatinine).
b. *Convulsions* in absence of hypertension, proteinuria, or facial edema.	CVA, epilepsy, drug toxicity; intracranial injury; diabetic complications; encephalopathy.	*Convulsion care:* 1. Oxygen/mask; drugs (magnesium sulfate IV). 2. Observe: a. Uterine tone, FHTs, fetal activity. b. Signs of labor. 3. Emotional support for woman and family.

Third Trimester

Assessment/Observations	Possible Problem	Nursing Plan/Implementation
Fluid-Gas Transport		
a. *Bleeding:* painless, bright red, vaginal. Contractions and/or uterine tone normal	Placenta previa.	**No vaginal exam.** Apply fetal monitor; assess for labor; *position:* semi- to high Fowler's.
b. *Pain:* abdomen rigid and tender to touch. Increased uterine tone; signs of shock disproportionate to visible blood loss; may have loss of FHTs; associated with: preeclampsia, multiparity, precipitous labor, oxytocin induction.	Abruptio placentae.	As for placenta previa. *Position:* Sims'.

c. Chronic diarrhea.

d. HIV positive.

e. Weight loss: 10 lb in 2 months.

f. Night sweats; lymphadenopathy.

g. Skin lesions; thrush.

3. **Analysis/nursing diagnosis:**

a. *Altered nutrition, less than body requirements,* related to general malaise.

b. *Fatigue,* related to altered health status, weight loss.

c. *Fear* related to progressively debilitating disease.

d. *Knowledge deficit* related to disease progression, treatment, life expectancy.

e. *Ineffective individual coping* related to disease progression.

4. **Nursing plan/implementation:**

a. Identify clients at risk.

b. Protect confidentiality.

c. Implement universal precautions.

d. Use proper gloves, gown.

e. Use protective eyewear and mask in labor, delivery.

5. **Evaluation**

a. No further transmission of virus.

b. Patient confidentiality maintained.

c. Universal precautions implemented.

d. Emotional support implemented.

e. Supportive groups contacted.

6. **HIV-positive women**—prenatal care:

a. *Antepartum*

(1) Increased incidence of other STD (gonorrhea, syphilis, herpes).

(2) Increased incidence of CMV.

(3) Differential diagnosis for all pregnancy-induced complaints.

(4) Counsel regarding nutrition.

(5) Advise about risk to infant.

(6) Counsel regarding safe sex.

b. *Intrapartum*

(1) Focus on prevention of transmission.

(2) EFM (electronic fetal monitoring) preferred.

(3) Mode of delivery not based on disease.

(4) Avoid use of fetal scalp electrodes or sampling.

c. *Postpartum*

(1) No remarkable alteration in disease progression.

(2) Breastfeeding contraindicated.

(3) Implement universal precautions for mother and infant.

(4) Refer to specialists in AIDS care and treatment.

7. **Newborn or neonate:**

a. *General aspects:* Neonatal AIDS—exact mode of transmission unknown, but possibly transplacental, contact with maternal blood at birth, and/or postnatal exposure to infected parent (i.e., breastfeeding). Classic signs evident in adult often not present. Common signs: lymphadenopathy, hepatosplenomegaly, oral candidiasis, bacterial infections, failure to thrive, craniofacial anomalies.

b. Provide supportive nursing care (thermoregulation, respiratory).

c. Encourage parent-infant contact.

d. Provide opportunities for sensory stimuli and touch.

e. Monitor intake and weight gain.

f. Observe for signs of infection.

g. Initiate social service consultation.

COMMON COMPLICATIONS OF PREGNANCY

First Trimester Complications

I. Complications affecting fluid-gas transport: ***hemorrhagic disorders***

A. General aspects (review Table 2.7)

1. **Assessment:**

a. Vital signs, output, general status.

b. Evidence of internal/external bleeding (pad count).

c. Pain.

d. Emotional response.

2. **Analysis/nursing diagnosis:**

a. *Knowledge deficit* related to diagnosis, prognosis, treatment, sequelae.

■ **TABLE 2.8** **Loss of Pregnancy**

Stage of Grief	Possible Maternal Response	Nursing Plan/Implementation
Shock, disbelief	Pulls back, withdraws: not interested in events around her; may stay in bed, staring at wall, with shades drawn.	Since mother cannot communicate effectively now, nurse demonstrates caring behaviors by staying with her, touching or massaging her; providing physical care; giving her opportunity to talk if she wants to. Do not make light of her situation.
Anger, fear	Verbal fault-finding and possible physical aggression, irritability, insomnia.	State that it is normal to be angry; help her identify her questions and concerns (guilt); be available to her (and her family).
Helplessness, despair, guilt	Dependent behaviors—may become demanding, may cry, may exhibit regressive behaviors; may see no purpose to anything; may feel very guilty, worthless.	Help her verbalize her actual and implied feelings: "It is hard to understand," "You probably feel you are to blame . . ."; "The way you feel may seem strange or even 'crazy' to you." Do provide physical care, give massage, keep her physically comfortable.
Reorganization (after discharge)	Begins to be interested in events around her, to have increased amounts of energy. Inquires again about events leading to the situation, the etiology, the medical and nursing management, as she tries to integrate the experience. Older siblings may show regressive behavior: fear of the dark, fear of school, or behavioral difficulties.	Community health or clinic nurse listens, clarifies, fills in gaps. Reexplain the grieving process—that her (their) behaviors were normal; that acute grief lasts 6 weeks, while the entire process lasts about 1 year. Talk about what older siblings or other family members may be feeling—a young child's return to bed-wetting may be a response to the parents' tension, etc.

b. *Anxiety/fear* related to loss of pregnancy, surgery.

c. *Fluid volume deficit, potential/actual,* related to excessive blood loss.

d. *Pain.*

e. *Ineffective coping, individual/family,* related to knowledge deficit and fear.

f. *Anticipatory/dysfunctional grieving,* related to loss of pregnancy.

g. *Disturbance in self-esteem, body image, role performance,* related to threat to self-image as woman and childbearer.

3. **Nursing plan/implementation:**

a. Goal: *minimize blood loss, stabilize physiologic status.*

(1) Facilitate prompt medical management.

▶ (2) Administer IV fluids, blood, as ordered.

(3) Administer analgesics, as needed.

b. Goal: *prevent infection.* Strict aseptic technique.

c. Goal: *emotional support.*

(1) Encourage verbalization of anxiety, fears, concerns.

(2) Supportive care for grief reaction (Table 2.8).

4. **Evaluation:**

a. Blood loss minimized; physiologic status stable.

b. Copes effectively with loss of pregnancy.

B. Spontaneous abortion: *before viable age of 24 weeks*

1. **Etiology:**

a. Defective products of conception.

b. Insufficient production of progesterone.

c. Acute infections.

d. Reproductive system abnormalities, e.g., incompetent cervical os.

e. Trauma (physical or emotional).

f. Rh incompatibility.

2. **Assessment:** types

a. *Threatened*—mild bleeding, spotting, cramping; cervix closed.

b. *Inevitable*—moderate bleeding, painful cramping; cervix dilated, positive Nitrazine test (membranes ruptured).

c. *Imminent*—profuse bleeding, severe cramping, urge to bear down.

d. *Incomplete*—fetal parts or fetus expelled; placenta and membranes retained.

e. *Complete*—all products of conception expelled; minimal vaginal bleeding.

f. *Habitual/recurrent*—history of spontaneous loss of three or more successive pregnancies.

g. *Missed*—fetal death with no spontaneous expulsion within four weeks.

(1) Anorexia, malaise, headache.

(2) Fundal height—inconsistent with gestational estimate.

(3) Laboratory—increased clotting time, due to resultant concurrent hypofibrinogenemia [disseminated intravascular coagulation (DIC), a major threat to mother].

h. *Induced* abortions (intentionally introduced loss of pregnancy).

3. **Analysis/nursing diagnosis:**
   a. *Altered family processes* related to pregnancy, circumstances surrounding abortion.
   b. *Sexual dysfunction* related to compromised self-image, altered interpersonal relationship, guilt feelings.
4. **Nursing plan/implementation:**
   a. *Threatened*—Goal: *health teaching.* Suggest: avoid coitus and orgasm, especially around normal time for menstrual period.
   b. *Incomplete, inevitable, imminent.*
      (1) Goal: *safeguard status.*
         (a) Save all pads, clots, tissue for expert diagnosis.
         (b) Report immediately any change in status, excessive bleeding, signs of infection, shock.
         (c) Prepare for surgery.
      (2) Goal: *comfort measures.*
         (a) Administer analgesics, as necessary.
         (b) Bedrest, quiet diversional activities.
      (3) Goal: *emotional support.*
         (a) Encourage verbalization of fear, concerns.
         (b) Reduce anxiety, as possible.
         (c) If pregnancy terminates, facilitate grieving process; assist in working through guilt feelings (Table 2.8).
         (d) Supportive care for grief reaction (Table 2.8).
      (4) Goal: *prevent isoimmunization.* See Rh incompatibility, p. 199.
      (5) *Medical management:*
         (a) Laboratory—blood type and Rh factor, direct Coombs, platelets, serum fibrinogen, clotting time.
         (b) Replace blood loss; maintain fluid levels with IV.
         (c) Dilatation and curettage or dilatation and evacuation.
         (d) *Habitual*—determine etiology.
5. **Evaluation:**
   a. *Threatened*—responds to medical/nursing regimen; abortion avoided, successfully carries pregnancy to term.
   b. *Spontaneous abortion*—after uterus emptied.
      (1) Bleeding controlled.
      (2) Vital signs stable.
      (3) Copes effectively with loss of pregnancy.
      (4) Expresses satisfaction with care.
   c. *Habitual abortion*—cause identified and corrected; carries subsequent pregnancy to successful termination.

C. Hydatidiform mole (complete)

1. **Pathophysiology**—chorionic villi degenerate into grapelike cluster of vesicles; may be antecedent to choriocarcinoma.
2. **Etiology**—genetic base; rare complication; more common in women over 45 years of age and Oriental women.
3. **Assessment:**
   a. Uterus—rapid enlargement; fundal height inconsistent with gestational estimate.
   b. Brownish discharge—beginning about week 12; may contain vesicles.
   c. Signs and symptoms of preeclampsia/eclampsia (before third trimester), increased incidence of hyperemesis gravidarum.
   d. *Medical evaluation*—procedures:
      ▶ (1) Sonography, X ray, amniography—no fetal parts present; "snow storm."
      (2) Laboratory test—for elevated Human Chorionic Gonadotropin (HCG) levels.
      (3) Follow-up surveillance of HCG levels for at least one year; persistent HCG level is consistent with choriocarcinoma; x-ray.
4. **Analysis/nursing diagnosis:**
   a. *Anxiety/fear* related to treatment, possible sequelae of hydatidiform mole (choriocarcinoma).
   b. *Potential for injury* related to hemorrhage, perforation of uterine wall, preeclampsia/eclampsia.
   c. *Fluid volume deficit* related to injury.
5. **Nursing plan/implementation:**
   a. *Medical management*
      (1) Monitor for PIH (pregnancy-induced hypertension).
      (2) Evacuate the uterus—hysterectomy may be necessary.
      (3) Strict contraception for at least one year to enable accurate assessment of status.
      (4) Choriocarcinoma—chemotherapy (methotrexate) and/or radiation therapy.
   b. *Nursing management*
      (1) Goal: *safeguard status.* Observe for hemorrhage, passage of retained vesicles and abdominal pain, or signs of infection (as at-risk for perforation of uterine wall).
      (2) Goal: *health teaching.*
         (a) Explain, discuss diagnostic tests; prepare for tests.
         (b) Discuss contraceptive options.
         (c) Importance of follow-up.
      (3) Goal: *preoperative and postoperative care.*
      (4) Goal: *emotional support.* Facilitate grieving (Table 2.8).
6. **Evaluation:**
   a. Verbalizes understanding of diagnosis, tests, and treatment.
   b. Complies with medical/nursing recommendations.
   c. Tolerates surgical procedure well.
      (1) Bleeding controlled.
      (2) Vital signs stable.

(3) Urinary output adequate.

d. Copes effectively with loss of pregnancy.

e. Returns for follow-up care/surveillance.

f. Selects and effectively implements method of contraception; avoids pregnancy for one year or more.

g. Tests for Human Chorionic Gonadotropin (HCG) remain negative for one year; no evidence of malignancy.

h. Achieves a pregnancy when desired.

i. Successfully carries pregnancy to term; normal, uncomplicated delivery of viable infant.

D. Ectopic pregnancy

1. **Pathology**—implantation outside of uterine cavity.
2. Types:
   a. Tubal (most common).
   b. Cervical.
   c. Abdominal.
   d. Ovarian.
3. **Etiology:**
   a. Pelvic Inflammatory Disease (PID)—pelvic salpingitis and endometriosis.
   b. Tubal or uterine anomalies, tubal spasm.
   c. Adhesions from pelvic inflammatory disease (PID) or past surgeries.
   d. Presence of IUD (intrauterine device).
4. **Assessment:** dependent on implantation site.
   a. *Early signs*—abnormal menstrual period (usually following a missed menstrual period), spotting, some symptoms of pregnancy; possible dull pain on affected side.
   b. *Impending or posttubal rupture*—sudden, acute, lower abdominal pain; nausea and vomiting; signs of shock; referred shoulder pain (*Kehr's sign*) or neck pain—due to blood in peritoneal cavity; blood in cul-de-sac may → rectal pressure.
   c. Sharp, localized pain when cervix is touched during vaginal exam; shock and circulatory collapse in some, usually following vaginal exam.
   d. Positive pregnancy test in many women.
5. **Analysis/nursing diagnosis:**
   a. *Fear* related to abdominal pain and pregnancy status.
   b. *Grief* related to pregnancy loss.
6. **Nursing plan/implementation:**
   a. *Medical management:* Surgical removal/repair.
   b. *Nursing management:*
      (1) Goal: *preoperative and postoperative care, health teaching.*
      (2) Goal: *supportive care for grief reaction;* encourage verbalization of anxiety and concerns of further pregnancies.
7. **Evaluation:**
   a. Uncomplicated postoperative course.
   b. Copes effectively with loss of pregnancy.

II. Complications affecting nutrition/elimination: *hyperemesis gravidarum*

A. Pathophysiology—pernicious vomiting during first 14–16 weeks (peak incidence around 10 weeks gestation); excessive vomiting at any time during pregnancy. Potential hazards include:

1. Dehydration with fluid and electrolyte imbalance.
2. Starvation, with loss of 5% or more of body weight; protein and vitamin deficiencies.
3. Metabolic acidosis—due to breakdown of fat stores to meet metabolic needs.
4. Hypovolemia and hemoconcentration; increased blood urea nitrogen (BUN); decreased urinary output.

B. Etiology:

1. Physiologic—secretion of HCG, decrease in free gastric HCl, decreased gastrointestinal motility. Increased incidence in hydatidiform mole and multiple pregnancy (due to high levels of HCG).
2. Psychologic—thought to be related to rejection of pregnancy and/or sexual relations.

C. Assessment:

1. Intractable vomiting.
2. Abdominal pain.
3. Hiccups.
4. Marked weight loss.
5. Dehydration—thirst, tachycardia, skin turgor.
6. Increased respiratory rate (metabolic acidosis).
7. Laboratory—elevated BUN.
8. *Medical evaluation:* rule out other causes (infection, tumors).

D. Analysis/nursing diagnosis:

1. *Altered nutrition, less than body requirements,* due to inability to retain oral feedings.
2. *Fluid volume deficit* due to dehydration.
3. *Ineffective individual coping* related to symptoms, insecurity in role, psychologic stress of unwanted pregnancy.
4. *Personal identity disturbance* related to symptoms and/or perception of self as inadequate in role, sick, socially unpresentable.

E. Nursing plan/implementation:

1. Goal: *minimize environmental stimuli.*
   a. Limit visitors and phone calls.
   b. Bedrest with bathroom privileges.
2. Goal: *emotional support.*
   a. Establish accepting, supportive environment.
   b. Encourage verbalization of anxiety, fears, concerns.
   c. Support positive self-image.

III. Complications affecting protective function: *sexually transmitted diseases*. This NCLEX category measures applications of knowledge about conditions related to client capacity to maintain defenses and prevent physical and chemical trauma, injury, infection, and threats to health status.

A. Vaginitis—inflammation of vagina.

1. **Pathophysiology**—local inflammatory reaction (redness, heat, irritation/tenderness, pain).

2. **Etiology:**
   a. Common causative organisms:
      (1) Bacteria—streptococci, *E. coli,* gonococci, chlamydia.
      (2) *Viruses*—herpes type II, CMV, HPV (human papillomavirus).
      (3) Protozoa—*Trichomonas vaginalis.*
      (4) Fungi—*Candida albicans.*
   b. Atrophic changes—due to declining hormone level (postmenopausal clients).
3. **Assessment:** differentiate among common vaginal infections:
   a. Vulvovaginal erythema.
   b. Pruritus, dysuria, dyspareunia.
   c. Vaginal discharge.
4. **Analysis/nursing diagnosis:** *pain* related to inflammation, discharge.
5. **Nursing plan/implementation:**
   a. Goal: *emotional support.*
   b. Goal: *health teaching.* Instruct client in self-care measures to promote comfort and healing:
      (1) Perineal care.
      (2) Sitz baths.
      (3) Douching (as ordered).
      (4) Exposure of vulva to air.
      (5) Cotton briefs.
      (6) Proper insertion of vaginal suppository.
   c. Goal: *prevent reinfection.*
      (1) Suggest sexual partner use condom until infection is eliminated—or abstain from intercourse.
      (2) Recommend sexual partner seek examination and treatment.
   d. Goal: *medical consultation/treatment.* Refer for diagnosis and treatment.
6. **Evaluation:**
   a. Asymptomatic; unable to recover organism from body fluids or tissue.
   b. Avoids reinfection.

B. Gonorrhea

1. **Pathophysiology:**
   a. Male—early infection usually confined to urethra, vestibular glands, anus, or pharynx. Untreated: ascending infection may involve testes, causing sterility.
   b. Female—early infection usually confined to vestibular glands, endocervix, urethra, anus (vagina is resistant). May ascend to involve pelvic structures, e.g., fallopian tubes, ovaries; scarring may cause sterility.
   c. Pregnant female—may result in premature rupture of membranes, amnionitis, premature labor, postpartum salpingitis.
   d. Sequelae (untreated):
      (1) May develop carrier state (asymptomatic; organism resident in vestibular glands).
      (2) Systemic spread may result in gonococcal:
         (a) Arthritis.
         (b) Endocarditis.
         (c) Meningitis.
         (d) Septicemia.
   e. Newborn—ophthalmia neonatorum (gonococcal conjunctivitis). Untreated sequelae: blindness.
2. **Etiology:** gram-negative diplococcus (*Neisseria gonorrhoeae*).
3. **Epidemiology:**
   a. Portal of entry—oral or genitourinary mucous membranes.
   b. Mode of transmission—usually sexual contact.
   c. Incubation period: 2–5 days; may be asymptomatic.
   d. Communicable period—as long as organisms are present; to 4 days after antibiotic therapy begun.
4. **Assessment:**
   a. History of known (or suspected) contact.
   b. *Male:*
      (1) Complaint of mucoid or mucopurulent discharge.
      (2) Medical diagnosis—procedure: urethral discharge gram stain.
   c. *Female:*
      (1) Often asymptomatic; acute infection: severe vulvovaginal inflammation, venereal warts, greenish-yellow vaginal discharge.
      (2) Medical diagnosis—procedure: endocervical culture.
   d. Gonococcal urethritis (male and female)—sudden severe dysuria, frequency, burning, edema.
   e. Salpingitis/oophoritis—severe, sudden abdominal pain, fever (with or without vaginal discharge).
5. **Analysis/nursing diagnosis:** *impaired tissue integrity* related to tissue inflammation.
6. **Nursing plan/implementation:**
   a. Goal: *emotional support.*
   b. Goal: *health teaching* to prevent transmission, sequelae, reinfection.
      (1) Need for accurate diagnosis and effective treatment, follow-up exam in 7–14 days, and culture.
      (2) All sexual partners need exam, treatment.
      (3) Possible sequelae/complications (sterility, carrier state).
   c. Goal: *medical consultation/treatment.*
      (1) Determine allergy to penicillin, erythromycin, probenecid.
      (2) Refer for diagnosis and treatment.
         (a) Diagnosis.
         (b) Treatment—aqueous penicillin G, 2.4 million units in each buttock (4.8 million units total dose) and Probenecid 1 gram po.
         (c) Follow-up culture before delivery.
         (d) Notification of sexual partners.

7. **Evaluation:**
   a. Verbalizes understanding of mode of transmission, prevention, importance of exam, treatment of sexual contacts.
   b. Informs sexual contacts of need for exam.
   c. Returns for follow-up examinations.
   d. Successfully treated; weekly follow-up cultures: negative on two successive visits.
   e. Avoids reinfection.

C. *Chlamydia trachomatis*

1. **Pathophysiology:**
   a. Most common sexually transmitted disease in U.S.
   b. Initial infection mild in females; inflammation of cervix with discharge.
   c. If untreated, may lead to urethritis, dysuria, PID, tubal occlusion, infertility.
2. **Etiology:**
   a. *Chlamydia trachomatis* has maternal-fetal effects.
   b. Bacteria can exist only within living cells.
   c. Transmission is by direct contact from one person to another.
3. **Assessment—maternal:**
   a. Inflamed cervix (may be asymptomatic).
   b. Cervical congestion, edema.
   c. Mucopurulent discharge.
4. **Assessment—fetal-neonatal:**
   a. Increased incidence of stillbirth.
   b. Preterm birth may result.
   c. Contact with infected mucus occurs during delivery.
   d. Newborn may be asymptomatic.
   e. Conjunctivitis may lead to scarring.
   f. Respiratory problems—tachypnea, dyspnea, apnea.
5. **Analysis/nursing diagnosis:**
   a. *Pain* related to inflamed reproductive organs.
   b. *Fatigue* related to inflammation.
   c. *Knowledge deficit* related to mode of treatment, disease transmission.
6. **Nursing plan/implementation:**
   a. Treatment with antibiotics, generally erythromycin, tetracycline.
   b. Provide pain relief, analgesics.
   c. Counsel regarding use of condoms, spermicidal agents to prevent reinfection.
7. **Evaluation:**
   a. Client understands treatment and shows compliance.
   b. Client understands portal of entry and risk for reinfection.

D. *Herpes genitalis*

1. **Pathophysiology**—initial infection: varies in severity of symptoms, may be local or systemic; duration: prolonged; morbidity: severe.
2. **Etiology**—Herpes virus type II.
3. **Epidemiology:**
   a. Portal of entry—skin, mucous membranes.
   b. Mode of transmission—usually sexual.
   c. Incubation: 3–14 days.
   d. Communicable period—while organisms are present.
4. **Assessment:**
   a. Lesions—painful, red papules; pustular vesicles that break and form wet ulcers that later crust; self-limiting (three weeks).
   b. Severe itching and/or pain.
   c. Discharge—copious; foul-smelling.
   d. Dysuria.
   e. Lymph nodes—enlarged, inflammatory, inguinal.
   f. Pregnant female—vaginal bleeding, spontaneous abortion, fetal death.
   g. May shed virus for seven weeks.
   ▶ h. Medical diagnosis: multinucleated giant cells in microscopic exam of lesion exudate; culture for herpes simplex virus.
5. **Analysis/nursing diagnosis:**
   a. *Pain* related to inflammation process.
   b. *Fear* related to longevity of disease.
   c. *Fear* related to no cure for disease.
   d. *Knowledge deficit* related to transmission to future partners.
6. **Nursing plan/implementation:**
   a. Goal: *emotional support.*
   b. Goal: *health teaching.*
      (1) Virus remains in body for life (dormant, noninfectious) in 25–30% of population; small percent have symptoms.
      (2) Recurrence probable; usually shorter and milder.
      ▶ (3) Annual Pap smear important—associated with later development of cervical cancer.
      (4) Need for close surveillance during pregnancy; cesarean section may be indicated if active lesions.
   c. Goal: *promote comfort.*
   d. Goal: *accurate definitive treatment.* Refer for diagnosis and treatment.
      ▶ (1) Diagnosis—cervical smears.
      (2) Treatment—acylovir ointment (Zovirax, but not in pregnancy).
7. **Evaluation:** asymptomatic.

E. Syphilis

1. **Pathophysiology:**
   a. *Primary stage:* nonreactive VDRL.
      (1) *Male:* three to four weeks after contact, painless, localized penile/anal ulcer (chancre); lymph nodes—enlarged, regional.
      (2) *Female:* often asymptomatic; labial, vaginal, or cervical chancre.

(3) Medical diagnosis—procedure: dark-field microscopic examination of lesion exudate.

b. *Secondary stage:* reactive VDRL.

(1) Six to eight weeks after infection.

(2) Rash—macular, papular; on trunk, palms, soles.

(3) Malaise, headache, sore throat, weight loss, low-grade temperature.

c. *Latent stage;* reactive serologic test for syphilis (STS). Asymptomatic; noninfectious.

d. *Tertiary stage:*

(1) Gumma formation in skin, cardiovascular or central nervous system.

(2) Psychosis.

2. **Etiology:** *Treponema pallidum* (spirochete).

3. **Epidemiology:**

a. Portal of entry—skin, mucous membranes.

b. Mode of transmission—usually sexual.

c. Incubation period—9 days to 3 months.

d. Communicable period—primary and secondary stages.

4. **Assessment:**

a. *Primary*—chancre, when detectable. Medical diagnosis—procedure: dark-field examination of lesion exudate.

b. *Secondary:*

(1) Malaise, lymphadenopathy, headache, elevated temperature.

(2) Macular, papular rash on palms and soles; may be disseminated.

(3) Medical diagnosis—see point d below.

c. *Tertiary:*

(1) Subcutaneous nodules (gumma).

(2) **Note:** Gumma formation may affect any body system; symptoms associated with area of involvement.

d. Medical diagnosis—procedures: stages other than primary—STS: VDRL, rapid plasma reagin (RPR), *Treponema pallidum* immobilization (TPI), fluorescent treponemal antibody absorption (FTA). *False positive STS* in: collagen diseases, infectious mononucleosis, malaria, systemic tuberculosis.

5. **Analysis/nursing diagnosis:**

a. *Pain* related to inflammation process.

b. *Knowledge deficit* related to treatment and transmission of the disease.

6. **Nursing plan/implementation:**

a. Goal: *emotional support*

(1) Nonjudgmental.

(2) Caring, supportive manner.

b. Goal: *health teaching.*

(1) Need for accurate diagnosis and treatment, follow-up examinations.

(2) All sexual partners need exam and treatment.

c. Goal: *medical consultation/treatment.*

(1) Refer for diagnosis and treatment. **Note:** In pregnancy—treatment by 18th gestational week prevents congenital syphilis in neonate; however, treat at time of diagnosis.

(2) Treatment:

(a) Primary, secondary—benzathine penicillin G, 2.4 million units.

(b) Other stages—7.2 million units over 3-week period.

(c) Erythromycin for penicillin-allergic clients.

7. **Evaluation:**

a. If treated by 18th week of pregnancy, congenital syphilis is prevented.

b. Appropriate treatment after 18th week cures both mother and fetus; however, any fetal damage occurring prior to treatment is irreversible.

c. Follow-up VDRL: nonreactive at 1, 3, 6, 9, and 12 months.

d. Tertiary—cerebrospinal fluid examination negative at six months and one year following treatment.

e. Verbalizes understanding of mode of transmission, potential sequelae without treatment, importance of exam/treatment of sexual contacts, preventive techniques.

f. Informs contacts of need for exam.

g. Returns for follow-up visit.

h. Avoids reinfection.

F. Pelvic inflammatory disease (PID)

1. **Pathophysiology**—ascending pelvic infection; may involve fallopian tubes (salpingitis), ovaries (oophoritis); may develop pelvic abscess (most common complication), pelvic cellulitis, pelvic thrombophlebitis, peritonitis.

2. **Etiology:**

a. *Chlamydia trachomatis.*

b. Gonococci.

c. Streptococci.

d. Staphylococci.

3. **Assessment:**

a. Pain: acute, abdominal.

b. Vaginal discharge: foul-smelling.

c. Fever, chills, malaise.

d. Elevated white blood count.

4. **Analysis/nursing diagnosis:**

a. *Pain* related to occluded tubules.

b. Infertility related to permanent block of tubes.

c. *Knowledge deficit* related to transmission of disease.

d. *Altered urinary elimination* due to dysuria.

5. **Nursing plan/implementation**—for hospitalized client:

a. Goal: *emotional support.*

b. Goal: *limit extension of infection.*

(1) Bedrest—position: semi-Fowler's, to promote drainage.

(2) Force fluids to 3000 mL/day.

(3) Administer antibiotics, as ordered.

c. Goal: *prevent autoinocculation/transmission.*

(1) Strict aseptic technique (handwashing, perineal care).

(2) Contact-item isolation.

(3) Health teaching: If untreated: high risk of tubal scarring, sterility, or ectopic pregnancy; pelvic adhesions; transmission of disease.

d. Goal: *promote comfort.*

(1) Analgesics, as ordered.

(2) External heat, as ordered.

6. **Evaluation:**

a. Responds to therapy; uneventful recovery.

b. Avoids reinfection.

Second Trimester Complications

See Table 2.7, p. 138.

I. Complications affecting comfort, rest, mobility: *Incompetent cervix*

A. Pathophysiology—inability of cervix to support growing weight of pregnancy; associated with repeated spontaneous second trimester abortion.

B. Etiology:

1. Unknown.
2. Congenital defect in cervical musculature.
3. Cervical trauma during previous birth, abortion; aggressive, deep, or repeated dilatation and curettage.

C. Assessment:

1. History of habitual, second trimester abortions.
2. Painless, progressive cervical effacement and dilatation during second trimester.
3. Signs of threatened abortion or (early third trimester) premature labor.

D. Analysis/nursing diagnosis:

1. *Pain* related to early dilatation.
2. *Fear* related to possible pregnancy loss.

E. Nursing plan/implementation:

1. *Medical management*

a. Cerclage surgical procedure (Shirodkar, McDonald).

2. *Preoperative nursing management*

a. Goal: *reduce physical stress on incompetent cervix.* Bedrest, supportive care.

b. Goal: *emotional support.* Encourage verbalization of anxiety, fear, concerns.

c. Goal: *health (preoperative) teaching.* Explain procedure—purse-string suture encircles cervix and reinforces musculature.

d. Goal: *preparation for surgery.*

3. *Postoperative nursing management*

a. Goal: *maximize surgical result.* Bedrest, supportive care.

b. Goal: *health teaching.*

(1) Avoid: strenuous physical activity; straining.

(2) Report promptly: signs of labor (vaginal bleeding, cramping).

(3) Need for continued, close health surveillance.

4. **Evaluation:** carries pregnancy to successful termination.

II. Complications affecting sensory/perceptual functions: *pregnancy-induced hypertension* (P.I.H.); preeclampsia—eclampsia

A. Pathophysiology

1. Generalized arteriospasm → increased peripheral resistance, decreased tissue perfusion, and hypertension.
2. *Kidney:*

a. Reduced renal perfusion and vasospasm → glomerular lesions.

b. Damage to membrane → loss of serum protein (albuminuria). **Note:** Reduced serum A/G (albumin/globulin) ratio alters blood osmolarity → edema.

c. Increased tubular reabsorption of sodium → increased water retention (edema).

d. Release of angiotensin contributes to vasospasm and hypertension.

3. *Brain:* decreased oxygenation, cerebral edema, and vasospasm → visual disturbances and hyperirritability, convulsions, and coma.
4. *Uterus:* decreased placental perfusion → increased risk of SGA baby, abruptio placentae.

B. Etiology: unknown. *Risk factors:*

1. Pregnancy—occurs only when a functioning trophoblast is present; more common in *first* pregnancies; develops after week 24 of gestation.
2. Age-related—under 17 and over 35 years of age.
3. Coexisting conditions—diabetes, multiple gestation, hydramnios.
4. Diet—low in protein.

C. Assessment—types:

1. *Preeclampsia—mild*

a. Hypertension—systolic increase of 30 mm Hg or more over baseline; diastolic rise of 15 mm Hg or more.

b. Proteinuria—1 g/day.

c. Edema—digital and periorbital; weight gain over 0.45 kg (1 lb) per week.

2. *Preeclampsia—severe*

a. Increasing hypertension—systolic at or above 160 mm Hg or more than 50 mm Hg over baseline; diastolic, 110 mm Hg or more.

b. Urine: proteinuria (5 g or more in 24 hours); oliguria (400 mL or less in 24 hours).

c. Hemoconcentration, hypoproteinemia, hypernatremia, hypovolemic condition.

d. Persistent vomiting.

e. Epigastric pain—due to edema of liver capsule.

f. Cerebral or visual disturbances (before convulsive state):

(1) Disorientation and somnolence.

(2) Severe frontal headache.

(3) Increased irritability; hyperreflexia.

(4) Blurred vision, halo vision, dimness, blind spots.

3. *Eclampsia*
   a. Tonic and clonic convulsions; coma.
   b. Renal shutdown—oliguria, anuria.

D. Assessment—hospitalized client:

1. Vital signs (blood pressure, pulse, respirations)—q 2–4 h, while awake (if mild to moderate preeclampsia) and/or as necessary. **Note:** record, report persistent hypertension.
2. Fetal heart tones at time of vital signs.
3. Deep tendon reflexes (DTR) and clonus—to identify/monitor CNS hyperirritability.
4. I&O—to identify diuresis. (**Note:** oliguria indicates pathologic progression.)
5. Urinalysis (clean-catch) for protein, daily or after each voiding, as necessary.
6. Signs of pathologic progression (see C. Assessment—types, above).
7. Signs of labor, abruptio placentae (**Note:** high blood pressure, or a rapid drop, may initiate abruptio), DIC.
8. Emotional status.
9. Daily weight, amount/distribution of edema (pitting; pedal, digital, periorbital)—to identify signs of mobilization of tissue fluid, diuresis.

E. Analysis/nursing diagnosis:

1. *Fluid volume excess:* hemoconcentration, edema related to altered blood osmolarity and sodium/water retention.
2. *Altered nutrition, less than body requirements:* protein deficiency related to dietary lack and/or loss through damaged renal membrane.
3. *Altered tissue perfusion* related to increased peripheral resistance and vasospasm in renal, cardiovascular system.
4. *Altered urinary elimination:* oliguria, anuria related to hypovolemia.
5. *Sensory/perceptual alterations:* visual disturbances, hyperirritability related to cerebral edema, decreased oxygenation to brain.
6. *Anxiety* related to symptoms, implications of pathophysiology.
7. *Diversional activity deficit* related to need for reduced environmental stimuli, bedrest.
8. *Potential for injury* related to seizure.

F. Prognosis:

1. *Good*—symptoms mild, respond to treatment.
2. *Poor*—convulsions (number and duration); persistent coma; hyperthermia, tachycardia (120 bpm); cyanosis.
3. *Terminal*—pulmonary edema, congestive heart failure, acute renal failure, cerebral hemorrhage. The earlier the symptoms appear, the poorer the outcome for the pregnancy.

G. Nursing plan/implementation: Goal: *health teaching.*

1. *Dietary counseling:* high-protein diet—to increase blood osmolarity, reduce movement of vascular fluid into interstitial space.
2. *Rest*—frequent naps in left Sims position.
3. Immediate report of danger signs.
   a. Digital and periorbital edema.
   b. Severe headache, irritability.
   c. Visual disturbances.
   d. Epigastric pain.
4. Do roll-over test (BP while on back and left positions).
5. Importance of regular prenatal visits.
6. Monitoring own blood pressure between prenatal visits.

H. Nursing plan/implementation—hospitalized client:

1. Goal: *reduce environmental stimuli.* To minimize stimulation of hyperirritable CNS. Limit visitors and phone calls.
2. Goal: *emotional support.*
   a. Encourage verbalization of anxiety, fears, concerns.
   b. Explain all procedures, seizure precautions.
3. Goal: *supportive care.*
   a. Encourage bedrest—to increase tissue perfusion, promote diuresis.
   b. Position: left Sims—to reduce risk of supine hypotensive syndrome.
4. Goal: *health teaching.* High protein diet—to replace protein lost in urine, to retain fluid in the intravascular compartment, to reduce edema; moderate sodium—reduce intake of high-sodium foods, no added salt.
5. Goal: *monitor and administer drugs as ordered.*
   a. Anticonvulsants (especially magnesium sulfate).
   b. Antihypertensives.
   c. Diuretics (rarely used).
   d. Blood volume expanders.
6. Goal: *seizure precautions.* To safeguard maternal/fetal status.
   a. Observe for signs and symptoms of *impending* convulsion:
      (1) Frontal headache.
      (2) Epigastric pain.
      (3) Sharp cry.
      (4) Eyes fixed; unresponsive.
      (5) Facial twitching.
   b. Emergency items (suction equipment, airway, drugs, IV fluids) immediately available.
7. Goal: *convulsion care* (eclamptic client).
   a. Maintain patent *airway;* administer oxygen.
   b. *Safety*—padded bed rails.
   c. Reduce environmental stimuli: dim lights, quiet.
   d. Observe, report, and record:
      (1) Onset and progression of convulsion.
      (2) If followed by coma and/or incontinence.
   e. Close observation for 48 hours postpartum, even if no further convulsions (or no convulsions to date). Check FHR; observe for labor.

TABLE 2.9 Comparison of Placenta Previa and Abruptio Placentae

Pathology	Etiology	Assessment	Nursing Plan/ Implementation
Placenta Previa			
Types: *Marginal*—low-lying. *Partial*—partly covers internal os. *Complete*—covers internal os.	Unknown. More common with multiparity, advanced maternal age. Fibroid tumors. Endometriosis. Old scars. Smoking. IVR.	Painless vaginal bleeding. Usually manifests in 8th month. *Postpartum:* signs of hemorrhage, infection.	*No* vaginal or rectal exams or enemas. Bedrest (high Fowler's if marginal previa). Continous fetal monitor. Maternal vital signs q 4 hours, or as needed. Note character and amount of bleeding. Emotional support.
Abruptio Placentae			
Types: *Partial*—small part separates. *Complete*—total placenta separates. *Retroplacental*—bleeding (concealed). *Marginal*—occurs at edges; external bleeding.	Preeclampsia/eclampsia. Prior to delivery of second twin. Traction on cord. Rupture of membranes. High parity. Chronic renal hypertension. Oxytocin induction/ augmentation of labor. Cocaine addiction.	Pain: sudden, severe. Abdomen: rigid. Uterus: very tender to touch. Fetal hyperactivity; bradycardia, demise. Shock: rapid, profound. Port wine amniotic fluid. Signs of DIC. *Postpartum:* signs of: atony, infection, pulmonary emboli.	Position: supine; elevate (R) hip. Monitor: vital signs, blood loss, fetus. I&O (anuria, oliguria; hematuria). Prepare for surgery. Emotional support.

I. Evaluation:

1. Complies with medical/nursing plan of care.
2. Symptoms respond to treatment; progression halted.
3. Carries uneventful pregnancy to successful termination.

Third Trimester Complications

See Table 2.7, p. 139.

I. Complications affecting fluid-gas transport

A. Placenta previa—abnormal implantation; near or over internal os. Increased incidence with smokers.

1. **Assessment:**
   a. Painless vaginal bleeding (may be intermittent); absence of contractions, abdomen soft.
   b. If in labor, contractions usually normal.
   c. Boggy lower uterine segment--palpated on vaginal exam. (**Note:** If placenta previa is suspected, internal exams are *contraindicated*.)
   ▶ d. *Medical diagnosis—procedure:* sonography—to determine placental site.
2. **Analysis/nursing diagnosis:**
   a. *Anxiety* related to bleeding, outcome.
   b. *Fluid volume deficit* related to excessive blood loss.
   c. *Altered tissue perfusion* secondary to blood loss.
   d. *Altered urinary elimination* related to hypovolemia.
   e. *Fear* related to fetal injury or loss.
3. **Nursing plan/implementation:**
   a. *Medical management*
      (1) Sterile vaginal exam under double set-up.
      (2) Vaginal delivery possible if bleeding minimal, marginal implantation; presenting part acts as tamponade.
      (3) Cesarean delivery for complete previa.
   b. *Nursing management.* Goal: *safeguard status.*
4. **Evaluation:** see Abruptio placentae below and Table 2.9.

B. Abruptio placentae—premature separation of normally implanted placenta.

1. **Assessment:**
   a. Sudden onset, severe abdominal pain.
   b. Increased uterine tone—may contract unevenly, fails to relax between contractions; very tender.
   c. Shock usually more profound than expected on basis of external bleeding or internal bleeding.
   d. *Medical evaluation—procedures:* DIC screening (bleeding time, platelet count, prothrombin time, activated partial thromboplastin time, fibrinogen).
2. **Analysis/nursing diagnosis:**
   a. *Fluid volume deficit* related to bleeding.
   b. *Potential for fetal injury* related to utero-placental insufficiency.
   c. *Fear* related to unknown outcome.
3. *Potential complications:*
   a. Afibrinoginemia and disseminated intravascular coagulation (DIC).
   b. Couvelaire uterus—bleeding into uterine muscle.
   c. Amniotic fluid embolus.
   d. Hypovolemic shock.
   e. Renal failure.

f. Uterine atony, hemorrhage, infection in postpartum.

4. **Nursing plan/implementation:**
   a. *Medical management*
      (1) Control: hemorrhage, hypovolemic shock, replace blood loss.
      (2) Cesarean delivery.
      (3) Fibrinogen, if necessary (avoided if possible, due to chance of hepatitis).
      (4) IV heparin—by infusion pump—to reduce coagulation and fibrinolysis.
   b. *Nursing management.* Goal: *safeguard status.*
5. **Evaluation:**
   a. Experiences successful termination of pregnancy.
      (1) Delivers viable newborn (via vaginal or cesarean method).
      (2) Minimal blood loss.
      (3) All assessment findings within normal limits.
      (4) Retains capacity for further childbearing.
   b. No evidence of complications (anemia, hypotonia, DIC) during postpartal period.

II. Complications affecting comfort, rest, mobility

A. Hydramnios—amniotic fluid in excess of 2000 mL (normal volume: 500–1200 mL).

1. **Etiology:** unknown. Risk factors:
   a. Maternal diabetes.
   b. Multiple gestation.
   c. Erythroblastosis fetalis.
   d. Preeclampsia/eclampsia.
   e. Congenital anomalies (e.g., anencephaly, upper GI anomalies, such as esophageal atresia).
2. **Assessment:**
   a. Fundal height: excessive for gestational estimate.
   b. Fetal parts: difficult to palpate, small in proportion to uterine size.
   c. Increased discomfort—due to large, heavy uterus.
   d. Increased edema in vulva and legs.
   e. Shortness of breath.
   f. GI discomfort—heartburn, constipation.
   g. Susceptibility to supine hypotensive syndrome—due to compression of inferior vena cava while in supine position.
   h. *Medical diagnosis—procedures:*
      ▶ (1) Sonography—to diagnose multiple pregnancy, gross fetal anomaly, locate placental site.
      (2) Amniocentesis—to diagnose anomalies, erythroblastosis.
3. *Potential complications:*
   a. Maternal respiratory embarrassment.
   b. Premature rupture of membranes (PROM) with prolapsed cord and/or amnionitis.
   c. Premature labor.
   d. Postpartum hemorrhage—due to overdistention and uterine atony.
4. **Analysis/nursing diagnosis:**
   a. *Pain* related to excessive size of uterus impinging on diaphragm, stomach, bladder.
   b. *Impaired physical mobility* related to increased lordotic curvative of back, increased weight on legs.
   c. *Altered tissue perfusion* related to decreased venous return from lower extremities, compression of body structures by overdistended uterus.
   d. *Potential fluid volume deficit* related to potential uterine atony in immediate postpartum, secondary to loss of contractility due to overdistention.
   e. *Sleep pattern disturbance* related to respiratory embarrassment and discomfort in side-lying position.
   f. *Anxiety* related to discomfort, potential for complications, associated with congenital anomalies.
   g. *Altered urinary elimination* frequency related to pressure of overdistended uterus on bladder.
5. **Nursing plan/implementation:**
   a. *Medical management*
      ▶ (1) Amniocentesis—remove excess fluid very slowly, to prevent abruptio placentae.
      (2) Termination of pregnancy—if fetal abnormality present *and* client desires.
   b. *Nursing management*
      (1) Goal: *health teaching.*
         (a) Need for left Sims position during resting; semi-Fowler's may alleviate respiratory embarrassment.
         (b) Explain diagnostic and/or treatment procedures.
         (c) Signs and symptoms to be reported immediately: bleeding, loss of fluid through vagina, cramping.
      (2) Goal: *prepare for diagnostic and/or treatment procedures.*
         (a) Force fluids—for sonography.
         (b) Permit for amniocentesis.
      (3) Goal: *emotional support for loss of pregnancy* (if applicable).
         (a) Encourage verbalization of feelings.
         (b) Facilitate grieving: permit parents to see, hold infant; if desired, take photograph, footprints for them.
6. **Evaluation:**
   a. Complies with medical/nursing management.
   b. Symptoms of respiratory embarrassment, etc. reduced; comfort promoted.
   c. Experiences normal, uncomplicated pregnancy, labor, delivery, and postpartum.

III. Diagnostic tests to evaluate fetal growth and well-being

▶ A. Daily fetal movement count (DFMC)

1. Assesses fetal activity.
2. Noninvasive test done by pregnant woman.
3. 3 movements/h normal activity.

4. 2 movements or less/h may indicate fetal jeopardy.
5. Assess for fetal sleep patterns; repeat after ingesting glucose.

B. Nonstress test (NST)

1. Correlates fetal movement with FHR. Requires electronic monitoring.
2. Reactive test—acceleration of FHR 15 bpm above baseline FHR, lasting for 15 sec or more.
3. Nonreactive test—acceleration less than 15 bpm above baseline FHR. May indicate fetal jeopardy.

C. Contraction stress test (CST); oxytocin challenge test (OCT)

1. Correlates fetal heart rate response to induced uterine contractions.
2. Requires electronic monitoring.
3. Indicator of utero-placental compatibility.
4. Identifies pregnancies at risk for fetal compromise from uteroplacental insufficiency.
5. Increasing doses of oxytocin are administered to stimulate uterine contractions.
6. Interpretation: *negative* results indicate absence of abnormal deceleration with all contractions.
7. *Positive* results indicate abnormal FHR decelerations with contractions.
8. Nipple stimulation (Breast self-stimulation test) may also release enough systemic oxytocin to contract uterus so as to obtain indicators of fetal well-being or fetal jeopardy.

D. Biophysical profile

1. Observation by ultrasound of 5 variables for 30 minutes:
   a. Fetal body movements.
   b. Fetal tone.
   c. Amniotic fluid volume.
   d. Response to non-stress testing.
   e. Fetal breathing movements.
2. Variables are scored at 2 if present; score of less than 6 is associated with perinatal mortality.

E. Ultrasound

1. Noninvasive procedure involving passage of high-frequency sound waves through uterus to obtain data regarding fetal growth, placental positioning, and the uterine cavity.
2. Purpose may include:
   a. Pregnancy confirmation.
   b. Fetal viability.
   c. Estimation of fetal age.
   d. BPD measurement (biparietal diameter).
   e. Placenta location.
   f. Detect fetal abnormalities.
   g. Confirm fetal demise.
   h. Identify multiple gestations.
3. No risk to mother with infrequent use. Fetal risk not determined on long-term basis.

F. Amniocentesis

1. Invasive procedure for amniotic fluid analysis to assess fetal growth and maturity; done after 14 weeks gestation.
2. Needle placed through abdominal-uterine wall; designated amount of fluid is withdrawn for examination.
3. Empty bladder if gestation greater than 20 weeks.
4. Risk of complications less than 1%. Ultrasound *always* precedes this procedure.
5. Possible complications: onset of contractions; infections (probably amnionitis); placental, cord puncture; bladder puncture.
6. Advise clients to observe and report to physician: fetal hypo- or hyperactivity, vaginal bleeding, vaginal discharge (clear or colored), signs of labor.

G. Analysis of amniotic fluid

1. Chromosomal studies to detect genetic aberrations.
2. Biochemical analysis of fetal cells to detect inborn errors of metabolism.
3. Determination of fetal lung maturity by assessing lecithin-sphingomyelin ratios.
4. Evaluation of phospholipids (PG and PI); aids in determining lung maturity; new and accurate.
5. Determination of creatinine levels, aids in determining fetal age. (Greater than 1.8 mg/100 cc indicates fetal maturity and the fetal age.)
6. Assesses isoimmune disease.
7. Assesses alfa-fetoprotein levels for determination of neural-tube defects.
8. Presence of meconium may indicate fetal hypoxia.

H. Chorionic villous sampling (CVS)

1. Cervically invasive procedure.
2. Advantage—results can be obtained after 6 weeks gestation due to fast-growing fetal cells.
3. Procedure—removal of small piece of tissue (chorionic villi) from fetal portion of placenta. Tissue reflects genetic makeup of fetus.
4. Determines some genetic aberrations and allows for earlier decision for induced abortion (if desired) from abnormal results. Does not diagnose neural tube defects; CVS patients need further diagnoses with ultrasound and serum AFP (alpha-fetoprotein) levels.
5. Protects "pregnancy privacy" since results can be obtained before the pregnancy is apparent and decisions can be made regarding abortion or carrying of gestation.
6. Risks involve spontaneous abortion, infection, hematoma, intrauterine death.

THE INTRAPARTAL EXPERIENCE

General overview: This review of the anatomic and physiologic determinants of successful labor provides baseline data against which the nurse compares findings of an ongoing assessment of the labor client. Nursing actions are planned and implemented to meet the present and emerging needs of the woman in labor.

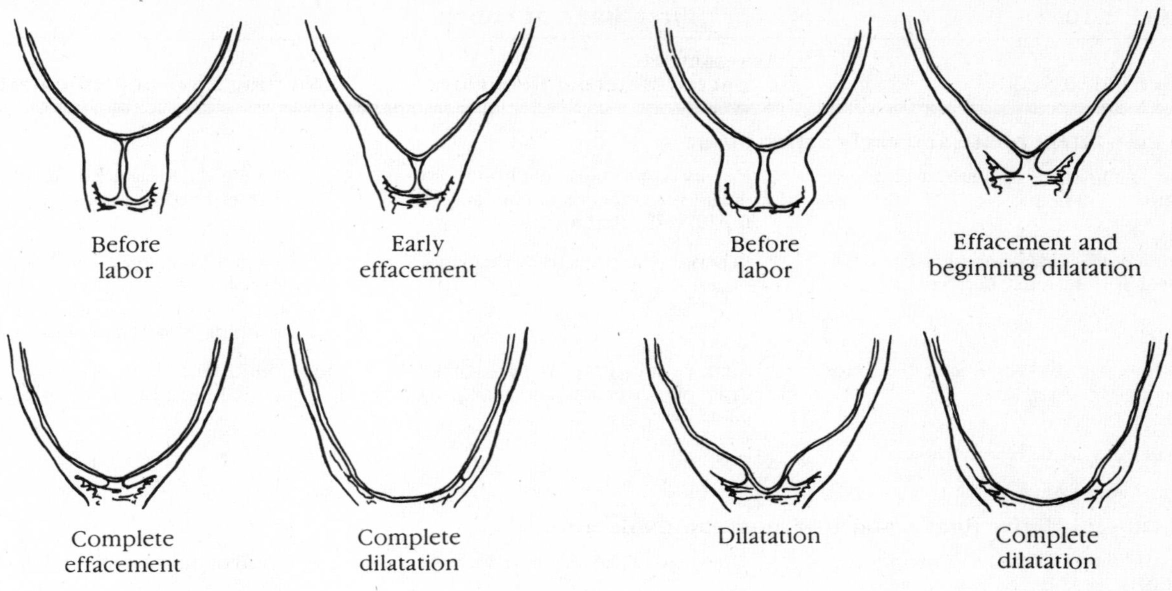

FIGURE 2.4
Comparison of nullipara (a) and multipara (b) dilatation and effacement. (Reprinted with permission of Ross Laboratories, Columbus, OH 43216, from Clinical Education Aid No. 13.)

I. Biologic foundations of labor

A. Premonitory signs

1. *Lightening*—process in which the fetus "drops" into the pelvic inlet.
   a. *Characteristics*
      (1) Nullipara—usually occurs 2–3 weeks prior to onset of labor.
      (2) Multipara—commonly occurs during labor.
   b. *Effects*
      (1) Relieves pressure on diaphragm—breathing is easier.
      (2) Increases pelvic pressure.
         (a) Urinary frequency returns.
         (b) Increased pressure on thighs.
         (c) Increased tendency to vulvar, vaginal, perianal, and leg varicosities.
2. *Braxton-Hicks contractions*—may become more uncomfortable.

B. Etiology: unknown. *Theories* include:

1. Uterine overdistention.
2. Placental aging—declining estrogen/progesterone levels.
3. Rising prostaglandin level.
4. Fetal cortisol secretion.
5. Maternal/fetal oxytocin secretion.

C. Overview of labor process—forces of labor (uterine contractions) overcome cervical resistance; cervix thins (*effacement*) and opens (0–10 cm *dilatation*) (Table 2.10 and Figure 2.4). Voluntary contraction of secondary abdominal muscles (e.g., pushing, bearing-down) forces fetal descent. Changing pelvic dimensions force fetal head to accommodate (*engagement, flexion, internal rotation, extension*), as shown in Figure 2.7, p. 155. *Stages of labor:*

1. *First*—begins with establishment of regular, rhythmic contractions; ends with complete effacement and dilatation (10 cm); divided into three phases:
   a. Latent and early active.
   b. Active.
   c. Transitional.
2. *Second*—begins with complete dilatation and ends with birth of infant.
3. *Third*—begins with birth of infant and ends with expulsion of placenta.
4. *Fourth*—begins with expulsion of placenta; ends when maternal status is stable (usually 1–2 hours postpartum).

D. Anatomic/physiologic determinants

1. *Maternal*
   a. *Uterine contractions*—expel products of conception, begin process of involution.
      (1) *Characteristics:* rhythmic; increasing tone (*increment*), peak (*acme*), relaxation (*decrement*).
      (2) *Effects:*
         (a) Decreases blood flow to uterus and placenta.
         (b) Dilates cervix during first stage of labor.
         (c) Raises maternal blood pressure during contractions.
         (d) With bearing-down efforts, expels fetus (second stage) and placenta (third stage).
         (e) Begins involution.
      (3) **Assessment:**
         (a) Frequently—time from beginning of one contraction to beginning of the next.

TABLE 2.10 First Stage of Labor

Phases of First Stage	Assessment: Expected Maternal Behaviors	Nursing Plan/Implementation
0 to 4 cm—latent phase and early active phase		
1. Time—nullipara 8–10 hours, average; multipara 5–6 hours.	1. Usually comfortable, euphoric, excited, talkative, and energetic, but may be fearful and withdrawn.	1. Provide encouragement, feedback for relaxation, companionship.
2. Contractions—regular, mild 5–10 minutes apart, 20–30 seconds' duration.	2. Relieved or apprehensive that labor has begun.	2. Coach during contractions: signal beginning of contraction, mark the seconds, signal end of contraction; "Follow my breathing," "Watch my lips," etc.
3. Low-back pain and abdominal discomfort with contractions.	3. Alert, usually receptive to teaching, coaching, diversion, and anticipatory guidance.	3. Comfort measures: position for comfort; praise; keep aware of progress.
4. Cervix thins; some bloody show.		
5. Station—Multipara: −2 to +1; nullipara: 0.		
4 to 8 cm—midactive phase, phase of most rapid dilatation		
1. Average time—nullipara 1–2 hours; multipara 1½–2 hours.	1. Tired, less talkative, and less energetic.	1. Coach during contractions; husband (coach) may need some relief.
2. Contractions—2–5 minutes apart, 30–40 seconds' duration, intensity increasing.	2. More serious, malar flush between 5 and 6 cm, tendency to hyperventilate, may need analgesia, needs constant coaching.	2. Comfort measures (to husband too—as needed): position for comfort while preventing hypotensive syndrome; encourage relaxation, focusing her on areas of tension; provide counterpressure to sacrococcygeal area, p.r.n.; praise; keep aware of progress; minimize distractions from surrounding environment (loud talking, other noises); offer analgesics and anesthetics, as appropriate; provide hygiene: mouth care, ice chips, clean perineum; warmth, as needed.
3. Membranes may rupture now.		3. Monitor progress of labor and maternal/fetal response.
4. Increased bloody show.		4. If monitors are in use, attention on mother; periodically check accuracy of monitor read-outs.
5. Station: −1 to 0.		
8 to 10 cm—transition, deceleration period of active phase		
1. Average time; nullipara—40 minutes to 1 hour; multipara—20 minutes.	1. If not under regional anesthesia, more introverted; may be amnesic between contractions.	1. Stay with woman (couple) and provide constant support.
2. Contractions—1½–2 minutes, 60–90 seconds' duration, strong intensity.	2. Feeling she cannot make it; increased irritability, crying, nausea, vomiting, and belching; increased perspiration over upper lip and between breasts; leg tremors; and shaking.	2. Continue to coach with contractions: may need to remind, reassure, and encourage her to reestablish breathing techniques and concentration with each contraction; coach panting or "he-he" respirations to prevent pushing.
3. Increased vaginal show; rectal pressure with beginning urge to bear down.	3. May have uncontrollable urge to push at this time.	3. Comfort measures: remind her and husband her behavior is normal and "OK"; coach breathing to quell nausea.
4. Station: +3 to +4.		4. Assist with countertension techniques woman requested: effleurage. Monitor contractions, FHR (after each contraction), vaginal discharge, perineal bulging, maternal vital signs; record every 15 minutes. Assess for bladder filling. Keep mother (couple) aware of progress. Prepare husband for birth (scrub, gown, etc.).

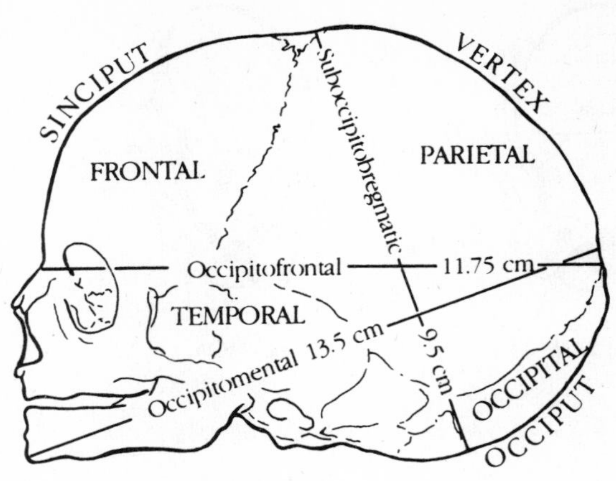

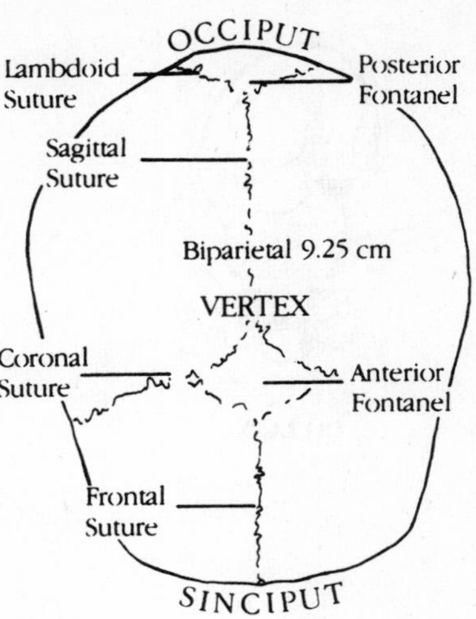

■ **FIGURE 2.5**
The fetal head. *Bones:* 2 frontal, 2 temporal, 1 occipital. *Sutures:* sagittal, frontal, coronal, lambdoid. *Fontanels:* anterior, posterior. (Reprinted with permission of Ross Laboratories, Columbus, OH, Clinical Education Aid No. 13.)

(b) Duration—time from beginning of contraction to relaxation.

(c) Strength (intensity)—resistance to indentation.

(d) False/true labor—differentiation (see Table 2.11).

(e) Signs of dysfunctional labor. See p. 167.

b. *Pelvic structures and configuration:*

(1) *False pelvis*—above linea terminalis (line travels across top of symphysis pubis around to sacral promontory); supports gravid uterus during pregnancy.

(2) *True pelvis*—lies below linea terminalis; divided into:

(a) Inlet—"brim," demarcated by linea terminalis.

(i) Widest diameter: transverse.

(ii) Narrowest diameter: anterior-posterior (true conjugate).

(b) Midplane—pelvic cavity.

(c) Outlet.

(i) Widest diameter: anterior-posterior (requires internal rotation of fetal head for entry).

(ii) Narrowest diameter: transverse (intertuberous); facilitates delivery in occiput anterior (OA) position.

(3) *Classifications*

(a) Gynecoid—normal female pelvis; rounded oval.

(b) Android—normal male pelvis; funnel-shaped.

(c) Anthropoid—oval.

(d) Platypelloid—flattened, transverse oval.

2. *Fetal*

a. *Fetal head* (Figure 2.5).

(1) Bones—1 occipital, 1 frontal, 2 parietals, 2 temporals.

(2) Suture—line of junction or closure between bones; sagittal (longitudinal), coronal (anterior), and lambdoidal (posterior); permit molding.

(3) Fontanels—membranous space between cranial bones during fetal life and infancy.

(a) *Anterior* "soft spot"—diamond-shaped; junction of coronal and sagittal sutures; closes (ossifies) in 12–18 months.

(b) *Posterior*—triangular; junction of sagittal and lambdoidal sutures; closes by 2 months of age.

b. *Fetal lie*—relationship of fetal long axis to maternal long axis (spine).

(1) Transverse—shoulder presents.

(2) Longitudinal—vertex or breech presents.

c. *Presentation*—fetal part entering inlet first (Figure 2.6).

■ **TABLE 2.11 Assessment: Differentiation of False/True Labor**

False Labor	True Labor
Contractions: Braxton-Hicks intensify (more noticeable at night). Short, irregular, little change.	*Contractions:* begin in lower back, radiate to abdomen ("girdling"). Become regular, rhythmic; frequency, duration, intensity increase.
Relieved by change of position or activity (e.g., walking).	*Unaffected* by change of position, activity, or moderate analgesia.
Cervical changes—none. *No* effacement or dilatation progress.	*Cervical changes*—*progressive* effacement and dilatation.

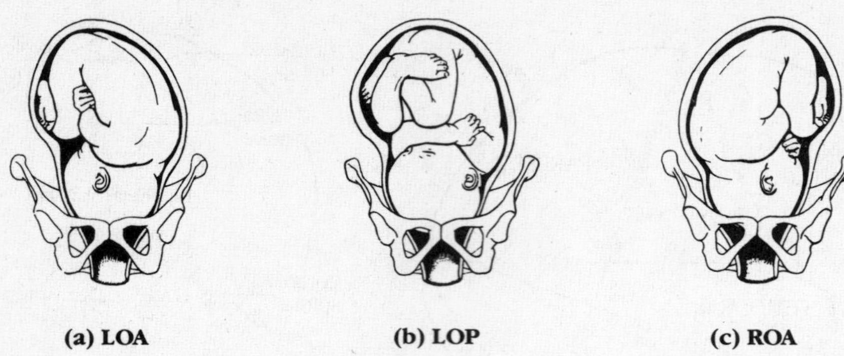

(a) LOA (b) LOP (c) ROA

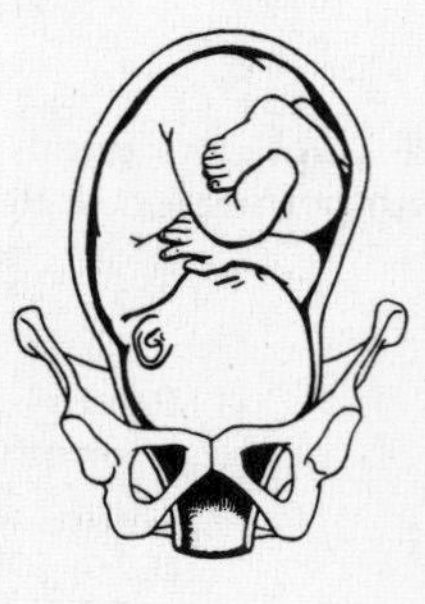

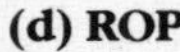

(d) ROP

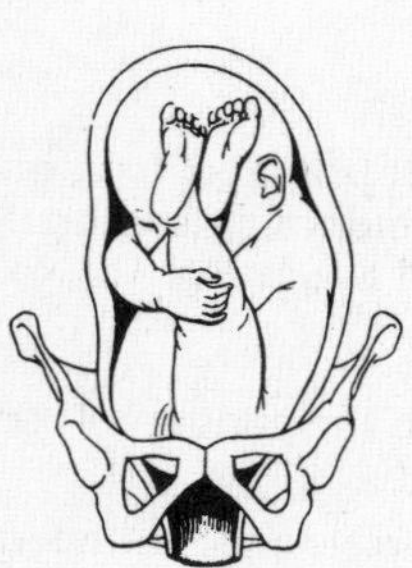

(e) LSP (Frank Breech)

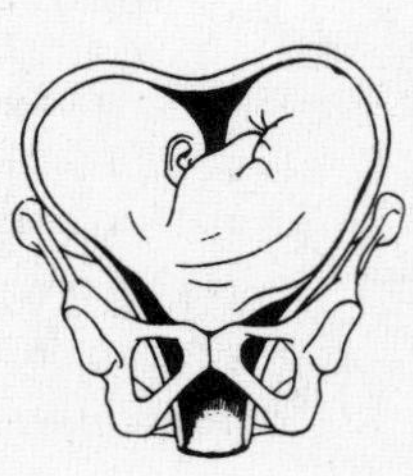

(f) Shoulder presentation

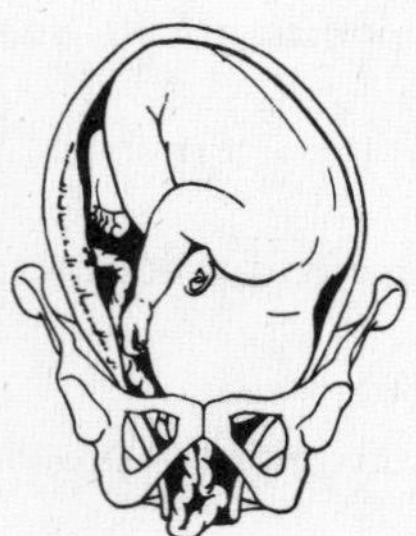

(g) Prolapse of cord

■ **FIGURE 2.6**
Categories of fetal presentation. (a) LOA: fetal occiput is in left anterior quadrant of maternal pelvis. (b) LOP: fetal occiput is in left posterior quadrant of maternal pelvis. (c) ROA: fetal occiput is in right anterior quadrant of maternal pelvis. (d) ROP: fetal occiput is in right posterior quadrant of maternal pelvis. (e) LSP: fetal sacrum is in left posterior quadrant of maternal pelvis. (f) Shoulder presentation with fetus in transverse lie. (g) Prolapse of umbilical cord with fetus in LOA position. (Reprinted with permission of Ross Laboratories, Columbus, OH, Clinical Education Aid No. 18.)

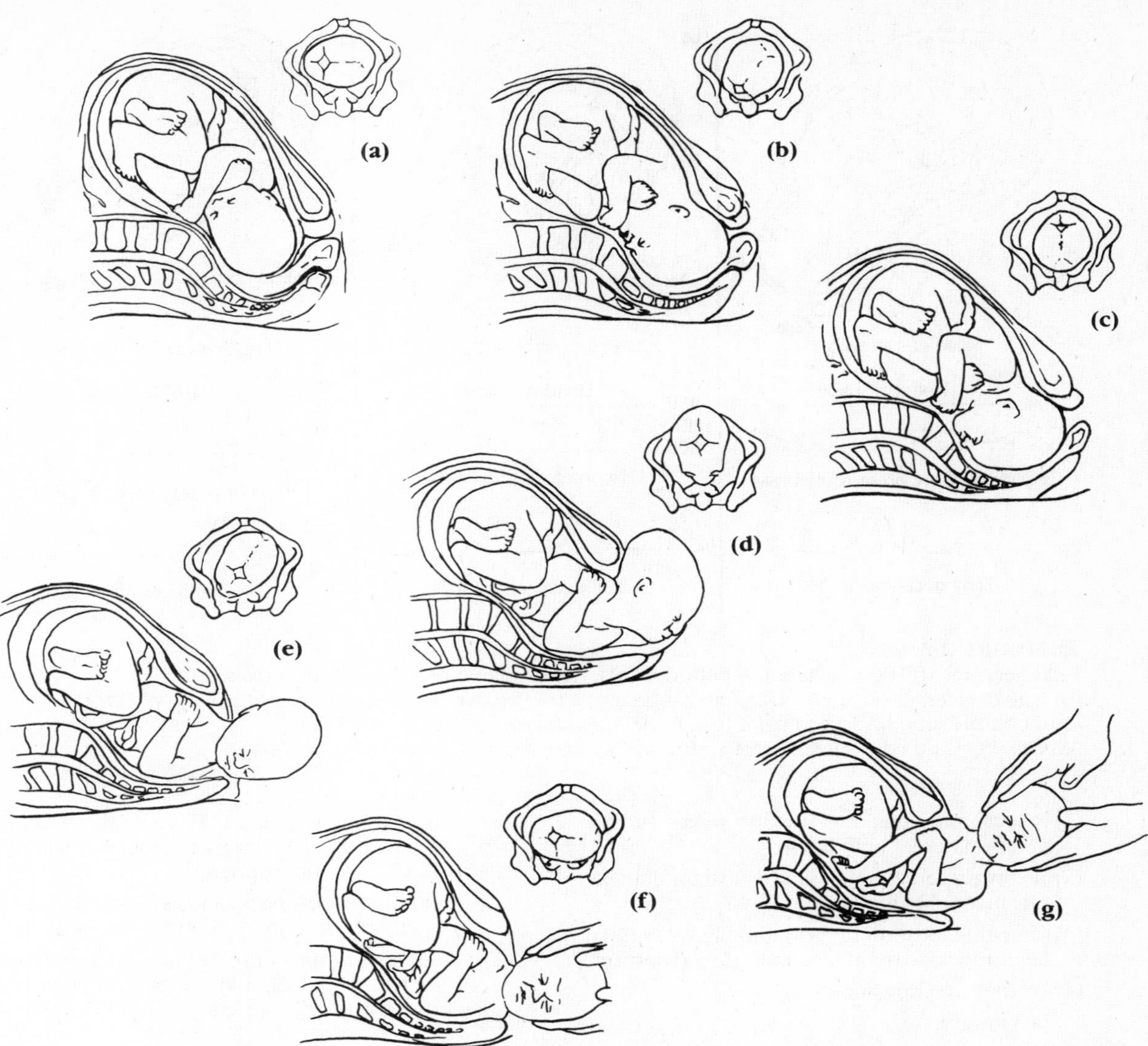

■ **FIGURE 2.7**
Cardinal movements in the mechanism of labor with the fetus in vertex presentation. (a) Engagement, descent, flexion. (b) Internal rotation. (c) Extension beginning (rotation complete). (d) Extension complete. (e) External rotation (restitution). (f) External rotation (shoulder rotation). (g) Expulsion. (Reprinted with permission of Ross Laboratories, Columbus, OH, Clinical Education Aid No. 13.)

(1) *Cephalic*—vertex (most common); face, brow.

(2) *Breech*

(a) *Complete*—feet and legs flexed on thighs; buttocks and feet presenting.

(b) *Frank*—legs extended on torso, feet up by shoulders; buttocks presenting.

(c) *Footling*—single (one foot), double (both feet) presenting.

d. *Attitude*—relationship of fetal parts to one another (e.g., head flexed on chest).

e. *Position*—relationship of presenting fetal part to quadrants of maternal pelvis; vertex most common, occiput anterior on maternal left side (LOA). See Figure 2.6.

3. **Assessment:** determine presentation and position.

a. *Leopold's maneuvers*—abdominal palpation.

(1) *First*—palms over fundus, breech feels softer, not as round as head would be.

(2) *Second*—palms on either side of abdomen, locates fetal back and small parts.

(3) *Third*—fingers just above pubic symphysis, grasp lower abdomen; if unengaged, presenting part is mobile.

(4) *Fourth*—facing mother's feet, run palms down sides of abdomen to symphysis; check for cephalic prominence (usually on right side), and if head is floating or engaged.

b. *Location of fetal heart tones*—heard best through fetal back or chest.

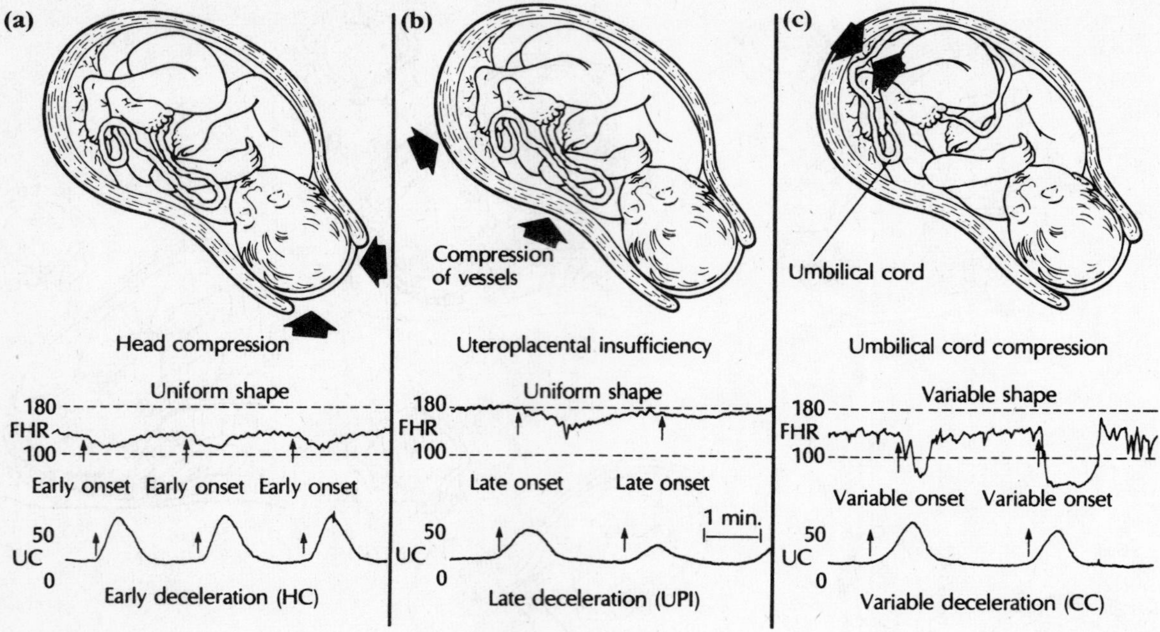

■ **FIGURE 2.8**
Fetal heart rate (FHR) deceleration patterns. (a) Early deceleration—head compression. (b) Late deceleration—uteroplacental insufficiency. (c) Variable deceleration—umbilical cord compression. (Adapted from Hon E: *An Introduction to Fetal Heart Rate Monitoring,* 2nd ed., University of Southern California School of Medicine, 1976.)

(1) *Breech* presentation—usually most audible *above* maternal umbilicus.

(2) *Vertex* presentation—usually most audible *below* maternal umbilicus.

(3) Changing location of most audible FHTs (fetal heart tones)—useful indicator of fetal descent.

(4) Factors affecting audibility:

(a) Obesity.

(b) Maternal position.

(c) Hydramnios.

(d) Maternal gastrointestinal activity.

(e) Loud uterine bruit—origin: hissing of blood through umbilical arteries; synchronous with maternal pulse.

(f) Loud funic souffle—origin: hissing of blood through umbilical arteries; synchronous with fetal heart rate (FHR).

(g) External noise, faulty equipment.

▶ c. *Vaginal examination:* palpable sutures, fontanels (triangular-shaped superior, diamond-shaped inferior = vertex presentation, OA position).

4. *Mechanisms of normal labor*—vertex presentation, positional changes of fetal head accommodate to changing diameters of maternal pelvis. See Figure 2.7.

a. *Descent*—head engages and proceeds down birth canal.

b. *Flexion*—head bent to chest; presents smallest diameter of vertex.

c. *Internal rotation*—during second stage of labor, transverse diameter of fetal head enters pelvis; occiput rotates 90° to bring back of neck under symphysis (e.g., LOT to LOA to OA); presents smallest diameter (biparietal) to smallest diameter of outlet (intertuberous).

d. *Extension*—back of neck pivots under symphysis, allows head to be born by extension.

e. *Restitution*—head returns to normal alignment with shoulders (with LOA, results in head facing right thigh), presents smallest diameter of shoulders to outlet.

f. *Expulsion*—delivery of neonate completed.

g. **Assessment:** relationship of fetal head to ischial spines (degree of descent).

(1) *Engagement*—widest diameter of presenting part has passed through pelvic inlet (e.g., biparietal diameter of fetal head).

(2) *Station*—relationship of presenting part to ischial spines (IS).

(a) *Floating*—presenting part above inlet, in false pelvis.

(b) Station −5 is at inlet (presenting part well above IS).

(c) Station 0—presenting part at IS (engaged).

(d) Station +4—presenting part at the outlet.

E. Danger signs during labor

1. *Contraction*—hypertonic, poor relaxation, or tetanic (greater than 90 seconds long).

2. *Abdominal pain*—sharp, rigid abdomen.

3. *Vaginal bleeding*—profuse.

4. *FHR*—late decelerations, prolonged variable decelerations, bradycardia, tachycardia (Figure 2.8). See also Table 2.14, p. 175.

5. *Maternal hypertension.*
6. *Meconium-stained amniotic fluid (MSAF).*
7. *Prolonged ROM.*

II. Participatory childbirth techniques

A. Psychoprophylaxis—Lamaze method

1. Premise—conditioned responses to stimuli occupy nerve pathways, reducing perception of pain. Emphasis is on childbirth as a natural event, with an informed client as the active participant. The ability to relax effectively reduces the perception of pain, and the involvement of the coach fosters the family concept.
2. Childbirth partners are taught:
   a. Anatomy and physiology of labor.
   b. Psychology of man and woman.
   c. What to expect in the hospital setting.
   d. Conditioned responses to labor stimuli.
      (1) Concentration on focal point.
      (2) Breathing techniques.
      (3) Need for active coaching to enable client to:
         (a) Use techniques appropriate to present stage of labor.
         (b) Avoid hyperventilation.
   e. Specific stage—appropriate techniques:
      (1) *First stage of labor—early:* slow, deep chest-breathing.
      (2) *Transition* (8–10 cm)—rapid, shallow breathing pattern, to prevent pushing prematurely.
         (a) Panting.
         (b) Pant-blow.
         (c) "He-he" pattern.
      (3) *Second stage of labor*
         (a) Pushing (or bearing-down)—aids fetal descent through birth canal.
         (b) Panting—aids relaxation between contractions; prevents explosive delivery of head.
   f. Effects on labor behaviors/coping:
      (1) Help mother cope with and assist contractions.
      (2) Prevent premature bearing-down; reduce possibility of cervical edema due to pushing on incompletely dilated cervix (panting).
      (3) When appropriate, improve efficiency of bearing-down efforts.

B. Other methods—include parent classes, classes for siblings, multiparas, and those who plan cesarean birth.

III. Nursing actions during first stage of labor

A. Assessment:—careful evaluation of:

1. *Antepartal history*
   a. EDD (expected date of delivery).
   b. Genetic and familial problems.
   c. Pre- and coexisting medical disorders, allergies.
   d. Pregnancy-related health problems (hyperemesis, bleeding, etc.).
   e. Infectious diseases (past and present herpes, etc.).
   f. Past obstetric history, if any.
   g. Pelvic measurements.
   h. Height.
   i. Weight gain.
   j. Laboratory results:
      (1) Blood type and Rh factor.
      (2) Serology.
      (3) Urinalysis.
   k. Prenatal care history.
   l. Use of medications.
2. *Admission findings*
   a. Emotional status.
   b. Vital signs.
   c. Present weight.
   d. Fundal height.
   e. Present fetal size.
   f. Edema.
   g. Urinalysis (for protein and sugar).
3. *Fetal heart rate (FHR)*—normal, 120–160/min (see Figure 2.8).
   a. Check and record every 30 minutes—to monitor fetal response to physiologic stress of labor.
   b. Bradycardia (mild, 100–119/min, or 30/min lower than baseline reading).
   c. Tachycardia (moderate, 160–179/min, or 30/min above baseline reading).
4. *Contractions*—every 15-30 minutes.
   a. Place fingertips over fundus, use gentle pressure; contraction felt as hardening or tensing.
   b. Time: frequency and duration.
   c. Intensity/strength at acme:
      (1) Weak—easily indent fundus with fingers.
      (2) Moderate—some tension felt, fundus indents slightly with finger pressure.
      (3) Strong—unable to indent fundus.
5. *Maternal response to labor*—assess for effective coping, cooperation and utilizing effective breathing techniques.
6. *Maternal vital signs*—between contractions.
   a. Response to pain or use of special breathing techniques alters pulse and respirations.
   b. B/P, P, RR—if normotensive: on admission, and then every hour and p.r.n.; after regional anesthesia: every 30 minutes (every 5 min first 20 min).
   c. Temp—if within normal range: on admission, and then every four hours and p.r.n. Every two hours after rupture of membranes.
   d. Prior to and after analgesia/anesthesia.
   e. After rupture of membranes (see Amniotic fluid embolism).
7. Character and amount of bloody show.
8. Bladder status: encourage voiding every 1–2 hours, monitor output.
   a. Determine bladder distention—palpate just above symphysis (full bladder may impede labor progress or result in trauma to bladder).

b. Admission urinalysis—check for protein and sugar.

9. Signs of deviations from normal patterns.

10. Status of membranes:

a. Intact.

b. Ruptured (nitrazine paper turns blue on contact with alkaline amniotic fluid). Note, record, and report:

(1) Time—danger of infection if ruptured more than 24 hours.

(2) FHR stat and 10 minutes later—to check for prolapsed cord.

(3) Character and color of fluid (see below).

11. Amniotic fluid.

a. Amount—hydramnios (>2000 mL)—associated with congenital anomalies.

b. Character—thick consistency and/or odor associated with infection.

c. Color—normally clear with white specks.

(1) Yellow—indicates fetal distress about 35 hours previous; Rh or ABO incompatibility.

(2) Green or meconium stained; if fetus in vertex position, indicates recent fetal hypoxia secondary to respiratory distress in fetus.

(3) Port wine—may indicate abruptio placentae.

12. Labor progress:

a. Effacement.

b. Dilatation.

c. Station.

d. Bulging membranes.

e. Molding of fetal head.

13. Perineum—observe for bulging.

B. Analysis/nursing diagnosis:

1. *Anxiety, fear* related to uncertain outcome, pain.

2. *Ineffective individual coping* related to lack of preparation for childbirth and/or poor support from coach.

3. *Altered nutrition: less than body requirements* related to physiologic stress of labor.

4. *Altered urinary elimination* related to pressure of presenting part.

5. *Altered thought processes* related to sleep deprivation, transition, analgesia.

6. *Fluid volume deficit* related to anemia, excessive blood loss.

7. *Impaired (fetal) gas exchange* related to impaired placental perfusion.

C. Nursing plan/implementation:

1. Goal: *comfort measures.*

a. Maintain hydration of oral mucosa. Encourage sucking on cool washcloth, ice chips, lollipops.

b. Reduce dryness of lips. Apply lip balm (Chapstick, petrolatum jelly).

c. Relieve backache. Apply sacral counterpressure [particularly with occiput posterior (OP) presentation].

d. Encourage significant other to participate.

e. Encourage ambulation when presenting part engaged.

2. Goal: *management of physical needs.*

a. Encourage frequent voiding—to prevent full bladder from impeding oncoming head.

b. Encourage ambulation throughout labor; left Sims position with head elevated to:

(1) Encourage relaxation.

(2) Allow gravity to assist in anterior rotation of fetal head.

(3) Prevent compression of inferior vena cava (supine hypotensive syndrome); (L) Sims c̄ head elevated.

(4) Promote placental perfusion.

c. Perineal prep, if ordered—to promote cleanliness.

d. Fleet's enema, if ordered—to stimulate peristalsis, evacuate lower bowel. **Note: contraindicated** if:

(1) Cervical dilatation (4 cm or more) with unengaged head—due to possibility of cord prolapse.

(2) Fetal malpresentation/malposition—due to possible fetal distress.

(3) Premature labor—may stimulate contractions.

(4) Painless vaginal bleeding—due to possible placenta previa.

3. Goal: *management of psychosocial needs. Emotional support:*

a. Encourage verbalization of feelings, fears, concerns.

b. Explain all procedures.

c. Reinforce self-concept ("You're doing well!").

4. Goal: *management of discomfort.*

a. Analgesia and/or anesthesia—may be required or desired—to facilitate safe, comfortable delivery.

b. Support/enhance/teach childbirth techniques.

(1) Reinforce appropriate breathing techniques for current labor status.

(a) If hyperventilating, to increase $Paco_2$, minimize fetal acidosis, and relieve symptoms of vertigo and syncope, suggest:

(i) Breathe into paper bag.

(ii) Breathe into cupped hands.

(b) Demonstrate appropriate breathing for several contractions—to reestablish rate and rhythm.

(2) Goal: *sustain motivation.*

(a) Offer support, encouragement, and praise, as appropriate.

(b) Keep informed of status and progress.

(c) Reassure that irritability is normal.

(d) Serve as surrogate coach when necessary (if no partner, prior to arrival of partner, while partner is changing clothes, during needed breaks); assist with effleurage, breathing, focusing.

(e) Discourage bearing-down efforts by pant-blow until complete (10 cm) dilatation—to avoid cervical edema.

(f) Facilitate informed decision-making regarding medication for relaxation or pain relief.

(g) Keep woman and family informed of her progress.

(h) Minimize distractions: quiet, relaxed environment; privacy.

D. Evaluation:

1. Manages own labor discomfort effectively.
2. Maintains control over own behavior.
3. Successfully completes first stage of labor without incident.

IV. Nursing actions during second stage of labor

A. Assessment:

1. Maternal (or couple's) response to labor.
2. FHR—continuous electronic monitoring, or after each contraction with fetoscope, Doppler.
3. Vital signs.
4. Time elapsed—average: 2 minutes to 1 hour; prolonged second stage increases risk of fetal distress, maternal exhaustion, psychologic stress, intrauterine infection.
5. Contraction pattern—average every 1½–3 min, lasting 60–90 seconds.
6. Vaginal discharge—increases.
7. Nausea, vomiting, disorientation, tremors, amnesia between contractions, panic.
8. Response to regional anesthesia, if administered.
   a. Signs of hypotension—reduces placental perfusion, increases risk of fetal hypoxia.
   b. Effect on contractions—note and report any slowing of labor.
9. Efforts to bear down—increases expulsive effects of uterine contractions.
10. Perineal bulging with contractions—fetal head distends perineum, crowns; head born by extension.

B. Analysis/nursing diagnosis:

1. *Pain* related to strong uterine contractions, pressure of fetal descent, stretching of perineum.
2. *Potential for injury:*
   a. Infection related to ruptured membranes, repeated vaginal examinations.
   b. Laceration related to pressure of fetal head exceeding perineal elasticity and uterine rupture related to fundal pressure.
3. *Impaired skin integrity* related to laceration, episiotomy.
4. *Fluid volume deficit* related to hypotension secondary to regional anesthesia.
5. *Anxiety* related to imminent delivery of fetus.
6. *Ineffective individual coping* related to prolonged sensory stimulation (contractions) and anxiety.
7. *Altered urinary elimination* related to anesthesia and contractions.
8. *Sleep pattern disturbance.*

C. Nursing plan/implementation:

1. Goal: *emotional support.*
   a. To sustain motivation/control:
      (1) Never leave mother and significant other alone now.
      (2) Keep informed of progress.
      (3) Direct bearing-down efforts without holding breath while pushing encourage pushing "out through vagina" and encourage mother to touch coming head; position mirror so client can see perineal bulging with effective efforts; minimize distractions.
   b. To allay significant other's anxiety: reassure regarding mother's behavior if she is not anesthetized.
   c. Support family choices.
2. Goal: *safeguard status.*
   a. Precautions when putting legs in stirrups:
      (1) If varicosities, **do not put legs in stirrups.**
      (2) Avoid pressure to popliteal veins; pad stirrups.
      (3) Assure proper, even alignment by adjusting stirrups.
      (4) Move legs simultaneously into or out of stirrups—to avoid nerve, ligament, and muscle strain.
      (5) Provide proper support to client not using stirrups.
   b. Support client in whatever position selected for birth, e.g., side-lying.
   c. Cleanse perineum, thighs, and lower abdomen, maintaining sterile technique.
3. Goal: *maintain a comfortable environment.*
   a. Free of unnecessary noise, light.
   b. Comfortable temperature (warm).
4. *Medical management*
   a. Episiotomy may be performed to facilitate delivery.
   b. Forceps may be applied to exert traction and expedite delivery.
   c. Vacuum attraction also used.
5. Birthing room delivery with alternative positions.

D. Evaluation:

1. Cooperative, actively participates in delivery; maintains control over own behavior.
2. Successful, uncomplicated delivery of viable infant.
3. All assessment findings within normal limits (vital signs, emotional status, response to birth).
4. Presence of significant other.

V. Nursing actions during third stage of labor

A. Assessment:

1. Time elapsed—average: 5 minutes; prolonged third stage (greater than 25 min) may indicate complications.
2. Signs of placental separation:
   a. Increase in bleeding.

b. Cord lengthens.

c. Uterus rises in abdomen, assumes globular shape.

3. Assess mother's level of consciousness.

4. Examine placenta for intactness and number of vessels in umbilical cord (normal: three. *Note:* two vessels only—associated with increased incidence of congenital anomalies); condition of placenta for calcification, infarcts, etc.

B. Analysis/nursing diagnosis:

1. *Family coping: potential for growth* related to bonding, beginning achievement of developmental tasks.

2. *Fluid volume deficit* related to blood loss during third stage.

C. Nursing plan/implementation:

1. Goal: *prevent uterine atony.* Administer oxytocin, as ordered.

2. Goal: *facilitate parent–child bonding.*

a. While protecting neonate from cold stress, encourage parents to see, hold, touch neonate.

b. Comment about neonate's individuality, characteristics, and behaviors.

c. After neonate assessed for congenital anomalies (cleft palate, esophageal atresia), encourage breastfeeding, if desired.

3. Goal: *health teaching.*

a. Describe, discuss common neonatal behavior in transitional period (periods of reactivity, sleep, hyperactivity).

b. Demonstrate removal of mucus by aspiration with bulb syringe.

c. Demonstrate ways of facilitating breastfeeding.

D. Evaluation:

1. Successful, uneventful completion of labor.

a. Minimal blood loss.

b. Vital signs within normal limits.

c. Fundus well contracted at level of umbilicus.

2. Parents express satisfaction with outcome, demonstrate infant attachment.

VI. Nursing actions during the fourth stage of labor—1–2 hours postpartum.

A. Assessment—every 15 minutes four times; then, every 30 minutes two times—or until stable—to monitor response to physiologic stress of labor/delivery.

1. Vital signs:

a. Temperature taken once; if elevated, requires follow-up—may indicate infection, dehydration, excessive blood loss. Note, record, report temperature of 100.4 °F (38 °C).

b. Blood pressure—every 15 minutes × 4.

(1) Returns to prelabor level—due to loss of placental circulation and increased circulating blood volume.

(2) Elevation may be in response to use of oxytocic drugs or preeclampsia (first 48 hours).

(3) Lowered blood pressure—may reflect significant blood loss during labor/delivery, or occult bleeding.

c. Pulse—every 15 minutes × 4.

(1) Physiologic bradycardia—due to normal vagal response.

(2) Tachycardia—may indicate excessive blood loss during labor/delivery, dehydration, exhaustion, or occult bleeding.

2. Location and consistency of fundus—every 15 minutes, to assure continuing contraction; prevent blood loss due to uterine relaxation.

a. Fundus—firm; at or slightly lower than the umbilicus; in midline.

b. May be displaced by distended bladder—due to normal diuresis; common cause of bleeding in immediate postpartum, uterine atony.

3. Character and amount of vaginal flow.

a. Moderate lochia rubra.

b. If perineal pad saturated in 15 minutes, or blood pools under buttocks, excessive loss.

c. Bright red bleeding may indicate cervical or vaginal laceration.

4. Perineum.

a. Edema.

b. Bruising—due to trauma.

c. Distention/hematoma, rectal pain.

5. Bladder fullness/voiding—to prevent distention.

6. Rate of IV, if present; response to added medication, if any.

7. Intake and output—to evaluate hydration.

8. Recovery from analgesia/anesthesia.

9. Energy level.

10. Verbal, nonverbal interaction between client and significant other.

a. Dialogue.

b. Posture.

c. Facial expressions.

d. Touching.

11. Interactions between parent(s) and newborn; signs of bonding.

a. Eye contact with newborn.

b. Calls by name.

c. Explores with fingertips, strokes, cuddles.

12. Signs of postpartal emergencies.

a. Uterine atony, hemorrhage.

b. Vaginal hematoma.

B. Analysis/nursing diagnosis:

1. *Fluid volume deficit* related to excessive intrapartal blood loss, dehydration.

2. *Altered urinary elimination* related to intrapartal bladder trauma, dehydration, blood loss.

3. *Impaired skin integrity* related to episiotomy, lacerations, cesarean birth.

4. *Altered family processes* related to role change.

5. *Altered parenting* related to interruption in bonding secondary to:

a. Compromised maternal status.

b. Compromised neonatal status.

6. *Knowledge deficit* regarding self-care procedures.

TABLE 2.12 **Apgar Score**

Sign	0	1	2
Heart rate	Absent.	Below 100.	Over 100.
Respiratory effort	Absent.	Slow and irregular.	Good and crying.
Muscle tone	Flaccid.	Some flexion of extremities.	Active motions, general flexion.
Reflex irritability	No response.	Weak cry or grimace.	Cry.
Color	Blue, pale.	Body pink, extremities blue.	Completely pink.

7. *Fatigue* related to sleep disturbances and anxiety.
8. *Anxiety* regarding status of self and infant.
9. *Altered nutrition, less than body requirements,* related to decreased food and fluid intake during labor.

C. Nursing plan/implementation:

1. Goal: *comfort measures.*
   a. Position, pad change.
   b. Perineal care—to promote healing; to reduce possibility of infection.
   c. Ice pack to perineum, as ordered—to reduce edema, discomfort, and pain related to hemorrhoids.
2. Goal: *nutrition/hydration.* Offer fluids, foods as tolerated.
3. Goal: *urinary elimination.*
   a. Encourage voiding—to avoid bladder distention.
   b. Record: time, amount, character.
   c. Anticipatory guidance related to nocturnal diuresis and increased output.
4. Goal: *promote bonding.*
   a. Provide privacy, quiet; encourage sustained contact with newborn.
   b. Encourage: touching, holding baby; breastfeeding (also promotes involution).
5. Goal: *health teaching.*
   a. Perineal care—front to back, labia closed (after *each* void/bm).
   b. Handwashing—before and after each pad change; after voiding, defecating; before and after baby care.
   c. Signs to report:
      (1) Cramping.
      (2) Increased bleeding, passage of large clots.
      (3) Nausea, dizziness.

D. Evaluation:

1. Expresses comfort, satisfaction in fourth stage.
2. Vital signs stable, fundus contracted, moderate lochia rubra, perineum undistended.
3. Tolerates food and fluids well.
4. Voids in adequate amount.
5. Demonstrates eye contact with infant, cuddles.
6. Verbalizes abnormal signs to report to physician.
7. Returns demonstration of appropriate perineal care.
8. Ambulates without pain, dizziness, numbness of legs.

VII. Nursing management of the newborn immediately after birth

A. Assessment:

1. Mucus in nasophyarynx, oropharynx.
2. Apgar score: note and record—at 1 and 5 minutes of age (Table 2.12).
   a. Score of 7–10: good condition.
   b. Score of 4–6: fair condition; assess for CNS depression; resuscitate, as necessary.
   c. Score of 0–3: poor condition; requires immediate resuscitative measures. *Asphyxia neonatorum*—fails to breathe spontaneously within 30–60 seconds after birth.
3. Number of vessels in umbilical stump.
4. Passage of meconium stool, urine.
5. General physical appearance/status.
   a. Signs of respiratory distress (nasal flaring, grunting, sternal retraction, cyanosis, tachypnea).
   b. Skin condition (meconium-stained, cyanosis, jaundice, lesions).
   c. Cry—presence, pitch, quality.
   d. Signs of birth trauma (lacerations, dislocations, fractures).
   e. Symmetry (absent parts, extra digits, gross malformations, ears, palm creases, sacral dimples).
   f. Molding, caput succedaneum, cephalohematoma.
   g. Assess gestational age.
6. Identify high-risk infant.

B. Analysis/nursing diagnosis:

1. *Ineffective airway clearance* related to excessive nasopharyngeal mucus.
2. *Ineffective breathing pattern* related to CNS depression secondary to intrauterine hypoxia narcosis, prematurity, and lack of pulmonary surfactant.
3. *Impaired gas exchange* related to respiratory distress.
4. *Fluid volume deficit* related to birth trauma; hemolytic jaundice.
5. *Impaired skin integrity* related to cord stump.
6. *Potential for injury* (biochemical, metabolic) related to impaired thermoregulation.
7. *Ineffective thermoregulation* related to environmental conditions.

C. Nursing plan/implementation:

1. Goal: *ensure patent airway.*

a. Suction mouth first, then nose; when stimulated, sensitive receptors around entrance to nares initiate gasp, causing aspiration of mucus present in mouth.

b. Suction with bulb syringe.

(1) If deeper suctioning necessary, use DeLee mucus trap attached to suction. Oral use of DeLee is discouraged due to risk of contact with baby's secretions.

(2) Avoid prolonged, vigorous suctioning.

(a) Reduces oxygenation.

(b) May traumatize tissue, cause edema, bleeding, laryngospasm, and cardiac arrhythmia.

c. Assist gravity drainage of fluids, Position: head-dependent (Trendelenberg), and side-lying.

2. Goal: *maintain body temperature*—to conserve energy, preserve store of brown fat, decrease oxygen needs; prevent acidosis. Prevent chilling:

a. Minimize exposure, dry quickly.

b. Warm, apply hat.

c. Take temperature hourly until stable.

3. Goal: *identify infant:*

a. Apply Identiband or name beads.

b. Take infant's footprints and maternal fingerprints.

4. Goal: *prevent eye infection* (gonorrheal and chlamydial ophthalmia neonatorum). Within 2 hours of birth apply antibiotic drops (two drops in each eye).

5. Goal: *facilitate prompt identification/vigilance for potential neonatal complications.*

a. Record significant data from mother's chart:

(1) History of pregnancy, diabetes, hypertension, current drug abuse, excessive caffeine, medications, alcohol, malnutrition.

(2) Course of labor, evidence of fetal distress, medications received in labor.

(3) Delivery history of anesthesia.

(4) Apgar; resuscitative efforts.

b. Goal: *facilitate prompt identification/intervention in hemolytic problems of the newborn.*

(1) Collect and send cord blood for appropriate tests:

(a) Blood type and Rh factor.

(b) Coombs test.

(2) Give vitamin K to facilitate clotting.

D. Evaluation: successful transition to extrauterine life.

1. Status satisfactory; all assessment findings within normal limits.

2. Responsive in bonding process with parents.

VIII. Nurse-attended emergency delivery (precipitate birth). When presents without prenatal care to ER, may represent drug abuse.

A. Assessment: identify signs of imminent delivery:

1. Strong contractions.

2. Bearing-down efforts.

3. Perineal bulging; crowning.

4. Mother states, "It's coming."

B. Analysis/nursing diagnosis:

1. *Pain* related to:

a. Strong, sustained contractions.

b. Descent of fetal head.

c. Stretching of perineum.

2. *Anxiety/fear* related to imminent birth.

3. *Ineffective individual coping* related to circumstances surrounding birth; anxiety, fear for self and infant.

4. *Injury* (mother) related to:

a. Lacerations (vaginal, perineal).

b. Infection secondary to unsterile birth.

5. *Fluid volume deficit* related to:

a. Lacerations.

b. Uterine atony.

c. Retained placental fragments.

6. *Impaired gas exchange* (infant) related to intact membranes during birth.

7. *Potential for injury* (infant) related to:

a. Precipitate birth.

b. Trauma.

c. Hypoxia.

C. Nursing plan/implementation:

1. Goal: *reduce anxiety/fear*—reassure mother.

2. Goal: *delay birth,* as possible.

a. Discourage bearing-down.

b. Encourage panting.

c. Side-lying position to slow descent and allow for more controlled birth.

3. Goal: *prevent infection.*

a. Provide sterile (or clean) field for birth.

b. Avoid touching birth canal without gloved hands.

c. Support perineum (and advancing head) with sterile (or clean) towel.

4. Goal: *prevent, or minimize, infant hypoxia* and perineal lacerations.

a. If membranes intact as head emerges, tear at neck to facilitate first breath.

b. Feel for cord around neck (if present, and if possible, slip cord over head; if tight, *and* sterile equipment at hand, clamp cord in two places, cut between clamps, unwrap cord). If unsterile environment, keep fetus and placenta attached—do not cut cord.

5. Goal: *facilitate/assist birth.*

a. Hold head in both hands.

b. After restitution, apply gentle downward pressure to bring anterior shoulder under pubic symphysis.

c. Gently lift head to deliver posterior shoulder.

d. Support infant as body slips free of mother's body.

6. Goal: *facilitate drainage of mucus and fluid* → patent airway.

a. Hold infant in head-dependent position.

b. Clear mucus with bulb syringe (if available), or use fingertip, wipe with towel.

7. Goal: *prevent placental transfusion*—hold infant level with placenta until cord stops pulsating.
8. Goal: *prevent chilling.*
   a. Wrap infant in towel or other clean material.
   b. Place infant on side, head-dependent, on mother's abdomen.
   c. Dry head, cover with cap or material.

D. Assessment—*third stage:* identify signs of placental separation.

E. Nursing plan/implementation:

1. Goal: *avoid/minimize potential for complications* (everted uterus, tearing of placenta with fragments remaining, separation of cord from placenta).
   a. Avoid traction (pulling) on cord.
   b. Avoid vigorous fundal massage.
   c. Discourage maternal bearing-down efforts unless placenta visible at introitus.
   d. With fundus well contracted, and placenta visible at introitus, encourage mother to bear down to deliver placenta.
2. Goal: *stimulate respiration.* If neonate fails to breathe spontaneously:
   a. Maintain body temperature—dry and cover.
   b. Clear airway.
      (1) Position: head down.
      (2) Turn head to side.
   c. Stimulate.
      (1) Rub back gently.
      (2) Flick soles of feet.
   d. If no response to stimulation:
      (1) Slightly extend neck to "sniffing" position.
      (2) Place mouth over newborn's nose and mouth and exhale air in cheeks, saying "ho" (prevents excessive pressure).
   e. Goal: begin *cardiopulmonary resuscitation (CPR)* if no heart rate.
      (1) Place infant on firm surface.
      (2) With 2–3 fingers on sternum depress ½–1 inch 80–100 times/min.
      (3) Assist ventilation on upstroke of every third compression (3:1 ratio).
      (4) Go immediately to emergency room.
3. Goal: *maintain infant's body temperature.*
   a. Wrap placenta with baby, if cord intact.
   b. Place infant in mother's arms.
4. Goal: *prevent maternal hemorrhage* (uterine atony).
   a. Encourage breastfeeding, or stimulate nipple.
   b. Gently massage fundus, express clots when uterus is contracted.
   c. Encourage voiding if bladder is full.
   d. Get to a medical facility.
5. Goal: *encourage bonding/stimulate uterine contractions.* Encourage breastfeeding.
6. Goal: *legal accountability* as birth attendant. Record date, time, birth events, maternal and fetal status.

F. Evaluation:

1. Experiences normal spontaneous birth of viable infant over intact perineum.
2. Uncomplicated fourth stage—status satisfactory for both mother and infant.
3. Expresses satisfaction in management and result.

IX. Alterations affecting protective function

A. Induction of labor—deliberate initiation of uterine contractions.

1. Indications for:
   a. History of rapid or silent labors, precipitate birth.
   b. Client resides some distance from hospital (controversial).
   c. Coexisting medical disorders:
      (1) Uncontrolled diabetes.
      (2) Progressive preeclampsia.
      (3) Severe renal disease.
   d. Premature rupture of membranes (PROM)—spontaneous rupture of membranes prior to onset of labor and less than 37 weeks from last menstrual period. **Hazards:**
      (1) Maternal—intrauterine infection (amnionitis, endometritis).
      (2) Fetal—sepsis; prolapsed cord.
   e. Rh or ABO incompatibility, fetal hemolytic disease.
   f. Congenital anomaly (e.g., anencephaly).
   g. Postterm pregnancy with nonreactive NST (nonstress test).
   h. Intrauterine fetal demise.
2. Criteria for induction:
   a. Absence of CPD, malpresentation, or malposition.
   b. Engaged vertex of single gestation.
   c. Nearing, or at, term.
   d. Fetal lung maturity.
      (1) Survival rate—better at 32 weeks or more.
      (2) Lecithin/spingomelin ratio greater than 2:1.
      (3) Diabetic mother—phosphatidylglycerol is present in amniotic fluid.
   e. "Ripe" cervix—softening, partially effaced, or ready for effacement/dilatation (if not already present). *Note:* Intravaginal or paracervical application of prostaglandin gel, or laminaria, may be used to prepare cervix for labor.
3. *Methods*
   a. Amniotomy—artificial rupture of membranes with fetal head engaged.
   b. Intravenous oxytocin infusion.
4. *Potential complications*
   a. Amniotomy—irrevocably committed to delivery.
      (1) Prolapsed cord.
      (2) Infection.
   b. IV oxytocin infusion.
      (1) Overstimulation of uterus.
      (2) Decreased placental perfusion/fetal distress.

(3) Precipitate labor and delivery.
(4) Cervical/perineal lacerations.
(5) Uterine rupture.
(6) Water intoxication—if large doses given in D/W over prolonged period (antidiuretic effect increases water reabsorption).
(7) Hypertensive crisis.

5. **Assessment**—*prior to induction:*
   a. Estimate of gestation (EDD, fundal height, cervical status).
   b. General health status:
      (1) Weight, vital signs, FHR, edema.
      (2) Status of membranes.
      (3) Vaginal bleeding.
      (4) Coexisting disorders.
   c. History of previous labors, if any.
   d. Emotional status.
   e. Knowledge/understanding of anticipated procedures:
      (1) Amniotomy (artificial rupture of membranes).
      (2) IV oxytocin infusion.
      (3) Fetal monitoring.
   f. Preparation for childbirth (Lamaze, etc.); coping strategies. Identify support person.
6. **Analysis/nursing diagnosis:**
   a. *Knowledge deficit* related to process of induction.
   b. *Anxiety/fear* related to need for induction of labor.
   c. *Ineffective individual coping* related to psychologic stress.
   d. *Pain* related to uterine contractions.
7. **Nursing plan/implementation:**
   a. Goal: *health teaching.*
      (1) Explain rationale for procedures:
         (a) Amniotomy.
            (i) Induces labor.
            (ii) Relieves uterine overdistention.
            (iii) Increases efficiency of contractions, shortening labor.
         (b) Oxytocin infusion.
            (i) Induces labor.
            (ii) Stimulates uterine contractions.
         (c) Internal fetal monitor.
            (i) Provides continuous assessment of uterine response to oxytocin stimulation.
            (ii) Provides continuous assessment of fetal response to physiologic stress of labor.
      (2) *Describe procedure*—to reduce anxiety and increase cooperation.
      (3) *Explain advantages/disadvantages*—to ensure "informed consent."
   b. Goal: *emotional support*—encourage verbalization of concerns, reassure, as possible.
8. **Evaluation:** verbalizes understanding of process, rationale, procedures, and alternatives.
9. **Assessment**—*during induction and labor:*
   a. *Amniotomy*—same as for spontaneous rupture of membranes:
      (1) Observe fluid—note color, amount.
      (2) Monitor FHR; assess for fetal distress.
      (3) Observe for signs of prolapsed cord.
      (4) Assess fetal activity.
         (a) Excessive activity may indicate distress.
         (b) Absence of activity may indicate distress or demise.
   b. *IV oxytocin infusion:*
      (1) Continually assess response to oxytocin stimulation/flow rate; always given via controlled infusion.
         (a) Uterine contractions.
         (b) Maternal vital signs, FHR.
      (2) Identify signs of:
         (a) *Deviation* from normal patterns:
            (i) Lack of response to increasing flow rate.
            (ii) Uterine hyperirritability (contractions —less than 2 minutes apart).
            (iii) Lack of adequate uterine relaxation between contractions.
         (b) *Side effects* of oxytocin: diminished output—potential water intoxication.
         (c) **Hazards** to mother or fetus:
            (i) Sustained (over 90 seconds duration) or tetanic (strong, spasmlike) contractions—potential abruptio placentae, uterine rupture, fetal hypoxia/anoxia/demise.
            (ii) *Fetal* arrhythmias, decelerations.
            (iii) *Maternal* hypertension—potential for hypertensive crisis, cerebral hemorrhage.
10. **Nursing plan/implementation:**
   a. Same as for other women in labor.
   b. If indications of deviations from normal patterns:
      (1) Stop oxytocin infusion, maintain IV with 5% D/W or other (Ringers lactate, etc.).
      (2) Oxygen per mask; up to 8–10 L/min.
      (3) Position change (see Table 2.13, p. 173).
      (4) Notify physician promptly.
   c. Anticipatory guidance: may have strong contractions soon after induction starts.
11. **Evaluation:**
   a. Demonstrates response to oxytocin stimulation.
      (1) Establishes desired contraction pattern, not hyperstimulated.
      (2) Progress through labor—within normal limits:
         (a) Normotensive.
         (b) Voids in adequate amounts.
         (c) No evidence of deviation from normal contraction patterns.

b. No evidence of fetal distress.

c. Experiences normal vaginal delivery of viable infant.

B. Operative obstetrics—procedures employed to prevent trauma/reduce hazard to mother and/or infant during the birth process.

1. *Episiotomy*—incision of perineum to facilitate infant's birth.

a. Rationale:

(1) Surgical incision reduces possibility of laceration.

(2) Heals more easily than a laceration.

(3) Protects infant's head from pressure exerted by resistant perineum.

(4) Shortens second stage of labor.

b. Types:

(1) Midline—chance of extension into anal sphincter greater than with mediolateral.

(2) Mediolateral—healing is more painful than midline.

c. **Assessment:**

(1) Suture line intact, separated.

(2) Healing.

(3) Edema.

(4) Bruised; hematoma.

(5) Signs of infection.

(6) Tenderness; pain. *Note:* evaluate complaints of pain carefully. If intense, and unrelieved by usual measures, report promptly. May indicate vulvar, paravaginal, or ischiorectal abscess or hematoma.

d. **Analysis/nursing diagnosis:**

(1) *Pain* related to labor process.

(2) *Impaired skin integrity* related to surgical incision.

(3) *Fluid volume deficit* related to hematoma.

(4) *Sexual dysfunction* related to discomfort.

e. **Nursing plan/implementation:**

(1) Goal: *prevent/reduce edema, promote comfort and healing.*

(a) Ice pack during immediate postpartum.

(b) Administer analgesics, topical sprays, ointments, witch hazel pads.

(c) Encourage use of Sitz bath or rubber ring.

(d) Kegal exercises.

(e) Health teaching:

(i) Instruct in tightening gluteal muscles before sitting.

(ii) Avoid sitting on one hip.

(2) Goal: *minimize potential for infection.*

(a) Perineal care during fourth stage of labor.

(b) Health teaching: instruct in self-perineal care after voiding, defecation, and with each pad change.

f. **Evaluation:**

(1) Incision heals by primary intention.

(2) Demonstrates appropriate self-perineal care.

(3) Evidences no signs of hematoma, infection, or separation of suture line.

(4) Experiences minimal discomfort.

2. *Forceps assisted birth*—use of instruments to assist birth of infant.

a. Indications:

(1) Fetal distress.

(2) Maternal need:

(a) Exhaustion.

(b) Coexisting disease, such as cardiac disorder.

(c) Poor progress in second stage.

(d) Persistent fetal OT or OP position.

b. Criteria for forceps application:

(1) Engaged fetal head.

(2) Ruptured membranes.

(3) Full dilatation.

(4) Absence of cephalopelvic disproportion.

(5) Some anesthesia has been given; usually, episiotomy has been performed.

(6) Empty bladder.

c. Types:

(1) Low—outlet forceps.

(2) Mid—applied after head is engaged (rarely used).

(3) High—applied before engagement (rarely done, very hazardous).

(4) Pipers—applied to after-coming head in selected breech deliveries.

d. Potential complications:

(1) Maternal:

(a) Lacerations of: birth canal, rectum, bladder.

(b) Uterine rupture/hemorrhage.

(2) Neonatal:

(a) Cephalohematoma.

(b) Skull fracture.

(c) Intracranial hemorrhage, brain damage.

(d) Facial paralysis.

(e) Direct tissue trauma (abrasions, ecchymosis).

(f) Umbilical cord compression.

e. **Assessment:**

(1) FHR immediately before—and after—forceps application (forceps blade may compress umbilical cord); suction.

(2) Observe mother/newborn for injury or signs of complications.

f. **Analysis/nursing diagnosis:**

(1) *Self-esteem disturbance* related to inability to deliver without surgical assistance.

(2) *Anxiety/fear* related to infant's appearance (forceps marks) or awareness of potential complications.

g. **Nursing plan/implementation:**

(1) Goal: *minimize feelings of failure due to inability to deliver "naturally."*

(a) Explain, discuss reasons/indications for forceps delivery.

(b) Emphasize no maternal control over circumstances.

(2) Goal: *reduce parental anxiety, maternal guilt over infant bruising/forceps marks.* Explain condition is temporary and has no lasting effects on child's appearance.

h. **Evaluation:**

(1) Verbalizes understanding of reasons for forceps delivery.

(2) Evidences no interruption in bonding with infant.

(3) Experiences uncomplicated recovery.

3. Vacuum cap and pump delivery.

4. *Cesarean birth*—incision through abdominal wall and uterus to deliver products of conception.

a. Indications for elective cesarean delivery:

(1) Known cephalopelvic disproportion (CPD).

(2) Previous uterine surgery (e.g., myomectomy), repeated cesarean births (depends on type of incision done).

(3) Active maternal genital herpes II infection.

(4) Breech presentation (*Note:* to reduce infant morbidity/mortality, elective cesarean delivery is common method of choice).

(5) Neoplasms of cervix, uterus, or birth canal.

(6) Maternal diabetes with placental aging; fetal macrosomia (cephalopelvic disproportion).

b. Criteria for elective cesarean delivery: L/S ratio greater than 2:1—indicates presence of pulmonary surfactant; less risk of respiratory distress syndrome.

c. Indications for emergency cesarean birth:

(1) Fetal:

(a) *Fetal distress:* prolapsed cord.

(b) *Fetal jeopardy:* Rh or ABO incompatibility.

(c) *Fetal malposition*/malpresentation.

(d) *Medical evaluation:* fetal blood sampling—low O_2, elevated CO_2, pH below 7.20 (indicates fetal hypoxia, acidosis).

(2) Maternal:

(a) Uterine dysfunction.

(b) Placental disorders:

(i) Placenta previa.

(ii) Abruptio placentae, with Couvelaire uterus.

(c) Severe maternal preeclampsia/eclampsia.

(d) Fetopelvic disproportion.

(e) Sudden maternal death.

(f) Carcinoma.

(g) Failed induction.

d. Types:

(1) Low segment—method of choice:

(a) Transverse incision through abdominal wall and lower uterine segment.

(b) Transverse incision through abdominal wall, with vertical incision of lower uterine segment.

(c) Advantages—fewer complications:

(i) Less blood loss.

(ii) More comfortable convalescence.

(iii) Less adhesion formation.

(iv) Lower risk of uterine rupture in subsequent pregnancy/labor and delivery.

(v) Cosmetically more acceptable.

(2) Classical—vertical incision through abdominal wall and uterus. Necessary for anterior placenta previa and transverse lie.

(3) Porro's—hysterotomy followed by hysterectomy. Necessary in presence of:

(a) Hemorrhage from uterine atony.

(b) Placenta previa, accreta.

(c) Large uterine myomas.

(d) Ruptured uterus.

(e) Cancer of uterus or ovary.

e. **Assessment:**

(1) Maternal physical status.

(a) Vital signs.

(b) Labor status, if any.

(c) Contractions (if any).

(d) Membranes (intact; ruptured).

(e) Signs of complications.

(2) Fetal status.

(a) FHR pattern.

(b) Color and amount of amniotic fluid.

(3) Maternal emotional status.

(4) Understanding of procedure, indications for, implications.

(5) Other—as for any abdominal surgery (see Unit 4).

f. **Analysis/nursing diagnosis:**

(1) *Self-esteem disturbance* related to perceived failure to delivery vaginally.

(2) *Anxiety/fear* related to impending surgery and/or reasons for cesarean birth.

(3) *Ineffective individual coping* related to anxiety and fear for self, infant.

(4) *Fluid volume deficit* related to abdominal surgery and/or reason for cesarean delivery.

(5) *Pain* related to abdominal surgery.

(6) *Constipation* related to decreased bowel activity.

(7) *Altered urinary elimination* related to fluid volume deficit.

g. **Nursing plan/implementation:**

(1) *Preoperative:*

(a) Goal: *safeguard fetal status.*

(i) Monitor fetal heart rate continually.

(ii) Notify neonatology and NICU of scheduled surgical delivery.

(b) Goal: *health teaching.*

(i) Describe, discuss anticipated anesthesia.

(ii) Explain rationale for preoperative antacid (sodium citrate)—to reduce gastric acidity; to minimize effects of aspiration.

(iii) Describe, explain anticipated procedures—abdominal shave, indwelling catheter, intravenous fluids to patient and support person.

(c) Other—as for any abdominal surgery.

(d) Prepare for cesarean section.

(2) *Postoperative:*

(a) Same as for other abdominal surgical clients (see Unit 4).

(b) Same as for other postpartum clients.

h. **Evaluation:**

(1) Verbalizes understanding of reasons for cesarean delivery.

(2) Successful delivery of viable infant.

(3) Evidences no surgical/delivery complications.

(4) Evidences no interference with bonding.

(5) Expresses satisfaction with procedure and result.

5. *Vaginal birth after cesarean (VBAC)*

a. Candidates for VBAC.

(1) Previous C/S low cervical.

(2) Head well-engaged in pelvis.

(3) Soft anterior cervix.

(4) Preexisting reason for C/S not apparent.

(5) No history of sepsis with previous C/S, which may hinder scar from healing properly.

b. **Assessment:**

(1) Monitor FHR carefully during trial of labor.

(2) Monitor contractions carefully for adequate progress of labor.

(3) Observe mother for signs of complications.

c. **Analysis/nursing diagnosis:**

(1) *Knowledge deficit* re trial of labor.

(2) *Fear* related to outcome for fetus.

(3) *Ineffective individual coping* related to labor progress and outcome.

COMPLICATIONS DURING THE INTRAPARTAL PERIOD

I. General aspects

A. Pathophysiology—interference with normal processes and patterns of labor/delivery result in maternal and/or fetal jeopardy (e.g., premature labor, dysfunctional labor patterns; prolonged (over 24 hours) labor; hemorrhage: uterine rupture/inversion, amniotic-fluid embolus).

B. Etiology:

1. Preterm labor—unknown.

2. Dysfunctional labor (dystocia: see page 170):

a. Physiologic response to anxiety/fear/pain—results in release of catecholamines, increasing physical/psychologic stress → myometrial dysfunction; painful and ineffectual labor.

b. Iatrogenic factors: premature or excessive analgesia, particularly during latent phase.

c. Maternal factors:

(1) Pelvic contractures.

(2) Uterine tumors (e.g., myomas, carcinoma).

(3) Congenital uterine anomalies (e.g., bicornate uterus).

(4) Pathologic contraction ring (Bandl's ring).

(5) Rigid cervix, cervical stenosis/stricture.

(6) Hypertonic/hypotonic contractions.

(7) Prolonged rupture of membranes.

(8) Prolonged first or second stage.

(9) Medical conditions: diabetes, hypertension.

d. Fetal factors:

(1) Macrosomia (large for gestational age babies).

(2) Malposition/malpresentation.

(3) Congenital anomaly (e.g., hydrocephalus, anencephaly).

(4) Multiple gestation (e.g., interlocking twins).

(5) Prolapsed cord.

(6) Post-term.

e. Placental factors:

(1) Placenta previa.

(2) Inadequate placental function with contractions.

(3) Abruptio placentae.

(4) Placenta accreta.

f. Physical restrictions: when confined to bed, flat position, etc.

C. Assessment:

1. Antepartal history.

2. Emotional status.

3. Vital signs, FHR.

4. Contraction pattern (frequency, duration, intensity).

5. Vaginal discharge.

D. Analysis/nursing diagnosis:

1. *Anxiety/fear* for self and infant related to implications of prolonged or complicated labor/delivery.

2. *Pain* related to hypertonic contractions/dysfunctional labor.

3. *Ineffective individual coping* related to physical/psychologic stress of complicated labor/delivery, lowered pain threshold secondary to fatigue.

4. *Potential for injury* related to prolonged rupture of membranes, infection.

5. *Fluid volume deficit* related to excessive blood loss secondary to placenta previa, abruptio placentae, Couvelaire uterus, DIC (disseminated intravascular coagulopathy).

E. Nursing plan/implementation:

1. Goal: *minimize physical/psychologic stress during labor/delivery.* Assist client in coping effectively:
   a. Reinforce relaxation techniques.
   b. Support couple's effective coping techniques/mechanisms.
2. Goal: *emotional support.*
   a. Encourage verbalization of anxiety/fear/concerns.
   b. Explain all procedures—to minimize anxiety/fear, encourage cooperation/participation in care.
   c. Provide quiet environment conducive to rest.
3. Goal: *continuous monitoring of maternal/fetal status and progress through labor*—to identify early signs of dysfunctional labor, fetal distress; facilitate prompt, effective treatment of emerging complications.
4. Goal: *minimize effects of complicated labor on mother, fetus.*
   a. Position change: left Sims'—to reduce compression of inferior vena cava.
   b. Oxygen per mask, as indicated.
   c. Institute interventions appropriate to emerging problems (see specific disorder).

F. Evaluation:

1. Successful delivery of viable infant.
2. Maternal/infant status stable, satisfactory.

II. Disorders affecting protective functions. *Preterm labor*—occurs post twenty weeks gestation and prior to beginning of week 38.

A. Pathophysiology—physiologic events of labor (i.e., contractions, spontaneous rupture of membranes, cervical effacement/dilatation) occur prior to completion of normal, term gestation.

B. Etiology—unknown. Theory: may be due to fetal factors released when placental function begins to diminish and intrauterine environment is hostile to continuing fetal well-being.

C. *Coexisting disorders:*

1. Infections that may cause premature rupture of membranes (PROM).
2. PROM of unknown etiology.
3. Hypertension (preeclampsia/eclampsia).
4. Uterine overdistention.
   a. Hydramnios.
   b. Multiple gestation.
5. Maternal diabetes, renal or cardiovascular disorder.
6. Severe maternal illness (e.g., pneumonia, acute pyelonephritis).
7. Abnormal placentation.
   a. Placenta previa.
   b. Abruptio placentae.
8. Iatrogenic: miscalculated EDD for repeat cesarean delivery.
9. Fetal demise.
10. Incompetent cervical os (small percentage).
11. Uterine anomalies (rare).
    a. Intrauterine septum.
    b. Bicornate uterus.
12. Uterine fibroids.

D. *Prevention:*

1. Primary—close obstetric supervision; education in signs/symptoms of labor.
2. Secondary—prompt, effective treatment of associated disorders (see point C above).
3. Tertiary—suppression of premature labor.
   a. Bedrest.
   b. Position: side-lying—to promote placental perfusion.
   c. Hydration.
   d. Pharmacologic (may require "informed consent"; follow hospital protocol). Beta-adrenergic agents (take ECG first) to reduce sensitivity of uterine myometrium to oxytocic and prostaglandin stimulation; increase blood flow to uterus.
   e. May be maintained at home with adequate follow-up and health teaching.

E. Contraindications for suppression: Don't suppress in presence of:

1. Placenta previa or abruptio placentae.
2. Chorioamnionitis.
3. Erythroblastosis fetalis.
4. Severe preeclampsia.
5. Severe diabetes (e.g., "brittle").
6. Increasing placental insufficiency.
7. Cervical dilatation of 4 cm or more.
8. Ruptured membranes (depends on cause and if sepsis).

F. Assessment:

1. Maternal vital signs. Response to medication:
   a. Hypotension.
   b. Tachycardia, arrhythmia.
   c. Dyspnea, chest pain.
   d. Nausea and vomiting.
2. Signs of infection:
   a. Increased temperature.
   b. Tachycardia.
   c. Diaphoresis.
   d. Malaise.
   e. Increased baseline heart rate.
3. Contractions: Frequency, duration, strength.
4. Emotional status—signs of denial, guilt, anxiety, exhaustion.
5. Signs of continuing and progressing labor. **Note:** vaginal exam *only* if indicated by other signs of continuing labor progress.
   a. Effacement.
   b. Dilatation.
   c. Station.
6. Status of membranes.
7. Fetal heart rate, activity (continuous monitoring).

G. Analysis/nursing diagnosis:

1. *Anxiety/fear* related to possible outcome.
2. *Self-esteem disturbance* related to feelings of guilt, failure.
3. *Impaired physical mobility* related to imposed bedrest.
4. *Knowledge deficit* related to medication side effects.
5. *Ineffective individual coping* related to possible outcome.
6. *Impaired gas exchange* related to side effects of medication (circulatory overload; pulmonary edema).
7. *Diversional activity deficit* related to imposed bedrest, decreased environmental stimuli.
8. *Altered urinary elimination* related to bedrest.
9. *Constipation* related to bedrest.

H. Nursing plan/implementation:

1. Goal: *inhibit uterine activity.* Administer medications as ordered—Ritodrine (Yutopar), Terbutaline, or magnesium sulfate.
2. Goal: *safeguard status.*
   a. Continuous maternal/fetal monitoring.
   b. I&O—to identify early signs of possible circulatory overload.
   c. Position: left Sims'—to increase placental perfusion, prevent supine hypotension.
   d. Report promptly to physician:
      (1) Maternal pulse of 110 or more.
      (2) Diastolic pressure of 60 mm Hg or less.
      (3) Respirations of 24 or more; rales.
      (4) Complaint of dyspnea.
      (5) Contractions: Assess frequency, strength, duration, or cessation of contractions.
      (6) Rupture of membranes.
      (7) Fetal distress.
3. Goal: *comfort measures.*
   a. Basic hygienic care—bath, mouth care, cold washcloth to face, perineal care.
   b. Backrub, linen change—to promote relaxation.
4. Goal: *emotional support.*
   a. Encourage verbalization of guilt feelings, anxiety, fear, concerns; provide factual information.
   b. Support positive self-concept.
   c. Keep informed of progress.
5. Goal: *provide quiet diversion.* Television, reading materials, handcrafts.
6. Goal: *health teaching.*
   a. Explain, discuss proposed management to suppress premature labor.
   b. Describe, discuss side effects of medication.
   c. Explain rationale for bedrest, position.
   d. Signs to be reported **promptly:**
      (1) Increasing strength, frequency, duration of contractions.
      (2) Rupture of membranes.
      (3) Vaginal bleeding.
      (4) Intermittent back and thigh pain.

I. *If labor continues to progress:*

1. Goal: *facilitate infant survival.*
   a. Administer betamethasone, as ordered, 24 hours before delivery—to increase/stimulate production of pulmonary surfactant.
   b. Notify perinatal team—to increase chances for fetal survival, assure prompt, expert management of neonate and provide information and support to parents.
   c. Monitor progress of labor to identify signs of impending delivery. **Note:** May deliver before complete (10 cm) dilatation.
   d. Consider transfer to high-risk facility.
   e. Prepare for delivery, or cesarean birth if infant less than 34–36 weeks gestation.
2. Goal: *emotional support.*
   a. Do not leave client (or couple) alone.
   b. Encourage verbalization of anxiety, fear, concern.
   c. Explain all procedures.
3. Goal: *comfort measures. Note:* analgesics contraindicated—to prevent depression of fetus/neonate.
4. Goal: *support effective coping techniques.* Encourage/support Lamaze (or other) techniques—coach, as necessary; discourage hyperventilation.
5. Goal: *health teaching*—for preterm birth.
   a. Discuss need for episiotomy, possibility of outlet forceps delivery—to reduce stress on fetal head, *or*
   b. Prepare for cesarean birth—to reduce possibility of fetal intraventricular hemorrhage.
   c. Rationale for avoiding use of medications to reduce contraction pain.

J. *Immediate care of neonate:*

1. Goal: *safeguard status.*
   a. Stabilize environmental temperature—to prevent chilling (isolette or other controlled-temperature bed).
   b. Oxygen, as needed; may need intubation.
   c. Parenteral fluids, as ordered—to support normal acid–base balance, pH; administer antibiotics, as necessary.
   d. Arrange transport to high-risk facility, as necessary.
2. Goal: *continuous monitoring of status.*
   a. Electronic monitors—to observe respiratory and cardiac functions.
   b. Blood samples—to monitor blood gases, pH, hypoglycemia.

K. *Postpartum care:* Goal: *emotional support.*

1. Facilitate attachment.
2. If couple, foster sense of mutual experience and closeness.
3. Help her/them maintain a positive self-image.
4. Encourage touching of infant before transport to nursery or high-risk facility; father may accompany infant and report back to mother.
5. Encourage early contact—to facilitate maternal need to ventilate her feelings.

6. Assist parent(s) with grieving process, if necessary.
7. Refer to support group if necessary.

L. *Other*—as for any postpartum client.

M. Evaluation:

1. Verbalizes understanding of medical/nursing recommendations and treatments.
2. Complies with medical/nursing regimen.
3. Experiences no discomfort from side effects of therapy.
4. Experiences successful outcome—labor inhibited.
5. Carries pregnancy to successful termination.
6. If preterm delivery occurs, copes effectively with outcome (physiologically compromised neonate, neonatal demise).

III. Grief and childbearing experience. The loss of a pregnancy or a newborn, or the birth of a physiologically compromised child (premature, congenital disorder), is a crisis situation. The unexpected outcome can cause the parent(s) to suffer a sense of loss of self-esteem, self-concept, positive body image, feelings of worth (see Table 2.8, p. 140).

A. Assessment:

1. Response to loss of the "fantasy child"/real child.
   a. Behavioral—anger, hostility, depression, disinterest in activities of daily living, withdrawal.
   b. Biophysical—somatic complaints (stomach pain, malaise, anorexia, nausea).
   c. Cognitive—feelings of guilt.
2. Knowledge/understanding/perception of situation.
3. Coping abilities, mechanisms.
4. Support system.

B. Analysis/nursing diagnosis:

1. *Ineffective family coping: compromised* due to psychologic stress related to fear for infant, guilt feelings, impact on self-image.
2. *Ineffective individual coping* related to anxiety, stress.
3. *Ineffective family coping: disabling* related to disturbance in intrafamily relations secondary to individual coping deficits, recriminations.
4. *Altered parenting* related to lack of effective bonding secondary to emotional separation from infant, feelings of guilt.
5. *Dysfunctional grieving* related to guilt feelings, impact of loss on self-concept.
6. *Disturbance in body image, self-esteem, role performance* related to perceived failure to complete gestational task, produce perfect, healthy infant, sleep deprivation.
7. *Social isolation* related to severe coping deficit, dysfunctional grieving, disturbance in self-esteem.

C. Nursing plan/implementation:

1. Goal: *emotional support.*
   a. Provide privacy; encourage open expression/verbalization of feelings, fears, concerns, perceptions.
   b. Crisis intervention techniques.
2. Goal: *facilitate bonding, effective coping, and/or anticipatory grieving processes.*
   a. Encourage contact and participation in care of premature or compromised infant.
   b. Keep informed of infant's status.
   c. Provide realistic data.
3. Goal: *health teaching.*
   a. Clarify misperceptions, as appropriate.
   b. Discuss, demonstrate infant care techniques (e.g., feeding infant who has cleft lip and/or palate).
   c. Refer to appropriate community resources.

D. Evaluation:

1. Verbalizes recognition and acceptance of diagnosis.
2. Verbalizes understanding of relevant information regarding treatment, prognosis.
3. Makes informed decision regarding infant care.
4. Demonstrates comfort and increasing participation in care of neonate.
5. Evidence of bonding (eye contact, cuddles, calls by name).

IV. Disorders affecting comfort, rest, mobility: *dystocia*

A. Definition—difficult labor.

B. General aspects (*MOTHER: P*sych, *P*lacenta, *P*osition):

1. **Pathophysiology**—see specific disorders.
2. **Etiology**—due to effects of factors that affect the:
   a. *P*OWER: forces of labor (uterine contractions, use of abdominal muscles).
      (1) Premature analgesia/anesthesia.
      (2) Uterine overdistention (multiple pregnancy, fetal macrosomia).
      (3) Uterine myomas.
   b. *P*ASSAGEWAY: resistance of cervix, pelvic structures.
      (1) Rigid cervix.
      (2) Distended bladder.
   c. Dimensions of the bony pelvis: pelvic contractures.
   d. *P*ASSENGER: accommodation of the presenting part to pelvic diameters.
      (1) Fetal malposition/malpresentation.
         (a) Transverse lie.
         (b) Face, brow presentation.
         (c) Breech presentation.
         (d) C.P.D.
      (2) Fetal anomalies.
         (a) Hydrocephalus.
         (b) Conjoined twins.
         (c) Myelomeningocele.
3. **Hazards:**
   a. Maternal:
      (1) Fatigue, exhaustion, dehydration—due to prolonged labor.
      (2) Lowered pain threshold, loss of control—due to prolonged labor, continued uterine contractions, anxiety, fatigue, lack of sleep.
      (3) Intrauterine infection—due to prolonged rupture of membranes.

(4) Uterine rupture—due to obstructed labor.

(5) Cervical, vaginal, perineal lacerations—due to obstetric interventions.

(6) Postpartum hemorrhage—due to uterine atony and/or trauma.

b. Fetal:

(1) Hypoxia, anoxia, demise—due to decreased O_2 concentration in cord blood.

(2) Intracranial hemorrhage—due to changing intracranial pressure.

C. Hypertonic dysfunction

1. **Pathophysiology**—increased resting tone of uterine myometrium; diminished refractory period; prolonged latent phase:

a. *Nullipara*—more than 20 hours.

b. *Multipara*—more than 14 hours.

2. **Etiology**—unknown. Theory—ectopic initiation of incoordinate uterine contractions.

3. **Assessment:**

a. Onset—early labor (latent phase).

b. Contractions:

(1) Continuous fundal tension, incomplete relaxation.

(2) Painful.

(3) Ineffectual—no effacement or dilatation.

c. Signs of fetal distress

(1) Meconium-stained amniotic fluid.

(2) Fetal heart rate irregularities.

d. Maternal vial signs.

e. Emotional status.

f. Medical evaluation: vaginal exam, X-ray pelvimetry, ultrasonography—to rule out CPD.

4. **Analysis/nursing diagnosis:**

a. *Pain* related to hypertonic contractions, incomplete uterine relaxation.

b. *Anxiety/fear* for self and infant related to strong, painful contractions without evidence of progress.

c. *Ineffective individual coping* related to fatigue, exhaustion, anxiety, tension, fear.

d. *Impaired gas exchange (fetal)* related to incomplete relaxation of uterus.

e. *Sleep pattern disturbance* related to prolonged ineffectual labor.

5. **Nursing plan/implementation:**

a. Medical management:

(1) Short-acting barbiturates (see Unit 6)—to encourage rest, relaxation.

(2) Intravenous fluids—to restore/maintain hydration and fluid–electrolyte balance.

(3) If CPD, cesarean delivery.

b. Nursing management:

(1) Goal: *emotional support*—assist coping with fear, pain, discouragement.

(a) Encourage verbalization of anxiety, fear, concerns.

(b) Explain all procedures.

(c) Reassure. Keep couple informed of progress.

(2) Goal: *comfort measures.*

(a) Position: left Sims—to promote relaxation and placental perfusion.

(b) Bath, backrub, linen change, clean environment.

(c) Environment: quiet, darkened room—to minimize stimuli and encourage relaxation, warmth.

(d) Encourage voiding—to relieve bladder distention; to test urine for ketones.

(3) Goal: *prevent infection.* Strict aseptic technique.

(4) Goal: *prepare for cesarean delivery* if necessary.

6. **Evaluation:**

a. Relaxes, sleeps, establishes normal labor pattern.

b. Demonstrates no signs of fetal distress.

c. Successfully completes uneventful labor.

D. Hypotonic dysfunction during labor

1. **Pathophysiology**—after normal labor at onset, contractions diminish in frequency, duration and strength; lowered uterine resting tone; cervical effacement and dilatation slows/ceases.

2. **Etiology:**

a. Premature or excessive analgesia/anesthesia (caudal or epidural block).

b. CPD.

c. Overdistention (hydramnios, fetal macrosomia, multiple pregnancy).

d. Fetal malposition/malpresentation.

e. Maternal fear/anxiety.

3. **Assessment:**

a. Onset—may occur in latent phase; most common during active phase.

b. Contractions: normal previously, demonstrate:

(1) Decreased frequency.

(2) Shorter duration.

(3) Diminished intensity (mild to moderate).

(4) Less uncomfortable.

c. Cervical changes—slow or cease.

d. Signs of fetal distress—rare.

(1) Usually occur late in labor due to infection secondary to prolonged rupture of membranes.

(2) Tachycardia.

e. Maternal vital signs may indicate infection (↑ temp).

f. Medical diagnosis—procedures: vaginal exam, X-ray pelvimetry, ultrasonography—to rule out CPD (most common cause).

4. **Analysis/nursing diagnosis:**

a. *Knowledge deficit* related to limited exposure to information.

b. *Anxiety/fear* related to failure to progress as anticipated; fear for fetus.

c. *Potential for injury* (infection) related to prolonged labor and/or ruptured membranes.

5. **Nursing plan/implementation:**

a. Medical management:

(1) Amniotomy—artificial rupture of membranes.

(2) Oxytocin augmentation of labor—intravenous infusion of oxytocin to increase frequency, duration, strength, and efficiency of uterine contractions (see Induction of labor, p. 163).

(3) If CPD, cesarean delivery.

b. Nursing management:

(1) Goals: *emotional support, comfort measures, prevent infection*—as for Hypertonic dysfunction, point C5b above.

(2) Other—see Induction of labor, p. 163.

6. **Evaluation:**

a. Reestablishes normal labor pattern.

b. Experiences successful delivery of viable infant.

V. Disorders affecting fluid-gas transport: *maternal*

A. Uterine rupture

1. **Pathophysiology**—stress on uterine muscle exceeds its ability to stretch.

2. **Etiology:**

a. Overdistention—due to large baby, multiple gestation.

b. Old scars—due to previous cesarean deliveries.

c. Contractions against CPD, fetal malpresentation, pathologic retraction ring (Bandl's).

d. Injudicious obstetrics—malapplication of forceps (or application without full effacement/dilatation).

e. Tetanic contraction—due to hypersensitivity to oxytocin (or excessive dosage) during induction/augmentation of labor.

3. **Assessment:**

a. Identify predisposing factors early.

b. *Complete rupture*

(1) Pain: sudden, sharp, abdominal; followed by cessation of contractions; tender abdomen.

(2) Signs of shock; vaginal bleeding.

(3) Fetal heart tones—absent.

(4) Presenting part—not palpable on vaginal examination.

c. *Incomplete rupture*

(1) Contractions: continue, accompanied by abdominal pain and failure to dilate.

(2) Signs of shock.

(3) May demonstrate vaginal bleeding.

(4) Fetal heart tones—absent.

4. *Prognosis*

a. Maternal—guarded.

b. Fetal—grave.

5. **Analysis/nursing diagnosis:**

a. *Pain* related to rupture of uterine muscle.

b. *Fluid volume deficit* related to massive blood loss secondary to uterine rupture.

c. *Anxiety/fear* related to concern for self, fetus.

d. *Altered tissue perfusion* related to blood loss secondary to uterine rupture.

e. *Altered urinary elimination* related to necessary conservation of intravascular fluid secondary to blood loss.

f. *Anticipatory grieving* related to expected loss of fetus; inability to have more children.

6. **Nursing plan/implementation:**

a. Medical management:

(1) Surgical—laparotomy, hysterectomy.

(2) Replace blood loss—transfusion, packed cells.

(3) Reduce possibility of infection—antibiotics.

b. Nursing management:

(1) Goal: *safeguard status.*

(a) Report *immediately;* mobilize staff.

(b) Prepare for immediate laparotomy.

(c) Oxygen per mask—to increase circulating oxygen level.

(d) Order stat type and crossmatch for blood —to replace blood loss.

(e) Establish intravenous line—to infuse fluids, blood, medications.

(f) Insert indwelling catheter—to deflate bladder.

(g) Abdominal prep—to remove hair, bacteria.

(h) Surgical permit for hysterectomy.

(2) Goal: *emotional support*—to allay anxiety (client and family).

(a) Encourage verbalization of fears, anxiety, concerns.

(b) Explain all procedures.

(c) Keep family informed of progress.

7. **Evaluation:**

a. Experiences successful termination of emergency; minimal blood loss.

b. Postoperative status stable.

B. Amniotic fluid embolus

1. **Pathophysiology:** acute cor pulmonale—due to embolus blocking vessels in pulmonary circulation; massive hemorrhage—due to DIC resulting from entrance of thromboplastin-like material into bloodstream.

2. **Etiology**—amniotic fluid (with any meconium, lanugo, or vernix) enters maternal circulation through open venous sinuses at placental site; travels to pulmonary arterioles.

a. Rare.

b. Associated with: tumultuous labor, abruptio placentae.

3. *Prognosis*—poor; often fatal to mother.

4. **Assessment:**

a. May occur during labor or immediate postpartum.

b. Sudden dyspnea and cyanosis.

c. Chest pain.

d. Hypotension, tachycardia.

e. Frothy sputum.

f. *Signs of DIC:*

(1) Purpura—local hemorrhage.

(2) Increased vaginal bleeding—massive.

(3) Rapid evolution of shock.

5. **Analysis/nursing diagnosis:**

a. *Impaired gas exchange* related to pulmonary edema.

b. *Potential fluid volume deficit* related to DIC.

c. *Anxiety/fear* for self and fetus related to severity of symptoms, perception of jeopardy.

6. **Nursing plan/implementation:**

a. Medical management:

(1) IV heparin, whole blood.

(2) Delivery: immediate, by forceps, if possible.

(3) Digitalize, as necessary.

b. Nursing management:

(1) Goal: *assist ventilation.*

(a) Position: semi-Fowler's.

(b) Oxygen under positive pressure.

(c) Suction p.r.n.

(2) Goal: *facilitate/expedite administration of fluids, medications, blood.*

(a) Establish intravenous line.

(b) Administer heparin, fluids, as ordered.

(3) Goal: *restore cardiopulmonary functions, if needed.* Cardiopulmonary resuscitation techniques.

(4) Goal: *emotional support* of client, family.

(a) Allay anxiety, as possible.

(b) Explain all procedures.

(c) Keep informed of status.

7. **Evaluation:**

a. Dyspnea relieved.

b. Bleeding controlled.

c. Successful delivery of viable infant.

d. Uneventful postpartum course.

VI. Disorders affecting fluid-gas transport: *fetal*

A. Fetus in jeopardy—general aspects:

1. **Pathophysiology**—maternal hypoxemia, anemia, ketoacidosis, Rh isoimmunization, or decreased uteroplacental perfusion.

2. **Etiology**—maternal:

a. Preeclampsia/eclampsia.

b. Heart disease.

c. Diabetes.

d. Rh or ABO incompatibility.

e. Insufficient uteroplacental/cord circulation due to:

(1) Maternal hypotension/hypertension.

(2) Cord compression.

(3) Hemorrhage.

TABLE 2.13 Abnormal Fetal Heart Rate Patterns (also see Fig. 2.8, p. 156; Table 2.14, p. 175)

Early Decelerations

1. FHR begins to slow with the onset of the uterine contraction (UC) and returns to baseline when contraction is over.
2. Fetal head compression occurs.
3. Vagal nerve stimulation.
4. Transient slowing FHR.
5. No intervention required.

Late Decelerations

1. FHR begins to fall at height of the UC and returns to baseline after contraction has ceased.
2. FHR usually remains within normal range.
3. Indicates some degree of uteroplacental insufficiency.
4. Interventions—*required:* position on left side, begin oxygen by mask; turn off Pitocin; notify MD.

Variable Decelerations

1. Slowing of FHR either with a contraction or in between contractions. Unrelated pattern of FHR and uterine contraction.
2. Pattern may be U shaped or V shaped.
3. Returns immediately to baseline.
4. Usually indicates cord compression.
5. Interventions: change position to alleviate cord pressure; begin oxygen by mask; notify MD.

(4) Malformation of the placenta/cord.

(5) Postterm gestation.

(6) Premature "aging" of placenta.

(7) Maternal infection.

(8) Hydramnios.

(9) Hypertonic uterine contractions.

(10) Placental infarcts.

(11) Maternal spotting.

f. PROM (premature rupture of membrane) with chorioamnionitis.

g. Dystocia (e.g., from CPD).

3. **Assessment**—intrapartal:

a. Amniotic fluid examination—at/or after rupture of membranes. *Signs of fetal distress:* meconium-stained, vertex presentation—due to relaxation of fetal anal sphincter secondary to hypoxia/anoxia. **Note:** Fetus "gasps" in utero—may aspirate meconium and amniotic fluid.

b. Fetal activity:

(1) Hyperactivity—due to hypoxemia, elevated CO_2.

(2) Cessation—possible fetal demise.

c. Methods of monitoring FHR:

(1) Stethoscope or fetoscope.

(2) Phonocardiography with microphone application.

(3) Internal fetal electrode—attached directly to fetus through dilated cervix after membranes ruptured.

(4) Doppler probe using ultrasound flow.

(5) Cardiotocograph—transducer on maternal abdomen transmits sound.

d. Abnormal fetal heart rate (FHR) patterns (Table 2.13 and Figure 2.8, p. 156).

(1) Persistent irregularity.

(2) Persistent tachycardia of 160 or more beats per minute.

(3) Persistent bradycardia of 100 or fewer beats per minute.

(4) *Early deceleration*—due to vagal response to head compression.

(5) *Late deceleration*—due to uteroplacental insufficiency.

(6) *Variable deceleration*—due to cord compression.

(7) Decreased or loss of variability in FHR pattern.

e. Medical evaluation—procedures: fetal blood gases, pH.

(1) Purpose—to identify fetal acid–base status.

(2) Requirements for:

(a) Ruptured membranes.

(b) Cervical dilatation.

(c) Engaged head.

(3) Procedure—under sterile condition, sample of fetal scalp blood obtained for analysis.

(4) Signs of fetal distress:

(a) pH below 7.20 (normal range is 7.3–7.4).

(b) Increased CO_2.

(c) Decreased Po_2.

4. **Analysis/nursing diagnosis:**

a. *Impaired gas exchange, fetal,* related to decreased placental perfusion/insufficient cord circulation.

b. *Altered tissue perfusion* related to hemolytic anemia.

c. *Potential for injury* related to hypoxia.

B. Prolapsed umbilical cord

1. **Pathophysiology**—cord descent in advance of presenting part; compression interrupts blood flow, exchange of fetal/maternal gases → fetal hypoxia, anoxia, demise (if unrelieved).

2. **Etiology:**

a. Spontaneous or artificial rupture of membranes before presenting part engaged.

b. Excessive force of escaping fluid, as in hydramnios.

c. Malposition—breech, compound presentation, transverse lie.

d. Premature or small for gestational age (SGA) fetus—allows space for cord descent.

3. **Assessment:**

a. Visualization of cord outside (or inside) vagina.

b. Palpation of pulsating mass on vaginal examination.

c. Fetal distress—variable deceleration and persistent bradycardia.

4. **Analysis/nursing diagnosis:**

a. *Impaired gas exchange, fetal,* related to interruption of blood flow from placenta/fetus.

b. *Anxiety/fear, maternal,* related to knowledge of fetal jeopardy.

5. **Nursing plan/implementation:**

a. Goal: *reduce pressure on cord.*

(1) Position: knee to chest; left Sims with hips elevated; modified Trendelenberg.

(2) With gloved hand, support fetal head off cord.

b. Goal: *increase maternal/fetal oxygenation:* oxygen per mask (8–10 liters/min).

c. Goal: *protect exposed cord:* cover cord with sterile wet saline dressing.

d. Goal: *identify fetal response* to above measures, reduce threat to fetal survival: monitor FHR continuously.

e. Goal: *expedite termination of threat to fetus:* prepare for immediate vaginal/cesarean birth.

f. Goal: *support mother and significant other* by staying with them and explaining.

6. **Evaluation:**

a. FHR returns to normal rate and pattern.

b. Uncomplicated birth of viable infant.

VII. Summary of danger signs during labor

A. Contractions—strong, every 2 minutes or less, lasting 90 seconds; poor relaxation between contractions.

B. Sudden sharp abdominal pain followed by boardlike abdomen and shock—abruptio placentae or uterine rupture.

C. Marked vaginal bleeding.

D. FHR periodic pattern decelerations—late; variable; absent (see Table 2.14).

E. Baseline.

1. Bradycardia (<100 bpm).

2. Tachycardia (>160 bpm).

F. Amniotic fluid.

1. Amount: excessive; diminished.

2. Odor.

3. Color: meconium-stained; port-wine; yellow.

4. 24 hours or more since rupture of membranes.

G. Maternal hypotension.

■ THE POSTPARTAL PERIOD

General overview: This review of the normal physiologic and psychologic changes occurring during the postpartal period (birth to 6 weeks after) provides the data base necessary for assessing the client's progress through involution, planning and implementing care, anticipatory guidance, health teaching, and evaluating the results. Emerging problems are identified by comparing client status against established standards.

I. Biologic foundations of the postpartal period

A. Uterine involution—integrated processes by which the uterus returns to normal size, shape, and consistency. **Assessment:**

1. Contractions ("after pains")—shorten muscles, close venous sinuses, restore normal tone.

a. Frequency, intensity, and discomfort decrease after first 24 hours.

■ TABLE 2.14 Nursing Care During Fetal Distress

Fetal distress is caused primarily by a decrease in the fetal oxygen supply. Interference with oxygen may be maternal or fetal in origin.

Maternal-Related Causes	Fetal-Related Causes	Fetal Distress Signs
Anemia	Prolapsed cord.	Hyperactivity of the fetus.
Hypertension or hypotension	Knotted cord.	Meconium-stained amniotic fluid, except in a known breech presentation.
Preeclampsia	Nuchal cord.	Persistent fetal bradycardia (below 100 beats/minute) or tachycardia (above 180 beats/minute) or loss of beat-to-beat variability.
Abruptio placentae		
Placenta previa		
Medication		
Prolonged contraction		
Pressure on the placenta		

Fetal Distress Pattern Graphs

Continuous electronic monitoring can identify fetal heart rate patterns that indicate fetal distress and its possible cause.

Early deceleration (related to head compression)

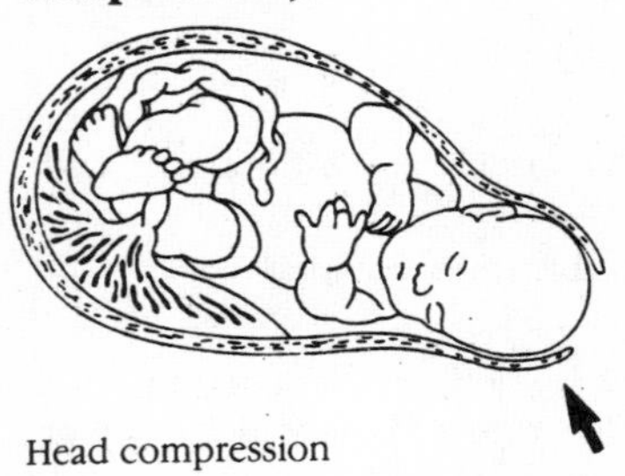

Head compression

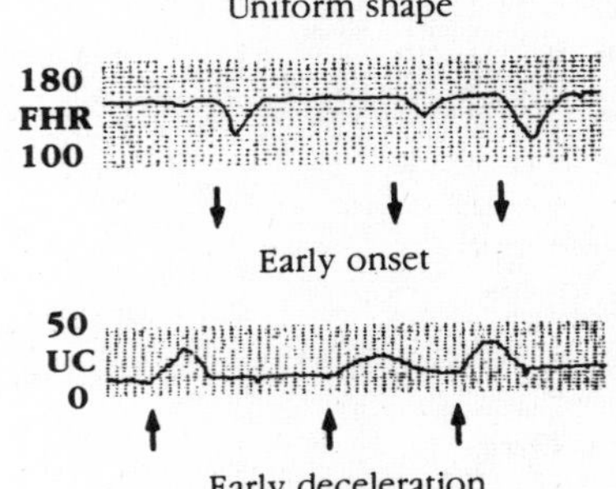

Early deceleration

Nursing Interventions

Continue observation. This pattern usually indicates head compression as the fetal head passes through the birth canal.

Late deceleration (related to uteroplacental compression)

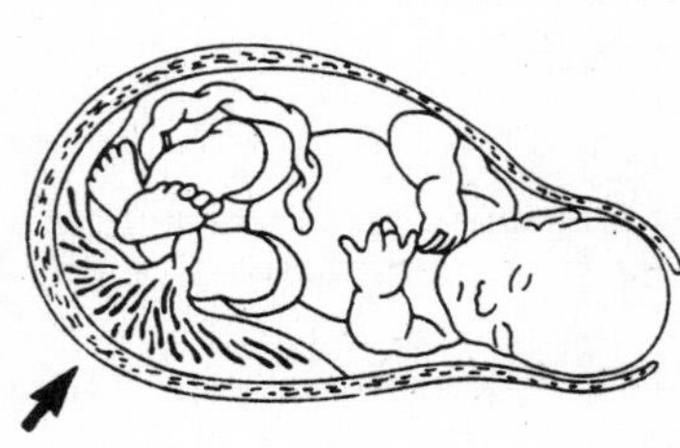

Compression of vessels

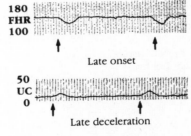

Uniform shape

180
FHR
100

Late onset

50
UC
0

Late deceleration

Nursing Interventions

Stop oxytocin if in progress, and replace IV fluid.

Change the client's position to the preferred left side-lying position.

Check blood pressure and pulse rate.

Administer oxygen.

Notify the doctor.

Variable deceleration (related to umbilical cord compression)

The first deceleration is U-shaped; the second, V-shaped. Transitory acceleration precedes or follows the deceleration. The fetal heart rate may fall to fewer than 100 beats/minute.

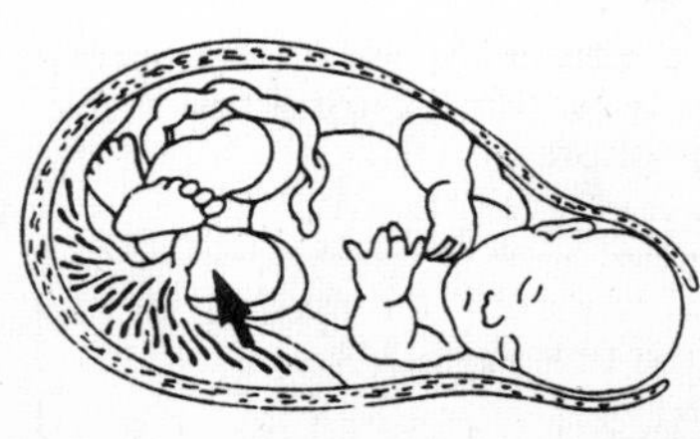

Umbilical cord compression

Variable shape

180
FHR
100

Variable onset

50
UC
0

Variable deceleration

Nursing Interventions

Stop oxytocin if in progress, and replace IV fluid.

Change maternal position.

Check for prolapsed cord.

Check blood pressure and pulse rate.

Administer oxygen.

Notify the doctor.

Prepare to assist with drawing blood sample from fetal scalp.

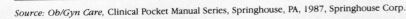

Source: Ob/Gyn Care, Clinical Pocket Manual Series, Springhouse, PA, 1987, Springhouse Corp.

Uterus	Nonpregnant	Pregnant (At Term)
Length	6.5 cm	32 cm
Width	4 cm	24 cm
Depth	2.5 cm	22 cm
Weight	50 g	1,000 g

Fundal height measurement landmarks

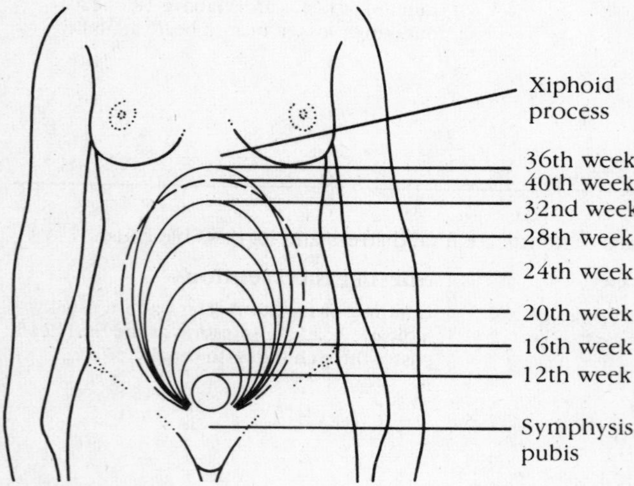

FIGURE 2.9
Uterine changes during pregnancy. (From *Ob/Gyn Care,* Clinical Pocket Manual Series, Springhouse Corp., Springhouse, PA, 1987.)

b. More common in: multiparas, and after delivery of a large baby; primiparous uterus remains contracted.

c. Increased by breastfeeding.

2. Autolysis—breakdown and excretion of muscle protein (decreasing size of myometrial cells). Lochia—sloughing of decidua and blood.
3. Formation of *new endometrium*—4–6 weeks until placental site healed.
4. *Cervix*
   a. Immediately following delivery—bruised, small tears; admits one hand.
   b. Eighteen hours after delivery—becomes shorter, firmer; regains normal shape.
   c. One week postpartum—admits two fingers.
   d. Never returns fully to prepregnant state.
      (1) Parous os is wider and not perfectly round.
      (2) Lacerations heal as scars radiating out from the os.
5. *Fundal height and consistency* (Figure 2.9)
   a. After delivery—at umbilicus; size and consistency of firm grapefruit.
   b. Day 1 (first 12 hours)—one finger above umbilicus.
   c. Descends by one finger-breadth daily until day 10.
   d. Day 10—behind symphysis pubis, nonpalpable.
6. *Lochia*
   a. Character:
      (1) Days 1–3; rubra (red).
      (2) Days 3–7; serosa (pink to brown).
      (3) Day 10; alba (creamy white).
   b. Amount:
      (1) Moderate: 4–8 pads/day (average 6 pads/day).
      (2) Cesarean birth clients: less lochia—due to manipulation during surgery.
   c. Odor: normal lochia has characteristic "fresh" odor; foul odor is characteristic of infection.
   d. Clots: normal: a few small clots, most commonly on arising—due to pooling. *Note:* Clots and *heavy* bleeding are associated with uterine atony, retained placental fragments.

B. Birth canal

1. *Vagina*—never returns fully to prepregnant state.
   a. First few weeks postpartum—thin-walled, due to lack of estrogen; few rugae.
   b. Week 3: rugae may reappear.
   c. Hymen—if torn, may heal.
2. *Pelvic floor*
   a. Immediately after delivery—infiltrated with blood, stretched, torn.
   b. Month 6: considerable tone regained.
3. *Perineum*
   a. Immediately following delivery—edematous; may have episiotomy (or repaired lacerations); hemorrhoids.
   b. Healing, incisional line clean; no separation.
   c. Hematoma—blood in connective tissue beneath skin; complains of pain, unrelieved by mild analgesia or heat; perineal distention; painful, tense, fluctuant mass.

C. Abdominal wall

1. Overdistention during pregnancy may → rupture of elastic fibers, persistent striae, and diastasis of the rectus muscles.
2. Usually takes 6–8 weeks to retrogress, dependent on previous muscle tone, obesity, and amount of distention during pregnancy.
3. Strenuous exercises discouraged until 8 weeks postpartum.

D. Cardiovascular system—characteristic changes:

1. Immediately after delivery—*increased* cardiac load, due to:
   a. Return of uterine blood flow to general circulation.
   b. Diuresis of excess interstitial fluid.
2. Volume—returns to prepregnant state (4 liters) in about 3 weeks. Major reduction—during first week, due to diuresis and diaphoresis.
3. Blood values (see Table 2.15)
   a. High WBC during labor (25,000/mL); drops to normal level in first few days.
   b. Week 1—Hgb, RBC, Hct, elevated fibrinogen return to normal.
4. Blood coagulation

■ **TABLE 2.15 Blood Values**

Component	Pregnant	Prepregnant
WBC	9–16,000 (25,000–labor).	4–11,000.
RBC volume	1900 mL.	1600 mL.
Plasma volume	3700 mL.	2400 mL.
Hct (PCV)	32–42%.	37–47%.
Hgb (at sea level)	10–14 g/dL.	12–16 g/dL.
Fibrinogen	400 mg/dL.	250 mg/dL.

a. During labor: rapid consumption of clotting factors.

b. During postpartum: increased consumption of clotting factors. Hypercoagulability maintained during first few days postpartum; predisposes to thrombophlebitis, pulmonary embolism.

5. **Assessment: potential complications**—vital signs:

a. Temperature—elevated in:

(1) Excessive blood loss, dehydration, exhaustion, infection.

(2) Elevation: 100.4 °F (38 °C) after first day postpartum suggests puerperal infection.

b. Pulse—physiologic bradycardia (50–70) common through second day postpartum; may persist 7–10 days; etiology: unknown. *Tachycardia*—associated with: excessive blood loss, dehydration, exhaustion, infection.

c. Blood pressure—generally unchanged. *Elevation*—associated with: preeclampsia, essential hypertension.

E. Urinary tract—characteristic changes:

1. Output—increased due to: diuresis (12 hours to 5 days postpartum); daily output to 3000 mL.

2. Urine constituents:

a. Sugar—primarily lactose.

b. Acetonuria—after prolonged labor; dehydration.

c. Proteinuria—first 3 days in response to the catalytic process of involution.

3. Dilatation of ureters—subsides in first few weeks.

4. **Assessment: potential complications**—measure first few voidings, palpate bladder to determine emptying.

a. Edema, trauma, and/or anesthesia may → retention with overflow.

b. Overdistended bladder—common cause of excessive bleeding in immediate postpartum.

F. Integument (skin)—characteristic changes:

1. Striae—persist as silvery lines.

2. Diastasis recti abdominis—some midline separation may persist.

3. Diaphoresis—excessive perspiration for first few (approximately 5) days.

4. Breast changes—see II.A.3. *Breasts,* following.

G. Legs

1. Should have no redness, tenderness, local areas of increased skin temperature, or edema.

2. May have some soreness from delivery position.

3. Homans' sign should be negative (no calf pain when knee is extended and gentle pressure applied to dorsiflex the foot).

H. Weight—characteristic changes:

1. Initial weight loss—fetus, placenta, amniotic fluid, excess tissue fluid.

2. Weighs more than in prepregnant state (weight maintained in breasts).

3. Week 6—weight loss is individualized.

I. Menstruation and ovarian function—first menstrual cycle may be anovulatory.

1. Nonnursing—ovulation at 4–6 weeks; menstruation at 6–8 weeks.

2. Nursing—anovulatory period varies (39 days to 6 months or more); some for duration of lactation; contraceptive value: *very unreliable.*

II. Nursing management during the postpartal period

A. Assessment—minimum of twice daily.

1. Vital signs.

2. Emotional status, response to baby.

3. *Breasts*

a. Observe: size, symmetry, placement and condition of nipples, leakage of colostrum. Normal: although one breast is usually larger than the other, breasts are essentially symmetrical in shape; nipples: in breast midline, erectile, intact (no signs of fissure); bilateral leakage of colostrum is common.

b. Note: reddened areas, elevations, supernumerary nipples, inverted nipples, cracks.

c. Observe for signs of (normal) engorgement (i.e., tenderness, distention, prominent veins). Transient; normally occurs shortly before lactation is established—due to venous and lymphatic stasis.

d. Palpate for: local heat, edema, tenderness, swelling (signs of localized infection).

e. *Lactation-suppressed mothers* (i.e., those who elect to bottlefeed their infants). Lactosuppression—hormone-limited production of milk; less common today. [*Note:* FDA (1977) specifies client must sign an informed consent prior to receiving estrogens for any reason.]

(1) Bromocriptine mesylate (Parlodel) inhibits prolactin secretion; withhold for all preeclamptics *and* until vital signs stable.

(2) Dosage: 2.5 mg PO bid for 14 days. (Controversial because of side effects).

4. Fundus, lochia, perineum.

5. Voiding and bowel function.

6. Legs (see point G above).

7. Signs of complications.

B. Analysis/nursing diagnosis: (See VI B, Nursing actions during the fourth stage of labor, p. 160.)

C. Nursing plan/implementation:

1. Goal: *comfort measures.*

a. Perineal care—to promote healing, prevent infection.
b. Sitz baths—to promote healing.
c. Apply topical anesthetics, witch hazel to episiotomy area, hemorrhoids.
d. Administer mild analgesia, as ordered.
e. Instruct in tensing buttocks on position change—to reduce stress on suture line, discomfort.

2. Goal: *encourage normal bowel function.* (Normal to take 1–3 days for function to resume).
a. Administer stool softeners, as ordered.
b. Encourage ambulation.
c. Increase dietary fiber (salads, fresh fruit, vegetables, bran cereals).
d. Provide adequate fluid intake.

3. Goal: *health teaching.*
a. Reinforce appropriate perineal self-care.
b. Reinforce handwashing (see Nursing actions during the fourth stage of labor, p. 160).
c. Infant care
(1) Bathing, cord care, circumcision care, diapering.
(2) Feeding, burping, scheduling.
(3) Assessment—temperature, skin color, newborn rash, jaundice.
(4) Normal stool cycle and voiding pattern.
(5) Common sleep/activity patterns.
(6) Signs to report immediately:
(a) Fever, vomiting, diarrhea.
(b) Signs of inflammation and/or infection at cord stump.
(c) Bleeding from circumcision site.
d. Self-care
(1) Adequate rest, nutrition, hydration.
(2) Breast self-exam; wear bra to support breasts, and promote comfort.
(3) Normal process of involution; lochial patterns.
e. Resumption of intercourse approximately 4 weeks postpartum (wait until discharge and lochia stops).
(1) Explain that time interval varies as to first postpartal ovulation.
(2) Family planning options may resume if desired:
(a) If not breastfeeding, oral contraceptives after first menstrual period (low dose given to breastfeeding mothers).
(b) Use of IUD or diaphragm decided at 6-week postpartal check-up.
(c) Emphasize need to recheck size and fit of diaphragm.
(d) Other options: condom plus spermacides.
f. Exercises—to restore muscle tone, relieve tension.
(1) Mild exercise during first few weeks.
(a) Deep abdominal breathing.
(b) Supine head-raising.
(c) Stretching from head to toe.
(d) Pelvic tilt.
(e) Kegel's—to regain perineal muscle tone.
(2) Strenuous exercises (sit-ups, leg lifts)—deferred until later in postpartum.
g. Maternal signs to report immediately:
(a) Prolonged lochia rubra.
(b) Cramping.
(c) Signs of infection.
(d) Excessive fatigue, depression.
(e) Dysuria.

4. Goal: *anticipatory guidance*—discharge planning: mothers are discharged earlier in their postpartum recovery today—(24–48 hours after delivery if asymptomatic).
a. Discuss, assist in organizing time schedule. Nap, when possible, when infant asleep—to minimize fatigue.
b. Common maternal emotional/behavior changes, feelings.
(1) Jealous of infant; guilt feelings.
(2) "Baby blues"—due to hormonal fluctuations, fatigue, change of life-style.
(3) Feelings of inadequacy.
c. Discuss support groups, aid in identifying supportive people.

D. Evaluation:
1. Experiences normal, uncomplicated postpartal period. All assessment findings within normal limits.
2. Returns demonstrations of appropriate self-care measures/techniques:
a. Perineal care, pad change, handwashing.
b. Breast care, breast self-exam.
3. Verbalizes understanding of:
a. Need for adequate rest and diversion.
b. Appropriate time for resumption of intercourse and exercise.
c. Appropriate nutritional intake to meet needs (own and, if breastfeeding, infant).
d. Signs to be reported immediately.
e. Returns demonstration of appropriate infant care measures.
f. Evidences beginning comfort and increasing confidence in parenting role.

E. Postpartal assessment—6 weeks after delivery:
1. Weight, vital signs, urine for protein, complete blood count.
2. Breast exam—lactating or not.
3. Pelvic exam—involution and position of uterus; perineal healing; tone of pelvic floor.
4. Desire for selection of method of contraception.

III. Psychologic/behavioral changes* *Achievement of developmental tasks*—progress in assumption of maternal role.

---

* This section is based on a study written by R. Rubin.

A. Assessment:

1. *Taking-in* phase: 1–3 days following delivery.
   a. Talkative; verbally relives labor/delivery experience.
   b. Passive, dependent, concerned with own needs (eating, sleeping, elimination).
2. *Taking-hold*—day 3 to 2 weeks.
   a. Impatient to control own bodily functions, care for self.
   b. Expresses interest/concern in learning how to care for baby (desire to assume "mothering" role).
   c. Responds to positive reinforcement.
3. *Letting-go*—mother "lets go" of former self-concept, role, life-style; begins to integrate new role and self-concept as "mother."
   a. Feelings of insecurity, inadequacy.
   b. Hesitancy in approaching infant-care tasks.
4. "Baby blues"—may appear on day 4 or 5. (*Note:* often, father experiences same feelings.)
   a. Thought to result from fatigue (sleep deprivation), realization of need for role change, recognition of new responsibilities.
   b. Mild depression, cries without provocation.
   c. Frightened—intimidated by own perceptions of responsibilities.
5. Lag in experiencing "maternal feelings"—usually resolved within 6 weeks.
   a. May contribute to "baby blues."
   b. Guilt regarding lack of "maternal feelings."
   c. Diminished by prompt bonding experience.

B. Analysis/nursing diagnosis:

1. *Ineffective family coping: compromised,* related to achieving developmental tasks.
2. *Situational low self-esteem* related to perceived inadequacy in acceptance of maternal role.
3. *Ineffective individual coping* related to "baby blues," lag in experiencing maternal feelings.

C. Nursing plan/implementation:

1. *Taking-in.* Goal: *emotional support.*
   a. Encourage verbalization of labor/delivery experiences; compliment parents on "how well" they did.
   b. Explore feelings of disappointment, if any.
   c. Meet dependency needs; comment on appearance, hair, personal gowns.
   d. Encourage rooming in.
2. *Taking-hold.* Goal: *health teaching.*
   a. Discuss self-care, postpartal physiologic/psychologic changes.
   b. Demonstrate infant care; mother returns demonstration.

D. Evaluation:

1. Demonstrates beginning comfort in maternal role.
2. Develops confidence and competence in infant care.
3. Expresses satisfaction with self, infant; eager to return home.
4. Successful in breastfeeding. (Tension inhibits let-down reflex; baby nurses poorly.)

IV. Breastfeeding and lactation

A. Biologic foundations:

1. Antepartal alterations
   a. High estrogen/progesterone levels—stimulate proliferation and development of breast ducts.
   b. High progesterone levels—also → development of mammary lobules and alveoli.
2. Postpartum alterations
   a. Rapid drop in estrogen/progesterone levels.
   b. Increased secretion of prolactin—stimulates alveolar cells → milk.
   c. Suckling—stimulates release of oxytocin → contraction of ducts → milk ejection (let-down reflex).
   d. Engorgement—due to venous and lymphatic stasis.
      (1) Immediately precedes lactation.
      (2) Lasts about 24 hours.
      (3) Frequent feeding reduces engorgement.

B. Assessment:

1. Colostrum (yellowish fluid)—continues for first 2–3 days; may have some antibiotic, immunologic, and nutritive value.
2. Milk (bluish-white, thin, consistency)—secreted on about third day.

C. Analysis/nursing diagnosis:

1. *Knowledge deficit* related to breastfeeding techniques.
2. *Pain* related to engorgement.
3. *Personal identity disturbance* related to problems in breastfeeding.
4. *Sleep pattern disturbance.*

D. Nursing plan/implementation:

1. Goal: *promote successful breastfeeding.*
   a. Encourage first feeding right after delivery.
   b. Encourage emptying both breasts at each feeding and prior to engorgement to stimulate milk production, prevent mastitis.
   c. Encourage rest, relaxation, fluids.
   d. Nutritional counseling (see Unit 5).
      (1) Additional 500 calories daily—may be supplied via one extra pint of milk, one extra egg, and one extra serving of meat, citrus fruit, and vegetable.
      (2) Increase fluid intake to 3000 mL daily.
2. Goal: *prevent or relieve engorgement.*
   a. Pain: relieved by warm packs, emptying breasts.
   b. Wear good, supportive bra.
   c. Administer analgesics, as ordered/necessary.
3. Goal: *health teaching.*
   a. Instruct, demonstrate rooting reflex and putting infant to breast. Infant must grasp nipple and areola over location of milk sinuses.
   b. Demonstrate burping techniques, what to do if infant chokes; removing infant from breast.

c. Instruct in basic nipple care.
   (1) Teach good handwashing.
   (2) Nurse on each breast making sure areola is in mouth, alternating position of infant.
   (3) Alternate "beginning" breast.
   (4) Break suction before removing infant from breast.
   (5) Air-dry nipples after each feeding and apply lanolin if abrased.
   (6) Teach daily hygiene of breasts.

d. Instruct in care of cracked or fissured nipples.
   (1) Encourage and support mothers.
   (2) Air-dry nipples after each feeding.
   (3) Use nipple shield if nipples extremely sore.
   (4) Discontinue nursing for 48 hours; maintain milk supply by expressing milk with pump.

e. Discuss avoiding use of any drugs except under medical supervision—may affect infant or suppress lactation.

f. Discuss possibility of sexual stimulation during breastfeeding.
   (1) Validate normalcy and acceptability.
   (2) *Note:* During orgasm, milk may squirt from nipples.

g. Explain that contraceptive value of nursing is unpredictable; time ovulation is inhibited varies widely.

h. Explain contraindications to breastfeeding:
   (1) Active tuberculosis.
   (2) Severe chronic maternal disease.
   (3) Mastitis (temporary interruption may be necessary).
   (4) Narcotic addiction, therapeutic drug dependence.
   (5) Severe cleft lip or palate in newborn (may pump and give in special bottles).
   (6) AIDS.
   (7) Drug abusers (must be drug-free 3 months).

E. Evaluation:

1. Verbalizes understanding of breastfeeding techniques, nutritional requirements for successful lactation.
2. Successfully demonstrates breastfeeding; infant nurses well.
3. Demonstrates appropriate burping techniques; clears excessive mucus from infant's mouth without incident.
4. Verbalizes understanding of basic breast-care techniques:
   a. Self-exam.
   b. Clear water bath.
   c. Drying nipples after bathing, feeding.
   d. Care of cracked or irritated nipples.

COMPLICATIONS DURING THE POSTPARTAL PERIOD

I. Disorders affecting fluid-gas transport

A. Postpartum hemorrhage

1. Definition—loss of 500 mL or more during first 24 postpartal hours in vaginal delivery; 1000 mL in cesarean delivery.
2. **Pathophysiology**—excessive loss of blood secondary to trauma, decreased uterine contractility; results in hypovolemia.
3. **Etiology** (in order of frequency):
   a. Uterine atony
      (1) Uterine overdistention (multiple pregnancy, hydramnios, fetal macrosomia).
      (2) Multiparity.
      (3) Prolonged or precipitous labor.
      (4) Anesthesia—deep inhalation or regional (particularly saddle block).
      (5) Myomata (fibroids).
      (6) Oxytocin induction of labor.
      (7) Overmassage of uterus in postpartum.
      (8) Distended bladder.
   b. Lacerations—cervical, vagina, perineal.
   c. Retained placental fragments—usually delayed postpartum hemorrhage.
   d. Hematoma—deep pelvic, vaginal, or episiotomy site.
4. **Assessment:**
   a. Uterus—boggy, flaccid; excessive vaginal bleeding (dark; seepage, large clots)—due to uterine atony, retained placental fragments.
   b. Signs of shock—air hunger; anxiety/apprehension, tachycardia, tachypnea, hypotension.
   c. Blood values (admission and postpartal) Hgb, Hct, clotting time.
   d. Estimated blood loss: during labor/delivery; in early postpartum.
   e. Pain: vulvar, vaginal, perineal.
   f. Perineum: distended—due to edema; discoloration—due to hematoma. May complain of rectal pressure.
   g. Lacerations—bright red vaginal bleeding with firm fundus.
5. **Analysis/nursing diagnosis:**
   a. *Fluid volume deficit* related to excessive blood loss secondary to uterine atony, retained placental fragments.
   b. *Anxiety/fear* related to unexpected complication.
   c. *Altered tissue perfusion* related to decreased oxygenation secondary to blood loss.
   d. *Activity intolerance* related to fatigue.
6. **Nursing plan/implementation:**
   a. Medical management:
      (1) Intravenous oxytocin infusion; intravenous or oral ergot preparations.

(2) Order blood work: clotting time, fibrinogen level, hemoglobin, hematocrit, CBC.

(3) Type and crossmatch for blood replacement.

(4) Surgical:

(a) Repair of lacerations.

(b) Evacuation, ligation of hematoma.

(c) Curettage—retained placental fragments.

b. Nursing management:

(1) Goal: *minimize blood loss.*

(a) Notify physician promptly of abnormal assessment findings.

(b) Order lab work stat, as directed—to determine blood loss and etiology.

(c) Fundal massage.

(2) Goal: *stabilize status.*

(a) Establish IV line—to enable administration of medications and rapid absorption/action. Administer whole blood (with larger catheter).

(b) Administer medications, as ordered—to control bleeding, combat shock.

(c) Prepare for surgery, as ordered.

(3) Goal: *prevent infection.* Strict aseptic technique.

(4) Goal: *continual monitoring.* Vital signs, bleeding (do pad count or weigh pads), fundal status.

(5) Goal: *prevent sequelae* (Sheehan's syndrome).

(6) Goal: *health teaching*—post episode: Reinforce appropriate perineal care and handwashing techniques.

7. **Evaluation:**

a. Maternal vital signs stable.

b. Bleeding diminished or absent.

c. Assessment findings within normal limits.

B. Subinvolution—delayed return of uterus to normal size, shape, position.

1. **Pathophysiology**—inability of inflamed uterus (endometritis) to contract effectively → incomplete uterine involution; failure of contractions to effect closure of vessels in site of placental attachment → bleeding.

2. **Etiology**

a. PROM with secondary amnionitis, endometritis.

b. Retained placental fragments.

c. Stimulation of overdistended uterine muscle may interfere with involution.

d. Full, distended bladder.

3. **Assessment:**

a. Uterus: large, flabby; lack of uterine tone; failure to progressively decrease in size.

b. Discharge: persistent lochia; painless fresh bleeding, hemorrhagic episodes.

4. **Analysis/nursing diagnosis:**

a. *Pain* related to tender, inflamed uterus secondary to endometritis.

b. *Anxiety/fear* related to change in physical status.

c. *Knowledge deficit* related to diagnosis, treatment, prognosis.

d. *Potential for injury* related to infection.

e. *Fluid volume deficit* related to excessive bleeding.

5. **Nursing plan/implementation:**

a. Medical management:

(1) Have client void or catheterize; massage.

(2) Surgical (curettage)—to remove placental fragments.

(3) Antibiotic therapy—to treat intrauterine infection.

(4) Oxytocics—to stimulate/enhance uterine contractions.

b. Nursing management:

(1) Goal: *health teaching.*

(a) Explain condition and treatment.

(b) Describe, demonstrate perineal care, pad change, handwashing.

(2) Goal: *emotional support.* Encourage verbalization of anxiety regarding return to normal, separation from newborn.

(3) Goal: *promote healing.*

(a) Encourage rest, complicance with medical/nursing regimen.

(b) Administer oxytocics, antibiotics, as ordered.

6. **Evaluation:**

a. Verbalizes understanding of condition and treatment.

b. Complies with medical/nursing regimen.

c. Demonstrates normal involutional progress.

d. All assessment findings (vital signs, fundal height, consistency, lochial discharge) within normal limits.

e. Expresses satisfaction with care.

C. Hypofibrinogenemia

1. **Pathophysiology**—decreased clotting factors, fibrinogen; may be accompanied by DIC.

2. **Etiology:**

a. Missed abortion.

b. Fetal death, delayed delivery.

c. Abruptio placentae; Couvelaire uterus.

d. Amniotic fluid embolism.

3. **Assessment:**

a. Observe for bleeding from injection sites, epistaxis, purpura.

b. See DIC assessment, p. 173.

c. Maternal vital signs, color.

d. I&O.

e. Medical evaluation—procedures.

(1) Thrombin clot test—important: size and persistence of clot.

(2) Prothrombin time—prolonged.

(3) Bleeding time—prolonged.

(4) Platelet count—decreased.
(5) Activated partial thromboplastin time—prolonged.
(6) Fibrinogen (Factor I concentration)—decreased.
(7) Fibrin degradation products—present.

4. **Analysis/nursing diagnosis:**
   a. *Fluid volume deficit* related to uncontrolled bleeding secondary to coagulopathy.
   b. *Anxiety/fear* related to unexpected critical emergency.
   c. *Altered tissue perfusion* related to decreased oxygenation secondary to blood loss.
5. **Nursing plan/implementation:**
   a. Medical management:
      (1) IV heparin—to inhibit conversion of fibrinogen to fibrin.
      (2) Replace blood loss.
   b. Nursing management:
      (1) Goal: *continuous monitoring.*
         (a) Vital signs.
         (b) I&O hourly.
         (c) Skin: color, emergence of petechiae.
         (d) Note, measure (as possible), record and report blood loss.
      (2) Goal: *control blood loss.*
         (a) Establish IV line, administer fluids or blood products as ordered.
         (b) Position: supine—to maintain blood supply to vital organs.
      (3) Goal: *emotional support.*
         (a) Encourage verbalization of anxiety, fear, concerns.
         (b) Explain all procedures.
         (c) Remain with client continuously.
         (d) Keep client and family informed.
6. **Evaluation:**
   a. Bleeding controlled.
   b. Laboratory studies—returning to normal values.
   c. Status stable.

II. Disorders affecting protective functions: postpartal infection (see Table 2.16).

A. General aspects

1. Definition—genital tract infection occurring during the postpartal period.
2. **Pathophysiology**—bacterial invasion of birth canal; most common: localized infection of the lining of the uterus (endometritis).
3. **Etiology:**
   a. Anaerobic nonhemolytic streptococci.
   b. *E. coli.*
   c. *Chlamydia trachomatis* (bacteroides).
   d. Staphylococci.
4. Predisposing conditions:
   a. Anemia.
   b. Premature or prolonged rupture of membranes (PROM).
   c. Prolonged labor.
   d. Repeated vaginal examinations during labor.
   e. Intrauterine manipulation—e.g., manual extraction of placenta.
   f. Retained placental fragments.
   g. Postpartum hemorrhage.
5. **Assessment:**
   a. Fever 38 °C (100.4 °F) or more on two or more occasions, but not within one 24-hour period; after first 24 hours postpartum.
   b. Other signs of infection: pain, malaise, dysuria, subinvolution, foul odor.
6. **Analysis/nursing diagnosis:**
   a. *Fluid volume deficit* related to excessive blood loss, anemia.
   b. *Knowledge deficit* related to danger signs of postpartum period.
   c. *Potential for injury* related to infection.
7. **Nursing plan/implementation:** prevention
   a. Goal: *prevent anemia.*
      (1) Minimize blood loss—accurate postpartal assessment and management of bleeding.
      (2) Diet: high-protein, high-vitamin.
      (3) Vitamins, iron—suggest continuing prenatal pattern until 6-week check-up.
   b. Goal: *prevent entrance/transport of microorganisms.*
      (1) Strict aseptic technique during labor, delivery, and postpartum (universal precautions).
      (2) Minimize vaginal examinations during labor.
      (3) Perineal care.
   c. Goal: *health teaching.*
      (1) Handwashing—before and after each pad change, after voiding and/or defecating.
      (2) Perineal care—from front to back; use clear, warm water or mild antiseptic solution as a cascade; do NOT separate labia.
      (3) Maintain sterility of pads; apply from front to back.
      (4) Avoid use of tampons until normal menstrual cycle resumes.
8. **Evaluation:**
   a. Assessment findings within normal limits:
      (1) Vital signs.
      (2) Rate of involution (fundal height, consistency).
      (3) Lochia: character, amount, odor.
   b. Avoids infection.

B. Endometritis—infection of lining of uterus.

1. **Pathophysiology**—see General aspects, point A above.
2. **Etiology**—most common: invasion by normal body flora (e.g., anaerobic streptococci).
3. Characteristics:

TABLE 2.16 Postpartum Complications

Alterations Related to	Causes	Signs and Symptoms	Nursing Interventions
Postpartum infection (one of the most common causes of maternal death)	Traumatic labor and delivery and postpartum hemorrhage make client more susceptible to invasion by such bacteria as nonhemolytic streptococci, *Escherichia coli,* and *Staphylococcus* species.	Depend on location and severity of infection and usually include fever, pain, swelling, and tenderness. Temperature of 100.4 °F (38 °C) or more after first 24 hours postpartum on two or more occasions in different 24-hour periods indicates puerperal infection.	Monitor for signs and symptoms and drainage (such as uterine); perform culture and sensitivity studies, as ordered. Administer antibiotic therapy, as ordered. Keep client comfortable and quiet. Prevent spread of infection. Force fluids and provide a high-calorie diet. Keep parents and family informed of the mother's and infant's progress. Promote maternal-infant contact as soon as possible. Maintain follow-up care after discharge.
Perineal infection	Laceration and trauma of perineum facilitates the invasion of bacteria.	Localized pain, fever, swelling, redness, and seropurulent drainage.	Administer antibiotics and analgesics; recommend Sitz baths or other heat applications.
Endometritis	Bacteria invade placental site and may spread to entire endometrium.	Temperature, chills, anorexia, malaise, boggy uterus, foul-smelling lochia, and cramps.	Administer antibiotics and ergonovine maleate, as ordered. Recommend Fowler's position to promote drainage. Force fluids.
Pelvic cellulitis or parametritis	Lymphatically spread bacteria invade tissues surrounding uterus.	Fever, chills, lower abdominal pain, and tenderness.	Administer antibiotics and analgesics as ordered. Encourage bed rest. Force fluids.
Thrombophlebitis	Infected pelvic or femoral thrombi.	Chills and fever. *Femoral:* Stiffness of affected area or part and positive Homan's sign. *Pelvic:* Severe chills and wide fluctuations in temperature.	*Femoral:* Rest and elevate leg; apply heat or ice to leg; administer antibiotics, analgesics, and anticoagulants, as ordered. *Pelvic:* Encourage bed rest and force fluids; administer anticoagulants and antibiotics, as ordered.
Mastitis	Usually, *Staphylococcus aureus* from nose and mouth of infant invades lactational system if there are lesions or fissures of nipples. With stasis, breast milk is a good medium for growth of organism.	Marked engorgement, pain, chills, fever, tachycardia. If untreated, single or multiple breast abscesses may form.	Arrange culture and sensitivity studies of mother's milk. Administer antibiotics and analgesics, as ordered. Locally apply heat; assist with incising and draining abscesses. Perform meticulous handwashing.

Source: Ob/Gyn Care, Clinical Pocket Manual Series, Springhouse, PA, 1987, Springhouse Corp.

a. Mild, localized—asymptomatic, or low-grade fever.

b. Severe—may lead to ascending infection, parametritis, pelvic abscess, pelvic thrombophlebitis.

c. If remains localized, self-limiting; usually resolves within 10 days.

4. **Assessment:**
   a. Signs of infection: fever, chills, malaise, anorexia, headache, backache.
   b. Uterus: large, boggy, extremely tender.
      (1) Subinvolution.
      (2) Lochia: dark brown; foul odor.

5. **Analysis/nursing diagnosis:**
   a. *Anxiety/fear* regarding self and newborn.
   b. *Self-esteem disturbance and altered role performance* related to inability to meet own expectations regarding parenting, secondary to unexpected hospitalization.
   c. *Pain* related to inflammation/infection.
   d. *Ineffective individual coping* related to physical discomfort and psychologic stress associated with self-concept disturbance; worry, guilt, concern regarding newborn at home.
   e. *Altered family processes*—interruption of adjustment to altered life pattern related to postpartal infection/hospitalization.
6. **Nursing plan/implementation:**
   a. Goal: *prevent cross-contamination.* Contact-item isolation.
   b. Goal: *facilitate drainage.* Position: semi-Fowler's.
   c. Goal: *nutrition/hydration.*
      (1) Diet: high-calorie, high-protein, high-vitamin.
      (2) Push fluids to 4000 mL/day (oral and/or IV, as ordered).
      (3) I&O.
   d. Goal: *increase uterine tone/facilitate involution.* Administer medications, as ordered (e.g., oxytocics, antibiotics).
   e. Goal: *minimize energy expenditure, as possible.*
      (1) Bedrest.
      (2) Maximize rest, comfort.
   f. Goal: *emotional support.*
      (1) Encourage verbalization of anxiety, concerns.
      (2) Keep informed of progress.
7. **Evaluation:** responds to medical/nursing regimen.
   a. Vital signs stable, within normal limits.
   b. All assessment findings within normal limits.
   c. Unable to recover organism from discharge.

C. Urinary tract infections

1. **Pathophysiology**—normal physiologic changes associated with pregnancy (e.g., ureteral dilatation) and the postpartal period (e.g., diuresis, increased bladder capacity with diminished sensitivity of stretch receptors) → increased susceptibility to bacterial invasion and growth → ascending infections (cystitis, pyelonephritis).
2. **Etiology:** usually bacterial.
3. Predisposing factors:
   a. Birth trauma to bladder, urethra, or meatus.
   b. Bladder hypotonia with retention (due to intrapartal anesthesia or trauma).
   c. Repeated or prolonged catheterization, or poor technique.
4. **Assessment:**
   a. Maternal vital signs (fever, tachycardia).
   b. Dysuria, frequency (flank pain—with pyelonephritis).
   c. Feeling of "not emptying" bladder.
   d. Cloudy urine; frank pus.
5. **Analysis/nursing diagnosis:**
   a. *Altered urinary elimination* related to diuresis, dysuria, inflammation/infection.
   b. *Pain* related to dysuria secondary to cystitis.
   c. *Knowledge deficit* related to self-care (perineal care).
6. **Nursing plan/implementation:**
   a. Goal: *minimize perineal edema.* Perineal icepack in fourth stage—to limit swelling secondary to trauma, facilitate voiding.
   b. Goal: *prevent overdistention of bladder.*
      (1) Monitor level of fundus, lochia, bladder distention. (*Note:* Distended bladder displaces uterus, limits ability to contract—boggy fundus, increased vaginal bleeding.)
      (2) Encourage fluids and voiding; I&O.
      (3) Aseptic technique for catheterization.
      (4) Slow emptying of bladder on catheterization—to maintain tone.
   c. Goal: *identification of causative organism*—to facilitate appropriate medication (antibiotics). Obtain clean-catch (or catheterized) specimen for culture and sensitivity.
   d. Goal: *health teaching.* See previous discussion re: fluids, general hygiene, diet, and medications.
7. **Evaluation:**
   a. Voiding: quantity sufficient (although small, frequent output may mean overflow with retention).
   b. Urine character: clear, amber, or straw-colored.
   c. Vital signs: within normal limits.
   d. No complaints of frequency, urgency, burning on urination, flank pain.

D. Mastitis—inflammation of breast tissue:

1. **Pathophysiology**—local inflammatory response to bacterial invasion; suppuration may occur; organism can be recovered from breast milk.
2. **Etiology**—most common: *Staphylococcus aureus;* source—most common: infant's nose, throat.
3. **Assessment:**
   a. Signs of infection (may occur several weeks postpartum).
      (1) Fever.
      (2) Chills.
      (3) Tachycardia.
      (4) Malaise.
      (5) Abdominal pain.
   b. Breast
      (1) Reddened area(s).
      (2) Localized/generalized swelling.
      (3) Heat, tenderness, palpable mass.
4. **Analysis/nursing diagnosis:**
   a. *Impaired skin integrity* related to nipple fissures, cracks.
   b. *Pain* related to tender, inflamed tissue secondary to infection.
   c. *Disturbance in body image, self-esteem* related to association of breastfeeding with feminine identity and role.

d. *Anxiety/fear* related to sexuality; impact on breastfeeding, if any.

5. **Nursing plan/implementation:**
   a. Goal: *prevent infection.* Health teaching in early postpartum:
      (1) Handwashing.
      (2) Breast care—wash with warm water only (no soap)—to prevent removing protective body oils.
      (3) Let breast milk dry on nipples to prevent drying of tissue.
      (4) Clean bra (with no plastic pads or liners) to support breasts, reduce friction, minimize exposure to microorganisms.
      (5) Good breastfeeding techniques, gradual increase in nursing time.
      (6) Alternate position of infant for nursing to change pressure areas.
   b. Goal: *comfort measures.*
      (1) Encourage bra or binder—to support breasts, reduce pain from motion.
      (2) Ice packs as ordered—to reduce engorgement, pain.
      (3) Administer analgesics, as necessary.
   c. Goal: *emotional support.*
      (1) Encourage verbalization of feelings, concerns.
      (2) If breastfeeding discontinued, reassure of ability to resume nursing.
   d. Goal: *promote healing.*
      (1) Discourage nursing—to promote healing of nipples; may pump.
      (2) Administer antibiotics as ordered.
6. **Evaluation:**
   a. Promptly responds to medical/nursing regimen.
      (1) Symptoms subside.
      (2) Assessment findings within normal limits.
   b. Successfully returns to breastfeeding.

E. Thrombophlebitis:

1. **Pathophysiology**—inflammation of a vein secondary to lodging of a clot.
2. **Etiology:**
   a. Extension of endometritis with involvement of pelvic and femoral veins.
   b. Clot formation in pelvic veins following cesarean delivery.
   c. Clot formation in femoral (or other) veins secondary to poor circulation, compression, and venous stasis.
3. **Assessment:**
   ▶ a. Pelvic—pain: abdominal or pelvic tenderness.
   b. Calf—pain: positive Homans' sign (pain elicited by flexion of foot with knee extended).
   c. Femoral
      (1) Pain.
      (2) Malaise, fever, chills.
      (3) Swelling—"milk leg."
4. **Analysis/nursing diagnosis:**
   a. *Pain* in affected region related to local inflammatory response.
   b. *Anxiety/fear* related to outcome.
   c. *Ineffective individual coping* related to unexpected postpartum complications, hospitalization, separation from newborn.
   d. *Impaired physical mobility* related to imposed bedrest to prevent emboli formation.
5. **Nursing plan/implementation:**
   a. Goal: *prevent clot formation.*
      (1) Encourage early ambulation.
      (2) Position: avoid prolonged compression of popliteal space, use of knee gatch.
      (3) Apply TED hose, as ordered, preoperatively and/or postoperatively for cesarean delivery.
   b. Goal: *reduce threat of emboli.*
      (1) Bedrest, with cradle to support bedding.
      (2) Discourage massaging "leg cramps."
   c. Goal: *prevent further clot formation.* Administer anticoagulants, as ordered.
   d. Goal: *prevent infection.*
      (1) Administer antibiotics, as ordered.
      (2) Push fluids.
   e. Goal: *facilitate clot resolution.* Heat therapy, as ordered.
6. **Evaluation:**
   a. Symptoms subside; all assessment findings within normal limits.
   b. No evidence of further clot formation.

III. Disorders affecting psycho-social-cultural functions

A. General aspects

1. Can occur in both new parents.
2. Usually occurs within 2 weeks of delivery.
3. Increased incidence among single parents.
4. Most common symptomatology: affective disorders.
5. Psychiatric intervention required in small percent of cases; if underlying cause unresolved, increased risk in subsequent pregnancies.

B. Etiology—theory: birth of child may emphasize:

1. Unresolved role conflicts.
2. Unachieved normal development tasks.

C. Assessment:

1. Withdrawal.
2. Paranoia.
3. Anorexia, sleep disturbance, mood swings.
4. Depression—may alternate with manic behavior.
5. Potential for self-injury or child abuse/neglect.

D. Analysis/nursing diagnosis:

1. *Ineffective individual coping* related to perceived inability to meet role expectations ("mother") and ambivalence related to dependence/independence.
2. *Self-esteem disturbance and altered role performance* related to "femaleness" and reaction to responsibility for care of newborn.

3. *Potential for violence*, self-directed or directed at newborn related to anger or depression.
4. *Ineffective family coping* related to lack of support system in early postpartum.
5. *Altered family processes* related to psychologic stress, interruption of bonding.
6. *Altered parenting* related to hormonal changes and stress.

E. Nursing plan/implementation:

1. Goal: *emotional support.*
   a. Encourage verbalization of feelings, fears, anxiety, concerns.
   b. Support positive self-image, feelings of adequacy, self-worth.
      (1) Reinforce appropriate comments and behaviors.
      (2) Encourage active participation in self-care, comment on accomplishments.
      (3) Reduce threat to self-image, fear of failure. Maintain support, gradually increase tasks.
2. Goal: *safeguard status of mother/newborn.*
   a. Unobtrusive, protective environment.
   b. Stay with client when with infant.
3. Goal: *nutrition/hydration.*
   a. Encourage selection of favorite foods—to aid security in decision-making; counteract anorexia, refusal to eat by tempting appetite.
   b. Push fluids (juices, soft drinks, milkshakes)—to maintain hydration.
4. Goal: *minimize stress, facilitate effective coping.* Administer therapeutic medications, as ordered.
   a. Schizophrenia—phenothiazines.
   b. Depression—mood elevators.
   c. Manic behaviors—sedatives, tranquilizers.

F. Evaluation:

1. Increases interaction with infant.
2. Expresses interest in learning how to care for infant.
3. Evidences no agitation, depression.
4. Actively participates in caring for self and infant.
5. Demonstrates increasing comfort in mothering role.
6. Positive family interactions.

■ THE NEWBORN INFANT

General overview: Effective nursing care of the newborn infant is based on: (1) knowledge of the conditions present during fetal life; (2) requirements for independent extrauterine life; and (3) alterations needed for successful transition. The first 24 hours are the most hazardous.

I. Biologic foundations of neonatal adaptation—*general aspects:*

A. *Fetal anatomy and physiology*

1. *Fetal circulation*—four intrauterine structures, differ from extrauterine structures:
   a. *Umbilical vein*—carries oxygen and nutrient-enriched blood from placenta to ductus venosus and liver.
   b. *Ductus venosus*—connects to inferior vena cava; allows most blood to bypass liver.
   c. *Foramen ovale*—allows fetal blood to bypass fetal lungs by shunting it from right atrium into left atrium.
   d. *Ductus arteriosus*—allows fetal blood to bypass fetal lungs by shunting it from pulmonary artery into aorta.
   e. *Umbilical arteries* (two)—allow return of deoxygenated blood to the placenta.
2. *Umbilical cord*—extends from fetus to center of placenta; usually 50 cm (18–22 inches) long and 1–2 cm (½–1 inch) in diameter. Contains:
   a. *Wharton's jelly*—protects umbilical vessels from pressure, cord "kinking," and interference with fetal-placental circulation.
   b. Umbilical vein—carries oxygen and nutrients from placenta to fetus.
   c. Two umbilical arteries—carry deoxygenated blood and fetal wastes from fetus to placenta. *Note:* Absence of one artery indicates need to rule out intraabdominal anomalies.
3. *Characteristics of fetal blood*
   a. Fetal hemoglobin (Hb_f)
      (1) Higher oxygen-carrying capacity than adult hemoglobin.
      (2) Releases oxygen easily to fetal tissues.
      (3) Ensures high fetal oxygenation.
      (4) Normal range at term: 12–22 g/dL; average: 15–20 g/dL.
   b. Total blood volume at term: 85 mL/kg body weight; Hct: 38–62%, average 53%; RBC 3–7 million, average 4.9 million/unit.

B. *Extrauterine adaptation: tasks*

1. Establish and maintain ventilation, successful gas transfer—requires patent airway and adequate pulmonary surfactant.
2. Modify circulatory patterns—requires closure of fetal structures.
3. Absorb and utilize fluids and nutrients.
4. Excrete body wastes.
5. Establish and maintain thermal stability.

C. *Nursing goals*

1. Facilitate successful transition to independent life.
2. Protect infant from physiologic stress and environmental hazards.
3. Encourage development of a strong family unit.

II. Admission to nursery

A. Admission assessment of normal, term neonate

1. Color and reactivity.
2. General appearance, symmetry.
3. Length and weight.
4. Head and chest circumference.
5. Vital signs:

■ **TABLE 2.17 Physical Assessment of the Term Neonate**

Criterion	Average Values and Normal Variations	Deviations from Normal
Vital Signs		
Heart rate	120–140/minute, irregular, especially when crying, and functional murmur.	Faint sound—pneumomediastinum; and heart rate under 100 or over 180/minute.
Respiratory rate	30–60/minute with short periods of apnea, irregular; cry—vigorous and loud.	Distress—flaring of nares, retractions, tachypnea, grunting, excessive mucus, under 30 or over 60/ minute; cyanosis.
Temperature	Stabilizes about 8 to 10 hours after birth; 36.5–37 °C (97.7–98.6 °F) axillary.	Unreliable indicator of infection.
Blood pressure	80/46; varies with change in activity level.	Hypotension: with RDS. Hypertension: coarctation of aorta.
Measurements		
Weight	3400 g (7½ lb).	Birth weight <2500 g: preterm or SGA infant; >4000 g; LGA infant, evaluate mother for gestational diabetes.
Length	50 cm (20 inches).	
Chest circumference	2 cm (¾ inch) less than head circumference.	If relationship varies, check for reason.
Head circumference	33–35 cm (13–14 inches).	Check for microcephalus and macrocephalus.
General Assessment		
Muscle tone	Good tone and generalized flexion; full range of motion; spontaneous movement.	Flaccid, and persistent tremor or twitching; movement limited; asymmetric.
Skin color	Mottling, acrocyanosis, and physiologic jaundice. Petechia (over presenting part), milia, mongolian spotting, lanugo, and vernix caseosa.	Pallor, cyanosis, or jaundice within 24 hours of birth. Petechiae or ecchymoses elsewhere; all rashes, except erythema toxicum; pigmented nevi; hemangioma; and yellow vernix.
Head	Molding of fontanels and suture spaces; comprises ¼ of body length.	Cephalohematoma, caput succedaneum, sunken or bulging fontanels, closed sutures; excessively wide sutures.
Hair	Silky, single strands; lies flat; grows toward face and neck.	Fine, wooly; unusual swirls, patterns, hair line; coarse.
Eyes	Edematous eyelids, conjunctival hemorrhage; grayish-blue to grayish-brown in color; blink reflex; usually no tears; uncoordinated movements may focus for a few seconds; good placement on face; cornea is bright and shiny; pupillary reflex equal and reactive to light; eyebrows distinct.	Epicanthal folds (in non-Orientals); discharges; agenesis; opaque lenses; lesions; strabismus; "doll's eyes" beyond 10 days; absence of reflexes.
Nose	Appears to have no bridge; should have no discharge; obligate nose breathers; sneezes to clear nose.	Discharge and choanal atresia; malformed; flaring of nares beyond first few moments of life.
Mouth	Epstein's pearls on gum ridges; tongue does not protrude and moves freely, symmetrically; uvula in midline; reflexes present: sucking, rooting, gag, extrusion.	*Cleft lip or palate;* teeth, cyanosis, circumoral pallor; asymmetric lip movement; excessive saliva; thrush; incomplete or absent reflexes.
Ears	Well formed, firm; notch of ear should be on straight line with outer canthus.	Low placement, clefts; tags; malformed; lack of cartilage.
Face	Symmetric movements and contours.	Facial palsy (7th cranial nerve); looks "funny."
Neck	Short, freely movable; some head control.	Wry neck, webbed neck; restricted movement; masses; distended veins; absence of head control.
Chest	Enlarged breasts, "witch's milk"; barrel-shaped; both sides move synchronously; nipples symmetrical.	Flattened, funnel-chested, asynchronous movement; lack of breast tissue; fracture of clavicle(s); supernumerary or widely spaced nipples; bowel sounds.
Abdomen	Dome-shaped, abdominal respirations; soft; may have small umbilical hernia; umbilical cord well formed, containing 3 vessels; dry around base; bowel sounds within 2 hours of birth; voiding; passage of meconium.	Scaphoid-shaped, omphalocele, diastasis recti, and distention; umbilical cord containing 2 vessels; redness or drainage around base of cord.
Genitalia		
Female	Large labia; may have pseudomenstruation, smegma; vaginal orifice open; increased pigmentation; ecchymosis and edema following breech birth; pink-stained urine (uric acid crystals).	Agenesis and imperforate hymen; ambiguous labia widely separated, fecal discharge per vagina; *epispadias or hypospadias.*
Male	Pendulous scrotum covered with rugae, and testes usually descended; voids with adequate stream; increased pigmentation; edema and ecchymosis following breech birth.	*Phimosis, epispadias,* or *hypospadias;* ambiguous; scrotum smooth and testes undescended. Hydrocele: collection of fluid in the sac surrounding the testes.

continued

■ **TABLE 2.17 *(Continued)*** **Physical Assessment of the Term Neonate**

Criterion	Average Values and Normal Variations	Deviations from Normal
General Assessment (cont.)		
Extremities	Synchronized movements, freely movable through full range of motion; legs appear bowed, and feet appear flat; attitude of general flexion; arms longer than legs; grasp reflex; palmar and sole creases; normal contour.	Fractures, brachial nerve palsy, *clubbed foot,* phocomelia or amelia, unusual number or webbing of digits, and abnormal palmar ceases; poor muscle tone; asymmetry; hypertonicity; unusual hip contour and click sign (*hip dysplasia*); hypermobility of joints.
Back	Spine straight, easily movable, and flexible; may have small pilonidal dimple at base of spine; may raise head when prone.	Fusion of vertebrae; pilonidal dimple with tuft of hair; *spina bifida,* agenesis of part of vertebral bodies; limitation of movement; weak or absent reflexes.
Anus	Patent, well placed; "wink" reflex.	Imperforate, and absence of "wink" (absence of sphincter muscle); fistula.
Stools	Meconium within first 24 hours; transitional—days 2 to 5; *breastfed:* loose, golden yellow; *bottlefed:* formed, light yellow.	Light-colored meconium (dry, hard), or absent with distended abdomen (*cystic fibrosis* or *Hirschsprung's disease*); diarrhetic.
Laboratory Values		
Hemoglobin (cord)	13.6–19.6 g/dL.	Evaluate for anemia and persistent polycythemia.
Serum bilirubin	2–6 mg/dL.	Hyperbilirubinemia (*term:* 12 mg or more; *preterm:* 15 mg or more).
Blood glucose	Over 30–40 mg/dL for *term;* over 20 mg/dL for *preterm.*	Identify hypoglycemia prior to overt or asymptomatic hypoglycemia—do Dextrostix on all suspects (large- or small-for-gestational-age neonates, or neonates of diabetic mothers).
Neurologic Examination*	Specific to gestational age and state of wakefulness.	
1. Behavioral patterns		
a. Feeding	Variations in interest, hunger. Usually feeds well within 48 hours.	Lethargic. Poor suck, poor coordination with swallow, choking, cyanosis.
b. Social	Crying is lusty, strong, and soon indicative of hunger, pain, attention-seeking. Responds to cuddling, voice by quietness and increased alertness.	Absent; no focusing on person holding him/her; unconsolable.
c. Sleep–wakefulness	Two periods of reactivity: at birth, and 6–8 hours later. Stabilization, with wakeful periods about every 3–4 hours.	Lethargy, drowsiness. Disorganized pattern.
d. Elimination	Stooling: see Stools. Urination: first few days: 3–4 q.d. end of first week: 5–6 q.d. later: 6–10 q.d., with adequate hydration.	See Stools. Diminished number: dehydration.
2. Reflex response	Bilateral, symmetric response (see Table 2.18).	Absent, hyperactive, incomplete, asynchronous.
3. Sensory capabilities		
a. Vision	Limited accommodation, with clearest vision within 7–8 inches. Focuses and follows by 15 minutes of age. Prefers patterns to plain.	Absence of these responses may be due to absence of or diminished acuity or to sensory deprivation.
b. Hearing	By 2 minutes of age, can move in direction of sound: responds to high pitch by "freezing," followed by agitation; to low pitch (crooning) by relaxing.	Absence of response: deafness.
c. Touch	Soothed by massaging, warmth, weightlessness (as in water bath).	Unable to be comforted: possible drug dependence. Cocaine-addicted newborns have no eye contact.
d. Smell	By 5th day, can distinguish between mother's breasts and those of another woman.	
e. Taste	Can distinguish between sweet and sour.	
f. Motor	Coordinates body movement to parent's voice and body movement.	Absence.

*Based on Brazelton's method.

■ TABLE 2.18 Assessment: Normal Newborn Reflexes*

Reflex	Description	Implications of Deviations from Normal Pattern
Moro (startle)	Symmetric *abduction* and *extension* of arms with fingers extended in response to sudden movement or loud noise.	Asymmetric reflex may indicate brachial (Erb's) palsy or fractured clavicle.
Tonic neck (fencing)	When head turned to one side, arm and leg on *that* side *extend,* and *opposite* arm and leg *flex.*	Asymmetry may indicate cerebral lesion, if persistent.
Rooting and sucking	With stimulus to cheek, turns *toward* stimulus, opens mouth, sucks.	Absence of response may indicate prematurity, neurologic problem, or depressed infant (or not hungry).
Palmar grasp	If palm stimulated, fingers *curl;* holds adult finger briefly.	Asymmetry may indicate neurologic involvement.
Plantar grasp	Pressure on sole will elicit *curling* of toes.	Absence/asymmetry associated with defects of lower spinal column.
Stepping/dancing	If held in upright position with feet in contact with hard surface, alternately raises feet.	Asymmetry may indicate neurologic problem.
Babinski	Stroking the sole in a upward fashion elicits *hyperextension* of toes.	Same as for plantar grasp.
Crawling	When placed in prone position, attempts to crawl.	Absence may indicate prematurity or depressed infant.

* *Note:* Reflexes are good indicators of the neurological system in well infants but not in sick neonates. Infants with infections may not show normal reflexes yet have an intact neurological system.

a. Axillary temperature.

b. Respirations (check rate, character, rhythm).

c. Apical pulse.

6. General physical assessment (Table 2.17) and reflexes (Table 2.18).
7. Estimate of gestational age (Table 2.19).

B. Analysis/nursing diagnosis:

1. *Altered health maintenance* related to separation from maternal support system.
2. *Impaired skin integrity* related to umbilical stump, incontinence of urine and meconium stool.
3. *Ineffective airway clearance* related to excessive mucus.
4. *Pain* related to environmental stimuli.
5. *Ineffective thermoregulation* related to immature temperature regulation mechanism.

C. Nursing plan/implementation:

1. Goal: *promote effective gas transport.*
   a. Maintain patent airway—to promote effective gas exchange and respiratory function.
   b. Position: right side-lying, head-dependent (gravity drainage of fluid, mucus).
   c. Suction p.r.n. with bulb syringe for mucus.
2. Goal: *establish/maintain thermal stability.*
   a. Avoid chilling—to prevent metabolic acidosis.
   b. Dry, wrap, and apply hat.
   c. Place in heated crib.
   d. Monitor vital signs hourly until stable.
3. Goal: *reduce possibility of blood loss.*
   a. Check cord clamp for security.
   b. Administer vitamin K injection, as ordered, in anterior or lateral thigh muscle—to stimulate blood coagulability.
4. Goal: *prevent infection.*
   a. Administer antibiotic treatment to eyes (if not performed in delivery room)—to prevent ophthalmia neonatorum.
   b. Treat cord stump (alcohol, Triple Dye antibiotic ointment), as ordered.
5. Goal: *promote comfort and cleanliness.* Admission bath when temperature stable.
6. Goal: *promote nutrition, hydration, elimination.*
   a. Encourage breastfeeding immediately after birth.
   b. Check blood sugar (Dextrostix or Chemstrip) at 30 minutes, 1, 2, and 4 hours postdelivery for infants at risk for hypoglycemia (e.g., SGA, LGA).
   c. First feeding at 1–4 hours of age with sterile water if permissible, and if not breastfeeding.
   d. Note voiding and/or meconium stool; report failure to void or defecate within 24 hours.
7. Goal: *promote bonding.*
   a. Encourage parent–infant interaction (holding, touching, eye contact, talking to infant).
   b. Encourage breastfeeding within 1 hour of birth, if applicable.
   c. Encourage parent participation in infant care—to develop confidence and competence in caring for newborn.
      (1) Assist with initial efforts at feeding.
      (2) Discuss and demonstrate positioning and burping techniques.

MATERNAL-INFANT NURSING

■ **TABLE 2.19** **Estimation of Gestational Age—Common Clinical Parameters**

Characteristic	Preterm	Term
Head	Oval—narrow biparietal (35 cm, 13 inches); large in proportion to body; face looks like "old man." Soft, flat, shapeless.	Square-shaped biparietal prominences; one-fourth body length.
Ears: form, cartilage	Soft, flat, shapeless.	Pinna firm; erect from head.
Hair: texture, distribution	Fine, fuzzy, or wooly; clumped; appears at 20 weeks.	Silky; single strands apparent.
Sole creases	Starting at ball of foot, one-third covered with creases by 36 weeks; two-thirds by 38 weeks.	Entire sole heavily creased.
Breast nodules	0 mm at 36 weeks; 4 mm at 37 weeks.	10 mm or more.
Nipples	No areolae.	Formed; raised above skin level.
Genitalia:		
Female	Clitoris large, labia gaping.	Labia larger, meet in midline.
Male	Small scrotum, rugae on inferior surface only, and testes undescended.	Scrotum pendulous, covered with rugae; testes usually descended.
Skin: texture, opacity	Visible abdominal veins; thin, shiny.	Few indistinct larger veins; thick, dry, cracked, peeling.
Vernix	Covers body by 31–33 weeks.	Small amount or absent at term; postterm: dry, wrinkled.
Lanugo	Apparent at 20 weeks; by 33–36 weeks, covers shoulders.	Minimal or no lanugo.
Muscle tone	Hypotonia; extension of arms and legs.	Hypertonia; well flexed.
Posture	Froglike.	Attitude of general flexion.
Head lag	Head lags; arms have little or no flexion.	Head follows trunk; strong arm flexion.
Scarf sign	Elbow capable of extension to opposite axilla.	Elbow to midline only; infant resists.
Square window	90 degrees.	0 degrees.
Ankle dorsiflexion	90 degrees.	0 degrees.
Popliteal angle	180 degrees.	Less than 90 degrees.
Heel-to-ear maneuver	Touches ear easily.	90 degrees.
Ventral suspension	Hypotonia; "rag-doll."	Good caudal and cephalic tone.
Reflexes:		
Moro	Apparent at 28 weeks; good, but no adduction.	Complete reflex with adduction; disappears 4 months postterm.
Grasp	Fair at 28 weeks; arm is involved at 32 weeks.	Strong enough to sustain weight for a few seconds when pulled up; hand, arm, shoulder involved.
Cry	24 weeks: weak; 28 weeks: high-pitched; 32 weeks: good.	Lusty; can persist for some time.
Length	Under 47 cm (18½ inches), usually.	50 cm (20 inches).
Weight	Under 2500 g (5 lb 5 oz).	3400 g (7½ lb).

(3) Demonstrate/assist with basic care procedures, as necessary:
   (a) Bath.
   (b) Cord care.
   (c) Diapering.
   (d) Aid parents in distinguishing normal vs abnormal newborn characteristics.

8. Goal: *health teaching*—to provide anticipatory guidance for discharge.
   a. Facilitate sibling bonding.
   b. Describe/discuss normal newborn behavior.
      (1) *Sleeping*—almost continual (wakes only to feed) or 12–16 hours daily.
      (2) *Feeding*—from every 2–3 hours to longer intervals; establish own pattern; breastfed babies feed more often.
      (3) *Weight loss*—5–10% in first few days; regained in 7–14 days.

TABLE 2.20 Infant Stool Characteristics

Age	Bottlefed	Breastfed	Implications of Abnormal Patterns
1 day	Meconium.	Meconium.	Absence may indicate obstruction, atresia.
2–5 days (transitional)	Greenish yellow; loose.	Greenish yellow; loose, frequent.	*Note*—At any time: *Diarrhea*—greenish, mucus or blood-tinged, or forceful expulsion, may indicate infection; *constipation*—dry, hard stools or infrequent or absent stools may indicate obstruction.
>5 days	Yellow to brown; firm; 2–4 daily; foul odor.	Bright golden yellow, loose; 6–10 daily.	

(4) *Stools*—see Table 2.20.

(5) *Cord care*—drops off in 7–10 days.

(a) Keep clean and dry.

(b) Alcohol to stump.

(c) HIV precautions

(6) *Circumcision care*

(a) Keep clean and dry; heals rapidly.

(b) Watch for bleeding.

(c) Petroleum jelly, gauze p.r.n., if ordered.

(d) Do not remove yellowish exudate.

(7) *Physiologic jaundice*—occurs 24–72 hours postbirth.

(a) Nonpathologic.

(b) Need for hydration.

(8) Identify need for PKU test (done routinely at 24 hours of age and later).

(9) Describe suggested sensory *stimulation* modalities (mobiles, color, music).

(10) Discuss *safety* precautions:

(a) Infant seat for travel and home safety.

(b) Maintaining contact/control over infant to prevent falls, drowning in bath.

(c) Instruct parents in infant CPR.

(11) Describe signs of *common health problems* to be reported promptly:

(a) Diarrhea, constipation.

(b) Colic, vomiting.

(c) Rash, jaundice.

(d) Differentiation from normal patterns.

D. Evaluation:

1. Infant demonstrates successful transition to independent life:
   a. Nurses well.
   b. Normal feeding, sleeping, elimination patterns.
   c. No evidence of infection or abnormality.
2. Mother/family evidence bonding.
   a. Eye contact.
   b. Stroking, cuddling.
   c. Crooning, calling baby by name, talking to infant.
3. Mother demonstrates comfort and skill in basic newborn care.
4. Mother verbalizes understanding of subjects discussed:
   a. Safety precautions.
   b. Health maintenance actions.
   c. Signs of normal infant behavior and health.

COMPLICATIONS DURING THE NEONATAL PERIOD: THE HIGH-RISK NEWBORN

I. General overview—successful newborn adaptation to the demands of independent extrauterine life may be complicated by environmental insults during the *prenatal* period and/or those arising in the period immediately surrounding birth. The nursing role focuses on minimizing the effect of present and emerging health problems and on facilitating and supporting a successful transition to extrauterine life.

II. General aspects—common neonatal risk factors:

A. Gestational age profile (see Tables 2.17 and 2.19):

1. Prematurity.
2. Dysmaturity.
3. Postmaturity.

B. Congenital disorders.

C. Birth trauma.

D. Infections.

III. Disorders affecting protective functions: neonatal infections

A. Assess for intrauterine infections.

B. Oral thrush (mycotic stomatitis).

1. **Pathophysiology**—local inflammation of oral mucosa due to fungal infection.
2. **Etiology:**
   a. Organism—*Candida albicans.*
   b. More common in vulnerable newborn, i.e., sick, debilitated; those receiving antibiotic therapy.
3. Mode of transmission—direct contact with:
   a. Maternal birth canal, hands, and linens.
   b. Contaminated feeding equipment, staff's hands.
4. **Assessment:**
   a. Appearance of white patches on oral mucosa, gums, and tongue that bleed when touched.

b. Occasional difficulty swallowing.

5. **Analysis/nursing diagnosis:**
   a. *Pain* related to irritation of oral mucous membrane secondary to oral moniliasis.
   b. *Altered nutrition, less than body requirements* related to irritability and poor feeding.
6. **Nursing plan/implementation:** Goal: *prevent cross-contamination.*
   a. Aseptic technique; good handwashing.
   b. Chemotherapy, as ordered:
      (1) Aqueous gentian violet, 1–2%: apply to infected area with swab.
      (2) Nystatin (Mycostatin)—instill into mouth with medicine dropper, or apply to lesions with swab, *after* feedings. **Note:** *prior* to medicating, feed sterile water to rinse out milk.
7. **Evaluation:** responds to medical/nursing regimen.
   a. Oral mucosa intact, lesions healed, no evidence of infection.
   b. Feeds well; maintains weight or regains weight lost, if any.

C. Neonatal sepsis

1. *Pathophysiology*—generalized infection; may overwhelm infant's immature immune system.
2. *Etiology:*
   a. Prolonged rupture of membranes.
   b. Long, difficult labor.
   c. Resuscitation procedures.
   d. Maternal infection (i.e., Beta strep vaginosis).
   e. Aspiration—amniotic fluid, formula, mucus.
   f. Iatrogenic (nosocomial)—caused by infected health personnel or equipment.
3. **Assessment:**
   a. Respirations—irregular, periods of apnea.
   b. Irritability or lethargy.
4. **Analysis/nursing diagnosis:**
   a. *Fatigue* related to increased oxygen needs.
   b. *Potential for infection* related to septic condition.
5. **Nursing plan/implementation:**
   a. Cultures (spinal, urine, blood).
   b. Check vitals.
   c. Monitor respirators.
6. **Evaluation:**
   a. Responds to medical/nursing regimen (all assessment findings within normal limits).
   b. Parent(s) verbalize understanding of diagnosis, treatment; demonstrate appropriate techniques in participating in care (as possible).
   c. Parent(s) demonstrate effective coping with situation; express satisfaction with care.

IV. Disorders affecting nutrition: infant of the diabetic mother (IDM)

A. Pathophysiology—hyperplasia of pancreatic beta cells → increased insulin production → excessive deposition of glycogen in muscles, subcutaneous fat, and tissue growth. Results in fetal:

1. *Macrosomia*—large for gestational age (LGA).
2. *Enlarged internal organs*—common.
   a. Cardiomegaly.
   b. Hepatomegaly.
   c. Splenomegaly.
3. Neonatal—inadequate carbohydrate reserve to meet energy needs.
4. Associated with *increased incidence of:*
   a. Congenital anomalies (five times average incidence)—includes cardiac, pelvic, and spinal anomalies.
   b. Preterm birth. Respiratory distress syndrome (RDS). Increased insulin needs prenatally lead to decreased surfactant production.
   c. Maternal dystocia—due to CPD.
   d. Neonatal metabolic problems:
      (1) Hypoglycemia.
      (2) Hypocalcemic tetany.
      (3) Metabolic acidosis.
      (4) Hyperbilirubinemia.

B. Etiology—high circulating maternal glucose levels during fetal growth and development; loss of maternal glucose supply following birth; decreased hepatic gluconeogenesis.

C. Assessment:

1. Characteristics of IDM.
2. Hypoglycemia—apply Dextrostix or Chemstrip to heel stick at:
   a. 30 minutes.
   b. 1, 2, 4, 6, 9, 12, and 24 hours of age.
   c. Hypoglycemia lab values for term infant: under 30–40 mg/dL.
   d. Hypoglycemia lab values for preterm infant: under 20 mg/dL.
   e. Behavioral signs—tremors, twitching, hypotonia, seizures.
3. Gestational age, since macrosomia may mask prematurity.
4. Hypocalcemia—usually within first 24 hours
   a. Irritability.
   b. Coarse tremors, twitching, convulsions.
5. Birth injuries
   a. Fractures: clavicle, humerus.
   b. Brachial palsy.
   c. Intracranial hemorrhage/signs of increased intracranial pressure.
   d. Cephalohemotoma.
6. Respiratory distress
   a. Nasal flaring.
   b. Sternal retraction.
   c. Costal breathing.
   d. Cyanosis.
   e. Expiratory grunt.
7. Jaundice.

D. Analysis/nursing diagnosis:

1. *Potential for injury* related to CPD, dystocia.
2. *Altered cardiopulmonary tissue perfusion* related to placental insufficiency, respiratory distress syndrome (RDS).
3. *Impaired gas exchange* related to RDS.
4. *Altered nutrition, less than body requirements,* related to hypoglycemia, hypocalcemia.
5. *Altered thought processes* related to hyperbilirubinemia and kernicterus.

E. Nursing plan/implementation:

1. Hypoglycemia—administer oral or intravenous glucose, as ordered (may cause rebound effect).
2. Premature/immature—institute premature-care p.r.n.
3. Hypocalcemia—administer oral or intravenous calcium gluconate, as ordered.
4. Inform pediatrician immediately of signs of:
   a. Jaundice.
   b. Hyperirritability.
   c. Birth injury.
   d. Increased intracranial pressure/hemorrhage.

F. Evaluation:

1. Makes successful transition to extrauterine life.
2. Responds to medical/nursing regimen. Experiences minimal or no metabolic disturbances (hypoglycemia, hypocalcemia, hyperbilirubinemia).
3. Exhibits normal respiratory function and gas exchange.

V. Hypoglycemia

A. Pathophysiology—low serum-glucose level → altered cellular metabolism → cerebral irritability, cardiopulmonary problems.

B. Etiology:

1. Loss of maternal glucose supply.
2. Normal physiologic activities of respiration, thermoregulation, muscular activity exceed carbohydrate reserve.
3. Decreased hepatic ability to convert amino acids into glucose.
4. More common in:
   a. Infants of diabetic mothers.
   b. Preterm, postterm infants.
   c. Small for gestational age (SGA).
   d. Smaller twin.
   e. Infant of preeclamptic mother.
   f. Birth asphyxia.

C. Assessment:

1. Jitteriness, tremors, convulsions; lethargy and hypotonia.
2. Sweating; unstable temperature.
3. Tachypnea; apneic episodes; cyanosis.
4. High-pitched, shrill cry.
5. Difficulty feeding.

D. Analysis/nursing diagnosis:

1. *Altered tissue perfusion (fetal)* related to placental insufficiency associated with maternal diabetes, preeclampsia, renal and/or cardiac disorders; erythroblastosis.
2. *Altered thought processes* related to high incidence of morbidity associated with birth asphyxia.
3. *Impaired gas exchange* related to coexisting RDS.
4. *Altered nutrition, less than body requirements,* related to hypoglycemia.
5. *Potential for injury* related to coexisting infection, metabolic acidosis.

E. Nursing plan/implementation: see IV., Infant of the diabetic mother.

F. Evaluation: see IV., Infant of the diabetic mother.

VI. Disorders affecting psycho-social-cultural functions: drug-dependent (heroin) neonate

A. General aspects

1. Maternal drug addiction has been associated with:
   a. Prenatal malnutrition and vitamin deficiencies.
   b. Increased risk of antepartal infections.
   c. Higher incidence of antepartal and intrapartal complications.
2. Infant at risk for:
   a. Intrauterine growth retardation (IUGR).
   b. Prematurity.
   c. Congenital anomalies.
   d. Fetal distress.
   e. Perinatal death.
   f. Child abuse.

B. Pathophysiology—withdrawal of accustomed drug levels → physiologic deprivation response.

C. Etiology—repeated intrauterine absorption of heroin/cocaine/methadone from maternal bloodstream → fetal drug dependency.

D. Assessment—degree of withdrawal depends on type and duration of addiction, and maternal drug levels at delivery.

1. Irritability, hyperactivity, hypertonicity, exaggerated reflexes, tremors, high-pitched cry, difficult to comfort:
   a. "Step" reflex (dancing)—infant places both feet on surface; assumes rigid stance—does not "step" or dance.
   b. "Head-righting" reflex—holds head rigid; fails to demonstrate head-lag.
2. Nasal stuffiness and sneezing; respiratory distress, tachypnea, cyanosis and/or apnea.
3. Exaggerated acrocyanosis and/or mottling in the warm infant.
4. Sweating.
5. Hunger—sucks on fists; feeding problems—regurgitation, vomiting, poor feeding, diarrhea and increased mucus production.
6. Convulsions with abnormal eye-rolling and chewing motions.
7. Developmental lags/mental retardation.

E. Analysis/nursing diagnosis:

1. *Potential for injury* related to convulsions secondary

to physiologic response to withdrawal, CNS hyperirritability.

2. *Impaired gas exchange* related to respiratory distress secondary to inhibition of reflex clearing of fluid by the lungs.
3. *Altered nutrition, less than body requirements,* related to feeding problems secondary to respiratory distress and GI hypermotility.
4. Potential for *impaired skin integrity* related to scratching secondary to withdrawal symptoms.

F. Nursing plan/implementation:

1. Goal: *prevent/minimize respiratory distress.*
   a. Position: side-lying, head-dependent—to facilitate mucus drainage.
   b. Suction p.r.n. with bulb syringe for excess mucus—to maintain patent airway.
   c. Monitor respirations and apical pulse.
2. Goal: *minimize possibility of convulsions.*
   a. Decrease environmental stimuli—quiet, touch only when necessary, offer pacifier.
   b. Keep warm, swaddle for comfort.
3. Goal: *maintain nutrition/hydration.*
   a. Food/fluids—oral or IV, as ordered.
   b. I&O.
   c. Daily weight.
4. Goal: *assist in diagnosis of drug and drug level.* Collect all urine during first 24 hours for toxicologic studies.
5. Goal: *maintain/promote skin integrity.*
   a. Mitts over hands—to minimize scratching.
   b. Keep clean and dry.
   c. Medicated ointment/powder, as ordered, q 2–4 h, to excoriated areas.
   d. Expose excoriated areas to air.
6. Goal: *minimize withdrawal symptoms.* Administer medications, as ordered.
   a. Paregoric elixir—to wean from drug.
   b. Phenobarbital—to reduce CNS hyperirritability, hyperbilirubinemia.
   c. Chlorpromazine (Thorazine), diazepam (Valium) —to tranquilize, reduce hyperirritability. *Note:* Valium is **contraindicated** for jaundiced neonate because it predisposes to hyperbilirubinemia.
   d. Methadone.
7. Goal: *emotional support to mother.*
   a. Encourage verbalization of feelings of guilt, anxiety, fear, concerns.
   b. Refer to social service.

G. Evaluation:

1. Responds to medical/nursing regimen.
   a. Maintains adequate respirations.
   b. Feeds well, gains weight.
   c. No evidence of CNS hyperirritability, convulsions; demonstrates normal newborn reflexes.
2. Evidences bonding with parent(s). Responsive to mother's voice.

VII. Disorders affecting psycho-social-cultural function: fetal alcohol syndrome. *General aspects:*

A. Maternal alcohol abuse has been associated with:

1. Malnutrition, vitamin deficiencies.
2. Bone marrow suppression.
3. Liver disease.
4. Child abuse.

B. Infant at risk for:

1. Congenital anomalies.
2. Mental deficiency.
3. IUGR, intrauterine growth retardation.

C. Pathophysiology—permanent damage to developing embryonic/fetal structures; cardiovascular anomalies (ventricular septal defects).

D. Etiology—high circulating alcohol levels are lethal to the embryo; lover levels cause permanent cell damage.

E. Assessment:

1. Characteristic craniofacial abnormalities:
   a. Short, palpebral fissure.
   b. Epicanthal folds.
   c. Maxillary hypoplasia.
   d. Micrognathia.
   e. Long, thin upper lip.
2. Short stature.
3. Irritable, hyperactive, poor feeding.
4. High-pitched cry, difficult to comfort.

F. Nursing plan/implementation:

1. Goal: *reduce irritability.*
   a. Reduce environmental stimuli.
   b. Wrap, cuddle.
   c. Administer sedatives, as ordered.
2. Goal: *maintain nutrition/hydration.*
3. Goal: *emotional support to mother.*

G. Evaluation—see Drug-dependent (heroin) neonate, p. 193.

1. No respiratory distress.
2. Infant feeding properly.
3. Maternal bonding apparent.
4. Social service—home involvement.

VIII. Classification of infants by weight and gestational age

A. Terminology

1. *Preterm, or premature*—37 weeks gestation or less [usually 2500 g (5 lb) or less].
2. *Term*—38–42 weeks gestation.
3. *Postterm*—over 42 weeks.
4. *Postmature*—gestation greater than 42 weeks.
5. *Appropriate for gestational age (AGA)*—for each week of gestation, there is a normal range of expected weight.
   a. Term infants weighing 2500 g or more are usually mature in physiologic functions.
   b. If respiratory distress occurs, it is usually related to aspiration syndrome

6. *Small for gestational age (SGA), or dysmature*—weight falls below normal range for age. *Etiology:*
   a. Preeclampsia.
   b. Malnutrition.
   c. Smoking.
   d. Placental insufficiency.
   e. Alcohol syndrome.
   f. Rubella.
   g. Syphilis.
   h. Multiple gestation (twins, etc.).
   i. Genetic.
   j. Cocaine abuse.
7. *Large for gestational age (LGA)*—above expected weight for age. **Note:** If **preterm,** at risk for **respiratory distress syndrome.** If **postterm,** at risk for **aspiration** and **sudden intrauterine death.**
   a. *Etiology:*
      (1) Maternal diabetes or prediabetes.
      (2) Maternal weight gain over 35 lb.
      (3) Maternal obesity.
      (4) Genetic.
   b. *Associated problems:*
      (1) Hypoglycemia.
      (2) Hypocalcemia.
      (3) Hyperbilirubinemia.
      (4) Birth injury.

B. *Estimation of gestational age*—planning appropriate care for the newborn requires accurate assessment to differentiate between premature and term infants.

Premature Infant

Born at 37 weeks gestation or less.

A. Pathophysiology—anatomic and physiologic immaturity of body systems compromises ability to adapt to extrauterine environment and independent life.

1. *Interference with protective functions*
   a. *Heat regulation*—unstable, due to:
      (1) Lack of subcutaneous fat.
      (2) Large body surface area in proportion to body weight.
      (3) Small muscle mass.
      (4) Absent sweat or shiver responses.
      (5) Poor capillary response to changes in environmental temperature.
   b. *Resistance to infection*—low, due to:
      (1) Lack of immune bodies from mother (these cross placenta *late* in pregnancy).
      (2) Inability to produce own immune bodies (immature liver).
      (3) Poor white blood cell response to infection.
   c. *Immature liver*
      (1) Inability to conjugate bilirubin liberated by normal breakdown of red blood cells → increased susceptibility to hyperbilirubinemia and kernicterus.
      (2) Immature production of clotting factors and immune globulins.
      (3) Inadequate glucose stores → increased susceptibility to hypoglycemia.
2. *Interference with elimination:* immature *renal* function—unable to concentrate urine → precarious fluid/electrolyte balance.
3. *Interference with sensory-perceptual functions:* central nervous system—immature → weak or absent reflexes and fluctuating primitive control of vital functions.

B. Etiology: (often unknown); premature labor.

1. *Iatrogenic*—EDD miscalculated for repeat cesarean delivery.
2. *Placental factors*
   a. Placenta previa.
   b. Abruptio placentae.
   c. Placental insufficiency.
3. *Uterine factors*
   a. Incompetent cervix.
   b. Overdistention (multiple gestation, hydramnios).
   c. Anomalies (e.g., myomas).
4. *Fetal factors*
   a. Malformations.
   b. Infections (rubella, toxoplasmosis, AIDS, cytomegalic inclusion disease).
   c. Multiple gestations (twins, triplets).
5. *Maternal factors*
   a. Severe physical or emotional trauma.
   b. Coexisting disorders (preeclampsia, hypertension, heart disease, diabetes, malnutrition).
   c. Infections (strep, syphilis, pyelonephritis, pneumonia, influenza, leukemia).
6. *Miscellaneous factors*
   a. Close frequency of pregnancies.
   b. Advanced parental age.
   c. Heavy smoking.
   d. High-altitude environment.
   e. Cocaine use.

C. Factors influencing survival:

1. Gestational age.
2. Lung maturity.
3. Anomalies.
4. Size.

D. Causes of mortality (in order of frequency):

1. Abnormal pulmonary ventilation.
2. Infection.
   a. Pneumonia.
   b. Septicemia.
   c. Diarrhea.
   d. Meningitis.
3. Intracranial hemorrhage.
4. Congenital defects.

E. Disorders affecting fluid-gas transport: respiratory distress syndrome (RDS)

1. **Pathophysiology**—insufficient pulmonary surfactant (lecithin) and insufficient number/maturity of alveoli predispose to atelectasis; alveolar ducts and terminal bronchi become lined with fibrous, glossy membrane.
2. **Etiology:**
   a. Primarily associated with prematurity.
   b. Other *predisposing* factors:
      (1) Fetal hypoxia—due to decreased placental perfusion secondary to maternal bleeding (e.g., abruptio) or hypotension.
      (2) Birth asphyxia.
      (3) Postnatal hypothermia, metabolic acidosis, or hypotension.
3. Factors *protecting* neonate from RDS:
   a. Chronic fetal stress—due to maternal hypertension, preeclampsia, or heroin addiction.
   b. Premature rupture of membranes (PROM).
   c. Maternal steroid ingestion (i.e., betamethasone).
   d. Low-grade chorioamnionitis.
4. **Assessment:**
   a. Usually appears during first or second day after birth.
   b. Signs of *respiratory distress:*
      (1) Nasal flaring.
      (2) Sternal retractions.
      (3) Tachypnea (60/minute or more).
      (4) Cyanosis.
      (5) Expiratory grunt.
      (6) Increasing number and length of apneic episodes.
      (7) Increasing exhaustion.
   c. *Respiratory acidosis*—due to hypercapnea and rising O_2 level.
   d. *Metabolic acidosis*—due to increased lactic acid levels and falling pH.
5. **Analysis/nursing diagnosis:**
   a. *Impaired gas exchange* related to lack of pulmonary surfactant secondary to preterm birth, intrapartal stress and hypoxia, infection, postnatal hypothermia, metabolic acidosis, or hypotension.
   b. *Altered nutrition, less than body requirements,* related to poor feeding secondary to respiratory distress.
6. **Nursing plan/implementation:**
   a. Goal: *reduce metabolic acidosis, increase oxygenation, support respiratory efforts.*
      (1) Ensure warmth (isolette at 97.6°F).
      (2) Warmed, humidified O_2 at lowest concentration required to relieve cyanosis, via hood, nasal prongs, or endotracheal tube.
      (3) Monitor continuous positive airway pressure (CPAP)—oxygen–air mixture administered under pressure during inhalation *and* exhalation to maintain alveolar patency.
      (4) *Position:* side-lying or supine with neck slightly extended ("sniffing" position); arms at sides.
      (5) Suction p.r.n. with bulb syringe—for excessive mucus.
   b. Goal: *modify care for infant with endotracheal tube.*
      (1) Disconnect tubing at adaptor.
      (2) Inject 0.5 mL sterile normal saline.
      (3) Insert sterile suction tube, start suction, rotate tube, withdraw.
      (4) Suction up to 5 seconds.
      (5) Ventilate with bag and mask during procedure.
      (6) Reconnect tubing securely to adaptor.
      (7) Auscultate for breath sounds and pulse.
   c. Goal: *maintain nutrition/hydration.*
      (1) Administer: fluids, electrolytes, calories, vitamins, minerals PO or IV, as ordered.
      (2) I&O.
   d. Goal: *prevent secondary infections.*
      (1) Strict aseptic technique.
      (2) Handwashing.
   e. Goal: *emotional support of infant.*
      (1) Gentle touching.
      (2) Soft voices.
      (3) Eye contact.
      (4) Rocking.
   f. Goal: *emotional support of parents.*
      (1) Keep informed of status and progress.
      (2) Encourage contact with infant—to promote bonding, understanding of treatment.
   g. Goal: *minimize possibility of iatrogenic disorders associated with oxygen therapy* (see point F below).
7. **Evaluation:**
   a. Respiratory distress treated successfully; infant breathes without assistance.
   b. Completes successful transition to extrauterine life.

F. Iatrogenic (oxygen toxicity) disorders: retinopathy of prematurity

1. **Pathophysiology**—intraretinal hemorrhage → fibrosis → retinal detachment → loss of vision.
2. **Etiology**—prolonged exposure to high concentrations of oxygen.
3. **Assessment**—only perceptible retinal change is vasoconstriction. *Note:* arterial blood (PaO_2) gas readings less than 50 or more than 70 mm Hg.
4. **Nursing plan/implementation:** Goal: *prevent disorder.* Maintain PaO_2 of 50–70 mm Hg.
5. **Evaluation:**
   a. Successful recovery from respiratory distress.
   b. No evidence of disorder.

G. Iatrogenic (oxygen toxicity) disorders: bronchopulmonary dysplasia (BPD)

1. **Pathophysiology**—damage to alveolar cells results in focal emphysema.
2. **Etiology**—positive pressure ventilation (CPAP and PEEP) and prolonged administration of high concentrations of oxygen.

3. **Assessment**—monitor for signs of:
   a. Tachypnea.
   b. Increased respiratory effort.
   c. Respiratory distress.
4. **Nursing plan/implementation:** Goal: *prevent disorder.*
   a. Use of *negative* pressure devices.
   b. Maintain oxygen concentration *below* 70%.
   c. Supportive care.
   d. Wean off ventilator, as possible.
5. **Evaluation:**
   a. Successful recovery from respiratory distress.
   b. No evidence of disorder.

H. Intraventricular hemorrhage

1. **Pathophysiology**—rupture of thin, fragile capillary walls within ventricles of the brain (more common in preterm).
2. **Etiology:**
   a. Hypoxia.
   b. Respiratory distress.
   c. Birth trauma.
   d. Birth asphyxia.
   e. Hypercapnia.
3. **Assessment:**
   a. Hypotonia.
   b. Lethargy.
   c. Hypothermia.
   d. Bradycardia.
   e. Bulging fontanels.
   f. Respiratory distress or apnea.
   g. Seizures.
   h. Cry: high pitched whining
4. **Nursing plan/implementation:** Goal: *supportive care*—to promote healing.
   a. Monitor vital signs.
   b. Maintain thermal stability.
   c. Assure adequate oxygenation (may be placed on CPAP).
5. **Evaluation:**
   a. Condition stable, all assessment findings within normal limits.
   b. No evidence of residual damage.

I. Disorders affecting nutrition

1. **Pathophysiology**—underdeveloped feeding abilities, small stomach capacity, immature enzyme system, fat intolerance.
2. **Etiology**—immature body systems associated with preterm delivery.
3. **Assessment:**
   a. Weak suck, swallow, gag reflexes—tendency to aspiration.
   b. Signs of malabsorption and fat intolerance (abdominal distention, diarrhea, weight loss, or failure to gain weight).
   c. Signs of vitamin E deficiency (edema, anemia).
4. **Analysis/nursing diagnosis:**
   a. *Altered nutrition, less than body requirements,* related to poor feeding reflexes, reduced stomach capacity, inability to absorb needed nutrients.
   b. *Impaired gas exchange* related to aspiration.
5. **Nursing plan/implementation:** Goal: *maintain/increase nutrition.*
   a. Frequent, small feedings—to avoid exceeding stomach capacity, facilitate digestion.
   b. Frequent "burping" during feeding—to avoid regurgitation/aspiration.
   c. Supplement vitamin E (alpha-tocopherol) intake, as ordered, in formula-fed infants (**Note:** intake adequate in breastfed babies.)
   d. Vitamin E actions:
      (1) Antioxidant.
      (2) Maintains structure and function of smooth, skeletal, and cardiac muscle.
      (3) Maintains structure and function of vascular tissue, liver, and red blood cell integrity.
      (4) Coenzyme in tissue respiration.
      (5) Treatment for malnutrition with macrocytic anemia.
   e. Encourage patient participation.
6. **Evaluation:**
   a. Feeds well without regurgitation/aspiration.
   b. Maintains/gains weight.
   c. No evidence of malabsorption, vitamin deficiency.

J. Disorders affecting nutrition/elimination: necrotizing enterocolitis (NEC)

1. **Pathophysiology**—intestinal thrombosis, infarction, autodigestion of mucosal lining, and necrotic lesions; incidence increased in preterm.
2. **Etiology**—intestinal ischemia, due to blood shunt to brain and heart in response to:
   a. Fetal distress.
   b. Fetal/neonatal asphyxia.
   c. Neonatal shock.
   d. After birth, may result from:
      (1) Low cardiac output.
      (2) Infusion of hyperosmolar solutions.
   e. Complicated by action of enteric bacteria on damaged intestine.
3. **Assessment**—early identification is **vital.**
   a. Abdominal distention and/or erythema.
   b. Poor feeding, vomiting.
   c. Blood in stool.
   d. Systemic signs associated with sepsis that may need temporary colostomy or iliostomy:
      (1) Lethargy or irritability.
      (2) Hypothermia.
      (3) Labored respirations or apnea.
      (4) Cardiovascular collapse.
   e. Medical diagnosis:
      (1) Increased gastric residual.
      (2) X ray shows ileus, air in bowel wall.

4. **Analysis/nursing diagnosis:**
   a. *Altered nutrition, less than body requirements,* related to inability to tolerate oral feedings and gastrointestinal dysfunction secondary to ischemia, thrombosis, and/or necrosis.
   b. *Constipation* related to paralytic ileus with stasis; diarrhea related to water loss.
   c. *Potential for injury* related to infection, thrombosis, metabolic alterations (acidosis, osmotic diuresis, dehydration, hyperglycemia) due to hyperalimentation.
   d. *Altered parenting* related to physiologic compromise and prolonged hospitalization.
   e. *Impaired skin integrity* when colostomy is necessary.
5. **Nursing plan/implementation:**
   a. Goal: *supportive care.*
      (1) Rest GI tract: no oral intake—to achieve gastric decompression.
      (2) IV fluids, as ordered—to maintain hydration.
   b. Goal: *prevent infection.* Administer antibiotics, as ordered.
   c. Goal: *Prevent trauma to skin surrounding stoma.*
6. **Evaluation:**
   a. Tolerates oral feedings.
   b. Demonstrates weight gain.
   c. Normal stool pattern.
   d. Parents are accepting and knowledgeable about care of infant.

Postterm Infant

Over 42 weeks gestation.

A. General aspects
1. Labor may be hazardous for mother and fetus because:
   a. Large size of infant contributes to maternal dystocia; diagnosis by: ultrasound, X ray.
   b. Placental insufficiency → fetal hypoxia; diagnosis by:
      (1) Contraction stress test.
      (2) Nonstress test
      (3) Maternal urine estriols.
   c. Meconium passage (common physiologic response) increases chance of meconium aspiration.

B. Assessment:
1. If postmature skin: dry, wrinkled—due to metabolism of fat and glycogen reserves to meet en utero energy needs.
2. Long limbs, fingernails, and toenails—due to continued growth en utero.
3. Lanugo and vernix—absent.
4. Expression: wide-eyed, alert—probably due to chronic hypoxia (oxygen hunger).
5. Placenta—signs of aging.

C. Analysis/nursing diagnosis: *potential for injury* related to high incidence of morbidity and mortality due to dystocia and/or hypoxia.

D. Nursing plan/implementation:
1. During labor:
   a. Goal: *emotional support of mother*—may require cesarean delivery due to CPD or fetal distress.
   b. Goal: *Continuous electronic monitoring of FHR.* Report *late* or *variable* decelerations immediately (indicate fetal distress).
2. After birth:
   a. Goal: *if delivered vaginally, prompt identification of birth injuries, respiratory distress.* Continual observation.
   b. Goal: *early identification/treatment of emerging signs of complications.*
      (1) *Hypoglycemia*—Dextrostix readings and behavior.
      (2) Administer oral or intravenous glucose, as ordered.

E. Evaluation: successful transition to extrauterine life (all assessment findings within normal limits).

CONGENITAL DISORDERS

I. *General overview:* Genetic abnormalities and environmental insults often lead to congenital disorders of the newborn. Successful transition to independent extrauterine life may pose a major challenge to infants compromised by anatomic and/or physiologic disorders. Knowledge regarding the implications of the neonate's structural and/or metabolic problems enables the nurse to identify early signs of health problems and to plan, provide, and evaluate appropriate goal-directed care to safeguard the status of the infant with a congenital disorder.

II. Disorders affecting fluid-gas transport: congenital heart disease

A. Pathophysiology—altered hemodynamics, due to persistent fetal circulation or structural abnormalities.
1. *Acyanotic defects*—no mixing of blood in the systemic circulation.
   a. *Patent ductus arteriosus.*
   b. *Atrial septal defect.*
   c. *Ventricular septal defect.*
   d. *Coarctation of the aorta.*
2. *Cyanotic defects*—unoxygenated blood enters systemic circulation.
   a. *Tetralogy of Fallot.*
   b. *Transposition of the great vessels.*

B. Etiology—unknown. Associated with maternal:
1. Prenatal viral disease (e.g., rubella, coxsackie).
2. Malnutrition; alcoholism.
3. Diabetes.
4. Ingestion of lithium salts.

C. Assessment:
1. Patent ductus arteriosus (Figure 3.3, p. 228)
   a. Characteristic machine murmur, mid to upper left sternal border (cardiomegaly); persists throughout systole and most of diastole; associated with a "thrill."
   b. Widened pulse pressure.
   c. Bounding pulse, tachycardia, "gallop" rhythm.

2. Atrial septal defect (Figure 3.1, p. 228)
   a. Characteristic crescendo/decrescendo systolic ejection murmur.
   b. Fixed S_2 splitting.
   c. Dyspnea, fatigue on normal activity.
   d. Medical diagnosis—cardiac catheterization, X ray.
3. Ventricular septal defect (Figure 3.2, p. 228)
   a. Loud, harsh, pansystolic murmur; heard best at left lower sternal border; radiates throughout precordium. (**Note:** may be absent—due to high pulmonary vascular resistance → equalization of interventricular pressure).
   b. Medical diagnosis—cardiac catheterization, ECG, chest X ray.
4. Coarctation of the aorta (Figure 3.4, p. 228)
   a. Absent femoral pulse.
   b. Late systolic murmur.
   c. Decreased blood pressure in *lower* extremities.
   d. Medical diagnosis: X ray.
5. Tetralogy of Fallot ("blue" baby) (Figure 3.5)
   a. Acute hypoxic/cyanotic episodes.
   b. Limp, sleepy, exhausted; hypotonic extended position—postepisode.
   c. Medical diagnosis—cardiac catheterization.
6. Transposition of the great vessels (Figure 3.6)
   a. Cyanotic after crying or feeding.
   b. Progressive tachypnea—attempt to compensate for decreased PaO_2, metabolic acidosis.
   c. Heart sounds vary, consistent with defect.
   d. Signs of congestive heart failure.
   ▶ e. Medical diagnosis—cardiac catheterization, X ray, ECG.

D. Analysis/nursing diagnosis:

1. *Fluid volume excess* related to persistent fetal circulation, structural abnormalities.
2. *Impaired gas exchange* related to abnormal circulation, secondary to above pathology.
3. *Altered nutrition, less than body requirements,* related to exhaustion, dyspnea.

E. Nursing plan/implementation:

1. Goal: *minimize cardiac workload.*
   a. Minimize crying—snuggle; pacifier—to meet psychologic needs.
   b. Keep clean and dry.
2. Goal: *maintain thermal stability*—to reduce body need for oxygen.
3. Goal: *prevent infection.*
   a. Strict aseptic technique.
   b. Handwashing.
4. Goal: *parental emotional support.*
   a. Encourage verbalization of anxiety, fears, concerns.
   b. Keep informed of status.
5. Goal: *health teaching*—explain, discuss:
   a. Diagnostic procedures.
   b. Treatment procedures.
   c. Basic care modalities.
6. Goal: *promote bonding.* Encourage to participate in infant care, as possible.
7. Medical/surgical management: surgical intervention/repair of congenital cardiac abnormality.

F. Evaluation:

1. Experiences no respiratory embarrassment in immediate postnatal period.
2. Completes transfer to high-risk center without incident, if applicable.
3. Surgical intervention successful, where applicable.

III. Disorders affecting fluid-gas transport: hemolytic disease of the newborn

A. Rh incompatibility

1. **Pathophysiology**—see Figure 2.10.
2. **Etiology**—see Rh isoimmunization, Figure 2.10.
3. **Assessment:**
   a. *Prenatal*—maternal Rh titers, amniocentesis.
   b. *Intrapartal*—amniotic fluid color:
      (1) Straw-colored: mild disease.
      (2) Golden: severe fetal disease.
   c. Direct Coombs test on cord blood; positive test demonstrates Rh antibodies in fetal blood.
4. **Nursing plan/implementation**—exchange transfusion:
   a. Goal: *health teaching.*
      (1) Explain purpose and process to parents.
      (2) Removes anti-Rh antibodies and fetal cells that are coated with antibodies.
      (3) Reduces bilirubin levels—indicated when 20 mg/dL in term neonate and 15 mg/dL in preterm.
      (4) Corrects anemia—supplies red blood cells that will not be destroyed by maternal antibodies.
      (5) Rh-negative type O blood elicits no reaction; maximum exchange is 500 mL; duration of exchange: 45–60 minutes.
   b. Goal: *minimize transfusion hazards.*
      (1) Warm blood to room temperature, as cold blood may precipitate cardiac arrest.
      (2) Use only fresh blood—to reduce possibility of hypocalcemia, tetany, convulsions.
      (3) Give calcium gluconate, as ordered, after each 100 mL of transfusion.
   c. Goal: *prepare for transfusion procedure.* Ready necessary equipment—monitor, resuscitation equipment, radiant heater, light.
   d. Goal: *assist with exchange transfusion.*
      (1) Continuous monitoring of vital signs; record baseline, and every 15 minutes during procedure.
      (2) Record: time, amount of blood withdrawn; time and amount injected; medications given.
      (3) Observe for: dyspnea, listlessness, bleeding from transfusion site, cyanosis, cardiovascular irregularity or arrest; coolness of lower extremities.

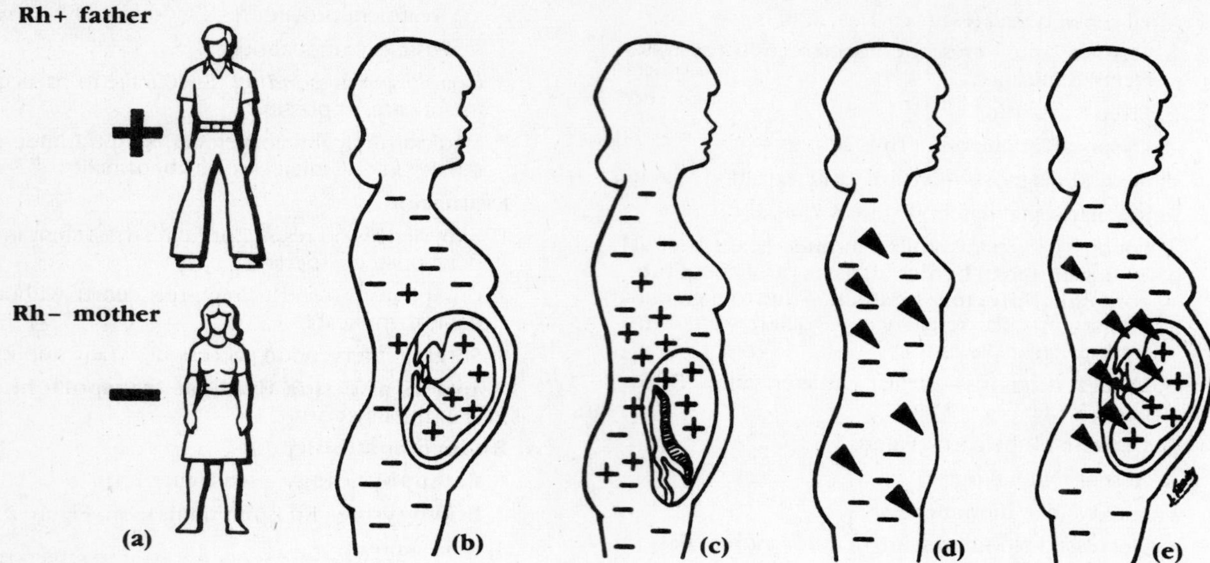

■ **FIGURE 2.10**
Erythroblastosis fetalis. Rh isoimmunization sequence. (a) Rh-positive father and Rh-negative mother. (b) Pregnancy with Rh-positive fetus. Some Rh-positive blood enters the mother's blood. (c) As placenta separates, further inoculation of mother by Rh-positive blood. (d) Mother sensitized to Rh-positive blood; anti–Rh-positive antibodies are formed. (e) With subsequent pregnancies with Rh-positive fetus, Rh-positive red blood cells are attacked. (From Olds SB, et al.: *Maternal Newborn Nursing,* 2nd ed., Addison-Wesley, Menlo Park, CA, 1984.)

e. Goal: *posttransfusion care.*

(1) **Assessment:**

(a) Observe for dyspnea, cyanosis, cardiac arrest or irregularities, jaundice, hypoglycemia; frequent vital signs.

(b) Signs of sepsis—fever, tachycardia, dyspnea, chills, tremors.

(2) **Nursing plan/implementation:**

(a) Maintain thermal stability—to reduce physiologic stress, possibility of metabolic acidosis.

(b) Give oxygen—to relieve cyanosis.

(c) Keep cord moist—to facilitate repeat transfusion, if necessary.

(d) Maintain nutrition/hydration—feed per schedule.

5. **Evaluation:**

a. Hemolytic process ceases; bilirubin level drops.

b. Infant makes successful transition to extrauterine life.

c. Experiences no complications of therapeutic regimen.

d. Evidence of bonding.

B. ABO incompatibility

1. **Pathophysiology**—fetal blood carrying antigens A/B enters maternal type O bloodstream → antibody formation → antibodies cross placenta → hemolyze fetal red cells. *Note:* less severe than Rh reaction.

2. **Etiology:**

a. Type O mother carries anti-A and anti-B antibodies.

b. Even first pregnancy is jeopardized if fetal blood enters maternal system.

c. Reaction possible if fetus is type A, type B or type AB and mother is type O.

3. **Assessment:**

a. Jaundice within first 24 hours.

b. Rising bilirubin levels.

c. Enlarged liver and spleen.

4. **Nursing plan/implementation:** Goal: *reduce hazard to newborn.*

a. Prepare for exchange transfusion with O negative blood.

b. Phototherapy may be ordered if bilirubin 10 mg/100 mL, and anemia is mild or absent.

c. Close monitoring of status.

d. Supportive care.

5. **Evaluation:**

a. Responds to medical/nursing regimen.

b. All assessment findings within normal limits.

C. Hyperbilirubinemia

1. **Pathophysiology**—bilirubin, a breakdown product of hemolyzed red blood cells, appears at increased levels; exceeds 13–15 mg/dL. Bilirubin is safe when bound with albumin and conjugated by user for body excretion; danger is when unconjugated and deposits in CNS.

a. **WARNING:** There is no "safe" serum-bilirubin level; kernicterus is a function of the bilirubin level *and* age and condition of the neonate; poor fluid-and-caloric balance subjects the infant (especially the premature) to kernicterus at low serum-bilirubin levels.

b. Kernicterus—high bilirubin levels result in deposition of yellow pigment in basal ganglia of brain → irreversible retardation.

2. **Etiology:**

a. Rh or ABO incompatibility, during first 48 hours.

b. Resolution of an enclosed hemorrhage (e.g., cephalohematoma).

c. Infection.

d. Drug-induced—vitamin K injection, maternal ingestion of sulfisoxazole (Gantrisin).

e. Bile duct blockage.

f. Albumin-binding capacity is exceeded.

g. "Breastfeeding jaundice" (e.g., pregnandiol in milk). Breastfeeding is *not* dangerous and not a cause of physiologic jaundice.

h. Dehydration.

i. Immature liver (interferes with conjugation).

3. **Assessment:**

a. Jaundice noted after blanching skin to suppress hemoglobin color; noted in sclera or mucosa in dark-skinned neonates; make sure light is adequate; spreads from head down, with increasing severity.

b. Pallor.

c. Concentrated, dark urine.

d. Blood level determination—hemoglobin or indirect bilirubin (unconjugated, unbound bilirubin deposits in CNS).

e. Kernicterus—similar to intracranial hemorrhage.

(1) Poor feeding and/or sucking.

(2) Regurgitation, vomiting.

(3) High-pitched cry.

(4) Temperature instability.

(5) Hypertonicity/hypotonicity.

(6) Progressive lethargy; diminished Moro reflex.

(7) Respiratory distress.

(8) Cerebral palsy, mental retardation.

(9) Death.

4. **Analysis/nursing diagnosis:**

a. *Fluid volume (red blood cell) deficit* related to hemolysis secondary to blood incompatibility.

b. *Potential for injury* (brain damage) related to kernicterus.

c. *Altered thought processes* (mental retardation) related to brain damage secondary to kernicterus.

d. *Knowledge deficit (parental)* related to infant condition.

5. **Nursing plan/implementation:**

a. Medical management:

(1) Prenatal—amniocentesis.

(2) Postnatal—exchange transfusion, phototherapy.

b. Goal: *assist bilirubin conjugation via phototherapy.*

(1) Cover closed eyelids while under light; remove eyepads when not under light (feeding, cuddling, during parental visits)—to protect eyes.

(2) Expose as much skin as possible—to maximize exposure of circulating blood to light. Remove for only brief time periods.

(3) Change position q1h—to maximize exposure of circulating blood to light.

(4) Note: any loose green stools as bile is cleared through gut; watch for skin breakdown on buttocks.

(5) Monitor temperature—to identify hyperthermia.

(6) Push fluids (to 25% more than average) between feedings—to counteract dehydration. Breast milk has natural laxative effects that help clear bile.

c. Goal: *health teaching.* Explain, discuss phototherapy, bilirubin levels, implications.

d. Goal: *emotional support.*

(1) Encourage verbalization of anxiety, fears, concerns.

(2) Encourage contact with infant.

(3) Reassure, as possible.

6. **Evaluation:**

a. Hemolytic process ceases; bilirubin level drops.

b. Infant makes successful transition to extrauterine life.

c. Experiences no complications of therapeutic regimen.

d. Evidence of effective bonding.

EMOTIONAL SUPPORT OF THE HIGH-RISK INFANT

I. General aspects

A. The high-risk infant has the same *developmental needs* as the healthy term infant:

1. Social and tactile stimulation.

2. Comfort and removal of discomfort (hunger, soiling).

3. Continuous contact with a consistent, parenting person.

B. Treatment for serious physiologic compromise may result in:

1. Isolation.

2. Sensory deprivation or noxious stimuli.

3. Emotional stress.

II. Assessment—signs of neonatal emotional stress:

A. Does not look at person performing care.

B. Does not cry or protest.

C. Poor weight gain; failure to thrive.

III. Analysis/nursing diagnosis: *sensory/perceptual alterations* related to isolation in isolette, oxygen hood.

IV. Nursing plan/implementation:

A. Goal: *provide consistent parenting contact.* Assign same nurses whenever possible.

B. Goal: *emotional support.*

1. Comfort when crying.
2. Provide positive sensory stimulation. Arrange time to:
   a. Stroke skin.
   b. Hold hand.
   c. Hum, sing, talk.
   d. Hold in en-face position (nurse looking into infant's eyes).
   e. Hold when feeding, if possible.

C. Goal: *encourage parents to participate in care*—to:

1. Reduce their psychologic stress, anxiety, fear.
2. Promote bonding.
3. Reduce possibility of later child abuse (higher incidence of child abuse against children who have been high-risk infants).

V. Evaluation:

A. Successful resolution of physiologic problems.

B. Parents and infant evidence bonding.

C. Parents express satisfaction with care and result.

GENERAL ASPECTS: NURSING CARE OF THE HIGH-RISK INFANT AND FAMILY

I. *General overview:* The birth of a physiologically compromised neonate is psychologically stressful for both infant and family, and physiologically stressful for the neonate. Effective, goal-directed nursing care is directed toward:

A. Minimizing physiologic and psychologic stress.

B. Facilitating/supporting successful coping and/or adaptation.

C. Encouraging parental attachment/separation/grieving, as appropriate.

II. Assessment—directed toward determining present and projected status of neonate:

A. Determine current physical status of neonate.

B. Identify specific status and diagnosis-related problems and needs.

C. Describe family psychologic status, strengths, and coping mechanisms/skills.

D. Determine medical/surgical/nursing approach to problems—and prognosis.

III. Analysis/nursing diagnosis:

A. Parental *anxiety/fear* related to physiologic compromise of neonate.

B. *Self-esteem disturbance* related to feelings of guilt and/or anger.

C. *Ineffective individual coping* related to severe psychologic stress.

D. *Knowledge deficit* related to diagnosis, treatment, prognosis of infant.

E. *Potential altered parenting* related to concern about infant.

IV. Nursing plan/implementation:

A. Goal: *preoperative and postoperative care.*

1. Maintain/improve physiologic stability.
   a. Temperature stabilization—keep warm.
   b. Oxygenation:
      (1) Position.
      (2) Administer oxygen, as ordered and/or necessary.
   c. Nutrition/hydration:
      (1) Administer/monitor intravenous fluids.
      (2) Oral fluids, as ordered.
      (3) Feed, as status permits.
2. Assist with diagnostic testing.

B. Goal: *emotional support of parents.*

1. Encourage exploring and ventilating feelings.
2. Involve parents in decision-making process.

C. Goal: *health teaching.*

1. Determine knowledge/understanding of problem.
2. Explain/simplify/clarify, as needed, physician's discussions with parents.
3. Describe/explain/discuss neonate's present status and any auxiliary equipment; teach CPR to family.
4. Refer, as needed, to hospital/community resources.

D. Goal: *promote bonding.* Encourage parental participation in care of the neonate.

V. Evaluation:

A. Parents verbalize understanding of relevant information; make informed decisions regarding infant care.

B. Parents demonstrate comfort and increasing participation in care of neonate.

C. Infant maintains/increases adequacy of adaptation to extrauterine life.

D. If relevant, parents demonstrate progress in grieving process.

■ QUESTIONS

Select the one answer that is best for each question, and fill in the answer circle beside the answer number.

Ruth Fara has come to clinic for family planning counseling. She states, "I want to postpone getting pregnant again for at least a year." Her history notes two episodes of thrombophlebitis with her previous pregnancy, repeated Candida infections, and gestational diabetes. Questions 1 through 3 refer to family planning.

1. Which of the following contraceptive methods is most appropriate for this client?

○ 1. Oral contraceptive pill. **IMP**
○ 2. Tubal ligation. **5**
○ 3. Diaphragm. **HPM**
○ 4. Intrauterine device.

2. Ruth states she is interested in "natural" methods for family planning. To aid Ruth in decision-making, the nurse discusses modern adaptations of the rhythm method. The success of these methods is dependent upon determining the time of ovulation by use of the basal body temperature (BBT) graph. Which of the following identifies the BBT change characteristic of ovulation?

○ 1. Falls slightly, then increases by about 0.5°C. **IMP**
○ 2. Rises slightly, then falls by about 0.5°C. **5**
○ 3. Is affected by a surge of FSH. **HPM**
○ 4. Is due to an estrogen surge.

3. Ruth asks the nurse about what causes the temperature change. The nurse correctly responds by stating that the postovulation temperature reading is due to the high blood level of which of the following hormones?

○ 1. FSH. **IMP**
○ 2. HCS/HPL (growth hormone). **5**
○ 3. Estrogen. **HPM**
○ 4. Progesterone.

Jana Wile is seen in clinic for the first time. When asked the reason for this visit, Jana tells the nurse her last menstrual period (LMP) was over 2 months ago, and she thinks she may be pregnant. Jane is 19, unmarried, and works days as a waitress. Questions 4 through 12 refer to this situation.

4. Objectives for the initial prenatal visit include determining the client's present health status, validating pregnancy, and identifying factors that may affect or be affected by a pregnancy. Which of the following assessment findings indicates a need for further evaluation of Jana's present health?

○ 1. Urinary frequency, nausea, fatigue. **AS**
○ 2. Vital signs—T 98.2, P 92, R 20, BP 110/70. **1**
○ 3. Urine—negative for sugar, trace of albumin. **HPM**
○ 4. Marked vaginal discharge with itching for the past few days.

5. Jana is anxious to know how soon a pregnancy test can be done and how reliable it is. She states that she used a urine-test kit she bought at the drugstore 1 month ago, and it was negative. Health teaching should include which of the following information?

○ 1. False negative tests may be due to dilute urine secondary to diuresis and inaccurate technique. **IMP** **5** **HPM**
○ 2. Urine tests are classed as presumptive signs of pregnancy.
○ 3. Levels of progesterone from the corpus luteum are sufficient to diagnose pregnancy as early as the fourth week.
○ 4. Urine tests are classed as positive signs of pregnancy.

6. Jana tells the nurse she is afraid of the pelvic examination. Which of the following nursing actions will *increase* her discomfort during the examination?

○ 1. Explaining why the exam is being done and what she may expect. **IMP** **5**
○ 2. Offering your hand for her to squeeze. **HPM**
○ 3. Suggesting breathing techniques to help her relax.
○ 4. Asking her to empty her bladder before the exam.

7. If Jana is pregnant, which of the following findings is inconsistent with an 8-week gestation?

○ 1. Chadwick's sign. **AS**
○ 2. Hegar's sign. **5**
○ 3. Goodell's sign. **HPM**
○ 4. Ballottement.

8. Jana's vaginal discharge is thick, white, cheeselike, and pruritic. The nurse's therapeutic and educational actions should be based on which of the following theories?

○ 1. No action needed. This is normal leukorrhea of pregnancy. **IMP** **1**
○ 2. Metronidazole (Flagyl) is the drug of choice to treat this condition. **HPM**
○ 3. Even if untreated, this condition presents no hazard to the neonate.
○ 4. This condition is more likely to occur in women who are pregnant or taking oral contraceptives or antibiotics, or who are diabetic.

9. Assessment findings are consistent with a pregnancy of 8-weeks gestation. When she asks when her baby is due, the nurse calculates from her last normal menstrual period, August 5. Which of the following accurately states Jana's estimated date of delivery (EDD)?

○ 1. May 12. **AS**
○ 2. May 30. **5**
○ 3. June 8. **HPM**
○ 4. June 12.

10. Jana's history reveals a pregnancy at age 15 that was terminated by elective abortion at 10 weeks, delivery of twin girls at 37 weeks, and a spontaneous abortion at 12 weeks last year. Analyzing these data, the nurse selects which of the following to describe Jana's present gravidity and parity?

○ 1. Gravida 5 Para 2. **AS**
○ 2. Gravida 5 Para 1. **5**
○ 3. Gravida 4 Para 2. **HPM**
○ 4. Gravida 4 Para 1.

11. According to the TPAL system, which of the following also describes Jana's present parity?

○ 1. 0-2-2-2. **AS**
○ 2. 2-0-2-2. **5**
○ 3. 0-1-2-2. **HPM**
○ 4. 1-0-2-2.

12. The client complains of severe "morning sickness": "I can hardly stand the smell of food in the morning. What can I do? I have to work to support myself and my family, and I can make more money on the breakfast shift." Which of the following plans should the nurse recommend to her for her morning nausea?

○ 1. Try a high-protein snack at bedtime. **IMP**
○ 2. Eat two dry crackers or toast before arising. **4**
○ 3. Eat a high-protein breakfast yourself. **HPM**
○ 4. Drink a glass of orange juice immediately on awakening.

You have been asked to present a short program on "You and Your Baby—Pregnancy, the First Nine Months" as part of a neighborhood health fair. Your goal is to help expectant couples actively participate in their own pregnancy-related care. Topics you plan to include are: (1) What's new with you?—normal maternal adaptations; (2) How your baby grows; (3) Dos and Don'ts; and (4) When to call the doctor/

Key to codes following questions Nursing process: **AS**, Assessment; **AN**, Analysis; **PL**, Plan; **IMP**, Implementation; **EV**, Evaluation. Category of human function: **1**, Protective; **2**, Sensory-perceptual; **3**, Comfort, Rest, Activity, and Mobility; **4**, Nutrition; **5**, Growth and Development; **6**, Fluid-Gas Transport; **7**, Psycho-Social-Cultural; **8**, Elimination. Client need: **SECE**, Safe, Effective Care Environment; **PhI**, Physiological Integrity; **PsI**, Psychosocial Integrity; **HPM**, Health Promotion/Maintenance. See frontmatter for full explanation.

nurse-midwife—signs of trouble. Questions 13 through 22 refer to this situation.

13. Your objective is to actively involve participants in the discussion. In answer to your question "What's new with you?" Rita Nole replies, "Indigestion, heartburn, and constipation. Why?" Your answer and subsequent health teaching are based on an understanding of the normal physiologic alterations during pregnancy. Which of the following *best* explains Rita's symptoms?

○ 1. Progesterone, produced by the placenta, causes reduced motility of smooth muscle, e.g., intestinal tract. **AS 4 HPM**
○ 2. Stress due to developmental tasks of pregnancy results in increased gastric acidity and reflux.
○ 3. Pressure from the growing uterus displaces the stomach and intestines.
○ 4. Increased pancreatic activity results in digestive-tract fat-intolerance.

14. Plans to minimize Rita's symptoms include suggesting which of the following?

○ 1. High-carbohydrate diet and decreased fluid intake, to stimulate peristalsis. **IMP 4 HPM**
○ 2. Pelvic rock-and-tilt exercises, to increase tone of her abdominal muscles.
○ 3. Symptomatic relief by over-the-counter antacids and mild laxatives.
○ 4. Increased fluid intake and small, frequent, high-bulk meals.

15. Clio Jones complains, "I waddle like a duck, and after even a short walk, my back and legs ache. Why? What can I do about that?" Which of the following theories provides the basis for appropriate health teaching?

○ 1. Relaxation of pelvic joint articulations and strain on supporting muscles due to the growing uterus cause these symptoms. **AS 3 HPM**
○ 2. An increased metabolic rate in pregnancy results in excess production of lactic acid in back muscles.
○ 3. Progesterone causes striated muscle-stretching and pain on motion.
○ 4. Decreased venous return from the legs and the pressure of the heavy uterus cause waddling and discomfort.

16. Which of the following actions should the nurse recommend to reduce Clio's normal discomforts of pregnancy?

○ 1. Avoid walking whenever possible; get bedrest in left Sim's position several times daily. **IMP 3 HPM**
○ 2. Perform pelvic tilt-and-rock exercises; get rest whenever possible, legs elevated.
○ 3. Wear a maternity girdle to provide support.
○ 4. Increase calcium intake, perform stretching exercises, and rest frequently during the day.

17. Nina Alb complains of urinary frequency and says, "It even wakes me up at night. Is there anything I can do about that?" Which of the following is the appropriate response to her question?

○ 1. "Placental progesterone causes irritability of the bladder sphincter. Your symptoms will go away after the baby comes." **IMP 8 HPM**
○ 2. "Frequency is due to bladder irritation from concentrated urine and is normal in pregnancy. Increase your daily fluid intake to 3000 mL."
○ 3. "Pregnant women void frequently to get rid of fetal wastes. Limit fluids to 1000 mL daily."
○ 4. "Try using Kegel's (perineal) exercises and limiting fluids before bedtime. If you have frequency associated with fever, pain on voiding, or blood in the urine, call your doctor/nurse-midwife."

18. Nora Ryan says, "My doctor says I'm five months (20 weeks) pregnant. What does my baby look like now?" Your response is based on knowledge of normal fetal development. Which of the following describes the average fetus at 20-weeks gestation?

○ 1. Viable, able to survive outside of the uterus with minimal assistance. **AS 5 HPM**
○ 2. About 10 inches long, weight about 10 ounces, and covered with fine, downy hair and vernix.
○ 3. Beginning sex differentiation, kidney function, and detectable movements.
○ 4. Shedding lanugo and vernix, growing rapidly, weighs about 1½ pounds.

19. In discussing "dos and don'ts," which of the following health teaching aspects should be emphasized as important for health maintenance during pregnancy?

○ 1. Keeping appointments for prenatal visits, remembering to ask questions when necessary, and following the medical/nursing recommendations. **IMP 5 HPM**
○ 2. Taking Lamaze (or other) preparation for childbirth classes.
○ 3. Moderate exercise, high-carbohydrate diet, and adequate rest.
○ 4. Taking multivitamins and iron, drinking six glasses of milk daily, and minimizing physical exertion.

20. During the coffee break at your presentation, Bob Hay says, "My wife, Lili, is a heavy smoker—three packs a day. She won't listen to me. Will you talk to her?" Which of the following is an appropriate approach to this problem?

○ 1. Tell Lili that, if she continues to smoke that much, the baby will be small and have a greater chance of childhood respiratory infections. **IMP 6 HPM**
○ 2. Teach Lili to substitute snacking on cheese, dried apricots, or raisins to curb her desire to smoke.
○ 3. Discuss with Lili current thoughts about the effects of smoking during pregnancy, and ask her if she can think of ways to cut down.
○ 4. Ask her how she plans to cut down to 10 cigarettes daily.

21. Anticipatory guidance during the prenatal period includes instructions enabling the expectant couple to recognize signs and symptoms requiring immediate medical evaluation. Which of the following should be included in this part of the teaching presentation?

○ 1. Excessive saliva, "bumps" around her areolae, and increased vaginal mucus. **IMP 6 HPM**
○ 2. Fatigue, nausea, and urinary frequency at any time during pregnancy.
○ 3. Ankle edema, enlarging varicosities, and heartburn.
○ 4. Severe abdominal pain and/or fluid discharge from the vagina.

22. In addition to the above, which of the following signs and symptoms should the nurse teach as possible danger signs?

○ 1. Edema of the lower extremities, vulvar varices, and copious, clear vaginal discharge. **IMP 2**
○ 2. Heartburn, shortness of breath, change in appetite. **HPM**
○ 3. Leg cramps, back pain, and increased pigmentation over the bridge of the nose and the cheeks.
○ 4. Headache, visual disturbances, and/or feeling of fullness in face and hands.

Lisa Catz is in her 34th week of pregnancy. She states that her legs become swollen by late afternoon, she is uncomfortable with heartburn, hemorrhoids, and constipation, and she can feel her womb tighten and relax "a lot." Questions 23 through 27 refer to this situation.

23. Which of the following normal assessment findings should the nurse expect Lisa to demonstrate?
○ 1. Braxton-Hicks contractions, joint hypermobility, and backache. **AS 3**
○ 2. Dysuria, constipation, hemorrhoids, and lightening. **HPM**
○ 3. Feeling of tranquillity and heightened introspection.
○ 4. Morning sickness, breast tenderness.

24. Which of the following should the nurse suggest Lisa try to relieve her heartburn symptoms?
○ 1. Eat dry bread products before rising. **IMP 4**
○ 2. Bend at the knees when reaching down, not at the waist. **HPM**
○ 3. Eat fewer, larger meals and avoid nibbling.
○ 4. Do pelvic-rock exercise in standing position.

25. Assessing for the normal psychologic changes in the third trimester, the nurse would expect Lisa to exhibit which of the following normal behaviors?
○ 1. Ambivalence about the pregnancy. **AS 4**
○ 2. Eagerness to begin Lamaze classes. **HPM**
○ 3. Fantasizing about her child.
○ 4. Withdrawal from other relationships.

26. In reviewing with Lisa those symptoms that require prompt medical evaluation, which of the following would the nurse include?
○ 1. Increasing pedal edema. **AS 2**
○ 2. Feelings of dizziness on arising. **HPM**
○ 3. Epigastric pain.
○ 4. Spotting within 24 hours of vaginal exam.

27. Lisa also complains of groin pain, which seems worse on her right side. Which of the following is the *most* likely cause of this symptom?
○ 1. Bladder infection. **AS 3**
○ 2. Constipation. **HPM**
○ 3. Tension on the round ligament.
○ 4. Beginning of labor.

Gigi Port, age 16, tells the nurse she has no idea when her last menstrual period occurred. "My periods are so crazy that I haven't paid much attention to dates. Just sort of take it as it comes. This is the first time something like this (pregnancy) has happened." Questions 28 through 32 refer to this situation.

28. On assessment, the nurse observes that Gigi has marked chloasma and secondary pigmented areolae and that her umbilicus is flush with her skin at the level of the umbilicus. During which trimester are these physical changes of pregnancy commonly found?
○ 1. First. **AS 5**
○ 2. Second. **HPM**
○ 3. Third.
○ 4. Fourth.

29. Which of the following assessment findings indicate that Gigi has a 20-weeks gestation?
○ 1. Lightening, FHR audible by fetoscope, fundus palpable at the umbilicus. **AS 5**
○ 2. Braxton-Hicks contractions, ballottement, and fundus at umbilicus. **HPM**
○ 3. Quickening noted, FHR audible by fetoscope, fundus just below the umbilicus.
○ 4. Goodell's, Hegar's, and Chadwick's signs present, fundus halfway between symphysis and umbilicus.

30. Gigi has been recently diagnosed as a diabetic and will be managed by diet. She says, "I just can't understand it. I've been fine all my life." Which of the following theories provides the basis for the nurse's explanation and patient teaching regarding gestational diabetes?
○ 1. Anti-insulin effect of human chorionic somatomammotropin HCS/HPL (Human Placental Lactogen). **AS 4 HPM**
○ 2. Proinsulin effect of HCS.
○ 3. Increased maternal tissue sensitivity to insulin.
○ 4. Diabetes is unrelated to pregnancy; size and production of the islets of Langerhans are unaffected.

31. During her last month of pregnancy, Gigi tells you, "I am sick and tired of this whole thing. I can hardly wait for it to be over." Comparing Gigi's statement to the normal psychologic responses of other pregnant women during the last trimester, the nurse responds appropriately with which of the following statements?
○ 1. "I think you should see May Harris, the psychiatric social worker. You should be feeling more positive about the baby by now." **IMP 7 HPM**
○ 2. "I know exactly how you feel. I've seen it a thousand times. It'll pass."
○ 3. "Well, sounds like you're ready for labor. Do you have any questions about your coming labor?"
○ 4. "Your pregnancy is getting a bit tiresome and the time is dragging?"

32. Gigi wants to give her baby up for adoption. Which of the following plans will be of most help to her?
○ 1. Provide a safe environment, encourage ventilation of her feelings, give no answers or direction so that she makes her own decisions. **IMP 7 HPM**
○ 2. Make sure she has all the information she needs to understand the situation, place it in perspective in terms of her life goals, and begin to plan for the future.
○ 3. Support her choice whatever her decision.
○ 4. Help her see ways of not making the same error again so she can grow in self-esteem and self-respect.

Peri Wynn, gravida 1 para 0, has been admitted to the labor suite at 38-weeks gestation. She states she has been having moderate contractions every 3–5 minutes, lasting "almost a minute." Her membranes are intact, and she reports no show of blood. Questions 33 through 42 refer to this situation.

33. Peri states she came to the hospital because the clinic nurse told the prenatal class not to worry about coming too soon. Health teaching during the prenatal period should emphasize that expectant mothers need to go to the hospital when which of the following patterns is evident?

○ 1. Contractions are 2–3 minutes apart, lasting 90 seconds, and membranes have ruptured. **IMP 5**
○ 2. Contractions are 3–5 minutes apart, accompanied by rectal pressure and bloody show. **HPM**
○ 3. Contractions are 5 minutes apart, lasting 60 seconds, and increasing in intensity.
○ 4. Contractions are 5–10 minutes apart, lasting 30 seconds, and are felt as strong menstrual cramps.

34. Assessment findings of Leopold maneuvers reveal a soft, rounded mass in the fundus, irregular nodules on Peri's right side, and a hard prominence on her right, just above the symphysis. Which of the following accurately describes the fetal presentation and position?

○ 1. RSP. **AS**
○ 2. LSA. **5**
○ 3. ROP. **HPM**
○ 4. LOA.

35. Continuing the admission assessment, in which of the following locations should the nurse anticipate finding the fetal heart tones?

○ 1. Below the umbilicus on Peri's left side. **AS**
○ 2. Below the umbilicus on Peri's right side. **5**
○ 3. Above the umbilicus on her left side. **HPM**
○ 4. Above the umbilicus on her right side.

36. Which of the following techniques should the nurse use to assess the frequency, duration, and intensity of Peri's contractions?

○ 1. Spreads fingers of one hand lightly over the fundus. **AS 4**
○ 2. Moves the fingers of one hand over the uterus, pressing into the muscle. **HPM**
○ 3. Holds her hand (fingers and palm) over the area just below the umbilicus.
○ 4. Indents the uterus in several places, during and between contractions.

37. Peri appears excited, euphoric, and eager to learn about her labor status. Her behavior supports the nursing assessment that she is progressing through which phase of labor?

○ 1. Latent. **AS**
○ 2. Active. **5**
○ 3. Transitional. **HPM**
○ 4. Prodromal.

38. In order to assess Peri's labor progress, a vaginal examination is done. Which of the following assessments can be determined by vaginal examination?

○ 1. Fetal weight. **AS**
○ 2. Cervical dilatation. **5**
○ 3. Strength of contractions. **HPM**
○ 4. Fetal head circumference.

39. The decision is made to encourage Peri to walk around the unit for a while, and to then reassess her status. Which of the following assessments distinguishes between true and false labor?

○ 1. Confirmation of spontaneous rupture of membranes. **AS 5**
○ 2. Signs and symptoms of increasing discomfort. **HPM**
○ 3. Evidence of cervical dilatation.
○ 4. Presence of copious bloody vaginal discharge.

40. Continuing assessment notes Peri is becoming more serious, evidences a malar flush, and has a tendency to hyperventilate with contractions. These signs occur most commonly when the client enters which of the following phases?

○ 1. Latent. **AS**
○ 2. Active. **5**
○ 3. Transitional. **HPM**
○ 4. Pushing.

41. Jon Wynn arrives to stay with Peri. As she progresses through labor, she becomes increasingly irritable with her husband, complaining of lower-back pain and fatigue. Which of the following nursing interventions is most appropriate now?

○ 1. Have Peri turn on her side and give her a backrub. **IMP 5**
○ 2. Ask her if she would like you to get an order for something for her discomfort. **HPM**
○ 3. Reassure Jon that Peri's irritability is normal, and teach him to apply sacral pressure with contractions.
○ 4. Send Jon for a coffee break, and encourage Peri to try to get some rest.

42. Peri continues to progress. Fifteen minutes later, the nursing assessment notes marked introspection, irritability, and inability to focus. Peri is diaphoretic, and cries, "I can't make it!" These behaviors are characteristic of which of the following stages or phases of labor?

○ 1. Active phase. **AS**
○ 2. Transitional phase. **5**
○ 3. Second stage. **HPM**
○ 4. Third stage.

Dana Tate is admitted at 36 weeks directly from clinic, with a blood pressure of 146/98. Dana complains her face and hands feel "puffy" and, lately, she has been having "awful headaches and problems seeing." Admission note states: Admit stat for preeclampsia. Questions 43 through 49 refer to this situation.

43. Which of the following nursing orders should be questioned?

○ 1. Assess reflexes and amount and distribution of edema every shift. **IMP 2**
○ 2. Up as desired. **HPM**
○ 3. Admission and daily weight.
○ 4. Test urine for protein every 4 hours.

44. When preparing the room for a preeclamptic patient, which of the following equipment items is most important to have ready?

○ 1. Suction and oxygen apparatus. **IMP**
○ 2. Foley catheter and drainage bag. **5**
○ 3. Electronic blood pressure monitor. **SECE**
○ 4. Padded tongue blade and airway.

45. For which of the following reasons must Dana be carefully assessed for fluid intake and urine output?

○ 1. Oliguria is a grave sign. **AS**
○ 2. Daily intake should never exceed 2000 mL. **2**
○ 3. Sudden diuresis can precipitate convulsion. **HPM**
○ 4. If urine output is less than 100 mL/4 h, repeat dose of magnesium sulfate is needed.

46. Dana is now considered a severe preeclamptic. Close observation and continuous nursing assessment are necessary to facilitate prompt identification and management of which of the following?

○ 1. Abruptio placentae. **AS**

○ 2. Placenta previa. 6
○ 3. Hydramnios. HPM
○ 4. Breech presentation.

47. The physician orders a magnesium sulfate infusion. Which of the following assessments is most important when administering this drug to Dana?
○ 1. Monitoring the serum magnesium level every eight hours. IMP 1
○ 2. Evaluating the apical heart rate every four hours. PhI
○ 3. Counting the respiratory rate every hour.
○ 4. Auscultating bowel sounds before meals.

48. Ongoing evaluation of Dana reveals 4 plus deep tendon patellar reflexes with two beats of clonus. The most appropriate nursing diagnosis related to her current status would be:
○ 1. *Pain* related to hyperreflexia and clonus. AS
○ 2. *Potential for injury* related to possible eclamptic seizures. 1 SECE
○ 3. *Impaired physical mobility* related to alterations in lower limbs.
○ 4. *Sensory/perceptual alterations* related to sensory overload.

49. Which of the following influences the planning and implementation of Dana's postpartum care?
○ 1. Even if she has had no convulsions during the antepartal and intrapartal periods, she remains at risk for convulsions for the first 48 hours postpartum. AN 6 HPM
○ 2. Preeclampsia is associated only with pregnancy. Once the baby has been born, she is cured.
○ 3. Dana should be advised she may be left with chronic renal damage.
○ 4. Since subsequent pregnancy is extremely hazardous, family planning should be implemented as soon as possible.

Both Sue Hoyt and her sister-in-law Judi Hill are pregnant with their first babies. Both are Rh negative. Sue is a 25-year-old diabetic who has been well controlled on insulin for the past 10 years. Judi is 20 years old, with a history of rheumatic fever at age 8. For both women, close observation and ongoing assessment are important to detect early signs of problems and assure prompt, appropriate management. Their estimated dates of confinement are 2 weeks apart. They come to their prenatal visits together. Questions 50 through 56 refer to this situation.

50. Appropriate prenatal assessments are based on the nurse's understanding of the normal physiology of pregnancy and the interactive effects of coexisting disorders during pregnancy. For which of the following complications of pregnancy are Sue and Judi at equal risk?
○ 1. Spontaneous abortion. AN
○ 2. Preeclampsia. 6
○ 3. Dystocia. PhI
○ 4. Erythroblastosis fetalis.

51. To enhance the pregnancy experience for both Sue and Judi, health teaching could be planned and implemented to meet both shared and individual needs. When discussing common complaints arising from normal maternal adaptations to pregnancy, which of the following normal physiologic changes has greater implications for Sue and requires more teaching about danger signs requiring prompt medical evaluation?
○ 1. Increased venous pressure in lower extremities. IMP
○ 2. Placental production of HPL (human placental lactogen). 4 PhI
○ 3. Increased cardiac output.
○ 4. Relaxation of the cardiac sphincter.

52. Which of these normal physiologic changes has greater implications for Judi and requires more teaching about danger signs requiring prompt medical evaluation?
○ 1. Increased venous pressure in lower extremities. IMP
○ 2. Placental production of HPL. 6
○ 3. Increased cardiac output. PhI
○ 4. Relaxation of the cardiac sphincter.

53. The physician has told Sue she may require hospitalization during the pregnancy for treatment of any problems associated with her pregnancy and/or for diagnostic tests. When asked to verbalize her understanding of the discussion, which of Sue's responses indicates a need for further health teaching?
○ 1. "Pregnancy may change the amount of insulin I need for regulation of my diabetes." EV 4
○ 2. "I may need to be hospitalized to evaluate how well my placenta is functioning." PhI
○ 3. "If this awful morning sickness keeps up, the doctor may put me in to control it."
○ 4. "The doctor said he might take a sample of my water (amniocentesis) to see if the baby has the gene for diabetes."

54. Individualizing Judi's health teaching requires discussing and explaining actions that will reduce the risk of further heart compromise during pregnancy. Which of the following should be emphasized as the most important factor in safeguarding Judi's heart during her pregnancy?
○ 1. Adequate exercise. IMP
○ 2. Adequate rest. 5
○ 3. Low-salt diet. PhI
○ 4. Ferrous sulfate.

55. Judi is admitted for evaluation of her cardiac status at 24-weeks gestation. During the evening, she complains of dyspnea and shortness of breath while ambulating. She has a moist cough. Her physician orders her placed on complete bedrest. Which of the following nursing interventions is most appropriate to prevent further deterioration in Judi's condition?
○ 1. Place Judi in Trendelenberg position to encourage venous return to the heart. IMP 3
○ 2. Assist Judi with activities of daily living to reduce energy expenditures. PhI
○ 3. Encourage frequent coughing and deep breathing to prevent pulmonary complications of immobility.
○ 4. Initiate a regimen of lower limb exercises to prevent venous stasis and leg thrombosis.

56. Which of the following nursing interventions is most likely to be included in the plan of care for the cardiac patient during the first postpartum day?
○ 1. Push oral and intravenous fluid to stimulate diuresis and prevent fluid volume overload. IMP 1
○ 2. Encourage early ambulation and exercise to reduce the risk of thrombophlebitis. PhI
○ 3. Monitor vital signs, skin color, and pulmonary status to identify cardiac decompensation.
○ 4. Encourage patient to defer breastfeeding on the first day to reduce the cardiac workload.

June West had a difficult labor and had a forceps delivery under general anesthesia. She has her baby, Kip, for the first time since the birth. Kip is June's first child, and she is both excited and nervous. Questions 57 through 62 refer to this situation.

57. June asks the nurse about the "lump" on the side of Kip's head. The nursing assessment reveals the lump does not cross suture lines. Which of the following should the nurse tell June is the cause of the lump?

○ 1. Bleeding between the periosteum and parietal bone occurred due to pressure against the bony pelvis during delivery. **IMP 5 HPM**
○ 2. Edema of the scalp occurred due to pressure of the vertex against the cervix during the first stage of labor.
○ 3. Intracranial hemorrhage occurred due to pressure from the forceps during delivery.
○ 4. Simple swelling of a common hemangioma occurred due to prolonged pushing in the second stage of labor.

58. June wants to breastfeed Kip. She has had no previous experience or instruction. Which of the following should the nurse include in teaching June about good nipple care?

○ 1. Washing nipples and breasts every day with soap and water to prevent infection. **IMP 5**
○ 2. Keeping nipples clean with warm water and then air-drying to reduce irritation. **HPM**
○ 3. Applying dilute alcohol solution to nipples after each feeding, to toughen them.
○ 4. Covering the nipples with a plastic-lined breast shield to protect clothing.

59. June tells the nurse she is breastfeeding Kip because she can't stand the thought of his being vaccinated. Which of the following responses demonstrates effective health teaching?

○ 1. "That's great. Vaccinations aren't needed if you breastfeed him." **IMP 5**
○ 2. "Oh, you still need to have him vaccinated against DPT, measles, and polio before he is 6 months old." **HPM**
○ 3. "You can only give temporary protection to the infant against the diseases you have had yourself."
○ 4. "The most protection comes from colostrum just after birth. Unfortunately, you didn't start feeding him until today."

60. June complains she is having severe cramping after nursing Kip. Which of the following would be the first action taken by the nurse to reduce June's discomfort?

○ 1. Administer pain medication as per order. **IMP**
○ 2. Have her lie on her abdomen with a rolled towel at the level of her fundus. **3 HPM**
○ 3. Ask her to walk around for a few minutes.
○ 4. Ask her to empty her bladder.

61. In assessing June's response to Kip's birth on the first postpartum day, which of the following behaviors should the nurse expect to find present?

○ 1. Talkativeness, dependency, passivity. **AS**
○ 2. Autonomy and independence. **7**
○ 3. Disinterest in her own body functions. **HPM**
○ 4. Interest in learning to bathe the baby.

62. June tells the nurse she is planning to breastfeed Kip until he is 2 years old so she won't have to worry about getting pregnant. Which of the following responses demonstrates appropriate health teaching?

○ 1. "Lactation does suppress ovulation, so you'll be pretty safe." **IMP 5**
○ 2. "You are safe only as long as you don't menstruate." **HPM**
○ 3. "It's best to use some other form of birth control. You may not menstruate, but you may ovulate, and could get pregnant."
○ 4. "You'll find you won't be interested in intercourse until you wean your baby."

Toni Home delivered twins one-half hour ago. The first two assessments of her postpartum status have been within normal limits. During this assessment, the nurse finds that Toni's fundus is "boggy" and her lochial flow has increased. Questions 63 through 65 refer to this situation.

63. The nurse expresses several large clots with moderate fundal massage. Toni's fundus becomes firmer with the fundal massage. Which of the following actions should the nurse take next?

○ 1. Notify the physician because the site of her bleeding must be located. **IMP 6**
○ 2. Notify the physician because Toni needs surgery. **HPM**
○ 3. Administer oxytocin according to p.r.n. order.
○ 4. Reapply perineal pad and tell her to keep her thighs together.

64. Fifteen minutes later Toni's perineal pad is saturated. Her fundus is firm and smooth and there is a constant trickle of blood from the vagina. No clots can be expressed when the fundus is massaged. Which of the following should the nurse suspect on the basis of these findings?

○ 1. Atonic bleeding. **AN**
○ 2. Traumatic bleeding. **6**
○ 3. Retained placental fragments. **PhI**
○ 4. Inverted uterus.

65. Based on the assessment findings, which of the following actions should the nurse take immediately?

○ 1. Notify the physician because Toni needs surgery. **IMP 6**
○ 2. Notify the physician because the site of her bleeding must be located. **PhI**
○ 3. Administer oxytocin according to p.r.n. order.
○ 4. Reapply perineal pad and evaluate bleeding in fifteen minutes.

Baby Tall is born by normal spontaneous delivery at 42-weeks gestation. Rina Tall is a suspected drug user who was admitted to the labor unit 2 hours prior to the birth. Variable decelerations were evident on two occasions during Rina's labor, but they responded to maternal position change. Questions 66 through 71 refer to this situation.

66. When calculating the 1-minute Apgar, the nurse adds the following assessment findings: heart rate—over 100; respiratory effort—slow and irregular; muscle tone—flaccid response to slap on soles of feet; weak cry; color—body pink, extremities blue. In view of these assessment findings, which of the following Apgar scores should the nurse record?

○ 1. 5. **AS**
○ 2. 6. **5**
○ 3. 7. **SECE**
○ 4. 8.

67. While performing the newborn assessment, the nurse notes the vernix on Baby Tall is yellowish. The nurse promptly calls this to the physician's attention because this may be a sign of which of the following?

○ 1. Rh or ABO incompatibility or maternal ingestion of sulfisoxazole. **AN 6 PhI**
○ 2. An intrauterine gonorrheal infection.
○ 3. Maternal diabetes mellitus.
○ 4. Fetal postmaturity.

68. Four hours after birth, Baby Tall begins to show signs of respiratory distress. On the basis of the history and assessment data, which of the following should the nurse suspect?
○ 1. Aspiration syndrome. **AN 6 PhI**
○ 2. Respiratory distress syndrome.
○ 3. Oxygen toxicity.
○ 4. Bronchopulmonary dysplasia.

69. When the baby is 2 days old, Rina tells the nurse she is frightened because the baby, who weighed 7 lb at birth, now weighs 6 lb 8 ounces. Implementing health teaching for Rina, the nurse tells Rina the percent of birth weight usually lost by normal, healthy babies. Which of the following represents the maximum amount of normal weight loss for Baby Tall?
○ 1. 6 ounces (170 g). **AN 5 PsI**
○ 2. 8 ounces (227 g).
○ 3. 11 ounces (317 g).
○ 4. 16 ounces (454 g).

70. Rina is also distressed because the baby looks a little yellow. She says, "The other nurse said she has 'physical' jaundice. What's that? Is it bad?" The nurse's explanation is based on knowledge of the normal physiologic changes of the newborn. Which of the following is responsible for the baby's jaundice?
○ 1. Liver immaturity and fetal polycythemia. **AN 6 PsI**
○ 2. Oliguria and kidney immaturity.
○ 3. Infection.
○ 4. Dehydration.

71. Rina tells the nurse, "I am afraid the baby will have something wrong with her because I was bad while I was carrying her. Is she really okay?" If observed, which of the following would the nurse note as unusual?
○ 1. Enlarged breasts and some pink drainage from the baby's vagina. **AS 5 PsI**
○ 2. A dark line between the baby's umbilicus and symphysis.
○ 3. Little "blackheads" covering her nose and chin.
○ 4. A dark discoloration over her sacrum and lower back.

Dian and Ben Kind have been married for 5 years. For the past 2 years, they have expected Dian to get pregnant and have used no contraception. However, Dian has not achieved a pregnancy, and she asks the nurse what tests can be done to find out why. Questions 72 through 78 refer to this situation.

72. An infertility assessment begins with a thorough health history. Which of the following factors is likely to be implicated in female infertility?
○ 1. Moderate alcohol intake. **AS 5 PhI**
○ 2. Menstrual cycle of 26 to 28 days.
○ 3. History of pelvic inflammatory disease.
○ 4. Past use of diaphragm and spermicide for contraception.

73. The physician determines that Dian's inability to conceive is due to anovulatory cycles. An expected emotional response to this diagnosis indicating that Dian understands the underlying problem would be:
○ 1. Guilt for past sexual behaviors. **AS 7 HPM**
○ 2. Grief because she will never be able to conceive.
○ 3. Fears regarding the need for corrective surgery.
○ 4. Anxiety regarding the side effects of clomiphen citrate (Clomid).

74. Dian's husband is also evaluated for possible problems related to the couple's inability to conceive. A semen analysis is ordered. Which of the following instructions regarding collection of a sperm specimen is appropriate?
○ 1. Collect specimen at night, refrigerate, and bring to clinic the next morning. **IMP 1 HPM**
○ 2. Collect specimen in the morning after 24 hours of abstinence and bring to clinic immediately.
○ 3. Collect specimen after 48 to 72 hours of abstinence and bring to clinic within 2 hours.
○ 4. Collect a specimen at the clinic, place in iced container, and give to lab personnel immediately.

75. Dian successfully achieves a pregnancy. She talks with the nurse about her desire to have a natural childbirth. In health teaching for Dian, which of the following statements should the nurse explain is a myth?
○ 1. Medication may be used to reduce tension and pain during labor. **IMP 5 HPM**
○ 2. Labor and delivery under Lamaze techniques are almost painless.
○ 3. Labor is easier for women who are self-assured, relaxed, and cooperative during the process.
○ 4. Preparation for childbirth may include bodybuilding exercises, breathing techniques, and comfort aids.

76. At 37 weeks, Dian calls the office to say she awoke in a pool of blood and is dizzy and nauseated. But she denies any abdominal pain or cramping. On the basis of this assessment, the nurse suggests she go to the hospital immediately and meet the doctor. The nurse established a nursing diagnosis of *potential fluid volume deficit* associated with which of the following?
○ 1. Placenta previa. **AN 6 PhI**
○ 2. Abruptio placentae.
○ 3. Preeclampsia.
○ 4. Uterine rupture.

77. When Dian is admitted to the hospital, she is having sufficient bleeding for blood to trickle down her leg. Her blood pressure is 102/68, pulse 92. Which of the following nursing actions will the admitting nurse perform based on her assessment of Dian?
○ 1. Vaginal examination to assess fetal presentation, position, station, effacement, and dilatation. **IMP 6 PhI**
○ 2. Position her on her left side with a small pillow under her head.
○ 3. Adjust the bed in semi-Fowler's position.
○ 4. Prepare her for immediate cesarean delivery.

78. Dian gives birth to a viable baby boy. Nursing assessments during the fourth stage of labor will include close monitoring for signs of hemorrhage. This nursing decision is based on which of the following rationales?
○ 1. Placenta was implanted in lower uterine segment, where there are fewer muscle fibers to contract the placental site. **AN 6 PhI**
○ 2. The area under an abrupted placenta never contracts as strongly as when there is no premature separation.
○ 3. Since the placenta was surgically removed, the uterine muscle does not contract as efficiently.
○ 4. Dian lost 250 cc of blood during the third stage of labor.

Mona Watt is admitted in active labor. In answer to the assessment questions, Mona responds she has never been pregnant before and is excited about having twins. She declares she wants to use Lamaze for her labor. Questions 79 through 85 refer to this situation.

79. Mona makes progress in labor using the Lamaze technique. She is examined and found to be in transition stage. Which of the following breathing patterns used at this time would indicate a need for nursing intervention?
- ○ 1. Rapid, shallow chest breathing. **EV**
- ○ 2. Slow, deep, abdominal breathing. **3**
- ○ 3. Use of intercostal muscles with diaphragm relaxed. **HPM**
- ○ 4. Begins and ends each contraction with two cleansing breaths.

80. Following the amniotomy, the nurse remains alert for any signs of complications. In addition to the FHR, which of the following may indicate fetal distress?
- ○ 1. Crowning and increased fetal activity. **AS**
- ○ 2. Crowning and hypotonic contractions. **5**
- ○ 3. Increased fetal activity and meconium-stained amniotic fluid. **HPM**
- ○ 4. Baseline variability on the monitor strip.

81. Mona insists on remaining in a supine position in bed. Which of the following responses should the nurse make regarding Mona's behavior?
- ○ 1. "It's best for the babies if you lie on your side." **IMP**
- ○ 2. "These two pillows under your knees will be good for the babies and more comfortable for you." **5** **HPM**
- ○ 3. "You will get nauseated and light-headed if you stay in that position."
- ○ 4. "This rolled-up towel under your hip will do the job just as well."

82. Mona delivers viable twin baby boys. After the physician has cut the cord, and before the babies are given to her, the nurse does all of the following. Which should the nurse do *first?*
- ○ 1. Confirm identification of the infants and apply bracelets to mother and infants. **IMP** **5**
- ○ 2. Examine the infants for any observable abnormalities. **HPM**
- ○ 3. Wrap the infants in a prewarmed blanket and cover their heads.
- ○ 4. Instill prophylactic medication in the infants' eyes.

83. In assessing Mona's babies, which of the following should elicit the Moro reflex in healthy newborns?
- ○ 1. Sudden or loud noises. **IMP**
- ○ 2. Stroking the soles of the feet. **5**
- ○ 3. Turning each newborn's head to one side. **HPM**
- ○ 4. Stroking each newborn's cheek.

84. In assessing the twins, which of the following would the nurse note as a deviation from the normal characteristics of the term neonate?
- ○ 1. Head circumference larger than chest circumference. **AN** **5**
- ○ 2. Diaphragmatic breathing. **HPM**
- ○ 3. Passage of meconium stool.
- ○ 4. Epicanthal folds.

■ ANSWERS/RATIONALE

1. (3) Of the family planning options presented, a diaphragm and jelly is the optimum choice for this client. (1) is incorrect because oral contraceptives are contraindicated with a history of thrombophlebitis. (2) is incorrect because Ruth has stated she is interested only in postponing pregnancy. (4) is incorrect because of a strong relative contraindication to use of intrauterine devices by clients with impaired responses to infection, such as diabetics (Hatcher, 1984).

2. (1) Basal body temperature falls slightly immediately before ovulation, then rises approximately 0.5 °C. This characteristic finding aids women in identifying the fertile period of their cycle. (2) is incorrect because the pattern described is reversed. (3) is wrong because ovulation is related to an LH surge. (4) is wrong because progesterone levels do not rise until after ovulation.

3. (4) High circulating levels of progesterone released by the corpus luteum are thought to be responsible for the immediate postovulation rise in body temperature. (1) is incorrect because FSH is responsible for maturation of the follicle prior to ovulation. (2) is wrong because HCS/HPL is produced by the placenta and is not present at this time. (3) is wrong because estrogen is not implicated in the rise in body temperature postovulation.

4. (4) Marked vaginal discharge with itching for the past few days indicates a need for further assessment. Itching is most commonly associated with vaginal infections, and the cause should be identified and treated. Altered vaginal pH in pregnancy contributes to increased susceptibility to infection. (1) is incorrect because urinary frequency, nausea, and fatigue are common complaints in early pregnancy. (2) is wrong because vital signs are within normal limits. (3) is wrong because normally increased vaginal discharge in pregnancy may contaminate voided urine and result in a nonpathologic trace of albumin.

5. (1) The most common cause of false negative findings in urine testing for signs of pregnancy (presence of HCG) is faulty technique; further, dilute urine secondary to diuresis may contain too little hormone to register in the routine over-the-counter (or office) pregnancy tests. *Note:* HCG levels peak approximately 50–60 days postconception. (2) is incorrect because urine tests are classed as "probable" signs of pregnancy. (3) is incorrect because pregnancy tests identify presence/levels of HCG. (4) is wrong because urine tests are classed as "probable" signs of pregnancy.

6. (2) Offering your hand to squeeze encourages her to tense her muscles, including the pubococcygeus muscle of the pelvic floor, increasing the discomfort of a pelvic exam. (1) is incorrect because explaining what she may expect and the reasons for examination procedures is an appropriate nursing action designed to *reduce* Jana's anxiety and tension. (3) is wrong because suggesting and demonstrating breathing techniques is an appropriate nursing action designed to assist her to *relax* during the procedures. (4) is wrong because asking her to empty her bladder is appropriate anticipatory guidance designed to *reduce* the stress of the pelvic exam.

7. (4) The finding of ballottement is more consistent with a pregnancy of 19 or more weeks. (1) is incorrect because

Chadwick's sign (bluish discoloration of the vagina) is usually present at 8-weeks gestation. (2) is wrong because Hegar's sign (softening of the lower uterine segment) is present by 8 weeks. (3) is wrong because Goodell's sign (softening of the cervix) is usually present at this point in gestation.

8. (4) Her discharge is characteristic of a monilial (yeast) infection. This infection is more common in women whose vaginal pH has changed because of pregnancy or diabetes or who are taking oral contraceptives. Antibiotic therapy is also associated with increased risk for developing an infection by *Candida albicans*. (1) is incorrect because normal leukorrhea associated with pregnancy is thin, colorless, and nonpruritic. (2) is wrong because Nystatin is the drug of choice for treating vaginal yeast infections; metronidazole (Flagyl) is used in treating trichomonal infections. (3) is wrong because, if present during the baby's birth, this organism causes neonatal thrush.

9. (1) Using Nägele's rule to calculate the EDD, the correct date is arrived at by taking the date of the first day of the last menstrual period (LMP) and subtracting 3 months and adding 7 days. (2) is wrong because 7 days have been *subtracted* from her LMP. (3) is wrong because calculations have erroneously included August as one of the 3 months, and only 3 days have been added to the date of LMP. (4) is wrong because, although calculations added 7 days, again August was erroneously included as one of the 3 months subtracted.

10. (4) Gravidity is defined as the number of pregnancies; she has been pregnant three previous times and is now pregnant for the fourth time. Parity is defined as the number of *pregnancies* carried to viability. Jana has had two pregnancies terminated before viability (abortions) and has carried *one* pregnancy, which resulted in viable twin girls. (1) is incorrect because this counts the twins as two pregnancies carried to viability. (2) is wrong because, although it correctly identifies the twins as one parity, it counts them as two pregnancies. (3) is wrong because, although it correctly identifies Jana as gravida 4, it counts the twins twice.

11. (3) 0-1-2-2 describes her present status. She has not carried a pregnancy to term: one pregnancy terminated in the birth of preterm twins, two pregnancies ended in abortion, and she has two living children. (1) is incorrect because only one was a preterm pregnancy. (2) is incorrect because it describes her as having delivered two term infants and no preterm infants. (4) is wrong because it describes her as having carried one pregnancy to term and having *no* preterm infants.

12. (2) Carbohydrates taken before arising seem to reduce symptoms of morning nausea; dry crackers may absorb stomach acid and raise blood sugar. (1) is incorrect because high-protein snacks at bedtime appear to have no effect on nausea in the morning. (3) is wrong because nausea is present prior to eating and may be so severe as to prevent eating. (4) is wrong because orange juice on an empty stomach may precipitate emesis in the client with "morning sickness."

13. (1) The effects of progesterone on the GI tract include relaxation of the cardiac sphincter and delayed gastric emptying, which contribute to indigestion and heartburn, and slowed intestinal peristalsis, which increases water reabsorption and predisposes to constipation. (2) is incorrect because the major cause of her symptoms is described in (1). (3) is wrong because displacement due to pressure from the uterus is secondary to the effects of reduced smooth muscle tone. (4) is wrong because increased pancreatic activity does not cause fat intolerance.

14. (4) Increasing her fluid and roughage intake will assist in reducing her symptoms of constipation. (1) is incorrect because a high-carbohydrate diet and reduced fluid intake may make her constipation worse. (2) is wrong because exercise does not counteract the effects of progesterone. (3) is wrong because many over-the-counter antacids contain sodium and frequent use of laxatives may result in further loss of tone leading to constipation.

15. (1) Shifting the center of gravity to compensate for the weight of the growing uterus places strain on supporting musculature and contributes to low-back ache during pregnancy; relaxation of joint articulations is responsible for the waddling gait. (2) is wrong because vigorous exercise contributes to the production of lactic acid; the increased metabolic rate during pregnancy has no effect. (3) is wrong because progesterone affects smooth muscle. (4) is wrong because decreased venous return and pressure from the growing uterus contribute to development of varicosities.

16. (2) Exercises like the pelvic tilt and rock strengthen the abdominal and back muscles, which support the mother in an erect position—and the growing uterus; rest while elevating the legs reduces stress on these muscles and the legs and decreases symptoms. (1) is incorrect because walking is an excellent mild exercise recommended for the pregnant woman. (3) is wrong because a girdle may contribute to decreased venous return from the extremities. (4) is wrong because symptoms are due to strain on supporting muscles and are unrelated to the level of circulating calcium.

17. (4) Progesterone also reduces smooth muscle motility in the urinary tract and predisposes the pregnant woman to urinary tract infections. Clients should contact their doctors if they exhibit signs of infection. Kegel exercises will help strengthen the perineal muscles; limiting fluids at bedtime reduces the possibility of being awakened by the necessity of voiding. (1) is incorrect because progesterone does not cause irritability of the bladder sphincter. (2) is wrong because frequency in early and late pregnancy is due to pressure on the bladder from the growing uterus. (3) is wrong because hydration is important in maintaining normal digestion and nutrient transport to body cells, removing wastes, and regulating body temperature. During pregnancy, eight glasses of fluid daily are recommended.

18. (2) These are the characteristics of the fetus at 20-weeks gestation. (1) is incorrect because, although 20 weeks has been identified as viability, most such fetuses are too immature to survive independent extrauterine existence successfully. (3) is wrong because sex differentiation begins at conception and is discernible at 12 weeks, and kidneys begin secreting urine at 11 weeks. (4) is wrong because the fetus begins to exhibit these characteristics at 31 weeks.

19. (1) The most important factor in reducing morbidity and mortality associated with pregnancy is close health supervision and prompt management of emerging problems and complications. (2) is incorrect because the primary goal of Lamaze classes is to prepare the couple for labor and delivery. (3) is wrong because high-protein diets are recommended during pregnancy to reduce the possibility of pregnancy-induced hypertension. (4) is wrong because the pregnant woman should drink one quart of milk and increase her intake during lactation.

20. (3) Encouraging her to consider ways to reduce her smoking implies your respect for her ability to deal with the problem and encourages her active participation in her own pregnancy-related care. (1) is incorrect because such comments generate guilt and may threaten her self-image. (2) is wrong because telling her to substitute even "good foods" implies lack of respect for her judgment and the assumption that she will comply with your choices for her behavior. (4) is wrong because it implies she has no choice in the matter; client goals are best established mutually.

21. (4) Severe abdominal pain may indicate complications of pregnancy such as abortion, ectopic pregnancy, and abruptio placentae; fluid discharge from the vagina may indicate premature rupture of the membranes; these signs should be evaluated by the health professional promptly to safeguard the mother and her infant. (1) is incorrect because ptyalism, elevated Montgomery tubercles, and leukorrhea are normal physiologic responses during pregnancy. (2) is wrong because fatigue, nausea, and frequency are normal in early pregnancy. (3) is wrong because ankle edema, varicosities, and heartburn are normal during pregnancy.

22. (4) Headache and feeling of fullness in face and hands may indicate preeclampsia. (1) is wrong because pedal edema, varicosities, and vaginal discharge are related to decreased venous return and increased vascularity in pregnancy. (2) is wrong because heartburn, shortness of breath, and change in appetite are normal responses in pregnancy. (3) is wrong because leg cramps, low-back ache, and chloasma are associated with normal physiologic changes of pregnancy.

23. (1) Braxton-Hicks contractions, hypermobility of joints, and backache are all normal findings at this point in pregnancy. (2) is incorrect because complaints of dysuria should be explored due to the tendency to urinary tract infection in pregnancy. (3) is wrong because a feeling of tranquillity and heightened introspection are common in the second trimester. (4) is wrong because these symptoms are most common in the first trimester.

24. (2) Bending at the waist facilitates movement of food out of the stomach through a relaxed cardiac sphincter. (1) is incorrect because this is the treatment for morning sickness. (3) is wrong because this tends to aggravate heartburn. (4) is wrong because the pelvic rock relieves backache, not heartburn.

25. (2) During the third trimester, the mother becomes ready to begin learning techniques for her use during labor. (1) is wrong because ambivalence about the pregnancy is usually seen in early pregnancy. (3) is wrong because fantasizing is typical during the second trimester. (4) is wrong because the period of introspection and introversion occurs in the second trimester.

26. (3) Epigastric pain is associated with edema of the liver capsule in preeclampsia. (1) is incorrect because dependent edema is common in late pregnancy, due to reduced venous return from the lower extremities. (2) is wrong because orthostatic hypotension may be a common occurrence during the third trimester. (4) is wrong because brown spotting is a normal finding within 24 hours of vaginal examination, due to the increased friability of the cervix during pregnancy.

27. (3) Tension on the round ligaments occurs because of the erect human posture and pressure exerted by the growing uterus. (1) is incorrect because bladder infection is accompanied by frequency and dysuria. (2) is wrong because discomfort from constipation is accompanied by other symptoms, and the location of the discomfort differs. (4) is wrong because groin pain is not characteristic of beginning labor.

28. (2) Chloasma, secondary pigmented areolae, and umbilicus flush with the skin are characteristic changes in the second trimester. (1) is wrong because these signs are not present during the normal first trimester. (3) is wrong because, although present during the third trimester, these changes begin during the second. (4) is wrong because these signs diminish during the fourth trimester.

29. (3) Quickening, audible FHR with fetoscope, and fundal height just below the umbilicus are present in most clients by the 20th week of pregnancy. (1) is wrong because lightening usually occurs at 36–38 weeks gestation. (2) is wrong because Braxton-Hicks contractions are palpable around the 30th week and the fundus is at the umbilicus at approximately the 22nd week. (4) is wrong because Goodell, Hegar, and Chadwick signs are first noted about the 6th week of pregnancy, and this fundal height is consistent with the 16th week of gestation.

30. (1) The anti-insulin effects of the placental hormone HCS and reduced maternal tissue sensitivity to insulin often may result in development of gestational diabetes in women who previously had no symptoms of diabetes. (2) is wrong because the effect of HCS is antagonistic to insulin, not proinsulin. (3) is wrong because there is decreased maternal tissue sensitivity to insulin. (4) is wrong because the size and production of the islets of Langerhans increase during pregnancy.

31. (4) She does need support for her feelings at this point in pregnancy, and validation that they are normal. (1) is incorrect because she is evidencing only normal responses to later pregnancy. (2) is wrong because such statements tend to inhibit further exploration of the client's feelings and convey that such feelings are unimportant to the nurse. (3) is wrong because it neither validates the normalcy of her feelings nor encourages any further ventilation.

32. (2) is correct because the nurse can best fulfill the role of client advocate by providing all essential information the adolescent needs to make informed decisions; this allows opportunity for introspection and growth. (1) is incorrect because adolescents require and desire some guidance or assistance with major life decisions from supportive adults. (3) is incorrect because it may not be appropriate or ethical to support some decisions the adolescent makes. (4) is incorrect because such actions are judgmental, tend to destroy rapport, and nullify possible growth.

33. (3) Although instructions vary from birth center to birth center, primigravidas should seek care when regular contractions are felt about 5 minutes apart, becoming longer and stronger. (1) is incorrect because she should have sought care earlier. (2) is incorrect because she should have sought care earlier. Rectal pressure may be a sign of impending birth. (4) is incorrect because this pattern may reflect "false labor" or very early latent phase labor.

34. (4) Of the choices given, if the breach is in the fundus, the occiput must be the presenting part; if the irregular nodules (elbows, knee, feet) are on Peri's right side, the fetal back is to the maternal left. (1) is incorrect because the "S" refers to the fetal sacrum and describes a breech presentation. (2) is wrong because this also describes a breech presentation. (3) is wrong because the fetal back is on the maternal left side, as is the occiput.

35. (1) FHR is heard best through the fetal back, which, in LOA presentations, is below the umbilicus on the maternal left side. (2) is incorrect because the fetal back is as described, i.e., on maternal left. (3) is wrong because, in a vertex presentation, the heart tones are more audible below the umbilicus. (4) is wrong because it describes the placement of FHR in breech presentations.

36. (1) The frequency, duration, and intensity of uterine contractions are assessed by light palpation of the contractile part, i.e., the fundus. (2) is incorrect because moving the hand over the uterus may reduce the accuracy of perceiving contractions; pressure into the muscle may contribute to uterine dysfunction due to manipulation. (3) is wrong because the most contractile part of the uterus is the fundus, not the corpus. (4) is wrong because uterine manipulation between contractions may contribute to uterine dysfunction.

37. (1) These behaviors are typical of the client during the latent phase of labor. (2) is incorrect because, as labor progresses, internal stimuli demand more focus. (3) is wrong because clients in transitional phase are irritable and increasingly aware of their labor as contractions increase in strength, length, and discomfort. (4) is wrong because, in the prodromal period of labor, contractions are mild and irregular and the major client question may be "Am I really in labor?"

38. (2) Cervical dilatation is determined by vaginal exam. (1) is incorrect because fetal weight can only be indirectly estimated by fundal height measurement and sonography. (3) is incorrect because strength of contractions is evaluated by palpation of the uterine fundus. (4) is incorrect because head circumference cannot be determined until after birth.

39. (3) The criterion used to distinguish true from false labor is evidence of cervical change. (1) is incorrect because spontaneous rupture of membranes can occur before initiation of labor. (2) is incorrect because clients who are not in true labor may experience increasing pain due to obstetric complications. (4) is incorrect because copious bloody vaginal discharge can occur without labor (placental problems).

40. (2) These behaviors are characteristic of the active phase of the first stage of labor; client is about 5 cm dilated. (1) is wrong because clients are more excited and relaxed during the latent phase when labor is less uncomfortable. (3) is wrong because behaviors during transition reveal the woman's focus on completing the process rapidly; irritability is common. (4) is wrong because the woman uses sustained inhalations to increase the force of her pushing.

41. (3) Reassurance that her behavior is normal for this point in labor helps reduce the mate's feelings of guilt and helplessness and fosters the sense of a mutual, shared experience; sacral pressure reduces her discomfort. (1) is wrong because it does not address the partner's feelings. (2) is wrong because it does not facilitate the shared experience and may result in feelings of failure in some women. (4) is wrong because Peri is progressing well and needs/wants her mate's support.

42. (2) These behaviors are characteristic of the transitional phase of labor. (1) is incorrect because the woman shows a more intense, serious demeanor and may hyperventilate with contractions in the active phase. (3) is incorrect because the second stage of labor is characterized by sustained inhalations and expulsive efforts. (4) is incorrect because in the third state of labor, the placenta is expelled and the woman is often euphoric and focuses on the infant.

43. (2) If avoidable, clients hospitalized for treatment of preeclampsia should be in a quiet environment to minimize stimuli. (1) is incorrect because the amount and distribution of edema should be assessed by the nurse. (3) is wrong because weight is an indicator of edema and diuresis and should be assessed in the preeclamptic woman. (4) is wrong because intake and output relationships are important in assessing the status of the preeclamptic woman, and the presence and amount of protein in the urine is another important indicator of her status.

44. (1) is correct as the primary responsibility of the nurse is to prepare for respiratory and cardiac support in the event the woman experiences an eclamptic seizure. (2) is incorrect because not all preeclamptics require bladder catheterization. (3) is incorrect because the nurse may monitor blood pressures using the standard sphygmomanometer and arm cuff. (4) is incorrect because tongue blades are never used in the management of seizures today.

45. (1) Oliguria is an ominous sign in preeclampsia. (2) is incorrect because daily intake is individualized for the preeclamptic client. (3) is wrong because sudden diuresis is a good prognostic sign. (4) is wrong because urinary output must *exceed* 100 mL/4 h before magnesium sulfate, if needed, can be given again.

46. (1) Abruptio placentae may be a complication of severe preeclampsia and places both mother and fetus in serious jeopardy. (2) is incorrect because placenta previa is due to low implantation, not pathophysiologic changes in preeclampsia. (3) is wrong because hydramnios is most commonly associated with maternal diabetes, and although it may coexist with preeclampsia, it is not a contributing factor. (4) is wrong because hyperemesis gravidarum occurs earlier in pregnancy and is not associated with development or progression of preeclampsia.

47. (3) is correct because respiratory depression is a cardinal sign of magnesium toxicity. (1) is incorrect because individual variations in respiratory depression are observed at the same serum magnesium level. (2) is incorrect because respiratory compromise normally precedes depressed cardiac function and is a late sign of magnesium toxicity. (4) is incorrect because, although decreased peristalsis can occur with a magnesium infusion, it is not the most important assessment to make.

48. (2) is correct because deep tendon reflexes indicate the degree of central nervous system irritability and the potential for seizure activity. (1) is incorrect because hyperreflexia and clonus are not associated with pain or discomfort. (3) is incorrect because hyperreflexia and clonus do not interfere with motor activity in the lower extremities. (4) is incorrect because women with preeclampsia are placed in environments with reduced stimuli to decrease the risk of seizure activity.

49. (1) The possibility of postpartum eclampsia, while high, is often overlooked. Nursing care should be planned to maintain ongoing status assessments and minimize environmental stimuli. (2) is wrong because, although the risk decreases subsequent to delivery, eclamptic convulsions have been known to occur in the postpartum. (3) is wrong because chronic renal disease is not a sequela to preeclampsia. (4) is wrong because preeclampsia does not necessarily occur in subsequent pregnancies.

50. (4) Both women are Rh-negative nulliparas and are at some risk for Rh incompatibility; erythroblastosis fetalis results from hemolysis of fetal cells by maternal antibodies. (1) is wrong because Sue is at greater risk for spontaneous abortion due to her diabetes. (2) is wrong because the incidence of preeclampsia is higher in the pregnant diabetic. (3) is wrong because fetal macrosomia in infants of diabetic mothers may result in dystocia.

51. (2) Human placental lactogen (HPL) is an insulin antagonist and may complicate management of Sue's diabetes during pregnancy. (1) is incorrect because fatigue and varicosities are common complaints associated with decreased venous return from the lower extremities. (3) is wrong because increased cardiac output places additional work on the heart. (4) is wrong because relaxation of the cardiac sphincter is associated with heartburn and gastric reflux.

52. (3) Increased cardiac output has greater implications for Judi because her heart has been compromised by rheumatic fever. Judi should understand and be able to recognize signs of complications associated with her heart function. (1) is wrong because increased venous pressure in the lower extremities presents little more than an annoyance to either woman. (2) is wrong because placental production of HPL presents a greater problem for *Sue* (because of her diabetes). (4) is wrong because relaxation of the cardiac sphincter results in minor complaints for both women.

53. (4) Amniocentesis does not provide evidence as to whether or not the fetus is a potential diabetic, but it may be performed on diabetic women to test for fetal lung maturity or on Rh-negative women to monitor Rh-sensitized fetuses. (1) is incorrect because her statement indicates understanding of the interrelationship between her pregnancy and her diabetes. (2) is wrong because pregnant diabetics may be hospitalized for testing for placental function. (3) is wrong because nausea and vomiting in the pregnant diabetic may lead to acidosis.

54. (2) The most important single factor in maintaining good health for the pregnant cardiac client is adequate rest. The pregnant cardiac client should have approximately 8–10 hours rest each night and should lie down for one-half hour after each meal (Williams, 1980). (1) is incorrect because *reduced* activity reduces fatigue and supports preservation of cardiac reserve. (3) is wrong because moderate sodium intake (2000 mg) is allowable for the average class I cardiac; nutritional counseling focuses on increasing dietary intake of iron, protein, and essential nutrients to meet the increased demands of pregnancy. (4) is wrong because ferrous sulfate is prescribed to meet the increased demands for hemoblogin synthesis and to combat nutritional anemia.

55. (2) Activities of daily living will increase energy expenditures in the cardiac patient and may contribute to further decompensation. (1) is incorrect because dyspnea and shortness of breath will be exacerbated in the head-down position. (3) is incorrect because any activity that causes the patient to perform a Valsalva maneuver (coughing) will cause a sudden increase in blood return to the heart, which is contraindicated in cardiac disease. (4) is incorrect because the major goal of care is to reduce all energy expenditures.

56. (3) is correct because major cardiovascular changes that occur with the termination of pregnancy can result in sudden cardiac decompensation in the first postpartum day. (1) is incorrect because pushing fluids can result in fluid volume overload and cardiac decompensation. (2) is incorrect because the postpartum cardiac patient is encouraged to rest in the first day to minimize cardiac stressors while major cardiovascular changes occur. (4) is incorrect because breastfeeding is not contraindicated.

57. (1) Cephalohematoma is caused by subperiosteal bleeding, and the "lump" is limited by the suture lines. (2) is incorrect because edema of the scalp is caput succedaneum. (3) is wrong because a cephalohematoma is outside the skull. (4) is wrong because hemangiomas are benign blood vessel tumors.

58. (2) Nipples cleansed with plain water and air-dried carefully are less likely to develop fissures. (1) is incorrect because soap is drying and removes natural oils. (3) is incorrect because alcohol would be too drying and promotes fissure development. (4) is wrong because a plastic shield would retain body heat and moisture, irritating nipples.

59. (3) Only disease-specific antibodies produced by the mother in response to that infection can be passed through breast milk to the baby. (1) is incorrect because vaccinations would be needed to develop active immunity. (2) is wrong because measles vaccination is not effective if given before 1 year of age. (4) is wrong because maternal antibodies confer only short-lived passive immunity.

60. (4) A full bladder may be the major source of her discomfort. (1) is incorrect because medication should be given for minor discomforts only after trying other comfort measures. (2) is wrong because this measure would be used only after she has voided. (3) is wrong because walking does not relieve afterpains.

61. (1) Talkativeness, dependency, and passivity are all signs of the "taking-in" phase of the postpartum. (2) is incorrect because the mother needs to have her needs for nurturing and positive reinforcement met at this time. (3) is wrong because she is most interested in her own body functions, her return to normal, and her ability to void and defecate. (4) is wrong because she is not ready to "take hold."

62. (3) Although lactation does suppress ovulation, time of ovulation varies widely, making this an unreliable birth-control method (bottlefeeding mothers have ovulated as early as 36 days postpartum; nursing mothers, as early as 39 days postpartum). (1) is incorrect because of the unpredictability of the time of inhibition of ovulation. (2) is wrong because the mother may have anovulatory or ovulatory menses or may ovulate in the absence of menstruation. (4) is wrong because the couple may desire to resume intercourse when lochia stops.

63. (3) The most common cause of bleeding in the immediate postpartum is uterine atony, and bleeding may be controlled with fundal massage and oxytocic stimulation. (1) is incorrect because Toni has responded to the nursing measures. (2) is wrong because her bleeding does not appear associated with lacerations that might require surgery. (4) is wrong because perineal pressure is effective only in treating superficial tears.

64. (2) Traumatic bleeding is characterized by a firm, smooth uterus and a continuous trickle. (1) is incorrect because the uterus remains well contracted. (3) is wrong because bleeding from retained placental fragments occurs most commonly later in the postpartum period. (4) is wrong because inverted uterus is characterized by profuse vaginal bleeding and collapse.

65. (2) The laceration must be located and treated before bleeding will stop. (1) is incorrect because, if the laceration is accessible, bleeding may be controlled by insertion of vaginal packing. (3) is wrong because bleeding is not related to uterine atony. (4) is wrong because perineal pressure would be ineffective with a vaginal laceration.

66. (1) Heart rate—2; respiratory effort—1; muscle tone—0; reflex response—1; color—1. Total Apgar score is 5. (2), (3), and (4) are incorrect because of inaccurate allocation of points for behaviors described.

67. (1) Yellow vernix results from the breakdown of hemoglobin and/or bile pigments in meconium. Both maternal anti–Rh-antigen antibodies and ingestion of Gantrisin are implicated in hemolysis of fetal RBCs. (2) is incorrect because gonorrheal infection renders amniotic fluid opaque, thick, and odorous without discoloring vernix. (3) is wrong because diabetes does not have any effect on the color of vernix. (4) is wrong because the postmature fetus does not have vernix.

68. (1) Aspiration syndrome occurs commonly among postterm newborns, especially if they are postmature. Hypoxia accompanies progressive placental insufficiency with advancing gestational age. Physiologic response to hypoxia is relaxation of the anal sphincter, with release of meconium into amniotic fluid, and the fetal gasp reflex. (2) is incorrect because RDS is associated most commonly with prematurity and insufficient pulmonary surfactant. (3) is wrong because oxygen toxicity occurs over a longer period of time. (4) is wrong because bronchopulmonary dysplasia is associated with prolonged administration of oxygen at high concentrations; the time since birth is too short for the baby to develop BPD.

69. (3) Term infants may lose 5–10% of their birth weight. Arithmetic: 7×16 oz = 112 oz; 10% of 112 = 11.2 oz (317.5g). (1), (2), and (4) are wrong because of inaccurate computation.

70. (1) Physiologic jaundice is related to the inability of the liver to conjugate bilirubin liberated by normal hemolysis of fetal RBCs and polycythemia. (2) is incorrect because jaundice associated with kidney immaturity is pathologic. (3) is wrong because jaundice occurring secondary to infection is also pathologic. (4) is wrong because, although dehydration may be associated with the jaundice, it also is pathologic.

71. (3) Is unusual because milia (unopened sebaceous glands) look like *white*-heads. (1) is *typical* because enlarged breasts and pink spotting (pseudomenstruation) are effects of high circulating levels of maternal hormones. (2) is *typical* because the linea nigra *is evident* due to maternal hormones. (4) is *typical* because "mongolian spots" *are found* on the lower back and sacrum of darker-skinned people.

72. (3) Pelvic inflammatory disease is associated with adhesions and blockage of the fallopian tubes, preventing transport and joining of the ovum and sperm. (1) is incorrect because moderate alcohol intake is not implicated in female infertility. (2) is incorrect because a normal menstrual cycle is not associated with infertility. (4) is incorrect because use of a diaphragm and spermicidal jelly is not implicated in infertility.

73. (4) is correct as clomiphen citrate (Clomid) is used in infertility caused by anovulatory cycles. It increases the secretion of FSH and LH and stimulates ovulation. Side effects include vasomotor flushes, bloating, nausea, vomiting, headache, hair loss, and visual disturbances. (1) is incorrect because anovulatory cycles are not caused by past patterns of sexual behavior. (2) is incorrect because many women who experience anovulatory cycles may successfully conceive after treatment. (3) is incorrect because anovulatory cycles are not treated with surgical intervention.

74. (3) is correct because semen analysis requires that a freshly masturbated specimen be obtained after a rest period of 48 to 72 hours. (1) is incorrect because an accurate sperm count and evaluation of motility require that the specimen be examined within two hours. Refrigeration will kill sperm. (2) is incorrect because 24 hours of abstinence are insufficient for adequate production of sperm. (4) is incorrect because ice will kill sperm and reduce motility.

75. (2) Lamaze techniques, although helpful, do not guarantee freedom from discomfort throughout the labor process. (1) is incorrect because medication may be used to assist the woman in controlling her response to the childbearing process and to facilitate a successful experience. (3) is wrong because labor is easier for the woman who understands what is happening and is able to relax and cooperate. (4) is wrong because many preparation-for-childbirth courses utilize these aids.

76. (1) Painless vaginal bleeding is associated with placenta previa. (2) is wrong because abdominal pain and a tense abdomen are signs of possible abruptio placentae. (3) is wrong because painless vaginal bleeding is not indicative of preeclampsia. (4) is wrong because the uterine rupture is characterized by sudden sharp abdominal pain, signs of internal bleeding, and shock.

77. (3) Semi-Fowler's position allows the presenting part to apply pressure to the placenta. (1) is incorrect because a vaginal or rectal examination is likely to increase the separation and hemorrhage. (2) is wrong because this position does not use the presenting part as a tamponade. (4) is wrong because some women with placenta previa are able to deliver vaginally.

78. (1) The lower uterine segment does not contract as effectively as the fundus. Postpartum bleeding is more common in women with placenta previa. (2) is incorrect because this client did not have abruptio placentae. (3) is wrong because surgical removal of the placenta does not inhibit uterine contraction. (4) is wrong because a loss of 250 mL during the third stage is within normal limits.

79. (2) is the best choice because *intervention* is needed since the breathing technique recommended for transition is rapid, shallow chest breathing. (1) is not the best choice because slow, deep abdominal breathing *is advised* in the latent and early active phases of labor. (3) is not the best choice because the use of intercostal muscles with a relaxed diaphragm *is recommended*. (4) is not the best choice because each contraction *should* begin and end with two cleansing breaths in the Lamaze method.

80. (3) Significantly increased fetal activity and meconium-stained amniotic fluid are signs of fetal distress. (1) is incorrect because crowning is followed rapidly by delivery and because any fetal distress can be treated promptly. (2) is wrong because crowning is shortly followed by birth. (4) is wrong because baseline variability is a normal fetal pattern.

81. (4) Tilting the hip moves the heavy uterus off the vena cava, preventing supine hypotension, reduced placental perfusion, and fetal bradycardia. (1) is incorrect because the statement denies the need for comfort at this time. (2) is wrong because the pillows may increase her comfort but will affect supine hypotension. (3) is wrong because the statement may be perceived as a threat and does not recognize the woman's need for comfort and emotional support.

82. (3) The first priority (beside maintaining each newborn's patent airway) is body temperature. (1) is incorrect because, although important, identification of the newborns may be delayed until each infant's status is stable. (2) is wrong because the second priority is to note any abnormalities. (4) is wrong because eye prophylaxis may be delayed for 2 hours.

83. (1) The Moro reflex occurs in response to sudden stimulation of the newborn's central nervous system by noise, falling, or jolting. (2) is incorrect because this action elicits the Babinski reflex. (3) is wrong because this action elicits the tonic neck reflex. (4) is wrong because this elicits rooting.

84. (4) Epicanthal folds are associated with a diagnosis of Down syndrome. (1) is incorrect because the head is the largest part of the newborn's body and is larger than the chest. (2) is wrong because diaphragmatic breathing is the normal newborn pattern of respiration. (3) is wrong because passage of meconium stool immediately following birth is within the normal pattern for newborns.

■ UNIT

3

Nursing Care of Children and Families

■ GROWTH AND DEVELOPMENT

PEDIATRIC NURSING

I. Infant (28 days–1 year)

A. Erikson's theory of personality development

1. *Central task:* basic trust vs mistrust; central person: primary caretaker.
2. *Behavioral indicators*
   a. Crying is only means of communicating needs.
   b. Quieting usually means needs are met.
   c. Fear of strangers at 6–8 months.
3. **Parental guidance/teaching**
   a. Must meet infant's needs consistently—cannot "spoil" infant by holding, comforting.
   b. Neonatal *reflexes* fade between 4 and 6 months, replaced with increase in purposeful behavior, e.g., babbling, reaching.
   c. *Fear of strangers* is normal—indicates attachment between infant and primary caretaker.
   d. Child may repeat over and over newly learned behaviors, e.g., sitting or standing.
   e. *Weaning* can begin around the time child begins walking.
4. Additional information about behavioral concerns for each age group may be found in Tables 3.3 and 3.4.

B. Physical growth

1. *Height* (length): 50% increase by first birthday.
2. *Weight*
   a. Doubles by 6 months, triples by 1 year.
   b. Gains 5–7 oz/week in first 6 months of life.
   c. Gains 3–5 oz/week in second 6 months of life.
3. *Vital signs:* see Table 3.1.
4. *Fontanels*
   a. *Posterior*—closed by 6–8 weeks.
   b. *Anterior*—remains open through first 12 months.
5. *Teething*
   a. Generally begins around 6 months.

■ **TABLE 3.1 Normal Vital Sign Measurements, Variations With Age**

Age	Heart Rate	Respiratory Rate	Blood Pressure
Birth	140	40–90	78/42
1 year	110	20–40	96/65
3 years	105	20–30	99/65
5–6 years	95	20–25	100/65
10 years	85	17–22	110/60
15 years	82	15–20	118/60
18 years	82	15–20	120/65

Source: Lowrey GH: *Growth and Development of Children,* 7th ed., Yearbook, 1978, p. 450. St. Louis: Mosby, 1978.

TABLE 3.2 Facts About the Denver Developmental Screening Test (DDST)

Parents' Questions	Nurse's Best Response
"Will this be used as a measure of my child's IQ?"	"No, it is a screening test for your child's development."
"What ages can be tested?"	"Infants through preschoolers, *or* from birth to 6 years."
"What will they test?"	"There are four areas: personal-social, fine motor-adaptive, language, gross motor."
"Can I stay with my child?"	"Yes, in fact it is preferred you be there."
"If my child fails, does it mean he is retarded?"	"No, this is not a diagnostic tool but rather a screening test."
"If he fails, what do we do?"	"Repeat the test in a week or two."
"Why didn't my child accomplish everything?"	"He is not expected to."
"Why did my child score so poorly?"	"Perhaps it's a bad day for the child, he isn't feeling up to par, etc."

b. First two teeth: lower central incisors.

c. By 1 year: 6–8 teeth.

C. Denver Developmental Screening Test (DDST): see Table 3.2.

1. *Birth–3 months*
   a. Personal-social: smiles responsively, then spontaneously.
   b. Fine motor-adaptive:
      (1) Follows 180°, past midline.
      (2) Grasps rattle.
      (3) Reaches for objects, missing them.
   c. Language: laughs/squeals; vocalizes without crying.
   d. Gross motor: while on stomach, lifts head 45°–90°, able to hold head steady and erect; rolls over, from stomach to back.
2. *4–6 months*
   a. Personal-social: resists toy pull.
   b. Fine motor-adaptive: palmar grasp.
   c. Language: turns toward voice.
   d. Gross motor: some weight-bearing on legs; no head lag when pulled to sitting; sits with support.
3. *7–9 months*
   a. Personal-social
      (1) Initially shy with strangers.
      (2) Feeds self crackers.
      (3) Plays peek-a-boo.
      (4) Works for toy out of reach.
   b. Fine motor-adaptive: takes two cubes in hands and bangs them together; passes cube hand to hand.
   c. Language: "dada," "mama," nonspecific, babbles.
   d. Gross motor: gets self up to sitting; pulls self to standing; stands holding on.
4. *10–12 months*
   a. Personal-social
      (1) Plays pat-a-cake, ball.
      (2) Indicates wants without crying.
      (3) Drinks from cup.
   b. Fine motor-adaptive: neat pincer grasp.
   c. Language: "dada," "mama," specific.
   d. Gross motor: stands alone well; walks holding on; stoops and recovers.

D. Nursing interventions/parental guidance, teaching:

1. *Play*
   a. First year—generally solitary.
   b. Visual stimulation
      (1) Best color: red.
      (2) Toys: mirrors, brightly colored pictures.
   c. Auditory stimulation
      (1) Talk and sing to infant.
      (2) Toys: musical mobiles, rattles, bells.
   d. Tactile stimulation
      (1) Hold, pat, touch, cuddle, swaddle/keep warm; rub body with lotion, powder.
      (2) Toys: various textures; nesting and stacking; plastic milk bottle with blocks to dump in, out.
   e. Kinesthetic stimulation
      (1) Cradle, stroller, carriage, infant seat, car rides, wind-up infant swing, jumper seat, walker, furniture strategically placed for walking.
      (2) Toys: cradle gym, push-pull.
2. *Safety*
   a. *Note:* Most common accident during first twelve months is the aspiration of foreign bodies.
      (1) Keep small objects out of reach.
      (2) Use one-piece pacifier only.
      (3) *No* nuts, raisins, hot dogs.
      (4) *No* toys with small, removable parts.
      (5) *No* balloons or plastic bags.
   b. *Falls*
      (1) Raise crib rails.
      (2) *Never* place child on high surface unsupervised.
      (3) Use restraining straps in seats, swings, highchairs, etc.

c. *Poisoning*
   (1) Check that paint on toys/furniture is *lead-free.*
   (2) Treat all medications as drugs, never as "candy."
   (3) Store all poisonous substances in locked cabinet, closet.
   (4) Have phone number of poison control center on hand.
   (5) Instruct in use of syrup of ipecac (see p. 251).

d. *Burns*
   (1) *Never* use microwave oven to heat bottles.
   (2) Check temperature of bath water; *never* leave alone in bath.
   (3) Special care with cigarettes, hot liquids.
   (4) Do *not* leave infant in sun.
   (5) Cover all electrical sockets.
   (6) Keep electrical wires out of sight/reach.
   (7) Avoid tablecloths with overhang.
   (8) Put guards around heating devices.

e. *Motor vehicles*
   (1) Use only federally approved car seat for all car rides.
   (2) *Never* leave stroller behind parked car.
   (3) Do *not* allow infant to crawl near parked cars or in driveway.

II. Toddler (1–3 years)

A. Erikson's theory of personality development

1. *Central task:* autonomy vs shame and doubt; central person(s): parent(s)
2. *Behavioral indicators*
   a. Does not separate easily from parents.
   b. Negativistic.
   c. Prefers rituals and routine activities.
   d. Active physical explorer of environment.
   e. Begins attempts at self-assertion.
   f. Easily frustrated by limits.
   g. Temper tantrums.
   h. May have favorite "security object."
   i. Uses "mine" for everything—does not understand concept of sharing.
3. **Parental guidance/teaching**
   a. Avoid periods of prolonged separation if possible.
   b. Avoid constantly saying "no" to toddler.
   c. Avoid "yes"/"no" questions.
   d. Stress that child may use "no" even when he or she means "yes."
   e. Establish and maintain rituals, e.g., toilet training, going to sleep.
   f. Offer opportunities for play, *with* supervision.
   g. Allow child to feed self.
   h. Offer only allowable choices.
   i. Best method to handle temper tantrums: ignore them.
   j. Keep security object with child, if so desired.
   k. Do not force toddler "to share."
4. Additional information about behavioral concerns for each age group may be found in Tables 3.3 and 3.4.

B. Physical growth

1. *Height*
   a. Slow, steady growth at 2–4 in./year, mainly in *legs* rather than trunk.
   b. Adult height is roughly twice child's height at 2 years of age.
2. *Weight*
   a. Slow, steady growth at 4–6 pounds/year.
   b. Birth weight *quadruples* by 2½ years of age.
3. *Vital signs:* refer to Table 3.1.
4. *Anterior fontanel*—closes between 12 and 18 months.
5. *Teething*
   a. Introduce tooth brushing as a "ritual."
   b. By 30 months: all 20 primary teeth present.
   c. First dental check-up.
6. *Vision*
   a. Full binocular vision well-developed.
   b. Visual acuity of toddler: 20/40.
7. *Posture and gait*
   a. Lordosis: abdomen protrudes.
   b. Walks like a duck: wide-based gait, side-to-side.

C. DDST

1. *12–18 months*
   a. Personal-social
      (1) Imitates housework.
      (2) Uses spoon, spilling little.
      (3) Removes own clothes.
   b. Fine motor-adaptive
      (1) Scribbles spontaneously.
      (2) Builds tower with two cubes.
   c. Language
      (1) Three words other than "mama," "dada."
      (2) Points to at least one named body part.
   d. Gross motor
      (1) Kicks ball.
      (2) Walks up steps.
2. *19–24 months*
   a. Personal-social
      (1) Puts on clothing.
      (2) Washes and dries hands.
      (3) Helps with simple tasks.
   b. Fine motor-adaptive
      (1) Builds tower with four cubes.
      (2) Imitates vertical line.
   c. Language
      (1) Combines 2–3 words.
      (2) Names one picture.
      (3) Follows 2–3 directions.
   d. Gross motor

TABLE 3.3 Pediatric Behavioral Concerns: Nursing Implications and Parental Guidance

Behavioral Concern	Nursing Implications/ Parental Guidance
Teething	Begins around age 4 months—infant may seem unusually fussy and irritable but should *not* run a fever. Provide relief with teething rings, acetaminophen, topical preparations.
Thumb sucking	Need to "suck" varies: may be due to hunger, frustration, loneliness. Do *not* stop *infant* from doing this—usually stops by preschool years. If behavior persists, evaluate need for attention, peer play.
Temper tantrums	Normal in the *toddler*—occurs in response to frustration. Avoid abrupt end to play or making excessive demands. Offer only allowable choices. Once a decision is verbalized, *avoid* sudden changes of mind. Provide diversion to achieve cooperation. If it occurs, best means to handle is to *ignore* the outburst.
Toilet training	Assess child for readiness: awareness of body functions, form of mutual communication, physical control over sphincters. Use child-size seat. *No* distractions (food, toys, books). Offer praise for success *or* efforts (never shame accidents).
Discipline	*Not* for infant. Can begin with *toddler,* within limits. Be consistent and clear. *Avoid* excessively strict measures.
Sibling rivalry	Fairly common, normal. Allow older child to "help." Give each child "special" time, with individual attention.
Masturbation	Normal, common in *preschooler.* Set firm limits. Avoid overreacting.
Lying	*In preschooler:* not deliberate; child is often unable to differentiate between "real" and "lie," and by speaking something he often feels it makes a thing real. *In older child:* may indicate problems and need for professional attention if persists. Serve as role model—no "white lies."
Cursing	Avoid overreacting. Defuse use of "the word" by simply stating "not here, not now." Distract, change subject, substitute activity. Serve as role model by own language.
"Accidents" (enuresis)	*Occasional*—common and normal through preschool. *If frequent*—need complete physical exam to rule out pathology. "Training": after dinner—avoid fluids; before bed—toilet (perhaps awaken once during night). *Never* put back into diapers or attempt to shame.
Smoking/drinking	May begin in *older schoolage* child or adolescent. Serve as role model with own habits.

(1) Throws ball overhand.
(2) Jumps in place.

3. *2–3 years*
   a. Personal-social
      (1) Dresses with supervision.
      (2) Plays interactive games (e.g., tag).
   b. Fine motor-adaptive
      (1) Copies circle.
      (2) Builds tower of 8 cubes.
   c. Language
      (1) Uses plurals.
      (2) Gives first and last name.
   d. Gross motor
      (1) Balances on one foot briefly.
      (2) Pedals tricycle.

D. Nursing interventions/parental guidance:

1. *Play:* toddler years—generally parallel.
2. Toys—stimulate multiple senses simultaneously:
   a. Push-pull.
   b. Riding toys, e.g., straddle horse or car.
   c. Small, low slide or gym.
   d. Balls, in various sizes.
   e. Blocks—multiple shapes, sizes, colors.
   f. Dolls, trucks, dress-up clothes.
   g. Drums, horns, cymbals, xylophones, toy piano.
   h. Pounding board and hammer, clay.

■ **TABLE 3.4 Pediatric Sleep and Rest Norms: Nursing Implications and Parental Guidance**

Pediatric Sleep and Rest Norms	Nursing Implications/Parental Guidance
Infant: 16–20 hours/day	No set schedule can be predetermined.
3 months: nocturnal pattern.	If waking at night after age 3 months, investigate hunger as a probable cause.
6 months: 1–2 naps, with 12 hours at night.	Monitor behavior to determine sleep needs: alert and active? growing, developing?
12 months: 1 nap, with 12 hours at night.	Routine fairly well established.
Toddler: 12–14 hours/night	
"Dawdles" at bedtime.	Set firm, realistic limits.
Dependency on security object.	Place favorite blanket or toy in crib/bed.
May ask to sleep with bottle.	**Avoid** "bottle mouth syndrome" (caries).
May rebel against going to sleep.	Establish bedtime "ritual."
Preschool: 10–12 hours/night	May regress in behavior when tired.
Gives up afternoon nap.	Provide "quiet time" in place of nap.
Difficulty falling asleep/nighttime waking.	Avoid overstimulation in evening.
Fear of dark.	Leave night-light on, door open.
Enuresis.	Occasional accidents are normal.
May begin to have nightmares.	Comfort child but leave in own bed.
School-age: 8–12 hours/night	
Nightmares common.	Comfort child but leave in own bed.
Awakens early in morning.	Important that child play/relax before school.
May not be aware he/she is tired.	Remind about bedtime.
Likes to stay up late.	"Privilege" of later bedtime can be "awarded" as child gets older.
Slumber parties.	Permit, as good opportunity to socialize.
Adolescent: 10–14 hours/night	Needs vary greatly among individuals.
Need for sleep increases greatly.	Rapid growth rate.
May complain of excessive fatigue.	Related to rapid growth and overall increased activity.

i. Finger paints, chalk and board, thick crayons.
j. Wooden puzzles with large pieces.
k. Toy record player with kiddie records.
l. Talking toys: dolls, see 'n say, phones.
m. Sand, water, soap bubbles.
n. Picture books, photo albums.
o. Nursery rhymes, songs, music.

3. *Safety*
   a. Accidents are the number-one cause of death among toddlers.
   b. *Motor vehicles:* most accidental deaths in children under age 3 are related to motor vehicles.
      (1) Use only federally approved car seat for all car rides, through age 4 or 40 pounds.
      (2) Follow manufacturer directions carefully.
      (3) Make car seat part of routine for toddler.
   c. *Poisonings:* most common in 2-year-olds.
      (1) Consider every nonfood substance a hazard and place out of child's sight/reach.
      (2) Keep all medications, cleaning materials, etc. in clearly marked containers in locked cabinets.
      (3) Instruct in use of syrup of ipecac (see p. 251).
   d. *Burns*
      (1) Turn pot handles *in* when on stove top.
      (2) Do *not* allow child to play with electrical appliances.
      (3) Decrease water temperature in house to avoid scald burns.
   e. *Falls*
      (1) Provide barriers on open windows.
      (2) Avoid gates on stairs—child can strangle on gate.
      (3) Move from crib to bed.
   f. *Choking:* avoid food on which child might choke:
      (1) Fish with bones.
      (2) Fruit with seeds or pits.
      (3) Nuts, raisins.
      (4) Hot dogs.

(5) Chewing gum.
(6) Hard candy.

g. *Water safety*
(1) Always supervise child near water: tub, pool, jacuzzi, lake, ocean.
(2) Keep bathroom locked to prevent drowning in toilet.

III. Preschooler (3–5 years)

A. Erikson's theory of personality development

1. *Central task:* initiative vs guilt; central person(s): basic family unit.
2. *Behavioral indicators*
a. Attempts to perform activities of daily living (ADL) independently.
b. Attempts to make things for self/others.
c. Tries to "help."
d. Talks constantly: verbal exploration of the world ("Why?").
e. Extremely active, highly creative imagination: fantasy and magical thinking.
f. May demonstrate fears: "monsters," dark rooms, etc.
g. Able to tolerate short periods of separation.
3. **Parental guidance/teaching**
a. Encourage child to dress self by providing simple clothing.
b. Remind to go to bathroom (tends to "forget").
c. Assign small, simple tasks or errands.
d. Answer questions patiently, simply; do *not* offer child more information than he or she is asking for.
e. Normal to have "imaginary playmates."
f. Offer realistic support and reassurance with regard to fears.
g. Expose to a variety of experiences: zoo, train ride, shopping, sleigh riding, etc.
h. Enroll in preschool/nursery school program; kindergarten at 5 years.
4. Additional information about behavioral concerns for each age group may be found in Tables 3.3 and 3.4.

B. Physical growth

1. *Height and weight*
a. Continued slow, steady growth.
b. Generally grows more in *height* than weight.
c. Posture: appears taller and thinner; "lordosis" of toddler gradually *disappears*.
2. *Vital signs:* see Table 3.1.
3. *Teeth*
a. *All* 20 "baby teeth" present.
b. Annual dental check-ups, daily brushing.
4. *Vision*
a. Visual acuity: 20/30 between 3 and 5 years.
b. Do vision/hearing screening prekindergarten.

C. DDST/developmental norms

1. *3 years*
a. Personal-social
(1) Can button clothing.
(2) Separates from mother easily.
b. Fine motor-adaptive
(1) Picks longer of two lines.
(2) Copies circle, intersecting lines.
(3) Beginning to use scissors.
c. Language
(1) Comprehends "cold," "tired," "hungry."
(2) Comprehends prepositions: "over," "under."
(3) Recognizes colors.
d. Gross motor
(1) Broad jumps, jumps in place.
(2) Balances on one foot.
2. *4 years*
a. Personal-social
(1) Brushes own teeth, combs own hair.
(2) Dresses without supervision.
(3) Knows own age and birthday.
(4) Eats with fork.
(5) Ties own shoes.
b. Fine motor-adaptive
(1) Draws person with three body parts.
(2) Better use of scissors.
c. Language
(1) Knows opposite analogies (2 of 3).
(2) Defines words (6 of 9).
(3) Follows simple directions.
d. Gross motor
(1) Hops on one foot.
(2) Catches bounced ball.
(3) Can walk heel-to-toe.
3. *5 years*
a. Personal-social
(1) Interested in money.
(2) Knows days of week, seasons.
b. Fine motor-adaptive
(1) Prints name.
(2) Draws person with six body parts.
c. Language
(1) Counts to 10.
(2) Verbalizes number sequences (e.g., phone number).
d. Gross motor
(1) Attempts to ride bike.
(2) Rollerskates, jumps rope, bounces ball.
(3) Backward heel–toe walk.

D. Nursing interventions/parental guidance:

1. *Play:* preschool years—associative and cooperative.
a. Likes to play house, "work," school, firehouse.
b. "Arts and crafts": color, draw, paint, dot-to-dot, color by number, cut and paste, simple sewing kits.

PEDIATRIC NURSING

c. Ball, roller skate, jumprope, jacks.
d. Swimming.
e. Puzzles, blocks (e.g., Lego's).
f. Tricycle, then bike (with/without training wheels).
g. Simple card games and board games.
h. Costumes and dress-up: "make-believe."

2. *Safety:* Emphasis now shifts from protective supervision to teaching simple safety rules. Preschoolers are "the great imitators" of parents, who serve as role models now.
a. Teach child car/*street* safety rules.
b. Change to "child booster seat" in car at 4 years or 40 pounds.
c. Teach child not to go with strangers or accept gifts or candy from strangers.
d. Teach child danger of *fire,* matches, flame: "drop and roll."
e. Teach child rules of *water* safety; provide swimming lessons.
f. Provide adult supervision, frequent checks on activity/location. Despite safety teaching, preschooler is still a child and may be unreliable.

IV. School age (6–12 years)

A. Erikson's theory of personality development

1. *Central task:* industry vs inferiority; central person(s): school, neighborhood friend(s).
2. *Behavioral indicators*
a. Moving toward complete independence in ADL.
b. May be very competitive—wants to achieve in school, at play.
c. Likes to be alone occasionally, may seem shy.
d. Prefers friends and peers to siblings.
3. *Parental guidance/teaching*
a. Be accepting of the child as he or she *is.*
b. Offer consistent support and guidance.
c. Avoid authoritative or excessive demands on child.
d. Respect need for privacy.
e. Assign household tasks, errands, chores.
4. Additional information about behavioral concerns for each age group may be found in Tables 3.3 and 3.4.

B. Physical growth

1. *Height and weight*
a. Almost *doubles* in weight from 6–12 years.
b. Period of slow, steady growth.
c. 1–2 inches per year.
d. 3–6 pounds per year.
e. Girls and boys differ very little in size.
2. *Vital signs:* refer to Table 3.1.
3. *Teeth*
a. Begins to lose primary teeth.
b. Eruption of permanent teeth, including molars; 26 permanent teeth by age 12 years.
c. Dental screening annually, daily brushing.
4. *Vision and hearing*
a. Should be screened annually—usually in school.
b. 20/20 vision well established between 9 and 11 years.
5. *Pubescence* (preliminary physical changes of adolescence)
a. Average age of onset: girls at 10, boys at 12.
b. Beginning of growth spurt.
c. Some sexual changes may start to occur.

C. DDST/developmental norms

1. *6–8 years*
a. Dramatic, exuberant, boundless energy.
b. Alternating periods: quiet, private behavior.
c. Conscientious, punctual.
d. Wants to care for own needs but needs reminders, supervision.
e. Oriented to time and space.
f. Learns to read, tell time, follow map.
g. Interested in money—asks for "allowance."
h. Eagerly anticipates upcoming events, trips.
i. Can ride bike, swim, play ball.
2. *9–11 years*
a. Worries over tasks; takes things seriously, yet also developing sense of humor—likes to tell jokes.
b. Keeps room, clothes, toys relatively tidy.
c. Enjoys physical activity, has great stamina.
d. Very enthusiastic at work and play; has lots of energy—may fidget, drum fingers, tap foot.
e. Wants to work to earn money: mow lawn, babysit, deliver papers.
f. Loves secrets (secret clubs).
g. Very well behaved outside own home (or with company).
h. Uses tools, equipment; follows directions, recipes.
i. By twelfth birthday: paradoxical stormy behavior, onset of adolescent conflicts.

D. Nursing interventions/parental guidance:

1. *Play*
a. Wants to win, likes competitive games.
b. Prefers to play with same-sex children.
c. Enjoys group, team play.
d. Loves to do magic tricks and other "show-off" activities (e.g., puppet shows, plays, singing).
e. Likes to collect things: cards, records.
f. Simple scientific experiments, computer games.
g. Hobbies: needlework, woodwork, models.
h. Enjoys pop music, musical instruments, radio, audio tapes, videos, posters.
2. *Safety*—motor vehicles
a. As passenger: teach to wear safety belt, not distract driver.
b. As pedestrian: teach bike, street safety.
c. Teach how to swim, rules of water safety.
d. Sports: teach safety rules.
e. Adult supervision still necessary; serve as role model for safe activities.

f. Suggest Red Cross courses on first aid, water safety, babysitting, etc.

V. Adolescent (12–18 years)

A. Erikson's theory of personality development

1. *Central task:* identity vs role confusion; central person(s): peer group.
2. *Behavioral indicators*
   a. Changes in body image related to sexual development.
   b. Awkward and uncoordinated.
   c. Much interest in opposite sex: females become romantic.
   d. Wants to be exactly like peers.
   e. Becomes hostile toward parents, adults, family.
   f. Concerned with vocation, life after high school.
3. *Parental guidance, teaching*
   a. Offer firm but realistic limits on behavior.
   b. Continue to offer guidance, support.
   c. Allow child to earn own money, control own finances.
   d. Assist adolescent to develop positive self-image.
4. Additional information about behavioral concerns for each age group may be found in Tables 3.3 and 3.4.

B. Physical growth

1. *Height and weight*
   a. Adolescent growth spurt lasts 24–36 months.
   b. Growth in height commonly *ceases* at 16–17 years in girls, 18–20 years in boys.
   c. Boys gain more weight than girls, are generally taller and heavier.
2. *Vital signs* approximately those of the adult. See Table 3.1.
3. *Teeth:* 32 permanent teeth by 18–21 years.
4. *Sexual changes*
   a. *Females*
      (1) Increase in transverse diameter of pelvis.
      (2) Enlargement of breasts.
      (3) Change in vaginal secretions.
      (4) Growth of pubic hair.
      (5) Menstruation—12½ years (average).
      (6) Growth of axillary hair.
      (7) Ovulation.
   b. *Males*
      (1) Enlargement of genitalia.
      (2) Swelling of breasts.
      (3) Growth of pubic, axillary, facial, and body hair.
      (4) Lowering of voice.
      (5) Production of sperm—14½ years (average).

C. Developmental norms

1. *Motor development*
   a. *Early (12–15 years)*—awkward, uncoordinated, poor posture, decrease in energy and stamina.
   b. *Later (15–18 years)*—increased coordination and better posture; more energy and stamina.
2. *Cognitive*
   a. Academic ability and interest vary greatly.
   b. "Think about thinking"—period of introspection.
3. *Emotional*
   a. Same-sex best friend, leading to strong friendship bonds.
   b. Highly romantic period for boys and girls.
   c. May be moody, unpredictable, inconsistent.
4. *Social*
   a. Periods of highs and lows, sociability and loneliness.
   b. Turmoil with parents—related to changing roles, desire for increased independence.
   c. Peer group is important socializing agent—conformity increases sense of belonging.
   d. Friendships: same sex best friend advancing to heterosexual "relationships."

D. Nursing interventions/parental guidance:

1. *Play*
   a. School-related group activities and sports.
   b. Develops talents, skills, and abilities.
   c. Television—watches soap operas, romantic movies, sports.
   d. Develops interest in art, writing, poetry, musical instrument.
   e. Girls: increased interest in make-up and clothes.
   f. Boys: increased interest in mechanical and electrical devices.
2. *Safety*—motor vehicles (cars and motorcycles)—as *passenger* or as *driver*
   a. Encourage driver education; serve as positive role model.
   b. Teach rules of safety for water sports.
   c. Wants to earn money but still needs guidance: advocate safe job, reasonable hours.

DEVELOPMENTAL DISABILITIES

I. Down syndrome

A. *Introduction:* Down syndrome (trisomy 21; mongolism) is a chromosomal abnormality involving an extra chromosome #21 and resulting in 47 chromosomes instead of the normal 46 chromosomes. As a consequence, the child usually presents with varying degrees of mental retardation, characteristic facial and physical features, and other congenital anomalies. Down syndrome is the most common chromosomal disorder, occurring in approximately 1 of 650 live births. Perinatal risk factors include advanced maternal age, especially with the first pregnancy; paternal age has not been proven a related factor.

B. Assessment:

1. *Physical characteristics*
   a. Brachycephalic (small, round *head*) with oblique palpebral fissures (Oriental *eyes*) and Brushfield's spots (speckling of *iris*)—flat *nasal* bridge and small, low-set *ears*.
   b. Mouth

(1) Small oral cavity with protruding tongue causes difficulty sucking and swallowing.

(2) Delayed eruption/misalignment of teeth.

c. Hands

(1) Clinodactyly—in-curved little finger.

(2) Simian crease—transverse palmar crease.

d. Muscles: hypotonic ("floppy baby") with hyperextensible joints.

e. Skin: dry, cracked.

2. Genetic studies reveal an extra chromosome #21 ("trisomy 21").

3. *Intellectual characteristics*

a. Mental retardation—varying degrees.

b. Most fall within "trainable" range, or IQ = 36–51 ("moderate mental retardation").

4. *Congenital anomalies/diseases*

a. 40% have congenital heart defects: mortality rates highest in patients with Down syndrome and cyanotic heart disease.

b. GI: tracheoesophageal fistula, Hirschsprung's disease.

c. Visual defects: cataracts, strabismus.

d. Increased incidence of leukemia.

5. *Growth and development*

a. Slow growth, especially in height.

b. Delay in developmental milestones.

6. *Sexual development*

a. Delayed or incomplete.

b. Females—few have babies.

c. Males—assumed to be sterile.

7. *Aging*

a. Premature aging, with shortened life expectancy.

b. Death usually before age 40—generally related to respiratory complication: repeated infections, pneumonia, lung disease.

C. Analysis/nursing diagnosis:

1. *Ineffective airway clearance/potential for aspiration* related to hypotonia.

2. *Altered nutrition, more than or less than body requirements,* related to hypotonia and/or congenital anomalies.

3. *Altered growth and development* related to Down syndrome.

4. *Self-care deficit* related to Down syndrome.

5. *Altered family processes* related to birth of an infant with a congenital defect.

6. *Knowledge deficit* related to Down syndrome.

D. Nursing plan/implementation:

1. Goal: *prevent physical complications.*

a. Respiratory

(1) Use bulb syringe to clear nose, mouth.

(2) Vaporizer.

(3) Frequent position changes.

(4) Avoid contact with people with upper respiratory infections.

b. Aspiration

(1) Small, more frequent feedings.

(2) Burp well during/after infant feedings.

(3) Allow sufficient time to eat.

(4) *Position after meals*: head of bed elevated, right side—or on stomach, with head to side.

c. Observe for signs and symptoms of heart disease, constipation/GI obstruction, leukemia, skin breakdown.

2. Goal: *meet nutritional needs.*

a. Suction (before meals) to clear airway.

b. Adapt feeding techniques to meet special needs of infant/child; e.g., use long, straight-handled spoon.

c. Monitor height and weight.

d. As child grows, monitor caloric intake (tends toward obesity).

e. Offer foods high in bulk to prevent constipation related to hypotonia.

3. Goal: *promote optimal growth and development.*

a. Encourage parents to enroll infant/toddler in early stimulation program and to follow through with suggested exercises at home.

b. Preschool/school-age: special education classes.

c. Screen frequently, using DDST to monitor development.

d. Help parents focus on "normal" or positive aspects of infant/child.

e. Help parents work toward realistic goals with their child.

4. Goal: *health teaching.*

a. Explain that tongue-thrust behavior is normal and that food should be re-fed.

b. Before adolescence—counsel parents and child about delay in sexual development, decreased libido, marriage and family relations.

c. In severe cases assist parents to deal with issue of placement/institutionalization.

E. Evaluation:

1. Physical complications are prevented.

2. Adequate nutrition is maintained.

3. Child attains optimal level of growth and development.

II. Attention deficit disorder (ADD); behavioral disorder (DSM-III-R)

A. *Introduction:* As defined by the APA, this diagnostic term includes hyperactivity, learning disabilities, and minimal brain dysfunction. The exact cause and pathophysiology remain unknown. The major symptoms include a greatly shortened attention span and difficulty in integrating and synthesizing information. This disorder is most common in boys, with onset before age 7; the diagnosis is based on the child's history rather than any specific diagnostic test.

B. Assessment:

1. Hyperactivity

a. Greater than average degree of activity.

b. Behavior is random, disorganized, nongoal-directed.

c. Easily distracted.

d. "Clumsy"—poor motor coordination.

2. Impulsiveness

a. Acts before thinking.

b. Aggressive/destructive.

c. Accident prone.

d. Unable to wait.

e. Labile emotions.

3. Perceptual deficits: vision and hearing.

4. Negative self-concept, reinforced by family and/or school.

C. Analysis/nursing diagnosis:

1. *Altered thought processes* related to inattention and impulsiveness.

2. *Impaired physical mobility* related to hyperactivity.

3. *Potential for injury* related to impulsivity.

4. *Self-esteem disturbance* related to hyperactivity and impulsivity.

5. *Knowledge deficit* related to behavioral modification program, medications, and follow-up care.

D. Nursing plan/implementation:

1. Goal: *teach family and child about ADD.*

a. Provide complete explanation about disorder, probable course, treatment, and prognosis.

b. Answer questions directly, simply.

c. Encourage family to verbalize; offer support.

2. Goal: *provide therapeutic environment* using principles of behavior modification.

a. Reduce extraneous or distracting stimuli.

b. Reduce stress by decreasing environmental expectations (home, school).

c. Provide firm, consistent limits.

d. Special education programs.

e. Special attention to safety needs.

3. Goal: *reduce symptoms by means of prescribed medication.*

a. Medications: Ritalin and Cylert—both are CNS stimulants but have a paradoxical calming effect on the child's behavior.

b. Health teaching (child *and* parents).

(1) Need to take medication regularly, as ordered. Avoid taking medication late in the day as it may cause insomnia.

(2) Need for long-term administration, with decreased need as child nears adolescence.

4. Goal: *provide safe outlet for excess energy.*

a. Alternate planned periods of outdoor play with school work or quiet indoor play.

b. Channel energies toward safe, large-muscle activities: running track, swimming, bike riding, hiking.

E. Evaluation:

1. Family and child verbalize understanding of "attention deficit disorders."

2. Therapeutic environment enhances socially acceptable behavior.

3. Medication taken regularly, with behavioral improvements noted.

4. Excess energy directed appropriately.

5. Dietary modification implemented.

■ PSYCHO-SOCIAL-CULTURAL FUNCTIONS

Refer to Table 3.5 for information on the nursing care of hospitalized infants and children as it relates to key developmental differences.

■ DISORDERS AFFECTING FLUID-GAS TRANSPORT

CARDIOVASCULAR DISORDERS

Congenital Heart Disease (CHD)

I. *Introduction:* There are well over 100 documented types of congenital heart defects, which occur in 8 to 10 per 1000 live births. For the purpose of this review, only six *major* defects are given. These are presented in Figures 3.1 through 3.6. *Note:* The content has been synthesized for ease in review and recall; for additional study aids, the student may wish to refer to Tables 3.6 and 3.7. Unit 4 also contains information on congestive heart failure, and Unit 6 covers the most commonly used drugs, including digoxin and lasix.

II. Assessment:

A. Exact cause unknown, but related factors include:

1. Familial history of CHD, especially in siblings, parents.

2. Presence of other genetic defects in infant, e.g., Down syndrome, trisomy 13 or 18.

3. History of maternal prenatal infection with rubella, cytomegalovirus, etc.

4. High-risk maternal factors:

a. Age: under 18, over 40 years.

b. Weight: under 100, over 200 pounds.

5. Maternal history of drinking during pregnancy, with resultant "fetal alcohol syndrome."

B. Most frequent parental complaint: difficulty feeding.

1. Infant must be awakened to feed.

2. Has weak suck.

3. May turn blue when eating, especially with cyanotic defects.

4. Infant takes overly long time to feed.

5. Falls asleep during feeding, without finishing.

C. Nursing observations

1. Most frequent symptom—tachycardia, as body attempts to compensate for lack of oxygen (hypoxia), i.e., heart rate over 160 bpm.

■ TABLE 3.5 Nursing Care of Hospitalized Infants and Children: Key Developmental Differences

Age	Assessment: Reaction to Hospitalization	Nursing Plan/Implementation: Key Nursing Behaviors
Infant	Difficult to assess needs, pain.	Close observation, need to look at behavioral cues.
	Wants primary caretaker.	Rooming-in.
Toddler	Separation anxiety.	Rooming-in.
	Frustration, loss of autonomy.	Punching bag, pounding board, clay.
	Regression.	Behavior modification.
	Fears intrusive procedures.	Axillary temperatures.
Preschooler	Fearful.	Therapeutic play with puppets, dolls.
	Fantasy about illness/hospitalization (may feel punished, abandoned).	Therapeutic play with puppets, dolls.
	Peak of body mutilation fear.	Care with dressings, casts, IMs.
	Behavior problems: aggressive, manipulative.	Clear, consistent limits.
	Regression.	Behavior modification.
School age	Cooperative.	Use diagrams, models to teach.
	Quiet, may withdraw.	Indirect interview: tell story, draw picture.
	May complain of being bored.	Involve in competitive game with peer. Encourage peers to call, send get well cards, and visit.
	Fears loss of control.	Provide privacy; allow to make some decisions.
	Competitive—afraid of 'failing."	Provide tutor p.r.n.; get books and homework.
Adolescent	Difficulty with body image.	Provide own clothes; give realistic feedback.
	Does not want to be separated from peers.	Phone in room; liberal visiting; teen lounge.
	Rebellious behavior.	Set clear rules; form teen "rap groups."

2. Tachypnea, corresponding to heart rate, i.e., respirations over 60/minute.
3. Cyanosis due to hypoxia:
   a. Not with acyanotic defects (unless CHF is present).
   b. Always with cyanotic defects ("blue babies").
4. Failure to grow at a normal rate, i.e., slow weight gain, height and weight below the norm due to difficulty feeding and hypoxia.
5. Developmental delays related to weakened physical condition.
6. Frequent respiratory infections associated with increased pulmonary blood flow and/or aspiration.
7. Dyspnea on exertion due to hypoxia, shunting of blood.
8. Murmurs may or may not be present, e.g., PDA—machinery murmur.
9. Changes in blood pressure, e.g., coarctation-increased blood pressure in arms; decreased blood pressure in legs.
10. Possible congestive heart failure—refer to Unit 4. *Note:* infants may *not* demonstrate distended neck veins.
11. Cyanotic heart defects
    a. "Tet. spells"—choking spells with paroxysmal dyspnea: severe hypoxia, deepening cyanosis; relieved by squatting, or placing infant in knee-chest position, which alters cardiopulmonary dynamics, thus increasing the flow of blood to the lungs.
    b. Clubbing of fingers and toes—due to chronic hypoxia.
    c. Polycythemia (↑ RBC) with possible thrombi/emboli formation.

III. Analysis/nursing diagnosis:

A. *Ineffective breathing pattern* related to tachypnea and respiratory infection.

B. *Activity intolerance* related to tachycardia and hypoxia.

C. *Altered nutrition, less than body requirements,* related to difficulty in feeding.

D. *Potential for infection* related to poor nutritional status.

E. *Knowledge deficit* related to diagnostic procedures, condition, surgical/medical treatments, prognosis.

IV. Nursing plan/implementation:

A. Goal: *promote adequate oxygenation.*

1. Administer oxygen per physician's order/p.r.n.
2. Use loose-fitting clothing; pin diapers loosely to avoid pressure on abdominal organs, which could impinge on diaphragm and impede respiration.

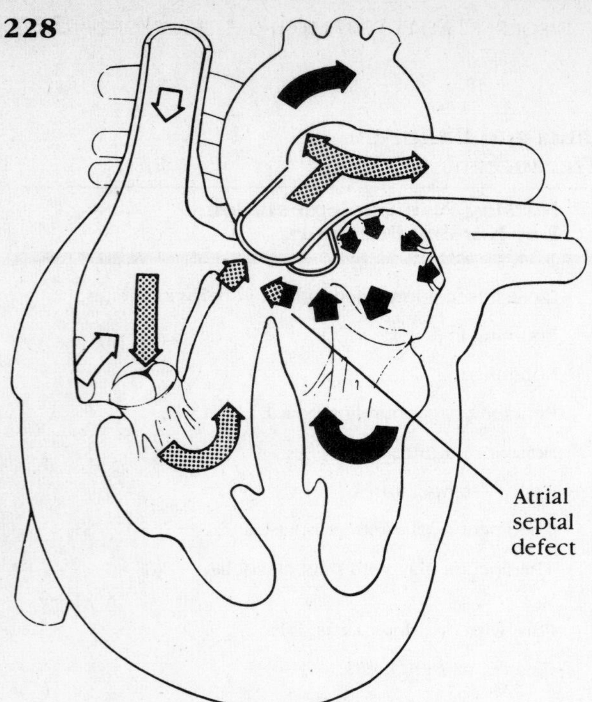

■ **FIGURE 3.1**
Atrial septal defect (ASD). A "hole in the heart," or an abnormal opening between the right and left atria. *White arrow,* unoxygenated blood; *solid arrow,* oxygenated blood; *speckled arrow,* mixed blood. (From Mott SR, Fazekas NF, James SR: *Nursing Care of Children and Families: A Holistic Approach,* Addison-Wesley, Menlo Park, CA, 1985, with permission.)

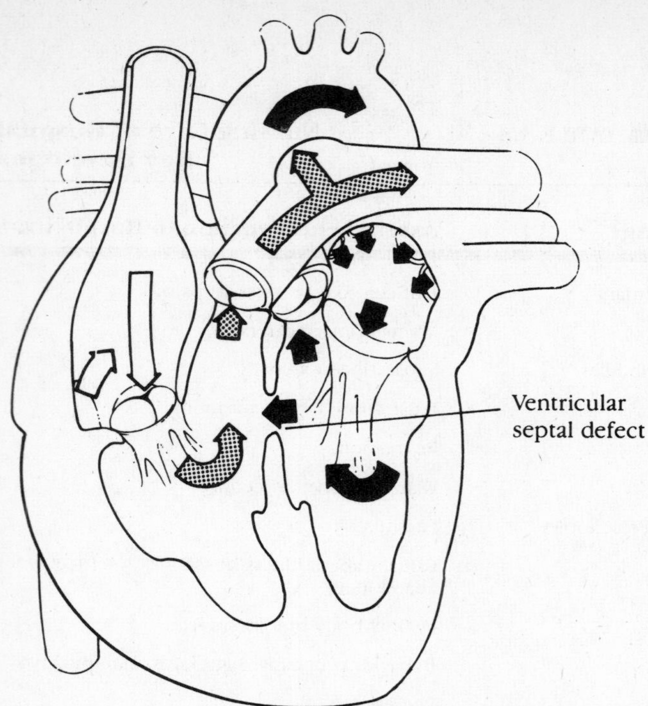

■ **FIGURE 3.2**
Ventricular septal defect (VSD). A "hole in the heart," or an abnormal opening between the right and left ventricles. *White arrow,* unoxygenated blood; *solid arrow,* oxygenated blood; *speckled arrow,* mixed blood. (From Mott SR, Fazekas, NF, James SR: *Nursing Care of Children and Families: A Holistic Approach,* Addison-Wesley, Menlo Park, CA, 1985, with permission.)

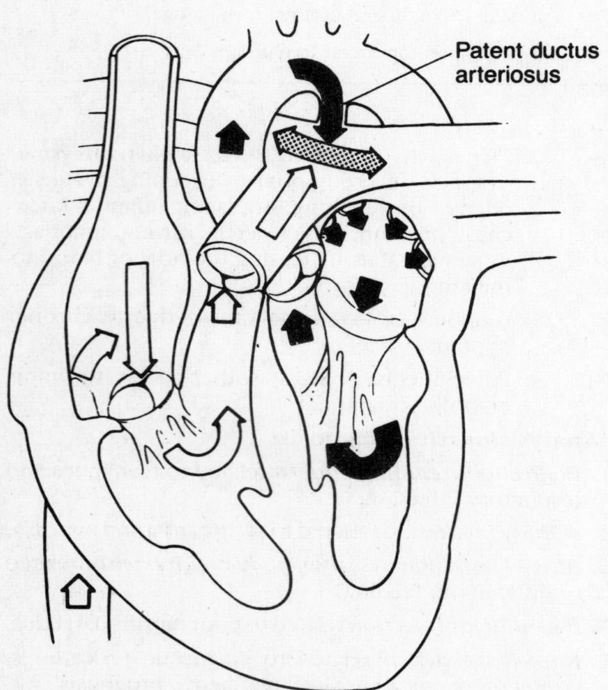

■ **FIGURE 3.3**
Patent ductus arteriosus (PDA). The ductus between the aorta and the pulmonary artery remains open (or patent). *White arrow,* unoxygenated blood; *solid arrow,* oxygenated blood; *speckled arrow,* mixed blood. (From Mott SR, Fazekas NF, James SR: *Nursing Care of Children and Families: A Holistic Approach,* Addison-Wesley, Menlo Park, CA, 1985, with permission.)

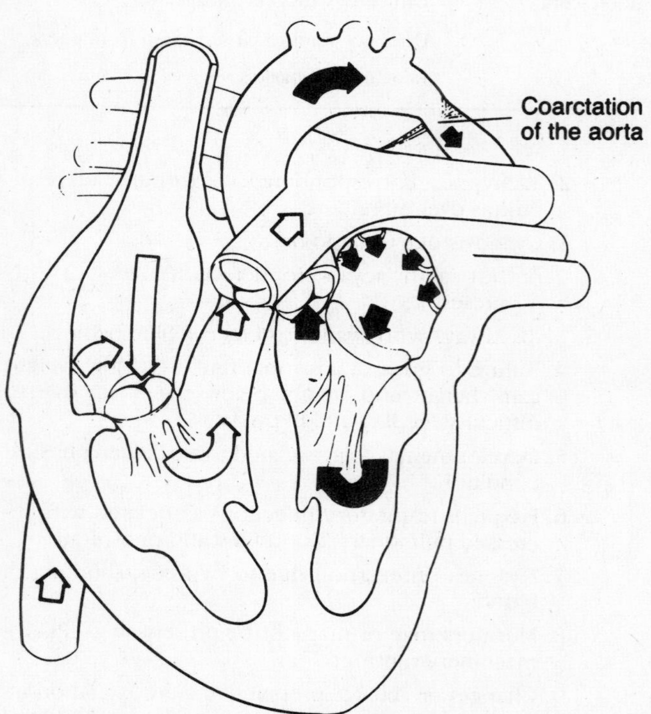

■ **FIGURE 3.4**
Coarctation of the aorta. A narrowing of the lumen of the vessel (the aorta). *White arrow,* unoxygenated blood; *solid arrow,* oxygenated blood; *speckled arrow,* mixed blood. (From Mott SR, Fazekas NF, James SR: *Nursing Care of Children and Families: A Holistic Approach,* Addison-Wesley, Menlo Park, CA, 1985, with permission.)

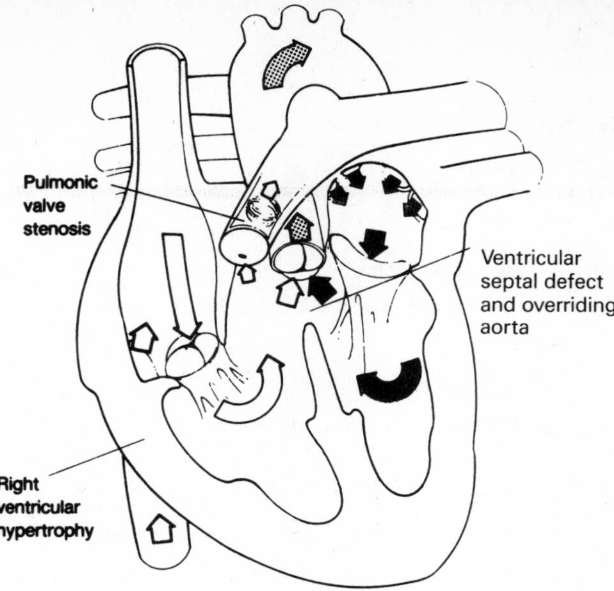

■ FIGURE 3.5
Tetralogy of Fallot. Four defects that occur together: ventricular septal defect, overriding aorta, pulmonic stenosis, right ventricular hypertrophy. *White arrow,* unoxygenated blood; *solid arrow,* oxygenated blood; *speckled arrow,* mixed blood. (From Mott SR, Fazekas NF, James SR: *Nursing Care of Children and Families: A Holistic Approach,* Addison-Wesley, Menlo Park, CA, 1985, with permission.)

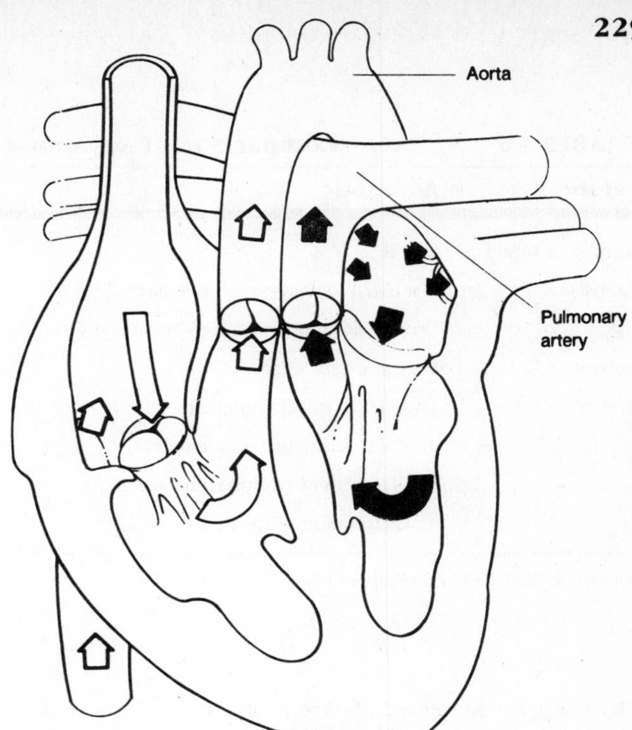

■ FIGURE 3.6
Transposition of the great arteries. The pulmonary artery arises from the left ventricle, and the aorta arises from the right ventricle. *White arrow,* unoxygenated blood; *solid arrow,* oxygenated blood (From Mott SR, Fazekas NF, James SR: *Nursing Care of Children and Families: A Holistic Approach,* Addison-Wesley, Menlo Park, CA, 1985, with permission.)

3. *Position*: neck slightly hyperextended to keep airway patent; place in knee–chest (squatting) position to relieve "Tet. spell" (choking spell).
4. Suction p.r.n. to clear the airway.
5. Administer digoxin, per physician's order, to slow and strengthen heart's pumping action (refer to Unit 6 and to Table 3.1 for pediatric pulse rate norms).

B. Goal: *reduce workload of heart to conserve energy.*

1. *Position*: infant seat, semi-Fowler's to provide maximum expansion of the lungs.
2. Provide pacifier to promote psychological rest.
3. Organize nursing care to provide periods of uninterrupted rest.
4. Adjust physical activity according to child's condition, capabilities to conserve energy.
5. Provide diversion, as tolerated, to meet developmental needs yet conserve energy.
6. Avoid extremes of temperature to avoid the stress of hypothermia/hyperthermia, which will increase the body's demand for oxygen.
7. Administer diuretics (lasix), per physician's order, to eliminate excess fluids, which increase the work load of the heart. *Note:* Refer to Unit 6.

C. Goal: *provide for adequate nutrition.*

1. Offer low-sodium formula (Lonalac) to minimize fluid retention.
2. Discourage foods with high or added sodium to minimize fluid retention.
3. I&O, daily/weekly weights, and monitor for rate of growth.
4. ▶ Supplement PO feeding with gavage feeding (p.r.n. with physician's order) to meet fluid and caloric needs.
5. Encourage foods high in potassium (prevent hypokalemia) and high in iron (prevent anemia). *Note:* refer to Unit 5.

D. Goal: *prevent infection.*

1. Universal precautions to prevent infection.
2. Use good handwashing technique.
3. Limit contact with staff/visitors with infections.
4. Monitor for early symptoms and signs of infection; report stat.

E. Goal: *meet teaching needs of patient, family.*

1. ▶ Explain diagnostic procedures: blood tests, X rays, urine, ECG, echocardiogram, cardiac catheterization.
2. Explain condition/treatment/prognosis. Refer to Table 3.7.
3. Review dietary restrictions, medications.
4. Discuss how to realistically adjust to life with congenital heart disease, activity restrictions, etc.

V. Evaluation:

A. Child's level of oxygenation is maintained, as evidenced by pink color in nailbeds and mucous membranes (for both light- and dark-skinned children) and ease in respiratory effort.

TABLE 3.6 Comparison of Acyanotic and Cyanotic Heart Disease

Feature	Acyanotic	Cyanotic
Shunting of blood	L → R.	R → L.
Cyanosis	Not usual (unless congestive heart failure).	Always; "blue babies."
Surgery	Usually done in one stage—technically simple.	Usually done in several stages—technically complex.
Prognosis	Very good/excellent.	Guarded.
Major types	1. ASD (atrial septal defect).	1. Tetralogy of Fallot.
	2. VSD (ventricular septal defect).	2. Transposition of the great vessels.
	3. PDA (Patent ductus arteriosus).	
	4. Coarctation of the aorta.	

B. Energy is conserved, thus reducing the workload of the heart, as evidenced by vital signs within normal limits.

C. The child's fluid and caloric requirements are met, allowing for physical growth to occur at normal or near-normal rate.

D. The family (and child, when old enough) verbalize their understanding of the type of CHD, its treatment and prognosis.

E. The family and child demonstrate adequate coping mechanisms to deal with CHD.

DISORDERS OF THE BLOOD

I. Leukemia

A. *Introduction:* Known as "cancer of the blood," leukemia is the most common form of childhood cancer, with an incidence of 4 per 100,000. Acute leukemia is basically a malignant proliferation of white-blood-cell (WBC) precursors triggered by an unknown cause and affecting all blood-forming organs and systems throughout the body. The onset is typically insidious, and the disease is most common in preschoolers (age 3–5 years).

B. Assessment

1. Major problem—leukopenia: ↓ WBC/↑ blasts (overproduction of immature, poorly functioning white blood cells).
2. Bone marrow dysfunction results in:
   a. *Neutropenia:* multiple prolonged infections.
   b. *Anemia:* pallor, weakness, irritability, shortness of breath.
   c. *Thrombocytopenia:* bleeding tendencies (petechiae, epistaxis, bruising).
3. Infiltration of reticuloendothelial system (RES): hepatosplenomegaly → abdominal pain, lymphadenopathy.
4. Leukemic invasion of CNS: ↑ ICP/leukemic meningitis.
5. Leukemic invasion of bone: pain, pathological fractures, hemarthrosis.

C. Analysis/nursing diagnosis:

1. *Potential for infection* related to neutropenia.
2. *Potential for injury* related to thrombocytopenia.
3. *Altered nutrition, less than body requirements,* related to loss of appetite, vomiting, mouth ulcers.
4. *Pain* related to disease process and treatments (e.g., hemarthrosis, bone pain, bone marrow aspiration).
5. *Activity intolerance* related to infection and anemia.
6. *Self-esteem disturbance* related to disease process and treatments (e.g., loss of hair with chemotherapy, moon face with prednisone).
7. *Anticipatory grieving* related to life-threatening illness.
8. *Knowledge deficit* related to diagnosis, treatment, prognosis.

D. Nursing plan/implementation:

1. Goal: *maintain infection-free state.*
   a. Universal precautions to prevent infection.
   b. Use good handwashing technique.
   c. Ongoing evaluation of sites for potential infection, e.g., gums.
   d. Provide meticulous oral hygiene.
   e. Keep record of vital signs, especially temperature.
   f. Provide good skin care.
   g. Screen staff and visitors—restrict anyone with infection.
   h. Protective isolation/reverse isolation to minimize exposure to potentially life-threatening infection.
   i. Discharge planning: return to school, but isolate from chickenpox or known communicable diseases.
2. Goal: *prevent injury.*
   a. Avoid IMs/IVs if possible, due to bruising and bleeding tendencies.
   b. Do *not* give aspirin or medications containing aspirin, which will interfere with platelet formation, thus increasing the risk of bleeding.

TABLE 3.7 Overview of the Most Common Types of Congenital Heart Disease

Type of Defect	Medical Treatment	Surgical Treatment	Prognosis
Acyanotic			
ASD (atrial septal defect)	None—supportive p.r.n.	Open chest/open heart surgery with closure via patch (recommended age: preschooler).	Excellent, with survival greater than 99%.
VSD (ventricular septal defect)	None—supportive p.r.n.	*Palliative treatment:* pulmonary banding; *definitive repair:* same as for ASD.	Excellent, with 96–99% survival rate.
PDA (patent ductus arteriosus)	In newborns—attempt pharmacologic closure with indomethacin (prostaglandin inhibitor).	Open chest: surgical ligation or division (recommended age: 1–2 years).	Excellent—*but* higher mortality among critically ill newborns.
Coarctation of the aorta	Infants or children with CHF: digitalis and diuretics.	Open chest: resection of coarcted portion of aorta with end-to-end anastamosis (recommended age: 4 years).	Excellent.
Cyanotic			
Tetralogy of Fallot	None—supportive p.r.n.	Often done in *stages* with definitive repair accomplished by 1–2 years of age.	Fair—5% mortality.
Transposition of the great vessels	None—supportive p.r.n.	Often done in *stages*. Examples: *palliative*—Rashkind procedure; *definitive repair* (before age 1 year)—Mustard procedure.	Guarded—8–15% mortality.

c. Use soft toothbrush to avoid trauma to gums, which may cause bleeding and infection.

d. *Avoid* "per rectum" suppositories, due to probable rectal ulcers.

e. Supervise play/activity carefully to promote safety and prevent excessive bruising or bleeding.

3. Goal: *promote adequate nutrition.*

a. Diet: high caloric, high protein, high iron.

b. Encourage extra fluids to prevent constipation or dehydration.

c. I&O, daily weights, to monitor fluid and nutritional status.

d. Allow child to be involved with food selection/preparation; allow child almost any food he or she tolerates, to encourage better dietary intake.

e. Serve frequent, small snacks to increase fluid and caloric consumption.

f. Offer dietary supplements to increase caloric intake.

g. Encourage viscous xylocaine "swished" around inside mouth before meals to allow child to eat without pain from oral mucous membrane ulcers.

4. Goal: *relieve pain.*

a. Offer supportive alternatives: extra company, back rub, etc.

b. Administer medications, regularly, before pain becomes excessive.

c. Use bean bag chair for positional changes.

d. *Avoid* excessive stimulation (noise, light), which may heighten perception of pain.

5. Goal: *promote self-esteem.*

a. Stress what child can still do to keep the child as independent as possible.

b. Encourage performance of ADL as much as possible to foster a sense of independence.

c. Provide diversion/activity as tolerated.

d. Give lots of positive reinforcement to enhance a sense of accomplishment.

e. Provide realistic feedback on child's appearance; offer suggestions, such as a wig or cap to cover alopecia secondary to chemotherapy.

f. Encourage early return to peers/school to avoid social isolation.

6. Goal: *prevent complications related to leukemia/prolonged immobility/treatments.*

a. Inspect skin for breakdown, especially over bony prominences, due to poor nutritional intake and limited mobility due to bone pain.

PEDIATRIC NURSING

▶ b. Anticipate need for and provide (per physician's order) multiple transfusions of platelets, packed red cells, etc.

c. Check for hemorrhagic cystitis; push fluids (especially with cytoxan).

d. Check for constipation and/or peripheral neuropathy (especially with vincristin). Refer to Unit 6 for specific information on chemotherapy.

7. Goal: *assist child and parents to cope with life-threatening illness.*

   a. Teach rationale for repeated hospitalizations, multiple invasive tests/treatments, long-term follow-up care.

   b. Encourage compliance with all aspects of therapy, to increase chances of survival.

   c. Be supportive of family and their coping mechanisms.

   d. Offer factual information regarding ultimate prognosis (60% "cure" for acute lymphocytic leukemia).

   e. If death appears imminent, assist family to cope with dying and death.

E. Evaluation:

1. Child is maintained in infection-free state.
2. Injuries are prevented or kept to a minimum.
3. Adequate nutrition is maintained.
4. Child is free from pain or can live with minimum level of pain.
5. Child's self-esteem is maintained; child is treated as living (not dying).
6. Complications are prevented or kept to a minimum.
7. Positive coping mechanisms are utilized by child and family to deal with illness.

II. Sickle cell anemia

A. *Introduction:* Sickle cell anemia is a congenital hemolytic anemia resulting from a defective hemoglobin molecule (hemoglobin S). It is most common in black Americans (1:400) and in people of Mediterranean descent. The diagnosis is usually made during the toddler or preschool years, during the first crisis episode following an infection. There is also the need to differentiate between *sickle cell trait* (sickledex test) and *sickle cell anemia* (hemoglobin electrophoresis). Sickle cell anemia has no known cure.

B. Assessment:

1. Increased susceptibility to infection (cause: unknown; most common cause of death in children under 5).
2. Inherited as autosomal recessive disorder (see Figure 3.7).
3. Precipitated by conditions of low oxygen tension and/or dehydration.
4. Signs of anemia:
   a. Pallor (in dark-skinned children, do not rely on pallor alone—check Hgb and Hct).
   b. Jaundice, due to excessive hemolysis.
   c. Irritability, lethargy, anorexia, malaise.
5. Vaso-occlusive crisis: severe pain (variable sites), fever, swelling of hands and feet, joint pain and swelling, all related to hypoxia, ischemia and necrosis at the cellular level.
6. Thrombocytic crisis: blood is sequestered (pooled) in liver and spleen; precipitous drop in B/P, ↑ pulse, profound anemia, shock, and ultimately death.

C. Analysis/nursing diagnosis:

1. *Altered tissue perfusion* related to anemia and occlusion of vessels.
2. *Pain* related to vaso-occlusion.
3. *Impaired physical mobility* related to pain, immobility.
4. *Knowledge deficit* related to disease process and treatment (e.g., prevention of sickling and/or infection; genetic counseling).

D. Nursing plan/implementation:

1. Goal: *prevent sickling.*
   a. *Avoid* conditions of low oxygen tension, which causes red blood cells (RBCs) to assume a sickled shape.
   b. Provide continuous extra fluids to prevent dehydration, which causes sluggish circulation.
   c. *Avoid* activities that may result in overheating, to prevent dehydration; suggest appropriate clothes; limit time in sun.
   d. If dehydrated due to acute illness, supplement with IV fluids and additional oral fluids to reestablish fluid balance.
2. Goal: *maintain infection-free state.*
   a. Universal precautions to prevent infection.
   b. Use good handwashing technique.
   c. Evaluate carefully, check continually for potential infection sites, which may either lead to death due to sepsis or precipitate sickle cell crisis.
   d. Teach importance of prevention: adequate nutrition; frequent medical check-ups; keep away from known sources of infection.
   e. Stress need to report early signs of infection promptly to physician.
   f. Need to balance prevention of infection with child's need for a "normal" life.
3. Goal: *provide supportive therapy during crisis.*
   a. Provide bedrest/hospitalization during crisis to decrease the body's demand for oxygen.
   b. Relieve pain by administering pain medications as ordered; handle gently and use proper positioning techniques.
   c. Apply heat (never cold) to affected painful areas to increase blood flow (vasodilation) and oxygen supply.
   ▶ d. Administer oxygen, as ordered, to relieve hypoxia and prevent further sickling.
   ▶ e. Administer blood transfusions, as ordered, to correct severe anemia.
   f. Monitor fluid and electrolyte balance: I&O, weight, electrolytes.

(a) Normal parent and parent who carries trait

	A	A
A	AA	AA
S	AS	AS

1:2 (or 2:4) chance offspring will carry trait.

(b) Two parents who carry trait

	A	S
A	AA	AS
S	AS	SS

1:4 chance offspring will be normal.
1:4 chance offspring will have sickle cell anemia.
1:2 (or 2:4) chance offspring will carry trait.

(c) Normal parent and parent with sickle cell anemia

	A	A
S	AS	AS
S	AS	AS

4:4 (100%) chance offspring will carry trait.

(d) Parent with sickle cell anemia and parent who carries trait

	A	S
S	AS	SS
S	AS	SS

1:2 chance offspring will carry trait.
1:2 chance offspring will have sickle cell anemia.

(e) Two parents with sickle cell anemia

	S	S
S	SS	SS
S	SS	SS

4:4 (100%) chance offspring will have sickle cell anemia.

Key AA normal hemoglobin
AS sickle cell trait
SS sickle cell disease (anemia)

Note: The odds cited here are for *each* pregnancy.

■ **FIGURE 3.7**
Genetic transmission of sickle cell anemia.

g. Perform ADL for child if unable to care for own needs; encourage self-care as soon as possible to promote independence.

4. Goal: *teach child and family about sickle cell anemia.*
   a. Provide factual information based on child's developmental level.
   b. When asked, offer information regarding prognosis (no known cure).
   c. Encourage child to live as normally as possible.
   d. Genetic screening and counseling (see Figure 3.7).

E. Evaluation:

1. Sickling is prevented or kept to a minimum.
2. Child is maintained in infection-free state.
3. Child/family verbalize that they can cope adequately with crisis.
4. Child/family verbalize their understanding about disease, its management and prognosis.

III. Hemophilia

A. *Introduction:* Hemophilia is a bleeding disorder inherited as a sex-linked (X-linked) recessive trait; that is, it occurs only in males but is transmitted by symptom-free female carriers (refer to Figure 3.8). Hemophilia results in a deficiency of one or more clotting factors, and there is a need to determine which clotting factor is deficient and to what extent. Classic hemophilia (hemophilia A) is a lack of clotting factor VIII and accounts for 75% of all cases of hemophilia.

B. Assessment:

1. Major problem is bleeding.
   a. In *newborn* male: abnormal bleeding from umbilical cord, prolonged bleeding from circumcision site.
   b. In *toddler* male: excessive bruising, possible intracranial bleeding, prolonged bleeding from cuts or lacerations.
   c. *General:* hemarthrosis, petechiae, epistaxis, frank hemorrhage anywhere in body, anemia.
2. Need to determine which clotting factor is deficient/missing and extent of deficiency:
   a. *Mild:* child has 5–25% of normal amount of clotting factor.
   b. *Moderate:* child has 1–5% of normal amount of clotting factor.
   c. *Severe:* child has less than 1% of normal amount of clotting factor.

(a) "Normal" male and female with trait

	X	Y
X•	X•X	X•Y
X	XX	XY

1:4 chance female will carry trait.
1:4 chance male will have hemophilia.
1:2 (or 2:4) chance will be "normal" female/male.

(b) Male with hemophilia and "normal" female

	X•	Y
X	XX•	XY
X	XX•	XY

1:2 (or 2:4) chance female will carry trait.
1:2 (or 2:4) chance will be "normal" male.

(c) Male with hemophilia and female with trait

	X•	Y
X•	X•X•	X•Y
X	X•X	XY

1:2 (or 2:4) chance female will carry trait.*
1:4 chance will be "normal" male.
1:4 chance male will have hemophilia.

Key XY = normal male
X•Y = male with hemophilia
XX = normal female
X•X = female carrying hemophilia trait
X•X• = female with possible relative lack of clotting factor—*not* a true hemophiliac

Note: The odds cited here are for *each* pregnancy.

FIGURE 3.8
Genetic transmission of hemophilia.

C. Analysis/nursing diagnosis:

1. *Potential for injury* related to bleeding tendencies.
2. *Pain* related to hemarthrosis.
3. *Impaired physical mobility* related to bleeding and pain.
4. *Knowledge deficit* related to home care and follow-up.

D. Nursing plan/implementation:

1. Goal: *prevent injury and possible bleeding.*
   a. Provide an environment that is as safe as possible, e.g., toys with no sharp edges, child's safety scissors.
   b. Use soft toothbrush to prevent trauma to gums.
   c. When old enough to shave, use only electric razor (no straight-edge razors).
   d. Avoid IMs/IVs—but when absolutely necessary, treat as arterial puncture; that is, apply direct pressure to the site for at least 5 minutes after withdrawing needle.
   e. Do **not** use aspirin or medication containing aspirin (prolongs bleeding/clotting time).
2. Goal: *control bleeding episodes when they occur.*
   a. Local measures: apply direct pressure, elevate, apply ice (vasoconstriction), keep immobilized during acute bleeding episodes only. For epistaxis: child should sit up and lean slightly forward.
   b. Systemic measures: administer clotting factor (Factorate, cryoprecipitate) via IV infusion. *Note:* This is a blood product, so a transfusion reaction is possible.
3. Goal: *prevent long-term disability related to joint degeneration.*
   a. Keep immobilized during period of acute bleeding and for 24–48 hours afterward to allow blood to clot and to prevent dislodging the clot.
   b. Begin passive range of motion as soon as possible after acute phase.
   c. Administer prescribed pain medications *before* physical therapy sessions.
   d. Begin prescribed exercise program, starting with passive range of motion (ROM) and gradually advancing to active ROM, then full exercise program, as tolerated, to maintain maximum joint function.
   e. **Avoid:** prolonged immobility, braces, splints—which can lead to permanent deformities and loss of mobility.
4. Goal: *promote independence in management of own care.*
   a. Encourage child to assume responsibility for choosing safe activities.
   b. Encourage child to attend regular school as much as possible; provide support via school nurse.
   c. Advise child to wear MedicAlert bracelet.
   d. Caution parents to avoid overprotection of child.
   e. Offer child chance to self-limit activities within appropriate limits (parents can offer guidance).
   f. Assist child to cope with life-threatening disorder with no known cure.
5. Goal: *health teaching.*
   a. Between 9 and 12 years of age: child can be taught to self-administer clotting factor intravenously (prior to this, family can perform).
   b. As child enters adolescence: begin to discuss issues such as realistic vocations, insurance coverage, genetic transmission (refer to Figure 3.8).

E. Evaluation:

1. Serious injuries are prevented; bleeding is kept to a minimum.
2. Episodes of bleeding controlled by prompt, effective intervention.
3. There are no long-term disabilities.
4. Child is able to manage own care independently, with minimum supervision.

PULMONARY DISORDERS

I. Cystic fibrosis (mucoviscidosis)

A. *Introduction:* Cystic fibrosis (mucoviscidosis) is a generalized dysfunction of the exocrine glands. Although the disorder is inherited as an autosomal recessive defect, the basic biochemical defect is unknown. However, its probable cause is an alteration in a protein or an enzyme, e.g., pancreatic enzyme deficiency. The basic problem is one of thick, sticky, tenacious mucous secretions that obstruct the ducts of the exocrine glands, thus affecting their ability to function. Cystic fibrosis is found in all races and socioeconomic groups, although there is a significantly lower incidence in black Americans. It is a chronic disease with no known cure and guarded prognosis; median age at death is 18–20 years.

B. Assessment:

1. Newborn: *meconium ileus.*
2. Frequent, recurrent *pulmonary infections:* bronchitis, bronchopneumonia, pneumonia, and ultimately chronic obstructive pulmonary disease (COPD) due to mechanical obstruction of respiratory tract caused by thick, tenacious mucous gland secretions.
3. *Malabsorption syndrome:* failure to gain weight, distended abdomen, thin arms and legs, lack of subcutaneous fat due to disturbed absorption of nutrients that results from the inability of pancreatic enzymes to reach intestinal tract.
4. *Steatorrhea:* bulky, foul-smelling, frothy, fatty stools in increased amounts and frequency (predisposed to rectal prolapse).
5. Parents may note that child *"tastes salty"* when kissed, due to excessive loss of sodium and chloride in sweat.
6. *Sweat test* reveals high sodium and chloride levels in child's sweat, unique to children with cystic fibrosis.
7. Sexual development
   a. *Male:* sterile (due to aspermia).
   b. *Female:* difficulty conceiving and bearing children (due to increased viscosity of cervical mucus, which acts as a plug and mechanically blocks the entry of sperm).

C. Analysis/nursing diagnosis:

1. *Ineffective breathing patterns* related to thick, viscid secretions.
2. *Altered nutrition, less than body requirements,* related to diarrhea and poor intestinal absorption of nutrients.
3. *Decreased cardiac output* related to COPD and decreased compliance of lungs.
4. *Activity intolerance* related to respiratory compromise.
5. *Self-esteem disturbance* related to body image changes.
6. *Knowledge deficit* related to disease process, treatments, medications, genetics.
7. *Noncompliance* (potential) related to complicated and prolonged treatment regimen.

D. Nursing plan/implementation:

1. Goal: *assist child to expectorate sputum.*
   ▶ a. Perform postural drainage as prescribed: first thing in morning, between meals, before bedtime.
   ▶ b. Administer nebulizer treatments, expectorants, mucolytics, bronchodilators.
   c. Provide for exercises that promote position changes and keep sputum moving up and out.
   d. Encourage high fluid intake to keep secretions liquefied.
   e. Suction, administer oxygen p.r.n.
2. Goal: *prevent infection.*
   a. Universal precautions to prevent infection.
   b. Evaluate carefully, check continually for potential infection (especially respiratory); report to MD promptly.
   c. Limit contact with staff or visitors with infection.
   d. Administer antibiotics as ordered, to treat respiratory infections and prevent overwhelming sepsis.
   e. May be placed on prophylactic antibiotic therapy between episodes of infection.
   f. Teach importance of prevention of infection at home: adequate nutrition, frequent medical check-ups, stay away from known sources of infection.
3. Goal: *maintain adequate nutrition.*
   a. Diet: low fat, high calorie and protein, to prevent malnutrition.
   b. Administer pancreatic enzyme (viokase, pancreatin) immediately before *every* meal and *every* snack to enhance the absorption of vital nutrients, especially fats.
   c. If child is unable to swallow tablets, mix pancreatic enzyme powder with cold applesauce.
   d. Administer water-miscible preparations of fat-soluble vitamins (A, D, E, K), multivitamins, and iron.
   e. Encourage extra salt intake to compensate for excessive sodium losses in sweat.
   f. Encourage extra fluid intake (e.g., Gatorade) to prevent dehydration/electrolyte imbalance.
   g. Daily I&O and weights to monitor nutritional and hydration status.
   h. Encourage child to assume gradually increasing responsibility for choosing own foods within dietary restrictions.
4. Goal: *teach child and family about cystic fibrosis.*
   ▶ a. Discuss diagnostic procedures: sweat test, stool specimens.
   b. Review multiple medications: use, effects, side/toxic effects.

PEDIATRIC NURSING

■ TABLE 3.8 Pediatric Respiratory Infections

Name	Definition	Age Group	Etiology	Definitive Clinical Signs and Symptoms	Specifics of Treatment	Prognosis
Bronchiolitis	Infectious disease of lower respiratory tract (small, low bronchioles), with resultant trapping of air.	Infants 2–12 months (peak at 6 months).	Viral.	Hyperinflation of alveoli. Scattered areas of atelectasis. Acute, severe respiratory distress for first 48–72 hours. Followed by rapid recovery.	Supportive care during acute phase: ■ hospitalization. ■ croup tent. ■ clear liquids.	Exellent (less than 1% mortality).
Croup (acute spasmodic laryngitis)	Paroxysmal attacks (spasms of larynx).	1–3 years.	Viral (possible allergy and/or psychogenic).	Most common onset at night. Inspiratory stridor. "Croupy" barking cough. Dyspnea. Anxiety.	Teach parents—turn on hot water in bathroom and close door (steam). Common to treat at home.	Excellent (but likely to recur).
LTB (laryngotracheo-bronchitis)	Acute infection of lower respiratory tract: larynx, trachea and bronchi.	Infants and toddlers (peak at 21 months).	Viral (possible secondary bacterial infection).	Inspiratory stridor. High fever. Signs and symptoms of severe respiratory distress. Hoarseness, progressing to aphonia and respiratory arrest without treatment.	Hospitalization: ■ Tracheostomy set at bedside. ■ Epinephrine/ steroids. ■ Antibiotics if cultures are positive.	Good.
Epiglottitis	Extremely acute, severe, and rapid, progressive swelling (due to infection) of epiglottis and surrounding tissue.	3–7 years.	Bacterial (*H. influenzae*, type B).	Abrupt onset—rapid progression. Dyspnea, dysphagia. Sit up/chin thrust/mouth open. Thick muffled voice. Cherry red, swollen epiglottis.	*Do not* visualize epiglottis unless airway support is immediately available. Will need endotracheal tube or tracheostomy for 24–48 hours to maintain patent airway. IV ampicillin for 10–14 days to treat bacterial infection. IV corticosteroids (e.g., Solucortef) to reduce inflammation.	Very good if detected and treated early.

c. Stress need to care for pulmonary systems (major cause of mortality/morbidity).

d. Teach various treatments: postural drainage, nebulizers, oxygen therapy, breathing exercise.

e. Encourage child to assume as much responsibility for own care as possible: medications, treatments, diet.

f. Promote development of healthy attitude toward disease/prognosis (no known cure).

g. Refer to appropriate community agencies for assistance with home care.

h. Assist with genetic counseling.

i. Discuss sexual concerns with adolescent.

5. Goal: *promote compliance with treatment regiment.*

a. Encourage child to verbalize anger or frustration at being "different"/body image alterations.

b. Suggest alternatives to postural drainage, e.g., yoga/standing on head.

c. Offer "rewards" for compliance: going swimming with friends or other types of peer activities.

E. Evaluation:

1. Child can clear own airway, expectorate sputum.
2. Child is maintained in infection-free state.
3. Adequate nutrition is maintained.
4. Child and family verbalize understanding of the disease.
5. Child complies with rigors of treatment.

II. Pediatric respiratory infections

A. Assessment: general assessment of infant/child with respiratory distress. *Note:* Additional information about specific respiratory infections may be found in Table 3.8.

1. Restlessness—*earliest* sign of hypoxia.
2. Difficulty sucking/eating—parents may state the infant or child has "poor appetite."
3. Expiratory grunt, flaring of nasal alae, retractions.
4. Changes in vital signs: fever, tachycardia, tachypnea.
5. Cough: productive/nonproductive.
6. Wheeze; expiratory/inspiratory.
7. Hoarseness or aphonic crying.
8. Dyspnea or prostration.
9. Dehydration—related to increase in sensible fluid loss and poor PO intake.
10. Color change (pallor, cyanosis)—*later* sign of respiratory distress.

B. Analysis/nursing diagnosis:

1. *Ineffective airway clearance* related to infection and/or obstruction.
2. *Fluid volume deficit* related to excessive losses through normal routes, discomfort and inability to swallow.
3. *Anxiety* related to hypoxia.
4. *Potential for injury* related to spread of infection.
5. *Knowledge deficit* related to disease process, infection control, home care, and follow-up.

C. Nursing plan/implementation:

1. Goal: *relieve respiratory distress by reducing swelling and edema and liquefying secretions.*

▶ a. Environment: cool, high-humidity croup tent (see Table 3.9).

b. Administer oxygen as ordered.

c. *Position*: semi-Fowler's or in infant seat to provide maximum expansion of the lungs; small blanket or diaper roll under neck to keep airway patent; change position at least q2h to prevent pooling of secretions.

▶ d. Suction/postural drainage p.r.n.

e. Pin diapers loosely and use only loose-fitting clothing to avoid pressure on abdominal organs, which could impinge on diaphragm and impede respirations.

f. Administer medications: antibiotics, bronchodilators, steroids.

g. Monitor temperature q4h/p.r.n.; reduce fever via acetaminophen, cool sponges, hypothermia blanket.

2. Goal: *observe for potential respiratory failure related to exhaustion or complete airway obstruction.*

a. Place in room near nurses' station for maximum observation.

b. Monitor vital signs: q1h during acute phase, then q4h.

▶ c. Place emergency equipment near bedside p.r.n.: endotracheal tube, tracheostomy set.

d. Monitor closely for signs of impending respiratory failure: ↑ rapid, shallow respirations, progressive hoarseness/aphonia, deepening cyanosis.

e. Report adverse changes in condition stat to physician.

3. Goal: *maintain normal fluid balance.*

a. May be NPO initially to prevent aspiration.

b. IVs until severe distress subsides and child is able to suck and swallow.

c. Monitor hydration status: I&O, urine specific gravity, weight.

d. When resuming PO fluids—start with sips of clear liquids, advance slowly as tolerated: "Pedialyte," clear broth, jello, popsicles, fruit juices, ginger ale, cola.

e. **Avoid** milk/milk products, which may cause increased mucus production.

4. Goal: *provide calm, secure environment.*

a. During acute distress: remain with child/family (do not leave unattended).

b. Keep crying to a minimum to prevent severe hypoxia and to reduce the body's demand for oxygen.

c. Avoid painful/intrusive procedures if possible.

d. Organize nursing care to provide planned periods of uninterrupted rest.

e. Allow parents to room-in, and encourage their participation in care of their child to keep the child relatively calm and reduce anxiety.

f. Allow child to keep favorite toy or security object.

TABLE 3.9 Nursing Care of the Child in a Croup Tent

Nursing Actions	Rationale
1. Explain purpose of tent to parents and child; stress it is temporary, to make breathing easier.	1. Relieves anxiety.
2. Inspect tent for cracks, tears. Repair or replace p.r.n.	2. Leaks will allow oxygen to escape.
3. Place unit at head of bed.	3. Child's upper torso and head must be inside tent.
4. Cover bed with rubber/plastic sheet.	4. Keeps mattress dry.
5. Apply extra linen to bed under tent.	5. Absorbs extra dampness, wetness.
6. Secure metal frame to bedspring, and fasten tent to frame.	6. Prevents collapse of tent and keeps it open.
7. Fill jar three-fourths with distilled *water*—check q 4h.	7. Provides *high humidity* to keep secretions moist and liquified.
8. Select "cool mode" by using the control switch.	8. Provides *cool air* to reduce swelling and edema.
9. Close zippers and tuck in edges tightly.	9. Prevents loss of oxygen.
10. "Flood" tent with oxygen for 5 minutes (flow rate = 15 liters per minute).	10. Raises oxygen concentration.
11. Adjust flow rate per physician's order.	11. Usual flow rate is 8–10 liters per minute to maintain 35% oxygen concentration.
12. Use oxygen analyzer to check concentration at least q 2h.	12. Oxygen is a drug and must be given per order.
13. Place child in tent—stay with child.	13. Relieves anxiety.
14. Place folded towel/blanket around child's head; stockinette cap for infant's head.	14. Keeps child dry and prevents heat loss.
15. Cover child with blanket.	15. Avoids chilling.
16. Selection of toys: ■ Nonflammable. ■ Items that can be wiped dry.	16. ■ Oxygen is highly combustible. ■ Avoids bacterial growth.
17. Change child's clothes and bed linens frequently (q 4h or p.r.n.).	17. High humidity in tent will cause moisture to collect on these items.

5. Goal: *provide parents with teaching, as necessary.*
   a. Short term: discuss equipment, treatments, procedures; offer frequent progress reports, answer parents' questions.
   b. Long term: how to handle recurrences, how to check temperature at home, medications for fever, when to call physician about respiratory problem.

D. Evaluation:

1. No further evidence of respiratory distress.
2. Resumption of normal respiratory pattern.
3. Normal fluid balance maintained/restored.
4. Parents verbalize their concerns and express confidence in their ability to care for their child after discharge.

III. Apnea-related disorders

A. Apnea of infancy

1. *Introduction:* Apnea of infancy is the unexplained cessation of breathing for 20 seconds or longer in an apparently healthy, full-term infant. It is usually diagnosed by the second month of life and is generally thought to resolve during the first 12–15 months of life. The exact cause is unknown. It is frequently accompanied by gastroesophageal reflux. The association between apnea of infancy and sudden infant death syndrome (SIDS) is still controversial. However, infants experiencing significant apnea without a known cause are thought to be at high risk for SIDS and must be treated accordingly.

2. **Assessment:**
   a. Unexplained cessation of breathing (apnea) for 20 seconds or longer.
   b. Bradycardia.
   c. Color change: cyanosis or pallor.
   d. Limp, hypotonic.

3. **Analysis/nursing diagnosis:**
   a. *Ineffective breathing patterns* related to apnea.
   b. *Anxiety, fear* related to apnea and threat of infant's death.
   c. *Knowledge deficit* regarding home care of infant on an apnea monitor and infant cardiopulmonary resuscitation (CPR).

4. **Nursing plan/intervention:**
   a. Goal: *maintain effective breathing pattern.*
   ▶ (1) Apnea monitor on infant at all times.
   (2) Place in room near nurses' station for maximum observation with a nurse or parent present at all times.

▶ (3) Suction, oxygen, and resuscitation equipment readily available if needed.

(4) Observe for apnea and/or bradycardia; note duration and associated symptoms—color change, change in muscle tone.

(5) If apnea occurs, use gentle stimulation to start infant breathing again. If ineffective, begin CPR (see Figure 3.9).

(6) If suctioning is needed, it should be done gently and for the shortest time and least number of times possible to maintain patent airway. Note that repeated, vigorous suctioning is associated with periods of apnea.

(7) Position: prone, to avoid regurgitation and apnea.

(8) Feedings: smaller and more frequent; avoid overfeeding, which can lead to reflux and apnea.

b. Goal: *teach parents how to care for their infant at home* (see Table 3.10).

(1) Thoroughly explain discharge plans to parents; encourage questions and discussion.

(2) Begin teaching use of apnea monitor and infant CPR techniques several days prior to discharge; allow parents to handle the monitor and become thoroughly familiar with its use.

(3) Provide parents with emergency response numbers and PHN referral.

(4) Stress need for at least one year of ongoing care with constant use of monitor.

(5) Discuss need for support and refer to local self-help/support group.

(6) Encourage parents to take time for themselves if a reliable caregiver is available who is trained in use of monitor and infant CPR.

5. **Evaluation:**

a. Effective breathing pattern is established.

b. Parents verbalize their concerns and express confidence in their ability to care for their infant at home.

B. Sudden infant death syndrome

1. *Introduction:* Sudden infant death syndrome (SIDS) is the *sudden, unexpected* death of an apparently healthy infant, which remains *unexplained* in the postmortem exam. Various theories have been suggested, none proven; research is ongoing.

2. **Assessment:**

a. Sudden, unexplained death in otherwise "normal" infant; occurs exclusively during sleep.

b. Note overall appearance of infant (differentiate from child abuse).

c. Obtain history from parents—note affect or how parents are dealing with grief.

3. **Analysis/nursing diagnosis:**

a. *Dysfunctional grieving* related to loss of infant.

b. *Knowledge deficit* related to SIDS.

4. **Nursing plan/implementation:**

a. *Immediate goal:* support grieving parents.

(1) Stress that nothing could have been done to prevent the death.

(2) Allow parents to express grief emotions; provide privacy.

(3) Offer parents opportunity to see, hold infant.

(4) Explain purpose of autopsy (physician to obtain consent).

■ **TABLE 3.10 Guidelines for Home Care of Infant on Apnea Monitor**

1. Demonstrate to the parents how to connect the monitor leads.
2. Remind parents to remove the leads unless they are connected to the infant.
3. Stress that the infant needs to be on the monitor whenever respirations are not being directly observed and that a trained person needs to be present in the home at all times in case the alarm sounds.
4. Explain that the infant will need direct observation whenever loud noises could obscure the monitor alarm, e.g., dishwasher, vacuum.
5. Teach parents what to look for when the alarm sounds, i.e., loose monitor leads vs apnea.
6. Teach parents how to assess the infant for an episode of apnea, i.e., lack of respirations, duration, color, muscle tone.
7. Teach the parents to first use gentle physical stimulation if the infant experiences an apnea spell, e.g., touching the face or stroking the soles of the feet.
8. Demonstrate infant CPR to be used if tactile stimulation is not effective in reestablishing respirations.
9. Encourage parents to keep emergency numbers posted near the phone.
10. Explain that monitor will not interfere with normal growth and development. Encourage the parents to promote normal growth and development as much as possible.

■ **TABLE 3.11 SIDS: What To Tell Families**

Concern	Facts
Etiology	Unknown (possibly related to delayed maturation of cardiorespiratory system).
Incidence	2 or 3/1000 live births (10,000/year); leading cause of death between ages of 1 week and 1 year.
When	Occurs during *sleep* (nap, night).
Age	90% of cases occur by age *6 months*.
Sex	More common in *males*.
Race	More common in *nonwhites*.
Season	More common in *winter*.
Family history	5 times more common in *siblings* of SIDS victims.
Perinatal	More common in *premature* infants, in *multiple* births, and in infants with *low Apgars*.

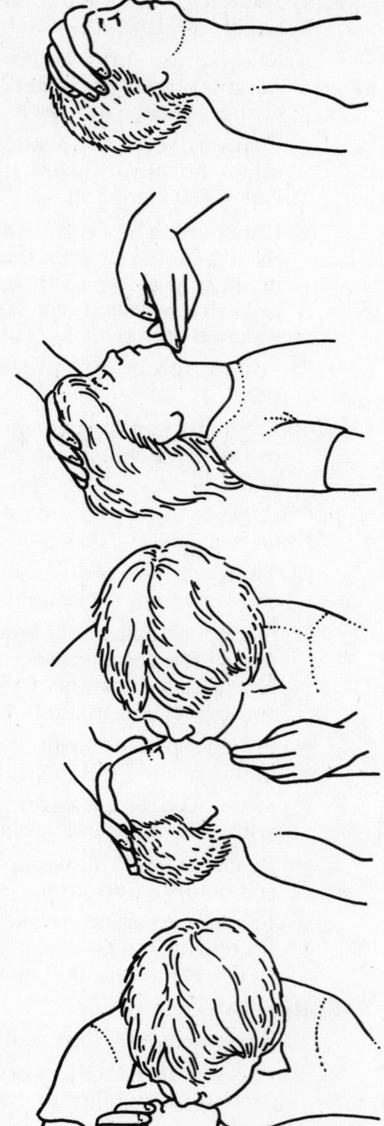

Problem: Child/infant is not breathing; cyanosis of lips and nail beds.
Procedure: Open airway

Infant

1. Pinch baby's feet or gently flick the base of the sternum.
2. Place infant on a flat, hard surface with hand on forehead.
3. Gently extend the head.
4. Place your cheek near the infant's nose and feel for exhalation.

Child (under age 8)

1. Tap or gently shake; ask if child is awake.
2. Tilt head back gently and lift chin to open airway.
3. Place child on a hard, flat surface.
4. Observe for respiration.

Problem: Child/infant is still not breathing after airway is open
Procedure: Attempt to resume respiration

Infant

1. Cover mouth and nose with your mouth, creating a seal.
2. Give 2 slow breaths.
3. Check for resumption of breathing.
4. If not breathing, check pulse at inner aspect of elbow; if pulse is present, continue breathing into infant's mouth.
5. Give 1 breath every 3 seconds, or 20 breaths per minute.

Child

1. Pinch nose and make a seal over the mouth only with your mouth.
2. Give 2 slow breaths, allowing for exhalation between breaths.
3. Check the carotid pulse for 5 seconds.
4. If pulse is present but child is not breathing, continue respirations.
5. Give 1 breath every 4 seconds, or 15 breaths per minute. For child over age 8, give 1 breath every 5 seconds, or 12 breaths per minute.
6. Check for rise and fall of chest, indicating that child is breathing.
7. Avoid getting air into child's stomach.

■ **FIGURE 3.9**
Cardiopulmonary resuscitation (CPR) in infants and children. (From James SR, Mott SR: *Child Health Nursing: Essential Care of Children and Families,* Addison-Wesley, Menlo Park, CA, 1988, p. 350.

(5) Contact spiritual advisor: priest, rabbi, minister.

(6) Assist parents to plan what to tell siblings.

b. *Ongoing goal:* provide factual information regarding SIDS.

(1) Offer information that is known about SIDS in simple, direct terms (see Table 3.11).

(2) Answer questions honestly.

(3) Give parents printed literature on SIDS.

(4) Refer to local/national SIDS foundation group.

c. *Long-term goal:* assist family to resolve grief.

(1) Track progress of other siblings.

(2) Refer to local perinatal bereavement group.

(3) Consider subsequent pregnancy to be at risk for:

(a) Attachment/bonding.

(b) SIDS recurrence.

5. **Evaluation:**

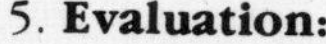

Problem: Absent pulse; cyanosis

Procedure: Restore circulation

Infant

1. Place index finger and middle fingers at 1 finger width below nipple line.
2. Depress from ½ ″ to 1 ″ (toward the backbone).
3. Give 100–120 compressions per minute. Give 1 breath for every 5 compressions.
4. Check for the resumption of heartbeat for 5 seconds after each 1 minute of CPR. **Do not stop CPR for more than 5 seconds.**

Child

1. Use the heel of one hand to compress sternum at the nipple line.
2. Depress from 1 ″ to 1½ ″.
3. Give 80–100 compressions per minute. Give 1 breath for every 5 compressions.
4. Check periodically for the resumption of heartbeat, but **do not stop CPR for more than 5 seconds.**

Older Child

1. Use 2 hands over lower portion of sternum at 2 finger widths from the xyphoid.
2. Depress from 1½ ″ to 2 ″.
3. Give 80 compressions per minute. Give 2 breaths after each 15 compressions.
4. Stop periodically to check for resumption of circulation. **Do not stop CPR for more than 5 seconds.**
5. *Two-person rescue:* Give 60 chest compressions with 1 breath after each 5 compressions.

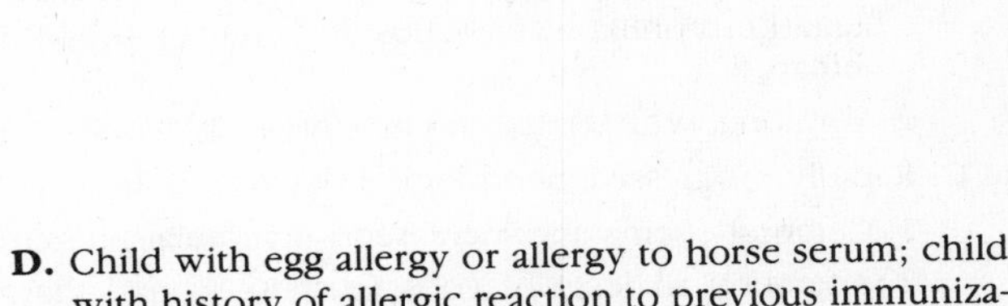

■ **FIGURE 3.9 (*Continued*)**

a. Parents are able to express their grief and receive adequate support.

b. Parents raise questions about SIDS and can understand answers.

c. Family's grief is resolved; in time, normal family dynamics resume.

■ DISORDERS AFFECTING PROTECTIVE FUNCTIONS

IMMUNITY AND COMMUNICABLE DISEASES

I. Recommended schedule for active immunization of normal infants and children (see Table. 3.12).

II. Side effects of immunizations and nursing care (see Table 3.13).

III. Contraindications to immunizations

A. Child who has an acute illness (e.g., upper respiratory infection (URI), gastroenteritis, or any fever).

B. Child with alteration in skin integrity: rash, eczema.

C. Child with alteration in immune system; steroids; chemotherapy, radiation therapy; HIV/AIDS (no live virus vaccine).

D. Child with egg allergy or allergy to horse serum; child with history of allergic reaction to previous immunization.

E. Pregnant female/female of childbearing age (rubella).

IV. Childhood communicable diseases (see Table 3.14). Basic principles of care:

A. Universal precautions to prevent communicability/infection.

B. Fever control.

C. Extra fluids for hydration.

D. General home care procedures.

REYE'S SYNDROME

I. *Introduction:* Reye's syndrome, first described as a disease entity in the mid 1960s, is a multi-system disorder primarily affecting children between 6 and 12 years of age. Although **not** truly a "communicable disease," studies have confirmed a relationship between aspirin administration during a viral illness (e.g., chickenpox, flu) and the onset of Reye's syndrome. The exact cause remains unknown. Reye's syndrome is characterized by acute metabolic encephalopathy and fatty degeneration of the visceral organs, particularly the liver. Earlier diagnosis, more sophisticated monitoring equipment, and more aggressive treatment have greatly improved the survival rate of children with Reye's syndrome; recovery is generally rapid in those children who do survive.

■ TABLE 3.12 Recommended Schedule for Active Immunization of Normal Infants and Children

Age	Recommended Immunization
2 months	DTP, OPV, and Hib
4 months	DTP, OPV, and Hib
6 months	DTP and Hib (third dose of OPV is given only if high risk of polio)
15 months	MMR, Hib
18 months	DTP, OPV
Pre-K (4–6 years)	DTP, OPV
11–12 years	MMR
14–16 years	Td

Source: Reprinted with permission from "Protecting Your Child Against Diphtheria, Tetanus, Pertussis." Copyright ©1992 American Academy of Pediatrics.

Key: DTP = diphtheria and tetanus toxoids with pertussis vaccine; OPV = oral poliovirus vaccine; MMR = live measles, mumps and rubella viruses in combined vaccine; Hib = *Haemophilus influenzae* type B conjugate vaccine. Td = adult tetanus-diphtheria toxoid.

Note: OPV given p.o.; DTP, Hib, and Td given I.M. MMR given S.C.

II. Assessment:

A. Onset typically follows a viral illness, just as child appears to be recovering.

B. Early signs and symptoms:

1. Rapidly progressing behavioral changes: irritability, agitation, combativeness, hostility, confusion, apathy, lethargy.
2. Vomiting, which becomes progressively worse.

C. Rapidly progressive neurological deterioration:

1. Cerebral edema and increased intracranial pressure.
2. Alteration in level of consciousness from lethargy through coma, decerebrate posturing, and respiratory arrest.

D. Liver dysfunction, necrosis and failure:

1. Elevated ALT[SGOT], AST[SGPT], LDH, serum ammonia levels.
2. Severe hypoglycemia.
3. Increased prothrombin time, coagulation defects, and bleeding.

III. Analysis/nursing diagnosis:

A. *Altered cerebral tissue perfusion* related to cerebral edema and increased intracranial pressure.

B. *Altered hepatic tissue perfusion* related to fatty degeneration of the liver.

C. *Potential for injury* related to coagulation defects and bleeding.

D. *Knowledge deficit* related to diagnosis, course of disease, treatment, and prognosis.

IV. Nursing plan/implementation:

A. Goal: *reduce intracranial pressure.*

1. Child is admitted to PICU for intensive nursing care, continuous observation and monitoring.
2. Monitor neurological status and vital signs continuously.
3. ▶ Assist with/prepare for numerous invasive procedures, including ET tube/mechanical ventilation and intracranial pressure monitor.
4. Monitor closely for the development of seizures; institute seizure precautions.
5. *Position*: elevate HOB 30–45 degrees.
6. Administer medications as ordered:
   a. Osmotic diuretics (e.g., mannitol) to ↓ ICP.
   b. Diuretics (e.g., Lasix) to ↓ CSF production.
   c. Anticonvulsants (e.g., dilantin, phenobarbital).

B. Goal: *restore and maintain fluid and electrolyte balance, including perfusion of liver.*

1. Administer IV fluids per MD order—usually 10% glucose (or higher).
2. Strict I&O.

■ TABLE 3.13 Immunizations: Assessment of Side Effects and Nursing Care

Immunization	Assessment: Side Effects	Nursing Care
Diphtheria	Crankiness, irritability.	*General teaching for DTP:*
	Moderate fever within 24–48 hours.	Prophylactic use of acetaminophen.
	Soreness, redness, swelling at injection site.	Apply ice/cool soak to injection site.
Tetanus	Lump at injection site.	Extra "TLC."
Pertussis	Seizures or changes in level of consciousness.	Notify physician promptly of any other side effects/severe side effects (seizures, temperature >101.5°F).
Polio	Essentially none.	—
Measles	Reaction is delayed until 7–10 days after immunization: fever, rash, coryza.	Teach parents about delay in side effects.
Mumps	Essentially none.	—
Rubella	Mild rash for 24–48 hours.	Teach parents about side effects, use mild analgesics; reassure that symptoms will subside.
	Arthralgia, arthritis—more common in older children and adults; may last weeks.	

■ TABLE 3.14 Childhood Communicable Diseases

Disease (Agent)	Incubation Period	Period of Communicability	Transmission	Nursing Assessment	Nursing Plan/ Implementation	Evaluation	Prevention
Diphtheria *(Corynebacterium diphtheria)*	2–5 days	2–4 weeks	Direct contact	Check anatomical location of pseudomembrane: smooth, adherent white or grayish membrane (most common in back of throat). Dyspnea, hoarseness, cough, retractions, potential complete airway obstruction and respiratory arrest. Fever, malaise, anorexia. Toxemia, septic shock, death in most severe cases.	Strict isolation. Medications as ordered: antitoxin IV; antibiotics, i.e., penicillin/ erythromycin. Tracheostomy set at bedside. Complete bedrest. Administer humidified oxygen as ordered. Suction p.r.n.	Child recovers completely, without lasting damage due to hypoxia.	Vaccination: series of three, begun at age 2 months, with boosters at 18 months and at 5 years → permanent immunity.
Pertussis (whooping cough) *(Bordetella pertussis)*	5–21 days	Precatarrhal stage to fourth week after onset of paroxysms	Direct contact; droplet infection; indirect contact	*Catarrhal stage:* 1–2 weeks; signs and symptoms of URI but with dry, hacking cough. *Paroxysmal stage:* Cough, typically worse at night Expiration—series of short, rapid coughs. Inspiration—"whoop" or high-pitched crowing sound. Accompanied by cyanosis, bulging eyes, protruding tongue. May be followed by vomiting of thick mucous plug.	Respiratory isolation. Bedrest with supportive care such as humidified oxygen, extra fluids: PO, IV. Observe for signs of ↑ respiratory distress; emergency equipment nearby. Administer antiobiotics as ordered, e.g., erythromycin.	Child recovers completely without complications such as pneumonia, atelectasis, hemorrhage.	Vaccination: series of three, begun at age 2 months, with boosters at 18 months and 5 years → permanent immunity.
Poliomyelitis (enteroviruses)	5–35 days	Unknown	Direct contact	"Paralytic"—fever, headache, malaise → pain and stiffness in back, legs, neck → complete CNS paralysis.	Complete bedrest. Assisted respiratory ventilation p.r.n. Supportive care. Physical therapy referral.	Determine degree of permanent, irreversible paralysis → child and family adjust to/cope with disability.	Vaccination: series of three, begun at age 2 months, with boosters at 18 months and at 5 years → permanent immunity.

continued

TABLE 3.14 *(Continued)* **Childhood Communicable Diseases**

Disease (Agent)	Incubation Period	Period of Communicability	Transmission	Nursing Assessment	Nursing Plan/ Implementation	Evaluation	Prevention
Measles (rubeola) (paramyxovirus)	10–20 days	Mainly during prodromal stage	Direct contact	*Prodromal stage:* fever, malaise, coryza, cough, Koplik's spots on buccal mucosa (fade in 18 hours). Rash: maculae to papules, fade with pressure, begins on hairline and face and spreads downward. *General:* photophobia, lymphadenopathy.	Isolate until fifth full day with rash. Bedrest until cough and fever subside. Antipyretics and/or tepid sponges to ↓ fever. Dim lights in room—rinse eyes with warm saline or water. Cool mist vaporizer. Antitussives for cough. Encourage additional fluids.	Child recovers completely without complications such as encephalitis.	Vaccine at 15 months of age → permanent immunity.
Mumps (parotitis) (virus)	14–21 days	Immediately before swelling begins until 9 days later	Direct contact; droplet infection	*Prodromal stage:* malaise, headache, with or without fever. *Parotitis:* swelling, unilateral or bilateral, of parotid glands accompanied by pain, tenderness and difficulty swallowing.	Isolate. Bedrest for duration of swelling. Analgesics for pain. Offer liquids or soft, bland foods. Use hot or cold compresses to neck, whichever is more comfortable.	Child recovers completely without complications such as meningoencephalitis, sterility (in adult males).	Vaccine at 15 months of age → permanent immunity.
German measles (rubella) (myxovirus)	14–21 days	7 days before to 5 days after rash appears	Direct contact; indirect contact	*Prodromal stage:* absent in children. *Rash:* first appears on face, spreads down to neck, arms, trunk, and legs; discrete pinkish red maculopapular exanthema; gone by third day. *General:* slight fever, mild coryza, arthritislike symptoms (older child and adult).	Antipyretics/ analgesics p.r.n. Bedrest until fever subsides. Avoid contact with pregnant female: greatest danger is teratogenic effect to fetus.	Child recovers completely without complications such as arthritis, encephalitis, purpura.	Vaccine at 15 months of age → permanent immunity.

continued

TABLE 3.14 *Continued*

Disease (Agent)	Incubation Period	Period of Communicability	Transmission	Nursing Assessment	Nursing Plan/Implementation	Evaluation	Prevention
Varicella (chickenpox) (varicella-zoster virus)	2–3 weeks	1 day before rash begins until vesicles have fully crusted over	Droplet infection; direct contact	*Prodromal stage:* fever, malaise, anorexia. *Rash:* highly pruritic; vesicular; begins on chest, spreading to trunk; mostly on face and trunk; stops appearing after fifth day. *General:* lymphadenopathy, irritability.	Isolate until all vesicles have fully crusted over. Relieve itching with benadryl or antihistamines. Administer skin care to prevent secondary infection: daily bath or p.r.n., change linens and clothing daily. Keep child from scratching: apply cornstarch or calamine lotion, keep nails cut short, apply mitts p.r.n., light clothing.	Child recovers completely without complications such as Reye's syndrome, secondary bacterial infection.	None (full-blown case of chickenpox imparts permanent immunity).
Scarlet fever (group-A beta hemolytic strep)	1–7 days	Approximately 10 days (carrier phase may last for months)	Direct contact; droplet infection; indirect contact	*Prodromal stage:* sudden high fever, chills, tachycardia; headache, vomiting, abdominal pain. *Enanthema:* red strawberry tongue; red, swollen tonsils; circumoral pallor and flushed cheeks. *Exanthema:* rash—red, pinhead size punctate lesions, ↑ in folds of skin; by end of first week desquamation begins, may last 3 weeks. Positive throat culture for strep. Elevated ASO titer.	Respiratory isolation. Bedrest until fever subsides. Administer penicillin (or erythromycin). Relieve sore throat: analgesics, gargles, lozenges, inhalation of cool mist. Encourage fluids and soft, bland diet.	Child recovers completely without complications such as rheumatic fever, acute glomerulonephritis.	None (permanent immunity with disease).

PEDIATRIC NURSING

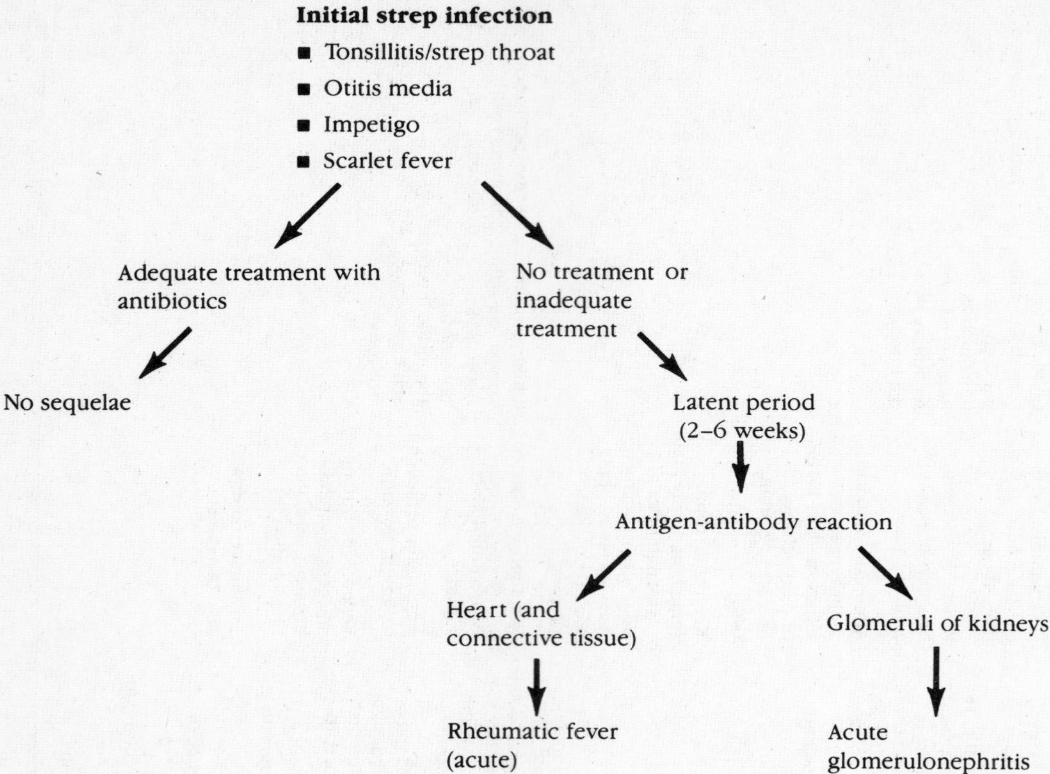

FIGURE 3.10
Sequelae of strep infections.

3. Prepare for/assist with Foley catheter placement, CVP, ICP monitor, NG tube, etc.
4. Monitor serum electrolyte lab values.

C. Goal: *prevent injury and possible bleeding.*

1. Observe child for petechiae, unusual bruising, oozing from body orifices or tubes, frank hemorrhage.
2. Check all urine and stool for occult blood.
3. Monitor lab values, including PT, PTT, platelets.
4. Administer blood products per MD order.

D. Goal: *provide parents with thorough understanding of Reye's syndrome.*

1. Primary nurse assigned to provide care and follow through with teaching.
2. Encourage parents' presence, even in PICU—explain all equipment and procedures in simple, direct terms.
3. Provide factual, honest and complete information re: disease, diagnosis, prognosis.

V. Evaluation:

A. Intracranial pressure is reduced and normal neurological functioning is restored.

B. Fluid and electrolyte balance is restored.

C. No clinical evidence of bleeding is found.

D. Parents express understanding of Reye's syndrome.

AUTOIMMUNE DISORDERS

Strep Infections/Sequelae

Introduction: Group A beta hemolytic strep is a common infectious organism that causes illness in children and is highly contagious. In themselves, the diseases caused by strep do not seem very serious: e.g., strep throat, otitis media, impetigo, or scarlet fever. The most common treatment for strep is a full course of antibiotic therapy: 10 days of penicillin (or, if allergic, erythromycin). With adequate therapy, generally no sequelae are seen. If the strep is *not* treated, or is only partially treated, the sequelae include serious systemic diseases, with potentially long-term effects. If the effect is manifested primarily in the heart (carditis), it is acute rheumatic fever. If the effect is manifested primarily in the kidneys, it is acute glomerulonephritis (see Figure 3.10).

I. Rheumatic fever

A. *Introduction:* Rheumatic fever is an acute, systemic, inflammatory disease affecting multiple organs and systems: heart, joints, CNS, collagenous tissue, etc. Thought to be autoimmune in nature, it most commonly follows a strep infection (see Figure 3.10) and occurs primarily in school-age children. In addition, it does tend to recur, and the risk of permanent heart damage increases with each subsequent attack of rheumatic fever.

B. Assessment:

1. Major manifestations (modified Jones criteria)
   a. Carditis: tachycardia, cardiomegaly, murmur, congestive heart failure (CHF).
   b. Migratory polyarthritis: swollen, hot, red, and excruciatingly painful large joints; migratory and reversible in nature.

c. Sydenham's chorea (St. Vitus Dance): purposeless, irregular, involuntary muscle spasms, loss of coordination, facial grimaces; completely reversible.

d. Subcutaneous nodules: small, round, freely movable, and painless swellings usually found over the extensor surfaces of the hands/feet or bony prominences; resolves without any permanent damage.

e. Erythema marginatum: reddish-pink-colored rash most commonly found on the trunk; nonpruritic, macular, clear center, wavy but clearly marked border; transient.

2. Minor manifestations

a. Clinical

(1) Previous history of rheumatic fever.

(2) Arthralgia.

(3) Fever—normal in morning, rises in mid-afternoon, normal at night.

b. Laboratory

(1) Increased erythrocyte sedimentation rate (ESR).

(2) Positive C-reactive protein.

(3) Leukocytosis.

(4) Anemia.

(5) Prolonged P–R/Q–T intervals on ECG.

3. Supportive evidence

a. Recent history of strep infection:

(1) Strep throat/tonsillitis.

(2) Otitis media.

(3) Impetigo.

(4) Scarlet fever.

b. Positive throat culture for strep.

c. Increased ASO titer: indicates presence of strep antibodies.

C. Analysis/nursing diagnosis:

1. *Decreased cardiac output* related to carditis.

2. *Pain* related to migratory polyarthritis.

3. *Potential for injury* related to chorea.

4. *Diversional activity deficit* related to lengthy hospitalization and recuperation.

5. *Knowledge deficit* related to preventing cardiac damage, relieving discomfort, and preventing injury.

6. *Noncompliance* with long-term antibiotic therapy and follow-up care.

D. Nursing plan/implementation:

1. Goal: *prevent cardiac damage.*

a. Hospitalization, with strict bedrest.

b. Monitor apical pulse for changes in rate, rhythm, murmurs.

c. Evaluate tolerance of increased activity via apical rate: if heart rate increases by more than 20 beats per minute over resting rate, child should return to bed.

d. Offer low-sodium diet to prevent fluid retention.

e. Administer oxygen, digoxin/lasix as ordered (if CHF develops). *Note:* Refer to Unit 4 for additional information on congestive heart failure.

2. Goal: *relieve discomfort.*

a. Use bed cradle to keep linens from resting on painful joints.

b. Administer aspirin as ordered to relieve pain.

c. Move child carefully, minimally—support joints.

d. *Do not* massage; *do not* perform ROM exercises; *do not* apply splints; *do not* apply heat/cold. All of these treatments will cause increased pain and are *not needed* since *no* permanent deformities will result from this type of arthritis.

3. Goal: *promote safety and prevent injury related to chorea.*

a. Use side rails: elevated, padded.

b. Restrain in bed if necessary.

c. *No* oral temperatures—child may bite thermometer.

d. Spoonfeed—no forks or knives, to prevent injury to oral cavity.

e. Assist with all aspects of ADL until child can care for own needs.

4. Goal: *provide diversion as tolerated.*

a. Encourage quiet diversional activities: hobbies, reading, puzzles.

b. Get homework, books; provide tutor as condition permits.

c. Encourage contact with peers: phone calls, letters, cards.

5. Goal: *encourage child and family to comply with long-term antibiotic therapy.*

a. Begin antibiotics immediately, to eradicate any lingering strep infection.

b. Prepare child/family for minimum of 5 years of intramuscular injections of penicillin.

c. Stress need for exact schedule: every 4 weeks.

d. Enlist child's cooperation with therapy, e.g., "hero" badge.

6. Goal: *health teaching.*

a. To encourage compliance with prolonged bedrest—stress that ultimate prognosis depends on amount of cardiac damage.

b. Teach necessity for long-term prophylactic therapy for 5 years initially (with lifetime follow-up), e.g., during dental work, childbirth, surgery (to prevent subacute bacterial endocarditis).

c. Teach rationale: permanent cardiac damage is more likely to occur with subsequent attacks of rheumatic fever.

E. Evaluation:

1. No permanent cardiac damage occurs.

2. Child is free from discomfort or is able to tolerate discomfort.

3. Injuries are avoided.

4. Child's need for diversional activity is met.

5. Child/family comply with long-term antibiotic therapy/prophylactic therapy.

II. Acute glomerulonephritis

A. *Introduction:* Acute glomerulonephritis (AGN) is a bilateral inflammation of the glomeruli of the kidneys and is the most common noninfectious renal disease of childhood. It occurs most frequently in boys ages 3–7 years, but it does occur in boys and girls ages 2–12 years. Like rheumatic fever, acute glomerulonephritis is thought to be the result of an antigen–antibody reaction to a strep infection (see Figure 3.10); however, unlike rheumatic fever, it does *not* tend to recur since specific immunity is conferred following the first episode of AGN. (Further information about AGN is found in Table 3.19, p. 264.)

B. Assessment:

1. Typical concerns from family about urine: change in color/appearance of urine (thick, reddish brown; decreased amounts).
2. Acute edematous phase—usually lasts 5–10 days.
   a. Lab examination of urine:
      (1) severe **hematuria.**
      (2) Mild proteinuria.
      (3) Increased specific gravity.
   b. **Hypertension**
      (1) Headache.
      (2) Potential hypertensive encephalopathy → seizures, increased intracranial pressure.
   c. Mild–moderate edema: chiefly periorbital; increased weight due to fluid retention.
   d. General:
      (1) Abdominal pain.
      (2) Malaise.
      (3) Anorexia.
      (4) Vomiting.
      (5) Pallor.
      (6) Irritability.
      (7) Lethargy.
      (8) Fever.
3. Diuresis phase:
   a. Copious diuresis.
   b. Decreased body weight.
   c. Marked clinical improvement.
   d. Decrease in gross hematuria, but miscoscopic hematuria may persist for weeks/months.

C. Analysis/nursing diagnosis:

1. *Fluid volume excess* related to decreased urine output.
2. *Pain* related to fluid retention.
3. *Altered nutrition, less than body requirements,* related to anorexia and vomiting.
4. *Impaired skin integrity* related to immobility.
5. *Activity intolerance* related to fatigue.
6. *Knowledge deficit* related to disease process, treatment, and follow-up care.

D. Nursing plan/implementation:

1. Goal: *monitor fluid balance, observing carefully for complications.*
   a. Check and record blood pressure at least every 4 hours to monitor hypertension.
   b. Monitor daily weights.
   c. Urine: strict I&O; specific gravity and dipstick for blood every void.
   d. Note edema: extent, location, progression.
   e. Adhere to fluid restrictions if ordered.
   f. Diet: low sodium, low potassium.
   g. Bedrest, chiefly due to hypertension: monitor for possible development of hypertensive encephalopathy (seizures, increased intracranial pressure); report any changes stat to physician.
   h. Administer medications as ordered:
      (1) Antibiotics—eradicate any lingering strep infection.
      (2) Antihypertensives, e.g., Apresoline.
      (3) Rarely use diuretics—limited value.
      (4) If CHF develops—may use digoxin.
      (5) Refer to Unit 6 for additional information on medications.
2. Goal: *provide adequate nutrition.*
   a. *Diet: low sodium, low potassium*—to prevent fluid retention and hyperkalemia; *high protein* to replace protein being lost via urine. Refer to Unit 5 for additional information on diets.
   b. Stimulate appetite: offer small portions, attractively prepared; meals with family or other children; offer preferred foods, if possible; encourage parents to bring in special foods, e.g., culturally related preferences.
3. Goal: *provide reasonable measure of comfort.*
   a. Encourage parental visiting.
   b. Provide for positional changes, give good skin care.
   c. Provide appropriate diversion, as tolerated.
4. Goal: *prevent further infection.*
   a. Use good handwashing technique.
   b. Screen staff, other patients, visitors to limit contact with infectious persons.
   c. Administer antibiotics if ordered (usually only for children with positive cultures).
   d. Keep warm and dry, stress good hygiene.
   e. Note possible sites of infection: ↑ skin breakdown secondary to edema.
5. Goal: *teach child and family about AGN/discharge planning.*
   a. Teach how to check urine at home: dipstick for protein and blood. (*Note:* Occult hematuria may persist for months.)
   b. Teach activity restriction: no strenuous activity until hematuria is completely resolved.
   c. Teach family how to prepare low-sodium, low-potassium diet.
   d. Arrange for follow-up care: physician, PHN.
   e. *Stress:* subsequent recurrences are *rare* because specific immunity is conferred.

E. Evaluation:

1. No permanent renal damage occurs.
2. Normal fluid balance maintained/restored.
3. Adequate nutrition is maintained.
4. No secondary infections occur.
5. Child/family verbalize their understanding of the disease, its treatment and prognosis.

Kawasaki Disease (Mucocutaneous Lymph Node Syndrome)

I. *Introduction:* Kawasaki disease (mucocutaneous lymph node syndrome) is an acute, febrile, multisystem disorder believed to be autoimmune in nature. Affecting primarily the skin and mucous membranes of the respiratory tract, lymph nodes, and heart, Kawasaki disease has a low fatality rate (<2%), although vasculitis and cardiac involvement (coronary artery changes) may result in major complications in as many as 20% of the children with this disease. The disease is not believed to be communicable, and the exact cause remains unknown; geographical (living near fresh water) and seasonal (late winter, early spring) outbreaks do occur. Kawasaki disease occurs in both boys and girls between 1 and 14 years of age; it is most common in boys between 2 and 4 years of age and in children of Japanese descent. It may be preceded by URI or exposure to a freshly cleaned carpet. A complete and apparently spontaneous recovery occurs within 3 to 4 weeks in the majority of cases. Treatment, which is primarily symptomatic, does not appear to either enhance recovery or prevent complications, although recent research indicates that life-threatening complications and long-term disability may be avoided or minimized with early treatment (i.e., gamma globulin) to reduce cardiovascular damage.

II. Assessment:

A. Abrupt onset with high fever (102°–106°F) lasting more than five days and does not remit with the administration of antibiotics.

B. Conjunctivitis—bilateral, nonpurulent.

C. Oropharnygeal manifestations:

1. Dry, red, cracked lips.
2. Oropharnygeal reddening and a "strawberry" tongue.

D. Peeling (desquamation) of the palms of the hands and the soles of the feet; begins at the fingertips and the tips of the toes; as peeling progresses, hands and feet become very red, sore, and swollen.

E. Cervical lymphadenopathy.

F. Generalized erythematous rash on trunk and extremities, without vesicles or crusts.

G. Irritability, anorexia.

H. Arthralgia and arthritis.

I. Panvasculitis of coronary arteries: formation of aneurysms and thrombi; CHF, myocarditis, pericardial effusion, arrhythmias, mitral insufficiency, myocardial infarction.

J. Lab tests:

1. Elevated: erythrocyte sedimentation rate.
2. Elevated: WBC count.
3. Elevated: platelet count.

III. Analysis/nursing diagnosis:

A. *Hyperthermia* related to high, unremitting fever.

B. *Altered oral mucous membrane and impaired swallowing* related to oropharyngeal manifestations.

C. *Impaired skin integrity* related to desquamation.

D. *Fluid volume deficit* related to high fever and poor oral intake.

E. *Altered tissue perfusion* (cardiovascular, potential/actual) related to vasculitis and/or thrombi.

F. *Knowledge deficit* related to disease course, treatment, prognosis.

IV. Nursing plan/implementation:

A. Goal: *reduce fever.*

1. Monitor rectal temperature every 2 hours or p.r.n.
2. Administer **aspirin** (not Tylenol) per MD order. (**Note:** aspirin is the drug of choice to reduce fever; also has anti-inflammatory effect and anti-platelet effect. Dose is 100 mg/kg/day. Monitor for signs of salicylate toxicity.)
3. ▶ Tepid sponge baths or hypothermia blanket per MD order.
4. Offer frequent cool fluids.
5. Apply cool, loose-fitting clothes; use cotton bed linens only (no heavy blankets).
6. Seizure precautions.

B. Goal: *provide comfort measures to oral cavity to ease the discomfort of swallowing.*

1. Good oral hygiene with soft sponge and diluted hydrogen peroxide.
2. Apply petroleum jelly to lips.
3. Topical anesthetic before meals (e.g., viscous xylocaine).
4. Bland foods in small amounts at frequent intervals.
5. Avoid hot, spicy foods.
6. Offer favorite foods from home or preferred foods from hospital selection.

C. Goal: *prevent infections and promote healing of skin.*

1. Monitor skin for desquamation, edema, rash.
2. Keep skin clean, dry, well lubricated.
3. Avoid soap to prevent drying.
4. Gentle handling of skin to minimize discomfort.
5. Provide sheepskin to lie on.
6. Prevent scratching and itching—apply cotton mittens if necessary.
7. Bedrest; elevate edematous extremities.

D. Goal: *prevent dehydration and restore normal fluid balance.*

1. Strict I&O.
2. Monitor urine specific gravity q8h for increase (dehydration) or decrease (hydration).
3. Monitor vital signs for fevers, tachycardia, arrhythmia.
4. Monitor skin turgor, mucous membranes, anterior fontanel for dehydration.
5. "Force" fluids.
6. IV fluids per MD order.

E. Goal: *prevent cardiovascular complications.*

1. ▶ ECG monitor—report arrhythmias or tachycardia.
2. Administer aspirin (see goal A, above).
3. Monitor for signs and symptoms of congestive heart failure: tachycardia, tachypnea, dyspnea, rales, orthopnea, distended neck veins, dependent edema.
4. Monitor circulatory status of extremities—check for possible development of thrombi.
5. ▶ Stress need for long-term follow-up, including ECGs and echocardiograms.

PEDIATRIC NURSING

V. Evaluation:

A. Fever returns to normal.

B. Oral cavity heals and child is able to swallow.

C. Skin heals and no infection occurs.

D. Normal fluid balance is restored.

E. Normal cardiovascular functioning is reestablished and no complications occur.

F. Parents/child verbalize their understanding of Kawasaki disease.

Bacterial Infections

Introduction: Acute bacterial ear infection *(acute otitis media)* is common in young children, primarily because their eustachian tube is shorter and straighter than the adult's; this allows for ready drainage of infected mucus from URIs directly into the middle ear. In *some* cases, acute otitis media precedes the onset of *bacterial meningitis,* an extremely serious and potentially fatal disease. Bacterial meningitis is a medical emergency, requiring early detection and prompt, aggressive therapy to prevent permanent neurologic damage or death. (Refer to section on Hydrocephalus, p. 268). Serous otitis (chronic) may result in hearing impairment or loss but is not likely to result in meningitis. Refer to Myringotomy, Table 3.15, p. 256.

I. Acute otitis media

A. Assessment:

1. Fever.
2. Pain in affected ear. Infant may not complain of pain but may tug at ear, cry, shake head, refuse to lie down.
3. Malaise, irritability, anorexia (possibly vomiting).
4. May have symptoms and signs of URI: rhinorrhea, coryza, cough.

B. Analysis/nursing diagnosis:

1. *Pain* related to pressure of pus/purulent material on eardrum.
2. *Potential for injury/infection* related to complication of meningitis.

C. Nursing plan/implementation:

1. Goal: *eradicate infection and prevent further complications (meningitis).* Administer antibiotics as ordered.
2. Goal: *relieve pain and promote comfort.*
   a. Administer decongestants as ordered.
   b. Offer analgesics/antipyretics to provide symptomatic relief and to decrease fever.
3. Goal: *health teaching.*
   a. Teach parents that the child needs to finish all medication, even though child will seem clinically better within 24–48 hours.
   b. Review appropriate measures to control fever: antipyretics, cool sponges.

D. Evaluation:

1. Infection is eradicated, no complications.
2. Child appears to be comfortable.

II. Bacterial meningitis

A. Assessment:

1. Abrupt onset: initial sign may be a seizure, following an episode of URI/acute otitis media.
2. Chills and fever.
3. Vomiting; may complain of headache, neck pain.
4. Photophobia.
5. Alterations in level of consciousness: delirium, stupor, increased intracranial pressure.
6. Nuchal rigidity.
7. Opisthotonus position: head is drawn backward into overextension.
8. Hyperactive reflexes related to CNS irritability.

B. Analysis/nursing diagnosis:

1. *Potential for infection* related to communicability of meningitis.
2. *Potential for injury* related to CNS irritability and seizures.
3. *Pain* related to nuchal rigidity, opisthotonus position, increased muscle tension.
4. *Sensory/perceptual alterations* related to seizures and changes in level of consciousness.
5. *Altered nutrition, less than body requirements,* related to fever and poor oral intake.
6. *Knowledge deficit* regarding diagnostic procedures, condition, treatment, prognosis.

C. Nursing plan/implementation:

1. Goal: *prevent spread of infection.*
   a. Institute universal precautions.
   b. Enforce strict handwashing.
   c. Institute and maintain respiratory isolation for minimum of 24 hours after starting IV antibiotics, at which time child is no longer considered to be communicable and can come off isolation.
   d. Supervise parents in isolation techniques.
   e. Identify family members and others at high risk: do cultures (*Haemophilus influenzae, E. coli,* etc.); possibly begin prophylactic antibiotics, e.g., Rifampin.
   f. Treat with IV antibiotics (as ordered) as soon as possible after admission (after cultures are obtained); continue 10–14 days (until cerebrospinal-fluid culture is negative and child appears clinically improved).
   g. Anticipate large-dose IV medications only—administer slowly in dilute form to prevent phlebitis.
   h. Restrain as needed to maintain IV.
2. Goal: *promote safety and prevent injury/seizures.*
   a. Maintain seizure precautions.
   b. Place child near nurses' station for maximum observation; provide private room for isolation.
   c. Minimize stimuli: quiet, calm environment.
   d. Restrict visitors to immediate family.
   e. *Position*: head of bed slightly elevated to decrease intracranial pressure. (If opisthotonus: side-lying, for comfort and safety.)
3. Goal: *maintain adequate nutrition.*
   a. NPO or clear liquids initially; supplement with IVs, as child may be unable to coordinate sucking and swallowing.
   b. Offer diet for age, as tolerated—child may experi-

ence anorexia (due to disease) or vomiting (due to increased intracranial pressure).

c. Monitor I&O, daily weights.

D. Evaluation:

1. No spread of infection noted.
2. Safety maintained.
3. Adequate nutrition and fluid intake maintained.
4. Child recovers without permanent neurologic damage, e.g., seizure disorders, hydrocephalus.

III. Infestations

A. Lice (Pediculosis)

1. *Introduction:* In children, the most common form of lice is the *Pediculosis capitis,* or head lice. This parasite feeds on the scalp, and its saliva causes severe itching. Head lice are frequently associated with the sharing of combs and brushes, hats, and clothing; thus, they are more common in girls, especially those with long hair. Lice are also associated with overcrowded conditions and poor hair hygiene.

2. **Assessment:**
   a. Severe itching of scalp.
   b. Visible eggs/nits on shafts of hair.

3. **Analysis/nursing diagnosis:**
   a. *Impaired skin integrity* related to infestation of scalp with lice.
   b. *Altered comfort* related to severe pruritus of scalp.
   c. *Knowledge deficit* related to transmission and prevention of disease and treatment regimen.

4. **Nursing plan/implementation:**
   a. Goal: *eradicate lice infestation.* Apply Kwell shampoo—rub in for 4–5 minutes, then comb with fine-tooth comb to remove dead lice and nits (eggs).
   b. Goal: *prevent spread of lice.*
      (1) Wear gloves and cap to protect self.
      (2) Inspect other family members; treat p.r.n. with Kwell.
      (3) Wash all clothes and linens to kill any lice that may have fallen off the child's hair.
      (4) Encourage short hair, if acceptable.
      (5) Teach preventive measures: don't share comb, brushes, hats.

5. **Evaluation:** lice eradicated and do not spread.

B. Pinworms (Oxyuriasis)

1. *Introduction:* In children, the most common parasitic infestation is pinworms. Infestation usually occurs when the child places fingers (and the pinworm eggs) into the mouth. Breaking the anus-to-mouth contamination cycle can best be accomplished by good hygiene, especially handwashing before eating and after toileting. If one family member has pinworms, it is highly likely that other family members are also infested; therefore, treat the entire family to eradicate the parasite. Pinworms are easily eradicated with anti-parasitic medications.

2. **Assessment:**
   a. Rectal itching.
   b. Visible pinworms in the stool.
   c. Vague abdominal discomfort.
   d. Anorexia and weight loss.

3. **Analysis/nursing diagnosis:**
   a. *Potential for infection/injury* related to the anus-to-mouth contamination cycle of pinworm infestation.
   b. *Altered comfort* related to severe rectal itching and abdominal pain.
   c. *Knowledge deficit* related to transmission and prevention of disease and treatment regimen.

4. **Nursing plan/implementation:**
   a. Goal: *eradicate pinworm infestation.* Treat all family members simultaneously with an anti-parasitic agent, e.g., pyramtel pamoate.
   b. Goal: *prevent spread of pinworms.*
      (1) Launder all underwear, bed linens, and towels in hot soapy water to kill eggs.
      (2) Teach family members the importance of good hygiene, especially handwashing before eating (or preparing food) and after toileting. Stress to children to keep their fingers out of their mouths.

5. **Evaluation:** Pinworms are eradicated and do not spread; reinfestation does not occur.

ACCIDENTS: INGESTIONS AND POISONINGS

I. General principles of treatment for ingestions and poisonings:

A. *Prevention:* refer to section on Toddler Safety, p. 221.

B. How to induce vomiting:

1. Drug of choice—syrup of ipecac (available over the counter; does not require an MD order). Families with young children should keep this medication on hand in case of accidental poisoning.
2. Dose:
   a. 30 mL for adolescents (12–18 years of age).
   b. 15 mL for children (1 year–11 years of age). *Note:* do not administer to infants less than 1 year of age without MD order.
3. Follow dose of ipecac with 4–8 ounces of tap water or as much water as child will drink. In young children, give water first as child may refuse to drink anything else after tasting the ipecac.
4. Monitor child for 15–30 minutes; the first dose of ipecac will produce vomiting within 30 minutes 90% of the time. If child does not vomit, give second dose of syrup of ipecac with additional water.
5. The child *must* vomit the syrup of ipecac to avoid it being absorbed and causing potentially fatal cardiotoxicity, i.e., cardiac arrhythmias, atrial fibrillation, severe heart block. If child does not vomit within 30 minutes of second dose, manually stimulate gag reflex (use spoon to touch back of throat) or assist with gastric lavage.

C. When **not** to induce vomiting:

1. Child is stuporous or comatose.
2. Poison ingested is a corrosive substance or petroleum distillate.
3. Child is having seizures.

II. Salicylate poisoning

A. Assessment:

1. Determine how much aspirin was ingested, when, which type.
2. Evaluate salicylate levels: normal, 0; therapeutic range = 15–30 mg/dL; *toxic,* 30 mg/dL.
3. *Early* identification of *mild toxicity:*
   a. Tinnitus (ringing in the ears).
   b. Changes in vision, dizziness.
   c. Sweating.
   d. Nausea, vomiting, abdominal pain.
4. *Immediate* recognition of salicylate *poisoning:*
   a. Hyperventilation (earliest sign).
   b. Fever—may be quite high (105°–106°F).
   c. Respiratory alkalosis and/or metabolic acidosis.
   d. *Late* signs: bleeding tendencies, severe electrolyte disturbances, liver and/or kidney failure.

B. Analysis/nursing diagnosis:

1. *Ineffective breathing patterns* related to hyperventilation/respiratory alkalosis.
2. *Fluid volume deficit* (dehydration) related to increased insensible loss of fluids via hyperventilation, increased loss of fluids via vomiting and increased need for fluids due to hyperpyrexia (fever).
3. *Potential for injury* related to bleeding.
4. *Anxiety* related to parental/child feelings of guilt, uncertainty as to outcome, invasive nature of treatments.
5. *Knowledge deficit* regarding accident prevention.

C. Nursing plan/implementation:

1. Goal: *promote excretion of salicylates.*
   a. If possible, induce vomiting using syrup of ipecac (save, bring to emergency room).
   ▶ b. Assist with gastric lavage, if appropriate.
   c. Administer activated charcoal after vomiting, as ordered, to absorb any salicylate remaining in stomach.
   ▶ d. Assist with dialysis, as ordered, to promote excretion of salicylates and fluids.
   e. Administer IV fluids, as ordered.
2. Goal: *restore fluid and electrolyte balance.*
   a. Monitor I&O, urinalysis, specific gravity.
   b. Prepare sodium bicarbonate, administer as ordered to correct metabolic acidosis.
   c. Monitor IV fluids and electrolytes.
   d. NPO initially (NG tube).
3. Goal: *reduce temperature.*
   a. **No** aspirin or acetaminophen, which might further complicate bleeding tendencies or lead to liver or kidney damage.
   ▶ b. Supportive measures: cool soaks, ice packs to armpits/groin, hypothermia blanket.
4. Goal: *prevent bleeding and possible hemorrhage.*
   a. Monitor urine and stools for occult blood.
   b. Insert NG tube to detect gastric bleeding.
   c. Observe for petechiae, bruising; monitor lab values for hematocrit and hemoglobin.
   d. Administer vitamin K as ordered to correct bleeding tendencies.
5. Goal: *health education to prevent another accidental poisoning:*
   a. Teach principles of poison prevention.
   b. Stress need to avoid accidental overdose with over-the-counter medications or dosage mix-ups.
   c. Allow child/parents to verbalize guilt, but avoid blaming or scapegoating.

D. Evaluation:

1. Aspirin is successfully removed from child's body without permanent damage.
2. Fluid and electrolyte balance is restored and maintained.
3. Child is afebrile.
4. Bleeding is controlled, no hemorrhage occurs.
5. No further episodes of poisoning occur.

III. Acetaminophen poisoning

A. Assessment:

1. Determine how much Tylenol was ingested, when, and which type.
2. Evaluate acetaminophen levels: normal = 0; therapeutic range = 15–30 μg/mL; toxic = 150 μg/mL 4 hours after ingestion.
3. *Phase I (first 24 hours):* anorexia, nausea, vomiting, diaphoresis, malaise, right upper quadrant (RUQ) tenderness.
4. *Phase II (1–3 days):* RUQ pain due to liver damage; elevated liver enzymes ALT (SGOT), AST (SGPT), increased bilirubin, increased prothrombin time and bleeding disorders.
5. *Late signs:* hepatic necrosis and failure, jaundice, renal failure, clotting disorders, hepatic encephalopathy.

B. Analysis/nursing diagnosis:

1. *Altered tissue perfusion* (liver) related to hepatic necrosis.
2. *Fluid volume deficit* related to increased loss of fluids secondary to vomiting and diaphoresis.
3. *Potential for injury* related to bleeding and clotting disorders.
4. *Anxiety* related to parental/child feelings of guilt, uncertainty as to outcome, and invasive nature of treatments.
5. *Knowledge deficit* regarding accident prevention.

C. Nursing plan/implementation:

1. Goal: *promote excretion of acetaminophen.*
   a. If possible, induce vomiting; save, bring to emergency room.
   b. Assist with gastric lavage, if appropriate.
   c. Assist with obtaining acetaminophen level 4 hours after ingestion.
   d. Administer N-acetylcysteine (Mucomyst) per MD order; this is the antidote.
2. Goal: *prevent permanent liver damage.*
   a. Treatment must begin as soon as possible; therapy

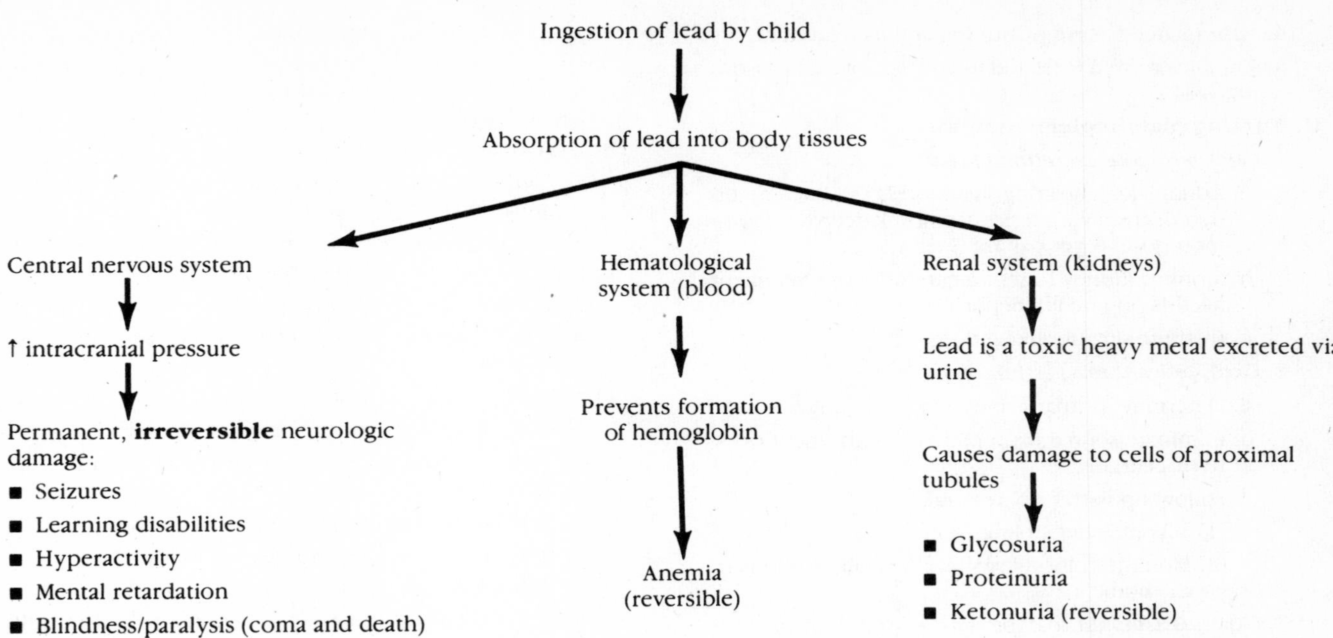

FIGURE 3.11
Pathophysiological effects of lead poisoning.

begun later than 10 hours after ingestion has no value.

b. Administer the antidote (Mucomyst) per MD order. Usually administered PO with cola or fruit juice; may be given via NG tube if necessary. If vomiting occurs within 1 hour, repeat the dose. Do **not** administer activated charcoal because it will bind the Mucomyst and make it ineffective.

c. Monitor hepatic functioning—assist with obtaining specimens and check results frequently; be aware that liver enzymes will rise and peak within 3 days and then should rapidly return to normal.

3. Goal: *restore fluid and electrolyte balance.*
   a. Monitor vital signs and perform neuro checks every 2–4 hours and p.r.n.
   b. Monitor I&O, urine analysis, including specific gravity, and weight.
   c. Monitor IV fluids as ordered.
4. Goal: *prevent bleeding.*
   a. Assist in monitoring child's prothrombin time; notify MD of significant changes.
   b. Monitor urine and stool for occult blood.
   c. Observe for and report any petechiae or unusual bruising.
5. Goal: *health education to prevent another accidental poisoning.* (See goal 5 nursing plan for Salicylate Poisoning, p. 252.)

D. Evaluation:

1. Acetaminophen is successfully removed from child's body.
2. Normal liver functioning is reestablished.
3. Fluid and electrolyte balance is restored and maintained.
4. No further episodes of poisoning occur.

IV. Lead poisoning (plumbism)

A. *Introduction:* Lead poisoning is a heavy-metal poisoning that occurs as a result of the ingestion or inhalation of lead. In children, this is most common in the toddler age group (1–3 years) and is usually a chronic type of poisoning that occurs as the result of repeated ingestions of lead. Children who engage in the practice of *pica,* the ingestion of nonnutritive substances, often ingest lead in flecks of lead-based paint from walls, furniture, or toys. In addition, research demonstrates that the parent–child relationship is a significant variable in lead poisoning; typically, there is a lack of adequate parental supervision that enables the child to engage in pica repeatedly over a fairly long period of time, until symptoms of lead poisoning become evident. (See Figure 3.11 for pathophysiologic effects of lead poisoning.)

B. Assessment:

1. Investigate history of pica (ingestion of nonnutritive substance).
2. Evaluate parent–child relationship.
3. Chronic lead poisoning: vague, crampy abdominal pain; constipation; anorexia and vomiting; listlessness.
4. Neurologic, renal, hematologic effects: see Figure 3.11.
5. "Blood-lead line"—bluish black line seen in gums.
6. X rays: lead lines in long bones and flecks of lead in GI tract.
7. Elevated serum-blood-lead levels: toxic ≥ 25 μg/dL

C. Analysis/nursing diagnosis:

1. *Altered thought processes* related to neurotoxicity.
2. *Activity intolerance* (and *potential for infection*) related to anemia.
3. *Altered urinary elimination* related to excretion of lead via kidneys.

PEDIATRIC NURSING

4. *Pain* related to lead poisoning and its treatment.
5. *Knowledge deficit* related to etiology of lead poisoning.

D. Nursing plan/implementation:

1. Goal: *promote excretion of lead.*
   a. Administer chelating agents (EDTA, BAL) as ordered: given via a series of painful, deep IMs (common dose: 6 per day for 5 days).
   b. Monitor kidney function carefully: the treatment itself is potentially nephrotoxic.
   c. Institute seizure precautions.
2. Goal: *prevent reingestion of lead.*
   a. Determine primary source of poisoning.
   b. Eliminate source from child's environment prior to discharge.
   c. Follow up with PHN referral.
      (1) Screen other siblings p.r.n.
      (2) Monitor "blood-lead level" of all children in the home.
3. Goal: *assist child to cope with multiple painful injections.*
   a. Prepare child for treatment regimen.
   b. Stress that this is **not** a punishment.
   c. Rotate sites as much as possible.
   d. May use a local anesthetic, e.g., procaine, injected simultaneously with chelating agent to decrease pain of injections.
   e. Apply warm soaks to injection sites: may help lessen pain.
   f. Encourage child to self-limit gross muscle activity (which increases pain).
   g. Offer child safe outlets for anger, fear, frustration—punching bag, pounding board, clay.
   h. Offer opportunity for medical play with empty syringes, etc.
4. Goal: *health teaching.*
   a. Stress (to child and parents) that getting the lead out is the only way to prevent permanent, irreversible neurologic damage (irreversible damage may have *already* occurred).
   b. Teach that the action of the chelating agent is to bind with the lead and to promote its excretion via the kidneys.

E. Evaluation:

1. Lead is successfully removed from child's body without permanent damage.
2. No further episodes of lead poisoning.
3. Child copes successfully with the disease and its treatment.

ALLERGIC RESPONSE: THREATS TO HEALTH STATUS

I. Infantile eczema (atopic dermatitis)

A. *Introduction:* Eczema is an allergic skin reaction, most commonly to foods, e.g., cow's milk or eggs. It is most common in infants and young children (under age 2 years). Infantile eczema generally undergoes permanent, spontaneous remission by age 3 years; however, approximately 50% of children who have had infantile eczema develop asthma during the preschool or school-age years.

B. Assessment:

1. Erythematous lesions, beginning on cheeks and spreading to rest of face and scalp.
2. May spread to rest of body, especially in flexor surfaces, e.g., antecubital space.
3. Lesions may ooze or crust over.
4. Severe pruritus, which may lead to secondary infection.
5. Lymphadenopathy near site of rash.
6. Unaffected skin tends to be dry and rough.
7. Systemic manifestations are rare—but child may be irritable, cranky.

C. Analysis/nursing diagnosis:

1. *Impaired tissue integrity* related to lesions.
2. *Pain* related to pruritus.
3. *Potential for (secondary) infection* related to breaks in the skin (first line of defense) and itching.
4. *Knowledge deficit* related to care of child with eczema, prognosis, how to prevent exacerbations.

D. Nursing plan/implementation:

1. Goal: *promote healing of lesions.*
   a. Give frequent baths in tepid water with cornstarch, to relieve pruritus, but with **no soap**—apply light coat of baby oil or mineral oil after bath.
   b. Apply wet soaks with Burow's solution (aluminum acetate solution; topical astringent/antiseptic).
   c. Protect child from possible sources of infection; universal precautions to prevent infection.
   d. Absolutely **no immunizations** during acute exacerbations of eczema because of the possibility of an overwhelming dermatitis, allergic reaction, shock, or even death.
   e. Apply topical creams/ointments as prescribed: A&D ointment, hydrocortisone cream to promote healing.
2. Goal: *provide relief from itching/keep child from itching.*
   a. Administer systemic medications as ordered, e.g., benadryl.
   b. Keep nails trimmed short—may need mittens (preferable not to use elbow restraints since the antecubital space is a common site for eczema).
   c. Use clothes and bedlinens that are nonirritating, i.e., pure cotton (**no** wool or blends).
   d. Institute elimination/hypoallergenic diet:
      (1) No milk or milk products.
      (2) Change to lactose-free formula, e.g., Isomil.
      (3) Avoid eggs, wheat, nuts, beans, chocolate.
   e. No stuffed animals or hairy dolls.
3. Goal: *provide discharge planning/teaching for parents and child.*
   a. Include all above information.

b. Include information on course of disease: characterized by exacerbations and remissions throughout early years.

c. Include information on prognosis: 50–60% will go into spontaneous (and permanent) remission during preschool years; 40–50% will develop asthma/hayfever during school-age years.

E. Evaluation:

1. Lesions heal well, without secondary infection.
2. Adequate relief from itching is achieved.
3. Parents verbalize understanding of eczema, prognosis, and how to prevent exacerbations.

II. Asthma

A. *Introduction:* Asthma is generally considered a chronic, reactive, lower airway disorder characterized by mucosal edema, ↑ viscid secretions, and small muscle contractions leading to bronchospasm and airway obstruction. The exact cause of asthma is unknown; however, it is believed to include an allergic reaction to one or more allergens, psychogenic factors, and perhaps other factors as well. The child usually exhibits other symptoms of allergy, such as infantile eczema or hayfever; in addition, 75% of children with asthma have a positive family history for asthma. The onset is usually before age 7 and remains with the child throughout life, although some children do experience dramatic improvement in their asthma with the onset of puberty.

B. Assessment:

1. Expiratory wheeze.
2. General signs and symptoms of respiratory distress, including anxiety, cough, shortness of breath, rales, cyanosis due to obstruction within the respiratory tract, use of accessory muscles of respirations.
3. Cough: hacking, paroxysmal, nonproductive.
4. Position of comfort for breathing: sitting straight up, leaning forward, which is the position for optimal lung expansion.

C. Analysis/nursing diagnosis:

1. *Ineffective airway clearance* related to bronchospasm.
2. *Anxiety* related to breathlessness.
3. *Knowledge deficit,* actual or potential, related to disease process, treatment, and prevention of future asthmatic attacks.
4. *Activity intolerance* related to dyspnea and bronchospasm.

D. Nursing plan/implementation:

1. Goal: *provide patent airway and effective breathing patterns.*

▶ a. Initiate oxygen therapy, as ordered, to relieve hypoxia, with high humidity (to liquify secretions).

b. Administer steroids as ordered to reduce inflammation.

c. Administer bronchodilators, as ordered, to relieve the obstruction: epinephrine, aminophylline, theophylline.

d. Carefully regulate flow of aminophylline IV to avoid giving too much medication in too little time.

e. Monitor vital signs closely while giving IV aminophylline, especially pulse and BP, as IV aminophylline can precipitate tachycardia or hypotension as side effects.

f. Observe for signs of aminophylline *toxicity:* prolonged increase in pulse, cardiac arrhythmias, or increasing restlessness.

g. Administer anti-inflammatory medications as ordered to relieve edema: prednisone, decadron.

2. Goal: *relieve anxiety.*

a. Provide relief from hypoxia (refer to goal 1), which is the chief source of anxiety.

b. Remain with child, offer support.

c. Administer sedation as ordered.

d. Encourage parents to remain with child.

3. Goal: *teach principles of prophylaxis.*

a. Review home medications, including cromolyn sodium. See Unit 6.

b. Review breathing exercises.

c. Discuss precipitating factors and offer suggestions as to how to avoid.

d. Introduce need for child to assume control over own care.

E. Evaluation:

1. Adequate oxygenation provided, as evidenced by pink color of nailbeds and mucous membranes and ease in respiratory effort.
2. Anxiety is relieved.
3. Child verbalizes confidence in, and demonstrates mastery of, skills needed to care for own asthma.

PEDIATRIC NURSING

PEDIATRIC SURGERY: NURSING CONSIDERATIONS

I. In general, basic care principles for children are the same as for adults having surgery.

II. Exceptions:

A. Children should be prepared according to their developmental level and learning ability.

B. Children cannot sign own surgical consent form; to be done by parent or legal guardian.

C. Parents should be actively involved in the child's care.

III. Table 3.15 reviews specific nursing care for the most common pediatric surgical procedures.

■ DISORDERS AFFECTING NUTRITIONAL FUNCTIONING

INSULIN-DEPENDENT DIABETES MELLITUS (IDDM)

IDDM was formerly called juvenile-onset diabetes. Since diabetes mellitus is fully covered in Unit 4, the information is not

■ TABLE 3.15 Pediatric Surgery: Nursing Considerations

Surgical Procedure	Specific Nursing Care
Tonsillectomy (the most frequently performed pediatric surgical procedure)	*Preoperative:* check bleeding and clotting times. *Postoperative:* ■ *Position*—place on abdomen or semi-prone with head turned to side to prevent aspiration. ■ *Observe for most frequent complication—hemorrhage* (frequent swallowing, emesis of bright red blood, shock). *Prevent bleeding:* ■ Do *not* suction—may cause bleeding. ■ Do *not* encourage coughing—may cause bleeding. ■ Minimize crying. *Decrease pain:* ■ Offer ice collar to decrease pain and for vasoconstriction, but do *not* force. ■ Acetaminophen for pain (*no* aspirin). *Nutrition:* ■ NPO initially, then cool, clear fluids such as ice water, "flat" ginger ale, apple juice. ■ **No** red fluids (punch, jello, icepops), citrus juices, warm fluids (tea, broth), toast, milk/ice cream/pudding, carbonated sodas. Progress to soft, bland. *Teach parents/discharge planning:* ■ Signs and symptoms of infection, call physician promptly. ■ 5–10 days postop, expect slight bleeding. ■ Continue soft, bland diet as tolerated.
Myringotomy ("tubes")	*Postoperative:* ■ *Position*—place with operated ear down, to allow for drainage. Expect moderate amount of purulent drainage initially. ■ Keep external ear canal clean and dry. *Teach parents/discharge planning:* ■ Need to keep water out of ear—use special ear plugs when bathing or swimming. ■ "Tubes" will remain in place 3–7 months and then fall out spontaneously (with healing of ear drum).
Appendectomy	(Observe same principles of preoperative and postoperative care as for adult GI surgery.) NPO until bowel sounds return (24–48 hours). If appendix ruptured pre- or intraoperatively, then *position* in semi-Fowler's and implement wound precautions; administer antibiotics as ordered. Monitor for signs and symptoms of peritonitis. Typical course: speedy recovery, with discharge in about 4–5 days and excellent prognosis.
Herniorrhaphy (umbilical/inguinal)	*Umbilical:* ↑ incidence in black infants. *Inguinal:* ↑ incidence in males. *Preoperative:* monitor for possible complications of strangulation. Routine postop GI surgery care. Prognosis—excellent, with discharge within 24–48 hours postop.

repeated here; please refer to Unit 4. Only the differences between the adult and the child are covered in Table 3.16.

UPPER GASTROINTESTINAL ANOMALIES

I. Cleft lip and cleft palate

A. *Introduction:* Cleft lip and cleft palate are congenital facial malformations resulting from faulty embryonic development; there appear to be multiple factors involved in the exact etiology: mutant genes, chromosomal abnormalities, teratogenic agents, etc. The infant may be born with cleft lip alone, cleft palate alone, or with both cleft lip and cleft palate. (See Table 3.1[illegible] for a comparison of these conditions.)

■ **TABLE 3.16** **Diabetes Mellitus: Differences Between the Child and the Adult**

IDDM: Insulin-Dependent Diabetes Mellitus (Child)	NIDDM: Non-Insulin-Dependent Diabetes Mellitus (Adult)
Absolute deficiency of insulin—pancreas produces *no* insulin at all.	*Relative* insufficiency of insulin rather than absolute deficiency.
Child is *totally dependent* on injections of exogenous insulin for the rest of his/her life.	Adult may control disease by *diet* and *oral* hypoglycemic agents or insulin injections.
Abrupt onset.	*Insidious* onset.
Age at onset—may begin at *any time* during childhood.	Age at onset—most common *between 40 and 60 years of age*.
Weight—*normal* or sudden *loss* of weight.	Weight—*obese,* or overweight.
Sex—boys and girls are *equally* affected.	Sex—more common in *females.*
Bed-wetting may be first clue.	First clue may be a complication rather than diabetes itself.
Insatiable thirst (polydipsia).	"3 p's": polyphagia, polydipsia; polyuria.
Very *unstable* or *difficult* to control—labile, brittle.	Relatively *more stable* and *easier* to control.
Prone to episodes of diabetic ketoacidosis.	Diabetic ketoacidosis is *rare.*
Honeymoon phase: a temporary, apparent remission—soon passes.	No honeymoon phase.
Due to young age at onset, *complications* seen at *younger* ages.	*Complications* often not seen until *later* adulthood—old age.

■ **TABLE 3.17** **Comparison of Cleft Lip and Cleft Palate**

Dimension	Cleft Lip Only	Cleft Palate Only	Both Cleft Lip and Cleft Palate
Incidence	1/1000. More common among males.	1/2500. More common among females.	Most common facial malformation. More common among males. More common among whites than blacks.
Surgical repair	"Cheiloplasty" (Logan bow)—see Figure 3.12. Often done in a single stage. Timing: age 6–12 weeks.	Palatoplasty. Often done in staged repairs. Timing: age 18 months	Lip always repaired before palate to enhance parent–infant attachment, bonding.
Position postoperatively	*Never* on abdomen.	*Always* on abdomen.	
Feeding postoperatively	*No* sucking. Use Breck feeder.	*No* sucking. Use wide-bowl spoon or plastic cup.	
Nursing care postoperatively	Elbow restraints. Lessen crying. Croup tent.	Elbow restraints. Lessen crying. Croup tent.	O.K. to show parents pictures of "before" and "after" repair.
Long-term concerns	Bonding, attachment. Social adjustment—potential threat to self-image.	Defective speech—refer to speech therapist. Abnormal dentition—refer to orthodontist. Hearing loss—refer to pediatric eye, ear, nose, throat specialist/ physician.	

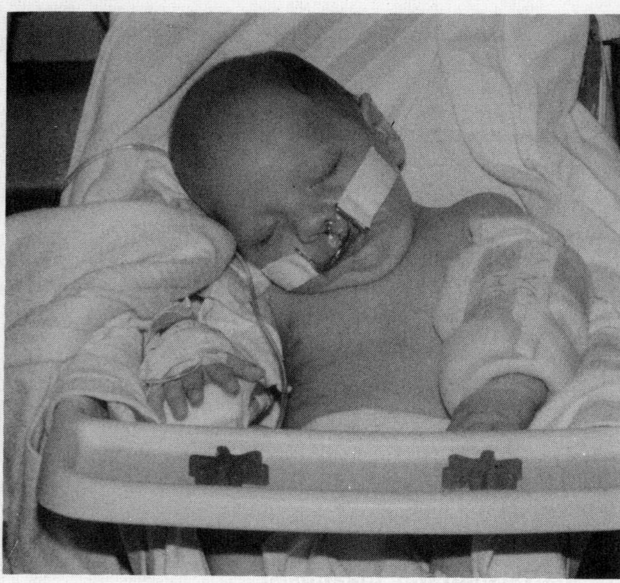

■ **FIGURE 3.12**
Logan bow—postop cleft lip repair. (Photo by Judy Koenig.)

B. Assessment:

1. *Cleft lip*—obvious facial defect, readily detectable at time of birth (see Figure 3.12).
2. *Cleft palate*—need to feel inside infant's mouth to check for presence of palatal defect and to note extent of defect: soft palate only or soft palate *and* hard palate.
3. *Both*—major problems with feeding: difficult to feed, noisy sucking, swallows excessive amounts of air, prone to aspiration. Also see Table 3.17.
4. Parent–infant attachment (bonding) may be adversely affected due to "loss of perfect infant," multiple hospitalizations: note amount and quality of parent–infant interaction.

C. Analysis/nursing diagnosis:

1. *Altered nutrition, less than body requirements,* related to difficulty feeding.
2. *Impaired physical mobility* (postop) related to post-op care requirements.
3. *Altered parenting* related to birth of child with obvious facial defect.
4. *Knowledge deficit,* actual or potential, related to treatment and follow-up.

D. Nursing plan/implementation:

1. Goal: *maintain adequate nutrition.*
   a. *Preoperative:* first encourage parents to watch nurse feed infant, then teach parents proper feeding techniques:
      (1) Use rubber-tipped medicine dropper (Breck-feeder).
      (2) Place tip to side of mouth, away from defect, to allow for sucking.
      (3) Rinse mouth with sterile water after feedings, to prevent infection.
      (4) Feed slowly, with child in sitting position, to prevent aspiration.
      (5) Burp frequently, as infant will swallow air along with formula due to the defect.
   b. *Postoperative*
      (1) Begin with clear liquids when child has fully recovered from anesthesia (see Table 3.17).
      (2) Monitor weight gain carefully, to assure adequate rate of growth.
2. Goal: *promote parent–infant attachment.*
   a. Show no discomfort handling infant.
   b. Stay with parents the first time they see/hold infant.
   c. Offer positive comments about infant.
   d. Give positive reinforcement to parents' initial attempts at parenting.
   e. Encourage parents to assume increasing independence in care of their infant.
   f. Allow rooming-in on subsequent hospitalizations.
3. Goal: *teach parents regarding feeding and need for long-term follow-up care.*
   a. Teach parents regarding long-term concerns (see Table 3.17).
   b. Make necessary referrals prior to discharge:
      (1) Specialists: speech, dentition, hearing.
      (2) Public health nurse.
      (3) Social service.
      (4) Disabled children's services for financial assistance.
      (5) Local facial-malformations support group.
   c. Refer parents to genetic counseling services due to mixed genetic/environmental etiology.
   d. Encourage parents to promote self-esteem in infant/child as child grows and develops.

E. Evaluation:

1. Adequate nutrition is provided, and infant grows at "normal" rate for age.
2. Parent–infant attachment is formed.
3. Parents verbalize confidence in their ability to care for infant.

II. Tracheoesophageal fistula

A. *Introduction:* Tracheoesophageal fistula (TEF) is a congenital anomaly resulting from faulty embryonic development; although there are numerous "types" of TEF, the major problem is an anatomical defect that results in an abnormal connection between the trachea (respiratory tract) and the esophagus (GI system). See Figure 3.13. No exact cause has been identified; however, infants born with TEF are often premature, with a maternal prenatal history of polyhydramnios. Diagnosis should be made in the immediate neonatal period, within hours after birth, and preferably before feeding (to avoid aspiration pneumonia).

B. Assessment:

1. Perinatal history: maternal polyhydramnios, premature infant.
2. *Most important system* affected is *respiratory:*
   a. Shortly after birth, infant has excessive amounts of mucus.

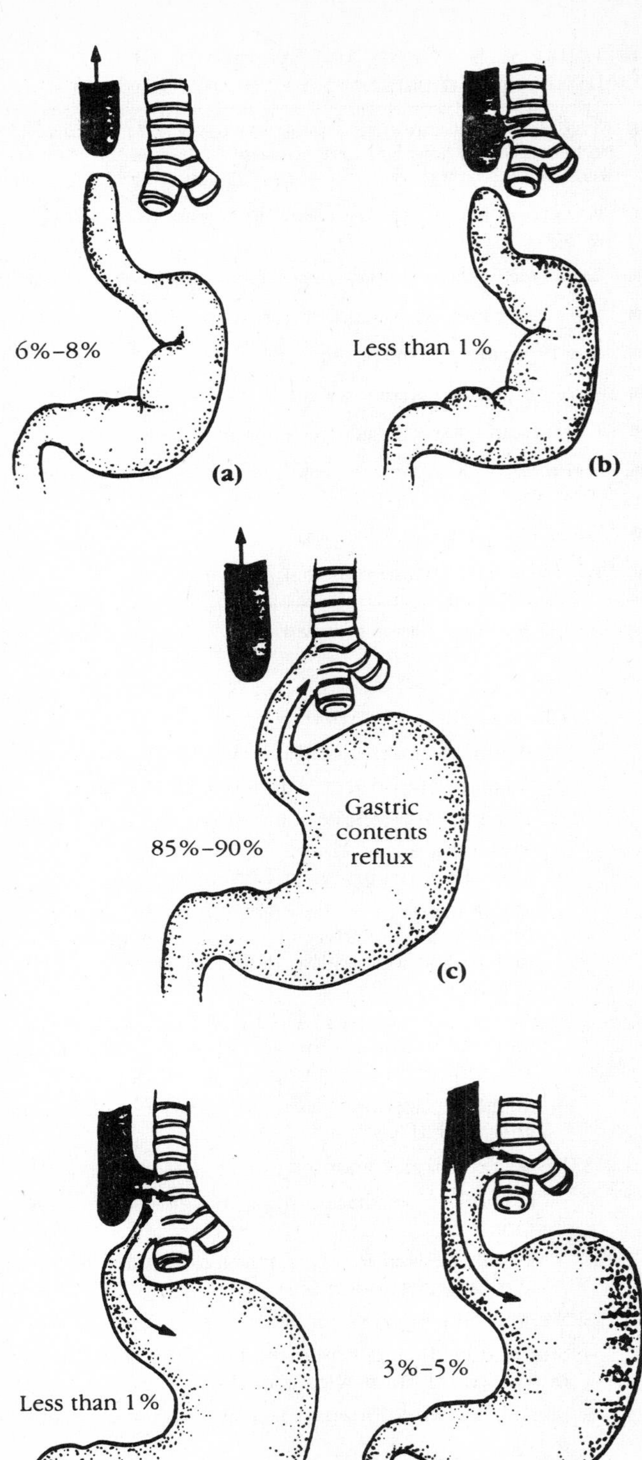

■ **FIGURE 3.13**
The five most frequently seen forms of tracheoesophageal fistulas and esophageal atresias, with their frequencies of occurrence. Arrows indicate what happens during infant feeding. (From James SR, Mott, SR: *Child Health Nursing*, Addison-Wesley, Menlo Park, CA, 1988, p. 902.)

b. Mucus bubbles or froths out of nose and mouth as infant literally "exhales" mucus.

c. *"3 c's": coughing, choking, cyanosis*—due to mucus accumulating in respiratory tract.

d. "Pinks up" with suctioning, only to experience repeated respiratory distress within a short time as mucus builds up again.

e. Aspiration pneumonia occurs early.

f. Respiratory arrest may occur.

3. *Second* system affected is GI:

a. Abdominal distention because excessive air enters stomach with each breath infant takes.

b. Inability to aspirate stomach contents when attempting to pass NG tube.

c. If all these signs are not correctly interpreted and feeding is attempted, infant takes 2–3 mouthfuls, coughs and gags, and forcefully "exhales" formula through nostrils.

C. Analysis/nursing diagnosis:

1. *Ineffective breathing pattern/ineffective airway clearance* related to excess mucus.
2. *Altered nutrition, less than body requirements,* related to inability to take fluids by mouth.
3. *Anxiety,* related to surgery, condition, premature delivery, and uncertain prognosis.
4. *Knowledge deficit* regarding discharge care of infant related to gastrostomy tube, feeding.

D. Nursing plan/implementation:

1. Goal: *prepare neonate for immediate surgery.*

a. Stress to parents that immediate surgery is *only* possible treatment; neonate is best surgical risk within *first 24 hours* of life.

b. Allow parents to see neonate prior to surgery to promote bonding and attachment.

c. Maintain NPO—provide IV fluids, monitor I&O.

d. *Position*: elevate head of bed (HOB) 20°–30° to prevent aspiration.

▶ e. Administer warmed, humidified oxygen, as ordered, to relieve hypoxia and to prevent cold stress.

2. Goal: *postoperative—maintain patent airway.*

a. *Position*: elevate HOB 20°–30°.

▶ b. Care of chest tubes (open-chest procedure).

▶ c. Care of endotracheal tube/ventilator (neonate frequently requires ventilatory assistance for 24–48 hours postop).

d. Monitor for symptoms and signs of pneumonia (most common postop complication):

(1) Aspiration.

(2) Hypostatic, secondary to anesthesia.

e. Monitor for symptoms and signs of RDS (premature infant).

f. Use special precautions when suctioning: "suction with marked catheter" to avoid exerting undue pressure on newly sutured trachea.

g. Administer prophylactic/therapeutic antibiotics, as ordered.

h. Administer warmed, humidified oxygen, as ordered; monitor ABGs.

3. Goal: *maintain adequate nutrition.*
   a. Maintain NPO for 10–14 days, until esophagus is fully healed (offer pacifier).
   b. 48–72 hours postop: IV fluids only.
   ▶ c. When condition is stable: begin gastrostomy tube feedings, as ordered.
      (1) Start with small amounts of clear liquids.
      (2) Gradually increase to full-strength formula.
      (3) Postop: leave G-tube open and elevated slightly above level of stomach to prevent aspiration if infant vomits.
      (4) Offer pacifier ad lib.
   d. Monitor weight, I&O.
   e. Between 10th and 14th postop day: begin oral feedings.
      (1) Start with clear liquids again.
      (2) Note ability to suck and swallow.
      (3) Offer small amounts at frequent intervals.
      (4) May need to supplement postop feeding with G-tube feeding p.r.n.
4. Goal: *prepare parents to successfully care for the infant after discharge.*
   a. Teach parents that infant will probably be discharged with G-tube in place; teach care of G-tube at home.
   b. Teach parents symptoms and signs of most common long-term problem, i.e., stricture formation.
      (1) Refusal to eat solids or swallow liquids.
      (2) Dysphagia.
      (3) Increased coughing or choking.
   c. Stress need for long-term follow-up care.
   d. Offer realistic encouragement, as prognosis is generally good.

E. Evaluation:

1. Neonate survives immediate surgical repair without untoward difficulties.
2. Patent airway is maintained; adequate oxygenation is provided.
3. Adequate nutrition is maintained; infant begins to gain weight and grow.
4. Parents verbalize confidence in ability to care for infant on discharge.

III. Pyloric stenosis

A. *Introduction:* Pyloric stenosis is a congenital anomaly of the upper GI tract, but the infant frequently does not present with symptoms until 2–4 weeks old. Basically the condition involves thickening, or hypertrophy, of the pyloric sphincter located at the distal end of the stomach; this causes a mechanical intestinal obstruction that becomes increasingly evident as the infant begins to consume larger amounts of formula during the early weeks of life. Pyloric stenosis is five times more common in males than females and is most often found in full-term white infants; the exact etiology remains unknown.

B. Assessment:

1. Classic symptom is *vomiting:*
   a. Begins as nonprojectile at 2–4 weeks of age.
   b. Advances to projectile at 4–6 weeks of age.
   c. Vomitus is nonbile-stained (stomach contents only).
   d. Most often occurs shortly after a feeding.
   e. Major problem is the mechanical obstruction of the flow of stomach contents to the small intestine due to the anatomical defect of stenosis of the pyloric sphincter.
   f. *No* apparent nausea or pain, as evidenced by the fact that infant eagerly accepts a second feeding after episode of vomiting.
   g. Metabolic alkalosis develops due to loss of hydrochloric acid.
2. Inspection of abdomen reveals:
   a. Palpable olive-shaped mass in right upper quadrant.
   b. Visible peristaltic waves, moving from left to right across upper abdomen.
3. Weight: fails to gain or loses.
4. Stools: constipated, diminished in number and size—due to loss of fluids with vomiting.
5. Signs of dehydration may become evident (see Table 3.18).
▶ 6. Upper GI series reveals:
   a. Delayed gastric emptying.
   b. Visible narrowing of pyloric sphincter at distal end of stomach.

C. Analysis/nursing diagnosis:

1. *Fluid volume deficit* related to vomiting.
2. *Altered nutrition, less than body requirements,* related to vomiting.
3. *Potential for injury/infection* related to altered nutritional state.

■ TABLE 3.18 Signs and Symptoms of Dehydration in Infants and Young Children

- *Weight loss* (most important variable to assess): *mild dehydration*—less than 5% weight loss; *moderate dehydration*—5–9% weight loss; *severe dehydration*—10–15% weight loss.
- *Skin:* gray, cold to touch, poor skin turgor (check skin across abdomen).
- *Mucous membranes:* dry oral buccal mucosa; salivation absent.
- *Eyes:* sunken eyeballs; absence of tears when crying.
- *Anterior fontanel* (in infant): sunken.
- *Shock:* ↑ pulse, ↑ respirations, ↓ BP.
- *Urine:* oliguria, ↑ specific gravity, ammonia odor.
- *Alterations in level of consciousness:* irritability, lethargy, stupor, coma, possible seizures.
- *Metabolic acidosis* (with diarrhea).
- *Metabolic alkalosis* (with vomiting).

4. *Impaired skin integrity* related to dehydration and altered nutritional state.
5. *Knowledge deficit* related to cause of disease, treatment and surgery, prognosis and follow-up care.

D. Nursing plan/implementation:

1. Goal (preoperative): *restore fluid and electrolyte balance.*
   a. Generally NPO, with IVs preop: IVs to provide fluids and electrolytes.
   b. Observe and record I&O, including vomiting and stool.
   c. Weight: check every 8 hours or daily.
   d. Monitor lab data.
2. Goal: *provide adequate nutrition.*
   a. Maintain NPO with IVs for 4–6 hours postop, as ordered (*can* offer pacifier).
   b. Follow specific feeding regimen ordered by doctor—generally start with clear fluids in small amounts on hourly basis, increasingly slowly as tolerated. Offer pacifier between feedings.
   c. Fed only by RN for 24–48 hours, as vomiting tends to continue in immediate postop period.
   d. Burp well—before, during, and after feeding.
   e. *Position* after feeding: high Fowler, turned to right side; minimal handling after feeding to prevent vomiting.
3. Goal (preop and postop): *institute preventive measures to avoid infection or skin breakdown.*
   a. Use good handwashing technique.
   b. Administer good skin care, especially in diaper area (urine is highly concentrated); special care to any reddened areas.
   c. Give mouth care when NPO or after vomiting.
   d. Tuck diaper down below suture line to prevent contamination with urine (postop).
   e. Note condition of suture line—report any redness or discharge immediately.
   f. Screen staff and visitors for any sign of infection.
4. Goal: *do discharge teaching to prepare parents to care for infant at home.*
   a. Teach parent that defect is anatomical and unrelated to their parenting behavior/skill.
   b. Demonstrate feeding techniques, and remind parent that vomiting may still occur.
   c. Stress that repair is complete; this condition will *never* recur.
   d. Instruct parents in care of the suture line: no baths for 10 days, tuck diaper down, report any signs of infection promptly.
   e. Offer follow-up referrals as indicated.

E. Evaluation:

1. Infant survives surgical repair without untoward difficulties (including infection/skin breakdown).
2. Adequate nutrition is maintained, and infant begins to grow and gain weight.
3. Parents verbalize confidence in their ability to care for their infant on discharge.

■ DISORDERS AFFECTING ELIMINATION

GASTROINTESTINAL DISORDERS

I. Lower gastrointestinal anomalies/obstruction

A. Hirschsprung's disease (congenital aganglionic megacolon)

1. *Introduction:* Hirschsprung's disease is a congenital anomaly of the lower GI tract, but the diagnosis is often not established until the infant is 6–12 months old. The major problem is a functional obstruction of the colon caused by the congenital anatomical defect of lack of nerve cells in the walls of the colon, resulting in the absence of peristalsis. Hirschsprung's disease is four times more common in males than females and is frequently noted in children with Down syndrome.
2. **Assessment:**
   a. In the newborn, failure to pass meconium (in addition to other signs and symptoms of intestinal obstruction).
   b. *Obstinate constipation*—history of inability to pass stool without stool softeners, laxatives, and/or enemas; persists in spite of all attempts to treat medically.
   c. Stools, while infrequent, tend to be thin and ribbonlike.
   d. Vomiting: bile stained, flecked with bits of stool (breath has fecal odor), due to GI obstruction and eventual backing-up of stools.
   e. Abdominal distention can be severe enough to impinge on respirations, due to GI obstruction and retention of stools.
   f. Anorexia, nausea, irritability due to severe constipation.
   g. Malabsorption results in anemia, hypoproteinemia, and loss of subcutaneous fat.
   h. Visible peristalsis and palpable fecal masses may also be detected.
3. **Analysis/nursing diagnosis:**
   a. *Constipation* related to impaired bowel functioning.
   b. *Altered nutrition, less than body requirements,* related to poor absorption of nutrients.
   c. *Potential for injury/infection* related to malnutrition.
   d. *Pain* related to surgery and treatments.
   e. *Knowledge deficit* regarding care of the child with a colostomy and follow-up care.
4. **Nursing plan/implementation:**
   a. Goal (preoperative): *promote optimum nutritional status, fluid and electrolyte balance.*
      (1) Monitor for signs and symptoms of progressive intestinal obstruction: measure abdominal girth daily.
      ▶ (2) Administer IV fluids, as ordered—may include hyperalimentation and/or intralipids.

PEDIATRIC NURSING

(3) Daily weights, I&O, urine specific gravity.

(4) Monitor for possible dehydration.

(5) Diet: *low* residue.

b. Goal (preoperative): *assist in preparing bowel for surgery.*

(1) Teach parents what will be done and why—enlist their cooperation as much as possible.

▶ (2) Insert NG tube, connect to low suction to achieve and maintain gastric decompression.

(3) *Position*: semi-Fowler's.

▶ (4) Bowel is cleansed via a series of isotonic saline (0.9%) enemas.

(5) Take axillary temperatures only.

(6) If child can understand, prepare for probable colostomy using pictures, dolls (usual age at surgery is 10–16 months).

c. Postoperative goals: Same as for adult having major abdominal surgery or a colostomy (see Unit 4).

d. Goal (postoperative): *discharge teaching to prepare parents to care at home for infant with a colostomy.*

(1) Home care of colostomy of infant is essentially same as for adult (see Unit 4).

(2) Teach parents to keep written records of stools: number, frequency, consistency.

(3) Teach parents to pin/tape diaper below colostomy to prevent irritation.

(4) Since colostomy is usually temporary, discuss:

(a) Second-stage repair (closure and pull-through) done between 2 and 3 years of age.

(b) Prepare parents for possible difficulties in toilet training.

(5) Stress need for long-term follow-up care.

(6) Make referral to public health nurse if indicated.

5. **Evaluation:**

a. Infant is prepared for surgery and tolerates procedure well.

b. Postop recovery is uneventful.

c. Parents verbalize confidence in ability to care at home for infant with a colostomy and verbalize their understanding that second surgery will be needed to effect closure of the colostomy.

B. Intussusception

1. *Introduction:* Intussusception is the apparently spontaneous telescoping of one portion of the intestine into another, resulting in a mechanical obstruction of the lower GI tract. There is no known cause, and intussusception is three times more common in males than females; the child with intussusception is usually between 6 and 24 months of age.

2. **Assessment:**

a. Typically presents with sudden onset in healthy, thriving child.

b. Pain: paroxysmal, abdominal, with intervals when the child appears normal.

c. Stools: "currant-jelly," bloody, mixed with mucus.

d. Vomiting due to intestinal obstruction.

e. Abdomen: distended, tender, with palpable, sausage-shaped mass over area of intussusception.

f. *Late signs:* fever, shock, signs of peritonitis as the compressed bowel-wall becomes necrotic and perforates.

3. **Analysis/nursing diagnosis:**

a. *Potential fluid volume deficit* related to diarrhea and vomiting.

b. *Pain* related to bowel-wall ischemia, necrosis, and death.

c. *Potential for injury/infection* related to bowel-wall perforation and peritonitis.

d. *Knowledge deficit* regarding the disease, medical and/or surgical treatment, and prognosis.

4. **Nursing plan/implementation:**

a. Goal: *assist with attempts at medical treatment.*

▶ (1) Explain to parents that a barium enema will be given to the child in an attempt to reduce the telescoping via hydrostatic pressure.

(2) Stress that, if this treatment is not successful, or if perforation of the bowel-wall has already occurred, surgery will be necessary.

(3) If medical treatment is apparently successful, monitor child for 24–36 hours for recurrence before discharge.

b. *Preoperative and postoperative goals:* same as for adult with major abdominal surgery (see Unit 4).

c. Goal: *discharge teaching to prepare parents for care of the child at home.*

(1) Stress that recurrence is rare (4–10%) and most often occurs within the first 24–36 hours after reduction.

(2) Other teaching: same as for adult going home after bowel surgery (see Unit 4).

5. **Evaluation:**

a. Infant tolerates medical-surgical treatment and completely recovers.

b. Parents verbalize confidence in ability to care for infant after discharge.

II. Acute gastroenteritis (AGE)

A. *Introduction:* In infants and young children, gastroenteritis is a very common acute illness that can rapidly progress to dehydration, hypovolemic shock, and severe electrolyte disturbances.

B. Assessment:

1. Diarrhea: often watery, green, explosive, contains mucus and blood.

2. Abdominal cramping and pain, often accompanied by bouts of diarrhea.

3. Dehydration: see Table 3.18.

4. Irritability, restlessness, alterations in level of consciousness.

5. Electrolyte disturbances: see Unit 4.

C. Analysis/nursing diagnosis:

1. *Fluid volume deficit* related to vomiting and diarrhea.

2. *Altered nutrition, less than body requirements,* related to AGE and its treatment, i.e., dietary restrictions.

3. *Pain* related to abdominal cramping, diarrhea.
4. *Impaired skin integrity* related to diarrhea.
5. *Altered tissue perfusion* related to dehydration and hypovolemia.
6. *Knowledge deficit* regarding diagnosis, dietary restrictions, treatment.

D. Nursing plan/implementation:

1. Goal: *prevent spread of infection.*
   a. Universal precautions to prevent infection.
   b. Enforce strict handwashing.
   c. Institute and maintain enteric precautions—follow policies regarding linens, excretions, specimens ("double bag, special tag").
   d. Pin diapers snugly; keep hands out of mouth.
   e. Obtain stool culture to identify causative organism; then administer antibiotics as ordered.
   f. Identify family members and others at high risk, obtain cultures.
2. Goal: *restore fluid and electrolyte balance.*
   a. Administer IV fluids and electrolytes as ordered.
   b. Monitor for appropriate response to therapy: decreased specific gravity, good skin turgor, normal vital signs.
   c. Monitor weight, I&O, specific gravity.
   d. Oral feedings—begin slowly with clear liquids, slow advance to "BRAT" diet: *b*ananas, *r*ice (cereal), *a*pplesauce, *t*ea or *t*oast; advance to regular diet as tolerated. **No milk/milk products** for 10 days, to prevent further diarrhea.
   e. Ongoing assessment of stools: note *a*mount, *c*olor, *c*onsistency, *t*iming ("ACCT").
3. Goal: *maintain or restore skin integrity.*
   a. Frequent diaper changes (use cloth diapers).
   b. Keep perineal area clean and dry.
   c. Apply protective ointments, e.g., petroleum jelly, A&D.
   d. If feasible, expose reddened buttocks to air (but *not* with explosive diarrhea).
4. Goal: *provide discharge teaching to parents.*
   a. Careful review of diet to be followed at home.
   b. Review principles of food preparation and storage to prevent infection.
   c. Instruct in disposal of stools at home.
   d. Emphasize importance of good hygiene.

E. Evaluation:

1. No spread of infection noted.
2. Fluid and electrolyte balance normal.
3. No skin breakdown noted.
4. Parents verbalize understanding of home care.

GENITOURINARY DISORDERS

I. Hypospadias

A. *Introduction:* Hypospadias is a congenital anatomical defect of the male genitourinary tract, readily detected at birth through simple visual examination. In hypospadias, the urethral opening is located on the ventral surface of the penile shaft; this makes voiding in the standing position virtually impossible and has the potential to cause serious psychologic difficulties. Although this condition should be detected in the delivery room/newborn nursery, staged surgical repairs often extend through the preschool years.

B. Assessment:

1. Urethral opening is located on ventral surface of penis.
2. May be accompanied by "chordee"—ventral curvature of the penis due to a fibrous band of tissue.
3. (Rare) ambiguous genitalia, resulting in need for chromosomal studies to determine sex of neonate.

PEDIATRIC NURSING

C. Analysis/nursing diagnosis:

1. *Altered urinary elimination* related to congenital anatomical defect of penis.
2. *Pain* related to surgery and treatments.
3. *Self-esteem disturbance* related to anatomical defect in penis and resulting disturbance in ability to void standing up.
4. *Knowledge deficit* related to condition, surgeries, outcome.

D. Nursing plan/implementation:

1. Goal: *promote normal urinary function.*
   a. Teach family that surgery is done in several stages, beginning at 2–3 years and finishing before kindergarten.
   b. Provide age-appropriate information to child regarding condition, surgery.
   c. *Preoperative* teaching with child should include: simulate anticipated postop urinary drainage apparatus and dressings on dolls; allow child to handle and play with them *now,* but stress need *not* to touch postoperatively.
   ▶ d. *Postoperatively:* Monitor urinary drainage apparatus; note hourly urine output, color, appearance (should be clear yellow, no blood).
2. Goal: *promote self-esteem.*
   a. Do not scold child if he exposes penis, dressings, catheters, etc.
   b. Reassure parents that preoccupation with penis is normal and will pass.
   c. Encourage calm, matter-of-fact acceptance of, and *avoid* strict discipline for, this behavior, which could negatively affect the child.

E. Evaluation:

1. Child is able to void in normal male pattern.
2. Child does not experience disturbances in self-concept and has normal self-esteem.

II. Wilm's tumor (nephroblastoma)

A. *Introduction:* Wilm's tumor is a malignant tumor of the kidney and is the most common form of renal cancer in children. Peak incidence occurs at 3 years of age, with a slightly higher incidence in males than females. Ninety percent of the cases occur unilaterally; the treatment of choice is nephrectomy (and adrenalectomy) followed by chemotherapy and radiation.

B. Assessment:

1. Most common sign: abdominal mass (firm, nontender).

TABLE 3.19 Comparison of Nephrosis and Acute Glomerulonephritis

Factor	Nephrosis (Nephrotic Syndrome)	Acute Glomerulonephritis
Illness type	Chronic.	Acute.
Illness course	Characterized by periods of exacerbations and remissions over many years.	Predictable, self-limiting, typically lasting 5–10 days (acute phase).
Cause	Unknown.	Group-A beta hemolytic strep.
Age at onset	2–5 years.	2–12 years (most common at 6 years).
Sex	More common among males.	More common among males.
Major signs and symptoms	Syndrome with variable pathology: massive proteinuria, hypoproteinemia, severe edema, hyperlipidemia.	Hematuria, hypertension.
Treatment	Symptomatic—no known cure.	Penicillin (EES), antihypertensives.
Diet	↓ sodium, ↑ protein.	↓ sodium, ↓ potassium, ↑ protein.
Fluid restrictions	Seldom necessary.	Frequently necessary (during acute phase).
Specific nursing care	Treat at home if possible; good skin care; prevent infection.	Treat in hospital during acute phase; monitor vital signs, especially BP; on discharge, stress need to restrict activity until microscopic hematuria is gone.
Prognosis	Fair; subject to long-term steroid treatment and social isolation related to frequent hospitalizations/confinement during relapses; 20% suffer chronic renal failure.	Good; stress that recurrence is *rare,* as specific immunity *is* conferred.

2. Most often first found by parent changing diaper; felt as a mass over the kidney area.
▶ 3. Intravenous pyelogram (IVP) confirms the diagnosis.
4. Metastasis occurs most frequently to the lungs: pain in chest, cough, dyspnea.

C. Analysis/nursing diagnosis: *altered urinary elimination* (other diagnoses depend on stage of tumor and presence of metastasis—similar to adult with cancer).

D. Nursing plan/implementation:

1. Goal: *promote normal urinary function.*
   a. Inform family that surgery is scheduled as soon as possible after confirmed diagnosis (within 24–48 hours).
   b. Explain to family that the preferred surgical approach is nephrectomy (and adrenalectomy).
   c. *Preoperative:* "Do not palpate abdomen" because the tumor is highly friable, and palpation increases the risk of metastasis.
   d. *Postoperative nursing care:* similar to care of adult with nephrectomy (see Unit 4).
   e. Postop care also includes long-term radiation therapy and chemotherapy (actinomycin D, vincristine, adriamycin; see Unit 6).
2. Goal: *discharge teaching to prepare parents to care for child at home.*
   a. Teach parents need for long-term follow-up care with specialists: oncologist, urologist.
   b. Answer questions regarding prognosis, offering realistic hope.
      (1) Child with localized tumor: 90% survival rate.
      (2) Child with metastasis: 50% survival rate.

E. Evaluation:

1. Child is able to maintain normal urinary elimination.
2. Parents verbalize their understanding of home care for the child.

III. Nephrosis. Nephrosis (idiopathic nephrotic syndrome) is a chronic renal disease having no known cause, variable pathology and no known cure. It is thought that several different pathophysiologic processes adversely affect the glomerular membranes of the kidneys, resulting in increased permeability to protein. This "leakage" of protein into the urine results in massive proteinuria, severe hypoproteinemia, and total body edema. A chronic disease, nephrosis often has its onset during the preschool years but is characterized by periods of exacerbation and remission throughout the childhood years.

The nursing care plan for the child with nephrosis is very similar to that for the adult with compromised renal functioning. The reader should refer to Units 5 and 6 for additional information about dietary restrictions and medications; also, refer to Table 3.19 for a chart comparing nephrosis and nephritis.

■ DISORDERS AFFECTING COMFORT, REST, ACTIVITY, AND MOBILITY

MUSCULOSKELETAL DISORDERS

Orthopedic conditions in infants and children are many and varied; but treatment is based on basic principles of nursing

TABLE 3.20 Common Pediatric Orthopedic Conditions

Condition	Definition	Age at Onset/Sex Difference	Treatment	Nursing Considerations
Club foot	Downward, inward rotation of one or both feet: talipes equinovarus (95%).	Newborn (congenital); twice as common among males.	Series of casts changed weekly followed by Denis Browne splint and then corrective shoes (severe cases—surgery).	Care of child in cast/brace. Stress need for follow-up. Encourage compliance.
Congenital hip dysplasia	Abnormal development of hip joint (most frequently unilateral).	Newborn (congenital); more common among females.	*Newborn*—double or triple diapers, Frejka pillow splint; *older infant or toddler*—possible surgery, spica cast.	Early identification (see Figure 3.14). Care of child in traction/cast. Encourage compliance. Check for other anomalies, e.g., spina bifida (see pp. 267–268).
Osteomyelitis	Most frequently occurring bone infection among children.	5–14 years; twice as common among males.	Blood cultures to diagnose causative organisms—select appropriate antibiotic; bedrest, immobilization with splint or cast.	Care of child in splint/cast. Provide diversion. Pain medications/antibiotics as ordered.
Legg-Calvé-Perthes	Aseptic necrosis of the head of the femur (cause unknown).	*Peak:* 4–8 years; *range:* 3–12 years; five times more common among males; ten times more common among whites than nonwhites.	Conservative therapy lasts 2–4 years, usually begins with bedrest and traction, followed by non–weight-bearing devices such as brace, cast.	Early identification. Care of child in traction/cast. Provide diversion. Assist child and family to cope with child's prolonged immobility.
Juvenile rheumatoid arthritis	Chronic systemic inflammatory disease (cause unknown).	*Peak:* 2–5 years and 9–12 years; more common among females.	Prevent joint deformity by exercise, splints, medications (steroids, ASA, IM gold); relieve symptoms (as per adult with arthritis).	Care of child in brace/splint. Provide diversion. Encourage compliance.
Scoliosis	Lateral curvature of the spine (cause unknown).	Adolescence; more common among females.	Milwaukee brace; halo-pelvic traction; Harrington rod.	Care of child in traction/cast/brace. Teach that brace is worn 23 hours per day, 7 days per week for 1–2 years (no exceptions). Encourage compliance. Promote positive self-image.
Osteosarcoma	Most frequently occurring bone cancer among children.	Adolescence (10–25 years); more common among males.	Amputation → prosthesis; intensive chemotherapy with high-dose methotrexate.	Prepare child for loss of limb. Help cope with prosthesis, life-threatening illness. Assist with grieving process.

care. Table 3.20 offers a quick review of the major pediatric orthopedic conditions. See also Figure 3.14.

NEUROMUSCULAR DISORDERS

I. Cerebral palsy (CP)

A. *Introduction:* Cerebral palsy is the most common permanent physical disability of childhood. It is a neuromuscular disorder of the pyramidal motor system resulting in the major problem of impaired voluntary muscle control. The damage appears to be fixed and nonprogressive, and the cause is unknown. However, although a variety of factors have been implicated in the etiology of CP, any perinatal incident that led to an episode of cerebral hypoxia/anoxia can usually be identified as a common link in its development.

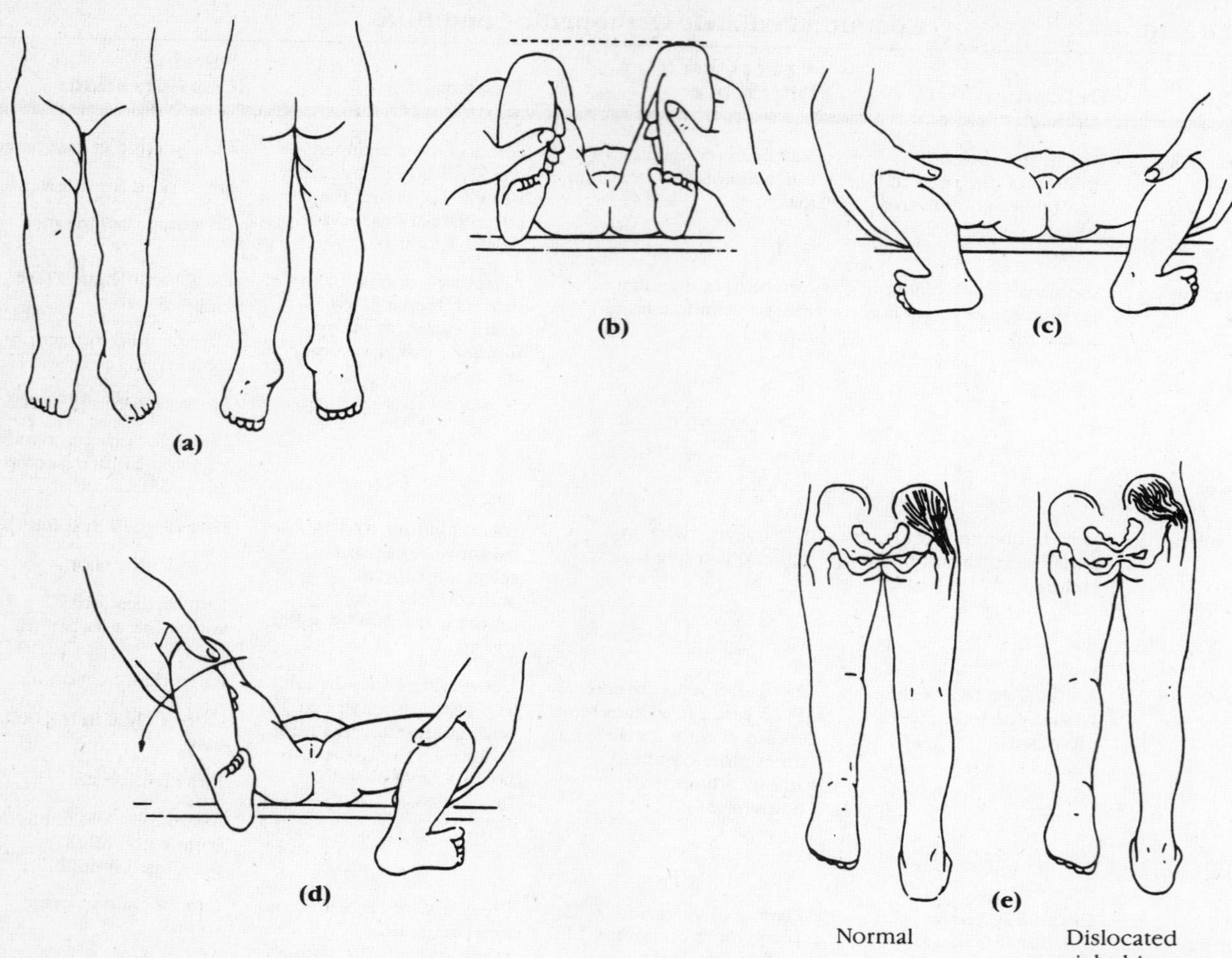

■ **FIGURE 3.14**
Signs of unilateral dislocated hip in an infant. (a) Unequal thigh folds. (b) Galleazzi's sign. (c) Normal abduction of the thighs. (d) Limited abduction of the thighs. (e) Trendelenburg's test. (From James SR, Mott, SR: *Child Health Nursing,* Addison-Wesley, Menlo Park, CA, 1988, p. 1038.)

B. Assessment:

1. Prenatal/perinatal history: incident that led to severe hypoxia or cerebral anoxia; also, low-birth-weight/premature infants.
2. Most common type of cerebral palsy—spastic.
   a. Hypertonicity (increased muscle tone).
   b. Persistent neonatal reflexes.
   c. "Scissoring" (legs crossed, with toes pointed).
   d. Tongue thrust, with difficulty sucking and swallowing → poor weight gain.
   e. Speech defects or difficulties.
3. IQ often normal (**not** necessarily mentally retarded) but difficult to "test" due to poor coordination, speech defects, and possible vision and hearing defects (occur in 50% of children with cerebral palsy).

C. Analysis/nursing diagnosis:

1. *Ineffective airway clearance* related to hyperactive gag reflex and possible aspiration.
2. *Altered nutrition, less than body requirements,* related to difficulty sucking and swallowing.
3. *Fluid volume deficit* related to difficulty sucking and swallowing.
4. *Impaired verbal communication* related to difficulty with speech.
5. *Sensory/perceptual alterations* related to potential vision and hearing defects.
6. *Potential for injury* related to difficulty controlling voluntary muscles.
7. *Self-esteem disturbance* related to disability.
8. **Note:** Because the level of disabilities with cerebral palsy can be varied, the nurse will need to select those diagnoses that apply, and clearly specify the individual child's limitations in any diagnostic statements.

D. Nursing plan/implementation:

1. Goal: *maintain patent airway.*
   a. Have suction and oxygen readily available.

b. Use feeding and positioning techniques to maintain patent airway.

c. Institute prompt, aggressive therapy for URIs, to prevent the possible development of pneumonia.

2. Goal: *promote adequate nutrition.*

a. Diet: high in calories (to meet extra energy demands).

b. Assure balanced diet of basic foods that can be easily chewed.

c. Provide feeding utensils that promote independence.

d. Relaxed mealtimes, decreased emphasis on manners, cleanliness.

e. Monitor I&O, weight gain.

3. Goal: *facilitate verbal communication.*

a. Refer to speech therapist.

b. Speak slowly, clearly to child.

c. Use pictures or actual objects to reinforce speech.

4. Goal: *prevent injury.* Refer to section on safety in growth and development.

a. Utilize individually designed chairs with restraints for positioning and safety.

b. Provide protective helmet to prevent head trauma.

c. Implement seizure precautions.

5. Goal: *provide early detection of and correction for vision and hearing defects.*

a. Arrange for screening tests.

b. Assist family with obtaining corrective devices: eyeglasses, hearing aids.

6. Goal: *promote locomotion.*

a. Encourage "infant stimulation" program to assist infant in reaching developmental milestones.

b. Refer to physical therapy for exercise program.

c. Incorporate play into exercise routine.

d. Use devices that promote locomotion: parallel bars, crutches, and braces.

e. Surgical approach may be needed to relieve contractures.

7. Goal: *encourage independence in ADL.*

a. Adapt clothing, feeding utensils, etc. to facilitate self-help.

b. Encourage child to perform ADL as much as possible; offer positive reinforcement.

c. Assist parents to have realistic expectations for their child; avoid excessively high expectations that might increase frustration.

8. Goal: *promote self-esteem.*

a. Praise child for each accomplishment or for sincere effort.

b. Help child dress and groom self daily in an attractive "normal" manner for developmental level and age.

c. Encourage child to form friendships with children with similar problems.

d. Enroll child in "special ed" classes to meet his or her needs.

e. Encourage parents to expose child to wide variety of experiences.

E. Evaluation:

1. Patent airway and adequate oxygenation maintained.
2. Adequate nutrition maintained, and child begins to grow and gain weight.
3. Child has an acceptable means of verbal communication.
4. Safety is maintained.
5. Vision and hearing within normal limits using corrective devices p.r.n.
6. Child is as mobile as possible, given disabilities.
7. Child is performing ADL, within capabilities.
8. Child has positive self-image/self-esteem.

PEDIATRIC NURSING

II. Spina bifidas (neural tube defects)

A. *Introduction:* Three different types of spina bifida:

1. Spina bifida occult—a "hidden"bony defect without herniation of the meninges or cord; no symptoms are present, no treatment is needed.
2. Meningocele—see Table 3.21.
3. Myelomeningocele—see Table 3.21. Most serious type of spina bifida and also most common.

The remainder of this section deals with *myelomeningocele* exclusively.

B. Assessment:

1. Congenital defect.
2. Readily detected by visual inspection in delivery room: round, bulging sac filled with fluid, usually in lumbosacral area.
3. Sensation and movement: complete lack below the level of the lesion.
4. Urinary: retention, with overflow incontinence.
5. Fecal: constipation, fecal impaction, oozing of liquid stool around impaction.
6. 90% develop signs and symptoms of hydrocephalus (see p. 268).
7. May have associated orthopedic anomalies: club foot, congenital hip dysplasia.

C. Analysis/nursing diagnosis:

1. *Potential for injury/infection* related to rupture of the sac.
2. *Altered urinary elimination* related to urinary retention and overflow incontinence.
3. *Impaired skin integrity* related to immobility.
4. *Constipation* related to fecal incontinence and impaired innervation.

D. Nursing plan/implementation:

1. Goal: *prevent rupture of the sac and possible infection (preoperative).*

a. *Position:* no pressure on sac; on abdomen to prevent contamination with urine or stool.

b. No clothing or diapers to avoid pressure on sac.

c. Place in heated isolette or warmer to maintain body temperature.

d. Keep sac covered with sterile moist soaks (normal saline) to prevent drying, cracking, and leakage of cerebrospinal fluid (CSF); change every 2–4 hours; document appearance of sac each dressing change to note signs and symptoms of infection.

TABLE 3.21 Comparison of Two Major Types of Spina Bifida

Dimension	Meningocele	Myelomeningocele
Contents of sac	Meninges and cerebrospinal fluid	Meninges, cerebrospinal fluid, spinal cord
Transillumination	Present	Absent
Percent of total cases	25%	75%
Motor function	Present	Absent
Sensory function	Present	Absent
Urinary/fecal incontinence	Absent	Present
Associated orthopedic anomalies	Rare	Congenital hip dysplasia, club foot
Other anomalies	Rare	Hydrocephalus (90%)
Treatment	Surgery	Surgery
Major short-term complication	Infection (meningitis)	Infection (meningitis)
Major long-term complication	None	Chronic urinary tract infection → renal disease/failure
Prognosis	Excellent	Guarded

e. Enforce strict aseptic tecnique to prevent infection (leading cause of morbidity/mortality in neonatal period).

2. Goal: *prevent infection in postoperative period.*
   a. *Position*: on abdomen, head 10° lower than hips to reduce pressure of circulating CSF on suture line.
   b. Use myelomeningocele apron (specific type of dressing) to prevent urine or stool from contaminating suture line.
   c. Administer antibiotics as ordered.
   d. Use strict aseptic techniques in dressing changes; universal precautions to prevent infection.
3. Goal: *prevent urinary retention and urinary tract infection.*
   a. Monitor I&O, offer extra fluids to flush kidneys.
   b. Keep urethral meatus clean of stool to prevent ascending bacterial infection.
   ▶ c. "Crede" bladder every 2–4 hours and p.r.n. to empty bladder per MD order.
4. Goal: *prevent complications of prolonged immobility and/or associated orthopedic anomalies.*
   a. *Position:* hips abducted.
   b. Use positional devices, rotating pressure mattress/flotation mattress.
   c. Refer to physical therapy for ROM exercises.
   d. Make necessary referrals for care of possible club feet/congenital hip dysplasia.
5. Goal: *monitor for possible development of hydrocephalus.* Occurs in 90% of infants born with myelomeningocele.

E. Evaluation:

1. Integrity of sac is maintained until surgery is done.
2. No infection occurs.
3. Adequate patterns of urinary and bowel elimination with necessary support.
4. Complications of immobility, orthopedic anomalies are prevented or treated promptly.

DISORDERS AFFECTING SENSORY-PERCEPTUAL FUNCTIONING

I. Hydrocephalus

A. *Introduction:* Hydrocephalus, known to the lay person as "water on the brain," is actually an abnormal increase in cerebrospinal fluid (CSF) within the intracranial cavity. The accumulation of this fluid causes enlargement and dilatation of the ventricles of the brain and increased intracranial pressure (ICP). If untreated, severe brain damage will result; treatment is a surgical shunting procedure that allows for the drainage of CSF from the ventricles of the brain to another, less harmful area within the body: jugular vein, right atrium of the heart, or peritoneal cavity. Hydrocephalus can develop as the result of a congenital malformation (e.g., Arnold-Chiari malformation), can be associated with other congenital defects (e.g., spina bifida), or can be acquired secondary to infection (e.g., meningitis) or trauma.

B. Assessment:

1. Head: increased circumference—earliest sign of hydrocephalus in the infant (more than 1 inch per month).
2. Fontanels: tense and bulging.
3. Veins: dilated scalp veins.
4. "Setting-sun" sign: sclera visible above iris.
5. Cry: shrill, high pitched.
6. Developmental milestones: delayed.
7. Reflexes: persistence of neonatal reflexes; hyperactive reflexes.

8. Signs of ↑ ICP:
   a. Vomiting.
   b. Irritability.
   c. Seizures.
   d. ↓ pulse.
   e. ↓ respirations.
   f. ↑ blood pressure.
   g. Widened pulse pressure.
9. History may reveal other CNS defects (e.g., spina bifida), infection (e.g., meningitis), or trauma.

C. Analysis/nursing diagnosis:

1. *Altered cerebral tissue perfusion* related to increased intracranial pressure.
2. *Impaired skin integrity* related to enlarged head size and lack of motor coordination.
3. *Altered nutrition, less than body requirements,* related to anorexia and vomiting.
4. *Anxiety* related to diagnosis and uncertain outcome.
5. *Knowledge deficit* regarding care of the child with a shunt and follow-up care.

D. Nursing plan/implementation:

1. Goal: *monitor neurologic status.*
   a. Measure head circumference daily, and note any abnormal increase.
   b. Perform neurologic checks at least every 4 hours to monitor for signs of ↑ ICP.
   c. Report signs of ↑ ICP **stat** to physician.
   ▶ d. Assist with diagnostic procedures/treatments: ventricular tap, CAT scan, etc.
2. Goal: *health teaching to reduce parental anxiety.*
   a. Do preoperative teaching regarding the shunt procedure: stress need to remove excessive cerebrospinal fluid to relieve pressure on brain; done as soon as possible after diagnosis is established.
   b. Stress early diagnosis and prompt shunting procedure to minimize the risk of long-term neurologic complications.
   c. Offer realistic information regarding prognosis:
      (1) Surgically treated, with continued follow-up care = 80% survival rate.
      (2) Of these survivors, 50% are completely normal and 50% have some degree of neurologic disability.
3. Goal: *provide postoperative shunt care.*
   a. *Position*:
      (1) Flat in bed for 24 hours, to prevent subdural hematoma.
      (2) Gradually increase the angle of elevation of head of bed, as ordered by surgeon.
      (3) On the unoperative side, to prevent mechanical pressure and obstruction to shunt.
   b. "Pump" the shunt as ordered: e.g., 10 times every 2 hours.
   c. Monitor head circumference daily to note any abnormal increase that might indicate malfunctioning shunt.
   d. Monitor vital signs; monitor for signs of ↑ ICP.
   e. Monitor for possible complications:
      (1) Infection.
      (2) Malfunction of shunt: ↑ ICP.
4. Goal: *provide discharge teaching to parents regarding home care of the child with a shunt.*
   a. Stress need for long-term follow-up care.
   b. Discuss feeding techniques, care of skin (especially scalp), need for stimulation.
   c. Prepare parents for shunt revisions to be done periodically as child grows.
   d. Teach parents signs and symptoms of shunt malfunctioning (i.e., of ↑ ICP or infection) and to report these promptly to physician.
   e. Encourage parents to enroll infant in "early infant stimulation" program to maximize developmental potential.
   f. Stress need to monitor development at frequent intervals, make referrals p.r.n.

E. Evaluation:

1. Neurologic functioning is maintained or improved.
2. Adequate nutrition is maintained.
3. No impairment of skin integrity occurs.
4. Parents' anxiety is relieved; they verbalize understanding of how to care for child after discharge.

II. Febrile seizures

A. *Introduction:* Febrile seizures are one of the most common neurologic disorders of childhood, affecting perhaps as many as 5% of all children. While the exact cause of febrile seizures remains uncertain, they seem to be a relatively transient problem that occurs exclusively in the presence of high, spiked fevers. Children in the infant and toddler stages (6 months–3 years) appear to be most susceptible to febrile seizures, and they are twice as common in males as in females. There also appears to be an increased susceptibility within families, suggesting a possible genetic predisposition. *Note:* Epilepsy is discussed in Unit 4.

B. Assessment:

1. History usually reveals presence of an upper respiratory infection or gastroenteritis.
2. Occurs with a sudden rise in fever: often spiked and quite high (102 °F or higher) versus prolonged temperature elevation.

C. Analysis/nursing diagnosis:

1. *Potential for injury* related to seizures.
2. *Knowledge deficit* related to prevention of future seizures, care of child having a seizure and possible long-term effects.

D. Nursing plan/implementation:

1. Goal: *reduce fever/prevent further increase in fever.*
   a. Administer antipyretics, as ordered: acetaminophen only (*not* aspirin).
   b. Use cool, loose, cotton clothes to decrease heat retention.
   c. Sponge with tepid water 20–30 minutes.
   d. Encourage child to drink cool fluids.
   e. Monitor temperature hourly.
   f. Minimize stimulation, frustration for child.

2. Goal: *teach parents regarding care of child who experiences febrile seizure.*
   a. Discuss how to prevent seizures from recurring: best method is to prevent temperature from rising over 102 °F (see goal 1).
   b. Discuss how to handle seizures if they do recur: prevent injury, maintain airway, etc.
   c. Answer questions simply and honestly:
      (1) 25% of children with one febrile seizure will experience a recurrence.
      (2) 75% of recurrences occur within 1 year.
      (3) As seizures recur, they also tend to increase in severity.
      (4) In children who experience numerous febrile seizures, there is an increased risk of epilepsy.

E. Evaluation:

1. Fever is kept below 102 °F; additional seizures are prevented.
2. Parents verbalize their understanding of how to care for child at home.

■ QUESTIONS

Following an uneventful 15-hour labor, 17-year-old primipara Mrs. Shirley Black delivers a live female infant. At birth, Baby Girl Black is found to have myelomeningocele at the lumbosacral area. Questions 1–8 refer to Baby Girl Black.

1. The best position for the delivery room nurse to place Baby Black in is:
○ 1. Prone. **IMP**
○ 2. Supine. **3**
○ 3. Side-lying. **SECE**
○ 4. Trendelenberg.

2. The nurse in the newborn nursery should plan any interventions with Baby Black based on the knowledge that the major *short-term* complication she is most likely to suffer is:
○ 1. Hydrocephalus. **AN**
○ 2. Meningitis. **3**
○ 3. Mental retardation. **PhI**
○ 4. Paraplegia.

3. When Mr. and Mrs. Black visit the nursery for the first time, they make no comments about the baby's spinal sac. Instead, they offer many positive observations about her size, color, hair, and appearance. The nurse would be most correct in interpreting the parents' behavior as:
○ 1. Attachment. **EV**
○ 2. Denial. **7**
○ 3. Immaturity. **PsI**
○ 4. Love.

4. The doctor attempts to shine a light through Baby Black's sac and notes "no transillumination." The nurse should interpret this finding to mean that the sac:
○ 1. Can be easily repaired. **AN**
○ 2. Cannot be evaluated via this technique. **3**
○ 3. Contains meninges and cerebrospinal fluid. **PhI**
○ 4. Contains meninges, cerebrospinal fluid, and the spinal cord.

5. The physician orders sterile moist soaks to the sac. The major reason for this treatment is to:
○ 1. Promote comfort. **AN**
○ 2. Prevent infection. **3**
○ 3. Relieve pressure. **SECE**
○ 4. Stimulate neural development.

6. Baby Girl Black is scheduled to have surgery to close the sac. Mrs. Black asks the nurse if the baby will be able to move her legs following this operation. The best response for the nurse to make would be:
○ 1. "Not usually, although we can always hope for a miracle." **IMP** **3**
○ 2. "There is no way to predict. All we can do is watch her closely." **HPM**
○ 3. "No, the surgery is done mainly to prevent infection."
○ 4. "Yes, the surgery will restore her ability to move her legs."

7. Following surgery to close the sac, Baby Girl Black returns to the nursery. In the absence of medical orders regarding positioning, the nurse should place Baby Black on her:
○ 1. Abdomen, with head 10° lower than hips. **IMP**
○ 2. Abdomen, with head of bed elevated 30°. **3**
○ 3. Abdomen, with hips 10° lower than head. **SECE**
○ 4. Abdomen, flat in bed.

8. The physician orders the nursing staff to monitor Baby Black for the possible development of hydrocephalus. In Baby Black, the earliest sign of hydrocephalus the nurse would observe is:
○ 1. Bulging anterior fontanel. **AN**
○ 2. Increasing head circumference. **3**
○ 3. Shrill, high-pitched cry. **PhI**
○ 4. Sunset eyes.

Craig Jefferson, 5 months old, is admitted to the pediatrics unit with a diagnosis of ventricular septal defect (VSD) and severe chronic congestive heart failure. Questions 9–18 refer to Craig.

9. While obtaining Craig's admission history from Ms. Jefferson, the nurse obtains all of the following information about Craig. Which one is the *most common complaint by parents* about infants with heart disease?
○ 1. Frequent, severe respiratory infections. **AN**
○ 2. "Slower" development. **6**
○ 3. "Stunted" growth. **PhI**
○ 4. Difficult to feed.

10. In doing Craig's admission exam, the nurse notes all of the following abnormal findings. Which one is the *most common sign* of heart disease the *nurse* should assess?

Key to codes following questions Nursing process: **AS**, Assessment; **AN**, Analysis; **PL**, Plan; **IMP**, Implementation; **EV**, Evaluation. Category of human function: **1**, Protective; **2**, Sensory-perceptual; **3**, Comfort, Rest, Activity, and Mobility; **4**, Nutrition; **5**, Growth and Development; **6**, Fluid-Gas Transport; **7**, Psycho-Social-Cultural; **8**, Elimination. Client need: **SECE**, Safe, Effective Care Environment; **PhI**, Physiological Integrity; **PsI**, Psychosocial Integrity; **HPM**, Health Promotion/Maintenance. See frontmatter for full explanation.

○ 1. Circumoral cyanosis. **AS**
○ 2. Hypertension. **6**
○ 3. Diastolic murmur. **PhI**
○ 4. Tachycardia.

11. Considering Craig's diagnosis, the formula the nurse should plan to offer him would be:
○ 1. Isomil. **PL**
○ 2. Lofenalac. **6**
○ 3. Lonalac. **SECE**
○ 4. Similac 27 with iron.

12. Craig takes 1¼ ounces of formula in 20 minutes. The doctor ordered 2 ounces of formula q3h. The *best* action for the nurse to take at this time would be to:
○ 1. Ask Craig's mother to feed him when she arrives. **IMP** **6**
○ 2. Burp Craig and try to stimulate him to suck. **PhI**
○ 3. Continue feeding Craig slowly, allowing him as much time as he needs to finish.
○ 4. Stop the feeding, and request an order for gavage feedings p.r.n.

13. Between meals, the nurse should place Craig in which position?
○ 1. In an infant seat with head elevated. **IMP**
○ 2. Prone with head turned to side. **6**
○ 3. Supine with head slightly hyperextended. **SECE**
○ 4. Side-lying with the head of the bed elevated 30°.

14. The nurse observes a nursing student fastening Craig's diaper snugly around his abdomen. The nurse should:
○ 1. Ask the student to loosen Craig's diaper. **EV**
○ 2. Do or say nothing, as this is expected behavior for a student. **6** **PhI**
○ 3. Loosen the diaper herself after the student leaves the room.
○ 4. Praise the student for her outstanding attention to detail.

15. Ms. Jefferson asks the nurse why Craig is sucking on a pacifier. The nurse would be most correct in telling her:
○ 1. "Craig seems to like it." **IMP**
○ 2. "Most infants, like Craig, prefer a pacifier to their thumb." **5/6** **PsI**
○ 3. "This is to keep Craig from crying."
○ 4. "We give all hospitalized infants, like Craig, a pacifier."

16. Considering Craig's developmental level and diagnoses, which one behavior should the nurse expect Craig to be capable of demonstrating?
○ 1. Rolling over from stomach to back. **AS**
○ 2. Sitting with support. **5/6**
○ 3. Pincer grasp. **HPM**
○ 4. Bearing some weight on legs.

17. Ms. Jefferson is getting ready to take Craig home. Which one visitor should the nurse discourage from touching or holding Craig?
○ 1. Craig's aunt, who has lupus. **IMP**
○ 2. Craig's grandmother, who has a slight cold. **6**
○ 3. Craig's father, who is a drug addict. **SECE**
○ 4. Craig's 3-year-old sister, who is in nursery school.

18. The nurse has completed her discharge teaching with Ms. Jefferson. Which one statement by the mother would indicate the need for additional teaching by the nurse?
○ 1. "I'll be sure to dress Craig in loose-fitting clothes." **EV** **6**
○ 2. "I'll try to keep my house as warm as I can for Craig." **HPM**
○ 3. "I'll be at the clinic in 3 days for Craig's appointment."
○ 4. "I'll put Craig in his playpen at least once a day."

Lureen White, 7 months old, is admitted to the pediatrics unit with moderate dehydration secondary to acute gastroenteritis (AGE). Questions 19–22 refer to Lureen.

19. The physician writes all the following orders for Lureen. Which one should the nurse implement *first?*
○ 1. Universal precautions. **AN**
○ 2. IV of 5% dextrose in ⅓ normal saline solution at 25 cc/hour. **3** **SECE**
○ 3. Urine specific gravity stat and q4h.
○ 4. Stool culture every shift × 3.

20. In doing the admission assessment, the nurse should expect to find which of the following signs of dehydration in Lureen?
○ 1. Fever and bradycardia. **AS**
○ 2. Irritability and sunken eyeballs. **8**
○ 3. Hypotension and anuria. **PhI**
○ 4. Dry mucous membranes and bulging anterior fontanel.

21. The best method to prevent the spread of infection from Lureen to other staff members or visitors would be:
○ 1. Double bagging all linens. **AN**
○ 2. Obtaining stool cultures. **8**
○ 3. Strict handwashing. **SECE**
○ 4. Wearing disposable gloves.

22. At 7 months of age, Lureen exhibits all of the following skills. The nurse should know that her most recently acquired skill is probably her ability to:
○ 1. Roll over. **AN**
○ 2. Sit up. **5**
○ 3. Bear some weight on legs. **HPM**
○ 4. Pick up objects with palmar grasp.

John Pace, 9 months old, is admitted to the pediatrics unit with a diagnosis of Hirschsprung's disease. Questions 23–27 refer to John.

23. While admitting John, the nurse notes all of the following abnormal findings. Which one is considered the classic sign of Hirschsprung's disease?
○ 1. Abdominal distention. **AN**
○ 2. Anorexia. **8**
○ 3. Constipation. **PhI**
○ 4. Vomitus flecked with feces.

24. In order to best perform a Denver Developmental Screening Test (DDST) on John, the nurse should:
○ 1. Take John from Mrs. Pace and ask her to wait in his room. **IMP** **5**
○ 2. Take John from Mrs. Pace and ask her to come with them to the testing area. **HPM**
○ 3. Briefly talk first with Mrs. Pace, then take John to the testing area alone.
○ 4. Ask Mrs. Pace to carry John to the testing area.

25. Mrs. Pace asks the nurse how John got Hirschsprung's disease. The nurse would be most correct in advising her that:
○ 1. John was born with this condition. **IMP**
○ 2. It is the result of the meconium ileus John experienced as a newborn. **8** **PhI**
○ 3. John spontaneously developed this condition at 9 months of age.

PEDIATRIC NURSING

○ 4. It often occurs following the introduction of solid foods due to a genetically inherited metabolic defect.

26. The surgeon orders a preoperative series of cleansing enemas for John. The nurse should expect the solution ordered for these enemas to be:
○ 1. SSE. **AN**
○ 2. Normal saline. **8**
○ 3. Pediatric Fleets. **SECE**
○ 4. Tap water.

27. Considering John's condition and his developmental level, the most appropriate person to administer these enemas would be John's:
○ 1. Primary nurse. **AN**
○ 2. Mother. **5/6**
○ 3. Student nurse. **HPM**
○ 4. Nursing assistant.

PEDIATRIC NURSING

Maria Lopez, 14 months old, is diagnosed at the child health clinic as having laryngotracheobronchitis (LTB). On admission she has a fever of 102°F. Questions 28–37 refer to Maria.

28. On admission, the nurse would expect Maria to demonstrate which two *early* signs of LTB?
○ 1. Dyspnea and cyanosis. **AN**
○ 2. Hoarseness and tachycardia. **6**
○ 3. Expiratory wheeze and low-grade fever. **PhI**
○ 4. Metallic cough and inspiratory stridor.

29. The physician orders Tylenol elixir for Maria. Considering her developmental level and her diagnosis, which would be the best approach by the nurse?
○ 1. Give Maria the medicine cup and tell her the "pretty red syrup" will taste sweet like candy. **IMP** **5**
○ 2. Mix the medication with 4 ounces of apple juice and allow her to drink it through a "crazy straw." **HPM**
○ 3. Put the medication into a brightly colored plastic cup and give Maria a chance to drink it herself.
○ 4. Raise Maria to a sitting position, bring the medicine cup to her lips, and tell her kindly but firmly to drink it.

30. Maria is to be placed in a croupette. The nurse should plan to perform which of the following nursing actions?
○ 1. Remove all toys from Maria's crib. **PL**
○ 2. Withhold all liquids and solids temporarily. **6**
○ 3. Monitor oxygen concentration daily and record in notes. **SECE**
○ 4. Evaluate Maria's reaction to oxygen therapy in terms of vital signs and color.

31. To "flood" the croupette with oxygen prior to placing Maria in the tent, the nurse should initially adjust the oxygen flow rate to:
○ 1. 2–3 liters per minute. **IMP**
○ 2. 4–5 liters per minute. **6**
○ 3. 8–10 liters per minute. **SECE**
○ 4. 15 liters per minute.

32. After flooding the tent for 5 minutes, the nurse should readjust the flow rate of oxygen. To maintain an oxygen concentration of 35–40%, the nurse should now adjust the oxygen flow rate to:
○ 1. 2–3 liters per minute. **IMP**
○ 2. 4–5 liters per minute. **6**
○ 3. 8–10 liters per minute. **SECE**
○ 4. 15 liters per minute.

33. After placing Maria in the croup tent, the nurse should adjust the plastic canopy so that:
○ 1. The edges are tucked tightly under the linen. **IMP**
○ 2. The edges are lying loosely on top of the linen. **6**
○ 3. The crib rails are raised and the canopy edges are over them. **SECE**
○ 4. The crib rails are lowered and the canopy edges are inside them.

34. Nursing care for Maria while she is in the croupette includes which of the following?
○ 1. Giving her a bald plastic doll. **IMP**
○ 2. Removing her blanket and pajamas. **6**
○ 3. Restraining her arms and legs. **SECE**
○ 4. Restricting visitors to her immediate family.

35. Maria cries and tries to cling to her mother. Ms. Lopez asks the nurse if she can climb into the crib and lie in the tent with Maria. The nurse's best response would be:
○ 1. "Do you always let Maria have her way like this?" **IMP** **5/6**
○ 2. "I'll have to check with Maria's doctor first." **PsI**
○ 3. "No, that would not be safe for you or Maria."
○ 4. "It may help Maria calm down; let's give it a try."

36. Three of the following signs or symptoms indicate an improvement in Maria's condition. Which one indicates a *worsening* and should be promptly reported to the physician?
○ 1. Apical pulse = 118. **EV**
○ 2. Increase in appetite. **6**
○ 3. Progressive hoarseness. **PhI**
○ 4. Pink nailbeds.

37. Prior to discharge, the nurse reviews Maria's immunizations with Ms. Lopez. If Maria is up to date on all her immunizations, the nurse should advise Ms. Lopez that the next immunization Maria is due to receive is:
○ 1. MMR (measles, mumps, rubella) at 15 months of age. **IMP** **1**
○ 2. MMR at 18 months of age. **HPM**
○ 3. DTP (diphtheria, tetanus, pertussis) at 15 months of age.
○ 4. DTP at 18 months of age.

Kelly John, 2 years old, is admitted to the hospital with acute bilateral otitis media. Her temperature is 103°F, and she has tremors in her arms and legs. The physician orders a spinal tap to rule out bacterial meningitis. Questions 38–44 refer to Kelly.

38. The doctor orders all of the following for Kelly. Which one should the nurse do *first?*
○ 1. Respiratory isolation. **AN**
○ 2. IV 5% dextrose in 0.45 normal saline solution at 35 cc/hour. **1** **SECE**
○ 3. Tylenol 120 mg PO q4h.
○ 4. Seizure precautions.

39. The doctor orders Kelly's IV to infuse at 35 cc/hour; a pediatric microdrip chamber is hanging. How many drops per minute should the nurse regulate the IV to infuse?
○ 1. 5–6. **IMP**
○ 2. 7–8. **1**
○ 3. 9–10. **SECE**
○ 4. 35.

40. Kelly tries to pull her IV out, and the nurse determines she must be restrained to maintain the IV site. Which restraint would the nurse be most correct in applying?

○ 1. Posey jacket. **IMP**
○ 2. Elbow. **1**
○ 3. Mummy. **SECE**
○ 4. Clove-hitch.

41. A lumbar puncture is performed by the doctor. After the procedure, the nurse should position Kelly:
○ 1. Flat in bed, with no pillow. **IMP**
○ 2. Flat in bed, with a small pillow. **1**
○ 3. In semi-Fowler's position. **SECE**
○ 4. Semi-prone, with head to the side.

42. The diagnosis of bacterial meningitis is confirmed; Kelly assumes an opisthotonus position. In which position should the nurse now place her?
○ 1. Prone. **IMP**
○ 2. Supine. **1**
○ 3. Side-lying. **SECE**
○ 4. Trendelenberg.

43. As Kelly recovers, the nurse should watch her carefully for which one of the following *long-term* complications of meningitis?
○ 1. Encephalitis. **AS**
○ 2. Hydrocephalus. **1**
○ 3. Learning disabilities. **PhI**
○ 4. Mental retardation.

44. If Kelly were to develop hydrocephalus, which would be the *earliest* sign(s) the nurse would most likely note?
○ 1. Irritability and poor feeding. **AN**
○ 2. Increasing head circumference. **1**
○ 3. Headache and diplopia. **PhI**
○ 4. Ruptured retinal vessels.

Arlene Major, 27 months old, was found sitting in the bathroom playing with an empty bottle of adult aspirin. Arlene had white powder around and in her mouth. Mrs. Major brought her to the emergency room. Questions 45–49 refer to Arlene.

45. After examining Arlene, the pediatrician orders syrup of ipecac for her. Generally, the nurse *should* administer this medication only if the child is:
○ 1. Alert and reactive. **AN**
○ 2. Convulsing. **1**
○ 3. Comatose. **SECE**
○ 4. Known to have swallowed a corrosive substance.

46. After the nurse administers the syrup of ipecac to Arlene, she should also give Arlene:
○ 1. Four ounces of warm milk. **IMP**
○ 2. Activated charcoal powder. **1**
○ 3. As much water as she will drink. **SECE**
○ 4. A slice of dry toast.

47. If Arlene has not vomited within 30 minutes, the nurse should:
○ 1. Stimulate the gag reflex using her fingers. **IMP**
○ 2. Wait another 30 minutes before doing anything else. **1** **SECE**
○ 3. Assume the danger is past and no further treatment is needed at this time.
○ 4. Repeat the dose a second time.

48. In monitoring Arlene for her response to the syrup of ipecac, the nurse should base any actions on the knowledge that ipecac is potentially:
○ 1. Cardiotoxic. **AN**
○ 2. Hepatotoxic. **1**
○ 3. Nephrotoxic. **PhI**
○ 4. Neurotoxic.

49. Before Arlene goes home, the *best* advice the nurse can give to Mrs. Major to handle Arlene's temper tantrums would be to:
○ 1. Allow Arlene to make her own choices. **IMP**
○ 2. Ignore this behavior. **5**
○ 3. Change the setting in which they occur. **HPM**
○ 4. Give in to Arlene's demands, to nurture her autonomy.

Teddy Quinn, age 3 years, is admitted to the hospital with classic hemophilia (Factor VIII deficiency). Questions 50–56 refer to Teddy.

50. Which admission procedure by the nurse will probably be the most frightening for Teddy?
○ 1. Blood pressure. **AN**
○ 2. Rectal temperature. **7**
○ 3. Urine specimen. **HPM**
○ 4. Weight.

51. In doing Teddy's admission history, the nurse notes all of the following signs of hemophilia. The hallmark, or classic sign, of hemophilia is:
○ 1. Excessive hematoma formation. **AN**
○ 2. Hemarthrosis. **6**
○ 3. Prolonged bleeding from lacerations. **PhI**
○ 4. Intracranial bleeding.

52. The nurse performs a Denver Developmental Screening Test (DDST) on Teddy. Which one of the following behaviors should the nurse expect Teddy to be capable of doing?
○ 1. Go up stairs on alternate feet. **AN**
○ 2. Pedal a bicycle. **6**
○ 3. Dress without supervision. **HPM**
○ 4. Tie shoelaces.

53. The first night that he is in the hospital, Teddy suffers an episode of epistaxis. In which position should the nurse place him?
○ 1. Prone, with head turned to side. **IMP**
○ 2. Semi-Fowler's with two pillows. **6**
○ 3. Sitting up with head tilted backward. **SECE**
○ 4. Sitting up and leaning forward slightly.

54. Teddy is to receive cryoprecipitate (Factorate). During the infusion of this medication, the nurse should plan to observe him for which one of the following potential complications?
○ 1. Emboli formation. **PL**
○ 2. Fluid volumes overload. **6**
○ 3. Onset of AIDS. **SECE**
○ 4. Transfusion reaction.

55. Teddy's mother tells the nurse that he is a very poor eater at home. The best recommendation the nurse can make to increase Teddy's nutritional intake would be:
○ 1. Provide Teddy with a child-size table. **IMP**
○ 2. Use plastic cups and plates with carton characters Teddy likes. **5** **HPM**
○ 3. Offer Teddy small portions of his favorite foods.
○ 4. Allow Teddy to feed himself.

56. Teddy is to be discharged, and the nurse has completed her teaching with Teddy's parents. Which one statement by Teddy's parents indicates they may have *misunderstood* the nurse's teaching regarding Teddy's care?
○ 1. "If Teddy gets a fever, we will only give him acetaminophen, not aspirin." **EV** **6**
○ 2. "We will be sure to supervise Teddy carefully so **HPM**

that he doesn't experience another bleeding episode."

○ 3. "I'll order a Medic-Alert bracelet for Teddy as soon as we get home."

○ 4. "It's a relief to know that Teddy's little sister will not get this disease too."

Martin Brown, 3 ½ years old, is admitted to the hospital with nephrosis. Questions 57–61 refer to Martin (Marty).

57. On admission, Marty is carrying a soiled and worn-looking "Cookie Monster" stuffed animal. Mrs. Brown states that this is his favorite toy. The most appropriate action for the nurse to take at this time is to:

○ 1. Offer Marty his choice of another stuffed animal from the hospital playroom. **IMP 7**

○ 2. Place Cookie Monster somewhere in Marty's room where he can see it but not touch it. **PsI**

○ 3. Suggest Marty's mother bring him a new Cookie Monster stuffed animal.

○ 4. Tell Marty that he can keep Cookie Monster in the bed with him.

58. In reviewing Marty's admission history and laboratory results, the nurse should know that the two most common findings in children with nephrosis are:

○ 1. Generalized edema and proteinuria. **AN**

○ 2. Hyperlipidemia and periorbital edema. **8**

○ 3. Hypertension and hematuria. **PhI**

○ 4. Oliguria and anorexia.

59. Marty is started on prednisone. If the prednisone is having the expected therapeutic effect, the nurse should expect that Marty will:

○ 1. Experience mood swings. **EV**

○ 2. Have sugar in his urine. **8**

○ 3. Gain weight. **SECE**

○ 4. Feel better.

60. Marty's scrotal sac is swollen. Which nursing action would be most effective in relieving discomfort?

○ 1. Apply zinc oxide to scrotum qid. **IMP**

○ 2. Cleanse scrotum with warm water only. **8**

○ 3. Sprinkle medicated powder on scrotum. **PhI**

○ 4. Support scrotum on folded diapers.

61. Marty is to be discharged, and the nurse has completed her teaching with his parents. Which statement by Mrs. Brown indicates that she has fully understood the nurse's teaching?

○ 1. "I will keep Marty away from other children so he doesn't get a relapse." **EV 8**

○ 2. "I'm so glad this is all over and we don't have to worry any more." **HPM**

○ 3. "When we get home, I'm going to find it hard to keep Marty in bed."

○ 4. "I will watch Marty for any signs of this starting up again."

Bradley Ross, 4 years old, experienced gradually increasing respiratory distress throughout the afternoon. At 5 P.M., his mother became alarmed and brought him to the emergency room. The admitting examination reveals that Brad is cyanotic, dyspneic, and dysphagic. The doctor makes a tentative diagnosis of epiglottitis. Questions 62–66 refer to Brad.

62. Mrs. Ross tells the nurse that she does not even know what epiglottitis is. The nurse would be most correct in telling her that it is:

○ 1. An infection of the upper respiratory tract related to allergy and excessive mucus production. **IMP 6 PhI**

○ 2. A potentially life-threatening infection that requires prolonged intensive care.

○ 3. A mild form of croup that is usually treated at home.

○ 4. A swelling in the throat that can lead to total airway obstruction if not treated promptly.

63. A medical student tells the nurse that she wants to look down Brad's throat to visualize the epiglottis. The nurse would be most correct in:

○ 1. Asking Brad's mother if she objects to a medical student checking her son. **IMP 6**

○ 2. Telling the medical student that she absolutely cannot do this. **PhI**

○ 3. Promising Brad a special treat if he opens his mouth real wide for the doctor.

○ 4. Helping restrain Brad so the medical student can get a better look.

64. Brad is admitted to the hospital and is to receive Solu-cortef 100 mg IV q6h. The main purpose for this medication is to:

○ 1. Provide mild sedation. **AN**

○ 2. Reduce swelling. **6**

○ 3. Relieve pain. **SECE**

○ 4. Treat infection.

65. After several days of treatment, Brad is recovering nicely. One night he wakes up crying at 2 A.M. and says, "I want my mommy now." The nurse should:

○ 1. Pick Brad up and rock him for a little while. **IMP**

○ 2. Talk softly to Brad while rubbing his back, but leave him in his crib. **7 PsI**

○ 3. Gently but firmly tell Brad to go back to sleep.

○ 4. Call Mrs. Ross and ask her for some suggestions as to how to handle this.

66. The nurse does discharge teaching with Mrs. Ross prior to Brad's discharge. Which statement by Mrs. Ross indicates that she has *correctly* understood the nurse's teaching?

○ 1. "I'm so glad that Brad is all better now." **EV**

○ 2. "I will keep Brad home from preschool for the rest of this month." **6 HPM**

○ 3. "I'm still worried that Brad will get sick again when we get home."

○ 4. "I will get a portable tank of oxygen for Brad before he comes home."

Kato Oo, 4 ½ years old, is admitted to the pediatrics unit for the third, and final, surgical procedure to correct his congenital hypospadias. Questions 67–71 refer to Kato.

67. When admitting Kato to the hospital, the nurse should assess all of the following. Which information will be most important to the nursing care planning for Kato?

○ 1. Kato's developmental level. **PL**

○ 2. Kato's knowledge level regarding hypospadias. **8**

○ 3. Kato's previous experience with illness and hospitalization. **PsI**

○ 4. Kato's parents' plans for rooming-in.

68. Kato's mother questions the need for another surgical procedure while Kato is still so young. The nurse should stress that:

○ 1. It is her right to refuse surgery at any time. **IMP**

○ 2. It's in Kato's best interest to follow the doctor's recommendations. **8 PhI**

○ 3. Kato can have this third, and final, surgery any time before the onset of puberty.

○ 4. This type of surgery is usually timed to precede kindergarten.

69. After the nurse completes preoperative teaching with Kato, which would be the one *best* method for evaluating the effectiveness of the teaching?
- ○ 1. Ask Kato to draw a picture of what he will look like after surgery. **EV 1 PsI**
- ○ 2. Using puppets, ask Kato to show the nurse what he has learned about his surgery.
- ○ 3. Tell Kato that this is a test and he must repeat what he has learned about his operation.
- ○ 4. Suggest Kato's parents check on their child's level of understanding and report back to the nurse.

70. The night before surgery, as he is getting ready for bed, Kato asks his father to "check under the bed for monsters." The nurse would be most correct in advising Kato's father to:
- ○ 1. Ask Kato to talk more about these monsters. **IMP 5 HPM**
- ○ 2. Leave a light on and let Kato check for himself.
- ○ 3. Make a game of checking under Kato's bed.
- ○ 4. Tell Kato that monsters are only make-believe.

71. When Kato returns to the unit following surgery, he has a Foley catheter in place. The nurse should expect the drainage to have:
- ○ 1. A clear yellow appearance. **EV 8 PhI**
- ○ 2. Small clots of blood or mucus.
- ○ 3. Gross hematuria in moderate amounts.
- ○ 4. A brownish tinge.

Jake Ellis, 6 years old, was admitted to the hospital two days ago with a diagnosis of cor pulmonale secondary to cystic fibrosis (CF). He is on a maintenance dose of digoxin, 0.125 mg PO bid. Questions 72–77 refer to Jake.

72. Prior to giving Jake his digoxin, which one of the following pulses would the nurse be most correct in assessing?
- ○ 1. Apical. **AS 6 SECE**
- ○ 2. Brachial.
- ○ 3. Pedal.
- ○ 4. Radial.

73. The nurse should withhold Jake's digoxin and notify the physician if Jake's pulse was *below*:
- ○ 1. 80 beats per minute. **EV 6 SECE**
- ○ 2. 90 beats per minute.
- ○ 3. 100 beats per minute.
- ○ 4. 110 beats per minute.

74. Jake is to receive the pancreatic enzyme viokase several times daily. The best time for the nurse to plan to administer this medication is:
- ○ 1. After every meal or snack. **PL 6 SECE**
- ○ 2. Between meals and after every snack.
- ○ 3. Immediately before meals or snacks.
- ○ 4. With meals and before snacks.

75. Jake refuses to swallow the viokase tablets. The best course of action for the nurse would be to:
- ○ 1. Check with the doctor about discontinuing this medication. **IMP 6/7 SECE**
- ○ 2. Crush the tablets and mix with 1 teaspoon of cold applesauce.
- ○ 3. Dissolve the tablets in 4 ounces of warm milk.
- ○ 4. Offer Jake a "special treat" if he swallows the tablets "like a big boy."

76. Jake's mother tells the nurse that she is thinking of getting pregnant again but is worried that her next child might also have cystic fibrosis. Because Jake does have this disease, the nurse should advise Jake's mother that a second child:
- ○ 1. Could be even more severely affected than Jake. **IMP 6 HPM**
- ○ 2. Might also have the disease.
- ○ 3. Should be "normal," or disease-free.
- ○ 4. Would only carry the trait.

77. Jake's mother asks the nurse if Jake will be allowed to participate in any team sports now that he is starting school. The nurse would be most correct in advising her that Jake can participate in:
- ○ 1. Softball. **IMP 5/6 HPM**
- ○ 2. Tennis.
- ○ 3. Soccer.
- ○ 4. Swimming.

Mary Jane Price, 7 years old, has had leukemia for 2 years. She was in primary remission for 18 months but recently experienced infections, epistaxis, and abdominal petechiae. The doctor suspects she is no longer in remission and admits her to the hospital. Questions 78–84 refer to Mary Jane.

78. In reviewing Mary Jane's admitting blood work, the nurse notes all of the following. Which finding should the nurse interpret as the probable cause of Mary Jane's infections?
- ○ 1. Anemia. **AN 1 PhI**
- ○ 2. Leukopenia.
- ○ 3. Neutropenia.
- ○ 4. Thrombocytopenia.

79. Mary Jane's parents tell the nurse that their daughter frequently has nightmares, and they wonder how to handle this. The nurse would be most correct in advising them to:
- ○ 1. Comfort Mary Jane, but leave her in her own bed. **IMP 5 HPM**
- ○ 2. Comfort Mary Jane by bringing her into their bed.
- ○ 3. Consult a child psychologist to determine why Mary Jane has recurring sleep disturbances.
- ○ 4. Encourage Mary Jane to keep a written record of her dreams and discuss them with her primary nurse during this hospitalization.

80. Mary Jane forgot her toothbrush at home, and she asks the nurse for one. Considering her diagnosis and her health teaching needs, the nurse would be most correct in advising Mary Jane to:
- ○ 1. Skip brushing her teeth at this time. **IMP 1/6 PhI**
- ○ 2. Brush her teeth with a soft toothbrush only.
- ○ 3. Brush her teeth with a firm toothbrush only.
- ○ 4. Rinse her mouth with an antiseptic solution instead of brushing her teeth.

81. In writing a nursing care plan for Mary Jane, the nurse should include all of the following goals. Which goal is *most* important and should receive *top* priority?
- ○ 1. Maintain infection-free state. **PL 1/6 SECE**
- ○ 2. Prevent injury.
- ○ 3. Promote adequate nutrition.
- ○ 4. Meet developmental needs.

82. Mary Jane is receiving vincristine. The nurse should observe her closely for the side effect of:
- ○ 1. Diarrhea. **IMP 6 PhI**
- ○ 2. Diplopia.
- ○ 3. Hemorrhagic cystitis.
- ○ 4. Peripheral neuropathy.

83. Mary Jane develops oral ulcers. The most appropriate nursing intervention would be to:
- ○ 1. Encourage Mary Jane to use viscous xylocaine before meals. **IMP 6**

○ 2. Offer Mary Jane lukewarm liquids, such as tea or broth. **PhI**
○ 3. Crush two tablets of aspirin in warm water and instruct Mary Jane to gargle with this solution.
○ 4. Allow Mary Jane to eat or drink foods of her own choosing.

84. Mary Jane is being discharged, and the doctor suggests an immediate return to school. The nurse should be sure to teach the parents to keep Mary Jane home if any of her classmates develops:
○ 1. Impetigo. **IMP**
○ 2. Strep throat. **1/6**
○ 3. Pneumonia. **PhI**
○ 4. Chickenpox.

PEDIATRIC NURSING

Lisa Fresh, 9 years old, is admitted to the hospital with her second attack of rheumatic fever. Questions 85–94 refer to Lisa.

85. In doing an admission assessment on Lisa, which group of symptoms would the nurse most likely find?
○ 1. Petechiae, malaise, and joint pain. **AS**
○ 2. Chorea, anemia, and hypertension. **1**
○ 3. Tachycardia, erythema marginatum, and fever in late afternoon. **PhI**
○ 4. Subcutaneous nodules, dependent edema, and conjunctivitis.

86. The number one priority during the nurse's admission assessment is Lisa's:
○ 1. Weight. **AN**
○ 2. Apical pulse rate. **1**
○ 3. Developmental level. **PhI**
○ 4. Erythrocyte sedimentation rate (ESR).

87. Lisa experiences all of the following signs or symptoms of rheumatic fever. The nurse should plan any interventions based on the knowledge that the only one that may result in *permanent* damage is:
○ 1. Sydenham's chorea. **PL**
○ 2. Migratory polyarthritis. **1**
○ 3. Carditis. **PhI**
○ 4. Erythema marginatum.

88. The best roommate for Lisa would be:
○ 1. An 8-year-old girl with impetigo. **IMP**
○ 2. A 9-year-old girl with a tonsillectomy. **1/5**
○ 3. A 10-year-old girl with a concussion. **HPM**
○ 4. An 11-year-old girl with a fractured elbow.

89. Lisa complains of severe joint pains in her knees and ankles. The best method to provide relief for Lisa would be for the nurse to:
○ 1. Give Lisa a warm bath or shower. **IMP**
○ 2. Apply splints to the affected joints. **1**
○ 3. Refer Lisa to physical therapy. **PhI**
○ 4. Place a bed cradle over Lisa's legs.

90. Lisa is very quiet and seldom talks to the staff. The nurse can best communicate with Lisa by saying:
○ 1. "I've noticed you seem very quiet. Is anything troubling you?" **IMP**
○ 2. "Let's tell each other a secret; you start by telling me what you are thinking." **7**
○ 3. "It must be awfully hard to be away from home. Let's call your mom!" **PsI**
○ 4. "Draw me some pictures of the things you've seen and done while you've been in the hospital."

91. Lisa develops heart failure and is placed on digoxin, lasix, and potassium. The chief purpose for Lisa's receiving potassium is to:
○ 1. Enhance the cardiogenic effect of digoxin. **AN**
○ 2. Potentiate the diuretic action of lasix. **1/5**
○ 3. Prevent hypokalemia. **PhI**
○ 4. Pharmacologically induce hyperkalemia.

92. Lisa and her roommate complain that they are "bored." The nurse should offer them:
○ 1. A game of "Monopoly" or "Life." **IMP**
○ 2. Workbooks, paper, and pencils. **7**
○ 3. Some books from the hospital library. **PsI**
○ 4. A chance to stay up late and watch TV.

93. The physician orders "increasing activity as tolerated." After getting Lisa up into an arm chair, the nurse should monitor how well Lisa tolerates this increase in activity by checking her:
○ 1. Apical pulse rate. **IMP**
○ 2. Breath sounds. **1/6**
○ 3. Degree of restlessness. **PhI**
○ 4. Lips and nailbeds.

94. Long-term follow-up care is being planned for Lisa prior to her discharge. This *must* include:
○ 1. Indefinite antibiotic therapy. **IMP**
○ 2. Immunization against future attacks. **1**
○ 3. Cardiac rehabilitation program. **PhI**
○ 4. Home-bound tutoring.

Beverly Snow, 12 years old, is admitted to the hospital in status asthmaticus. Beverly has had asthma since age 6 and has been hospitalized previously. Questions 95–101 refer to Beverly.

95. In planning for Beverly, the nurse must *first* assess:
○ 1. What Beverly knows about asthma. **AN**
○ 2. How Beverly usually cares for herself. **7**
○ 3. What Beverly knows about hospitalization. **PsI**
○ 4. How Beverly feels about becoming a teenager.

96. In what position should the nurse place Beverly?
○ 1. Knee-chest. **IMP**
○ 2. High Fowler's. **6**
○ 3. Lateral Sims'. **SECE**
○ 4. Supine, with neck hyperextended.

97. In reviewing her childhood history, which one factor should the nurse realize may be related to the development of her asthma?
○ 1. Strep throat/tonsillitis at age 2. **AN**
○ 2. Eczema at age 3½. **1/5**
○ 3. Paternal death at age 5. **SECE**
○ 4. Pneumonia at age 7.

98. Beverly's mother asks the nurse what causes asthma. The nurse would be most correct in telling her the cause is:
○ 1. Unknown. **IMP**
○ 2. Allergies. **1**
○ 3. Stress. **PhI**
○ 4. Multiple factors.

99. The nurse should review principles of care with Beverly's mother and with Beverly. Which one comment by Beverly would require additional teaching by the nurse?
○ 1. "I keep all my stuffed animals on my bookcase now." **EV**
○ 2. "I have aluminum mini-blinds on the windows in my room." **1** **HPM**
○ 3. "I gave my cat to my best friend."
○ 4. "I joined the swim team at school."

100. Beverly is prepubescent, and her mother asks the nurse about the normal time for the onset of menstruation.

The nurse would be most correct in advising her that menses usually begin at age:
○ 1. 11½. **IMP**
○ 2. 12 years. **5**
○ 3. 12½. **PsI**
○ 4. 13 years.

101. Beverly's roommate is discharged. Before the nurse assigns another client to this room, which one consideration about Beverly's developmental level should she or he keep in mind? Beverly will:
○ 1. Probably prefer another girl her own age. **AN**
○ 2. Most likely seek out opportunities to socialize with teenagers. **7** **PsI**
○ 3. Enjoy being with either a girl or boy, as long as they're the same age.
○ 4. Feel helpful if given the opportunity to look after a slightly younger child.

Jacklyn Rose, 13 years old, is admitted to the hospital in sickle cell crisis with severe pain in her legs and abdomen. Questions 102–106 refer to Jacklyn.

102. Jacklyn asks the nurse why the doctor ordered oxygen for her when she has no trouble breathing. The nurse would be *most* correct in telling her that the main therapeutic effect of oxygen for Jacklyn is to:
○ 1. Reverse sickling of RBCs. **IMP**
○ 2. Prevent further sickling. **6**
○ 3. Prevent respiratory complications. **PhI**
○ 4. Increase the oxygen-carrying capacity of RBCs.

103. In planning care for Jacklyn, the nurse should base any actions on the knowledge that pain in vaso-occlusive crisis is *primarily* due to:
○ 1. Increased RBC destruction. **PL**
○ 2. Hepatosplenomegaly. **6**
○ 3. Occlusion of small blood vessels. **PhI**
○ 4. Sequestration of blood.

104. In addition to administering oxygen, the nurse can also relieve Jacklyn's pain by:
○ 1. Applying warm compresses. **IMP**
○ 2. Applying cold compresses. **6**
○ 3. Performing passive ROM exercises. **SECE**
○ 4. Performing ADL as needed.

105. In teaching Jacklyn how to prevent further episodes of crisis, the nurse should stress the need to *avoid:*
○ 1. Moderate emotional stress. **IMP**
○ 2. Cool weather. **6**
○ 3. Swimming in public pools. **PsI/PhI**
○ 4. Extra fluid consumption.

106. Both of Jacklyn's parents have the sickle cell trait. In counseling the parents about having another child, the nurse would be most correct in telling them that future pregnancies will have a:
○ 1. 1:4 chance of producing a child with sickle cell anemia. **IMP** **6**
○ 2. 1:2 chance of producing a child with sickle cell anemia. **PhI**
○ 3. 1:4 chance of producing a child with sickle cell trait.
○ 4. 4:4 chance of producing a child with sickle cell anemia.

Lee Yu, 16 years old, is admitted to the hospital for a weight loss of 20 pounds over a 3-week period. Diagnostic studies confirm diabetes, and the nursing staff is to institute a teaching program for Lee and his family. Questions 107–112 refer to Lee.

107. When the nurse begins teaching Lee about insulin, which one fact should be stressed to Lee and his family?
○ 1. Properly controlled dietary management, along with hypoglycemic agents, may eventually be utilized by Lee. **IMP** **4** **PhI**
○ 2. Exogenous insulin will be necessary for the rest of Lee's life.
○ 3. Activity level, nutritional intake, and state of health will necessitate daily modifications in Lee's insulin dose.
○ 4. Due to his need for insulin, Lee should no longer participate in active sports.

108. The following morning Lee is preparing his first dose of insulin. The physician orders 14 units of NPH insulin; Lee draws up 13 units and shows it to the nurse. The nurse should base any response on the knowledge that:
○ 1. This is Lee's first attempt and he did come close to the exact dose. **EV** **4/5**
○ 2. At Lee's age, he cannot be expected to make such fine discriminations in dosage. **PsI**
○ 3. Lee must draw up the exact amount prior to administration.
○ 4. Teenagers like Lee often antagonize adults subconsciously.

109. Lee goes to the teen lounge and becomes very boisterous and aggressive, starting a fight with another teen. The *first* question the nurse should consider is:
○ 1. "Should Lee be sent to his room?" **AN**
○ 2. "Did Lee eat breakfast today?" **4**
○ 3. "What did the other teen do to Lee?" **PhI**
○ 4. "Does Lee miss his own friends?"

110. After several days of administering his own insulin, Lee's blood sugar drops quite low. The nurse should know that this most likely means that Lee:
○ 1. Has entered the "honeymoon" phase. **EV**
○ 2. Deliberately gave himself too much insulin to see what would happen. **4** **PhI**
○ 3. Accidentally gave himself too much insulin.
○ 4. Had transient diabetes and will no longer need insulin.

111. About a week after discharge, Lee and his mother return to the clinic for a check-up. Lee's mother states, "I'm worried Lee will make a mistake, so I've been giving him his insulin." The nurse should:
○ 1. Allow Lee and his mother to work this out on their own. **IMP** **5/7**
○ 2. Assist Lee's mother to understand that Lee must assume this responsibility. **HPM**
○ 3. Encourage Lee's mother to continue working closely with him.
○ 4. Realize that this is an appropriate response by the mother.

112. In reviewing what he would do if he experienced a hypoglycemic episode, Lee correctly states that he would eat a piece of candy or drink a glass of orange juice. The nurse should then instruct Lee to follow up this concentrated sweet with:
○ 1. A Dextrostix test. **IMP**
○ 2. A urine dipstick for glucose. **4**
○ 3. A glass of milk. **PhI**
○ 4. 5 units of regular insulin.

113. A mother who lost her first-born to SIDS tells the nurse that she plans to breastfeed her second baby to prevent this from happening again. The nurse should base any response on the knowledge that:

○ 1. Breastfeeding does *not* prevent SIDS. **IMP**
○ 2. Breastfeeding *does* seem to prevent SIDS. **5**
○ 3. SIDS occurs *more* frequently in infants who are bottlefed. **PhI**
○ 4. Breastfeeding is contraindicated for *siblings* of infants who died from SIDS.

114. Normally, an infant's birth weight doubles by the age of 6 months and triples by the age of 1 year. By what age should the nurse expect the birth weight to *quadruple?*
○ 1. 18 months. **EV**
○ 2. 2 years. **5**
○ 3. 2½ years. **PhI**
○ 4. 3 years.

115. A mother asks the nurse how tall her child will be when he grows up. What answer should the nurse offer?
○ 1. "This is virtually impossible to predict." **IMP**
○ 2. "It will be double the child's height at 2 years of age." **5** **HPM**
○ 3. "It will be triple the child's height at 18 months of age."
○ 4. "Add 2 feet to the child's height at 4 years of age."

116. The only childhood communicable disease for which there is *not* currently an available immunization is:
○ 1. Chickenpox. **AN**
○ 2. Smallpox. **1**
○ 3. Parotitis. **HPM**
○ 4. Rubeola.

117. In teaching principles of poison control to a group of mothers, the nurse would be most correct in stressing that the age group most likely to suffer from accidental ingestions is:
○ 1. 6 months to 18 months. **AN**
○ 2. 12 months to 2½ years. **1**
○ 3. 2 years to 4 years. **SECE**
○ 4. 3 years to 5 years.

118. In deciding which *one* type of accident prevention to discuss *first* with the parents of a toddler, the nurse should base the choice on the knowledge that most deaths in children under age 3 are caused by:
○ 1. Aspiration/suffocation. **AN**
○ 2. Falls. **1**
○ 3. Motor vehicles. **SECE**
○ 4. Poisonings.

119. The following four children are clients in the pediatrics unit. Which one should the nurse anticipate will be *most* affected by separation from parents?
○ 1. Tasha, a 6-week-old with pyloric stenosis. **AN**
○ 2. Lenore, a 19-month-old with salicylate poisoning. **7** **PsI**
○ 3. Sam, a 3½-year-old with hypospadias.
○ 4. Terry, a 5-year-old with hemophilia.

120. In assessing the development of a 5-year-old, the nurse would expect the child to be capable of all of the following *except:*
○ 1. Name primary colors. **AS**
○ 2. Count to 100. **5**
○ 3. Know the days of the week. **PsI**
○ 4. Give phone number and address.

■ ANSWERS/RATIONALE

1. (1) The infant with a myelomeningocele should be placed on her stomach in a prone position to avoid pressure on the sac, which could cause tears, leaks, and infection. The side-lying position (3) might be an acceptable second choice, depending on the exact size and location of the sac. Placing the infant on her back (2) is absolutely contraindicated, as this would lead to immediate rupture of the sac. Trendelenberg position (4) is unnecessary for this infant.

2. (2) The major short-term complication that infants with myelomeningocele face is infection following a tear or rupture of the sac. Hydrocephalus (1) does occur in 90% of these cases, usually following closure of the sac, but it is thought to be part of the CNS defect rather than a "complication." Likewise, paraplegia (4) is part of the symptom complex these patients present with, rather than a "complication." Finally, mental retardation (3) may or may not occur, but if it does occur it is a long-term complication.

3. (2) The usual response to the birth of a defective infant is denial, often manifest in the parents' "refusing" to acknowledge the problem; this is a normal response, at least initially. The Blacks' comments about their infant, in view of her serious defect, should not be interpreted as attachment (1), immaturity (3), or love (4).

4. (4) Transillumination, or the procedure of shining a light through the sac, is the usual means for evaluating the contents of the sac. When there is "no transillumination" (the light cannot shine through the sac), this indicates the presence of solid material, or the spinal cord, within the sac. Thus (2) and (3) are incorrect. Transillumination has no bearing on determining whether or not the sac can be easily repaired (1).

5. (2) The chief purpose of the moist soaks is to prevent tears or leaks in the sac, which could lead to infection, the number one cause of death during the neonatal period. Promoting comfort (1) and relieving pressure (3) are not reasons for ordering moist soaks for this infant. It is *not* possible to stimulate neural development (4), which is permanently and irreversibly arrested before birth.

6. (3) Parents often hope that the surgery done to close the sac will also help the infant move her legs; it is very important to stress the permanent, irreversible nature of the nerve damage. Surgery will *not* enable the infant to regain motor or sensory functioning; surgery is done primarily to prevent infection. Parents should not be told the infant will move her legs after surgery (4) or offered false hope (1 or 2).

7. (1) The infant is placed on her abdomen, postoperatively, to prevent trauma or pressure to the sutured area on her back. In addition, the infant's head should be positioned 10° lower than her hips to prevent the pressure of circulating CSF from affecting the suture line on the lower back. An obvious contraindication to this position is if increased intracranial pressure is present, in which case the infant would be positioned flat in bed (4). In general, the head is never higher than the hips (2 or 3) during the immediate postoperative period for this type of surgery.

8. (2) In infants, the earliest sign of hydrocephalus is increasing head circumference, which occurs as the suture lines separate and the fontanels widen to accommodate the extra fluid within the skull. Later signs would indicate that no further accommodation can occur and brain tissue is being destroyed; these signs might include bulging anterior fontanel (1), shrill, high-pitched cry (3), and sunset eyes (4).

9. (4) Typically, the majority of parents of infants with CHD will complain about the infant's being very difficult to feed: must be woken up to feed, has weak suck, may turn blue with feeding, takes an overly long time to feed but falls asleep before finishing. Because of the weak suck, and altered cardiopulmonary dynamics, the infant is also prone to aspiration, pneumonia, and various respiratory infections (1) as well, although parents often do not make the connection between these factors. In addition, because of the difficulty in feeding the infant, the infant typically presents with developmental delays (2) and a slow rate of growth (3), although again this is not what the majority of parents of infants with CHD complain about.

10. (4) The majority of infants with CHD present with tachycardia, or a heart rate above 160 bpm; this is often the first sign of CHD that the nurse can assess. Circumoral cyanosis (1), hypertension (2), and diastolic murmur (3) all may or may not be present, depending on the type and severity of the defect.

11. (3) Because Craig has heart failure (and VSD), he should be on a low-sodium formula, Lonalac. Isomil (1) is a lactose-free formula that contains a normal amount of sodium. Lofenalac (2) is the formula used to treat infants with PKU and also contains a normal amount of sodium. Similac 27 with iron (4) is most frequently used for premature infants and also contains a normal amount of sodium.

12. (4) Infants with CHD should be given about 15–20 minutes per feeding; if the infant is unable to finish the feeding, or if the infant becomes cyanotic or experiences respiratory distress during the feeding, gavage feeding should be used to avoid exhausting the infant and possibly precipitating an episode of apnea. No attempts should be made to continue the feeding (1, 2, or 3).

13. (1) As with an adult with CHF, the infant should be positioned in a chair/infant seat, in semi-Fowler's position, to provide for maximum expansion of the lungs and to assist the heart. Placing Craig on his stomach (2) might be an acceptable second choice, providing he can tolerate this position. Craig should never be placed on his back (3), even with his head slightly hyperextended, because of the possibility of aspiration and other respiratory complications. A side-lying position (4) would be difficult to maintain in a 5-month-old, especially with the head of the bed elevated; an infant seat is more appropriate.

14. (1) Craig should be wearing loose-fitting clothes, including diapers, to avoid pressure on the abdominal organs, which could impinge on Craig's diaphragm and impede his respiratory effort. The student nurse should loosen his diaper, and she should know the rationale for this action as well. The nurse should not take care of this herself (3), as the student will repeat the mistake without the nurse's intervention; in addition, pinning the diaper snugly is inappropriate for Craig (2, 4), and the nurse has the final responsibility for the care Craig receives.

15. (3) The use of a pacifier for Craig will promote true psychologic rest for him, thus reducing his body's demand for oxygen and reducing the workload of his heart. This is the *most* important reason that Craig should be offered the pacifier; while it may also be true that Craig seems to like the pacifier (1), this is not the main reason he should be given one. (2) and (4) are too generalized and not necessarily true.

16. (1) Considering Craig's diagnosis, the nurse should anticipate that Craig will most likely have at least some developmental delays; most infants would begin to roll over by 3 months of age, but Craig—5 months—should be doing this now. Sitting (2) is normally found around 6 months of age; Craig will most likely *not* be capable of this behavior at 5 months. A pincer grasp (3) is normally found at 9–12 months of age, and again Craig will most likely *not* be capable of this behavior either. Finally, weight bearing (4) is typically noted in healthy infants 4–6 months of age; but considering Craig's diagnosis, he may or may not be capable of this more strenuous behavior.

17. (2) Because Craig does have a tendency toward respiratory infections, he should have limited contact with visitors with URIs, such as the grandmother with her slight cold. In fact, her slight cold might mean an episode of pneumonia for Craig. Lupus (1) in the aunt is not contagious, nor is the father's drug addiction (3). Craig's sister (4) should be allowed to see and touch Craig, unless she herself is sick.

18. (2) Extremes of temperatures, either too warm or too cold, should be avoided for infants with CHD, as this increases the body's demand for oxygen, thus increasing the workload of the heart. The mother would need no further teaching if she correctly stated that Craig should be dressed in loose-fitting clothing (1), should be brought back to the clinic for regularly scheduled appointments (3), and should be placed in a safe play area to stimulate development (4).

19. (1) With a patient with a potentially contagious infection such as AGE, the nurse must *first* protect herself and other clients by observing appropriate infection control measures. Other interventions can then be safely implemented without risk of cross-contamination (2, 3, 4).

20. (2) Signs of dehydration in infants would include irritability and sunken, dry eyeballs due to fluid loss. Fever may be present, and tachycardia, not bradycardia (1) is also common. Low blood pressure often results, followed by oliguria; anuria (3) is rare and would be an ominous sign of renal failure. Finally, the oral buccal mucosa may be quite dry, and the anterior fontanel may be sunken, not bulging (4).

21. (3) The best means to prevent any type of infection in any type of setting is good handwashing. Other techniques are secondary (1, 2, 4).

22. (2) At 7 months of age, Lureen may either sit with some support or sit alone; either behavior is commonly acquired at this age. Rolling over (1) is usually found in infants around 3–4 months of age, whereas weight bearing (3) and the palmar grasp (4) are commonly found in infants between the ages of 4 and 6 months of age.

23. (3) The classic sign of Hirschsprung's disease is obstinate constipation that persists in spite of all efforts at treatment. Other symptoms may also occur but are not generally considered specific to Hirschsprung's disease as much as they indicate intestinal obstruction: abdominal distention (1), anorexia (2), and vomiting (4).

24. (4) The instruction manual of the DDST clearly states that the parent should accompany the child who is to have the DDST and that the examiner should do everything possible to establish rapport with the parent and the child. With a 9-month-old, such as John, this should include allowing the parent to hold the child rather than separating them for the purpose of testing (1, 2, 3).

25. (1) Hirschsprung's disease is a congenital condition. It does not "develop spontaneously," although the diagnosis may not be made until symptoms have been present for several months and some attempts at conservative medical treatment (enemas, stool softeners, etc.) have been made (3). In the newborn with Hirschsprung's disease, there may be an episode of meconium ileus (2), but this occurs as a result of the Hirschsprung's disease rather than as the cause of it. Finally, there is no known metabolic defect (4).

26. (2) The only solution that should be used in doing cleansing enemas for a child with Hirschsprung's disease is normal saline, because the child will retain some of this fluid, which will be absorbed through the bowel wall. As an isotonic solution, normal saline will not alter the fluid balance like a nonisotonic solution almost certainly would (1, 3, 4).

27. (2) As a 9-month-old with a chronic bowel problem, John has probably become accustomed to his mother's administering suppositories or enemas. In addition, fear of strangers is common in this age group. Considering these factors, John's mother should at least be offered the opportunity to administer or assist with the enemas. If this is not feasible, another qualified person could take her place (1, 3, 4).

28. (4) Early in the course of LTB, children most commonly exhibit inspiratory stridor, a harsh-pitched crowing sound made upon inspiration, and a croupy, barking, metallic cough. As the condition worsens and respiratory efforts increase, there may be dyspnea and cyanosis (1), tachycardia and hoarseness (2) progressing to aphonia. Fever up to 104 °F is also common, but an expiratory wheeze is not (3).

29. (4) As a toddler, Maria will probably assert her autonomy by refusing to take this medication. The best approach is to be firm yet kind, and always calm. No child should be told medicine is (like) candy (1). Medication should be mixed with no more than one teaspoon of any nonessential food or beverage (2). Maria will probably not drink this medication by herself, and the nurse should not offer her this choice because, if Maria refuses, then a "power" struggle will follow (3).

30. (4) If Maria responds well to oxygen therapy, she should show clinical improvement in terms of pink lips and nailbeds and normal vital signs, especially pulse. "All" toys do not have to be removed from Maria's crib (1), nor will she have to be NPO (2), although she will probably be somewhat anorexic and prefer clear, cool liquids initially. Oxygen concentrations should be monitored and recorded at least every 2 hours (3).

31. (4) To "flood" the croupette with oxygen means to raise the oxygen concentration to that level ordered by the physician; in general, the flow rate should be adjusted to 15 liters per minute, the tent should be closed and tucked in, and the nurse should wait about 15 minutes before checking the concentration and readjusting the flow. Lower flow rates (1, 2, 3) would result in lower-than-required oxygen concentrations.

32. (3) To maintain an oxygen concentration of 35–40%, the flow rate should now be adjusted to 8–10 liters per minute; this is the usual concentration ordered for a croup tent. Other flow rates would result in higher or lower concentrations (1, 2, 4).

33. (1) Because oxygen is heavier than room air, it will settle to the bottom of the croupette and leak out unless the edges are tucked in tightly. If the edges are lying loosely on top of the linens (2), the oxygen will escape, resulting in lower concentrations than ordered. The crib rails should be raised for safety, not lowered (4); and again the edges should be tucked in tightly, not draped over the rails (3).

34. (1) While in the croupette, Maria should be allowed only those toys that can be dried off easily; all stuffed animals, dolls with hair, etc. are not allowed, as they will harbor moisture and bacteria. While in the croupette, Maria and her linens will also get damp or wet, and the nurse should implement measures to prevent chilling. Pajamas and blankets should be changed q 4h or p.r.n. (2). There is no need to restrain a child in the croupette (3), as all working parts are safely outside the croupette. Finally, there is also no need to restrict visitors (4).

35. (4) As a toddler, Maria will suffer the most if separated from her mother; a croupette is a particularly frightening experience for her, as explanations are difficult. If Maria will calm down with mother in the croupette with her, this will decrease her body's need for oxygen. There is no need to check with the physician (2), nor would it be "unsafe" (3). Given Maria's present condition, there is no reason to question the parent's handling of the situation (1).

36. (3) Progressive hoarseness, followed by aphonia, is an ominous sign of impending airway obstruction and respiratory arrest secondary to edema and inflammation. This must be promptly reported to the physician, who will probably do an emergency tracheostomy. An apical pulse of 118 (1) is normal for a 14-month-old like Maria; pink nailbeds (4) indicate a satisfactory level of oxygenation. Finally, as Maria begins to improve, her appetite should also pick up (2).

37. (1) MMR is given as a combined immunization at age 15 months (2). DTP "booster" is given 3 months later, at age 18 months (3, 4).

38. (1) In caring for a client with a potentially contagious condition such as meningitis, the nurse must *first* protect him/herself and other patients by observing appropriate infection control measures, in this case, respiratory isolation. All other nursing care measures would then follow in the appropriate order (2, 3, 4).

39. (4) With a pediatric microdrip chamber, the number of cc/hour = number of drops/minute. Therefore, if the physician orders 35 cc/hour, the IV should infuse at 35 drops/minute. Any other flow rate would be incorrect (1, 2, 3).

40. (4) In order to restrain a toddler receiving IV therapy, clove-hitch restraint to two or more limbs is most effective in maintaining the IV site. A posey jacket (1) would allow Kelly use of her hands with which to pull at her IV. Elbow restraints (2) would still allow Kelly to stand and twist at the IV tubing. A mummy restraint (3) would be unnecessarily restrictive for Kelly.

41. (1) The best position for clients who have had a spinal tap is perfectly flat in bed, with no pillow at all. Such clients are prone to headaches due to the loss of CSF during the spinal tap; until the fluid is naturally replaced by the body, a flat position will minimize cerebral irritation and minimize headache; thus, (2) is incorrect. Elevating the head of the bed (3) will increase her headache and is not recommended. There is no need to place Kelly semi-prone (4) at this time.

42. (3) The opisthotonus position occurs in children with severe meningitis due to the pressure on the spinal cord; the child's head is drawn back and the spine is arched backward in an attempt to minimize pressure on the cord. When the child assumes this position, the nurse should place the child in a side-lying position for safety and comfort. Any other position would not work as well (1, 2, 4).

43. (2) As healing of the pathways of the CSF occurs following an episode of meningitis, scar tissue naturally forms; this may lead to noncommunicating hydrocephalus. The hydrocephalus might then lead to learning disabilities (3) or mental retardation (4). Encephalitis (1) may occur in conjunction with the meningitis, but it is not a complication.

44. (1) At 2 years of age, if Kelly were to develop hydrocephalus, the first sign she would most likely demonstrate would be irritability and poor feeding due to increased intracranial pressure. Her head circumference would not increase (2), as her fontanels have closed. Headaches or double vision might occur (3), but at 2 years of age, Kelly is not likely to complain of them. Ruptured retinal vessels (4) is a later sign of increased intracranial pressure.

45. (1) With a child who has suffered an ingestion, vomiting should be induced only if the child is fully alert and reactive. If the child has any alterations in level of consciousness, such as seizures (2) or coma (3), vomiting may cause an aspiration pneumonia. Further, if the child has swallowed a corrosive substance (4), the substance that burned once going down will burn a second time coming up if vomiting is induced.

46. (3) Syrup of ipecac is an emetic used to induce vomiting following ingestion of a harmful substance; the usual dose in children is 10–15 mL PO followed by at least 200 mL of water. The water is thought to enhance the emetic effect of ipecac and stimulate emptying of the stomach, thus ridding the body of the harmful substance. Activated charcoal (2) will neutralize the emetic effect and should not be given with ipecac, although in some cases it may be given after vomiting has occurred. Milk or toast (1, 4) have little or no effect and will neither help nor harm, although, if the child does vomit, they may increase the risk of aspiration.

47. (4) With children who have received a 10-mL dose of syrup of ipecac, if vomiting has not occurred within 30 minutes, the dose can and should be repeated once more. While the first dose is generally effective in the majority of cases, a second dose is almost always 100% effective. If the child does not vomit after a second dose, manual stimulation of the gag reflex and/or gastric lavage must be promptly initiated to avoid toxic effects of ipecac (see the next answer). The nurse should never use her fingers to stimulate the gag reflex (1), especially in a toddler, because of the danger of receiving a human bite. Ipecac works within 15–30 minutes, and waiting another 30 minutes will not be helpful (2). If the child does not vomit at all, thus not removing either the ipecac or the ingested substance(s), there is the danger of ipecac toxicity as well as poisoning from the ingested substance (3).

48. (1) The chief danger of ipecac's being absorbed into the body is potentially fatal cardiotoxicity, which can cause cardiac arrhythmias, atrial fibrillation, or severe heart block. There is minimal effect on the liver (2), kidneys (3), or CNS (4).

49. (2) The general recommendation to make to parents on how to handle temper tantrums is to ignore this behavior because attention to a tantrum can reinforce undesirable behavior. If a parent allows a child to make a choice (1) and then does not follow through with this choice either because of personal preference or because the choice is unsafe, then tantrums will increase. Changing settings (3) is often a catalyst for a tantrum as the child is moved from one area to another, e.g., from the park to home. Finally, giving in to a toddler's demands (4) is unrealistic; parents should offer only allowable choices to their toddler and then allow the toddler to follow through with these choices.

50. (2) Toddlers typically fear those procedures that are "intrusive," that is, where something goes into their bodies. Therefore, a rectal temperature would most likely evoke the most anxiety in a 3-year-old. Generally, a child Teddy's age would be relatively cooperative with getting weighed (4) and giving a urine specimen (3), although having BP taken might also be somewhat threatening (1).

51. (2) Hemarthrosis, or bleeding into a joint either spontaneously or following an injury, is considered the hallmark, or most typical sign, of hemophilia. If hemarthrosis is not treated properly or adequately, permanent joint deformities may result. Other signs of hemophilia include prolonged bleeding from a relatively minor injury (3), excessive or unusual hematoma formation (1), and intracranial bleeding following a closed head injury (4).

52. (1) At 3 years of age, Teddy should be able to coordinate the brain and gross motor activity necessary to go up stairs using alternate feet; he should also be able to pedal "Big Wheels" or a tricycle, but not a bicycle (2). Teddy should also be capable of getting dressed *with* supervision but not without it (3). Teddy should not be ready to master tying his shoelaces (4) for another year or two.

53. (4) Contrary to popular belief, the best position for the nurse to place Teddy in when he has a nosebleed is sitting up and leaning forward slightly, with head remaining above the level of the heart; this position will allow the blood to drain freely from his nose and prevent aspiration. Sitting up with his head tilted backward (3) will predispose Teddy to swallowing or aspirating blood, as will a semi-Fowler's position (2). The prone position (1) might be an acceptable second choice if Teddy were too weak to sit up by himself.

54. (4) Cryoprecipitate, or Factorate, is a blood product; a type and cross match may be ordered for the child prior to the IV administration of this medication. As with any blood product, the child should be closely observed for possible transfusion reaction. Given the relatively small volume of fluid to be administered, it would not usually cause fluid volume overload (2). Although there has been some discussion about the administration of multiple IV medications in the hemophiliac and the linkage to AIDS (3), this is not a concern during the actual administration of the medication but rather a long-term concern. Finally, emboli formation (1) can occur with any IV administration and is not specific to cryoprecipitate, although the nurse would need to take the necessary precautions to prevent this possibility.

55. (4) For a child just leaving the toddler period of autonomy and just entering the preschool period of initiative, the best suggestion to improve his nutritional intake would be to allow the child to feed himself. Other suggestions would supplement and enhance this one primary consideration (1, 2, 3).

56. (2) It would be impossible to supervise a hemophiliac child so carefully that any other bleeding episodes would be prevented; further, to attempt to do so would cause the parents to totally restrict the child, resulting in extreme overprotection. An acceptable alternative response would be to prevent "major" episodes of bleeding or to promptly recognize signs of a bleeding episode that would require medical intervention. The other statements (1, 3, 4) are all correct responses by the parents, indicating they have probably understood the nurse's teaching regarding Teddy's care.

57. (4) When a child like Marty has a favorite "security object," be it a blanket or a doll or a stuffed animal, that child should be allowed to keep the security object, even during hospitalization. This will promote the child's sense of trust and security, thus helping to make the hospitalization a more positive experience. Offering Marty another toy (1), putting the toy where he can see it but not touch it (2), or giving him a new Cookie Monster (3) will not take the place of Marty's old but well-loved original Cookie Monster.

58. (1) Nephrosis (nephrotic syndrome) is a chronic syndrome characterized by variable pathology and questionable prognosis. In general, most children with nephrosis do present with severe, total body edema and 4 + proteinuria, along with hypoproteinemia. Hypertension and hematuria (3), and hyperlipidemia and periorbital edema (2), are more common in acute glomerulonephritis. The child with nephrosis seldom presents with severe oliguria (4), although occasionally this may occur; anorexia (4) may or may not occur, depending on the severity of the exacerbation.

59. (4) There is no known cure for nephrosis; rather, treatment is aimed at providing symptomatic relief. To that effect, prednisone—an antiinflammatory corticosteroid—is given to relieve symptoms rather than effect a cure. If prednisone has the expected therapeutic effect, the patient should report "feeling better" as symptoms are relieved. *Side* effects of prednisone therapy may also include mood swings (1), glucosuria (2), and fluid retention with weight gain (3).

60. (4) As generalized edema progresses, in males the scrotal sac can become extremely swollen, tender, and painful. The best nursing intervention is to place soft, folded diapers under the scrotum while the child is lying in bed. Zinc oxide (1) or medicated powder (3) will have little beneficial effect because the problem is mechanical rather than on the skin itself. Cleansing the scrotum (2) is important to prevent infection, as all edematous tissue needs special care to prevent skin breakdown; however, this will not relieve Marty's discomfort.

61. (4) Nephrosis is characterized by periods of exacerbations and remissions that occur throughout the childhood years. Marty's parents should watch him closely for exacerbations, which should be reported promptly to the physician. Marty should be encouraged to play with other children, not to stay away from them (1) to avoid feelings of social isolation. It is not "over" (2), and Marty will need to be watched carefully for periods of exacerbation. Once Marty is discharged, he will generally not need to remain in bed (3) but rather can convalesce at home with alternating periods of activity and rest.

62. (4) Epiglottitis is a bacterial infection of the epiglottis resulting in swelling and obstruction; without prompt, aggressive treatment, it can progress rapidly, resulting in respiratory arrest within 6–8 hours of onset. Although this condition does require hospitalization and is potentially life-threatening, the ICU stay is usually less than 5 days (2, 3). There is no allergic cause of epiglottitis (1).

63. (2) In suspected cases of epiglottitis, the visualization of the epiglottis is strictly contraindicated, as it may precipitate laryngospasm and immediate respiratory arrest. It is a nursing responsibility to inform any less knowledgeable health care providers of this danger; any other action (1, 3, 4) would be inappropriate at this time.

64. (2) Solucortef is a corticosteroid/anti-inflammatory, used in epiglottitis to relieve swelling and edema. Solucortef does not provide sedation (1) or relieve pain (3), and the bacterial infection is treated with antibiotics (4).

65. (2) Hospitalized preschoolers often regress in their behavior and want "mommy," but this is obviously not practical all the time. The nurse should do her best to soothe the child back to sleep during the middle of the night. Calling the mother to come right in (4) would be inappropriate, as the family should not be called in the absence of a genuine emergency. The nurse should also not pick the child up (1), as hospitalized preschoolers frequently reject everyone except their "mommy." Simply insisting Brad go back to sleep (3) is not enough, as he needs some degree of comfort at this time.

66. (1) Although the abrupt onset and critical nature of this illness is very frightening for parents, the child is expected to make a total recovery prior to discharge. The parents should be aware of this very positive diagnosis. Although discharge instructions from the physician may include some rest at home, there is no need for Brad to miss almost a month of school (2). The parents should not worry about Brad's getting sick again (3) or having oxygen in the home (4); again, the excellent prognosis should be stressed.

67. (3) In working with children in hospitals, the most important factor for the nurse to assess first is what that child's experience with illness and hospitalization has been thus far. This is of special importance with Kato, who has previously had two hospitalizations and surgeries; the nurse needs to know if these were positive experiences for Kato and how he was able to cope with them. After this, the nurse would continue her admitting assessment by determining Kato's developmental level (1), what Kato already knows about hypospadias (2), and whether or not Kato's parents plan to room in with him (4).

68. (4) Because hypospadias interferes with the child's ability to void in the normal male standing position, the corrective surgery is usually timed to be completed prior to the child's entering kindergarten. The main reason is to avoid other children making fun of the little boy's having to sit to void. Developmental and psychologic factors thus play a crucial role in the timing of this surgery, and other explanations (1, 2, 3) are either incorrect or inappropriate for Kato.

69. (2) When doing preoperative teaching with preschoolers, the best method is to use puppets (doctor, nurse, hospital set-up) to "act out" what the child can expect to happen. For evaluating the teaching, the nurse can then ask the child to use puppets to give a return demonstration of what was learned; this enables the nurse to clarify any misconceptions or answer any lingering questions the child might still have. Most preschoolers will not be able to *accurately* draw pictures regarding the factual information of preop teaching (1), although this might be a good way to get at feelings about the surgery or hospital. At 4½, Kato probably has had limited experience with "tests" (3). The nurse should not rely on the parents to evaluate her preop teaching (4), as they are not professionals and are most likely too involved emotionally.

70. (3) As a preschooler, Kato is in the age of fantasy or magical thinking. By making a game of "checking for monsters," a potentially frightening situation is relieved, and Kato may even begin to realize that there "really" are no monsters. Asking Kato to talk about his monsters (1) may make him believe they are real and that the nurse also believes in them. It would be too frightening to Kato to have to look for these monsters by himself (2). Telling a preschooler that his fantasies are not real (4) would not be enough to convince him and might make him become even more convinced they are indeed real!

71. (1) The surgical repair for hypospadias is done on the urethra primarily and also on the urethral meatus. Postoperatively, a urinary drainage apparatus (foley or supra-pubic) will be in place, and the urine is expected to have a clear yellow appearance. There should normally be no blood or mucus (2, 3, 4), which would indicate hemorrhage or infection if present.

72. (1) Prior to administering digoxin to a child, the nurse should auscultate the apical pulse for a full minute to most accurately evaluate cardiac rate and rhythm. Other pulse sites (2, 3, 4) are less accurate in children.

73. (1) The lower limit of a normal pulse rate for a 6-year-old is 75–80 beats per minute; the nurse would be most correct in withholding Jake's digoxin and notifying his physician if Jake's pulse were below 80. A pulse rate of from 90 to 110 (2, 3, 4) would be considered within normal limits for a 6-year-old, and the nurse would be correct in administering the medication as ordered.

74. (3) To be most effective, viokase should be administered immediately before every meal and every snack; this will facilitate the absorption of fats and proteins contained within the meal. The enzyme will have little or no therapeutic value if given at other times (1, 2, 4).

75. (2) Viokase is an enzyme; as such, it will begin to break down whatever food or liquid it is mixed with. However, for maximum therapeutic effect, the enzymatic action should be delayed until the medication reaches the stomach. The best food to mix with viokase is the cold applesauce. The applesauce should be cold because cold delays the enzymatic action, which is most effective at 98.6°F. Applesauce is used because of its high fiber content, which also delays the enzymatic action of the viokase. Any other foods or liquids the viokase might be mixed with (1, 3, 4) would be less than ideal.

76. (2) Cystic fibrosis is inherited as an autosomal recessive disorder. The fact that Jake has the disease means that his parents are carriers of the trait, and each subsequent pregnancy might result in a child who also has CF, like Jake. It would not be correct to advise the mother that a second child would only carry the trait (4) or would be normal (3), although there is a possibility these might occur; the parents should be fully advised as to the odds of this happening. In addition, it would needlessly worry the parents to tell them a second child might be more severely affected (1), although this is also a possibility.

77. (4) The best exercise for a child with CF is swimming, which provides needed exercise at an activity level that is not overly taxing for the child. Softball, tennis, and soccer (1, 2, 3) are all generally thought to be too strenuous for a child with CF.

78. (3) Neutropenia is an abnormal decrease in the number of neutrophils, the specific type of white blood cell responsible for phagocytosis and bacterial destruction; as such, the infection in an leukemic patient is most commonly related to neutropenia. Leukemic clients may also suffer from anemia (1), leukopenia (2) or thrombocytopenia (4), although these blood dyscrasias will result in other signs or symptoms of leukemia.

79. (1) Most psychologists would recommend that a child be offered comfort in the form of a hug, kiss, or cuddle; however, the child should be left in his or her own bed to avoid overdependence on the parents or possible psychosexual conflicts caused by entering the parents' bed (2). For the school-age child, nightmares are a common occurrence and can be accepted as a normal part of growth and development; therefore, no professional intervention is necessary at this time (3). At 7 years of age, it would be very difficult for Mary Jane to keep written records of her dreams (4); in fact, such an expectation might lead to even more severe sleep disturbances for her.

80. (2) Children with leukemia often experience bleeding gums due to thrombocytopenia; in addition, chemotherapy may cause oral mucous membrane ulceration. Therefore, the nurse would be most correct in advising Mary Jane to brush her teeth with a soft toothbrush only. Using a firm toothbrush (3) might cause a break in the gums, leading to infection. Rinsing her mouth only (4) might also lead to infection, as this would not necessarily clean the gums and teeth adequately; likewise, infection might be caused by not brushing her teeth (1).

81. (1) The leading cause of morbidity and mortality in children with leukemia is infection; therefore, preventing infection is the most important nursing care plan goal. Preventing injury (2), promoting adequate nutrition (3), and meeting developmental needs (4) are other, less important goals for the leukemic child.

82. (4) Vincristine is an antineoplastic vinca alkaloid, which has the major side effect of peripheral neuropathy; this may be manifested in numbness, tingling, foot drop, paresthesia, etc. In addition, vincristine may also cause constipation, not diarrhea (1). Hemorrhagic cystitis (3) may be caused by cytoxan, not vincristine. Vincristine does not cause visual changes (2).

83. (1) Viscous xylocaine is a topical anesthetic that is often used with leukemic patients; by numbing the mouth, pain due to oral ulcers is relieved, and the child may eat better. The leukemic child with oral ulcers should not be offered lukewarm liquids, which may serve as media for bacterial growth (2). The leukemic child with bleeding tendencies should never be offered aspirin for pain (3). Allowing Mary Jane, at 7 years of age, to choose her own menu (4) would not necessarily relieve the pain due to her oral ulcers.

84. (4) While any infection can be life-threatening to a child with leukemia, chickenpox presents a particular danger, as the child may develop encephalitis or sepsis. Infections such as impetigo (1), strep (2), or pneumonia (3) are less specific dangers.

85. (3) The most common symptom in children with rheumatic fever is tachycardia due to cardiac involvement; in addition, these children may develop a rash, "erythema marginatum," and a characteristic fever, which spikes in the late afternoon. They do not usually present with petechiae (1), hypertension (2), or conjunctivitis (4).

86. (2) Carditis is the only manifestation of rheumatic fever that can lead to permanent damage; the best way to evaluate Lisa for the presence of carditis is to monitor her apical pulse at least q 4h. Her growth and development (1, 3) and her ESR (4) deserve secondary consideration after checking her apical pulse.

87. (3) Carditis can lead to permanent, irreversible cardiac damage, specifically, mitral valvular stenosis. The other manifestations of rheumatic fever (1, 2, 4) are transient and do not leave any permanent effects.

88. (4) Lisa will be in the hospital for a relatively longer period of time and will be confined to bed most of the time. The ideal roommate would be another child of the same sex and same developmental level who will also be in the hospital for some time and confined to bed. The best choice is the young girl with the fractured elbow, who will probably be in traction and also on bedrest. The child with a tonsillectomy (2) or the child with a concussion (3) will most likely be in the hospital for a very short time and will be out of bed. The child with impetigo, caused by strep (1), would be a most unsatisfactory roommate for Lisa, as she might reinfect Lisa with strep.

89. (4) For a child like Lisa, experiencing migratory polyarthritis, even the weight of a single sheet can cause excruciating pain; therefore, a bed cradle will help keep the linens off Lisa's joints and provide symptomatic relief. Lisa is most likely on absolute bedrest, thus making a bath or shower (1) out of the question. Splints or a referral to physical therapy (2, 3) are unnecessary, as this type of arthritis causes no permanent deformities.

90. (4) Projective techniques seem to work best with school-age children in getting them to share their thoughts, feelings, and experiences. Direct questioning (1) often proves too threatening, causing the child to become even quieter. Challenging the child directly to "tell secrets" (2) is also too threatening and will likely cause the child to refuse to speak about anything. Finally, calling the child's mother (3) will not necessarily assist the child to communicate with the nurse.

91. (3) Clients receiving digoxin in addition to lasix are particularly prone to developing hypokalemia, which can result in digoxin toxicity and potentially fatal cardiac dysrhythmias. Potassium supplements are frequently administered to avoid this problem rather than for any of the other reasons cited here (1, 2, 4).

92. (1) School-age children are notoriously competitive, and they particularly enjoy the challenge of board games such as "Monopoly" or "Life." While school work is important and should receive due consideration (2), it will not relieve the girls' boredom. Likewise, books or TV (3, 4) are less effective diversions for the school-age child.

93. (1) Due to Lisa's carditis, the best means for the nurse to evaluate how well she tolerates any increase in activity would be via monitoring her apical pulse rate. Any increase in Lisa's pulse rate over 15–20 beats per minute would indicate that Lisa is not tolerating the increase in activity and would be an indication for returning her to bed immediately. Any other method of evaluating Lisa's tolerance of increasing activity would be less effective (2, 3, 4).

94. (1) Long-term follow-up care for children with rheumatic fever most frequently includes antibiotic therapy with penicillin or erythromycin on an exact schedule for an indefinite period of time, or a minimum of 5 years. There is no way to immunize Lisa against future attacks (2). Lisa will be sent home on severely restricted activity, and cardiac rehabilitation programs are out of the question at this time (3). Home-bound tutoring would be fine, after a while, but it is not a priority at this time (4).

95. (3) In working with children in hospitals, the most important factor for the nurse to assess first is the child's experience with illness and hospitalization. This is of special importance with Beverly, who has been hospitalized previously. After this most important factor, the nurse would continue the admitting assessment by determining what Beverly knows about asthma (1), how she usually cares for herself (2), and how Beverly feels about becoming a teenager (4).

96. (2) The preferred position for asthmatics is high Fowler's, or sitting up straight, which allows for maximum expansion of the lungs. Other positions would not allow for the maximum expansion of the lungs (1, 3, 4) and would only contribute to Beverly's hypoxia.

97. (2) About half of the children with eczema during the toddler or preschool years develop asthma during the school-age or teenage years. Asthma seems to have little or no relation to strep throat or tonsillitis (1). The death of her father undoubtedly affected Beverly, but it occurred one year before the onset of her asthma (3). The pneumonia she experienced at age 7 might have been related to her asthma but was not the cause of it (4).

98. (4) There are multiple factors involved in the etiology of asthma, including an allergic predisposition (2), precipitation by severe emotional or physical stress (3), and other factors yet to be determined (1).

99. (1) Children with asthma should have no stuffed animals in their rooms, as they tend to collect dust. Additional measures to "allergy proof" Beverly's room and home should include using only aluminum mini-blinds rather than curtains (2), having no pets in the home (3), and exercising such as swimming (4).

100. (3) The average age for the onset of menstruation for American females is 12½ years of age; girls between 10 and 16 years can begin to menstruate within the normal range (1, 2, 4).

101. (1) Younger teenage girls in particular prefer the company of other young girls; this is the age of the "best friend," and a definite preference for same-sex, same-age companions. As such, Beverly would not necessarily seek out older or younger children (2, 4) nor would she have "no preference" regarding the sex of her companion (3).

102. (2) Sickling of RBCs occurs under conditions of low oxygen tension; giving Jacklyn oxygen will prevent further sickling of RBCs, but it will not reverse the sickling of cells that has already occurred (1). The oxygen is not given to prevent any respiratory complication (3), nor will the oxygen have an effect on the oxygen-carrying capacity of the RBCs (4).

103. (3) The pain in vaso-occlusive crisis is due primarily to the clumping together of RBCs, which blocks small blood vessels, thus causing tissue ischemia, necrosis, and death. Although there may be increased RBC destruction (1) and hepatosplenomegaly (2), this is not the primary cause of Jacklyn's pain. Sequestration of blood does not normally occur with sickle cell anemia (4).

104. (1) Warmth causes vasodilatation, thus relieving the occlusion of small vessels and preventing tissue damage. Cold (2) would never be used, as it causes vasoconstriction. Performing ROM exercises (3) or ADL (4) would not relieve pain.

105. (3) Crises are precipitated by conditions of low oxygen tension; this may include infection, which could easily be picked up by swimming in public pools. Other sources of low oxygen tension might include severe emotional stress (1), extremely cold or windy weather (2), or dehydration (4), as well as high altitudes.

106. (1) Because sickle cell anemia is inherited as an autosomal recessive disorder, if both of Jacklyn's parents have the trait, any future pregnancies would have a 1:4 chance of producing a child with sickle cell anemia (2, 4). In addition, each pregnancy would have a 1:2 chance of producing a child with the trait (3), or a 1:4 chance of producing a normal child.

107. (2) Because the beta cells of the islets of Langerhans of Lee's pancreas will never again produce a sufficient quantity of insulin, Lee will remain dependent on insulin injections (exogenous insulin) for the rest of his life. Lee, like all juvenile diabetics, can never rely on hypoglycemic agents to control his diabetes (1), as these drugs work by stimulating the pancreas, and in Lee's case the stimulation would have absolutely no effect. *Daily* modifications would generally not be necessary (3), although periodic adjustments in insulin dosage would be needed as Lee grows. Lee can continue to participate in sports (4), but he should be taught to take some extra foods on those days he is active in sports.

108. (3) From the very first attempt by the child to administer his or her own insulin, the nurse should stress the need to administer exact amounts as ordered by the physician. The child should learn from the start that "close" is not "correct" (1). At 16, Lee can and should be capable of drawing up the exact amount (2). Drawing up an incorrect dose does not mean Lee is trying to antagonize the nurse, consciously or subconsciously (4).

109. (2) Juvenile diabetics are extremely brittle, or difficult to control, and prone to episodes of hypoglycemia and/or ketoacidosis. If Lee were to experience a hypoglycemic episode, the earliest symptoms would often be behavioral: irritability, personality changes, etc. If Lee becomes disruptive, the nurse should first ask if Lee has eaten his breakfast, how much he ate, and when; other areas (1, 3, 4) would be appropriate to explore *after* this primary consideration.

110. (1) Juvenile diabetics may experience a "honeymoon" phase about 1–2 weeks after they are initially diagnosed; during this time, they seem to be "cured," no longer requiring insulin. What is actually happening is that the pancreas is pushing out the last bit of insulin left in it; after this relatively short period, Lee will go back to total dependence on exogenous insulin (4). It is not likely that Lee gave himself too much insulin, either deliberately or accidentally (2, 3), if the nurse is supervising his dosage as she should be during Lee's hospitalization.

111. (2) At 16, Lee must assume responsibility for his own care as soon as possible; diabetes is a chronic disease with no known cure that Lee will have to live with for the rest of his life. The nurse should discourage Lee's mother from being overly protective of him or from assuming this responsibility (1, 3, 4).

112. (3) Because concentrated sweets will cause a rise in blood sugar, followed by a precipitous drop, the nurse should teach Lee that he should follow up this concentrated sweet with a complex carbohydrate such as a glass of milk. The complex carbohydrate will help maintain a consistent level of blood sugar, thus avoiding the precipitous drop. Any other action would be inappropriate at this time (1, 2, 4).

113. (1) The most recent research indicates that there is no relationship, either positive or negative, between breastfeeding and the occurrence of SIDS; there is roughly the same incidence of SIDS in infants who are breastfed or bottlefed (2, 3, 4).

114. (3) Generally, infants who weigh 7 pounds at birth will weigh 28 pounds, or quadruple their birth weight, by 2½ years of age. Consequently the other listed ages are incorrect (1, 2, 4).

115. (2) The general rule of thumb to predict a child's height as an adult is to double the child's height at 2 years of age. The other answers (1, 3, 4) are incorrect.

116. (1) The only communicable childhood disease for which there is not currently a mass-produced, mass-available immunization is chickenpox, although there is some promising research in this area. Recently, the U.N. World Health Organization officially listed smallpox as "eradicated," making immunization no longer necessary, although a vaccine had been available (2). The immunization for measles (rubeola) (4), mumps (parotitis) (3), and rubella (german measles) is currently available and is recommended to be given at 15 months of age.

117. (2) Poisoning is most common in toddlers, who have the motor skills necessary to reach the poisons yet lack the intelligence to know not to ingest the poison. The other answers (1, 3, 4) are, therefore, incorrect.

118. (3) In children under 3, most accidental deaths are related to motor vehicles in which the child is a passenger; other types of accidents are not as common or not as likely to result in death (1, 2, 4).

119. (2) Toddlers always suffer when separated from their parents, more so than any other age group (1, 3, 4). In fact, the years between ages 1 and 3 are when children are most likely to suffer separation anxiety.

120. (2) Five-year-olds may count up to 20 or 25, but seldom beyond this. They should be capable of naming colors such as red, green, and blue (1). In addition, they should be able to give their phone number and address (4) and have a better sense of temporal relationships, as evidenced by their ability to name days of the week, months of the year, and seasons (3).

■ UNIT

4

Nursing Care of the Acutely Ill and the Chronically Ill Adult

■ ASSESSMENT, ANALYSIS, AND NURSING DIAGNOSIS OF THE ADULT

Assessment is the process of gathering a comprehensive data base about the client's present, past, and potential health problems, as well as a description of the client as a whole in his or her environment. It includes a comprehensive nursing history, a physical examination, and laboratory/X-ray data, and it concludes with the formulation of nursing diagnoses.

SUBJECTIVE DATA

Nursing History

The nursing history obtains data for planning and implementing nursing actions.

I. General information: reason for admission; duration of present illness; previous hospitalization; history of illnesses; diagnostic procedures prior to admission; allergies—type and severity of reactions; medications taken at home—over-the-counter and prescription.

II. Information relative to growth and development: age; menarche—age at onset; heavy menses; dysmenorrhea; vaginal discharge; date of last Pap smear; pregnancies; abortions; miscarriages.

III. Information relative to psychosocial functions: feelings (anger, denial, fear, anxiety, guilt, life-style changes); language barriers; family support; spiritual needs; history of trauma/rape.

IV. Information relative to nutrition: appetite—normal, changes; dietary habits; food preferences or intolerances; difficulty swallowing or chewing; dentures; use of caffeine/alcohol; weight changes; excessive thirst, hunger, sweating.

V. Information relative to fluid and gas transport: difficulty breathing; shortness of breath; history of cough/smoking; colds; sputum; swelling of extremities; chest pain; palpitations; varicosities; excessive bruising; blood transfusions; excessive bleeding.

VI. Information relative to protective functions: skin problems—rash, itch; current treatment; unusual hair loss.

VII. Information relative to comfort, rest, activity, mobility: usual activity (ADL); present ability and restrictions; rest and sleep pattern; weakness; joint or muscle stiffness, pain, or swelling; occupation; interests.

VIII. Information relative to elimination: bowel habits; changes—constipation, diarrhea; ostomy; emesis; nausea; voiding—retention, frequency, dysuria, incontinence.

IX. Information relative to sensory-perceptual functions: pain—verbal report; quality, location; precipitating factors; duration; limitations in vision (glasses), hearing, touch, smell; orientation to person, place, time; confusion; headaches; fainting; dizziness; convulsions.

OBJECTIVE DATA

I. Physical assessment—requires knowledge of normal findings, organization, and keen senses, i.e., visual, auditory, touch, smell. For abnormal findings, refer to the Assessment section of each health problem discussed under the categories of human functioning.

ADULT NURSING

A. *Inspection*—uses observations to detect deviations from normal.

B. *Auscultation*—to perceive and interpret sounds arising from various organs, particularly heart, lungs, and bowel.

C. *Palpation*—used to assess for discomfort, temperature, pulsations, size, consistency, and texture.

D. *Percussion*—technique used to elicit vibrations produced by underlying organ structures; used less frequently in nursing practice.

1. Flat—normal percussion note over muscle or bone.
2. Dull—normal percussion note over organs such as liver.
3. Resonance—normal percussion note over lungs.
4. Tympany—normal percussion note over stomach or bowel.

II. General—provides information on the client as a whole.

A. *Race, sex, apparent age* in relation to stated age.

B. *Nutritional status*—well hydrated and developed or obesity, cachexia—include weight.

C. *Apparent health status*—general good health or mild, moderate, severe debilitation.

D. *Posture and motor activity*—erect, symmetric, and balanced gait and muscle development or ataxic, circumducted, scissor, or spastic gait; slumped or bent-over posture; mild, moderate, or hyperactive motor responses.

E. *Behavior*—alert; oriented to person, time, place; hears and comprehends instructions, or tense, anxious, angry; uses abusive language; slightly or largely unresponsive; delusions, hallucinations.

F. *Odors*—noncontributory, or acetone, alcohol, fetid breath, incontinent of urine or feces.

III. Health assessment of the older adult

A. *Skin:*

1. Decrease in elasticity → wrinkles and lines, dryness.
2. Loss of fullness → sagging.
3. Wasting appearance due to generalized loss of adipose and muscle tissue.
4. Decrease of adipose tissue on extremities, redistributed to hips and abdomen in middle age.
5. Bony prominences become visible.
6. Excessive pigmentation → age spots.
7. Dry skin and deterioration of nerve fibers and sensory endings → pruritus.
8. Pallor and blotchiness because of decreased blood flow.
9. Overgrowth of epidermal tissue leads to lesions (some benign, some premalignant, some malignant).

B. *Nails:*

1. Dry, brittle.
2. Increased susceptibility to fungal infections.
3. Decreased growth rate.
4. Toe nails thick, difficult to cut.

C. *Hair:*

1. Loss of pigment → graying, white.
2. Decreased density of hair follicles → thinning of hair.
3. Baldness due to decreased blood flow to skin and decreased estrogen production.
   a. Hair distribution thin on scalp, axilla, pubic area, upper and lower extremities.
   b. Decreased facial hair in *men.*
4. Increased facial (chin, upper lip) hair in *women* due to decreased estrogen production.

D. *Eyes:*

1. Loss of soluble protein with loss of lens transparency → development of *cataracts.*
2. Decrease in pupil size limits amount of light entering the eye → elderly need more light to see.
3. Decreased pupil reactivity → decrease in rate of light changes to which a person can readily adapt.
4. Diminished night vision due to decreased accommodation to darkness and dim light.
5. Shrunken appearance due to loss of orbital fat.
6. Blink reflex—slowed.
7. Eyelids—loose.
8. Visual acuity—decreased.
9. Peripheral vision—diminished.
10. Visual fields—diminished.
11. Lens accommodation—decreased; requires corrective lenses.
12. *Presbyopia*—lens may lose ability to become convex enough to accommodate to nearby objects; starts at age 40 (*farsightedness*).
13. Color—fades.
14. Conjunctiva—thins, looks yellow.
15. Increased intraocular pressure leads to glaucoma.

E. *Ears:*

1. Changes in cochlea: decrease in average pitch of sound.
2. Hearing loss: greater in left ear than right; greater in higher frequencies than in lower.
3. Tympanic membrane: atrophied, thickened, causing hearing loss.
4. Presbycusis—progressive loss of hearing in old age.

F. *Mouth:*

1. Dental caries.
2. Poor-fitting dentures.
3. Cancer of the mouth—increased risk.
4. Decrease in taste buds → inability to taste sweet/salty foods.
5. Olfactory bulb atrophies → decreased ability to smell.

G. *Cardiovascular:*

1. Blood pressure increased due to lack of elasticity of vessels → increased resistance to blood flow; decreased diameter of arteries.
2. Atherosclerotic plaques → thrombosis.
3. Valves become sclerotic, less pliable → reduced filling and emptying.
4. Diastolic murmurs heard at base of heart.
5. Loss of elasticity, decreased contractility → decreased cardiac output.

6. Pumping action of the heart is reduced due to changes in the coronary arteries → pooling of blood in systemic veins and shortness of breath.
7. Dysrhythmias due to disturbance of the autonomic nervous system.
8. Extremities—pedal pulses weaker due to arteriosclerotic changes; colder extremities, mottled color.

H. *Respiratory:*

1. Efficiency reduced with age.
2. Greater residual air in lungs after expiration.
3. Decreased vital capacity.
4. Decreased capacity to cough because of weaker expiratory muscles.
5. Decreased ciliary activity → stasis of secretions → susceptibility to infections.
6. Dyspnea on exertion (DOE) due to oxygen debt in the muscles.
7. Reduced chest wall compliance.

I. *Breasts:*

1. Atrophy.
2. Cancer risk—increased with age.

J. *Gastrointestinal:*

1. Pernicious anemia due to lack of intrinsic factor.
2. Gastric motility—decreased.
3. Esophageal peristalsis—decreased.
4. Hiatal hernia—increased incidence.
5. Digestive enzymes—gradual decrease of ptyalin (which converts starch), pepsin and trypsin (which digest protein), lipase (fat-splitting enzyme).
6. Absorption—decreased.
7. Constipation due to improper diet.

K. *Endocrine:*

1. Basal metabolism rate lowered → decreased temperature.
2. Cold intolerance.
3. *Females:* decreased ovarian function → increased gonadotropins.
4. Decreased renal sensitivity to ADH → unable to concentrate urine as effectively as younger persons.
5. Decreased clearance of blood glucose after meals → elevated postprandial blood glucose.
6. Risk of diabetes mellitus increased with age.

L. *Urinary:*

1. Renal function—impaired due to poor perfusion.
2. Filtration—impaired due to reduction in number of functioning nephrons.
3. Urgency and frequency: *men*—often due to prostatic hypertrophy; *women*—due to perineal muscle weakness.
4. Nocturia—both men and women.
5. Urinary tract infection—increased incidence.
6. Incontinence—especially with dementia.

M. *Musculoskeletal:*

1. Muscle mass—decreased.
2. Bony prominences—increased.
3. Demineralization of bone.
4. Shortening of trunk due to narrowing of intervertebral space.
5. Posture—normal; some kyphosis.
6. Range of motion—limited.
7. Osteoarthritis—related to extensive physical activities and joint use.
8. Gait—altered.
9. Osteoporosis related to menopause, immobilization, elevated levels of cortisone.
10. Calcium, phosphorous, and vitamin D decreased.

N. *Neurological:*

1. Voluntary, automatic reflexes—slowed.
2. Sleep pattern—changes.
3. Mental acuity—changes.
4. Sensory interpretation and movement—changes.
5. Pain perception—diminished.
6. Dexterity and agility—lessened.
7. Reaction time—slowed.
8. Memory—past more vivid than recent memory.
9. Depression.
10. Alzheimer's disease.

O. *Sexuality:*

1. Women
   a. Estrogen production—decreased with menopause.
   b. Breasts atrophy.
   c. Vaginal secretions—reduced lubricants.
   d. Sexuality—drive continues; sexual activity declines.
2. Men
   a. Testosterone production—decreased.
   b. Testes—decrease in size; decreased sperm count.
   c. Libido and sexual satisfaction—no changes.

IV. Routine laboratory studies—see Appendix G for normal ranges.

A. *Hematology*

1. Complete blood count—detects presence of anemia, infection, allergy, and leukemia.
2. Prothrombin time—increase may indicate need for vitamin K therapy.
3. Serology (VDRL)—determines presence of syphilitic reagin; false positives may indicate collagen dysfunctions.

B. *Urinalysis*

1. Specific gravity—measures ability of kidney to concentrate urine. Fixed specific gravity indicates renal tubular dysfunction.
2. Albumin and pus—indicate renal infection.
3. Sugar and acetone—presence indicates metabolic disorder.

C. *Chest X ray*—detects tuberculosis or other pulmonary dysfunctions, as well as changes in size and/or configuration of heart.

D. *Electrocardiogram (ECG)*—detects rhythm and conduction disturbances, presence of myocardial ischemia or necrosis, and ventricular hypertrophy.

E. *Blood chemistries*—detect deviation in electrolyte balance, presence of tissue damage; and adequacy of glomerular filtration.

Assessment is followed by analysis of data and formulation of a nursing diagnosis. Possible nursing diagnoses for each category of human functioning are given in the following sections.

■ GROWTH AND DEVELOPMENT*

ADULT NURSING

YOUNG ADULTHOOD (20–30 YEARS OF AGE)

I. Stage of development—psychosocial stage: intimacy versus isolation.

II. Physical development

A. At the *height* of bodily vigor.

B. *Maximum* level of strength, muscular development, height, and cardiac and respiratory capacity; also, period of peak sexual capacity for males.

III. Cognitive development

A. Close to *peak* of intelligence, memory, and abstract thought.

B. Maximum ability to solve problems and learn new skills.

IV. Socialization

A. Has a vision of the future and imagines various possibilities for self.

B. Defines and tests out what can be accomplished.

C. Seeks out a mentor to emulate as a guiding, though transitional, figure; the mentor is usually a mixture of parent, teacher, and friend who serves as a role model to support and facilitate the developing vision of self.

D. Grows from a beginning to a fuller understanding of own authority and autonomy.

E. Transfers an interest into an occupation or profession; crucial work choice may be made after one has knowledge, judgment, and self-understanding, usually at the end of young adulthood; when the choice is deferred beyond these years, valuable time is lost.

F. Experiments with and chooses a life-style.

G. Forms mature peer relationships with the opposite sex.

H. Overcomes guilt and anxiety about the opposite sex and learns to understand the masculine and feminine aspects of self as well as the adult concept of roles.

I. Learns to take the opposite sex seriously and may choose someone for a long-term relationship.

J. Accepts the responsibilities and pleasures of parenthood.

*From Saxton et al.: *Addison–Wesley Manual of Nursing Practice* (Menlo Park, CA: Addison–Wesley Publishing Co., 1983), with permission.

ADULTHOOD (31–45 YEARS OF AGE)

I. Stage of development—psychosocial stage: generativity versus self-absorption.

II. Physical development

A. Gradual decline in biologic functioning, although in the late 30s the individual is still near peak.

B. Period of peak sexual capacity for females occurs during the mid-30s.

C. Distinct sense of bodily decline occurs around 40 years of age.

D. *Circulatory* system begins to slow somewhat after 40 years of age.

III. Cognitive development

A. Takes longer to memorize.

B. Still at peak in abstract thinking and problem solving.

C. Generates new levels of awareness.

D. Gives more meaning to complex tasks.

IV. Socialization

A. Achieves a realistic self-identity.

B. Perceptions are based on reality.

C. Acts on decisions and assumes responsibility for actions.

D. Accepts limitations while developing assets.

E. Delays immediate gratification in favor of future satisfaction.

F. Evaluates mistakes, determines reasons and causes, and learns new behavior.

G. Struggles to establish a place in society.

1. Begins to settle down.
2. Pursues long-range plans and goals.
3. Has a stronger need to be responsible.
4. Invests self as fully as possible in social structure, including work, family, and community.

H. Seeks advancement by improving and using skills, becoming more creative, and pursuing ambitions.

MIDDLE LIFE (46–64 YEARS OF AGE)

I. Stage of development—psychosocial stage: continuation of generativity versus self-absorption.

II. Physical development

A. Failing *eyesight,* especially for close vision, may be one of the first symptoms of aging.

B. Hearing loss is very gradual, especially for low sounds; hearing for high-pitched sounds is impaired more readily.

C. There is a gradual loss of *taste* buds in the 50s and gradual loss of sense of *smell* in the 60s, causing the individual to have a diminished sense of taste.

D. *Muscle strength* declines because of decreased levels of estrogen and testosterone; it takes more time to accomplish the same physical task.

- **E.** *Lung* capacity is impaired, which adds to decreased endurance.
- **F.** The *skin* begins to wrinkle, and hair begins graying.
- **G.** *Postural changes* take place because of loss of calcium and reduced activity.

III. Cognitive development

- **A.** *Memory* begins to decline slowly around the age of 50 years.
- **B.** It takes longer to *learn* new tasks, and old tasks take longer to perform.
- **C.** *Practical judgment* is increased due to experiential background.
- **D.** May tend to withdraw from mental activity or overcompensate by trying the impossible.

IV. Socialization

- **A.** The middle years can be very rewarding if previous stages have been fulfilled.
- **B.** The years of responsibility for raising children are over.
- **C.** Husbands and wives usually find a closer bond.
- **D.** There is less financial strain for those with steady employment.
- **E.** Individuals are usually at the height of their careers; the majority of leaders in their field are in this age group.
- **F.** Self-realization is achieved.
  1. There is more inner direction.
  2. There is no longer a need to please everyone.
  3. Individual is less likely to compare self with others.
  4. Individual approves of self without being dependent on standards of others.
  5. There is less fear of failure in life because past failures have been met and dealt with.

EARLY LATE YEARS (65–79 YEARS OF AGE)

I. Stage of development—psychosocial stage: ego integrity and acceptance versus despair and disgust.

II. Physical development

- **A.** Continues to decrease in vigor and capacity.
- **B.** Has more frequent aches and pains.
- **C.** Likely to have at least one major illness.

III. Cognitive development

- **A.** Mental acuity continues to slow down.
- **B.** Judgment and problem solving remain intact, but the processes may take longer.
- **C.** May have problems in remembering *names* and *dates*.

IV. Socialization

- **A.** Individual is faced with the reality of the experience of physical decline.
- **B.** Physical and mental changes intensify the feelings of aging and mortality.
- **C.** Increasing frequency of death and serious illness among friends, relatives, and associates reinforces further the concept of mortality.
- **D.** Constant reception of medical warnings to follow certain precautions or run serious risks adds to general feeling of decline.
- **E.** Individual is less interested in obtaining the rewards of society and is more interested in utilizing own inner resources.
- **F.** Individuals feel that they have earned the right to do what is important for self-satisfaction.
- **G.** Retirement allows time for expression of own creative energies.
- **H.** Overcomes the splitting of youth and age; gets along well with adolescents.
- **I.** Learns to deal with the reality that only old age remains.
- **J.** Provides moral support to grandchildren; more tolerant of grandchildren than was of own children.
- **K.** Tends to release major authority of family to children while holding self in the role of consultant.

LATER YEARS (80 YEARS OF AGE AND OLDER)

I. Stage of development—psychosocial stage: continuation of ego integrity and acceptance versus despair and disgust.

II. Physical development

- **A.** Additional sensory problems occur, including diminished sensation to *touch and pain.*
- **B.** Increase in loss of muscle tone occurs, including *sphincter* (urinary and anal) control.
- **C.** Individual is insecure and unsure about orientation to *space* and sense of *balance,* which may result in falls and injury.

III. Cognitive development

- **A.** Has better memory for the *past* than the present.
- **B.** *Repetition* of memories occurs.
- **C.** Individual may use *confabulation* to fill in memory gaps.
- **D.** Forgetfulness may lead to serious *safety* problems, and individual may require constant supervision.
- **E.** Increased arteriosclerosis may lead to mental illness (organic brain syndrome).

IV. Socialization

- **A.** Few significant relationships are maintained; death of friends, family, and associates causes isolation.
- **B.** Individual may be preoccupied with immediate bodily needs and personal comforts; the *gastrointestinal tract* frequently becomes the major focus.
- **C.** Individuals see they can provide others with an example of wisdom and courage.
- **D.** Individuals come to terms with themselves.
- **E.** Individuals are concerned with own immortality.
- **F.** Individuals come to terms with the process of dying and prepare for own death.

■ **TABLE 4.1** **Imbalances in Blood Pressure: Comparative Assessment of Hypotension and Hypertension**

	Hypotension	Hypertension
	Common Causes	**Common Causes**
	■ Angina pectoris.	■ Essential hypertension.
	■ Myocardial infarction.	■ Iron deficiency anemia.
	■ Acute and chronic pericarditis.	■ Pernicious anemia.
	■ Valvular defects.	■ Arteriosclerosis obliterans.
	■ Congestive heart failure.	■ Polycythemia vera.
Assessment		
Behavior	Anxiety, apprehension, decreasing mentation, confusion	Nervousness, mood swings, irritability, difficulty with memory, depression, confusion.
Neurologic	Essentially noncontributory.	Decreased vibratory sensations, increased/decreased reflexes, Babinski reflex, changes in coordination.
Head/neck	Distended neck veins, worried expression.	Bruits over carotids, distended neck veins, epistaxis, diplopia, ringing in ears, dull occipital headaches on arising.
Skin	Pale, cool, moist.	Dry, pale, glossy, flakey, cold; decreased or absent hair
GI	Anorexia, nausea, vomiting, constipation.	Anorexia, flatulence, diarrhea, constipation.
Respiratory	Dyspnea, orthopnea, paroxysmal nocturnal dyspnea, tachypnea, moist rales, cough.	Dyspnea, orthopnea, moist rales.
Cardiovascular	Tires easily.	Decreased exercise tolerance, weakness, palpitations.
	Blood pressure—decreased systolic, decreased systolic/diastolic.	Blood pressure—increased systolic, increased systolic and diastolic.
	Pulse—increased/decreased, weak, thready, irregular, arrhythmias.	Decreased or absent pedal pulses.
Renal	Oliguria.	Oliguria, nocturia, proteinuria.
Extremities	Dependent edema.	Tingling, numbness, or cold hands and feet, dependent edema, ulcers of legs or feet.

ADULT NURSING

■ FLUID-GAS TRANSPORT

CONDITIONS AFFECTING FLUID TRANSPORT

I. Hypertension: sustained, elevated, systemic, arterial blood pressure; diastolic elevation more serious, reflecting pressure on arterial wall during resting phase of cardiac cycle (see Table 4.1).

A. Pathophysiology: increased peripheral resistance leading to thickened arteriole walls and left ventricular hypertrophy.

B. Risk factors

1. Black race (2:1).
2. Use of birth control pills.
3. Overweight.
4. Smoking.
5. Stress.
6. Excessive sodium intake.
7. Lack of activity.

C. Classifications

1. *Primary* (essential): occurs in 90% of clients; etiology unknown; diastolic pressure is 90 mm Hg or higher and other causes of hypertension are absent. Benign hypertension (diastolic pressure up to 120 mm Hg) considered controllable; malignant hypertension (diastolic greater than 140–150 mm Hg) uncontrollable.
2. *Secondary:* occurs in remaining 10%; usually renal, endocrine, neurogenic, and/or cardiac in origin.
3. Labile (prehypertensive): a fluctuating blood pressure; increases during stress, otherwise normal or near normal.

D. Assessment:

1. Subjective data
   a. Early morning headache, usually occipital.
   b. Light-headedness, tinnitus.
   c. Palpitations.
   d. Fatigue, insomnia.
   e. Forgetfulness, irritability.
   f. Altered vision: white spots, blurring, or loss.

2. Objective data
   a. Epistaxis (nosebleeds).
   b. Elevated blood pressure: systolic >140 mm Hg, diastolic >90 mm Hg; narrowed pulse pressure.
   c. Retinal changes; papilledema.
   d. Shortness of breath on slight exertion.
   e. Cardiac, cerebral, and renal changes.

E. Analysis/nursing diagnosis:

1. *Altered peripheral tissue perfusion* related to increased peripheral resistance.
2. *Decreased cardiac output* related to ventricular hypertrophy.
3. *Potential for injury* related to altered vision.
4. *Potential activity intolerance* related to inadequate oxygenation.
5. *Fatigue* related to poor perfusion.

F. Nursing plan/implementation:

1. Goal: *provide for physical and emotional rest.*
   a. Rest periods before/after eating, visiting hours; avoid upsetting situations.
   b. Give tranquilizers, sedatives, as ordered.
2. Goal: *provide for special safety needs.*
   a. Monitor blood pressure: both arms; standing, sitting, lying positions.
   b. Limit/prevent activities that increase pressure (anxiety, anger, frustration, upsetting visitors, fatigue).
   c. Assist with ambulation; change position gradually to prevent dizziness and light-headedness (postural hypotension).
   d. Monitor for electrolyte imbalance when on low-sodium diet, diuretic therapy; I&O to prevent fluid depletion and arrhythmias from potassium loss.
   e. Observe for signs of hemorrhage, shock, and stroke, which may occur following surgery.
3. Goal: *health teaching* (client and family).
   a. Procedures to decrease anxiety; relaxation techniques, stress management.
   b. Side effects of hypotensive drugs: diuretics; adrenergic blockers; vasodilators, calcium channel blockers (faintness, nausea, vomiting, postural hypotension, sexual dysfunction). See Unit 6 for specific pharmacologic actions.
   c. Weight control to reduce arterial pressure.
   d. Restrictions: stimulants (tea, coffee, tobacco); sodium, calories, fat.
   e. Life-style adjustments: daily exercise needed; reduce occupational and environmental stress; importance of rest.
   f. Blood pressure measurement: daily, same conditions, position preference of physician.
   g. Signs, symptoms, complications of disease (headache, confusion, visual changes, nausea/vomiting, convulsions).
   h. Causes of intermittent hypotension: alcohol, hot weather, exercise, febrile illness, hot bath.

G. Evaluation:

1. Blood pressure within normal range for age (diastolic <90 mm Hg)—stable.
2. Minimal or no pathophysiologic or therapeutic complications (e.g., visual changes, CVA, drug side effects).
3. Reduces weight to reasonable level for height, bone structure.
4. Takes prescribed medications regularly, even when symptoms have resolved.
5. Complies with restrictions: no smoking, restricted sodium, fat.
6. Exercises regularly—program compatible with personal and health care goals.

II. Cardiac arrhythmias: any variation in normal rate, rhythm, or configuration of waves on electrocardiograph (see Figure 4.1).

A. Pathophysiology

1. Dysfunction of SA node, atria, AV node, or ventricular conduction.
2. Primary heart problem or secondary systemic problem.

B. Risk factors

1. Myocardial infarction.
2. Drug toxicity.
3. Stress.
4. Cardiac surgery.
5. Hypoxia.
6. See also Table 4.2.

C. Assessment: see Table 4.2 for specific arrhythmias.

D. Analysis/nursing diagnosis:

1. *Decreased cardiac output* related to abnormal ventricular function.
2. *Altered tissue perfusion* related to inadequate cardiac functioning.
3. *Potential for injury* (death) related to improper cardiac function.
4. *Potential activity intolerance* related to inadequate oxygenation.
5. *Anxiety* related to dependence, fear of death.

E. Nursing plan/implementation:

1. Goal: *provide for emotional and safety needs.*
   a. Document ECG tracing for presence of arrhythmia.
   b. Encourage discussion of fears, feelings.
   c. Bedrest; restricted activities; quiet environment; limit visitors.
   d. Oxygen, if ordered.
   e. Check vital signs frequently for shock, CHF, drug toxicity.
   f. Prepare for cardiac emergency: CPR.
   g. Give cardiac medications; check lab tests for digitalis and potassium levels, to prevent drug toxicity.
2. Goal: *prevent thromboemboli.*
   a. Apply antiembolic stockings (TED hose).
   b. Give anticoagulants as ordered. (Check for bleeding—gums, urine; monitor lab tests—Lee White clotting time and partial thromboplastin time with heparin; prothrombin time with coumarin.)
   c. Encourage flexion-extension of feet.

(a) Cardiac Cycle

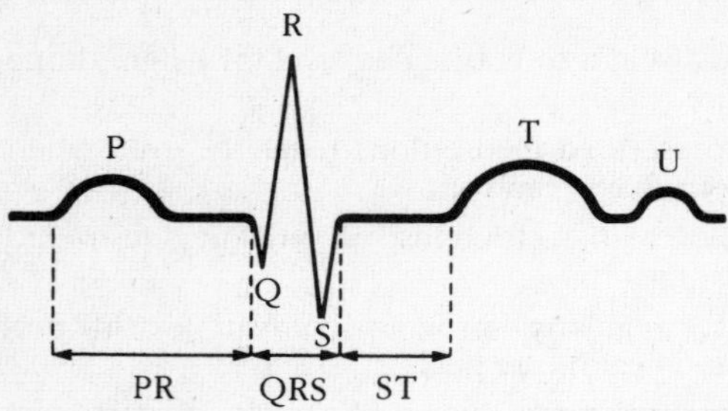

Components	Definition
1. P wave	Atrial depolarization
2. QRS wave	Ventricular depolarization
3. T wave	Ventricular repolarization
4. PR interval (normal range: 0.12–0.20 seconds)	Start of atrial depolarization to start of ventricular depolarization
5. QRS interval (normal range: 0.06–0.10 seconds)	Start to end of ventricular depolarization
6. QT interval	Duration of ventricular depolarization and repolarization
7. ST segment	Interval between the end of ventricular depolarization and the T wave

(b) Normal Sinus Rhythm

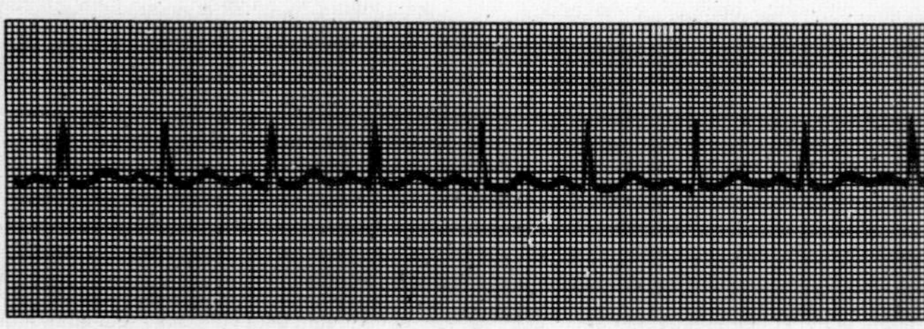

Description	
Regularity and rate	
Ventricular	Regular 60–100
Atrial	Same as ventricular
P waves	Rounded, symmetrical
P:QRS ratio	1:1
PR interval	0.12–0.20 seconds
QRS interval	0.06–0.10 seconds

FIGURE 4.1
Normal cardiac configuration. (From Holloway N: *Nursing the Critically Ill Adult,* 3rd ed., pp. 270, 277, Addison-Wesley, Menlo Park, CA, 1988.)

3. Goal: *provide for physical and emotional needs with pacemaker insertion.*
   a. *General concerns*
      (1) Report excessive bleeding/infection at insertion site—hematoma may contribute to wound infection.
      (2) Encourage verbalization of feelings.
      (3) Report prolonged hiccoughs, which may indicate pacemaker failure.
      (4) Know pacing mode: fixed-rate or demand (most common).
   b. *Temporary pacemaker*
      (1) Limit excessive activity of extremity if antecubital insertion, to prevent displacement; subclavian insertion increases catheter stability.
      (2) Secure wires to chest to prevent tension on catheter.
      (3) Do *not* defibrillate over insertion site, to avoid electrical hazards.
      (4) Electrical safety (grounding; disconnect electric beds/call lights; use battery-operated equipment).
   c. *Permanent pacemaker*
      (1) Limit activity of shoulder for 48–72 h with transvenous catheter to prevent dislodgement.
      (2) Postinsertion ROM (passive) at least once per shift after 48 h to prevent frozen shoulder.
   d. *Health teaching* following permanent pacemaker
      (1) Explain procedure: duration, equipment, purpose, type of pacemaker.
      (2) MedicAlert bracelet; pacemaker information card.
      (3) Daily pulse-taking upon arising (report variation of ± 5 beats).
      (4) Signs, symptoms of: malfunction (vertigo, syncope, dyspnea, slowed speech, confusion, fluid retention); infection (fever, heat, pain, skin breakdown at insertion site).
      (5) Restrictions: contact sports; electromagnetic interferences (few)—TV/radio transmitters, improperly functioning microwave ovens, certain cautery machines; may trigger airport metal-detector alarm.

F. Evaluation:

1. Regular cardiac rhythm; monitors own radial pulse.
2. No complications (e.g., pacemaker malfunction).
3. Returns for regular follow-up of pacemaker function.
4. Tolerates physical or sexual activity.
5. Wears identification bracelet; carries pacemaker identification card.

III. Cardiac arrest: sudden unexpected cessation of heartbeat and effective circulation leading to inadequate perfusion and sudden death.

■ **TABLE 4.2** **Comparison of Cardiac Arrhythmias**

Arrhythmia	Description	Causes	Significance	Treatment
Sinus tachycardia	P waves present, followed by QRS. Rhythm regular. Heart rate 100 to 180.	Normal heart. Tea, coffee, tobacco. Stress. Coronary heart disease.	Usually not significant, except in heart disease.	If asymptomatic, none; if symptomatic, treat underlying cause. Occasionally sedatives.
Sinus bradycardia	P waves present. Rhythm regular. Heart rate less than 60.	Decreased oxygen delivery; shock, hemorrhage, anemia. Physical fitness. Parasympathetic stimulation (sleep).	Prolonged episodes may lead to decreased cardiac output. Depends on rate. Very low rates may cause decreased cardiac output; light-headedness, faintness, chest pain.	None if asymptomatic; atropine if cardiac output is decreased. Isoproterenol. Pacemaker.
First degree AV block	P wave followed by normal QRS. Regular rhythm. PR interval constant but greater than 0.20 sec.	Normal heart. Vagal stimulation. Increased ICP. MI.		Usually none necessary. Possibly atropine.
Second degree AV block (Mobitz I) Wenckebach	Atrial rate faster than ventricular; ventricular rhythm irregular, but consistent pattern. Interval lengthens until one P wave not conducted; cycle repeats.	Normal heart. Coronary artery disease. Digitalis toxicity. Cardiac surgery.	Relatively benign; may progress to second- or third-degree block.	Usually none necessary. If symptomatic, atropine. Discontinue digitalis.
Second degree AV block (Mobitz II)	One P wave and one QRS, except for nonconducted P wave. Irregular ventricular rhythm with no consistent pattern.	Increased parasympathetic tone. Digitalis toxicity. Inferior wall MI.	Relatively benign; cardiac output unchanged. Usually transient.	Atropine. Isuprel. Prophylactic artificial pacemaker.
Complete heart block	Atria and ventricles beat independently. P waves have no relation to QRS. Heart rate 20 to 40.	Necrosis or fibrosis of conduction pathway. Anterior wall MI.	Often precedes sudden complete heart block.	Pacemaker. Isoproterenol to increase heart rate. Atropine.
Premature atrial beats (PAB)	Early P wave followed by normal QRS. Rhythm irregular.	Digitalis toxicity. Infectious disease. Coronary artery disease. Myocardial infarction.	Very low rates may cause decreased cardiac output; light-headedness, faintness, chest pain.	Sedation. Propranolol.
Premature ventricular beats	Early wide bizarre QRS, not associated with a P wave. Rhythm irregular.	Stress, ischemia, atrial enlargement, caffeine, nicotine.	May produce palpitations. May precede atrial tachycardia, flutter, or fibrillation.	Lidocaine. Procainamide (Pronestyl). Oxygen. Sodium bicarbonate. Potassium. Treat CHF.
Atrial flutter	More than one P wave to QRS complex; usually constant 2:1, 4:1 ratio; atrial rate 200–350/min.	Stress, acidosis. Electrolyte imbalance. Drug toxicity (digitalis). Hypoxemia, hypercapnia.	Same as for PAB.	Cardioversion. Verapamil. Digitalis. Propranolol. Quinidine.

continued

TABLE 4.2 *(Continued)* **Comparison of Cardiac Arrhythmias**

Arrhythmia	Description	Causes	Significance	Treatment
Atrial fibrillation	Rapid, irregular waves (atrial rate over 350/min). Ventricular rhythm irregularly irregular. Heart rate varies, may be increased to 160–180/min.	Coronary artery disease. Valvular disease. Cor pulmonale.	Carotid massage ineffective.	Digitalis. Quinidine. Cardioversion. Verapamil. Propranolol.
Ventricular tachycardia	Generally no P wave. Regular QRS pattern; wide configuration. Nonresponsive to vagal stimulation. Heart rate 130–150/min.	Rheumatic heart disease. Mitral stenosis. Atrial infarction.	Pulse deficit. Decreased cardiac output if rate is rapid. Promotes thrombus formation in atria.	If pulseless, treat as ventricular fibrillation. With pulse, lidocaine, procainamide, bretylium, cardioversion.
Ventricular fibrillation	Chaotic electrical activity. No recognizable QRS complex.	Acute MI, especially anteroseptal. Coronary artery disease.	Very low or no BP; generally absent central pulses. May progress to ventricular fibrillation, shock, cardiac failure.	Defibrillation. Lidocaine. Epinephrine. Bretylium. Sodium bicarbonate. CPR.
Ventricular asystole	Can only be distinguished from ventricular fibrillation by ECG. P waves *may* be present. No QRS. "Straight line."	Myocardial infarction. Electrocution. Freshwater drowning. Drug toxicity. Myocardial infarction. Chronic diseases of conducting system.	No cardiac output. Absent pulse or respiration. Cardiac arrest. Same as for ventricular fibrillation.	CPR. Pacemaker. Intracardiac epinephrine. Calcium chloride.

Source: Brown FR: Problems of the Heart and Major Blood Vessels, in *Medical/Surgical Nursing,* Phipps, Long, and Woods, eds. St. Louis: Mosby, 1987.

A. Risk factors:
1. Myocardial infarction.
2. Multiple traumas.
3. Respiratory arrest.
4. Drowning.
5. Electric shock.
6. Drug reactions.

B. Assessment—objective data:
1. Unresponsive to stimuli (i.e., verbal, painful).
2. Absence of: breathing, carotid pulse.
3. Pale or bluish: lips, fingernails, skin.
4. Pupils: dilated.

C. Analysis/nursing diagnosis:
1. *Decreased cardiac output* related to heart failure.
2. *Impaired gas exchange* related to breathlessness.
3. *Altered tissue perfusion* related to pulselessness.

D. Nursing plan/implementation:
1. Goal: *prevent irreversible cerebral anoxic damage:* initiate CPR within 4–6 min; continue until relieved; document assessment factors, effectiveness of actions; presence or absence of pulse at 1 min and every 4–5 min.
2. Goal: *establish effective circulation, respiration:* see Emergency Nursing Procedures, p. 444, for complete protocols.

E. Evaluation:
1. Carotid pulse present; check after 1 minute and every few minutes thereafter.
2. Responds to verbal stimuli.
3. Pupils constrict in response to light.
4. Return of spontaneous respiration; adequate ventilation.

IV. Arteriosclerosis: loss of elasticity, thickening, hardening of arterial walls; common type—atherosclerosis. Arteriosclerosis precedes angina pectoris and myocardial infarction.

A. Pathophysiology:
1. Atherosclerotic plaque, discrete lumpy thickening of arterial wall.
2. Narrows lumen, can occlude vessel.

B. Risk factors:
1. Increased serum cholesterol (low-density lipids).
2. Hypertension.
3. Cigarette smoking.
4. Diabetes mellitus.

(See V. Angina pectoris and VI. Myocardial infarction for nursing implications.)

V. Angina pectoris: transient paroxysmal episodes of substernal or precordial pain.

A. Pathophysiology:

1. Insufficient blood flow through coronary arteries.
2. Temporary myocardial ischemia.

B. Risk factors:

1. Cardiovascular:
   a. Atherosclerosis.
   b. Thromboangiitis obliterans.
   c. Aortic regurgitation.
   d. Hypertension.
2. Hormonal:
   a. Hyperthyroidism.
   b. Diabetes mellitus.
3. Blood disorders:
   a. Anemia.
   b. Polycythemia vera.

C. Assessment:

1. Subjective data:
   a. Pain (see Table 4.3).
      (1) *Type:* squeezing, pressing, burning.
      (2) *Location:* retrosternal, substernal, left of sternum, radiates to left arm.
      (3) *Duration:* short, usually 3–5 minutes, <30 min.
      (4) *Cause:* emotional stress, overeating, physical exertion, exposure to cold.
      (5) *Relief:* rest, nitroglycerin.
   b. Dyspnea.
   c. Palpitations.
   d. Dizziness; faintness.
   e. Epigastric distress; indigestion; belching.
2. Objective data:
   a. Tachycardia.
   b. Pallor.
   c. Diaphoresis.

D. Analysis/nursing diagnosis:

1. *Altered cardiopulmonary tissue perfusion,* related to insufficient blood flow.
2. *Pain* related to myocardial ischemia.
3. *Activity intolerance* related to onset of pain.

E. Nursing plan/implementation:

1. Goal: *provide relief from pain.*
   a. Rest until pain subsides.
   b. Nitroglycerin or amyl nitrite, as ordered.
   c. Identify precipitating factors: large meals, heavy exercise, stimulants (coffee, smoking), sex when fatigued, cold air.
   d. Vital signs; hypotension.
   e. Assist with ambulation; dizziness, flushing occur with nitroglycerin.
2. Goal: *provide emotional support.*
   a. Encourage verbalization of feelings, fears.
   b. Reassurance; positive self-concept.
   c. Acceptance of limitations.
3. Goal: *health teaching.*
   a. Pain: alleviation, differentiation of angina from myocardial infarction, precipitating factors (see Table 4.3).
   b. Medication: frequency, expected effects (headache, flushing); carry fresh nitroglycerin; loses potency after 6 months ("stings" under tongue when potent); may use nitroglycerin paste—instruct how to apply.
   c. Diet: restricted calories if weight loss indicated; restricted fat, cholesterol, gas-producing foods; small, frequent meals.
   ▶ d. Diagnostic tests if ordered (e.g., cardiac catheterization; see Unit 7).
   e. Exercise: regular, graded, to promote coronary circulation.
   f. Prepare for coronary bypass surgery, if necessary.
   g. Behavior modification to assist with life-style changes, i.e., stress-reduction, stop smoking.

F. Evaluation:

1. Relief from pain.
2. Fewer attacks.
3. No myocardial infarction.
4. Alters life-style; complies with limitations.
5. No smoking.

VI. Myocardial infarction (MI): localized area of necrotic tissue in myocardium from cessation of blood flow; leading cause of death in North America.

A. Pathophysiology:

1. Coronary occlusion due to thrombosis, embolism, or hemorrhage adjacent to atherosclerotic plaque.
2. Insufficient blood flow from cardiac hypertrophy, hemorrhage, shock, or severe dehydration.

B. Risk factors:

1. Age (35–70 yr).
2. Men more than women until menopause.
3. Life-style.
4. Stress.
5. High-cholesterol diet (specifically low-density lipoproteins).
6. Chronic illness (diabetes, hypertension).

C. Assessment:

1. Subjective data
   a. Pain (see Table 4.3).
      (1) *Type:* sudden, severe, crushing, heavy tightness.
      (2) *Location:* substernal; radiates to one or both arms, jaw, neck.
      (3) *Duration:* >30 minutes.
      (4) *Cause:* unrelated to exercise; frequently occurs when sleeping (REM stage).
      (5) *Relief:* oxygen, narcotics; *not* relieved by rest or nitroglycerin.

ADULT NURSING

TABLE 4.3 Comparison of Different Physical Causes of Chest Pain

Subjective Characteristics	Angina	Myocardial Infarction	Pericarditis
Onset	Gradual or sudden.	Sudden.	Sudden.
Precipitating factors	May be nothing specific; can occur at rest or after physical exertion, emotional stress, eating, exposure to cold or hot, humid weather, or during micturition or defecation.	May be nothing specific; can occur at rest or after physical exertion or emotional stress.	Not induced by activity but related to respiratory movement; increases with coughing.
Location	Substernal, anterior chest (not sharply localized).	Substernal, anterior chest, or midline.	Substernal (to left of midline) or precordial only.
Radiation	To back, neck, arms, or jaw; occasionally to upper abdomen or fingers.	Down one or both arms; to jaw, neck, or back.	To back or left supraclavicular area.
Quality	Deep, squeezing, or tight sensation; feeling of heavy pressure.	Deep, burning, stabbing, choking, squeezing, or viselike sensation; feeling of heavy pressure.	Sharp, stabbing, deep or superficial sensation.
Intensity	Mild to moderate; tends to build in intensity (crescendo pattern).	Asymptomatic to severe.	Moderate to severe pain or only an ache.
Duration	Usually less than 15 minutes (rarely more than 30 minutes); average duration is about 3 minutes.	Often 30 minutes, but usually 1 to 2 hours; residual soreness lasts 1 to 3 days.	Continual (may last for days); residual soreness.
Relieving factors	Rest, nitroglycerin.	Rest (but only temporarily); narcotics.	Shallow breathing, sitting up, leaning forward.
Aggravating factors	Physical or emotional stress, cold weather.	Physical or emotional stress.	Lying down, leaning forward, muscle movement, inspiration, laughter, coughing, or left lateral position.
Associated symptoms	Indigestion, dizziness, urge to void, belching.	Dizziness, nausea, fatigue.	Air hunger, tachypnea, dizziness, restlessness.
Emotional response	Anxiety, fear.	Anxiety, fear, feeling of impending doom.	Anxiety, fear.

Source: Smith, Carol. (1988). Assessing Chest Pain. *Nursing 88, 18*(5): 56–57.

b. Nausea.

c. Shortness of breath.

d. Apprehension, fear of impending death.

e. History of cardiac disease (family); occupational stress.

2. Objective data

a. Vital signs: shock; rapid (>100), thready pulse; fall in blood pressure; tachypnea, shallow respirations; elevated temperature within 24 h (100°–103°F).

b. Skin: cyanotic, ashen or clammy; diaphoretic.

c. Emotional: restless.

d. Lab data: *increased*—WBC (12,000–15,000/mm³), serum enzymes (CPK-MB, LDH, >LDH_2 "flipped LDH"); *changes*—ECG (elevated ST segment, inverted T wave, arrhythmia).

D. Analysis/nursing diagnosis:

1. *Decreased cardiac output* related to myocardial damage.
2. *Impaired gas exchange* related to poor perfusion, shock.
3. *Pain* related to myocardial ischemia.
4. *Activity intolerance* related to pain or inadequate oxygenation.
5. *Fear* related to possibility of death.

E. Nursing plan/implementation:

1. Goal: *reduce pain, discomfort.*

a. Narcotics—morphine, meperidine (Demerol) HCl; note response.

b. Humidified oxygen; mouth care—oxygen is drying.

c. *Position:* semi-Fowler's to improve ventilation.

■ **TABLE 4.3 *(Continued)***

Pleuropulmonary Disorders	Gastric Disorders
Gradual or sudden.	Gradual or sudden.
Pneumonia or other respiratory infection.	Esophagitis and gastritis often occur after eating or taking medication or when person leans over.
Over lung fields to side and back; substernal or retrosternal.	Epigastric, slightly to left of midline.
To anterior chest, shoulder, or neck; none with some disorders.	Under sternum or to back of neck, left shoulder, or lower thoracic spine.
Sharp, burning, stabbing, shooting, deep, crushing, or tearing sensation.	Gnawing, burning , or aching (sharp or dull) sensation; feeling of bloating or pressure.
Sharp ache (mild to severe).	Mild to severe.
Intermittent (may last for hours, days, or weeks).	Varies (may be intermittent or continous, lasting seconds, minutes, or hours).
Warm, moist air; rest; splinting; heat; sitting up.	Food, antacid, standing upright, belching.
Cold air or dry environment, high altitude, hypoxia, carbon monoxide, coughing, exertion, immobility.	Emotional stress; caffeine, protein, and some spices; constipation; heavy meal (or lying down after meal); carbonated beverage; cold liquids; exercise; aspirin; smoking.
Air hunger, dyspnea, restlessness, splinting.	Nausea, vomiting, dysphagia. restlessness, diaphoresis, foul breath, bad taste in mouth.
Anxiety, anger (over shortness of breath).	Anxiety, withdrawal.

2. Goal: *maintain adequate circulation.*
   a. Monitor vital signs and urine output; observe for cardiogenic shock.
   b. Monitor ECG for arrhythmias.
   c. Give medications as ordered: *antiarrhythmics*—lidocaine HCl, quinidine HCl, procainamide (Pronestyl), bretylium (Bretylol); propranalol (Inderal); verapamil; *anticoagulants*—heparin sodium, bishydroxycoumarin or dicoumarin; *fibrinolytic agents*—streptokinase, TPA.
   d. Recognize heart failure: edema, cyanosis, dyspnea, cough, rales.
   e. Check lab data—normal: serum enzymes (CPK 0–7 IU/L; LDH <115 IU/L; LDH, $<LDH_2$); blood gases (pH 7.35–7.45; CO_2 35–45; Po_2 80–100; HCO_3 22–26); electrolytes (K^+ 3.5–5.0 mEq/L); clotting time (APTT 30–40 sec; PT 11–15 sec).
   f. CVP—zero level at right atrium; fluctuates with respiration; normal range 5–15 cm H_2O; note trend; increases with heart failure.
   g. ROM of lower extremities; TED hose/antiembolic stockings.
3. Goal: *decrease oxygen demand/promote oxygenation.*
   a. O_2 as ordered.
   b. Activity: bedrest (24–48 h); planned rest periods; control visitors.
   c. Position: semi-Fowler's to facilitate lung expansion and decrease venous return.
   d. Anticipate needs of client: call light, water.
   e. Assist with feeding, turning.
   f. Environment: quiet, comfortable.
   g. Reassurance; stay with anxious client.
   h. Give medications as ordered: cardiotonics, calcium channel blockers, vasodilators, vasopressors.
4. Goal: *maintain fluid, electrolyte, nutritional status.*
   a. IV (keep vein open); CVP; vital signs; urine output—30 mL/h.
   b. Lab data within normal limits (Na^+ 135–145 mEq/L; K^+ 3.5–5.0 mEq/L).
   c. Monitor ECG—*hyperkalemia:* peaked T wave; *hypokalemia:* depressed T wave.
   d. Diet: progressive low calorie, low sodium, low cholesterol, low fat.
5. Goal: *facilitate fecal elimination.*
   a. Medications: stool softeners to prevent Valsalva (straining); mouth breathing during bowel movement; recognize complications of Valsalva—chest pain, cyanosis, diaphoresis, arrhythmias.
   b. Bedside commode if possible.
6. Goal: *provide emotional support.*
   a. Recognize fear of dying: denial, anger, withdrawal.
   b. Encourage expression of feelings, fears, concerns.
   c. Discuss rehabilitation, life-style changes: prevent cardiac-invalid syndrome by promoting self-care activities, independence.
7. Goal: *promote sexual functioning.*
   a. Encourage discussion of concerns re: activity, inadequacy, limitations, expectations—include partner (usually resume activity 5–8 wk following uncomplicated MI).
   b. Identify need for referral for sexual counseling.
8. Goal: *health teaching.*
   a. Diagnosis and treatment regimen.
   b. *Caution* about when to *avoid* sexual activity: following heavy meal, alcohol ingestion; when fatigued, tense, under stress; with unfamiliar partners; in extreme temperatures.
   c. Information about sexual activity: less fatiguing positions (side to side; noncardiac on top); vasodilators, if ordered, prior to intercourse; select comfortable, familiar environment.

d. Available community resources for information, support groups (e.g., American Heart Association, Stop Smoking Clinics).

e. Medications: administration, importance, untoward effects, pulse-taking.

f. Control risk factors: rest, diet, exercise, no smoking, weight control, stress-reduction techniques.

g. Need for follow-up care for regulation of medications, evaluating risk factors.

h. Prepare for coronary bypass if planned.

F. Evaluation:

1. No complications: stable vital signs; relief of pain.
2. Adheres to prescribed medication regimen, demonstrates knowledge about medications.
3. Activity tolerance is increased, participates in program of progressive activity.
4. Reduction or modification of risk factors. Plans to alter life-style (e.g., loses weight, quits smoking).

VII. Cardiac valvular defects: alteration in the structure of a valve; impedes flow of blood or permits regurgitation.

A. Pathophysiology:

1. *Stenosis*—narrowing of valvular opening due to adherence, thickening, and rigidity of valve cusp.
2. *Insufficiency* (incompetence)—incomplete closure of valve due to contraction of chordae tendinae, papillary muscles, or to calcification, scarring of leaflets.
3. *Mitral stenosis*
   a. Most common residual cardiac lesion of rheumatic fever.
   b. Affects *women* under 45 yr more often than men.
   c. Narrowing of mitral valve.
   d. Interferes with filling of left ventricle.
   e. Produces pulmonary hypertension, right-sided heart failure.
4. *Mitral insufficiency* (incompetence)
   a. Leaking/regurgitation of blood back into left atrium.
   b. Results from rheumatic fever, bacterial endocarditis; less common.
   c. Affects *men* more often.
   d. Produces pulmonary congestion, right-sided heart failure.
5. *Aortic stenosis*
   a. Fusion of valve flaps between left ventricle and aorta.
   b. Congenital or acquired from atherosclerosis or from rheumatic fever and bacterial endocarditis; seen in *men* more often; pulmonary circulation congested, cardiac output decreased.
6. *Aortic insufficiency*
   a. Incomplete closure of valve between left ventricle and aorta (regurgitation).
   b. Left ventricular failure leading to right-sided heart failure.

B. Risk factors:

1. Congenital abnormality.
2. History of rheumatic fever.
3. Atherosclerosis.

C. Assessment: see Table 4.4.

D. Analysis/nursing diagnosis:

1. *Decreased cardiac output* related to inadequate ventricular filling.
2. *Fluid volume excess* related to compensatory response to decreased cardiac output.
3. *Impaired gas exchange* related to pulmonary congestion.
4. *Activity intolerance* related to impaired cardiac function.
5. *Fatigue* related to poor oxygenation.

E. Nursing plan/implementation:

1. Goal: *reduce cardiac workload.*
2. Goal: *promote physical comfort and psychologic support.*
3. Goal: *prevent complications.*
4. Goal: *prepare client for surgery* (commissurotomy, valvuloplasty or valvular replacement, depending on defect and severity of condition).
5. See X. Cardiac surgery for specific nursing actions.

F. Evaluation:

1. Relief of symptoms.
2. Increase in activity level.
3. No complications following surgery.

▶ **VIII. Cardiac catheterization:** a diagnostic procedure to evaluate cardiac status. Introduces a catheter into the heart, blood vessels; analyzes blood samples for oxygen content, cardiac output, pulmonary blood flow; done prior to heart surgery; frequently combined with angiography to visualize coronary arteries; also provides access for specialized cardiac techniques (e.g., internal pacing and coronary angioplasty).

A. Approaches

1. *Right-heart* catheterization—venous approach (antecubital or femoral) → right atrium → right ventricle → pulmonary artery.
2. *Left-heart* catheterization—retrograde approach: right brachial artery or percutaneous puncture of femoral artery → ascending aorta → left ventricle.
   a. Transeptal: femoral vein → right atrium → septum → left atrium → left ventricle.
   ▶ b. Angiography/arteriography: done during left-heart catheterization.

B. Precatheterization

1. **Assessment:**
   a. Subjective data
      (1) Allergies: iodine, seafood.
      (2) Anxiety.
   b. Objective data
      (1) Vital signs: baseline data.
      (2) Distal pulses: mark for reference after catheterization.
2. **Analysis/nursing diagnosis:**
   a. *Anxiety* related to fear of unknown.
   b. *Knowledge deficit* related to difficulty learning or limited exposure to information.

TABLE 4.4 Comparison of Symptomatology for Valvular Defects

Assessment	Mitral Stenosis	Mitral Insufficiency	Aortic Stenosis	Aortic Insufficiency
Subjective Data				
Fatigue	✓	✓	✓	✓
Shortness of breath	✓			
Orthopnea	✓		✓	✓
Paroxysmal nocturnal dyspnea	✓		✓	✓
Cough	✓	✓		
Dyspnea on exertion		✓	✓	✓
Palpitations		✓	✓	
Syncope on exertion			✓	
Angina			✓	✓
Weight loss		✓		
Objective Data				
Vital Signs				
Blood pressure:				
Low or normal	✓	✓		
Normal or elevated			✓	✓
Pulse:				
Weak, irregular	✓	✓		
Rapid, "waterhammer"				✓
Respirations:				
Increased, shallow	✓			
Cyanosis	✓			
Jugular vein distention	✓			
Enlarged liver	✓		✓	
Dependent edema	✓		✓	
Murmur	✓	✓	✓	✓

3. **Nursing plan/implementation:**
   a. Goal: *provide for safety, comfort.*
      (1) Signed informed consent.
      (2) NPO (except for medications 6–8 h before).
      (3) Have client urinate before going to lab.
      (4) Give sedatives, as ordered, 30 min before procedure (e.g., Versed).
   b. Goal: *health teaching.*
      (1) Procedure: length (1–3 h).
      (2) Expectations (strapped to table for safety, must lie still, awake but mildly sedated).
      (3) Sensations (hot, flushed feeling in head with dye injection; thudding in chest from premature beats during catheter manipulation; desire to cough, particularly with right-heart angiography and contrast-medium injection).
      (4) Alert physician to unusual sensations (coolness, numbness, paresthesia).

C. Postcatheterization

1. **Assessment** (potential complications):
   a. Subjective data
      (1) Puncture site: increasing pain, tenderness.
      (2) Palpitations.
      (3) Affected extremity: tingling numbness, pain from hematoma or nerve damage.
   b. Objective data
      (1) Vital signs: shock, respiratory distress (related to pulmonary emboli, allergic reaction).
      (2) Puncture site: bleeding (hematoma).
      ▶ (3) ECG: arrhythmias, signs of MI.
      (4) Affected extremity: color, temperature, peripheral pulses.
2. **Analysis/nursing diagnosis:**
   a. *Decreased cardiac output* related to arrhythmias or MI.

b. *Altered tissue perfusion* related to bleeding following procedure.

c. *Pain* related to puncture site tenderness.

3. **Nursing plan/implementation:**

a. Goal: *prevent complications.*

(1) Bedrest: 3–6 h; with femoral approach, supine position, 12–24 h on bedrest; encourage ankle flexion, extention, and rotation.

(2) Vital signs: record q15min for 1 h, q 30min for 3 h or until stable; check BP on opposite extremity.

(3) Puncture site: observe for bleeding, swelling, inflammation, or tenderness; check pulse distal to insertion site to determine patency of artery; report complaints of coolness, numbness, or paresthesia in extremity.

(4) ECG: monitor, document rhythm.

(5) Give medications as ordered: sedatives; mild narcotics; antiarrhythmics.

b. Goal: *provide emotional support.*

(1) Explanations: brief, accurate; client anxious to learn results of test.

(2) Counseling: refer as indicated.

c. Goal: *health teaching.*

(1) Late complications: infection.

(2) Prepare for surgery if indicated.

(3) Follow-up medical care.

4. **Evaluation:** no complications (e.g., cardiac arrest, hematoma at insertion site).

IX. Percutaneous transluminal coronary angioplasty (PTCA): a balloon-tipped catheter is threaded to site of coronary occlusion and inflated repeatedly until blood flow increases distal to the obstruction; a nonsurgical alternative to bypass surgery for about 10% of clients with coronary artery occlusion; recommended in clients with poorly controlled angina and single vessel disease with a noncalcified, discrete, and proximal lesion that can be reached by the catheter; costs less and requires shorter hospitalization and rehabilitation period (see VIII. Cardiac catherization, for nursing process).

X. Cardiac surgery: done to alter the structure of the heart or vessels when congenital or acquired disorders interfere with cardiac functioning: septal defects; transposition of great vessels; tetralogy of Fallot; pulmonary/aortic stenosis; coronary artery bypass; valve replacement.

Cardiopulmonary bypass (open-heart surgery): blood from cardiac chambers and great vessels is diverted into a pump oxygenator; allows full visualization of heart during surgery; maintains perfusion and body functioning.

A. Preoperative

1. **Assessment:** see specific conditions for preoperative signs and symptoms, i.e., valvular defects, angina, MI; also see I. Preoperative preparation, p. 342. Establish complete baseline: daily weight; vital signs—integrity of all pulses, BP both arms; CVP or pulmonary artery pressures (Swan–Ganz); neurologic status; emotional status; nutritional and elimination ▶ patterns; lab values (urine, electrolytes, enzymes, coagulation studies); pulmonary function studies.

2. **Analysis/nursing diagnosis** (see also VI. Myocardial infarction, p. 297):

a. *Decreased cardiac output* related to myocardial damage.

b. *Activity intolerance* related to poor cardiac function.

c. *Knowledge deficit* related to insufficient time for teaching.

d. *Anxiety* related to fear of unknown.

e. *Fear* related to possible death.

f. *Spiritual distress* related to possible death.

3. **Nursing plan/implementation:**

a. Goal: *provide emotional and spiritual support.*

(1) Arrange for religious consultation if desired.

(2) Provide opportunity for family visit morning of surgery.

(3) Encourage verbalization/questions: fear, depression, despair frequently occur.

b. Goal: *health teaching.*

(1) Diagnostic procedures, treatments, specifics for surgery (i.e., leg incision with use of saphenous vein in coronary bypass surgery).

(2) Postoperative regimen: turn, cough, deep breathe, ROM, equipment used, medication for pain.

(3) Tour ICU; meet personnel.

(4) Alternative method of communication while intubated.

4. **Evaluation:**

a. Displays moderate anxiety level.

b. Verbalizes/demonstrates postoperative expectations.

c. Quits smoking before surgery.

B. Postoperative

1. **Assessment:**

a. Subjective data

(1) Pain.

(2) Fatigue—sleep deprivation.

b. Objective data

(1) Neurologic: level of consciousness; pupillary reactions; movement of limbs (purposeful, spontaneous).

(2) Respiratory: rate changes (increases occur with obstruction, pain; decreases occur with CO_2 retention); depth (shallow with pain, atelectasis); symmetry; skin *color;* patency/*drainage* from chest tubes; *sputum* (amount, color); endotracheal tube placement (bilateral breath sounds).

(3) Cardiovascular:

(a) BP—*hypotension* may indicate heart failure, tamponade, hemorrhage, arrhythmias, or thrombosis; *hypertension* may indicate anxiety, hypervolemia.

(b) Pulse: radial, apical, pedal; rate (>100 may indicate shock, fever, hypoxia, arrhythmias); rhythm, quality.

(c) CVP or Swan–Ganz (elevated in cardiac failure); temperature (normal postop: 98.6°–101.6°F oral).

(4) GI: nausea, vomiting, distention.

(5) Renal: urine—minimum output (30 cc/h); color; specific gravity (<1.010 occurs with *overhydration,* renal tubular damage; >1.020 present with *dehydration,* oliguria, blood in urine).

2. **Analysis/nursing diagnosis:**
   a. *Decreased cardiac output* related to decreased myocardial contractility or postoperative hypothermia.
   b. *Pain* related to incision.
   c. *Ineffective airway clearance* related to effects of general anesthesia.
   d. *Altered tissue perfusion* related to postoperative bleeding or thromboemboli.
   e. *Fluid volume deficit* related to blood loss.
   f. *Potential for infection* related to wound contamination.
   g. *Altered thought processes* related to anesthesia or stress.
   h. *Body image disturbance* related to incision or limitations.
   i. *Sleep pattern disturbance* related to ICU environment or pain.

3. **Nursing plan/implementation:**
   a. Goal: *provide constant monitoring to prevent complications.*
      (1) Respiratory:
         (a) Observe for respiratory distress: restlessness, nasal flaring, Cheyne-Stokes, dusky/cyanotic; assisted or controlled ventilation via endotracheal tube common first 24 h; supplemental O_2 after extubation.
         (b) Suctioning; cough, deep breathe.
         (c) Elevate head of bed.
         (d) Position chest tube to facilitate drainage; mediastinal sump tube maintains patency—"milking" not necessary. See also chest tube care in Table 7.5, p. 528.
      (2) *Cardiovascular:*
         (a) Vital signs: BP > 80–90 systolic; *CVP:* range 5–15 cm H_2O unless otherwise ordered; pulmonary artery line (Swan–Ganz): mean pressure 4–12 mm Hg; I&O: report <30 cc urine/h from indwelling urinary catheter.
         (b) ECG; PVCs occur most frequently following aortic valve replacement and bypass surgery.
         (c) Peripheral pulses if leg veins used for grafting.
         (d) Activity: turn q2h; ROM; progressive, early ambulation.
      (3) Inspect dressing for bleeding.
      (4) Medications according to therapeutic directives—cardiotonics (digoxin); coronary vasodilators (nitrates); antibiotics (penicillin); analgesics; anticoagulants (with valve replacements); antiarrhythmics (quinidine, Pronestyl).
   b. Goal: *promote comfort, pain relief.*
      (1) Medicate: Demerol or morphine sulfate, as severe pain lasts 2–3 days.
      (2) Splint incision when moving or coughing.
      (3) Mouth care: keep lips moist.
      (4) *Position:* use pillows to prevent tension on chest tubes, incision.
   c. Goal: *maintain fluid, electrolyte, nutritional balance.*
      (1) I&O; urine specific gravity.
      (2) Measure chest drainage—should not exceed 200 mL/h for first 4–6 h.
      (3) Give fluids as ordered; maintain IV patency.
      (4) Diet: clear fluids → solid food if no nausea, GI distention; sodium restricted, low fat.
   d. Goal: *promote emotional adjustment.*
      (1) Anticipate behavior disturbances (depression, disorientation often occur 3 days postop) related to medications, fear, sleep deprivation.
      (2) Calm, oriented, supportive environment, as personalized as possible.
      (3) Encourage verbalization of feelings (family and client).
      (4) Encourage independence to avoid cardiac-cripple role.
   e. Goal: *health teaching.*
      (1) Alterations in life-style; activity, diet, work.
      (2) Available community resources for cardiac rehabilitation (e.g., American Heart Association, Mended Hearts).
      (3) Drug regimen: purpose, side effects.
      (4) Potential complications: dyspnea, pain, palpitations common postoperatively.

4. **Evaluation:**
   a. No complications; incision heals.
   b. Activity level increases—no signs of overexertion (e.g., fatigue, dyspnea, pain).
   c. Relief of symptoms.
   d. Returns for follow-up medical care.
   e. Takes prescribed medications; knows purposes and side effects.

XI. Congestive heart failure (CHF): inability of the heart to meet the peripheral circulatory demands of body; cardiac decompensation; combined right- and left-sided heart failure.

A. Pathophysiology: increased cardiac workload or decreased effective myocardial contractility → decreased cardiac output (forward effects). Left ventricular failure → pulmonary congestion; right atrial and right ventricular failure → systemic congestion → peripheral edema (backward effects). Compensatory mechanisms in CHF include tachycardia, ventricular dilation, and hypertrophy of the myocardium.

B. Risk factors:

1. Decreased myocardial contractility:

ADULT NURSING

a. Myocarditis.
b. MI.
c. Tachyarrhythmias.
d. Bacterial endocarditis.
e. Acute rheumatic fever.

2. Increased cardiac workload:
a. Elevated temperature.
b. Physical/emotional stress.
c. Anemia.
d. Hyperthyroidism (thyrotoxicosis).
e. Valvular defects.

C. Assessment:

1. Subjective data
a. Shortness of breath.
(1) Orthopnea (sleeps on two or more pillows).
(2) Paroxysmal nocturnal dyspnea (sudden breathlessness during sleep).
(3) Dyspnea on exertion (climbing stairs).
b. Apprehension; anxiety; irritability.
c. Fatigue; weakness.
d. Reported weight gain; feeling of puffiness.

2. Objective data
a. Vital signs:
(1) BP: decreasing systolic; narrowing pulse pressure.
(2) Pulse: pulsus alternans (alternating strong-weak-strong cardiac contraction), increased.
(3) Respirations: moist rales.
b. Edema: dependent, pitting (1 + to 4 + mm).
c. Liver: enlarged, tender.
d. Neck veins: distended.
► e. Chest X ray:
(1) Cardiac enlargement.
(2) Dilated pulmonary vessels.
(3) Diffuse interstitial lung edema.

D. Analysis/nursing diagnosis:

1. *Decreased cardiac output* related to decreased myocardial contractility.
2. *Activity intolerance* related to generalized weakness and inadequate oxygenation.
3. *Fatigue* related to edema and poor oxygenation.
4. *Altered tissue perfusion* related to peripheral edema and inadequate blood flow.
5. *Fluid volume excess* related to compensatory mechanisms.
6. *Impaired gas exchange* related to pulmonary congestion.
7. *Anxiety* related to shortness of breath.
8. *Sleep pattern disturbance* related to paroxysmal nocturnal dyspnea.

E. Nursing plan/implementation:

1. Goal: *provide physical rest/reduce emotional stimuli.*
a. *Position:* sitting or semi-Fowler's until tachycardia, dyspnea, edema resolved; change position frequently; pillows for support.
b. Rest: planned periods; limit visitors, activity, noise.
c. Support: stay with anxious client; have supportive family member present; administer sedatives/tranquilizers as ordered.
d. Warm fluids if appropriate.

2. Goal: *provide for relief of respiratory distress; reduce cardiac workload.*
a. Oxygen: low flow rate; encourage deep breathing (5–10 min q2h); auscultate breath sounds for congestion, pulmonary edema.
b. *Position:* head of bed 20–30 cm (8–10 in.) alleviates pulmonary congestion.
c. Medications as ordered:
(1) *Digitalis* preparations.
(2) *Beta-adrenergics*—dobutamine, dopamine.
(3) *Diuretics*—thiazides, furosemide, ethacrynic acid.
(4) *Tranquilizers*—phenobarbital, diazepam (Valium), chlordiazepoxide (Librium) HCl.
(5) *Stool softeners* to avoid Valsalva maneuver.

3. Goal: *provide for special safety needs.*
a. Skin care:
(1) Inspect, massage, lubricate bony prominences.
(2) Use foot cradle, heel protectors; sheepskin.
b. Siderails up if hypoxic (disoriented).
c. Vital signs: monitor for signs of fatigue, pulmonary emboli.
d. ROM: active, passive; elastic stockings.

4. Goal: *maintain fluid and electrolyte balance, nutritional status.*
a. Urine output: 30 cc/h minimum; estimate insensible loss in diaphoretic client.
b. Daily weight; same time, clothes, scale.
c. IV: use microdrip to avoid circulatory overloading.
d. Diet:
(1) Low-sodium as ordered.
(2) Small, frequent feedings.
(3) Discuss food preferences with client.

5. Goal: *health teaching.*
a. Diet restrictions; meal preparation.
b. Activity restrictions, if any; planned rest periods.
c. Medications: schedule, purpose, dosage, side effects (importance of daily pulse-taking, daily weights, intake of potassium-containing foods).
d. Available community resources for dietary assistance, weight reduction, exercise program.

F. Evaluation:

1. Increase in activity level tolerance—fatigue decreased.
2. No complications—pulmonary edema, respiratory distress.

3. Reduction in dependent edema.

XII. Pulmonary edema: sudden transudation of fluid from pulmonary capillaries into alveoli.

A. Pathophysiology: increased pulmonary capillary permeability; increased hydrostatic pressure (pulmonary hypertension); and/or decreased blood colloidal osmotic pressure; fluid accumulation in alveoli → decreased compliance → decreased diffusion of gas → hypoxia, hypercapnea.

B. Risk factors:

1. Left-sided heart failure.
2. Pulmonary embolism.
3. Drug overdose.
4. Smoke inhalation.
5. CNS damage.
6. Fluid overload.

C. Assessment:

1. Subjective data
   a. Anxiety.
   b. Restlessness at onset progressing to agitation.
   c. Stark fear.
   d. Intense dyspnea, orthopnea, fatigue.
2. Objective data
   a. Vital signs:
      (1) Pulse: tachycardia; gallop rhythm.
      (2) Respiration: tachypnea, moist, bubbling, wheezing.
      (3) Temperature: normal to subnormal.
   b. Skin: pale, cool, diaphoretic, cyanotic.
   c. Auscultation: rales, coarse rhonchi.
   d. Cough: productive of large quantities of pink, frothy sputum.
   e. Right-sided heart failure: distended neck veins, peripheral edema, hepatomegaly, ascites.
   f. Mental status: restless, confused, stuporous.

D. Analysis/nursing diagnosis:

1. *Decreased cardiac output* related to decreased myocardial contractility.
2. *Impaired gas exchange* related to pulmonary congestion.
3. *Altered tissue perfusion* related to inadequate blood flow.
4. *Anxiety,* severe, related to difficulty breathing.
5. *Fear* related to pulmonary congestion.

E. Nursing plan/implementation:

1. Goal: *promote physical, psychologic relaxation measures to relieve anxiety.*
   a. Slow respirations: morphine sulfate, as ordered, to reduce respiratory rate, to sedate, and to produce vasodilation.
   b. Remain with client.
   c. Encourage slow, deep breathing; assist with coughing.
   d. Work calmly, confidently, unhurriedly.
   e. Frequent rest periods.
2. Goal: *improve cardiac function, reduce venous return, relieve hypoxia.*
   a. O_2: via mask; IPPB with 100% oxygen to slow respiratory rate, provide uniform ventilation, reduce venous return, and inhibit "leaky capillary" syndrome.
   b. Give aminophylline, as ordered, to lower venous pressure and increase cardiac output.
   c. *Position:* high Fowler's, extremities in dependent position, to reduce venous return and facilitate breathing.
   d. Medications as ordered: digitalis; diuretics—ethacrynic acid (Edecrin), furosemide (Lasix); beta adrenergics—dobutamine (Dobutrex).
   e. Vital signs; auscultate breath sounds.
   f. Diet: low-sodium; fluid restriction as ordered.
3. Goal: *health teaching* (include family or significant other).
   a. Medications.
      (1) Side effects.
      (2) Potassium supplements if indicated.
      (3) Pulse-taking.
   b. Exercise; rest.
   c. Diet: low-sodium.
   d. Signs of complications: edema; weight gain of 2–3 lb (0.9–1.4 kg) in a few days; dyspnea.

F. Evaluation:

1. No complications; vital signs stable; clear breath sounds.
2. No weight gain; weight loss if indicated.
3. Alert, oriented, calm.

XIII. Shock: a critically severe deficiency in nutrients, oxygen, and electrolytes delivered to body tissues, plus deficiency in removal of cellular wastes; results from cardiac failure, insufficient blood volume, and/or increased vascular bed size.

A. Types, pathophysiology, and risk factors:

1. *Hypovolemic* (hemorrhagic, hematogenic)—markedly decreased volume of blood (hemorrhage or plasma loss from intestinal obstruction, burns, physical trauma, or dehydration) → decreased venous return, cardiac output → decreased tissue perfusion.
2. *Cardiogenic*—failure of cardiac muscle pump (myocardial infarction) → generally decreased cardiac output → pulmonary congestion, hypoxia → inadequate circulation; high mortality.
3. *Distributive:*
   a. Neurogenic—massive vasodilatation from reduced vasomotor, vasoconstrictor tone (e.g., head injuries, anesthesia, pain); interruption of sympathetic nervous system; blood volume that is normal but inadequate for vessels → decreased venous return → tissue hypoxia.
   b. Vasogenic (anaphylactic, septic, endotoxic)—severe reaction to foreign protein (insect bites, drugs, toxic substances, aerobic, gram-negative organisms) → histamine release → vasodilatation, venous stasis → diminished venous return.

TABLE 4.5 Assessment Parameters According to Severity of Hypovolemic Shock

Shock	Respirations	Pulse	Blood Pressure	Skin	Urine	Level of Consciousness
Mild (Early)	Rapid, deep	Increased slightly	Normal or slightly decreased	Cool and pale	Normal, slight decrease	Alert, oriented, diffuse anxiety
Moderate (25% blood loss)	Rapid, becoming shallow	Rapid, thready	80–100 mm Hg systolic (frank hypotension)	Cool, pale, moist	Decrease to <30 cc/h	Agitated, mental cloudiness, or increased restlessness
Severe (40% blood loss)	Rapid, shallow, irregular	Very rapid, irregular, weak	Below 80 mm Hg systolic	Cold, clammy; cyanosis of lips and nails; mottled	Oliguric, <20 cc/h	Lethargy, reacts to noxious stimuli, disoriented
Irreversible	Irregular	Irregular apical pulse	None palpable	Cold, clammy, cyanotic, or pale	Anuric	Does not respond to stimuli; unconscious

Source: Saxton DF et al.: *The Addison-Wesley Manual of Nursing Practice*, Menlo Park, CA: Addison-Wesley, 1983.

ADULT NURSING

B. Assessment: varies, depending on degree of shock; see Table 4.5.

1. Subjective data
   a. Anxiety; restlessness.
   b. Dizziness; fainting.
2. Objective data
   a. Vital signs:
      (1) *BP*—hypotension (postural changes in early shock; systolic <70 mm Hg in late shock).
      (2) *Pulse*—tachycardia, thready; irregular (cardiogenic shock); could be slow if conduction system of heart damaged.
      (3) *Respirations*—increased depth, rate; wheezing (anaphylactic shock).
      (4) *Temperature*—decreased (elevated in septic shock).
   b. Skin:
      (1) Pale, cool, clammy (warm to touch in septic shock).
      (2) Urticaria (anaphylactic shock).
   c. Level of consciousness: alert, oriented → unresponsive.
   d. CVP:
      (1) *Below* 5 cm water with hypovolemic shock.
      (2) *Above* 15 cm water with cardiogenic, possibly septic shock.
   e. Urine output: decreased (<30 mL/h).

C. Analysis/nursing diagnosis:

1. *Altered tissue perfusion* related to vasoconstriction or decreased myocardial contractility.
2. *Impaired gas exchange* related to ventilation-perfusion imbalance.
3. *Decreased cardiac output* related to loss of circulating blood volume or diminished cardiac contractility.
4. *Altered urinary elimination* related to decreased renal perfusion.
5. *Fluid volume deficit* related to blood loss.
6. *Anxiety* related to severity of condition.
7. *Potential for injury* related to death.

D. Nursing plan/implementation: Goal: *promote venous return, circulatory perfusion.*

1. *Position:* foot of bed *elevated* 20° (12–16 inches), knees straight, trunk horizontal, head slightly elevated; *avoid* Trendelenburg position.
2. Ventilation: monitor respiratory effort, loosen restrictive clothing; O_2 as ordered.
3. Fluids: maintain intravenous infusions; give blood, plasma expanders as ordered (exception—*stop* blood immediately in anaphylactic shock).
4. Vital signs:
   a. CVP (↓ with hypovolemia) arterial line, Swan–Ganz (↑ pulmonary artery wedge pressure indicating cardiac failure).
   b. Urine output (insert catheter for hourly output).
   c. Monitor ECG (↑ rate, arrhythmias).
5. Medications (depending on type of shock) as ordered:
   a. *Antihypotensives*—epinephrine (adrenalin), norepinephrine (Levophed), metaraminol (Aramine), isoproterenol (Isuprel), dopamine (Intropin).
   b. *Antiarrhythmics.*
   c. *Cardiac glycosides.*
   d. *Adrenocorticoids.*
   e. *Antibiotics.*
   f. *Vasodilators* (nitroprusside).
   g. *Beta adrenergics* (dobutamine).
6. Mechanical support: medical antishock trousers (MAST) or pneumatic antishock garment (PASG); used to promote internal autotransfusion of blood from legs and abdomen to central circulation; *do not* remove (deflate) suddenly to examine underlying areas or BP will drop precipitously; compartment syndrome may result with prolonged use and high pressure; controversial.

E. Evaluation:

1. Vital signs stable, within normal limits.

2. Alert, oriented.
3. Urine output >30 cc/h.

XIV. Disseminated intravascular coagulation (DIC): diffuse or widespread coagulation initially within arterioles and capillaries leading to hemorrhage.

A. Pathophysiology: activation of coagulation system from tissue injury → fibrin microthrombin form in brain, kidneys, lungs → microinfarcts, tissue necrosis → red blood cells, platelets, prothrombin, other clotting factors trapped, destroyed in process → excessive clotting → release of fibrin split products → inhibition of platelet clotting → bleeding.

B. Risk factors:
1. Obstetrical complications.
2. Neoplastic disease.
3. Low perfusion states.

C. Assessment—objective data:
1. Skin, mucous membranes: petechiae, ecchymosis.
2. Extremities (fingers, toes): cyanosis.
3. Bleeding: venipuncture sites, wound, oral, rectal, vaginal.
4. Urine output: oliguria → anuria.
5. Level of consciousness: convulsions, coma.
6. Lab data: *prolonged*—prothrombin time (PT); *decreased*—platelets, fibrinogen level.

D. Analysis/nursing diagnosis:
1. *Altered tissue perfusion* related to peripheral microthrombi.
2. *Potential for injury* (death) related to bleeding.
3. *Potential impaired skin integrity* related to ischemia.
4. *Altered urinary elimination* related to renal tubular necrosis.

E. Nursing plan/implementation: Goal: *prevent and detect further bleeding.*
1. Carry out nursing measures designed to alleviate underlying problem (e.g., shock, delivery of fetus, surgery/irradiation for cancer).
2. Medications: heparin SO_4 IV, 1000 U/h, if ordered, to reverse abnormal clotting (controversial).
3. IVs: blood to lessen shock; platelets, cryoprecipitate, fresh plasma to restore clotting factors, fibrinogen.
4. Observe: vital signs, CVP (normal 5–15 mm Hg), PAP (normal 20–30 systolic and 8–12 diastolic), and intake and output for signs of shock or fluid overload from frequent infusions; specimens for occult blood (urine, stool).
5. Precautions: Avoid IM injections if possible; pressure 5 min to venipuncture sites; no rectal temperatures.

F. Evaluation:
1. Clotting mechanism restored (increased platelets, normal PT).
2. Renal function restored (urine output >30 cc/h).
3. Circulation to fingers, toes; no cyanosis.
4. No irreversible damage from renal, cerebral, cardiac, or adrenal hemorrhage.

XV. Pericarditis: inflammation of parietal and/or visceral pericardium; acute or chronic condition; may occur with or without effusion.

A. Pathophysiology: fibrosis or accumulation of fluid in pericardium → compression of cardiac pumping → decreased cardiac output → increased systemic, pulmonic venous pressure.

B. Risk factors:
1. Bacterial, viral, and/or fungal infections.
2. Tuberculosis.
3. Collagen diseases.
4. Uremia.
5. Transmural MI.
6. Trauma.

C. Assessment:
1. Subjective data
   a. Pain:
      (1) *Type*—sharp, moderate to severe.
      (2) *Location*—wide area of pericardium, may radiate; right arm, jaw/teeth.
      (3) *Precipitating factors*—movement, deep inspiration, swallowing.
   b. Chills; sweating.
   c. Apprehension; anxiety.
   d. Fatigue.
   e. Abdominal pain.
   f. Shortness of breath.
2. Objective data
   a. Vital signs:
      (1) BP: decreased pulse pressure; pulsus paradoxus—abnormal drop in systemic BP of >8–10 mm Hg during inspiration.
      (2) Pulse: tachycardia.
      (3) Temperature: elevated; erratic course; low grade.
   b. Pericardial friction rub.
   c. Increased CVP; distended neck veins; dependent pitting edema; liver engorgement.
   d. Restlessness.
   e. Lab data: elevated ALT[SGOT], WBC; chest X ray—cardiac enlargement.

D. Analysis/nursing diagnosis:
1. *Decreased cardiac output* related to impaired cardiac muscle contraction.
2. *Pain* related to pericardial inflammation.
3. *Anxiety* related to unknown outcome.
4. *Fatigue* related to inadequate oxygenation.
5. *Ineffective breathing pattern* related to discomfort during inspiration.

E. Nursing plan/implementation:
1. Goal: *promote physical and emotional comfort.*
   a. *Position:* semi-Fowler's (upright or sitting); bedrest.
   b. Vital signs: q2–4h and p.r.n.: apical and radial pulse; notify physician if heart sounds decrease in amplitude or if pulse pressure *narrows,* indicating cardiac tamponade; cooling measures as indicated.
   c. O_2 as ordered.

d. Medications as ordered:
(1) *Analgesics*—aspirin, morphine sulfate.
(2) *Nonsteroidal anti-inflammatory agents.*
(3) *Antibiotics.*
(4) *Digitalis* and *diuretics,* if heart failure present.

▶ e. Assist with aspiration of pericardial sac (pericardiocentesis) if needed: medicate as ordered; elevate head 60°; monitor ECG; have defibrillator and pacemaker available.

f. Prepare for pericardectomy (excision of constricting pericardium) as ordered.

g. Continual emotional support.

h. Enhance effects of analgesics: positioning; turning; warm drinks.

i. Monitor for signs of cardiac tamponade: tachycardia; tachypnea; hypotension; pallor; narrowed pulse pressure; pulsus paradoxus; distended neck veins.

2. Goal: *maintain fluid, electrolyte balance.*
a. Parenteral fluids as ordered; strict I&O.
b. Assist with feedings; low-sodium diet may be ordered.

F. Evaluation:
1. Relief of pain, dyspnea.
2. No complications (e.g., cardiac tamponade).
3. Return of normal cardiac functioning.

XVI. Arteriosclerosis obliterans: most common obstructive disorder of the arterial system (aorta, large and medium-size arteries); frequently involves the femoral artery.

A. Pathophysiology: fatty deposits in intimal, medial layer of arterial walls; plaque formation → narrowed arterial lumens; decreased distensibility → decreased blood flow; ischemic changes in tissues.

B. Risk factors:
1. Age (over 50).
2. Sex (men).
3. Diabetes mellitus.
4. Hyperlipidemia—obesity.
5. Cigarette smoking.
6. Hypertension.
7. Polycythemia vera.

C. Assessment:
1. Subjective data
a. Pain:
(1) *Type*—cramplike.
(2) *Location*—foot, calf, thigh, buttocks.
(3) *Duration*—variable, may be relieved by rest.
(4) *Precipitating causes*—exercise (intermittent claudication), but occasionally may occur when at rest.
b. Tingling, numbness in toes, feet.
c. Persistent coldness of one or both lower extremities.
2. Objective data
a. Lower extremities:
(1) Pedal pulses—absent or diminished.
(2) Skin—shiny, glossy, dry, cold, chalky white, decreased/absent hair, ulcers, gangrene.
b. Lab data: increased serum cholesterol, triglycerides, CBC, platelets

▶ c. Angiography—indicates location, nature of occlusion.

D. Analysis/nursing diagnosis:
1. *Altered tissue perfusion* related to peripheral vascular disease.
2. *Potential activity intolerance* related to pain and sensory changes.
3. *Pain* related to ischemia.
4. *Potential impaired skin integrity* related to poor circulation.
5. *Potential for injury* related to numbness of extremities.

E. Nursing plan/implementation:
1. Goal: *promote circulation; decrease discomfort.*
a. *Position:* elevate head of bed on blocks (3–6 in.), as gravity aids perfusion to thighs, legs; elevating legs increases pain.
b. Comfort: keep warm; avoid chilling or use of heating pads, which may burn skin; apply bed socks.
c. Circulation: check pedal pulses, skin color, temperature qid.
d. Medications:
(1) *Vasodilators.*
(2) *Anticoagulants*—heparin sodium, dicumarol, ASA.
(3) *Antihyperlipidemics*—clofibrate, cholestyramine resin, nicotinic acid.

2. Goal: *prevent infection, injury.*
a. Skin care: use bed cradle, sheepskin, heel pads; milk soap; dry thoroughly; lotion; do not massage, so as to prevent release of thrombus.
b. Foot care: wear properly fitting shoes, slippers when out of bed; inspect for injury or pressure areas; nail care by podiatrist.
c. Diet: high in vitamins B and C to improve cardiovascular functioning and skin integrity.

3. Goal: *health teaching.*
a. Skin care; inspect daily.
b. Activity: balance exercise, rest to increase collateral circulation; walk only until painful.
c. Exercises: walking, Buerger-Allen exercises (gravity alternately fills and empties blood vessels).
d. Diet: low in fat, high in vitamins B, C.
e. Avoid smoking.
f. Recognizes and reports signs of occlusion (e.g., pain, cramping, numbness in extremities, color changes—white or blue, temperature changes—cool to cold).

F. Evaluation:
1. Decreased pain.
2. Skin integrity preserved; no loss of limb.

3. Quits smoking.
4. Does exercises to increase collateral circulation.

XVII. Aneurysms (thoracic or abdominal aortic): localized or diffuse dilatations/outpouching of a vessel wall, usually an artery; exerts pressure on adjacent structures; affects primarily males over age 60; resected surgically, reconstructed with synthetic or vascular graft.

A. Risk factors:

1. Atherosclerosis.
2. Trauma.
3. Syphilis.
4. Congenital weakness.
5. Local infection.

B. Assessment:

1. Subjective data
   a. Pain:
      (1) Constant, boring, neuralgic, intermittent—low back, abdominal.
      (2) Angina—sudden onset may mean rupture or dissection, which are **emergency** conditions.
   b. Dyspnea; orthopnea.
   c. Dysphagia.
2. Objective data
   a. Vital signs:
      (1) Radial pulses differ.
      (2) Tachycardia.
      (3) Hypotension following rupture leading to shock.
   b. Pulsating mass: abdominal, chest wall pulsation; edema of chest wall (thoracic aneurysm); periumbilical (abdominal aneurysm); audible bruit over aorta.
   c. Cyanosis, mottled below level of aneurysm.
   d. Veins: dilated, superficial—neck, chest, arms.
   e. Cough: paroxysmal, brassy.
   f. Diaphoresis, pallor, fainting following rupture.
   g. Peripheral pulses:
      (1) Femoral present.
      (2) Pedal weak or absent.
   h. Stool bloody from irritation.

C. Analysis/nursing diagnosis:

1. *Altered tissue perfusion* related to distal arterial emboli.
2. *Pain* related to pressure on lumbar nerves.
3. *Anxiety* related to risk of rupture.

D. Nursing plan/implementation:

1. Goal: *provide emergency care prior to surgery for dissection or rupture.*
   a. Vital signs: at least every 5 min; (systolic BP <100 mm Hg and pulse >100 with rupture).
   b. IVs: may have 2–4 sites; lactated Ringer's may be ordered.
   c. Urine output: monitored every 15–30 min.
   d. O_2: usually via nasal prongs.
   e. Medications as ordered: antihypertensives to prevent extension of dissection.
   f. Transport to operating room quickly.
   g. See The Perioperative Experience, p. 342, for general preoperative care.
2. Goal: *prevent complications postoperatively.*
   a. *Position:* initially flat in bed; avoid sharp flexion of hip and knee, which places pressure on femoral and popliteal arteries; turn gently side to side; note erythema on back from pooled blood.
   b. Vital signs: CVP; hourly peripheral pulses distal to graft site, including neurovascular check of lower extremities; absent pulses for 6–12 h indicates occlusion; check with Doppler blood flow detector.
   c. Urine output: hourly from indwelling catheter.
      (1) Immediately report anuria or oliguria (<30 cc/h).
      (2) Check color for hematuria.
      (3) Monitor daily blood urea nitrogen (BUN) and creatinine.
   d. Observe for signs of atheroembolization (patchy areas of ischemia); report change in color, motor ability, or sensation of lower extremities.
   e. Observe for signs of bowel ischemia (decreased/absent bowel sounds, pain, guiac-positive diarrhea, abdominal distention); may have nasogastric tube.
   f. Measure abdominal girth; increase seen with graft leakage.
3. Goal: *promote comfort.*
   a. Position: alignment, comfort; prevent heel ulcers.
   b. Medication: narcotics.
4. Goal: *health teaching.*
   a. Minimize recurrence: avoid trauma, infection, smoking, high-cholesterol diet, obesity.
   b. Regular medical supervision.

E. Evaluation:

1. Surgical intervention before rupture.
2. No loss of renal function.

XVIII. Varicose veins: abnormally lengthened, tortuous, dilated superficial veins (saphenous); result of incompetent valves, especially in lower extremities; process is irreversible.

A. Pathophysiology: dilated vein → venous stasis → edema, fibrotic changes, pigmentation of skin, lowered resistance to trauma.

B. Risk factors:

1. Congenital defect of venous valves.
2. Trauma.
3. Deep vein thrombosis.
4. Pregnancy.
5. Abdominal tumors.
6. Chronic disease (heart, liver).
7. Occupations requiring long periods of standing.

C. Assessment:

1. Subjective data
   a. Dull aches; heaviness in legs.
   b. Pain; muscle cramping.
   c. Fatigue in lower extremities, increased with hot weather, high altitude, history of prolonged standing.
2. Objective data
   a. Nodular protrusions along veins.
   b. Edema.
   ▶ c. Diagnostic tests: Trendelenburg test; phlebography; Doppler flowmeter.

D. Analysis/nursing diagnosis:

1. *Altered tissue perfusion* related to venous valve incompetence.
2. *Pain* related to edema and muscle cramping.
3. *Potential activity intolerance* related to leg discomfort.
4. *Body image disturbance* related to disfigurement of leg.

E. Nursing plan/implementation:

1. Goal: *promote venous return from lower extremities.*
   a. Activity: walk every hour.
   b. Discourage prolonged sitting, standing, sitting with crossed legs.
   c. *Position:* elevate legs q2–3h; elastic stockings or ace wraps.
2. Goal: *provide for safety.*
   a. Assist with early ambulation.
   b. Surgical asepsis with wounds, leg ulcers.
   c. Observe for hemorrhage—if occurs: elevate leg, apply pressure, notify physician.
   d. Observe for allergic reactions if sclerosing drugs used; have antihistamine available.
3. Goal: *health teaching.*
   a. Weight-reducing techniques, dietary approaches if indicated.
   b. Preventive measures: leg elevation; avoiding prolonged standing, sitting, high chairs, tight girdles, constrictive clothing; wear support hose.
   ▶ c. Expectations for Trendelenburg test.
      (1) While client is lying down, elevate leg 65° to empty veins.
      (2) Apply tourniquet high on upper thigh (do not constrict deep veins).
      (3) Client stands with tourniquet in place.
      (4) Filling of veins is observed.
      (5) Normal response is slow filling from below in 20–30 sec, with no change in rate when tourniquet is removed.
      (6) Incompetent veins distend very quickly with back flow.
   d. Prepare for vein ligation and stripping.

F. Evaluation:

1. Relief or control of symptoms.
2. Activity without pain.

XIX. Vein ligation and stripping: surgical intervention for advancing varicosities, stasis ulcerations, and cosmetic needs of client. Procedure involves ligation of the saphenous vein at the groin, where it joins the femoral vein; saphenous stripping from the groin to the ankle; legs are wrapped with a pressure bandage.

A. See XVIII. Varicose veins for assessment data and nursing diagnosis of the client requiring surgery.

B. Nursing plan/implementation:

1. Goal: *prevent complications.*
   a. *Position:* elevate legs 18 out of 24 h above level of heart, for 1 week.
   b. Activity:
      (1) Assist with early, frequent ambulation; medicate for pain before ambulation.
      (2) No chair-sitting to prevent venous pooling, thrombus formation.
   c. Bleeding: check elastic bandages, dressings several times a day.
2. Goal: *health teaching* to prevent recurrence.
   a. Weight reduction.
   b. Avoid constricting garments.
   c. Change positions frequently.
   d. Wear support hose/stockings to enhance venous return.
   e. No crossing legs at knees.

C. Evaluation:

1. No complications—hemorrhage, infection, nerve damage, deep vein thrombosis.
2. No recurrence of varicosities.
3. Adequate circulation to legs: strong pedal pulses.
4. Resumes daily activities; free of pain.

XX. Thrombophlebitis: formation of a blood cot in an inflamed vein, secondary to phlebitis or partial obstruction; may lead to venous insufficiency and pulmonary embolism.

A. Pathophysiology: endothelial inflammation → formation of platelet plug (blood clot) → slowing of blood flow → increase in procoagulants in local area → initiation of clotting mechanisms.

B. Risk factors:

1. Immobility.
2. Venous disease.
3. Prolonged sitting—knees bent.
4. Childbirth.
5. Hypercoagulability of blood.
6. Venous trauma (IVs).
7. Fractures.

C. Assessment:

1. Subjective data
   a. Calf stiffness, soreness.
   b. Severe pain: walking, dorsiflexion of foot (Homans' sign).
2. Objective data
   a. Vein: redness, heat, hardness, threadiness.
   b. Limb: swollen, pale, cold.

■ **TABLE 4.6** **Nursing Responsibilities With Anticoagulant Therapy**

	Heparin	Coumadin
Monitor	PTT (2–3 times baseline).	PT (1½–2½ times baseline).
Inspect	Ecchymosis, bleeding gums, petechiae, hematuria.	Bleeding, ecchymosis.
Administer	With an infusion pump; never mix with other drugs; never aspirate; avoid massaging site.	Same time every day; PO.
Avoid	Salicylates and other anticoagulants, e.g., antacids, corticosteroids, penicillin, phenytoin.	Same as heparin.
Antidote	Protamine sulfate.	Vitamin K.

c. Vital signs: low-grade fever.

D. Analysis/nursing diagnosis:

1. *Altered peripheral tissue perfusion* related to venous stasis.
2. *Pain* related to inflammation.
3. *Activity intolerance* related to leg pain.

E. Nursing plan/implementation:

1. Goal: *provide rest, comfort, and relief from pain.*
   a. Bedrest.
   b. *Position:* as ordered; usually extremity *elevated;* watch for pressure points.
   c. Apply warm, moist heat to affected area as prescribed (cold may also be ordered).
   d. Assess progress of affected area: swelling, pain, soreness, temperature, color.
   e. Administer analgesics as ordered.
2. Goal: *prevent complications.*
   a. Observe for signs of embolism (pain at site of embolism); allergic reaction (anaphylactic shock) with streptokinase.
   b. Precautions: *no* rubbing or massage of limb.
   c. Medications: anticoagulants (sodium heparin, coumarin); streptokinase (Varidase). See Table 4.6.
   d. Bleeding: hematuria, epitaxis, ecchymosis.
   e. Skin care, to relieve increased redness/maceration from hot or cold applications.
   f. ROM: unaffected limb.
3. Goal: *health teaching.*
   a. Precautions: tight garters, girdles; sitting with legs crossed; oral contraceptives.
   b. Preventive measures: walking daily, swimming several times weekly if possible, wading, rest periods—with legs elevated, elastic stockings (may remove at bedtime).
   c. Medication side effects: anticoagulants—pink toothbrush, hematuria, easily bruised.
      (1) Carry MedicAlert card/bracelet.
      (2) Contraindicated drugs—aspirin, glutethimide (Doriden), chloramphenicol (Chloromycetin), neomycin, phenylbutazone (Butazolidin), barbiturates.
   d. Prepare for surgery (thrombectomy, vein ligation).

F. Evaluation:

1. No complications (e.g., embolism).
2. No recurrence of symptoms.
3. Free of pain—ambulates without discomfort.

XXI. Peripheral embolism: fragments of thrombi, globules of fat, clumps of tissue, calcified plaques, or air move in the circulation and lodge in vessel, obstructing blood flow; thrombic emboli most common; may be venous or arterial.

CONDITIONS AFFECTING TISSUE PERFUSION

I. Iron deficiency anemia (hypochromic microcytic anemia): inadequate production of red blood cells due to lack of heme (iron); common in infants, pregnant women, and premenopausal women.

A. Pathophysiology: decreased dietary intake, impaired absorption, or increased utilization of iron decreases the amount of iron bound to plasma transferrin and transported to bone marrow for hemoglobin synthesis; decreased hemoglobin in erythrocytes decreases amount of oxygen delivered to tissues.

B. Risk factors:

1. *Excessive menstruation.*
2. *Gastrointestinal bleeding*—peptic ulcer, hookworm, tumors.
3. *Inadequate diet*—anorexia, fad diets, cultural practices.
4. *Poor absorption*—stomach, small intestine disease.

C. Assessment:

1. Subjective data
   a. Fatigue: increasing.
   b. Headache.
   c. Change in appetite; difficulty swallowing due to pharyngeal edema/ulceration; heartburn.
   d. Shortness of breath on exercise.
   e. Extremities: numb, tingling.
   f. Flatulence.
   g. Menorrhagia.
2. Objective data
   a. Vital signs:
      (1) *BP*—increased systolic, widened pulse pressure.

(2) *Pulse*—tachycardia.

(3) *Respirations*—tachypnea.

(4) *Temperature*—normal or subnormal.

b. Skin/mucous membranes: pale, dry.

c. Sclera: pearly white.

d. Nails: brittle, spoon-shaped, flattened.

e. Lab data: *decreased*—hemoglobin (<10 g/100 mL blood), serum iron (<65 μg/100 mL blood); *increased* total iron-binding capacity.

D. Analysis/nursing diagnosis:

1. *Altered nutrition, less than body requirements,* related to inadequate iron absorption.
2. *Altered tissue perfusion* related to reduction in red cells.
3. *Potential activity intolerance* related to profound weakness.
4. *Impaired gas exchange* related to decreased oxygen-carrying capacity.

E. Nursing plan/implementation:

1. Goal: *promote physical and mental equilibrium.*

a. Position: optimal for respiratory excursion; deep breathing; turn frequently to prevent skin breakdown.

b. Rest: balance with activity, as tolerated; assist with ambulation.

c. Medication (hematinics):

(1) Oral iron therapy (ferrous sulfate)—give *with* meals.

(2) Intramuscular therapy (iron dextran)—use second needle for injection after withdrawal from ampule; use Z track method; inject 0.5 cc of air before withdrawing needle, to prevent tissue necrosis; use 2–3 in. needle; rotate sites; do not rub site or wear constricting garments after injection.

d. Keep warm: *no* hot water bottles, heating pads, due to decreased sensitivity.

e. Diet: high in protein, iron, vitamins (see Unit 5); assistance with feeding, if needed.

2. Goal: *health teaching.*

a. Dietary regimen.

b. Iron therapy: explain purpose, dosage, side effects (black or green stools, constipation, diarrhea); take with meals.

c. Activity: exercise to tolerance, with planned rest periods.

F. Evaluation:

1. Hemoglobin level returns to normal range.
2. Tolerates activity without fatigue.
3. Selects foods appropriate for dietary regimen.

II. Hemolytic anemia (normocytic normochromic anemia): unknown factor causes antibodies to destroy the body's own erythrocytes (autoimmune); may occur secondary to malignant lymphoma, ulcerative colitis, lupus erythematosus, or drug therapy; common in those over age 40.

A. Risk factors:

1. Malignant lymphoma.
2. Ulcerative colitis.
3. Lupus erythematosus.
4. Drug therapy.

B. Assessment:

1. Subjective data

a. Fatigue; physical weakness.

b. Dizziness.

c. Shortness of breath.

d. Diaphoresis on slight exertion.

2. Objective data

a. Skin: pallor, jaundice.

b. Posture: drooping.

c. Lab data:

(1) Decreased hemoglobin.

(2) Increased reticulocyte count.

(3) Direct Coombs test positive.

C. See I. Iron deficiency anemia for analysis, nursing plan/implementation, and evaluation.

III. Pernicious anemia (hyperchromic macrocytic anemia): lack of intrinsic factor found in gastric mucosa, which is necessary for vitamin B_{12} (extrinsic factor) absorption; slow developing, usually after age 50; may be an autoimmune disorder.

A. Pathophysiology: atrophy or surgical removal of glandular mucosa in fundus of stomach → degenerative changes in brain, spinal cord, and peripheral nerves from lack of vitamin B_{12}.

B. Risk factors:

1. Partial or complete gastric resection.
2. Prolonged iron deficiency.
3. Heredity.

C. Assessment:

1. Subjective data

a. Hands, feet: tingling, numbness.

b. Weakness, fatigue.

c. Sore tongue, anorexia.

d. Difficulties with memory, balance.

e. Irritability, mild depression.

f. Shortness of breath.

g. Palpitations.

2. Objective data

a. Skin: pale, flabby, jaundiced.

b. Sclera: icterus (yellow).

c. Tongue: smooth, glossy, red, swollen.

d. Vital signs:

(1) *BP*—normal or elevated.

(2) *Pulse*—tachycardia.

e. Nervous system:

(1) Decreased vibratory sense in lower extremities.

(2) Loss of coordination.

(3) *Babinski* present (flaring of toes with stimulation of sole of foot).

(4) Positive *Romberg* (loses balance when eyes closed).

(5) Increased or diminished reflexes.

f. Lab data:

(1) *Increased*—hemoglobin, bilirubin.

(2) *Decreased*—RBCs, platelets, gastric secretions, Shilling test (radioactive vitamin B_{12} urine test).

D. Analysis/nursing diagnosis:

1. *Altered nutrition, less than body requirements,* related to B_{12} deficiency.
2. *Impaired physical mobility* related to numbness of extremities.
3. *Fatigue* related to decreased oxygen-carrying capacity.
4. *Altered oral mucous membrane* related to changes in gastric mucosa.
5. *Altered thought processes* related to progressive neurologic degeneration.

E. Nursing plan/implementation:

1. Goal: *promote physical and emotional comfort.*
   a. Activity: bedrest or activity as tolerated—restrictions depend on neurologic or cardiac involvement.
   b. Comfort: keep extremities warm—light blankets, loose-fitting socks.
   c. Medication: vitamin B_{12} therapy as ordered.
   d. Diet:
      (1) Six small feedings.
      (2) Soft or pureed.
      (3) Organ meats, fish, eggs.
   e. Mouth care: before and after meals, to increase appetite and relieve mouth discomfort.
2. Goal: *health teaching.*
   a. Medication:
      (1) Lifelong therapy.
      (2) Injection techniques; rotation of sites.
   b. Diet.
   c. Rest; exercise to tolerance.

F. Evaluation:

1. No irreversible neurologic or cardiac complications.
2. Takes vitamin B_{12} for the rest of life—uses safe injection technique.
3. Returns for follow-up care.

IV. Polycythemia vera: abnormal increase in circulating red blood cells; considered to be a form of malignancy; occurs more frequently among middle-aged Jewish men.

A. Pathophysiology: unknown causes → massive increases of erythrocytes, myelocytes (bone marrow leukocytes), and thrombocytes → increased blood viscosity/volume and tissue/organ congestion; increased peripheral vascular resistance; intravascular thrombosis usually develops in middle age, particularly in Jewish males; in contrast, *secondary* polycythemia occurs as a compensatory response to tissue hypoxia associated with prolonged exposure to high altitude, chronic lung disease, and heart disease.

B. Assessment:

1. Subjective data
   a. Headache; dizziness; ringing in ears.
   b. Weakness; loss of interest.
   c. Feelings of abdominal fullness.
   d. Shortness of breath; orthopnea.
   e. Pruritus, especially after bathing.
   f. Pain: gouty-arthritic.
2. Objective data
   a. Skin: mucosal erythema, ruddy complexion (reddish purple).
   b. Ecchymosis; gingival (gum) bleeding.
   c. Enlarged liver, spleen.
   d. Hypertension.
   e. Lab data:
      (1) *Increased*—hemoglobin, hematocrit, RBCs, leukocytes, platelets, uric acid.
      (2) *Decreased* bone marrow iron.

C. Analysis/nursing diagnosis:

1. *Altered tissue perfusion* related to capillary congestion.
2. *Potential for injury* related to dizziness, weakness.
3. *Fluid volume excess* related to mass production of red blood cells.
4. *Potential impaired skin integrity* related to pruritus.
5. *Ineffective breathing pattern* related to shortness of breath, orthopnea.

D. Nursing plan/implementation:

1. Goal: *promote comfort and prevent complications.*
   a. Observe for signs of bleeding, thrombosis—stools, urine, gums, skin, ecchymosis.
   b. Reduce occurrence: avoid prolonged sitting, knee gatch.
   c. Assist with ambulation.
   d. *Position:* elevate head of bed.
   e. Skin care: cool-water baths to decrease pruritus; may add bicarbonate of soda to water.
   f. Fluids: force, to reduce blood viscosity and promote urine excretion; 1500–2500 mL/24 h.
   g. Diet: avoid foods high in iron, to reduce RBC production.
   h. Assist with venesection (phlebotomy), as ordered.
2. Goal: *health teaching.*
   a. Diet: foods to avoid (e.g., liver, egg yolks); fluids to be increased.
   b. Signs/symptoms[1] of complications: infections, hemorrhage.
   c. Avoid: falls, bumps; hot baths/showers (worsens pruritus).
   d. Drugs: myelosuppressive agents (Myleran, Cytoxan, chlorambucil, radioactive phosphorus); purpose; side effects.

ADULT NURSING

e. Procedures: venesection (phlebotomy) if ordered.

E. Evaluation:

1. Acceptance of chronic disease.
2. Reports at prescribed intervals for follow-up.
3. Remission: reduction of bone marrow activity, blood volume and viscosity (RBC < 6,500,000/mm³; Hgb < 18; Hct < 45%; WBC < 10,000).
4. No complications (e.g., thrombi, hemorrhage, gout, CHF, leukemia).

V. Leukemia (acute and chronic): a neoplastic disease involving the leukopoietic tissue in either the bone marrow or lymphoid areas; acute leukemia occurs in children, young adults; chronic forms occur in later adult life.

A. Types

1. Acute nonlymphocytic (ANLL)—formerly acute myelogenous leukemia (AML); seen generally in older age (>60 years).
2. Acute lymphocytic (ALL)—common in children 2–10 years.
3. Chronic lymphocytic (CLL)—generally affects the elderly.
4. Chronic myelogenous (CML)—also known as chronic granulocytic leukemia (CGL); more likely to occur between 25 and 60 years of age.

B. Pathophysiology: displacement of normal marrow cells by proliferating leukemic cells (abnormal, immature leukocytes) → normochromic anemia, thrombocytopenia.

C. Risk factors:

1. Viruses.
2. Genetic abnormalities.
3. Exposure to chemicals.
4. Radiation.
5. Treatment for other types of cancer (e.g., alkylating agents).

D. Assessment:

1. Subjective data
   a. Fatigue, weakness.
   b. Anorexia, nausea.
   c. Pain: joints, bones (acute leukemia).
   d. Night sweats, weight loss, malaise.
2. Objective data
   a. Skin: pallor due to anemia; jaundice.
   b. Fever: frequent infections; mouth ulcers.
   c. Bleeding: petechiae, purpura, ecchymosis, epistaxis, gingiva.
   d. Organ enlargement: spleen, liver.
   e. Enlarged lymph nodes; tenderness.
   f. Lab data:
      (1) WBC—15,000 to 500,000.
      (2) RBC—normal to severely decreased.
      (3) Hgb—low.

E. Analysis/nursing diagnosis:

1. *Potential for infection* related to immature or abnormal leukocytes.
2. *Activity intolerance* related to hypoxia and weakness.
3. *Fatigue* related to anemia.
4. *Altered tissue perfusion* related to anemia.
5. *Anxiety* related to diagnosis and treatment.
6. *Altered oral mucous membrane* related to susceptibility to infection.
7. *Fear* related to diagnosis.
8. *Ineffective individual or family coping* related to potentially fatal disease.

F. Nursing plan/implementation:

1. Goal: *prevent, control, and treat infection.*
   a. Protective isolation if indicated.
   b. Observe for early signs of infection:
      (1) Inflammation at injection sites.
      (2) Vital-sign changes.
      (3) Cough.
      (4) Obtain cultures.
   c. Give antibiotics as ordered.
   d. Mouth care: clean q2h, examine for new lesions, avoid trauma.
2. Goal: *assess and control bleeding, anemia.*
   a. Activity: restrict to prevent trauma.
   b. Observe for hemorrhage: vital signs; body orifices, stool, urine.
   c. Control localized bleeding: ice, pressure at least 3–4 min after needle sticks, positioning.
   d. Use soft-bristle or foam-rubber toothbrush to prevent gingival bleeding.
   e. Give blood/blood components as ordered; observe for transfusion reactions.
3. Goal: *provide rest, comfort, nutrition.*
   a. Activity: 8 h sleep; daily nap.
   b. Comfort measures: flotation mattress, bed cradle, sheepskin.
   c. Analgesics: without delay.
      (1) Mild pain (Tylenol, Darvon without aspirin).
      (2) Severe pain (codeine, Demerol).
   d. Diet: bland.
      (1) High in protein, minerals, vitamins.
      (2) Low roughage.
      (3) Small, frequent feedings.
      (4) Favorite foods.
   e. Fluids: 3000–4000 mL/day.
4. Goal: *reduce side effects from therapeutic regimen.*
   a. Nausea: antiemetics, usually half-hour *before* chemotherapy.
   b. Increased uric acid level: force fluids.
   c. Stomatitis: antiseptic anesthetic mouthwashes.
   d. Rectal irritation: meticulous toileting, Sitz baths, topical relief (i.e., Tucks).
5. Goal: *provide emotional/spiritual support.*
   a. Contact clergy if client desires.
   b. Allow, encourage client-initiated discussion of death (developmentally appropriate).

c. Allow family to be involved in care.

d. If death occurs, provide privacy, listening, sharing of grief for family.

6. Goal: *health teaching.*

a. Prevent infection.

b. Limit of activity.

c. Control bleeding.

d. Reduce nausea.

e. Mouth care.

f. Chemotherapy: regimen; side effects.

G. Evaluation:

1. Alleviate symptoms; obtain remission.
2. Prevent complications (e.g., infection).
3. Ventilates emotions—accepts and deals with anger.
4. Experiences peaceful death (e.g., pain-free).

VI. Idiopathic thrombocytopenia purpura (ITP): potentially fatal disorder characterized by spontaneous increase in platelet destruction; possible autoimmune response; remissions occur spontaneously or following splenectomy; in contrast, secondary thrombocytopenia (STP) is caused by viral infections, drug hypersensitivity (i.e., *quinidine, sulfonamides*), lupus, or bone marrow failure; treat cause.

A. Assessment:

1. Subjective data

a. Spontaneous skin hemorrhages—lower extremities.

b. Menorrhagia.

c. Epistaxis.

2. Objective data

a. Bleeding: GI, urinary, nasal; following minor trauma, dental extractions.

b. Petechiae; ecchymosis.

c. Lab data:

(1) *Decreased* platelets (<100,000/mm³).

(2) Increased bleeding time.

(3) Tourniquet test—positive, demonstrating increased capillary fragility.

B. Analysis/nursing diagnosis:

1. *Potential for injury* related to hemorrhage.
2. *Altered tissue perfusion* related to fragile capillaries.
3. *Impaired skin integrity* related to skin hemorrhages.

C. Nursing plan/implementation:

1. Goal: *prevent complications from bleeding tendencies.*

a. Precautions:

(1) Injections—use small-bore needles; rotate sites; apply direct pressure.

(2) Avoid bumping, trauma.

(3) Use swabs for mouth care.

b. Observe for signs of bleeding, petechiae following blood pressure reading, ecchymosis, purpura.

c. Administer steroids (e.g., prednisone) with ITP to increase platelet count; give platelets for count below 20,000–30,000/mm³ with STP.

2. Goal: *health teaching.*

a. Avoid traumatic activities:

(1) Contact sports.

(2) Violent sneezing, coughing, nose blowing.

(3) Straining at stool.

(4) Heavy lifting.

b. Signs of decreased platelets—petechiae, ecchymosis, gingival bleeding, hematuria, menorrhagia.

c. Use MedicAlert tag/card.

d. Precautions: self-medication; particularly avoid aspirin-containing drugs.

e. Prepare for splenectomy if drug therapy unsuccessful (prednisone, Cytoxan, Imuran).

D. Evaluation:

1. Returns for follow-up.
2. No complications (e.g., hemorrhage).
3. Platelet count >200,000/mm³.
4. Skin remains intact.
5. Resumes self-care activities.

VII. Splenectomy: removal of spleen following rupture due to acquired hemolytic anemia, trauma, tumor, or idiopathic thrombocytopenia purpura.

A. Analysis/nursing diagnosis:

1. *Potential fluid volume deficit* related to hemorrhage.
2. *Potential for infection* related to impaired immune response.
3. *Pain* related to abdominal distention.

B. Nursing plan/implementation:

1. Goal: *prepare for surgery.*

a. Give whole blood, as ordered.

b. Insert nasogastric tube to decrease postoperative abdominal distention, as ordered.

2. Goal: *prevent postoperative complications.*

a. Observe for:

(1) *Hemorrhage*—bleeding tendency with thrombocytopenia due to decreased platelet count.

(2) *Gastrointestinal distention*—removal of enlarged spleen may result in distended stomach and intestines, to fill void.

b. Recognize 101 °F temp as normal for 10 days.

c. Incision: splint when coughing, to prevent high incidence of atelectasis, pneumonia with upper abdominal incision.

3. Goal: *health teaching.*

a. Increased risk of infection postsplenectomy.

b. Report signs of infection *immediately.*

C. Evaluation:

1. No complications (e.g., respiratory, subphrenic abscess or hematoma, thromboemboli, infection).
2. Complete and permanent remission—occurs in 60–80% of patients.

FLUID AND ELECTROLYTE IMBALANCES

Imbalances in fluid and electrolytes may be due to changes in the total quantity of either substance (deficit or excess), protein deficiencies, and/or extracellular fluid volume shifts. Older clients and very young clients are particularly susceptible.

I. Fluid volume deficits: decreased quantities of fluid and electrolytes may be caused by deficient intake (poor dietary habits, anorexia, and nausea), excessive output (vomiting, nasogastric suction, and prolonged diarrhea), or failure of regulatory mechanism.

A. Pathophysiology: water moves out of the cells to replace a significant water loss; cells eventually become unable to compensate for the lost fluid, and cellular dehydration begins, leading to circulatory collapse.

B. Risk factors:

1. No fluids available.
2. Available fluids not drinkable.
3. Inability to take fluids independently.
4. No response to thirst; does not recognize the need for fluids.
5. Inability to communicate need; does not speak same language.
6. Aphasia.
7. Weakness, comatose.
8. Inability to swallow.
9. Psychological alterations.

C. Assessment:

1. Subjective data
   a. Thirst.
   b. Behavioral changes: apprehension, apathy, lethargy, confusion, restlessness.
   c. Dizziness.
   d. Numbness and tingling of hands and feet.
   e. Anorexia and nausea.
   f. Abdominal cramps.
2. Objective data
   a. Sudden weight loss of 5%.
   b. Vital signs:
      (1) *Decreased* blood pressure.
      (2) *Increased* temperature.
      (3) Irregular pulse.
      (4) Increased rate and depth of respirations.
   c. Skin: cool and pale in absence of infection; decreased turgor.
   d. Urine: oliguria to anuria, high specific gravity.
   e. Eyes: soft, shrunken.
   f. Tongue: furrows.
   g. Lab data:
      (1) Blood—increased hematocrit and BUN.
      (2) Urine—decreased 17 ketosteroids.

D. Analysis/nursing diagnosis:

1. *Fluid volume deficit* related to inadequate fluid intake.

E. Nursing plan/implementation:

1. Goal: *restore fluid and electrolyte balance*—increase fluid intake to hydrate client.
   a. IVs as ordered; small, frequent drinks by mouth.
   b. Daily weights (same time of day) to monitor progress of fluid replacement.
   c. I&O, hourly outputs (when in acute state).
   d. Avoid hypertonic solutions (may cause fluid shift when compensatory mechanisms begin to function).
2. Goal: *promote comfort.*
   a. Frequent skin care (lack of hydration causes dry skin, which may increase risk for skin breakdown).
   b. Position: change every hour to relieve pressure.
   c. Medications as ordered: antiemetics, antidiarrheal.
3. Goal: *prevent physical injury.*
   a. Frequent mouth care (mucous membrane dries due to dehydration; therefore, client is at risk for breaks in mucous membrane, halitosis).
   b. Monitor IV flow rate—observe for circulatory overload, pulmonary edema related to potential fluid shift when compensatory mechanisms begin, or client inability to tolerate rate of fluid replacement.
   c. Monitor vitals, including level of consciousness (decreasing BP and level of consciousness indicate continuation of fluid loss).
   d. Prepare for surgery if hemorrhage present (internal bleeding can only be relieved by surgical intervention).

F. Evaluation:

1. Mentally alert.
2. Moist, intact mucous membranes.
3. Urinary output approximately equal to intake.
4. No further weight loss.
5. Gradual weight gain.

II. Fluid volume excess: excessive quantities of fluid and electrolytes may be due to increased ingestion, tube feedings, intravenous infusions, multiple tap water enemas, or a failure of regulatory systems, resulting in inability to excrete excesses.

A. Pathophysiology: hyposmolar water excess in extracellular compartment leads to intracellular water excess because the concentration of solutes in the intracellular fluid is greater than in the extracellular fluid. Water moves to equalize concentration, causing swelling of the cells.

B. Risk factors:

1. Excessive intake of electrolyte-free fluids.
2. Increased secretion of ADH in response to stress, drugs, anesthetics.
3. Decreased or inadequate output of urine.
4. Psychogenic polydipsia.
5. Certain medical conditions: tuberculosis; encephalitis; meningitis; endocrine disturbances; tumors of lung, pancreas, duodenum.
6. Inadequate kidney function or kidney failure.

C. Assessment:

1. Subjective data
   a. Behavioral changes: irritability, apathy, confusion, disorientation.
   b. Headache.
   c. Anorexia, nausea, cramping.
   d. Fatigue.
   e. Dyspnea.
2. Objective data
   a. Vital signs: elevated blood pressure.
   b. Skin: warm, moist; edema—eyelids, facial, dependent, pitting.
   c. Sudden weight gain of 5%.
   d. Pink, frothy sputum; productive.
   e. Urine: polyuria, nocturia.
   f. Lab data:
      (1) Blood—*decreasing* hematocrit, BUN.
      (2) Urine—*decreasing* specific gravity.

D. Analysis/nursing diagnosis:

1. *Fluid volume excess* related to excessive fluid intake or decreased fluid output.

E. Nursing plan/implementation:

1. Goal: *maintain oxygen to all cells.*
   a. *Position:* semi-Fowler's or Fowler's to facilitate improved gas exchange.
   b. Vital signs: every four hours.
   c. Fluid restriction.
   d. Possible rotating tourniquets as needed (especially for interstitial-to-plasma shift).
2. Goal: *promote excretion of excess fluid.*
   a. Medications as ordered: diuretics.
   b. If in kidney failure: may need dialysis; explain procedure.
   ► c. Assist client during paracentesis, thoracentesis, phlebotomy.
      (1) Monitor vital signs to detect shock.
      (2) Prevent injury by monitoring sterile technique.
      (3) Prevent falling by stabilizing appropriate position during procedure.
      (4) Support client psychologically.
3. Goal: *obtain/maintain fluid balance.*
   a. Daily weights.
   b. Measure: all edematous parts, abdominal girth, I&O.
   c. Limit: fluids by mouth, IVs, sodium.
   d. Strict monitoring of IV fluids.
4. Goal: *prevent tissue injury.*
   a. Skin and mouth care as needed.
   b. Evaluate feet for edema and discoloration when client is out of bed.
   c. Observe suture line on surgical clients (potential for evisceration due to excess fluid retention).
   d. IV route preferred for parenteral medications; Z track if medications are to be given IM (otherwise injected liquid will escape through injection site).
5. Goal: *health teaching.*
   a. Improve nutritional status with low-sodium diet.
   b. Identify cause that put client at risk for imbalance, methods to avoid this situation in the future.
   c. Desired and side effects of diuretics and other prescribed medications.
   d. Monitor urinary output, ankle edema, and report to health care manager when fluid retention is noticed.
   e. Limit fluid intake when kidney/cardiac function impaired.

F. Evaluation:

1. Fluid balance obtained.
2. No respiratory, cardiac complications.
3. Vital signs within normal limits.
4. Urinary output improved, no evidence of edema.

III. Common electrolyte imbalances: electrolytes are taken into the body in foods and fluids; normally lost through sweat and urine. May also be lost through hemorrhage, vomiting, and diarrhea. Clinically important electrolytes are:

A. Sodium (Na^+): Normal 138–145 mEq/L. Most prevalent cation in extracellular fluid. Controls osmotic pressure; essential for neuromuscular functioning and intracellular chemical reactions. Aids in maintenance of acid-base balance. Necessary for glucose to be transported into cells.

1. *Hyponatremia*—sodium deficit, resulting from either a sodium loss or water excess. Serum-sodium level below 138 mEq/L.
2. *Hypernatremia*—excess sodium in the blood, resulting from either high sodium intake, water loss, or low water intake. Serum-sodium level above 145 mEq/L.

B. Potassium (K^+): Normal 3.5–5 mEq/L. Direct effect on excitability of nerves and muscles. Contributes to intracellular osmotic pressure and influences acid-base balance. Major cation of the cell. Required for storage of nitrogen as muscle protein.

1. *Hypokalemia*—potassium deficit related to dehydration, starvation, vomiting, diarrhea, diuretics. Serum-potassium level below 3.5 mEq/L.
2. *Hyperkalemia*—potassium excess related to severe tissue damage, renal disease, excess administration of oral or IV potassium. Serum-potassium level above 5 mEq/L.

C. Calcium (Ca^+): Normal 4.3–5.3 mEq/L. Essential to muscle metabolism, cardiac function and bone health. Controlled by parathyroid hormone; reciprocal relationship between calcium and phosphorus.

1. *Hypocalcemia*—loss of calcium related to inadequate intake, vitamin D deficiency, hypoparathyroidism, damage to the parathyroid gland, decreased absorption in the GI tract, excess loss through kidneys. Serum calcium level below 4.3 mEq/L.
2. *Hypercalcemia*—calcium excess related to hyperparathyroidism, immobility, bone tumors, renal failure, excess intake of Ca^{++} or Vitamin D. Serum calcium level above 5.3 mEq/L.

D. Magnesium (Mg^{++}): Normal 1.5–2.5 mEq/L. Essential to cellular metabolism of carbohydrates and proteins.

TABLE 4.7 Electrolyte Imbalances

Disorder and Related Condition	Assessment: Subjective Data	Assessment: Objective Data	Analysis/Nursing Diagnosis
Hyponatremia Addison's disease. Starvation. GI suction. Thiazide diuretics. Excess water intake, enemas. Fever. Fluid shifts. Ascites. Burns. Small-bowel obstruction. Profuse perspiration.	Apathy, apprehension, mental confusion, delirium. Fatigue. Vertigo, headache. Anorexia, nausea. Abdominal and muscle cramps.	*Pulse:* rapid and weak. *BP:* postural hypotension. Shock, coma. *GI:* weight loss, diarrhea, loss through NG tubes. Muscle weakness.	*Diarrhea.* *Fluid volume deficit.* *Altered nutrition: less than body requirements.* *Sensory/perceptual alteration (kinesthetic).*
Hypernatremia High sodium intake. Low water intake. Diarrhea. High fever with rapid respirations. Impaired renal functions. Acute tracheobronchitis.	Lethargy. Restlessness, agitation. Confusion.	*BP and temperature:* elevated. *Neuromuscular:* diminshed reflexes. *Skin:* flushed; firm turgor. *GI:* mucuous membrane dry, sticky. *GU:* decreased output.	*Fluid volume deficit.* *Fluid volume excess.* *Altered nutrition: less than body requirements.* *Sensory/perceptual alteration (kinesthetic).*
Hypokalemia *Decreased Intake:* Poor potassium food intake. Excessive dieting. Nausea. Alcoholism. IV fluids without added potassium. *Increased loss:* GI suctioning, vomiting, diarrhea. Ulcerative colitis. Drainage: ostomy, fistulas. Medications: potassium-losing diuretics, digoxin, cathartics. Increased aldosterone production. Renal disorders.	Apathy, lethargy, fatigue, weakness. Irritability, mental confusion. Anorexia, nausea. Leg cramps.	*Muscles:* flaccid paralysis, parasthesia. *Respirations:* shallow to respiratory arrest. *Cardiac:* decreased BP; elevated, weak, irregular pulse; arrhythmias. *ECG:* low, flat T waves; prolonged ST segment; elevated U wave; potential arrest. *GI:* vomiting, flatulence; decreased motility → distention → paralytic ileus *GU:* urine not concentrated; polyuria, nocturia; kidney damage. *Speech*—slow.	*Decreased cardiac output.* *Fatigue.* *Altered cardiopulmonary tissue perfusion.* *Ineffective breathing patterns.* *Constipation.* *Bathing/hygiene self-care deficit.* *Impaired home maintenance management.* *Sensory/perceptual alteration (gustatory).*
Hyperkalemia Burns. Crushing injuries.	Irritability. Weakness.	*Cardiac:* irregular pulse; arrhythmias; bradycardia.	*Decreased cardiac output.* *Altered urinary elimination.*

continued

■ TABLE 4.7 *(Continued)*

Nursing Plan/ Implementation	Evaluation
Obtain normal sodium level: identify cause of deficit, increase sodium intake PO (salty foods), IVs—hypertonic solutions. *Prevent further sodium loss:* irrigate NG tubes with saline; hourly I&O to monitor kidney output. *Prevent injury* related to shock, dizziness, decreased sensorium; dangle before ambulation. *Skin care.*	Na^+ 138–145 mEq/L. No complications of shock present. Return of muscle strength. Alert, oriented. Limits intake of plain water.
Obtain normal sodium level: decrease sodium intake. I&O to recognize signs and symptoms of complications, e.g., congestive heart failure, pulmonary edema.	Na^+ 138–145 mEq/L. No complaint of thirst. Alert, oriented. Relaxed in appearance. Identifies high-sodium foods to avoid.
Replace lost potassium: increase potassium in diet (see Unit 5); liquid PO potassium medications—dilute in juice to aid taste; give potassium only if kidneys functioning. *Prevent injury to tissues:* prevent infiltration, pain, tissue damage. *Prevent potassium loss:* irrigate NG tubes with saline, *not* water.	K^+ 3.5–5 mEq/L. Identifies cause of imbalance. Lists foods to include in diet. Lists signs and symptoms of imbalance. Return of muscle strength. No cardiac arrhythmias.
Decrease amount of potassium in body; identify and treat cause of imbalance; give foods low in K^+; avoid drugs or IV fluids containing K^+	K^+ 3.5–5 mEq/L. No complications (e.g., arrhythmias, acidosis, respiratory failure).

continued

1. *Hypomagnesemia*—magnesium deficit related to impaired absorption from GI tract, excess loss through kidneys, and prolonged periods of poor nutritional intake. Hypomagnesia leads to neuromuscular irritability. Serum magnesium level below 1.5 mEq/L.
2. *Hypermagnesemia*—magnesium excess related to renal insufficiency, overdose during replacement therapy, severe dehydration, repeated enemas with Mg^{++} sulfate (epsom salts). Serum magnesium level above 2.5 mEq/L.

E. See Table 4.7 for assessment, analysis, nursing plan/implementation, and evaluation of the various electrolyte imbalances.

IV. Acid-base balance: concentration of hydrogen ions in extracellular fluid is determined by the ratio of bicarbonate to carbonic acid. The normal ratio is 20:1. Even when arterial blood gases are abnormal, if the ratio remains at 20:1, no imbalance will occur. See Table 4.8 for blood-gas variations with acid-base imbalances.

A. Types of acid-base imbalance:

1. *Acidosis:* hydrogen ion concentration increases and pH decreases.
2. *Alkalosis:* hydrogen ion concentration decreases and pH increases.
3. *Metabolic imbalances:* bicarbonate is the problem. In primary conditions, the level of bicarbonate is directly *proportional* to pH.
   a. *Metabolic acidosis:* excessive acid is produced or added to the body, bicarbonate is lost or acid is retained due to poorly functioning kidneys. Deficit of bicarbonate.
   b. *Metabolic alkalosis:* excessive acid is lost or bicarbonate or alkali is retained. Excess of bicarbonate.
   c. As compensatory mechanism, P_{CO_2} will be low in metabolic acidosis, as the body attempts to eliminate excess carbonic acid and elevate pH. P_{CO_2} will become elevated in metabolic alkalosis.
4. *Respiratory imbalances:* carbonic acid is the problem. In primary conditions, P_{CO_2} is inversely proportional to the pH.
   a. *Respiratory acidosis:* pulmonary ventilation decreases, causing an elevation in the level of carbon dioxide or carbonic acid. Excess of P_{CO_2}.
   b. *Respiratory alkalosis:* pulmonary ventilation increases, causing a decrease in the level of carbon dioxide or carbonic acid. Deficit of P_{CO_2}.
   c. As a compensatory mechanism, the level of bicarbonate will increase in respiratory acidosis and decrease in respiratory alkalosis.

B. Assessment: see Table 4.9.

C. Analysis/nursing diagnosis:

1. *Impaired gas exchange* related to hyperventilation.
2. *Ineffective breathing pattern* related to decreased thoracic movements.
3. *Ineffective airway clearance* related to retained secretions.
4. *Potential for injury* related to poorly functioning kidneys.
5. *Altered renal tissue perfusion* related to dehydration.
6. *Altered urinary elimination* related to renal failure.

■ TABLE 4.7 *(Continued)* **Electrolyte Imbalances**

Disorder and Related Condition	Assessment: Subjective Data	Assessment: Objective Data	Analysis/Nursing Diagnosis
Hyperkalemia (cont.)			
Kidney disease. Excessive infusion or ingestion of K^+. Adrenal insufficiency. Mercurial poisoning.	Nausea, intestinal cramps.	*ECG:* high T waves; depressed ST segment; widened QRS complex; diminished or absent P waves; ventricular fibrilation. *GI:* diarrhea. *Kidney:* scanty to no urine.	*Activity intolerance.* *Ineffective breathing patterns.* *Diarrhea.* *Impaired home maintenance management.*
Hypocalcemia			
Acute pancreatitis. Diarrhea. Peritonitis. Damage to parathyroid during thyroidectomy. Hypothyroidism. Burns. Pregnancy and lactation. Low vitamin D intake. Multiple blood transfusions. Renal disorders. Massive infection.	Fatigue. Tingling/numbness; fingers and circumoral. Abdominal cramps. Palpitations.	Spasms: tonic muscles, carpopedal, laryngeal. Grimacing: hyperirritable facial nerves. Tetany → convulsions. Osteoporosis → fractures. Arrhythmias → arrest.	*Pain.* *Diarrhea.* *Altered nutrition: less than body requirements.* *Potential for injury.* *Sensory/perceptual alteration (gustatory).*
Hypercalcemia			
Parathyroid glands: overactive, tumor. Increased immobility. Decreased renal function. Bone cancer. Increased vitamin D and calcium intake. Milk alkali syndrome—self-administration of antacids; increased milk in diet to relieve GI symptoms.	*Pain:* flank, deep bone, shin splints. Muscle weakness, fatigue. Anorexia, nausea. Headache. Thirst → polyuria.	Relaxed muscles. Kidney stones. Increased milk intake. Constipation. Dehydration. Stupor → coma.	*Decreased cardiac output.* *Constipation.* *Activity intolerance.* *Altered urinary elimination.* *Pain.*
Hypomagnesemia			
Impaired GI absorption. Prolonged malnutrition or starvation. Alcoholism. Excess loss of magnesium through kidneys, related to increased aldosterone production. Prolonged diarrhea. Draining GI fistulas.	Agitation. Depression. Confusion. Paresthesia.	Muscles: irritable, tremors, spasticity, tetany → convulsions. Arrhythmias, tachycardia.	*Potential for injury related to seizure activity.* *Decreased cardiac output.*
Hypermagnesemia			
Renal failure. Diabetic ketoacidosis. Severe dehydration. Antacid therapy.	Drowsiness, lethargy.	Loss of deep-tendon reflexes. Hypotension. Respiratory depression. Cardiac arrest.	*Ineffective breathing pattern.* *Decreased cardiac output.* *Fluid volume deficit.* *Fluid volume excess.* *Altered cardiopulmonary tissue perfusion.*

■ **TABLE 4.7 *(Continued)***

Nursing Plan/ Implementation	Evaluation
If kidney failure present, may need to prepare for dialysis.	
Prevent tetany **(medical emergency):** calcium gluconate IV, 2.5–5 mL 10% solution; repeated q10 min to maximum dose of 30 mL.	Calcium level 4.5–5.7 mEq/L. No signs of tetany. Absent Trousseau's and Chvostek's signs.
Prevent tissue injury due to hypoxia and sloughing; administer slowly; avoid infiltration.	Lists foods high in vitamin D and calcium.
Prevent injury related to medication administration. Caution: drug interaction with carbonate, phosphate, digitalis; avoid hypercalcemia.	
In less acute condition: increase calcium intake—calcium gluconate or lactate.	
Reduce calcium intake: decrease foods high in calcium; identify cause of imbalance; give steroids, diuretics as ordered; isotonic saline IV.	Calcium 4.5–5.7 mEq/L. No pain reported. No fractures/calculi seen on X-ray exam.
Prevent injury: prevent pathologic fractures, (e.g., advanced cancer); prevent renal calculi by increasing fluid intake.	
Provide safety: prevent injury to disoriented client; administer magnesium salts PO or IV.	Serum magnesium level 1.5–2.5 mEq/L.
Health teaching: prevention; diet—high-magnesium foods, fruits, green vegetables, whole grain cereals, milk, meats, nuts.	
Obtain normal magnesium level: IV calcium; fluids; possible dialysis.	Magnesium 1.5–2.5 mEq/L. No complications (e.g., respiratory depression, arrhythmias). Identifies magnesium-based antacids (e.g., Gelusil). Deep-tendon reflexes 2 +.

7. *Fluid volume excess* related to altered kidney function.
8. *Fluid volume deficit* related to diarrhea or dehydration.
9. *Knowledge deficit* related to self-administration of antacid medications.

D. Nursing plan/implementation: see Table 4.9.

E. Evaluation: see Table 4.9.

CONDITIONS AFFECTING GAS TRANSPORT

I. Pneumonia: acute inflammation of lungs with exudate accumulation in alveoli and other respiratory passages that interferes with ventilation process.

A. Types:

1. *Typical/classic pneumonia:* related to diminished defense mechanisms, history of alcoholism, recent respiratory tract infection, viral influenza, increased age, and COPD.
2. *Atypical pneumonia:* related to contact with specific organisms.
   a. *Mycoplasma pneumoniae* or *Legionella pneumophelia,* if untreated, can lead to serious complications such as disseminated intravascular coagulation (DIC), thrombocytopenic purpura, renal failure, inflammations of the heart, neurologic disorders, or possible death.
   b. *Pneumocystis carinii* in conjunction with AIDS.
3. *Aspiration pneumonia:*
   a. *Noninfectious:* aspiration of fluids (gastric secretions, foods, liquids, tube feedings) into the airways.
   b. *Bacterial aspiration pneumonia:* related to poor cough mechanisms due to anesthesia, coma (mixed flora of upper respiratory tract cause pneumonia).
4. *Hematogenous pneumonia bacterial infections:* related to spread of bacteria from the blood stream.

B. Pathophysiology: caused by infectious or noninfectious agents, clotting of an exudate rich in fibrogen, consolidated lung tissue.

C. Assessment:

1. Subjective data
   a. Pain location: chest, referred to abdomen, shoulder, flank.
   b. Irritability, restlessness.
   c. Apprehensiveness.
   d. Nausea, anorexia.
   e. History of exposure.
2. Objective data
   a. Cough
      (1) Productive, rust or yellowish sputum (greenish with atypical pneumonia).
      (2) Splinting of affected side when coughing.
   b. Sudden increased fever, chills.
   c. Nasal flaring, circumoral cyanosis.
   d. Respiratory distress: tachypnea.

ADULT NURSING

TABLE 4.8 Blood-Gas Variations With Acid-Base Imbalances

Blood-Gas Feature	Normal Value	Value With: Respiratory Acidosis	Respiratory Alkalosis	Metabolic Acidosis	Metabolic Alkalosis
HCO_3 (bicarbonate)	22–26 mm Hg	Normal or ↑	Normal or ↓	↓	↑
P_{CO_2}	35–45 mm Hg	↑	↓	Normal or ↓	Normal or ↑
(Carbonic acid*)	(1.05–1.35)	↑	↓	Normal or ↓	Normal or ↑
pH (hydrogen-ion concentration)	7.35–7.45	↓	↑	↓	↑

*To obtain carbonic acid level, multiply P_{CO_2} value by 0.03. ↑, increased; ↓, decreased.

ADULT NURSING

e. Auscultation
   (1) Decreased breath sounds on *affected* side.
   (2) Exaggerated breath sounds on *unaffected* side.
   (3) Crepitant rales, bronchial breath sounds.
   (4) Dullness over consolidated area.
   (5) Possible pleural friction rub.

f. Chest retraction (air hunger in infants).

g. Vomiting.

h. Facial herpes simplex.

i. Diagnostic studies.
   ▶ (1) Chest X ray: haziness to consolidation.
   (2) Sputum culture: specific organisms, usually pneumococcus.

j. Lab data:
   (1) Blood culture: organism-specific except when viral.
   (2) WBC: leukocytosis.
   (3) Sedimentation rate: elevated.

D. Analysis/nursing diagnosis:

1. *Ineffective airway clearance* related to retained secretions.
2. *Activity intolerance* related to inflammatory process.
3. *Pain* related to continued coughing.
4. *Knowledge deficit* related to proper management of symptoms.
5. *Potential fluid volume deficit* related to tachypnea.

E. Nursing plan/implementation:

1. Goal: *promote adequate ventilation.*
   a. Deep breathe, cough.
   b. Remove respiratory secretions, suction p.r.n.
   c. High humidity with or without oxygen therapy.
   d. Intermittent positive pressure breathing (IPPB); incentive spirometry, chest physiotherapy, as ordered and needed to loosen secretions.
   e. Use of expectorants as ordered.
2. Goal: *control infection.*
   a. Monitor vital signs; hypothermia for elevated temperature.
   b. Administer *antibiotics* as ordered to control infection—cephalexin (Keflex), cephalothin (Keflin), erythromycin, gentamicin sulfate (Garamycin), penicillin G. *Note:* need cultures *before* starting on antibiotics.
3. Goal: *provide rest and comfort.*
   a. Planned rest periods.
   b. Adequate hydration by mouth, I&O.
   c. Diet: high carbohydrate, high protein to meet energy demands and assist in the healing process.
4. Goal: *prevent potential complications.*
   a. Cross infection: use good handwashing technique.
   b. Hyperthermia: tepid baths, hypothermia blanket.
   c. Respiratory insufficiency and acidosis: clear airway, promote expectoration of secretions.
   d. Assess cardiac and respiratory function.
5. Goal: *health teaching.*
   a. Proper disposal of tissues, cover mouth when coughing.
   b. Expected side effects of prescribed medications.
   c. Need for rest, limited interactions, increased caloric intake.
   d. Need to avoid future respiratory infections.
   e. Correct dosage of antibiotics and the importance of taking entire prescription at prescribed times (times evenly distributed throughout the 24-hour period to maintain blood level of antibiotic) for increased effectiveness.

F. Evaluation:

1. Adheres to medication regime.
2. Has improved gas exchange as shown by improved pulmonary function tests.
3. No acid-base or fluid imbalance: normal pH.
4. Energy level increased.
5. Sputum production decreased, normal color.

TABLE 4.9 Acid-Base Imbalances

Disorder and Related Conditions	Assessment: Subjective Data	Assessment: Objective Data	Nursing Plan/ Implementation	Evaluation
Respiratory Acidosis				
COPD. Emphysema. Respiratory obstruction. Atelectasis. Damage to respiratory center. Pneumonia. Asthmatic attack. Drug overdose.	Headache. Irritability. Disorientation. Weakness. Dyspnea on exertion. Nausea.	Increased respirations. Cyanosis. Tachycardia. Diaphoresis. Dehydration. Coma (CO_2 narcosis). Hyperventilation to compensate if no pulmonary pathology present. HCO_3 normal, P_{CO_2} elevated, pH below 7.35.	*Assist with normal breathing:* encourage coughing; suction airway; postural drainage; pursed-lip breathing; raise HOB. *Protect from injury:* oxygen at 2 L; encourage fluids; avoid sedation; medications as ordered—bicarbonates, antibiotics, bronchial dilators, detergent. *Health teaching:* identify cause, prevent future episodes; increase awareness regarding risk factors and early signs of impending imbalance; encourage compliance.	Normal acid-base balance obtained. Respiratory rate slows, <30. No signs of pulmonary infection (e.g., sputum colorless, breath sounds clear). Demonstrates breathing exercises (e.g., diaphragmatic breathing).
Metabolic Acidosis				
Diabetic ketoacidosis. Hyperthyroidism. Severe infections. Lactic acidosis in shock. Renal failure → uremia. Prolonged starvation diet; low-protein diet. Diarrhea, dehydration. Hepatitis. Burns.	Headache Restlessness. Apathy, weakness. Disorientation. Thirst. Nausea, abdominal pain.	Kussmaul's respirations: deep, rapid air hunger; ↑temperature. Vomiting, diarrhea. Dehydration. Stupor → convulsions → coma. HCO_3 below normal. P_{CO_2} normal, K^+ above 5; pH below 7.35.	*Restore normal metabolism:* correct underlying problem; sodium bicarbonate PO/IV; sodium lactate; fluid replacement, Ringer's solution; diet: high-calorie. *Prevent complications: regular* insulin for ketoacidosis; hourly outputs; prepare for dialysis if in kidney failure. *Health teaching:* identify signs and symptoms of primary illness; prevent complications, cardiac arrest; diet instructions.	Normal acid-base balance obtained. No rebound respiratory alkalosis following therapy. No tetany following return of normal pH. Alert, oriented. No signs of K^+ excess.
Respiratory Alkalosis				
Hyperventilation—CO_2 loss. Fever. Metabolic acidosis. Increased ICP, encephalitis. Salicylate poisoning. After intense exercise. Hypoxia, high altitudes.	Circumoral parasthesia. Weakness. Apprehension.	Increased respirations. Increased neuromuscular irritability; hyperreflexia, muscle twitching, tetany, positive Chvostek's sign. Convulsions. Unconsciousness. Hypokalemia. HCO_3 normal, P_{CO_2} decreased, pH above 7.45.	*Increase carbon dioxide level:* rebreathing into a paper bag; adjusting respirator for CO_2 retention and oxygen inspired. *Prevent injury:* safety measures for those who are unconscious; hypothermia for elevated temperature. *Health teaching:* recognize stressful events; counseling if problem is hysteria.	Normal acid-base balance obtained. Recognizes psychologic and environmental factors causing condition. Respiratory rate returns to normal limits. No cardiac arrhythmias. Alert, oriented.

continued

■ TABLE 4.9 *(Continued)* **Acid-Base Imbalances**

Disorder and Related Condition	Assessment: Subjective Data	Assessment: Objective Data	Nursing Plan/ Implementation	Evaluation
Metabolic Alkalosis				
Potassium deficiencies. Vomiting. GI suctioning. Intestinal fistulas. Inadequate electrolyte replacement. Increased use of antacids. Diuretic therapy, steroids. Increased ingestion/ injection of bicarbonates.	Lethargy. Irritability. Disorientation. Nausea.	*Respirations:* shallow; apnea, decreased thoracic movement; cyanosis. *Pulse:* irregular → cardiac arrest. Muscle twitching→ tetany, convulsions. Vomiting, diarrhea, paralytic ileus. HCO_3 elevated above 26, Pco_2 normal, K^+ below 3.5, pH above 7.45.	*Obtain, maintain acid-base balance:* irrigate NG tubes with saline; Monitor I&O; IV saline, potassium added; isotonic solutions PO; monitor vital signs. *Prevent physical injury:* monitor for potassium loss, side effects of medications. *Health teaching:* increase sodium when loss expected; instructions regarding self-administration of medications (e.g., baking soda).	Normal acid-base balance obtained. No signs of potassium deficit. Respiratory rate 16–20 No arrhythmias—pulse regular. Lists food sources high in potassium.

6. Vital signs stable.
7. Breath sounds clear.
8. Cultures negative.
9. Reports comfort level increased.

II. Atelectasis: (collapsed alveoli in part or all of the lung)

A. Pathophysiology: due to compression (tumor), airway obstruction, decreased surfactant production, or progressive regional hypoventilation.

B. Risk factors:

1. Shallow breathing due to pain, abdominal distension, narcotics, or sedatives.
2. Decreased ciliary action due to anesthesia, smoking.
3. Thickened secretions due to immobility, dehydration.
4. Aspiration of foreign substances.
5. Bronchospasms.

C. Assessment:

1. Subjective data: restlessness.
2. Objective data
   a. Tachypnea.
   b. Tachycardia.
   c. Dullness on percussion.
   d. Absent bronchial breathing.
   e. Tactile fremitus in affected area.
   ▶ f. X ray:
      (1) Patches of consolidation.
      (2) Elevated diaphragm.
      (3) Mediastinal shift.

D. Analysis/nursing diagnosis:

1. *Impaired gas exchange* related to shallow breathing.
2. *Pain* related to collapse of lung.
3. *Fear* related to altered respiratory status.

E. Nursing plan/implementation:

1. Goal: *relieve hypoxia.*
   a. Frequent respiratory assessment.
   b. Respiratory hygiene measures, cough, deep breathe.
   c. Oxygen as ordered.
   d. Monitor effects of respiratory therapy, ventilators, breathing assistance measures to ensure proper gas exchange.
   e. *Position* on unaffected side to allow for lung expansion.
2. Goal: *prevent complications.*
   a. Antibiotics as ordered.
   b. Sterile technique when tracheal bronchial suctioning to reduce risk of possible infection.
   c. Turn, cough and deep breathe.
   d. Increase fluid intake to liquefy secretions.
3. Goal: *health teaching.*
   a. Need to report signs and symptoms listed in assessment data for early recognition of problem.
   b. Importance of coughing and deep breathing to improve present condition and prevent further problems.

F. Evaluation:

1. Lung expanded on X ray.
2. Acid-base balance obtained and maintained.
3. No pain on respiration.
4. Activity level increased.

III. Pulmonary embolism: undissolved mass that travels in blood stream and occludes a blood vessel; can be thromboemboli, fat, air, or catheter. Constitutes a **critical medical emergency.**

A. Pathophysiology: obstructs blood flow to lung → increased pressure on pulmonary artery and reflex constriction of pulmonary blood vessels → poor pulmonary circulation → pulmonary infarction.

B. Risk factors:

1. Thrombophlebitis.
2. Recent surgery.
3. Invasive procedures.
4. Immobility.
5. Obesity.
6. Myocardial infarction, congestive heart failure.

C. Assessment:

1. Subjective data
   a. Chest pain: substernal, localized; type—crushing, sharp, stabbing upon respirations.
   b. Dyspnea.
   c. Restless, irritable, anxious.
   d. Sense of impending doom.
2. Objective data
   a. Respirations: either rapid, shallow or deep, gasping.
   b. Auscultation: friction rub, rhonchi, rales; diminished breath sounds.
   c. Shock
      (1) Tachycardia.
      (2) Hypotension.
      (3) Skin: cold, clammy.
   d. Cough: hemoptysis.
   e. X ray: area of density.
   f. Lab data:
      (1) Decreased P_{CO_2}.
      (2) Elevated WBC.

D. Analysis/nursing diagnosis:

1. *Ineffective breathing pattern* related to shallow respirations.
2. *Impaired gas exchange* related to dyspnea.
3. *Pain* related to decreased tissue perfusion.
4. *Altered peripheral tissue perfusion* related to occlusion of blood vessel.
5. *Fear* related to emergency condition.
6. *Anxiety* related to sense of impending doom.

E. Nursing plan/implementation:

1. Goal: *monitor for signs of respiratory distress.*
   a. Monitor blood coagulation studies, e.g., PTT.
   b. Ambulate as tolerated and indicated.
   c. Administer IVs, transfusions, and vasopressor medications.
   d. Fluids, by mouth, when able.
   e. Monitor signs: Homan's, acidosis.
   f. Prepare for surgery if peripheral embolectomy indicated.
2. Goal: *health teaching.*
   a. Prevent further occurrence.
   b. Decrease stasis.
   c. If history of thrombophlebitis, avoid birth control pills.
   d. Need to continue medication.
   e. Follow-up care.

F. Evaluation:

1. No complications; no further incidence of emboli.
2. Respiratory rate returns to normal.
3. Coagulation studies within normal limits (PTT 30–40 seconds).
4. Reports comfort achieved.

IV. Histoplasmosis: infection found mostly in central U.S. Not transmitted from human to human but from dust and contaminated soil. Progressive histoplasmosis, seen most frequently in middle-aged white males who have chronic obstructive pulmonary disease, is characterized by cavity formation, fibrosis, and emphysema.

A. Pathophysiology: spores of *Histoplasma capsulatum* (from droppings of infected birds and bats) are inhaled, multiply, and cause fungal infections of respiratory tract. Leads to necrosis and healing by encapsulation.

B. Assessment:

1. Subjective data
   a. Malaise.
   b. Chest pain, dyspnea.
2. Objective data
   a. Weight loss.
   b. Nonproductive cough.
   c. Fever.
   d. Positive skin test for histoplasmosis.
   e. Benign acute pneumonitis.
   ▶ f. Chest X ray: nodular infiltrate.
   g. Sputum culture shows *Histoplasma capsulatum*.
   h. Hepatomegaly, splenomegaly.

C. Analysis/nursing diagnosis:

1. *Ineffective airway clearance* related to pneumonitis.
2. *Ineffective breathing pattern* related to dyspnea.
3. *Pain* related to infectious process.

4. *Potential for infection* related to repeated exposure to fungal spores.
5. *Impaired gas exchange* related to chronic pulmonary disease.
6. *Knowledge deficit* related to prevention of disease.

D. Nursing plan/implementation:

1. Goal: *relieve symptoms of the disease:*
   a. Administer medications as ordered.
      (1) Amphotericin B (IV) and ketoconazole.
         (a) Monitor for drug side effects: local phlebitis, renal toxicity, hypokalemia, anemia, anaphylaxis, bone marrow depression.
         (b) Azotemia (presence of nitrogen-containing compounds in blood) is monitored by biweekly BUN or creatinine levels. BUN >40 or creatinine of 3.0 necessitate stopping amphotericin B until values return to within normal limits.
      (2) Aspirin, Benadryl, Phenergan, Compazine: used to decrease systemic toxicity of chills, fever, aching, nausea, and vomiting.
2. Goal: *health teaching:*
   a. Desired effects and side effects of prescribed medications; importance of taking medications for entire course of therapy (usually from 2 weeks to 3 months).
   b. Importance of follow-up laboratory tests to monitor toxic effects of drug.
   c. Identify source of contamination if possible and avoid future contact if possible.
   d. Importance of deep breathing, pursed lip breathing, coughing (see Emphysema, p. 328 for specific care).
   e. Signs and symptoms of chronic histoplasmosis, chronic obstructive pulmonary disease (COPD), drug toxicity, and drug side effects, as in (1)(a) above.

E. Evaluation:

1. Complies with treatment plan.
2. Respiratory complications avoided.
3. Symptoms of illness decreased.
4. No further spread of disease.
5. Source of contamination identified and removed.

V. Tuberculosis: inflammatory, communicable disease that commonly attacks the lungs, although may occur in other body parts.

A. Pathophysiology: exposure to causative organism *(Mycobacterium tuberculosis)* in the alveoli in susceptible individual leads to inflammation. Infection spreads by lymphatics to hilus; antibodies are released, leading to fibrosis, calcification, or inflammation. Exudate formation leads to caseous necrosis, then liquefication of caseous material leads to cavitation.

B. Risk factors:

1. Persons who have been exposed to tubercule bacillus.
2. Persons who have diseases or therapies known to suppress the immune system.
3. Immigrants from Latin America, Africa, Asia, and Oceania living in the United States for less than a year.
4. Americans living in those regions for a prolonged time.
5. Residents of overcrowded metropolitan cities.
6. Men over 65.
7. Women between ages 25–44 and over 65.
8. Children under 5 years.

C. Assessment:

1. Subjective data
   a. Loss of appetite, weight loss.
   b. Weakness, loss of energy.
   c. Pain: knifelike, chest.
   d. Though patient may be symptom free, the disease is found on screening.
2. Objective data
   a. Night sweats.
   b. Fever: low grade, late afternoon.
   c. Pulse: increased.
   d. Respiratory assessment:
      (1) Productive cough, hemoptysis.
      (2) Respirations: normal, increased depth.
      (3) Asymmetrical lung expansion.
      (4) Increased tactile fremitus.
      (5) Dullness to percussion.
      (6) Rales following short cough.
   e. Diagnostic tests:
      (1) Positive tuberculin test (Mantoux—reaction to test begins approximately 12 hours after administration with area of redness and a central area of induration. The peak time is 48 hours. Determination of positive or negative is made. A reaction is positive when it measures 10 mm. Contacts reacting from 5–10 mm may need to be treated prophylactically.)
      (2) Sputum: positive for acid fast (smear and culture).
      (3) X ray: infiltration cavitation.
   f. Lab data: blood: decreased RBC, increased sedimentation rate.
   g. Classification of tuberculosis.

Class	Description
0	No TB exposure, not infected.
1	TB exposure, no evidence of infection.
2	TB infection, no disease.
3	TB: current disease (person with completed diagnostic evidence of TB—both a significant reaction to tuberculin skin test and clinical and/or X-ray evidence of disease).
4	TB: no current disease (persons with previous history of TB or with abnormal X-ray films but no significant tubercuiin skin test reaction or clinical evidence).

TABLE 4.10 Respiratory Isolation

When Used:

- For infectious diseases that are transmitted through droplet transmission (i.e., tuberculosis).

Precautions:

- Isolate in private room (clients infected with same disease can be placed in same room).
- Client should wear mask if out of room for testing, etc.
- Masks to be worn by personnel when working within three feet of client.
- Gowns not necessary.
- Contaminated articles need to be labeled before being sent for decontamination.
- Provide adequate ventilation in the client's room.
- Careful handwashing.

5 TB: suspect (diagnosis pending) (used during diagnostic testing period of suspect persons, for no longer than a 3-month period).

D. Analysis/nursing diagnosis:

1. *Ineffective airway clearance* related to productive cough.
2. *Impaired gas exchange* related to asymmetrical lung expansion.
3. *Pain* related to unresolved disease process.
4. *Body image disturbance* related to feelings about tuberculosis.
5. *Social isolation* related to fear of spreading infection.
6. *Knowledge deficit* related to medication regime.

E. Nursing plan/implementation:

1. Goal: *reduce spread of disease.*
   a. Administer medications: isoniazid (INH), rifampin—most commonly used; ethambutol, streptomycin, aminosalicylate sodium (PAS).
   b. The following may need to take 300 mg of INH daily for 1 year as prophylactic measure: positive skin test reactors, including contacts; persons who have diseases or are receiving therapies that affect the immune system; persons who have leukemia, lymphoma, or uncontrolled diabetes or who have had a gastrectomy.
   c. *Avoid direct contact with sputum.*
      (1) Use good handwashing technique after contact with client, personal articles.
      (2) Have client cover mouth and nose when coughing and sneezing, and use disposable tissues to collect sputum.
   d. *Provide good circulation of fresh air* (Changes of air dilute the number of organisms. This plus chemotherapy provide protection needed to prevent spread of disease).
   e. Implement respiratory isolation procedure (see Table 4.10).
2. Goal: *promote nutrition.*
   a. Increased protein, calories to aid in tissue repair and healing.
   b. Small, frequent feedings.
   c. Increased fluids, to liquefy secretions so they can be expectorated.
3. Goal: *promote increased self-esteem.*
   a. Encourage client and family to express concerns regarding long-term illness and treatment protocol.
   b. Explain methods of disease prevention, and encourage contacts to be tested and treated if necessary.
   c. Encourage client to maintain role in family while home treatment is ongoing and to return to work and social contacts as soon as it is determined safe for progress of treatment plan.
4. Goal: *health teaching.*
   a. Desired effects and side effects of medications:
      (1) INH may affect memory and ability to concentrate. May result in peripheral neuritis, hepatitis, rash, or fever.
      (2) Streptomycin may cause 8th cranial nerve damage and vestibular ototoxity, causing hearing loss; may cause labyrinth damage, manifested by vertigo and staggering; also may cause skin rashes, itching, and fever.
      (3) Important for client to know that medication regime must be adhered to for entire course of treatment.
      (4) Discontinuation of therapy may allow organism to flourish and make the disease more difficult to treat.
   b. Need for follow-up, long-term care and contact identification.
   c. Importance of nutritious diet, rest, avoidance of respiratory infections.
   d. Identify community agencies for support and follow-up.
   e. Inform that this communicable disease must be reported.

F. Evaluation:

1. Complies with medication regime.
2. Lists desired effects and side effects of medications prescribed.
3. Gains weight, eats food high in protein and carbohydrates.
4. Sputum culture becomes negative.
5. Retains role in family.
6. No complications: (i.e., no hemorrhage, bacillus not spread to others).

VI. Emphysema: chronic disease with excessive inflation of the air spaces distal to the terminal bronchioles, alveolar ducts, and alveoli; characterized by increased airway resistance and decreased diffusing capacity. Emphysema, asthma, and chronic bronchitis together constitute chronic obstructive pulmonary disease (COPD).

A. Pathophysiology: increased airway resistance during expiration results in air trapping and hyperinflation → increased residual volumes. Increased dead space → unequal ventilation → perfusion of poorly ventilated alveoli → hypoxia and carbon dioxide retention (hypercapnia). Chronic hypercapnia reduces sensitivity of respiratory center; chemoreception in aortic arch and carotid sinus become principal regulators of respiratory drive (respond to hypoxia).

B. Risk factors:

1. Smoking.
2. Air pollution: fumes, dust.
3. Anti-enzymes and alpha 1 antitrypsin deficiencies.
4. Destruction of lung parenchyma.
5. Family history and increased age.

C. Assessment:

1. Subjective data
   a. Weakness, lethargy.
   b. History of repeated respiratory infections.
   c. Long-term smoking.
   d. Irritability.
   e. Inability to accept medical diagnosis and treatment plan.
   f. Refusal to stop smoking.
2. Objective data
   a. Increased BP, pulse.
   b. Dyspnea on exertion, dyspnea at rest.
   c. Nostrils: flaring.
   d. Cough: chronic, productive.
   e. Episodes of wheezing, rhonchi.
   f. Increased anterior-posterior diameter of chest (barrel chest).
   g. Use of accessory respiratory muscles, abdominal and neck.
   h. Asymmetric thoracic movements, decreased diaphragmatic excursion.
   i. Position: sits up, leans forward to compress abdomen and push up diaphragm, increasing intrathoracic pressure, producing more efficient expiration; pursed lips for greater expiratory breathing phase.
   j. Weight loss due to hypoxia.
   k. Skin: ruddy color, nail clubbing (pink puffer); when combined with bronchitis: cyanosis (blue bloater).
   l. Respiratory: early disease—alkalosis; late disease—acidosis, respiratory failure.
   m. Spontaneous pneumothorax.
   n. Cor pulmonale (emergency cardiac condition involving right ventricular failure due to increased pressure within pulmonary artery).
   ▶ o. X ray: hyperinflation of lung, flattened diaphragm.
   ▶ p. Pulmonary function tests:
      (1) Prolonged rapid, forced exhalation.
      (2) Decreased: vital capacity (below 4000 mL); forced expiratory volume.
      (3) Increased: residual volume (may be 200%); total lung capacity.
   q. Lab data:
      (1) Po_2 below 80 torr (mm Hg), pH below 7.35.
      (2) Pco_2 above 45 torr.

      Note: In clients whose compensatory mechanisms are functioning, lab values may be out of the normal range, but if a 20:1 ratio of bicarbonate to carbonic acid is maintained, then appropriate acid-base balance also will be maintained. (Carbonic acid value can be obtained by multiplying the Pco_2 value by 0.003).

D. Analysis/nursing diagnosis:

1. *Impaired gas exchange* related to thick pulmonary secretions.
2. *Ineffective breathing pattern* related to hyperinflated alveoli.
3. *Altered nutrition, less than body requirements,* related to weight loss due to hypoxia.
4. *Activity intolerance* related to increased energy demands used for breathing.
5. *Sleep pattern disturbance* related to changes in body positions necessary for breathing.
6. *Anxiety* related to disease progression.

E. Nursing plan/implementation:

1. Goal: *promote optimal ventilation.*
   a. Institute measures designed to decrease airway resistance and enhance gas exchange.
   b. *Position:* Fowler's or leaning forward to encourage expiratory phase.
   c. Oxygen with humidification, as ordered—no more than 2 L/minute to prevent depression of hypoxic respiratory drive (see Oxygen Therapy in Unit 7, p. 525).
   d. Intermittent positive pressure breathing (IPPB) with nebulization as ordered.
   e. Assisted ventilation.
   f. Postural drainage, chest physiotherapy.
   g. Medications, as ordered:
      (1) Bronchodilators to increase air flow through bronchial tree: aminophylline, theophylline, isoetharine (Bronkosol), isoproterenol (Isuprel).

(2) Antimicrobials to treat infection (determined by sputum cultures and sensitivity): tetracycline and ampicillin most common (condition deteriorates with respiratory infections).

(3) Steroids used when bronchodilators are ineffective or for short-term therapy in acute episodes: Prednisone, methylprednisolone sodium succinate (Solu-Medrol), dexamethasone (Decadron).

(4) Expectorants (increase water intake to achieve desired effect): glyceryl guaiacolate (Robitussin).

(5) Bronchial detergents/liquefying agents (Mucomyst).

2. Goal: *employ comfort measures and support other body systems.*
   a. Oral hygiene p.r.n.; frequently, client is mouth breather.
   b. Skin care: water bed, air mattress, foam pads to prevent skin breakdown.
   c. Active and passive ROM exercises to prevent thrombus formation; antiembolic stocking or ace bandages may be applied.
   d. Increase activities to tolerance.
   e. Adequate rest and sleep periods to prevent mental disturbances due to sleep deprivation and to reduce metabolic rate.
3. Goal: *improve nutritional intake.*
   a. High-protein, high-calorie diet to prevent negative nitrogen balance.
   b. Give small, frequent meals.
   c. Supplement diet with high-calorie drinks.
   d. Push fluids to 3000 mL per day, unless contraindicated—helps moisten secretions.
4. Goal: *provide emotional support for client and family.*
   a. Identify factors that increase anxiety:
      (1) Fears related to mechanical equipment.
      (2) Loss of body image.
      (3) Fear of dying.
   b. Assist family coping:
      (1) Do not reinforce denial or encourage overconcern.
      (2) Give accurate, up-to-date information on client's condition.
      (3) Be open to questioning.
      (4) Encourage client-family communication.
      (5) Provide appropriate diversional activities.
5. Goal: *health teaching.*
   a. Breathing exercises, such as pursed-lip breathing and diaphragmatic breathing.
   b. Stress management techniques.
   c. Methods to stop smoking.
   d. Importance of avoiding respiratory infections.
   e. Desired effects and side effects of prescribed medications, possible interactions with over-the-counter drugs.
   f. Purposes and techniques for effective bronchial hygiene therapy.
   g. Rest/activity schedule that increases with ability.
   h. Food selection for high-protein, high-calorie diet.
   i. Importance of taking 2500–3000 mL fluid per day (unless contraindicated by another medical problem).
   j. Importance of medical follow-up.

F. Evaluation:

1. Takes prescribed medication.
2. Participates in rest/activity schedule.
3. Improves nutritional intake, gains appropriate weight for body size.
4. No complications of respiratory failure, cor pulmonale.
5. No respiratory infections.

VII. Asthma: increased responsiveness of the trachea and bronchi to various stimuli, with difficulty in breathing; caused by narrowing of the airways. *Immunologic* asthma occurs in childhood and follows other allergic disease. *Nonimmunologic* asthma occurs in adulthood and is associated with history of recurrent respiratory tract infections.

A. Pathophysiology: bronchial smooth muscle constricts, bronchial secretions increase, mucosa swell, and there is a significant narrowing of air passages. Histamine is produced by the lung. Bronchospasm, production of large amounts of thick mucus, and inflammatory response all contribute to the respiratory obstruction.

1. *Immunologic,* or allergic, asthma in persons who are atopic (hypersensitivity state that is subject to hereditary influences); immunoglobulin E (IgE) usually elevated.
2. *Nonimmunologic,* or nonallergic, asthma in persons who have a history of repeated respiratory tract infections; age usually over 35.
3. *Mixed,* combined immunologic and nonimmunologic; any age, allergen or nonspecific stimuli.

B. Risk factors:

1. History of allergies to identified or unidentified irritants; seasonal and environmental inhalants.
2. Recurrent respiratory infection.
3. Decreased ability to effectively cope with emotional stress.

C. Assessment:

1. Subjective data
   a. History: URI, rhinitis, allergies, family history of asthma.
   b. Increasing tightness of the chest → dyspnea.
   c. Anxiety, restlessness.
   d. Attack history:
      (1) *Immunologic:* contact with allergen to which person is sensitive; seen most often in children and young adults.
      (2) *Nonimmunologic:* develops in adults over 35; aggravated by infections of the sinuses and respiratory tract.
2. Objective data
   a. Tachycardia, tachypnea.

b. Cough: dry, hacking, persistent.

c. Respiratory assessment: audible expiratory wheeze (also inspiratory) on auscultation; rales, coarse rhonchi, rib retraction, use of accessory muscles on inspiration.

d. General appearance: pallor, cyanosis, diaphoresis, chronic barrel chest, elevated shoulders, flattened molar bones, narrow nose, prominent upper teeth, dark circles under eyes, distended neck veins, orthopnea.

e. Expectoration of tenacious mucoid sputum.

▶ f. Diagnostic tests:

(1) Vital capacity: reduced.

(2) Forced expiratory volume: decreased.

(3) Residual volume: increased.

g. Lab data: Blood gases: elevated P_{CO_2}; decreased P_{O_2}, pH.

Emergency Note: Persons severely affected may develop *status asthmaticus,* a life-threatening asthmatic attack in which symptoms of asthma continue and do not respond to usual treatment. Could lead to respiratory failure and hypoxemia.

D. Analysis/nursing diagnosis:

1. *Ineffective airway clearance* related to tachypnea.
2. *Impaired gas exchange* related to constricted bronchioles.
3. *Anxiety* related to breathlessness.
4. *Activity intolerance* related to persistent cough.
5. *Knowledge deficit* related to causal factors.

E. Nursing plan/implementation:

1. Goal: *promote pulmonary ventilation.*

a. *Position:* high Fowler's for comfort.

b. Medications as ordered:

(1) Bronchodilators and expectorants to improve ventilation (monitor for alterations in BP and tachycardia).

(2) Antibiotics to control infection.

(3) Steroids to reduce inflammatory response.

c. Oxygen therapy with increased humidity as ordered.

d. Frequent monitoring for respiratory distress.

e. Rest periods and gradual increase in activity.

2. Goal: *facilitate expectoration.*

a. High humidity.

b. Increase fluid intake.

c. Monitor for dehydration.

d. Respiratory therapy: IPPB.

3. Goal: *health teaching to prevent further attack.*

a. Identify and avoid allergen.

b. Encourage medication compliance.

c. Medication side effects, withdrawals.

d. Postural drainage, percussion techniques to family.

e. Breathing techniques to increase expiratory phase.

f. Teach effective stress management techniques.

g. Recognition of precipitating factors.

F. Evaluation:

1. No complications.
2. Has fewer attacks.
3. Takes prescribed medications, avoids infections.
4. Adjusts life-style.

VIII. Bronchitis: acute or chronic inflammation of bronchus resulting as a complication from colds and flu. *Acute bronchitis* is caused by an extension of upper respiratory infection, such as a cold, and can be given to others. It can also result from an irritation from physical or chemical agents. *Chronic bronchitis* is characterized by hypersecretion of mucus and chronic cough for 3 months a year for 2 consecutive years.

A. Pathophysiology: bronchial walls are infiltrated with lymphocytes and macrophages; lumen becomes obstructed due to decreased ciliary action and repeated bronchospasms. Hyperventilation of alveolar sacs occurs. Long-term condition results in respiratory acidosis, recurrent pneumonitis, emphysema, and cor pulmonale.

B. Risk factors:

1. Smoking.
2. Repeated respiratory infections.
3. History of living in area where there is much air pollution.

C. Assessment:

1. Subjective data

a. History: recurrent, chronic cough, especially when arising in the morning.

b. Anorexia.

2. Objective data

a. Respiratory:

(1) Shortness of breath.

(2) Use of accessory muscles.

(3) Cyanosis, dusky complexion (blue bloater).

(4) Sputum: excessive, nonpurulent.

(5) Vesicular and bronchovesicular breath sounds.

b. Weight loss.

c. Fever.

▶ d. Pulmonary function tests:

(1) Decreased forced expiratory volume.

(2) P_{O_2} below 90 mm Hg; P_{CO_2} above 40 mm Hg.

e. Lab data:

(1) RBC: elevated to compensate for hypoxia (polycythemia).

(2) WBC: elevated to fight infection.

D. Analysis/nursing diagnosis:

1. *Ineffective airway clearance* related to excessive sputum.
2. *Ineffective breathing pattern* related to need to use accessory muscles for breathing.
3. *Impaired gas exchange* related to shortness of breath.
4. *Activity intolerance* related to increased energy used for breathing.

E. Nursing plan/implementation:

1. Goal: *assist in optimal respirations.*
   - a. Increase fluid intake.
   - b. IPPB, chest physiotherapy.
   - c. Administer medications as ordered:
     - (1) Bronchodilators.
     - (2) Antibiotics.
     - (3) Bronchial detergents, liquefying agents.
2. Goal: *minimize bronchial irritation.*
   - a. Avoid respiratory irritants—for example, smoke, dust, cold air, allergens.
   - b. Environment: air conditioned, increased humidity.
   - c. Encourage nostril breathing rather than mouth breathing.
3. Goal: *improve nutritional status.*
   - a. Diet: soft, high-calorie.
   - b. Small, frequent feedings.
4. Goal: *prevent secondary infections.*
   - a. Administer antibiotics as ordered.
   - b. Avoid exposure to infections, crowds.
5. Goal: *health teaching.*
   - a. Avoid respiratory infections.
   - b. Medications: desired effects and side effects.
   - c. Methods to stop smoking.
   - d. Rest and activity balance.
   - e. Stress management.

F. Evaluation:

1. Stops smoking.
2. Acid-base balance maintained.
3. Respiratory infections less frequent.

IX. Acute adult respiratory distress syndrome (ARDS) (formerly called by other names, including *shock lung):* noncardiogenic pulmonary infiltrations resulting in stiff, wet lungs and refractory hypoxemia in previously healthy adult. Acute hypoxemic respiratory failure without hypercapnea.

A. Pathophysiology: damage to alveolar capillary membrane, increased vascular permeability to pulmonary edema, and impaired gas exchange; decreased surfactant production and potential atelectasis; severe hypoxia → death.

B. Risk factors:

1. Primary
   - a. Shock, multiple trauma.
   - b. Infections.
   - c. Aspiration, inhalation of chemical toxins.
   - d. Drug overdose.
   - e. Disseminated intravascular coagulation (DIC).
   - f. Emboli, especially fat emboli.
2. Secondary
   - a. Overaggressive fluid administration.
   - b. Oxygen toxicity.

C. Assessment:

1. Subjective data
   - a. Restlessness, anxiety.
   - b. History of risk factors.
2. Objective data
   - a. Severe dyspnea → cyanosis.
   - b. Tachycardia.
   - c. Hypotension.
   - d. Hypoxemia, acidosis.
   - e. Rales.
   - f. Death if untreated.

D. Analysis/nursing diagnosis:

1. *Anxiety* related to serious physical condition.
2. *Ineffective breathing pattern* related to severe dyspnea.
3. *Impaired gas exchange* related to retention of carbon dioxide.
4. *Ineffective airway clearance* related to respiratory infection.
5. *Altered tissue perfusion* related to acidosis.

E. Nursing plan/implementation:

1. Goal: *assist in respirations.*
   - a. May require mechanical ventilatory support to maintain respirations.
   - b. May need to be transferred to ICU.
   - c. May need oxygen to combat hypoxia.
   - d. Suction p.r.n.
   - e. Monitor blood-gas results to detect early signs of acidosis/alkalosis.
   - f. If not on ventilator, assess vital signs and respiratory status every 15 minutes.
   - g. Cough, deep breathe every hour.
   - h. May need:
     - (1) Chest percussion, vibration.
     - (2) Postural drainage, suction.
     - (3) Bronchodilator medications.
2. Goal: *prevent complications.*
   - a. Decrease anxiety and provide psychological care:
     - (1) Maintain a calm atmosphere.
     - (2) Encourage rest to conserve energy.
     - (3) Emotional support.
   - b. Obtain fluid balance:
     - (1) Slow IV flow rate.
     - (2) Diuretics: rapid acting, low dose.
   - c. Monitor:
     - (1) Pulmonary artery and capillary wedge pressure.
     - (2) CVP (central venous pressure), cardiac output, peripheral perfusion.
     - (3) I&O.
     - (4) Assess for bleeding tendencies, potential for disseminated intravascular coagulation.
   - d. Protect from infection:
     - (1) Strict aseptic technique.
     - (2) Antibiotic therapy.
   - e. Provide physiological support:

(1) Maintain nutrition.

(2) Skin care.

3. Goal: *health teaching.*

a. Briefly explain procedures as they are happening (emergency situation can frighten client).

b. Give rationale for follow-up care.

c. Identify risk factors as appropriate for prevention of recurrence.

F. Evaluation:

1. Client survives and is alert.
2. Skin warm to touch.
3. Respiratory rate within normal limits.
4. Lab values and pressures within normal limits.
5. Urinary output greater than 30 mL/hour.

X. Pneumothorax: presence of air within the pleural cavity; occurs spontaneously or as a result of trauma.

A. Types:

1. *Closed:* rupture of a subpleural bulla, tuberculous focus, carcinoma, lung abscess, pulmonary infarction, severe coughing attack, or blunt trauma.
2. *Open:* communication between atmosphere and pleural space because of opening in chest wall.
3. *Tension:* positive pressure within chest cavity resulting from accumulated air that cannot escape during expiration. Leads to collapse of lung, mediastinal shift, and compression of the heart and great vessels.

B. Pathophysiology: pressure builds up in the pleural space, lung on the affected side collapses, and the heart and mediastinum shift toward the unaffected lung.

C. Assessment:

1. Subjective data

a. Pain

(1) Sharp, aggravated by activity.

(2) Location—chest; may be referred to shoulder, arm on affected side.

b. Restlessness, anxiety.

2. Objective data

a. Dyspnea, cough.

b. Cessation of normal movements on affected side.

c. Absence of breath sounds on affected side.

d. Pallor, cyanosis.

e. Shock.

f. Tracheal deviation to unaffected side.

▶ g. X ray; air in pleural space.

D. Analysis/nursing diagnosis:

1. *Ineffective breathing pattern* related to collapse of lung.
2. *Impaired gas exchange* related to abnormal thoracic movement.
3. *Pain* related to trauma to chest area.
4. *Fear* related to emergency situation.

E. Nursing plan/implementation:

1. Goal: *protect against injury during thoracentesis.*

a. Provide sterile equipment.

b. Explain procedure.

c. Monitor vital signs for shock.

d. Monitor for respiratory distress, mediastinal shift.

2. Goal: *promote respirations.*

a. *Position:* Fowler's.

b. Oxygen therapy as ordered.

c. Encourage slow breathing to improve gas exchange.

d. Careful administration of narcotics to prevent respiratory depression (avoid morphine).

3. Goal: *prepare client for closed chest drainage, physically and psychologically.*

a. Explain purpose of the procedure—to provide means for evacuation of air and fluid from pleural cavity; to reestablish negative pressure in pleural space; to promote lung reexpansion.

b. Explain procedure and apparatus (see Chest tubes in Table 7.5).

c. Cleanse skin at tube insertion site, place client in sitting position, assuring safety by having locked over-bed table for client to lean on, or have a nurse stay with client so appropriate position is maintained throughout the procedure.

4. Goal: *prevent complications with chest tubes.*

a. Observe for and immediately report crepitations (air under skin, also called subcutaneous emphysema), labored or shallow breathing, tachypnea, cyanosis, tracheal deviation, or signs of hemorrhage.

b. Monitor for signs of infection.

c. Assure that tubing stays intact.

d. Monitor for proper tube function (*fluctuation or oscillation* of water in the tube located in the water bottle will occur with respirations; water level will rise in the tube when client inhales or coughs; water level in tube will lower during exhalation). If no bubbling in water, check tubing for kinks or lack of patency. Manipulation of chest tube done only according to specific physician order.

e. Monitor for air leaks (continuous bubbling of water in the bottle).

f. Arm and shoulder ROM.

5. Goal: *health teaching.*

a. How to prevent recurrence by avoiding overexertion; avoid holding breath.

b. Signs and symptoms of condition.

c. Methods to stop smoking.

d. Encourage follow-up care.

F. Evaluation:

1. No complications noted.
2. Closed system remains intact until chest tubes are removed.
3. Lung reexpands, breath sounds heard, pain diminished, symmetrical thoracic movements.

XI. Hemothorax: *presence of blood* in pleural cavity related to trauma or ruptured aortic aneurysm. See X. Pneumothorax for assessment, analysis/nursing diagnosis, nursing plan/implementation, and evaluation.

XII. Chest trauma

Flail chest: multiple rib fractures resulting in instability of the chest wall, with subsequent paradoxical breathing (portion of lung under injured chest wall moves in on inspiration while remaining lung expands; on expiration the injured portion of the chest wall expands while unaffected lung tissue contracts).

Sucking chest wound: penetrating wound of chest wall with hemothorax and pneumothorax, resulting in lung collapse and mediastinal shift toward unaffected lung.

A. Assessment:

1. Subjective data
   a. Severe sudden, sharp pain.
   b. Dyspnea.
   c. Anxiety, restlessness, fear, weakness.
2. Objective data
   a. Vital signs:
      (1) Pulse: tachycardia, weak.
      (2) BP: hypotension.
      (3) Respirations: shallow, decreased expiratory force, tachypnea, stridor, accessory muscle breathing.
   b. Skin color: cyanosis, pallor.
   c. Chest:
      (1) Asymmetric chest expansion (paradoxical movement).
      (2) Chest wound, rush of air through trauma site.
      (3) Crepitus over trauma site (from air escaping into surrounding tissues).
      (4) Lateral deviation of trachea, mediastinal shift.
   d. Pneumothorax: documented by absence of breath sounds, X-ray examination.
   e. Hemothorax: documented by needle aspiration by physician, X-ray examination.
   f. Shock; blood and fluid loss.
   g. Hemoptysis.
   h. Distended neck veins.

B. Analysis/nursing diagnosis:

1. *Ineffective airway clearance* related to shallow respirations.
2. *Impaired gas exchange* related to asymmetric chest expansion.
3. *Pain* related to chest trauma.
4. *Fear* related to emergency situation.
5. *Potential for trauma* related to fractured ribs.
6. *Potential for infection* related to open chest wound.

C. Nursing plan/implementation:

1. Goal: *restore adequate ventilation and prevent further air from entering pleural cavity:* **MEDICAL EMERGENCY.**
   a. In emergency situation: place air-occlusive dressing or hand over open wound as client exhales forcefully against glottis (Valsalva maneuver helps expand collapsed lung by creating positive intrapulmonary pressures); or place client's weight onto *affected* side. Administer oxygen.
   b. Assist with endotracheal tube insertion; client will be place on volume controlled ventilator. (See discussion of ventilators under Oxygen Therapy, Unit 7.)
   c. Assist with thoracentesis and insertion of chest tubes with connection to water-seal drainage as ordered. (See Chest tubes section of Table 7.5).
   d. Monitor vital signs to determine early shock.
   e. Monitor blood gases to determine early acid-base imbalances.
   f. Pain medications given with caution, so as not to depress respiratory center.

D. Evaluation:

1. Respiratory status stabilizes, lung reexpands.
2. Shock and hemorrhage are prevented.
3. No further damage done to surrounding tissues.
4. Pain is controlled.

XIII. Thoracic surgery: used for bronchogenic and lung carcinomas, lung abscesses, tuberculosis, bronchiectasis, emphysematous blebs, and benign tumors.

A. Types:

1. *Thoracotomy*—incision in the chest wall, pleura is entered, lung tissue examined, biopsy secured. *Chest tube is needed postoperatively.*
2. *Lobectomy*—removal of a lobe of the lung. *Chest tube is needed postoperatively.*
3. *Pneumonectomy*—removal of an entire lung. *No chest tube is needed postoperatively.*

B. Analysis/nursing diagnosis:

1. *Potential for injury* related to chest wound.
2. *Impaired gas exchange* related to pain from surgical procedure.
3. *Ineffective airway clearance* related to decreased willingness to cough due to pain.
4. *Pain* related to surgical incision.
5. *Impaired physical mobility* related to large surgical incision and chest tube drainage apparatus.
6. *Knowledge deficit* related to importance of coughing and deep breathing to prevent complications.

C. Nursing plan/implementation:

1. *Preoperative*
   a. Goal: *minimize pulmonary secretions.*
      (1) Humidify air to moisten secretions.
      (2) Use IPPB, as ordered, to improve ventilation.
      (3) Administer bronchodilators, expectorants, and antibiotics as ordered.
      (4) Use postural drainage, cupping, and vibration to mobilize secretions.
   b. Goal: *preoperative teaching.*
      (1) Teach patient to cough against a closed glottis to increase intrapulmonary pressure for improved expiratory phase.
      (2) Instruct in diaphragmatic breathing and coughing.
      (3) Encourage to stop smoking.

(4) Instruct and supervise practice of postoperative arm exercises—flexion, abduction, and rotation of shoulder—to prevent ankylosis.

(5) Explain postoperative use of chest tubes, IV, and oxygen therapy.

2. *Postoperative.*

a. Goal: *maintain patent airway.*

(1) Auscultate chest for breath sounds; report diminished or absent breath sounds on unaffected side (indicates decreased ventilation → respiratory embarrassment).

(2) Turn, cough, and deep breathe, every 15 minutes to 1 hour first 24 hours and p.r.n. according to pulmonary congestion heard on auscultation.

b. Goal: *promote gas exchange.*

(1) Splint chest during coughing—support incision to help *cough up sputum (most important activity postoperatively).*

(2) *Position:* high Fowler's.

(a) Turn client who has had a *pneumonectomy* to operative side (avoid extreme lateral positioning and mediastinal shift) to allow unaffected lung expansion and drainage of secretions; can also be turned onto back.

(b) Client who has had a *lobectomy* or *thoracotomy* can be turned on either side or back because chest tubes will be in place.

c. Goal: *reduce incisional stress and discomfort*—pad area around chest tube when turning on operative side to maintain tube patency and promote comfort.

d. Goal: *prevent complications related to respiratory function.*

(1) Maintain chest tubes to water-seal drainage system.

(2) See Chest tubes section in Table 7.5.

(3) Observe for *mediastinal shift* (trachea should always be midline; movement toward either side indicates shift).

(a) Move client onto back or toward opposite side.

(b) **MEDICAL EMERGENCY:** Notify physician immediately.

e. Goal: *maintain fluid and electrolyte balance.*

(1) Administer parenteral infusion slowly (risk of pulmonary edema due to decrease in pulmonary vasculature with removal of lung lobe or whole lung).

f. Goal: *postoperative teaching.*

(1) Prevent ankylosis of shoulder—teach passive and active ROM exercises of operative arm.

(2) Importance of early ambulation, as condition permits.

(3) Importance of stopping smoking.

(4) Dietary instructions—nutritious diet to aid in healing process.

(5) Importance of deep breathing, coughing exercises, to prevent stasis of respiratory secretions.

(6) Importance of increased fluids in diet to liquefy secretions.

(7) Desired and side effects of prescribed medications.

(8) Importance of rest, avoidance of heavy lifting and work during healing process.

(9) Importance of follow-up care; give names of referral agencies where client and family can obtain assistance.

(10) Signs and symptoms of complications.

D. Evaluation:

1. Client and/or significant other will be able to:

a. Give rationale for activity restriction and demonstrate prescribed exercises.

b. Identify name, dosage, side effects, and schedule of prescribed medications.

c. State plans for necessary modifications in lifestyle, home.

d. Identify support systems.

2. Wound heals without complications.

3. Obtains range of motion in affected shoulder.

4. No complications of thoracotomy:

a. Respiratory—pulmonary insufficiency, respiratory acidosis, pneumonitis, atelectasis, pulmonary edema.

b. Circulatory—hemorrhage, hypovolemia, shock, myocardial infarction.

c. Mediastinal shift.

d. Renal failure.

e. Gastric distention.

XIV. Tracheostomy: opening into trachea, temporary or permanent. *Rationale:* airway obstruction due to foreign body, edema, tumor, excessive tracheobronchial secretions, respiratory depression, decreased gaseous diffusion at alveolar membrane, or increased dead space (e.g., severe emphysema).

A. Analysis/nursing diagnosis:

1. *Ineffective airway clearance* related to increased secretions and decreased ability to cough effectively.

2. *Ineffective breathing pattern* related to physical condition that necessitated tracheostomy.

3. *Impaired verbal communication* related to inability to speak when tracheostomy tube cuff inflated.

4. *Fear* related to need for specialized equipment to breathe.

B. Nursing plan/implementation:

1. **Preoperative**

a. Goal: *relieve anxiety and fear.*

(1) Explain purpose of procedure and equipment.

(2) Demonstrate suctioning procedure.

(3) Establish means of postoperative communication, e.g., paper and pencil, magic slate, picture cards, and call bell. Specialized tubes such as a fenestrated tracheostomy tube or a tracheostomy button allow the individual to talk when the external opening is plugged.

(4) Remain with client as much as possible.

TABLE 4.11 Tracheostomy Suctioning Procedure

1. Suction as necessary to facilitate respirations.
2. *Position:* semi-Fowler's to prevent forward flexion of neck, to facilitate respiration, to promote drainage, and to minimize edema.
3. Administer *mist* to tracheostomy since natural humidifying of oropharynx pathways has been eliminated.
4. Auscultate for moist, noisy respirations as nonproductive coughing may indicate need for suctioning.
5. Prevent hypoxia by administering *100% oxygen before suctioning* (unless contraindicated).
6. Use *strict aseptic technique* and sterile suctioning catheters with each aspiration; use sterile saline to clear catheter of secretions. Keep dominant hand gloved with sterile glove, nondominant hand with nonsterile glove to control thumb control of suction.
7. *Do not apply suction when inserting* suction catheter to prevent injury to respiratory tract and prevent loss of oxygen.
8. If client coughs during suctioning, gently remove catheter to permit ejection and suction of mucus.
9. Apply suction intermittently for *no longer* than 10 to 15 seconds as prolonged suction decreases arterial oxygen concentrations. Do not suction for more than 3–5 minutes.
10. Cuff deflation: if high volume, low-pressure cuffed tube is used, deflation not necessary. If other tracheostomy cuffed tube is used, deflate for five minutes every hour to prevent damage to trachea.
11. Use caution not to dislodge tube when changing dressing or ties that secure tube.

2. **Postoperative**
   a. Goal: *maintain patent airway.* See Table 4.11.
   b. Goal: *alleviate apprehension.*
      (1) Remain with client as much as possible.
      (2) Encourage client to communicate feelings using preestablished communication system.
   c. Goal: *improve nutritional status.*
      (1) Provide nutritious foods/liquids the client can swallow.
      (2) Give supplemental drinks to maintain necessary calories.
   d. Goal: *health teaching.*
      (1) Explain all procedures.
      (2) Teach alternative methods of communication (best if done before the tracheostomy if it is not an emergency situation).
      (3) Teach self-care of tracheostomy as soon as possible.

C. Evaluation:
1. Airway patent.
2. Acid-base balance maintained.
3. No respiratory infection/obstruction.

■ PROTECTIVE FUNCTIONS

I. Burns: wounds caused by exposure to excessive heat, chemicals, fire, steam, radiation, or electricity; most often related to carelessness or ignorance; 10,000–12,000 deaths annually; survival best at ages 15–45 years and in burns covering less than 20% of total body surface.

A. Pathophysiology:
1. *Emergent phase* (injury to 72 hours): shock due to pain, fright, or terror → fatigue, failure of vasoconstrictor mechanisms → hypotension. Capillary dilatation, increased permeability → plasma loss to blisters, edema → hemoconcentration → hypovolemia → hypotension → decreased renal perfusion → renal shutdown.
2. *Acute phase* (3–5 days): interstitial-to-plasma-fluid shift → hemodilution → hypervolemia → heart failure → pulmonary edema.

B. Assessment:
1. Subjective data: how the burn occurred.
2. Objective data.
   a. Extent of body surface involved: "rule of nines"—head and both upper extremities, 9% each; front and back of trunk, 18% each; lower extremities, 18% each; and perineum, 1%. Requires adjustment for variation in size of head and lower extremities according to age.
   b. *Location*—facial, perineal, and hand and foot burns have potentially more complications and fatalities because of poor vascularization.
   c. *Depth* of burn (see Table 4.12):
      (1) *First degree*—epidermal tissue only; not serious unless large areas involved.
      (2) *Second degree*—epidermal and dermal tissue; hospitalization required if over 25% of body surface involved (major burn).
      (3) *Third degree*—destruction of all skin layers; requires immediate hospitalization; involvement of 10% of body surface considered major burn.
      (4) *Fourth degree*—skin and structures underneath.
   d. Indications of airway burns, e.g., singed nasal hair, brassy cough, sooty expectoration, increased mortality; edema may occur in 1 hour.
   e. Poorer prognosis—*infants,* due to immature immune system and effects of fluid loss; *elderly,* due to degenerative diseases and poor healing.
   f. Medical history—presence of hypertension, diabetes, alcohol abuse, or chronic obstructive pulmonary disease increases complication rate.

C. Analysis/nursing diagnosis:
1. *Impaired skin integrity* related to thermal injury.
2. *Pain* (depending on type of burn) related to exposure of sensory receptors.

TABLE 4.12 Characteristics of First-, Second-, Third-, and Fourth-Degree Burns

Characteristic	First-Degree (Superficial)	Second-Degree (Shallow or Deep Partial Thickness)	Third-Degree (Full Thickness)	Fourth-Degree (Deep Penetrating)
Depth of involvement (erythema)	Epidermis	Epidermis: dermal elements	All elements of skin	All elements of skin, fat, muscle, and bone
Color	Pink or red (erythema)	Cherry red, white, mottled	Tan, brown, black, marble white	Black
Skin surface	Dry; flaking or peeling within 2–3 days	Moist; blisters; minor scar tissue formation	Charred; dry; leathery; scar tissue formation	Charred; dry; leathery; scar tissue formation
Pain	Mild pain	Pain	No pain	No pain
Healing period	3–5 days	14–21 days	Grafting needed	Grafting needed

Source: From Saxton et al.: *The Addison-Wesley Manual of Nursing Practice,* Menlo Park, CA: Addison-Wesley, 1983.

ADULT NURSING

3. *Fluid volume excess or deficit* related to hemodynamic changes.
4. *Potential for infection* related to destruction of protective skin.
5. *Body image disturbance* related to scarring, disfigurement.
6. *Impaired gas exchange* related to airway injury.
7. *Ineffective individual or family coping* related to traumatic experience.

D. Nursing plan/implementation:

1. Goal: *alleviate pain, relieve shock, and maintain fluid and electrolyte balance.*
   a. Medications: give narcotic while physical exam is being completed and removing burned clothing.
   b. Fluids: IV therapy (see Unit 7); colloids, crystalloids, or 5% dextrose according to burn formula.
   c. Monitor hydration status:
      (1) Insert in-dwelling catheter.
      (2) Note color, odor, and amount of urine; report fixed specific gravity—may indicate kidney problems.
      (3) *Strict* intake and output.
      (4) Check hematocrit (normal: men >54%; women >47%).
      (5) Weigh daily.
   d. Soak: small burns may be soaked in cool saline.
2. Goal: *prevent physical complications.*
   a. Vital signs: hourly; central venous pressure (CVP) for signs of shock or fluid overload.
   b. Assess respiratory function (particularly with head, neck burns); patent airway; breath sounds.
   c. Give medications as ordered—*tetanus booster; antibiotics* to prevent infection; *sedatives* and *analgesics; steroids; antipyretics*—avoid aspirin.
   d. Isolation: protective; *strict* surgical asepsis (handwashing, protective clothing).
   e. *Positioning:* turn q2h; prevent contractures—stryker frame or circle bed if circumferential trunk burns present.
      (1) Head and neck burns—use pillows under shoulders only for hyperextension of neck.
      (2) Hand burns—use towel rolls or sandbags to align hands.
      (3) Upper-body burns—keep arms at 90° angle from body and slightly above shoulders.
      (4) Ankle and foot burns—allow feet to hang at 90° angle from ankles in prone position; use footboards to maintain angle in supine position; elevate to prevent edema.
      (5) Traction and splints to maintain positions.
      (6) ROM exercises according to therapy guidelines; usually several times per day; active exercises most beneficial.
   f. Diet: initially NPO; begin oral fluids after bowel sounds return; do *not* give ice chips or free water, as these may contribute to electrolyte imbalance; food as tolerated—high-protein, high-calorie for energy and tissue repair (promote positive nitrogen balance).
   g. Observe for:
      (1) Curling's (stress) ulcer—sudden drop in hemoglobin, melena (give antacids, cimetidine as ordered).
      (2) Constriction due to eschar (circumferential or chest wall)—prepare for escharotomy, (lengthwise incisions), painless procedure.
3. Goal: *promote emotional adjustment and provide supportive therapy.*
   a. Care by same personnel as much as possible, to develop rapport and trust.
   b. Involve client in care plans.
   c. Answer questions clearly, accurately.
   d. Encourage family involvement and participation.
   e. Provide diversional activities and change furnishings or room adornments when possible, to prevent perceptual deprivation related to immobility.
   f. Point out signs of progress (e.g., decreased edema, healing) as client and family tend to become discouraged and cannot see progress.
   g. Encourage self-care to highest level tolerated.
   h. Anticipate psychologic changes:
      (1) *Acute period*—severe anxiety, mental confusion: orient to person, place, time; maintain eye contact; explain procedures.

(2) *Intermediate period*—reactions associated with pain, dependency, depression, anger: give medications to decrease pain; explain procedures; use other clients as models; have open, nonjudgmental attitude; use consistent approaches to care; contract with client regarding division of responsibilities; encourage self-care.

(3) *Recuperative period*—grief process reactivated. Anxiety, depression, anger, bargaining, as client tries to cope with altered body image, leaving security of hospital, finances. Encourage verbalization; refer to self-help group to assist adaptation.

4. Goal: *promote wound healing*—wound care:

a. *Open method*—exposure of burns to drying effect of air; useful in burns of neck, face, trunk, and perineum; eliminates painful dressing changes; protective isolation may be required.

b. *Closed method*—pressure dressings applied to burned areas, particularly extremities; changed 1–3 times/day; if ordered, give pain medication 30 min before change; tubbing facilitates removal.

c. *Topical therapies* (see Table 4.13).

d. *Tubbing and debridement:*

(1) Hydrotherapy—body temperature bath water; loosens dressings so they float off; soak 20–30 min; encourage limb exercises; do not leave unattended; loss of body heat may occur, with chilling and poor perfusion resulting.

(2) Removal of eschar (debridement)—done with forceps and curved scissors; medicate for pain before; use sterile technique; only loose eschar removed, to prevent bleeding; examine wound for infection, color change, decreased granulation—report changes immediately.

e. Wound coverage, to decrease chances of infection:

(1) Biological dressings (see Table 4.14).

(2) *Autograft*—client donates skin for wound coverage.

(a) Types—free (unattached to donor site) and pedicle grafts (attached to donor site).

(b) Procedure—general anesthesia; donor sites shaved and prepared; graft applied to granulation bed; face, hands, and arms grafted first.

(c) *Post–skin-graft care:*

(i) Roll graft with cotton-tipped applicator to remove excess exudate, maintaining dressings, and with aseptic technique using heat lamps to dry donor sites.

(ii) Third to fifth day—graft takes on pink appearance if it has taken.

(iii) Skeletal traction may be applied, to prevent contractures.

(iv) Elastic bandages may be applied 6 months to 1 year, to prevent hypertrophic scarring.

5. Goal: *health teaching.*

a. Mobility needs: exercise; physical therapy; splints, braces.

b. Community resources: mental health practitioner or psychotherapist if needed for problems with self-image or sexual role; referrals as needed.

c. Techniques to camouflage appearance: slacks, turtlenecks, long sleeves, wigs, makeup.

E. Evaluation:

1. Return of vital signs to preburn levels.
2. Minimal to no hypertrophic scarring.
3. Free of infection; demonstrates wound care.
4. Maintains functional mobility of limbs; no contractures.
5. Adjusts to changes in body image; no depression.
6. Regains independence; returns to work, social activities.

II. Lyme disease: a spirochetal illness (syndrome) carried by infected ticks; incidence greatest during May through August when out of doors and wearing fewer clothes; only a small percentage of people hospitalized.

A. Stages:

(I) Rash at site of tick bite; bullseye or target pattern; may appear as hives or cellulitis; common in moist areas (groin, armpit, behind knees). Flulike symptoms may occur (joint pain, chills, fever).

(II) If untreated, may progress to cardiac problems (10% of patients) or neurologic disturbances—Bell's palsy (10% of patients); occasionally meningitis, encephalitis, and eye damage may result.

(III) From four weeks to a year after the tick bite, "arthritis" develops in half the patients. If untreated, chronic neurologic problems may develop.

B. Assessment (depends on stage):

1. Subjective data:
   a. Malaise (I).
   b. Headache (I).
   c. Joint, neck, or back pain (I and III).
   d. Weakness (II and III).
   e. Chest pain (II).
   f. Lightheadedness (II).
   g. Numbness, pain in arms or legs (III).
2. Objective data:
   a. Rash—erythema migrans (I).
   b. Dysrhythmias; heart block (II).
   c. Facial paralysis (II).
   d. Conjunctivitis, iritis, optic neuritis (II).
   e. Lab data: Lyme titer—elevated (II and III).
   f. Diagnostic tests: Joint aspiration—fibrous exudate, WBCs, immune complexes; Synovium biopsy—lymphocytic infiltrates.

C. Analysis/nursing diagnosis:

1. *Anxiety* related to diagnosis.
2. *Pain* related to joint inflammation.
3. *Fatigue* related to viral illness.
4. *Impaired physical mobility* related to joint pain.
5. *Altered thought processes* related to neurologic deficit.

TABLE 4.13 Topical Preparations Used in Burn Care

Preparation	Advantages	Disadvantages	Nursing Actions
Silver sulfadiazine (Silvadene)	Wide-spectrum antimicrobial. Antifungal. Nonstaining. Relatively painless. Usable without dressings. No systemic metabolic abnormalities.	Less eschar penetration than Sulfamylon. Decreased granulocyte formation.	Check for allergy to sulfa; sometimes causes rash.
Mafenide acetate (Sulfamylon)	Eschar penetration. Effective with *Pseudomonas.* Topical of choice for electrical burns. Suitable for open method of treatment. Used for gram-negative organisms.	Severe pain and burning sensation (lasts 30 min). Acidic breakdown product. Carbonic anhydrase inhibitor. Ineffective against fungi. May cause hypersensitivity rash.	Administer pretreatment analgesic. Monitor for metabolic acidosis and hyperventilation. Check for allergy to sulfa; observe for rash.
Povidone-iodine (Betadine)	Antifungal. Wide-spectrum microbicidal.	Iodine absorption. Staining of clothing. Dressing necessary. Metabolic acidosis.	Assess for allergy to iodine. Check serum iodine levels.
Bismuth tribromphenate (Xeroform)	On Vaseline gauze, so conforms to wound.	Painful removal.	Alert patient to discomfort before removing. Keep dressings wet. Perform active debridement.
Silver nitrate	Low cost.	Continuous wet soaks. Superficial penetration. Black staining. Stinging. Electrolyte imbalances (low sodium, low chloride, low calcium), alkalosis.	Check serum electrolytes daily.
Enzymatic Debriding Agents			
Fibrinolysin and deoxyribonuclease (Elase)	Digestion of necrotic material.	Burning sensation.	Remove dry eschar before applying.
Sutilains (Travase)	Digestion of necrotic material.	Refrigeration necessary. Irritation of wound and skin. Can cause some bleeding. Can cause fluid loss. Painful on partial-thickness burn.	Limit use to 10–15% of burn surface at one time. Observe for infection. Cross-hatch eschar if necessary to allow optimal penetration. Monitor fluid balance. Assess need for analgesic.

Source: Holloway N: *Nursing the Critically Ill Adult,* 3rd ed., p. 566. Addison-Wesley, Menlo Park, CA, 1988.

ADULT NURSING

■ TABLE 4.14 Types of Burn Dressings

Preparation	Advantages	Disadvantages
Poly-2-hydroxyethylmethacrylate (Hydron)	Spray powder. Flexible. Conforms to wound.	Fluid loss via oozing.
Pigskin	Relief of pain. Reduction of water and heat loss. Available in several forms. Can be meshed.	Costly. Can provoke rejection.
Cadaver skin	Relief of pain. Reduction of water and heat loss. Can be meshed.	Expensive. Scarce and not always available.
Amniotic membrane	Biologic dressing. Relief of pain. Reduction of water and heat loss.	Difficult to apply at times.
Op-site (polyurethane)	Permeable to air. Not permeable to fluid or bacteria—promotes wound healing in moist environment. No scab formation. No debridement necessary. Immediate pain reduction. Painless removal. Transparent. Significantly shortens healing time.	Time-consuming application. Self-adhesive—can be difficult to apply. Not suitable for full-thickness burns.

Source: Conkle W: Op-site dressing: New approach to burn care. *J Emer Nurs* (January/February) St. Louis, C. V. Mosby, 1981; 9–16; and Holloway N: *Nursing the Critically Ill Adult,* 3rd ed., p. 567. Addison-Wesley, Menlo Park, CA, 1988.

6. *Decreased cardiac output* related to dysrhythmias.
7. *Knowledge deficit* related to treatment and course of disease.

D. Nursing plan/implementation:

1. Goal: *minimize irreversible tissue damage and complications.*
   a. Medications: *Stage I*—oral antibiotics for 21 days (doxycycline and Pen V K); *Stages II and III*—intravenous antibiotics for 14 days (penicillin or ceftriaxone).
   b. If hospitalized, monitor vital signs q4h for increased temperature, signs of heart failure; check level of consciousness and cranial nerve functioning.
   c. Note treatment response: worsening of symptoms during first 24 h; redder rash, higher fever, greater pain (Jarisch-Herxheimer reaction).
2. Goal: *alleviate pain, promote comfort.*
   a. Medications: salicylates, nonsteroidal anti-inflammatory agents or other analgesic, as ordered; observe for side effects (GI irritation).
   b. Rest: give instructions on relaxation techniques; create a quiet environment.
3. Goal: *maintain physical and psychological well-being.*
   a. Activity: ROM at regular intervals; medicate for pain prior to exercise; encourage proper posture to reduce joint stress; rest periods between activities and treatments.
   b. Referral: occupational and/or physical therapy as appropriate.
   c. Reassurance: give psychological support; encourage discussion of feelings.
4. Goal: *health teaching.*
   a. Information on disease.
   b. Instructions for home IV antibiotics with heparin lock, if ordered.
   c. Side effects of antibiotics (drug-specific); importance of completing therapy.
   d. Signs of disease recurrence (later stages of disease; less severe attacks).
   e. Preventing subsequent infections: wear proper clothing and tick repellent on clothing; conduct "tick checks" of self, children, and pets.

E. Evaluation:

1. Achieves reasonable comfort.
2. Regains normal physiologic and psychologic functioning—no irreversible complications; vital signs within normal limits.
3. Resumes previous activity level; returns to work.
4. Adheres to follow-up care recommendations.
5. Knows ways to minimize risk of reinfection.

III. Rheumatoid arthritis: chronic, systemic, collagen, inflammatory disease; etiology unknown; may be autoimmune, viral, or genetic; affects primarily women 20–40 years of age; present in 2–3% of total population; follows a course of exacerbations and remissions.

A. Pathophysiology: synovitis with edema → proliferation of various blood material (formation of pannus) → destruction and fibrosis of cartilage (fibrous ankylosis); calcification of fibrous tissue (osseous ankylosis).

B. Assessment:

1. Subjective data
   a. Joints: pain; stiffness; swelling.
   b. Easily fatigues; malaise.
   c. Anorexia; weight loss.
2. Objective data
   a. Subcutaneous nodules over bony prominences.
   b. Bilateral symmetric involvement of joints: crepitation, creaking, grating.
   c. Deformities: contractures, muscle atrophy.
   d. Lab data: blood: *decreased*—RBCs; *increased*—WBCs (12,000–15,000), sedimentation rate (>20 mm/h), rheumatoid factor.

C. Analysis/nursing diagnosis:

1. *Pain* related to joint destruction.
2. *Impaired physical mobility* related to joint contractures.
3. *Potential for injury* related to the inflammatory process.
4. *Body image disturbance* related to joint deformity.
5. *Self-care deficit* related to musculoskeletal impairment.
6. *Potential activity intolerance* related to fatigue and stiffness.
7. *Altered nutrition, less than body requirements,* related to anorexia and weight loss.
8. *Self-esteem disturbance* related to chronic illness.

D. Nursing plan/implementation:

1. Goal: *prevent or correct deformities.*
   a. Activity:
      (1) Bedrest during exacerbations.
      (2) Daily ROM—active and passive exercises *even* in acute phase 5–10-min periods; avoid fatigue and persistent pain.
      (3) Heat and/or pain medication before exercise.
   b. Medications: *aspirin* (high dosages); *nonsteroidals; steroids; antacids* given for possible GI upset with ASA, steroids.
   c. Fluids: at least 1500 mL liquid daily to avoid renal calculi; milk for GI upset.
2. Goal: *health teaching.*
   a. Side effects of medications: tarry stools (GI bleeding); tinnitus (ASA).
   b. Psychosocial aspects: possible need for early retirement; financial hardship; loss of libido; unsatisfactory sexual relations.
   c. Prepare for joint repair or replacement if indicated.

E. Evaluation:

1. Remains as active as possible; limited loss of mobility; performs self-care activities.
2. No side effects from drug therapy (e.g., GI bleeding).
3. Copes with necessary life-style changes; complies with treatment regimen.

IV. Systemic lupus erythematosus (SLE): chronic inflammatory disease of connective tissue; may affect or involve any organ; vague etiology, but genetic factors, viruses, hormones, or drugs are being investigated; occurs primarily in women ages 18–35.

A. Pathophysiology: possible toxic effects from immune complexes deposited in tissue—fibrinoid necrosis of collagen in connective tissue, small arterial walls (kidneys and heart particularly) → cellular death, obstructed blood flow.

B. Assessment:

1. Subjective data
   a. Pain: joints.
   b. Anorexia; weight loss.
   c. Photophobia; sensitivity to sun.
   d. Weakness.
   e. Nausea, vomiting.
2. Objective data
   a. Fever.
   b. Rash: butterfly distribution across nose, cheeks.
   c. Ulcerations: oral or nasopharyngeal.
   d. Lab data:
      (1) Blood: *increased* LE cells; *decreased*—RBCs, WBCs, thrombocytes.
      (2) *Urine*—hematuria, proteinuria (nephritis).

C. Analysis/nursing diagnosis:

1. *Potential for injury* related to possible autoimmune disorder.
2. *Pain* related to joint inflammation.
3. *Potential activity intolerance* related to extreme fatigue, anemia.
4. *Impaired skin integrity* related to sunlight sensitivity and rashes.
5. *Altered nutrition, less than body requirements,* related to anorexia, nausea, vomiting.
6. *Altered oral mucous membrane* related to ulcerations.

D. Nursing plan/implementation:

1. Goal: *minimize or limit immune response and complications.*
   a. Activity: rest; 8–10 hours sleep; unhurried environment; assist with stressful activities; ROM to prevent joint immobility and stiffness.

b. Skin care: hygiene; topical steroid cream as ordered for inflammation, pruritus, scaling.

c. Mouth care: several times daily if stomatitis present; soft, bland or liquid diet to prevent irritation.

d. Diet: low sodium if edematous; low protein with renal involvement.

e. Observe for signs of complications:

(1) *Cardiac* (tachycardia, tachypnea, dyspnea, orthopnea).

(2) *GI* (diarrhea, abdominal pain, distention).

(3) *Renal* (increased weight, oliguria, decreased specific gravity).

(4) *Neurologic* (ptosis, ataxia).

(5) *Hematologic* (malaise, weakness, chills, epitaxis); report immediately.

f. Medications, as ordered:

(1) *Analgesics*.

(2) *Anti-inflammatory* agents (aspirin, prednisone) and *immunosuppressive* drugs (Imuran, Cytoxan) to control inflammation.

(3) *Anti-malarials* for skin and joint manifestations.

2. Goal: *health teaching*.

a. Disease process: diagnosis, prognosis, effects of treatment.

b. *Avoid* precipitating factors:

(1) Sun (aggravates skin lesions; thus, cover body as much as possible).

(2) Altering dosage of medications.

(3) Pregnancy needs medical clearance.

(4) Fatigue, stress.

(5) Infections.

c. Medications: side effects of immunosuppressives and corticosteroids.

d. Regular exercise: walking, swimming; but avoid fatigue.

e. Wear MedicAlert bracelet.

E. Evaluation:

1. Attains a state of remission.
2. No organ involvement (e.g., cardiac, renal complications).
3. Keeps active within limitations.
4. Continues follow-up medical care—recognizes symptoms requiring immediate attention.

V. Acquired immune deficiency syndrome (AIDS): the terminal stage of the disease continuum caused by human immunodeficiency virus (HIV), a retrovirus; typically progresses from asymptomatic seronegative status to asymptomatic seropositive status to subclinical immune deficiency to lymphadenopathy to AIDS-related complex (ARC) to AIDS; hallmarks of HIV infection include opportunistic infections: *Pneumocystis carinii* pneumonia (PCP); cytomegalovirus (CMV); *Mycobacterium tuberculosis;* hepatitis B; herpes simplex or zoster; candidiasis; may take 3–5 years before signs and symptoms occur.

A. High-risk populations:

1. Males, homosexual or bisexual.
2. Intravenous substance abusers.
3. Hemophiliacs and multiple transfusion recipients (particularly before 1985).
4. Sexual partners of persons with HIV infection or at risk for infection.
5. Infants of HIV-infected women.

B. Pathophysiology: abnormal response to foreign antigen stimulation (acquired immunity) → deficiency in cell-mediated immunity—T lymphocytes, specifically helper cells (T4 cells) and hyperactivity of the humoral system (B cells).

C. Assessment:

1. Subjective data

a. Fatigue: prolonged; associated with headache or light-headedness.

b. Unexplained weight loss: >10%.

2. Objective data

a. Fever: prolonged or night sweats >2 weeks.

b. Lymphadenopathy.

c. Skin or mucous membrane lesions: purplish, nodules, or plaques.

d. Cough: persistent, heavy, dry.

e. Diarrhea: persistent.

f. Tongue/mouth "thrush"; oral hairy leukoplakia.

▶ g. Diagnostic tests (with permission of patient): enzyme-linked immunosorbent assay (ELISA); Western blot test.

h. Lab data: *Decreased*—T4 count, serum cholesterol, platelets; *elevated*—LDH, serum globulin, erythrocyte sedimentation rate; seropositive—syphilis, hepatitis B; enzyme-linked immunosorbent assay (ELISA)—positive; Western blot test—positive (mean time for seroconversion is 6 weeks after infection).

D. Analysis/nursing diagnosis:

1. *Potential for infection* related to immunocompromised state.
2. *Fatigue* related to anemia.
3. *Altered nutrition, less than body requirements,* related to anorexia.
4. *Impaired skin integrity* related to nonhealing viral lesions, Kaposi sarcoma.
5. *Diarrhea* related to infection or parasites.
6. *Potential activity intolerance* related to shortness of breath.
7. *Ineffective airway clearance* related to pneumonia.
8. *Visual sensory/perception alteration* related to retinitis.
9. *Potential altered body temperature* (fever) related to opportunistic infections.
10. *Social isolation* related to stigma attached to AIDS.
11. *Powerlessness* related to inability to control disease progression.
12. *Altered thought processes* related to dementia.
13. *Ineffective individual coping* related to poor prognosis.
14. *Potential for violence, self-directed,* related to anger, panic, or depression.

TABLE 4.15 Universal Precautions

1. Wash hands before and after all patient or specimen contact.
2. Handle blood or body fluids of all patients as potentially infectious.
3. Wear gloves for potential contact with blood and body fluids.
4. Wear protective eyewear and mask if splatter with blood and body fluids is possible.
5. Wear gowns when splash with blood and body fluids is anticipated.
6. Place used needles and syringes in impermeable container in the patient's room. DO NOT recap or manipulate needles. Replace container when full.
7. Handle all linen soiled with blood or body secretions as potentially infectious.

E. Nursing plan/implementation:

1. Goal: *reduce risk of infection; slow disease progression.*
   a. Observe signs of opportunistic infections: weight loss, diarrhea, skin lesions, sore throat.
   b. Monitor vital signs (including temperature).
   c. Note secretions and excretions: changes in color, consistency, or odor indicating infection.
   d. Diet: monitor fluid and electrolytes; strict measurement; encourage adequate dietary intake (high calorie, high nutrient, low bulk); 5–10 times RDA for water-soluble vitamins (B complex, C); favorite foods from home; enteral feedings.
   e. Protective isolation, if indicated, for severe immunocompromise.
   f. Medications, as ordered: zidovudine (Retrovir), trimethaprim-sulfametherazole (Septra), acyclovir (Zovirax), and/or pentamidine; do not give at mealtime; may need antinauseants or antiemetics to control side effects.
2. Goal: *prevent the spread of disease.*
   a. Frequent handwashing, even after wearing gloves.
   b. Avoid exposure to blood, body fluids of client; wear gloves, gowns; proper disposal of needles, IV catheters (see Table 4.15).
3. Goal: *provide physical and psychological support.*
   a. Oral care: frequent.
   b. Cooling bath: 1:10 concentration of isopropyl alcohol in tepid water; avoid plastic-backed pads with night sweats.
   c. Encourage verbalization of fears, concerns without condemnation; may suffer loss of job, lifestyle, significant other.
   d. Determine status of support network: arrange contact with support group.
   e. Observe for severe emotional symptoms (suicidal tendencies).
   f. Address issues surrounding death to ensure quality of life: designation of durable power of attorney for health care; code blue status; reassurance of comfort and pain control.
4. Goal: *health teaching.*
   a. Avoidance of environmental sources of infection (kitty litter, bird cages, tub bathing).
   b. Precautions following discharge: risk-reducing behaviors; condoms (latex), limit number of sexual partners, avoid exposure to blood or semen during intercourse.
   c. Family counseling; availability of community resources.
   d. Information on disease progression and life span.
   e. Stress reduction techniques: visualization, guided imagery, meditation.
   f. Expected side effects with drug therapy; importance of compliance.

F. Evaluation:

1. Relief of symptoms (e.g., afebrile, gains weight).
2. Resumes self-care activities; returns to work; improved quality of life.
3. Accepts diagnosis; participates in support group.
4. Progression of disease slows; improved survival probability.
5. Retains autonomy, self-worth.
6. Permitted to die with dignity.

THE PERIOPERATIVE EXPERIENCE

I. Preoperative preparation

A. Assessment:

1. Subjective data
   a. Understanding of proposed surgery—site, type, extent of hospitalization.
   b. Previous experiences with hospitalization.
   c. Concerns or feelings about surgery:
      (1) Exaggerated ideas of surgical risk, i.e., fear of colostomy when none is being considered.
      (2) Nature of anesthesia, i.e., fears of going to sleep and not waking up, saying or revealing things of a personal nature.
      (3) Degree of pain, i.e., may be incapacitating.
      (4) Misunderstandings regarding prognosis.
   d. Identification of significant others as a source of client support and/or care responsibilities postdischarge.
2. Objective data
   a. Speech patterns indicating anxiety—repetition, changing topics, avoiding talking about feelings.
   b. Interactions with others—withdrawn or involved.
   c. Physical signs of anxiety, i.e., increased pulse, respirations; clammy palms, restlessness.
   d. Baseline physiologic status: vital signs; breath sounds; peripheral circulation; weight; hydration status (hematocrit, skin turgor, urine output); degree of mobility; muscle strength.

B. Analysis/nursing diagnosis:

1. *Anxiety* related to proposed surgery.
2. *Knowledge deficit* related to incomplete teaching or lack of understanding.

3. *Fear* related to threat of death or disfigurement.
4. *Potential for injury* related to surgical complications.
5. *Ineffective individual coping* related to anticipatory stress.

C. Nursing plan/implementation:

1. Goal: *reduce preoperative and intraoperative anxiety and prevent postoperative complications.*
   a. *Preoperative teaching:*
      (1) Provide information about hospital and nursing routines to reduce fear of unknown.
      (2) Explain purpose of diagnostic procedures to enhance ability to cooperate and tolerate procedure.
      (3) What will occur and what will be expected in the postoperative period:
         (a) Will return to room, recovery room, or intensive care unit.
         (b) Special equipment—monitors, tubes, suction equipment.
2. Goal: *instruct in exercises to reduce complications.*
   a. *Diaphragmatic breathing*—refers to flattening of diaphragm during inspiration, which results in enlargement of upper abdomen; during expiration the abdominal muscles are contracted, along with the diaphragm.
      (1) The client should be in a *flat, semi-Fowler's,* or *side* position, with knees flexed and hands on the midabdomen.
      (2) Have the client take a deep breath through nose and mouth, letting the abdomen rise.
      (3) Have client exhale through nose and mouth, squeezing out all air by contracting the abdominal muscles.
      (4) Repeat 10 to 15 times, with a short rest after each five to prevent hyperventilation.
      (5) Inform client that this exercise will be repeated 5 to 10 times every hour postoperatively.
   b. *Coughing*—helps clear chest of secretions and, although uncomfortable, will not harm incision site.
      (1) Have client lean forward slightly from a sitting position, and place client's hands over incisional site; this acts as a splint during coughing.
      (2) Have client inhale and exhale several times.
      (3) Have client inhale deeply and cough sharply three times as exhaling—client's mouth should be slightly open.
      (4) Tell client to inhale again and to cough deeply once or twice.
   c. *Turning and leg exercises*—help prevent circulatory stasis, which may lead to thrombus formation and postoperative flatus, or "gas pains," as well as respiratory problems.
      (1) Tell client to turn on one side with uppermost leg flexed; use side rails to facilitate the movement.
      (2) In a supine position, have client bend the knee and lift the foot; this position should be held for a few seconds, then the leg should be extended and lowered; repeat five times, and do the same with the other leg.
      (3) Teach client to move each foot through full range of motion.
3. Goal: *reduce the number of bacteria on the skin to eliminate incision contamination.* Skin preparation:
   a. Prepare area of skin wider and longer than proposed incision in case a larger incision is necessary.
   b. Gently scrub with an antiseptic agent such as Betadine. Note possibility of allergy to iodine.
      (1) Hexachlorophene should be left on the skin for 5–10 minutes.
      (2) If Zephiran Cl solution is ordered, do *not* soap skin prior to use; soap reduces effectiveness of Zephiran by causing it to precipitate.
   c. Use clean safety razor with a new blade if shaving ordered; shave against grain of hair shaft.
   d. Note any nicks, cuts, or irritations, potential infection sites.
   e. Depilatory creams: if ordered, leave on skin for 10 minutes, then wash off along with the hair; occasional side effect—transient rashes.
   f. Clipping of hair, rather than shaving or depilatories, may be ordered.
   g. Skin prep may be done in surgery.
4. Goal: *reduce the risk of vomiting and aspiration during anesthesia; prevent contamination of abdominal operative sites by fecal material.* Gastrointestinal tract preparation:
   a. No food or fluid at least 4 hours prior to surgery.
   b. Remove food and water from bedside.
   c. Place NPO signs on bed or door.
   d. Inform kitchen and oncoming nursing staff that patient is NPO for surgery.
   e. Give IV infusions up to time of surgery if dehydrated or malnourished.
   f. Enemas: two or three may be given the evening prior to surgery with intestinal, colon, or pelvic surgeries; 3 days of cleansing with large-intestine procedures.
   g. Possible antibiotic therapy to reduce colonic flora with large-bowel surgery.
   h. Gastric or intestinal intubation may be inserted the evening prior to major abdominal surgery.
      (1) Types of tubes:
         (a) Levin: single-lumen; sufficient to remove fluids and gas from stomach; suction may damage mucosa.
         (b) Salem-sump: large lumen; prevents tissue–wall adherence.
         (c) Miller-Abbott: long single- or double-lumen; required to remove the contents of jejunum or ileum.
      (2) Pressures: low setting with Levin and intestinal tubes; high setting with Salem-sump; ex-

cessive pressures will result in injury to mucosal lining of intestine or stomach.

5. Goal: *promote rest and facilitate reduction of apprehension.*
   a. Medications as ordered: on evening prior to surgery may give barbiturate—pentobarbital (Nembutal), secobarbital (Seconal).
   b. Quiet environment: eliminate noises, distractions.
   c. Position: reduce muscle tension.
   d. Back rub.
6. Goal: *protect from injury; ensure final preparation for surgery.* Day of surgery:
   a. Operative permit signed and on chart.
   b. Shower or bathe.
      (1) Dress: hospital pajamas.
      (2) Remove: hair pins (cover hair); nail polish, to facilitate observation of peripheral circulation; jewelry (tape wedding bands securely); pierced earrings; contact lenses; dentures (store and give mouth care); give valuable personal items to family; chart disposition of items.
   c. Proper identification—check band for secureness and legibility.
   d. Vital signs—baseline data.
   e. Void, to prevent distention and possible injury to bladder.
   f. Give preoperative medication to ensure smooth induction and maintenance of anesthesia:
      (1) Administered 45–75 minutes before anesthetic induction.
      (2) Siderails up (client will begin to feel drowsy and lightheaded).
      (3) Expect complaint of dry mouth if atropine SO_4 given.
      (4) Observe for side effects—morphine SO_4 and meperidine (Demerol) HCl may cause nausea and vomiting or drop in blood pressure.
      (5) Quiet environment until transported to operating room.
   g. Note completeness of chart:
      (1) Surgical checklist completed.
      (2) Vital signs recorded.
      (3) Routine laboratory reports present.
      (4) Preoperative medications given.
      (5) Significant client observations.
   h. Assist client's family in finding proper waiting room.
      (1) Inform them that the surgeon will contact them after the procedure is over.
      (2) Explain length of time client is expected to be in recovery room.
      (3) Prepare family for any special equipment or devices that may be needed to care for client postoperatively—oxygen, monitoring equipment, ventilator, or blood transfusions.

II. Intraoperative preparation—anesthesia: blocks transmission of nerve impulses, suppresses reflexes, promotes muscle relaxation, and in some instances achieves reversible unconsciousness.

A. Regional anesthesia—purpose is to block pain reception and transmission in a specified area. Commonly used drugs are lidocaine HCl, tetracaine HCl, cocaine HCl, and procaine HCl. Types of regional anesthetics:

1. *Topical*—applied to mucous membranes or skin; drug anesthetizes the nerves immediately *below* the area. May be used for bronchoscopic or laryngoscopic examinations. Side effects: rare anaphylaxis.
2. *Local infiltration*—used for minor procedures; anesthetic drug is injected directly into the area to be incised, manipulated, or sutured. Side effects: rare anaphylaxis.
3. *Peripheral nerve block*—regional anesthesia is achieved by injecting drug into or around a nerve after it passes from vertebral column; procedure is named for nerve involved, such as brachial-plexus block. Requires a high degree of anatomic knowledge. *Side effects:* may be absorbed into bloodstream. Observe for signs of excitability, twitching, changes in vital signs, or respiratory difficulties.
4. *Field block*—a group of nerves is injected with anesthetic as the nerves branch from a major or main nerve trunk. May be used for dental procedures, plastic surgery. Side effects: rare.
5. *Epidural anesthesia*—anesthetizing drug is injected into the epidural space of vertebral canal; produces a bandlike anesthesia around body. Frequently used in obstetrics. Rare complications.
6. *Spinal anesthesia*—anesthetizing drug is injected into the subarachnoid space and mixes with spinal fluid; drug acts on the nerves as they emerge from the spinal cord, thereby inhibiting conduction in the autonomic, sensory, and motor systems.
   a. Advantages: rapid onset; produces excellent muscle relaxation.
   b. Utilization: surgery on lower limbs, perineum, and lower abdomen.
   c. Disadvantages:
      (1) Loss of sensation below point of injection for 2–8 hours—watch for signs of *bladder distention;* prevent injuries by maintaining alignment, keeping bedclothes straightened.
      (2) Client awake during surgical procedure—avoid light or upsetting conversations.
      (3) Leakage of spinal fluid from puncture site—keep flat in bed for 8 hours to prevent headache. Keep well hydrated to aid in spinal-fluid replacement.
      (4) Depression of vasomotor responses—frequent checks of vital signs.
7. *Intravenous regional anesthesia*—used in an extremity whose circulation has been interrupted by a tourniquet; the anesthetic is injected into vein, and blockage is presumed to be achieved from extravascular leakage of anesthetic near a major nerve trunk. Precautions as for peripheral nerve block.

B. General anesthesia—a reversible state in which the client loses consciousness due to the inhibition of neuronal impulses in the brain by a variety of chemical agents; may be given intravenously, by inhalation, or rectally.

1. *Side effects:*
   a. Respiratory depression.
   b. Nausea, vomiting.
   c. Excitement.
   d. Restlessness.
   e. Laryngospasm.
   f. Hypotension.
2. **Nursing plan/implementation**—Goal: *prevent hazardous drug interactions.*
   a. *Notify anesthesiologist* if client is taking any of the following drugs:
      (1) *Antibiotics,* such as neomycin SO_4, streptomycin SO_4, polymyxin A and B SO_4, colistin SO_4, and kanamycin SO_4—when mixed with curariform muscle relaxant they interrupt nerve transmission and may cause *respiratory paralysis and apnea.*
      (2) *Antidepressants*—particularly MAO (monoamine oxidase) inhibitors, which increase *hypotensive* effects of anesthetic agents.
      (3) *Diuretics*—particularly thiazide diuretics, which may induce *potassium depletion;* a potassium deficit may lead to *respiratory depression* during anesthesia.
      (4) *Antihypertensives,* such as reserpine, hydralazine, and methyldopa—*potentiate* the hypotensive effects of anesthetic agents.
      (5) *Anticoagulants,* such as heparin, Coumadin—increase bleeding times, which may result in excessive *blood loss* and/or hemorrhage.
      (6) *Aspirin*—decreases platelet aggregation and may result in increased *bleeding.*
      (7) *Steroids,* such as cortisone—anti-inflammatory effect may *delay* wound-healing.
   b. *Stages of inhalation anesthesia and nursing goals:*
      (1) Stage I—extends from beginning of induction to loss of consciousness. Nursing goal: *reduce external stimuli,* as all movement and noises are exaggerated for the client and can be highly distressing.
      (2) Stage II—extends from loss of consciousness to relaxation; stage of delirium and excitement. Nursing goal: *prevent injury* by assisting anesthesiologist to restrain client if necessary; maintain a quiet, nonstimulating environment.
      (3) Stage III—extends from loss of lid reflex to cessation of voluntary respirations. Nursing goal: *reduce risk of untoward effects* by preparing the operative site, assisting with procedures, and observing for signs of complications.
      (4) Stage IV—indicates overdose and consists of respiratory arrest and vasomotor collapse due to medullary paralysis. Nursing goal: *promote restoration of ventilation and vasomotor tone* by assisting with cardiac arrest procedures and by administering cardiac stimulants or narcotic antagonists as ordered.

C. Muscle relaxants—given to supplement general anesthetic agents, i.e., curare, succinylcholine Cl (Anectine).

1. **Actions:**
   a. Facilitates endotracheal intubation.
   b. Relaxes abdominal muscles.
   c. Facilitates the administration of lower doses of potent general anesthetic.
2. **Nursing plan/implementation:**
   a. Goal: *observe for respiratory depression*—respiratory rate >30, shallow, quiet, use of accessory muscles.
   b. Goal: *document observations.*

D. Hypothermia—a specialized procedure in which the client's body temperature is lowered to 28°–30°C (82°–86°F).

1. Reduces tissue metabolism and oxygen requirements.
2. Used in heart surgery, brain surgery, and surgery on major blood vessels.
3. **Nursing plan/implementation:**
   a. Goal: *prevent complications:*
      (1) Monitor vital signs for shock.
      (2) Note levels of consciousness.
      (3) Record intake and output accurately.
      (4) Maintain good body alignment; reposition to prevent edema, pressure, or discoloration of skin.
      (5) Maintain patent IV.
   b. Goal: *promote comfort.*
      (1) Apply blankets to rewarm and prevent shivering.
      (2) Mouth care.

E. Evaluation: complete reversal of anesthetic effects (e.g., spontaneous respirations, pupils react to light).

III. Postoperative experience

A. Assessment:

1. Subjective data
   a. Pain: location, onset, intensity.
   b. Nausea.
2. Objective data
   a. Operative summary:
      (1) Type of operation performed.
      (2) Pathologic findings if known.
      (3) Anesthesia and medications received.
      (4) Problems during surgery that will affect recovery, i.e., arrhythmias, bleeding (estimated blood loss).
      (5) Fluids received: type, amount.
      (6) Needs for drainage or suction apparatus.
   b. Observations:
      (1) Patency of airway.
      (2) Vital signs.

(3) Skin color and dryness.

(4) Level of consciousness.

(5) Status of reflexes.

(6) Dressings.

(7) Type and rate of IV infusion and blood transfusion.

(8) Tubes/drains: urinary, chest, penrose, hemovac; note color and amount of drainage.

B. Analysis/nursing diagnosis:

1. *Ineffective breathing pattern* related to general anesthesia.
2. *Ineffective airway clearance* related to absent or weak cough.
3. *Potential for aspiration* related to vomiting.
4. *Pain* related to surgical incision.
5. *Altered tissue perfusion* related to shock.
6. *Potential fluid volume deficit* related to blood loss.
7. *Potential for injury* related to disorientation.
8. *Potential for wound infection* related to disruption of skin integrity.
9. *Urinary retention* related to anesthetic effects.
10. *Constipation* related to decreased peristalsis.

C. Nursing plan/implementation—*immediate post-anesthesia nursing care:* refers to time following surgery that is usually spent in the recovery room (1–2 h).

1. Goal: *promote a safe, quiet, nonstressful environment.*
   a. Siderails up at all times.
   b. Nurse in constant attendance.
2. Goal: *promote lung expansion and gas exchange.*
3. Goal: *Prevent aspiration and atelectasis.*
   a. *Position:* side or back, with head turned to side to prevent obstruction of airway by tongue; allows for drainage from mouth.
   b. Airway: leave the oropharyngeal or nasopharyngeal airway in place until client awakens and begins to eject; gagging and vomiting may occur if not removed before pharyngeal reflex returns.
   c. After removal of airway: turn on side in a lateral position; support upper arm with pillow.
   d. Suction: remove excessive secretions from mouth and pharynx.
   e. Encourage coughing and deep breathing: aids in upward movement of secretions.
   f. Give humidified oxygen as necessary: reduces respiratory irritation and keeps bronchotracheal secretions soft and moist.
   g. Mechanical ventilation: Bird or Bennet respirators if needed (see Ventilators in Unit 7, p. 525).
4. Goal: *promote and maintain cardiovascular function.*
   a. Vital signs, as ordered: usually q15min until stable.
      (1) Compare with preoperative vital signs.
      (2) Immediately report: systolic blood pressure that *drops 20* mm Hg or more, a pressure *below 80* mm Hg, or a pressure that continually drops 5–10 mm Hg over several readings; pulse rates *under 60* or *over 110* beats per minute, or irregularities; respirations *over 30* per minute; becoming shallow, quiet, slow; use of neck and diaphragm muscles (symptoms of *respiratory depression*).
   b. Observe for other alterations in circulatory function—pallor; thready pulse; cold, moist skin; decreased urine output; restlessness.
      (1) Immediately report to physician.
      (2) Initiate oxygen therapy.
      (3) Place client in shock position unless contraindicated—feet elevated, legs straight, head *slightly* elevated to increase venous return.
   c. Intravenous infusions: time, rate, orders for added medications.
   d. Monitor blood transfusions if ordered: observe for signs of *reaction* (chills, elevated temperature, urticaria, laryngeal edema, and wheezing). See Table 4.16, p. 349, for nursing plan/implementation.
   e. If reaction occurs, immediately stop transfusion and notify physician. Send STAT urine to lab.
5. Goal: *promote psychologic equilibrium.*
   a. Reassure on awakening—orient frequently.
   b. Explain procedures even though client does not appear alert.
   c. Answer client's questions briefly and accurately.
   d. Maintain quiet, restful environment.
   e. Comfort measures:
      (1) good body alignment.
      (2) Support dependent extremities to avoid pressure areas and possible nerve damage.
      (3) Check for constriction: dressings, clothing, bedding.
      (4) Check IV sites frequently for patency and signs of infiltration (swelling, blanching, cool to touch).
6. Goal: *maintain proper function of tubes and apparatus.* (See Table. 7.5).

D. General postoperative nursing care: refers to period of time from admission to the general nursing unit until anticipated recovery and discharge from the hospital. Table 4.16 reviews postoperative complications.

1. Goal: *promote lung expansion, gaseous exchange, and elimination of bronchotracheal secretions.*
   a. Turn, cough, and deep breathe every two hours.
   b. Use incentive spirometer as ordered to enable client to observe depth of ventilation.
   c. Administer nebulization as ordered to help mobilize secretions.
   d. Encourage hydration to thin mucous secretions.
   e. Assist in ambulation as soon as allowed.
2. Goal: *provide relief of pain.*
   a. Assess type, location, intensity, and duration; possible causative factors, such as poor body alignment or restrictive bandages.
   b. Observe and evaluate reaction to discomfort.

■ **TABLE 4.16** **Postoperative Complications**

Condition and Etiology	Assessment: Signs and Symptoms	Nursing Plan/ Implementation
Respiratory Complications—Most Common Are Atelectasis, Pneumonias (Lobar, Bronchial, and Hypostatic), and Pleuritis; Other Complications Are Hemothorax and Pneumothorax		
Atelectasis—undetected preoperative upper respiratory infections, aspiration of vomitus; irritation of the tracheobronchial tree with increased mucous secretions due to intubation and inhalation anesthesia, a history of heavy smoking or chronic obstructive pulmonary disease; severe postoperative pain or high abdominal or thoracic surgery, which inhibits deep breathing; and debilitation or old age, which lowers the client's resistance.	Dyspnea; ↑ temperature; absent or diminished breath sounds over affected area, asymmetrical chest expansion, ↑ respirations and pulse rate; tracheal shift to affected side when severe; anxiety and restlessness.	1. *Position:* unaffected side. 2. Turn, cough, and deep breathe. 3. Postural drainage. 4. Nebulization. 5. Force fluids if not contraindicated.
Pneumonia—see *Atelectasis* for etiology.	Rapid, shallow, painful respirations; rales; rhonchi; diminshed or absent breath sounds; asymmetrical lung expansion; chills and fever; productive cough, rust-colored sputum; and circumoral and nailbed cyanosis.	1. *Position* of comfort—semi- to high-Fowler's. 2. Force fluids to 3000 mL/day. 3. Provide humidification of air and oxygen therapy. 4. Oropharyngeal suction p.r.n. 5. Assist during coughing. 6. Administer antibiotics and analgesics as ordered. 7. Diet: high-calorie, as tolerated. 8. Cautious disposal of secretions; proper oral hygiene.
Pleuritis—see *Atelectasis* for etiology.	Knifelike chest pain on inspiration; intercostal tenderness; splinting of chest by patient; rapid, shallow respirations; pleural friction rub; ↑ temperature; malaise.	1. *Position: affected* side to splint the chest. 2. Manually splint client's chest during cough. 3. Apply binder or adhesive strapping as ordered. 4. Administer analgesics as ordered.
Hemothorax—chest surgery, gunshot or knife wounds, and multiple fractures of chest wall.	Chest pain; increased respiratory rate; dyspnea, decreased or absent breath sounds; decreased blood pressure; tachycardia, and mediastinal shift may occur (heart, trachea, and esophagus great vessels are pushed toward unaffected side).	1. Observe vital signs closely for signs of shock and respiratory distress. 2. Assist with thoracentesis (needle aspiration of fluid). 3. Assist with insertion of thoracostomy tube to closed chest drainage (see care of water-sealed drainage system).
Pneumothorax, closed or tension—thoracentesis (needle nicks the lung), rupture of alveoli or bronchi due to accidental injury, and chronic obstructive lung disease.	Marked dyspnea, sudden sharp chest pain, subcutaneous emphysema (air in chest wall tissue); cyanosis; tracheal shift to unaffected side; hyperresonance on percussion, decreased or absent breath sounds; increased respiratory rate, tachycardia; asymmetrical chest expansion, feeling of pressure within chest; *mediastinal shift*—severe dyspnea and cyanosis, deviation of larynx and trachea toward unaffected side, deviation either medially or laterally of apex of heart, decreased blood pressure; distended neck veins; increased pulse and respirations.	1. Remain with client—keep as calm and quiet as possible. 2. *Position:* high-Fowler's (sitting). 3. Notify physician through another nurse, and have thoracentesis equipment brought to bedside. 4. Administer oxygen as necessary. 5. Take vital signs to evaluate respiratory and cardiac function. 6. Assist with thoracentesis. 7. Assist with initiation and maintenance of closed-chest drainage.
Circulatory Complications—Shock, Thrombophlebitis, Pulmonary Embolism, and Disseminated Intravascular Coagulation		
Shock—hemorrhage, sepsis, decreased cardiac contractility (myocardial infarction, cardiac failure, tamponade), drug sensitivities, transfusion reactions, pulmonary embolism and emotional reaction to pain or deep fear.	Dizziness; fainting; restlessness; anxiety. *BP:* ↓ or falling. *Pulse:* weak, thready. *Respirations:* ↑, shallow. *Skin:* pale, cool, clammy, cyanotic. ↓ temperature; oliguria; CVP below 5 cm; thirst.	1. *Position:* foot of bed raised 20°, knees straight, trunk horizontal, head slightly elevated; *avoid* Trendelenburg's position. 2. Administer blood transfusions, plasma expanders, and intravenous infusions as ordered; medications specific to type of shock. 3. Check: vital signs, CVP, temperature. 4. Insert urinary catheter to monitor hourly urine output. 5. Administer oxygen as ordered.

continued

TABLE 4.16 *(Continued)* **Postoperative Complications**

Condition and Etiology	Assessment: Signs and Symptoms	Nursing Plan/ Implementation
Circulatory Complications (cont.)		
Thrombophlebitis—injury to vein wall by tight leg straps or leg holders during gynecologic surgery; hemoconcentration due to dehydration or fluid loss; and stasis of blood in extremities due to postoperative circulatory depression.	Calf pain or cramping, redness and swelling (the left leg is affected more frequently than the right); slight fever, chills; Homans' sign and tenderness over the anteromedian surface of thigh.	1. Maintain complete bedrest, *avoiding positions* that restrict venous return. 2. Apply elastic stockings or wrap legs from toes to groin with elastic bandages to prevent swelling and pooling of venous blood. 3. Apply warm, moist soaks to area as ordered. 4. Administer anticoagulants as ordered. 5. Use bed cradle over affected limb. 6. Provide active and passive ROM exercises in unaffected limb.
Pulmonary embolism—obstruction of a pulmonary artery by a foreign body in bloodstream, usually a blood clot that has been dislodged from its original site.	*Sudden,* severe stabbing chest pain; *severe* dyspnea; cyanosis; *rapid* pulse; anxiety and apprehension; pupillary dilatation; *profuse* diaphoresis; and *loss* of consciousness.	1. Administer oxygen and inhalants while client is sitting upright. 2. Maintain bedrest and frequent reassurance. 3. Administer heparin sodium, as ordered. 4. Administer analgesics, such as morphine SO_4, to reduce pain and apprehension.
Wound Complications—Infection, Dehiscence, and Evisceration		
Wound infection—*obesity* or *undernutrition,* particularly protein and vitamin deficiencies; *decreased* antibody production in aged; *decreased* phagocytosis in newborn; metabolic disorder, such as diabetes mellitus, Cushing's syndrome, malignancies, and shock; breakdown in aseptic technique.	Redness, tenderness, and heat in area of incision; wound drainage; ↑ temperature; ↑ pulse rate.	1. Assist in cleansing and irrigation of wound and insertion of a drain. 2. Apply hot, wet dressings as ordered. 3. Give antibiotics as ordered; observe responses.
Wound dehiscence and evisceration—obesity and undernutrition, particularly protein and vitamin C deficiencies; immunosuppression; metabolic disorders; cancer; liver disease; common site is midline abdominal incision, frequently about 7 days postoperatively; and precipitating factors include abdominal distention, vomiting, coughing, hiccups, and uncontrolled motor activity.	Slow parting of wound edges with a gush of pinkish serous drainage; or rapid parting with coils of intestines escaping onto the abdominal wall; the latter is accompanied by pain and often by vomiting.	1. *Position:* bedrest, low-Fowler's or horizontal position. 2. Notify physician stat. 3. Cover exposed coils of intestines with sterile towels or dressing and keep moist with sterile normal saline. 4. Monitor vital signs frequently. 5. Remain with client, reassure that physician is coming. 6. Prepare for physician's arrival; set up IV, suction equipment, and nasogastric tube; obtain sterile gown, mask, gloves, towels, and warmed normal saling. 7. Notify surgery that client will be returning to operating room.
Urinary Complications—Retention and Infections		
Urinary retention—obstruction in bladder or urethra; neurologic disease; mechanical trauma as in childbirth or gynecologic surgery; psychologic conditioning that inhibits voiding in bed; prolonged bedrest; pain with lower abdominal surgery.	Inability to void *10–18* hours postsurgery, despite adequate fluid replacement; palpable bladder, frequent voiding of small amounts of urine or dribbling; suprapubic pain.	1. Assist client to stand, or use bedside commode if not contraindicted. 2. Provide privacy. 3. Reduce tension, provide support. 4. Use warm bedpan. 5. Run tap water. 6. Place client's feet in warm water. 7. Pour warm water over perineum. 8. Catheterize if conservative measures fail.
Urinary infections—urinary retention, bladder distension, repeated or prolonged catheterization.	*Urinary:* burning and frequency. *Pain:* low-back or flank. Pyuria,hematuria; ↑ temperature, chills; anorexia; positive urine culture.	1. Push fluids to 3000 mL daily, unless contraindicated. 2. *Avoid* stimulants such as caffeine. 3. Give antibiotics, sulfonamides, or acidifying agents as ordered. 4. Give perianal care after each bowel movement.

continued

■ **TABLE 4.16 *(Continued)*** **Postoperative Complications**

Condition and Etiology	Assessment: Signs and Symptoms	Nursing Plan/ Implementation
Gastrointestinal Complications—Gastric Distention, Paralytic Ileus, and Intestinal Obstruction		
Gastric distention—depressed gastric motility due to sympathoadrenal stress response; idiosyncrasy to drugs; emotions, pain, shock; fluid and electrolyte imbalances.	Feeling of fullness, hiccups, overflow vomiting of dark, foul-smelling liquid; severe retention leads to decreased blood pressure (due to pressure on vagus nerve) and other symptoms of shock syndrome.	1. Report signs to physician *immediately.* 2. Insert or assist in insertion of NG tube; attach to intermittent suction. 3. Irrigate nasogastric tube with *saline* (water will deplete electrolytes and result in metabolic alkalosis). 4. Administer IV infusions with electrolytes as ordered.
Paralytic ileus—see *Gastric distention.*	Greatly decreased or absent bowel sounds, failure of either gas or feces to be passed by rectum; nausea and vomiting; abdominal tenderness and distention; fever; dehydration.	1. Notify physician. 2. Insert or assist with insertion of NG tube; attach to low, intermittent suction. 3. Insert rectal tube. 4. Administer IV infusion with electrolytes as ordered. 5. Irrigate nasogastric tube with saline. 6. Assist with insertion of Miller-Abbott tube if indicated. 7. Administer medications to increase peristalsis as ordered.
Intestinal obstruction—due to poorly functioning anastomosis, hernia, adhesions, and fecal impaction.	Severe, colicky abdominal pains, mild to severe abdominal distention, nausea and vomiting, anorexia and malaise; fever; lack of bowel movement; electrolyte imbalance; high-pitched tinkling bowel sounds.	1. Assist with insertion of nasoenteric tube and attach to intermittent suction. 2. Maintain IV infusions with electrolytes. 3. Encourage nasal breathing to avoid air swallowing. 4. Check abdomen for distention and bowel sounds every 2 hours. 5. Encourage verbalization. 6. Plan rest periods for client. 7. Administer oral hygiene frequently.
Transfusion Reactions—Allergic, Febrile, and Hemolytic		
Allergic and febrile reactions—unidentified antigen or antigens in donor blood or transfusion equipment; previous reaction to transfusions; small thrombi; bacteria; and lysed red cells.	Fever to 103 °F, may have *sudden* onset; chills; itching; erythema; urticaria; nausea; vomiting; dyspnea and wheezing, occasionally.	1. *Stop* transfusion and notify physician. 2. Administer *antihistamines,* as ordered. 3. Send stat urine to lab for analysis. 4. Institute *cooling* measures if indicated. 5. Maintain *strict* input and output records. 6. Send remaining blood to lab for analysis, and order recipient blood sample for analysis.
Hemolytic reaction—infusion of incompatible blood.	*Early* chills and fever; feeling of burning in face; hypotension; tachycardia; chest, back, or flank pain; nausea, vomiting; feeling of doom; spontaneous and diffuse bleeding; icterus; oliguria; anuria; hemoglobinuria.	1. *Stop* infusion immediately; take vital signs and notify physician. 2. Send client blood sample and unused blood to lab for analysis. 3. Send stat urine to lab. 4. Save *all* urine for observation of discoloration. 5. Administer parenteral infusions to combat shock, as ordered. 6. Administer medications as ordered—*diuretics, sodium bicarbonate, hydrocortisone,* and *vasopressors.*
Emotional Complications		
Emotional disturbances—grief associated with loss of body part or loss of body image; previous emotional problems; decreased sensory and perceptual input; sensory overload; fear and pain; decreased resistance to stress as a result of age, exhaustion, or debilitation.	Restlessness, insomnia, depression, hallucinations, delusions, agitation, and suicidal thoughts.	1. Report symptoms to physician. 2. Encourage verbalization of feelings; give realistic assurance. 3. Orient to time and place as necessary. 4. Provide safety measures, such as siderails. 5. Keep room lit, to reduce incidence of visual hallucinations. 6. Administer tranquilizers as ordered. 7. Use restraints as a *last* resort.

c. Utilize comfort measures, such as back rubs and proper ventilation, staying with client and encouraging verbalization.

d. Reduce incidence of pain: change position frequently; support dependent extremities with pillows, sandbags, and footboards; keep bedding dry and straight.

e. Give analgesics or tranquilizers as ordered; assure patient that it will help.

f. Observe for desired and untoward effects of medication.

3. Goal: *promote adequate nutrition and fluid and electrolyte balance.*

a. Parenteral fluids, as ordered.

b. Monitor blood pressure, I&O to assess adequate, deficient, or excessive extracellular fluid volume.

c. Diet: liquid when nausea and vomiting stop and bowel sounds are established, progress as ordered.

4. Goal: *assist client with elimination.*

a. Encourage voiding within 8–10 hours after surgery.

(1) Allow client to stand or use commode, if not contraindicated.

(2) Run tap water or soak feet in warm water to promote micturition.

(3) Catheterization if bladder is distended and conservative treatments have failed.

b. Maintain accurate I&O records.

c. Expect bowel function to return in 2–3 days.

5. Goal: *facilitate wound-healing and prevent infection.*

a. Incision care: avoid pressure to enhance venous drainage and prevent edema.

b. Elevate injured extremities to reduce swelling and promote venous return.

c. Support or splint incision when coughing.

d. Check dressings every 2 hours for drainage.

e. Change dressings on draining wounds p.r.n.; aseptic technique; protective ointments to reduce skin irritation may be ordered.

f. Carefully observe wound suction (e.g., Jackson-Pratt), if applied, for kinking or twisting of the tubes.

6. Goal: *promote comfort and rest.*

a. Recognize factors that may cause restlessness—fear, anxiety, pain, oxygen lack, wet dressings.

b. Comfort measures: analgesics or barbiturates; apply oxygen as indicated; change positions; encourage deep breathing; massage back to reduce restlessness.

c. Allow rest periods between care-group activities.

d. Give antiemetic for relief of nausea and vomiting, as ordered.

e. Vigorous oral hygiene (brushing) to prevent "surgical mumps" or parotitis from preop atropine or general anesthesia.

7. Goal: *encourage early movement and ambulation to prevent complications of immobilization.*

a. Turn or reposition q2h.

b. ROM: passive and active exercises.

c. Encourage leg exercises.

d. Assist with standing or use of commode if allowed.

e. Encourage resumption of personal care as soon as possible.

f. Assist with ambulation in room as soon as allowed. Avoid chair-sitting as it enhances venous pooling and may predispose to thrombophlebitis.

E. Evaluation:

1. Incision heals without infection.
2. No complications, i.e., atelectasis, pneumonia, thrombophlebitis.
3. Normal bowel and bladder functions resume.
4. Carries out activities of daily living, self-care.
5. Accepts possible limitations: dietary, activity, body image (e.g., no depression, complies with treatment regimen).

■ NUTRITION

I. General nutritional deficiencies

A. Assessment:

1. Subjective data

a. Mental irritability or confusion.

b. History of poor dietary intake.

c. History of lack of adequate resources to provide adequate nutrition.

d. Lack of knowledge about proper diet, food selection, or preparation.

e. History of eating disorders.

f. Paresthesia (burning and tingling): hands and feet.

2. Objective data

a. *Appearance:* listless; *posture:* sagging shoulders, sunken chest, poor gait.

b. *Muscle:* weakness, fatigue, wasted appearance.

c. *GI:* indigestion, vomiting, enlarged liver, spleen.

d. *Cardiovascular:* tachycardia on minimal exertion; bradycardia at rest; enlarged heart, elevated BP.

e. *Hair:* brittle, dry, thin, sparse; lack of natural shine; color changes; can be easily plucked out.

f. *Skin:* dryness (xerosis), scaly, dyspigmentation, petechiae, lack of fat under skin.

g. *Mouth:*

(1) *Teeth:* missing, abnormally placed, caries.

(2) *Gums:* bleed easily, receding.

(3) *Tongue:* swollen, sore.

(4) *Lips:* red, swollen, angular fissures at corners.

h. *Eyes:* pale conjunctiva, corneal changes.

i. *Nails:* brittle, ridged.

j. *Nervous system:* abnormal reflexes.

■ TABLE 4.17 **Common Mineral Deficiencies**

Mineral	Function	Deficiency Leads To
Calcium	Aids in formation and maintenance of bones and teeth; permits healthy nerve functioning and normal blood-clotting.	↑ neuromuscular irritability, impaired blood-clotting.
Phosphorus	Bone building.	Rickets.
Magnesium	Cellular metabolism of carbohydrates and protein.	↓ cellular metabolism of carbohydrates and protein; tetany.
Sodium	Fluid and electrolyte balance; acid-base balance; electrochemical impulses of nerves and muscles.	Fluid and electrolyte imbalance; ↓ muscle contraction.
Potassium	Osmotic pressure and water balance.	Fluid and electrolyte imbalance; ↓ cardiac and skeletal muscular contractility.
Chloride	Fluid and electrolyte balance; acid–base balance; digestion.	Fluid imbalances; alkalosis.
Iron	Hemoglobin formation; cellular oxidation.	Anemia.
Iodine	Synthesis of thyroid hormone; overall body metabolism.	Goiter.
Zinc	Constituent of cell enzyme system; CO_2 carrier in RBC.	↓ metabolism of protein and carbohydrates; delayed wound healing.

k. Lab data: blood: *decreased* albumin, iron binding capacity, lymphocyte, hemoglobin, and hematocrit.

l. Anthropometric measurements document nutritional deficiencies.

B. Analysis/nursing diagnosis:

1. *Altered nutrition, less than body requirements,* related to poor dietary intake.
2. *Knowledge deficit* related to nutritional requirements.
3. *Altered health maintenance* related to inability to provide own nutritional care.
4. *Ineffective individual coping* related to eating disorders.
5. *Ineffective family coping, disabling,* related to inadequate resources or knowledge to provide appropriate family nutrition.

C. Nursing plan/implementation:

1. Goal: *prevent complications of specific deficiency.*
   a. Identify etiology of nutritional deficiency.
   b. Recognize signs of nutritional deficiencies (see Table 4.17).
   c. Identify foods high in deficient nutrient (see Unit 5).
   d. Evaluate economic resources to purchase appropriate foods.
   e. Identify community resources for assistance.
   f. Monitor progress for potential additional illnesses.
2. Goal: *health teaching.*
   a. Effects of nutritional deficiencies on health.
   b. Foods to include in diet to avoid deficits.

D. Evaluation:

1. Complications do not occur.
2. Client gains weight.
3. Client selects appropriate foods to alleviate deficiency.

II. Celiac disease (nontropical sprue): gluten-induced intestinal disease affecting adults and children, characterized by inability to digest and utilize sugars, starches and fats.

A. Pathophysiology: intolerance to the gliadin fraction of grains causing degeneration of the epithelial surface of the intestine, atrophy of the intestinal villi, and impaired absorption of essential nutrients.

B. Risk factors:

1. Possible genetic or familial factors.
2. Hypersensitivity response.
3. History of childhood celiac disease.

C. Assessment:

1. Subjective data: family history.
2. Objective data
   a. Loss: weight, fat deposits, musculature.
   b. Anemia.
   c. Vitamin deficiencies.
   d. Abdomen distended with flatus.
   e. Stools: diarrhea, foul smelling, bulky, fatty, float in commode.
   f. History of acute attacks of fluid/electrolyte imbalances.
   ▶ g. Diagnostic tests: small bowel biopsy, stool for fat.
   h. Gluten-free diet leads to remission of symptoms.

D. Analysis/nursing diagnosis:

1. *Altered nutrition, less than body requirements,* related to inability to digest and utilize sugars, starches, and fats.
2. *Diarrhea* related to intestinal response to gluten in diet.

3. *Fluid volume deficit* related to loss through excessive diarrhea.
4. *Knowledge deficit* related to dietary restrictions to control symptoms.

E. Nursing plan/implementation:

1. Goal: *prevent weight loss.*
   a. Diet: high in calories, protein, vitamins, and minerals, and gluten-free.
      (1) Avoid wheat, rye, oats, barley.
      (2) All other foods permitted.
   b. Daily weights to monitor weight changes.
2. Goal: *health teaching.*
   a. Nature of disease.
   b. Dietary restrictions and allowances.
   c. Complications of noncompliance.

F. Evaluation:

1. No further weight loss.
2. Normal stools.
3. Fluid/electrolyte balance obtained and maintained.

III. Hepatitis: inflammation of the liver

A. Pathophysiology:

1. Infection with either hepatitis A (infectious hepatitis), hepatitis B (serum hepatitis), non-A, non-B hepatitis (caused by at least two unidentified viruses), or delta hepatitis (infection caused by a defective RNA virus that requires HBV to multiply) → inflammation, necrosis, and regeneration of liver parenchyma. Hepatocellular injury impairs clearance of urobilinogen → elevated urinary urobilinogen; and, as injury increases → conjugated bilirubin not reaching the intestines → decreased urine and fecal urobilinogen → increased serum bilirubin → jaundice.
2. Failure of liver to detoxify products → increased toxic products of protein metabolism → gastritis and duodenitis.

B. Risk factors:

1. Exposure to virus.
2. Exposure to carriers of virus.
3. Exposure to hepatotoxins such as dry cleaning agents.
4. Nonimmunized.

C. Assessment:

1. Subjective data
   a. Anorexia, nausea.
   b. Malaise, dull ache in upper right quadrant.
   c. Repugnance to food, cigarette smoke, strong odors, alcohol.
   d. Headache.
2. Objective data
   a. Fever.
   b. Liver: enlarged (hepatomegaly), tender, smooth.
   c. Skin: icterus in sclera of eyes, jaundice; rash; pruritus; petechiae, bruises.
   d. Urine: normal, dark.
   e. Stool: normal, clay-colored, loose.
   f. Vomiting, weight loss.
   g. Lymph nodes: enlarged.
   h. Lab data:
      (1) Blood—leukocytosis.
      (2) Increased SGOT, SGPT, and bilirubin levels, alkaline phosphatase.
      (3) Urine—increased urobilinogen.
   i. See Table 4.18.

D. Analysis/nursing diagnosis:

1. *Pain* related to inflammation of liver.
2. *Impaired skin integrity* related to pruritus.
3. *Activity intolerance* related to malaise.
4. *Potential for infection* to others related to incubation/infectious period.
5. *Altered nutrition, less than body requirements,* related to repugnance of food.
6. *Social isolation,* related to isolation precautions.

E. Nursing plan/implementation:

1. Goal: *promote comfort.*
   a. Bedrest to combat fatigue and reduce metabolic needs until hepatomegaly subsides.
   b. Oral hygiene q1h to q2h to decrease nausea.
   c. ROM exercises to maintain muscle strength.
   d. Measures to reduce pruritus:
      (1) Mild, oil-based lotion to reduce itching.
      (2) Nails cut short, cotton gloves, long-sleeved clothing to prevent skin injury from scratching.
      (3) Environment: cool and dry.
      (4) Cool wet soaks to skin.
      (5) Diversional activities.
      (6) Medications as ordered:
         (a) Emollients to relieve dry skin.
         (b) Topical corticosteroids to reduce inflammation.
         (c) Antihistamines to reduce itch.
         (d) Tranquilizers and sedatives to allow rest and prevent exhaustion.
2. Goal: *prevent spread of infection to others.*
   a. Isolation according to type
      (1) *Infectious hepatitis A:*
         (a) Enteric precautions.
         (b) Private room preferred.
         (c) Gown/gloves for direct contact with feces.
         (d) Handwashing when indirect contact with feces.
      (2) *Serum hepatitis B:* blood and body fluid precautions
         (a) Needle/dressing precautions.
         (b) Private room not necessary.
         (c) Gown: only if enteric precautions also necessary.
         (d) Handwashing: use gloves when in direct contact with blood.
      (3) Non-A, non-B:

ADULT NURSING

■ TABLE 4.18 Etiology, Incidence, and Epidemiologic Comparison of Hepatitis A, Hepatitis B, Non-A, Non-B Hepatitis, and Delta Hepatitis

	Infectious Hepatitis A	Serum Hepatitis B	Non-A, Non-B	Delta
Incubation	2–6 weeks	4 weeks–6 months	Variable: 14–160 days; average, 50 days	6 weeks–6 months
Communicable	Until 7–9 days after jaundice occurs	Several months—as long as virus present in blood	As long as virus present in blood	As long as virus present in blood
Transmission	Fecal-oral	Parenteral; sexual	Percutaneous, via contaminated blood, parenteral drug abuse; some fecal-oral form of this non-A, non-B found in Southeast Asia, North Africa	Parenteral
Sources	Crowding; contaminated food, milk or water	Contaminated needles, syringes, surgical instruments	Persons who have received 15 or more blood transfusions; IV drug users; persons traveling to contaminated areas	Contaminated needles, syringes
Portal of entry	GI tract; asymptomatic carriers	Integumentary: blood plasma or transfusions	Blood	Integumentary: blood
HB antigen	Not present	Present	Not present	Present as with Hepatitis B
Incidence	Sporadic epidemics; increased in children and young adults	Increased in ages 15–29, particularly in heroin addiction; occupational hazard for laboratory workers, nurses, physicians	All age groups; higher in adults because of exposure to risk factors	Same as Hepatitis B
Immunity	*Preexposure:* Immune globulin 0.02 mL/kg *Postexposure:* Within two weeks of exposure, as above	*Preexposure:* Hepatitis B vaccine *Postexposure:* Immune globulin with high amounts of anti-HBs (HBIG); Hepatitis B vaccine	None	Same as Hepatitis B
Prevention	Handwashing, use of gloves	Care when handling products contaminated by blood, use of gloves	Same as Hepatitis B	Same as Hepatitis B

(a) Same as B, except when in countries with fecal-oral form of non-A, non-B exposure, then use hepatitis A precautions also.

(4) *Delta*

(a) Same as hepatitis B.

b. Passive immunity for contacts

(1) *Infectious hepatitis A:* immune serum globulin (ISG).

(2) *Serum hepatitis B:* hepatitis serum globulin (HGIB) or immune serum globulin (ISG).

(3) *Non-A, non-B:* prophylaxis not as effective; IG may be given.

(4) *Delta:* same as for hepatitis B.

c. Goal: *promote healing.*

(1) Diet as tolerated:

(a) NPO with parenteral infusions, when in acute stage.

(b) High-protein, high-carbohydrate, low-fat, offered in frequent small meals.

(c) Push fluids, if not contraindicated; I&O.

d. Goal: *monitor for increase in disease process, failure to respond to prescribed treatment.*

(1) Observe urine—dark due to presence of bile and stool, clay colored.

(2) Observe sclera, lab tests for increasing jaundice.

(3) Mental confusion, unusual somnolence may indicate decreased liver function.

(4) Weigh daily—increase indicates fluid retention and possible ascites.

e. Goal: *health teaching.*

(1) Diet and fluid intake to promote liver regeneration.

(2) Importance of rest and limited activity to reduce metabolic workload of liver.

(3) Personal hygiene practices to prevent contamination.

(4) Avoid alcohol, blood donations, and contact with communicable infections.

(5) Follow-up case referral.

(6) Teach contacts about available immunizations.

F. Evaluation:

1. Tolerates food; nausea and vomiting decreased.
2. Signs of infection/inflammation absent.
3. No complications, hemorrhage, liver damage, ascites.
4. No jaundice noted.

IV. Pancreatitis: inflammatory disease of the pancreas; caused by alcoholism or alcohol consumption, biliary tract disease, carcinoma, adenoma, infections, drugs, metabolic diseases, hypercalcemia, and trauma.

A. Pathophysiology: proteolytic enzymes within the pancreas are activated by endotoxins, exotoxins, ischemia, anoxia, or trauma. Pancreatic enzymes begin process of autodigestion of pancreas and surrounding tissues; also activate other enzymes that digest cellular membranes. Autodigestion leads to edema, hemorrhage, vascular damage, coagulation necrosis, and fat necrosis.

B. Risk factors:

1. Obesity.
2. Alcoholism.
3. Biliary tract disease.
4. Abdominal trauma.
5. Surgery.
6. Drugs.
7. Metabolic problems.
8. Intestinal disease.

C. Assessment:

1. Subjective data
   a. Pain:
      (1) Sudden onset; severe, widespread, constant, and incapacitating.
      (2) Location—epigastrium, rest of the abdomen; radiates to back, flanks, and substernal area.
   b. Nausea.
   c. History of risk factors.
   d. Dyspnea.
2. Objective data
   a. *Elevated:* temperature, pulse, respirations, BP (unless in shock).
   b. Decreased breath sounds related to atalectasis/pleural effusion.
   c. Increased rales, cyanosis.
   d. Hemorrhage, shock.
   e. Vomiting.
   f. Fluid and electrolyte imbalances, dehydration.
   g. Decreased bowel sounds; abdominal tenderness with guarding.
   h. Stools: bulky, pale, foul smelling.
   i. Skin: pale, moist, cold; may be jaundiced.
   j. Muscle rigidity.
   k. Supine position leads to increased pain.
   l. Lab data:
      (1) *Elevated:*
         (a) Amylase, serum, and urine.
         (b) Serum lipase, SGOT.
         (c) Alkaline phosphatase.
         (d) Bilirubin, glucose; serum and urine.
         (e) Urine protein, WBC.
         (f) Leukocytes.
         (g) BUN.
      (2) *Decreased:*
         (a) Serum calcium.
         (b) Protein.

D. Analysis/nursing diagnosis:

1. *Altered nutrition, less than body requirements,* related to nausea and vomiting.
2. *Pain* related to inflammatory and autodigestive processes of pancreas.
3. *Fluid volume deficit* related to inflammation, decreased intake and vomiting.
4. *Ineffective breathing pattern* related to pain and pleural effusion.
5. *Knowledge deficit* related to risk factors and disease management.

E. Nursing plan/implementation:

1. Goal: *control pain.*
   a. Medications: analgesics—meperidine (not morphine or codeine due to spasmodic effect).
   b. Position: sitting with knees flexed.
2. Goal: *rest injured pancreas.*
   a. NPO.
   b. NG tube to low suction.
   c. Medications:
      (1) Antacids.
      (2) Antibiotics.
      (3) Antiemetics.
      (4) Antispasmotics.
3. Goal: *prevent fluid and electrolyte imbalance.*
   a. Monitor: vitals, CVP.
   b. IVs, fluids, blood, albumin, plasma.
4. Goal: *prevent respiratory and metabolic complications.*
   a. Cough, deep breathe, change position.
   b. Monitor: sugar and acetone q4h.
   c. Monitor calcium levels: Chvostek's and Trousseau's sign positive when calcium deficit exists (see XVI. Thyroidectomy, p. 419, for description of tests).
5. Goal: *provide adequate nutrition.*
   a. Low-fat diet.
   b. Bland, small, frequent meals.
   c. Vitamin supplements.
   d. Avoid alcohol.

6. Goal: *prevent complications.*
   a. Monitor for signs of:
      (1) Peritonitis.
      (2) Bowel obstruction, perforation.
      (3) Respiratory complications.
      (4) Hypotension, shock.
      (5) D.I.C.
      (6) Hemorrhage from ulcers, varicies.
      (7) Anemia.
      (8) Encephalopathy.
7. Goal: *health teaching.*
   a. Food selections for low-fat, bland diet.
   b. Necessity of vitamin therapy.
   c. Importance of avoiding alcohol.
   d. Signs and symptoms of recurrence.
   e. Importance of rest, to prevent relapse.
   f. Desired effects and side effects of prescribed medications:
      (1) Narcotics for pain.
      (2) Antiemetics for nausea and vomiting.
      (3) Pancreatic hormone and enzymes to replace enzymes not reaching duodenum.

F. Evaluation:

1. Pain is relieved.
2. No complications, e.g., peritonitis, respiratory.
3. States dietary allowances and restrictions.
4. Takes medications as ordered; states purposes, side effects.

V. Cirrhosis: chronic inflammation and fibrosis of the liver in which some liver cells (hepatocytes) undergo necrosis and others undergo proliferative regeneration.

A. Pathophysiology: progressive destruction of hepatic cells → loss of normal metabolic function of the liver and formation of scar tissue. Regeneration and proliferation of fibrous tissue → obstruction of the portal vein → increased portal hypertension, ascites, liver failure, and eventual death.

B. Risk factors:

1. Alcohol abuse most common cause.
2. Nutritional deficiency with decreased protein intake.
3. Hepatotoxins.
4. Virus.

C. Assessment:

1. Subjective data
   a. Chronic feeling of malaise.
   b. Anorexia, nausea.
   c. Abdominal pain.
   d. Pruritus.
2. Objective data
   a. GI:
      (1) Malnutrition, weight loss.
      (2) Vomiting.
      (3) Flatulence.
      (4) Ascites.
      (5) Enlarged liver and spleen.
      (6) Glossitis.
      (7) Fetid breath (sweet, musty odor).
   b. Blood—coagulation defects, possible esophageal varicosities, portal hypertension, bleeding from gums and injection sites.
   c. Skin and hair—edema, jaundice, spider angioma, palmar erythemia, decreased pubic and axillary hair.
   d. Reproductive—menstrual abnormalities, gynecomastia, testicular atrophy, impotence.
   e. Neurological deficits, including memory loss, hepatic coma, decreased level of consciousness; flappy tremor, grimacing.
   f. Lab data:
      (1) *Decreased:* albumin, potassium, magnesium, BUN.
      (2) *Elevated:* prothrombin time, globulins, ammonia, SGOT, BSP, alkaline phosphate, uric acid, blood sugar.

D. Analysis/nursing diagnosis:

1. *Altered nutrition, less than body requirements,* related to decreased intake, nausea, and vomiting.
2. *Potential for injury* related to decreased prothrombin production.
3. *Activity intolerance* related to fatigue.
4. *Fatigue* related to anorexia and nutritional deficiencies.
5. *Self-esteem disturbance* related to physical body changes.
6. Potential for *impaired skin integrity* related to pruritus.

E. Nursing plan/implementation:

1. Goal: *provide for special safety needs.*
   a. Monitor vitals (including neurologic) frequently for hemorrhage from esophageal varicies (may have Sengstaken-Blakemore or Linton tube inserted).
   b. Prepare client for Le Veen shunt surgery for portal hypertension as needed.
   c. Assist with paracentesis performed for ascites; monitor vitals to prevent shock during procedure.
2. Goal: *relieve discomfort caused by complications.*
   a. *Position:* semi-Fowler's or Fowler's to decrease pressure on diaphragm due to ascites.
   b. Deep breathing q2h to prevent respiratory complications.
   c. Skin care, topical mediations to relieve pruritus; nail care to decrease possibility of further skin injury.
   d. Frequent oral hygiene related to nausea, vomiting, and fetid breath.
3. Goal: *improve fluid and electrolyte balance.*
   a. IV fluids and vitamins.
   b. I&O, hourly urines during acute attacks.

c. Daily: girths, weights to monitor fluid balance.

d. Diuretics as ordered to decrease edema.

e. May receive serum albumin to promote adequate vascular volume, prevent azotemia and encephalopathy, and promote diuresis (observe carefully, as albumin could escape quickly through cell walls and cause increase in ascites).

4. Goal: *promote optimum nutrition within dietary restrictions.*

a. NPO during acute episodes.

b. Small, frequent meals when able to eat.

c. Low protein (to decrease the amount of nitrogenous materials in the intestines) and sodium (to decrease fluid retention).

d. Moderate carbohydrate (to meet energy demands) and fat (to make diet more palatable to anorexic clients).

5. Goal: *provide emotional support.*

a. Quiet environment during acute episodes to decrease external stimuli.

b. Identify community agencies for assistance for client, e.g., Alcoholics Anonymous; for family, Alanon/Ala-teen.

6. Goal: *health teaching.*

a. Avoid alcohol, exposure to infections.

b. Dietary allowances, restrictions (see IV. Sodium-restricted diet and VII. Purine-restricted diet, pp. 474, 475).

c. Drugs: names, purposes.

d. Signs, symptoms of disease and complications.

e. Stress-management techniques.

F. Evaluation:

1. No complications.
2. Nutritional status improves; lists dietary restrictions.
3. No alcohol consumption.
4. Lists signs and symptoms of increased disease process and complications.
5. Complies with discharge plan, becomes involved with an alcohol treatment program.

VI. Esophageal varicies: life-threatening hemorrhage from tortuous dilated, thin-walled veins in submucosa of lower esophagus. May rupture when chemically or mechanically irritated or when pressure is increased because of sneezing, coughing, use of the Valsalva maneuver, or excessive exercise.

A. Pathophysiology: portal hypertension related to cirrhosis of the liver → distended branches of the azygos and vena cava veins where they join the smaller vessels of the esophagus.

B. Risk factors for hemorrhage:

1. Exertion that increases abdominal pressure.
2. Trauma from ingestion of coarse foods.
3. Acid pepsin erosion.

C. Assessment:

1. Subjective data

a. Fear.

b. Dysphagia.

c. History: alcohol ingestion, liver dysfunction.

2. Objective data

a. Hematemesis.

b. Hemorrhage: sudden, often fatal.

c. Decreased BP; increased pulse, respirations.

d. Melena (occult blood in stool).

D. Analysis/nursing diagnosis:

1. *Fluid volume deficit* related to blood loss.
2. *Potential for injury* related to hemorrhage.
3. *Fear* related to massive blood loss.
4. *Ineffective individual coping* related to complications of cirrhosis.

E. Nursing plan/implementation:

1. Goal: *provide safety measures related to hemorrhage.*

a. Recognize signs of shock; vitals q15min.

b. Assist with insertion of Sengstaken-Blakemore or Linton tube (tube is large and uncomfortable for client during insertion); explain procedure briefly to decrease fear and attempt to gain client's cooperation.

c. While tube in place, observe for respiratory distress; if present, *deflate the balloon by releasing pressure; do not cut the tube.*

d. Deflate the balloon as ordered to prevent necrosis.

e. NG tube to low gastric suction; monitor for amount of bright red blood; irrigate only as ordered using tepid, *not* iced, solutions.

f. Vitamin K as ordered to control bleeding.

2. Goal: *promote fluid balance.*

a. IV fluids, expanders, blood.

b. Fresh blood as ordered to avoid increased ammonia; aids in coagulation.

3. Goal: *prevent complications of hepatic coma.*

a. Saline cathartics as ordered to remove old blood from GI tract.

b. Antibiotics as ordered to prevent infection.

4. Goal: *provide emotional support.*

a. Stay with client.

b. Calm atmosphere.

5. Goal: *health teaching.*

a. Explain use of tube to client and family.

b. Bland diet instructions.

c. Recognize signs of bleeding.

d. Avoid straining at stool.

e. Avoid aspirin because of increased bleeding tendency.

F. Evaluation:

1. Survives acute bleeding episode.
2. Further episodes prevented by avoiding irritants, especially alcohol.
3. Improves nutritional status.
4. Recognizes symptoms of complications, e.g., bleeding.
5. Demonstrates knowledge of medications by avoiding aspirin.

ADULT NURSING

VII. Diaphragmatic hernia (hiatus hernia): protrusion of part of stomach through diaphragm and into thoracic cavity. *Types:* sliding (most common); paraesophageal "rolling."

A. Pathophysiology: weakening of the musculature of the diaphragm, aggravated by increased intra-abdominal pressure → protrusion of the abdominal organs through the esophageal hiatus → reflux of gastric contents → esophagitis.

B. Risk factors:

1. Congenital abnormality.
2. Penetrating wound.
3. Age (middle-aged or elderly).
4. Women more than men.
5. Obesity.
6. Ascites.
7. Pregnancy.
8. History of constipation.

C. Assessment:

1. Subjective data
   a. Pressure: substernal.
   b. Pain: epigastric, burning.
   c. Eructation, heartburn after eating.
   d. Dysphagia.
   e. Symptoms aggravated when recumbent.
2. Objective data
   a. Cough, dyspnea.
   b. Tachycardia, palpitations.
   c. Bleeding: hematemesis, melena, signs of anemia due to gastroesophageal irritation, ulceration, and bleeding.
   ▶ d. Diagnostic tests:
      (1) Chest X rays, showing protrusion of abdominal organs into thoracic cavity.
      (2) Barium swallow (upper GI) to show presence of hernia.

D. Analysis/nursing diagnosis:

1. *Pain* related to irritation of lining of GI tract.
2. *Altered nutrition, less than body requirements,* related to dysphagia.
3. *Sleep pattern disturbance* related to increase in symptoms when recumbent.
4. *Potential for aspiration* related to reflux of gastric contents.
5. *Activity intolerance* related to dyspnea.
6. *Anxiety* related to palpitations.

E. Nursing plan/implementation:

1. *Presurgical*
   a. Goal: *promote relief of symptoms.*
      (1) Diet:
         (a) Small, frequent feedings of soft, bland foods, to reduce abdominal pressure and reflux.
         (b) Large amounts of fluid when swallowing solids; may push food into stomach.
         (c) Avoid eating 2 hours before bedtime.
         (d) High-protein, low-fat foods to decrease heartburn.
      (2) *Positioning:* head elevated to increase movement of food into stomach. Symptoms may decrease if head of bed at home is elevated on 8-inch blocks.
      (3) Weight reduction to decrease abdominal pressure.
      (4) Medications as ordered:
         (a) 30 mL antacid 1 h after meals and at bedtime.
         (b) Avoid anticholinergic drugs, which decrease gastric emptying.
2. *Postsurgical*
   a. Goal: *provide for postoperative safety needs.*
      (1) Respiratory: deep breathing, coughing, splint incision area.
      (2) *Nasogastric tube:* check patency
         (a) Drainage: should be small amount.
         (b) Color: dark brown 6–12 h after surgery, changing to greenish yellow.
         (c) Do *not* disturb tube placement to avoid traction on suture line.
      (3) *Position:* initially head of bed elevated slightly, then semi-Fowler's; turn side to side frequently, to prevent pressure on diaphragm.
      (4) Maintain closed chest drainage if indicated (see Table 7.5).
      (5) Check for return of bowel sounds.
   b. Goal: *promote comfort and maintain nutrition.*
      (1) IVs for hydration and electrolytes.
      (2) Initiate feeding through *gastrostomy* tube if present.
         (a) Usually attached to intermittent, low suction after surgery.
         (b) Aspirate gastric contents before feeding—delay if 75 mL or more is present; report these findings to physician.
         (c) Feed in *high-Fowler's* or sitting position; keep head elevated for 30 minutes after eating.
         (d) Warm feeding to room temperature; dilute with H_2O if too thick.
         (e) Give 50 mL H_2O before feeding; 200–500 mL feeding by gravity over 10–15 minutes; follow with 50 mL H_2O.
         (f) Give frequent mouth care.
   c. Goal: *health teaching.*
      (1) Avoid constricting clothing and activities that increase intra-abdominal pressure, e.g., lifting, bending, straining at stool.
      (2) Weight reduction.
      (3) Dietary needs: small, frequent, soft, bland meals; chew thoroughly; upright position for at least 1 hour after meals.

F. Evaluation:

1. Relief from symptoms, comfortable.
2. Receiving adequate, balanced nutrition.
3. Describes dietary changes, recommended positioning, and activity limitations to prevent recurrence.

VIII. Peptic ulcer disease: circumscribed loss of mucosa, submucosa, or muscle layer of the gastrointestinal tract caused by a decreased resistance of gastric mucosa to acid-pepsin injury. *Peptic ulcer disease* is a chronic disease and may occur in the distal esophagus, stomach, upper duodenum, or jejunum. *Gastric ulcers,* located on the lesser curvature of stomach, are larger, deeper than duodenal ulcers and tend to become *malignant. Duodenal ulcers* are located on the first part of the duodenum; they are more common than gastric ulcers. *Stress ulcers,* an acute problem, occur after a major insult to the body.

A. Pathophysiology: failure of the body to regenerate mucous epithelium at a sufficient rate to counterbalance the damage to tissue during the breakdown of protein; decrease in the quantity and quality of the mucus; poor local mucosal blood flow, along with individual susceptibility to ulceration.

B. Risk factors:

1. *Gastric ulcers*
   a. Decreased resistance to acid-pepsin injury.
   b. Gastritis.
   c. Increased histamine release → inflammatory reaction.
   d. Cigarette smoking, increased caffeine/alcohol use.
   e. Family history.
   f. Difficulty coping with high-stress environment.
   g. Ulcerogenic drugs that aggravate preexisting condition.
   h. Increased hydrogen ion back-diffusion.
   i. Age: over 50.
2. *Duodenal ulcers*
   a. Elevated gastric acid secretory rate.
   b. Elevated gastric acid levels postprandially (after eating).
   c. Increased rate of gastric emptying → increased amount of acid into duodenum → irritation and breakdown of duodenal mucosa.
   d. Men more than women; possible influence of endocrine factors such as estrogen and adrenal steroids.
   e. Seasonal influence: spring and fall.
   f. Cigarette smoking; increased caffeine/alcohol use.
   g. Family history.
   h. Difficulty coping with high-stress environment.
   i. Ulcerogenic drugs that aggravate preexisting condition.
   j. Persons with blood type O.
   k. Age 25–50.
3. *Stress ulcers*
   a. Severe trauma or major illness.
   b. Severe burns (Curling's ulcer); develop in 72 hours with majority of persons with burns over more than 35% of their body surface.
   c. Head injuries or intracranial disease (Cushing's ulcers).
   d. Medications in large doses: corticosteroids, salicylates, ibuprofen, indomethacin, phenylbutazone (Butazolidin).
   e. Shock.
   f. Sepsis.

C. Assessment:

1. Subjective data
   a. *Gastric ulcers*
      (1) Pain
         (a) Type: gnawing, aching, burning.
         (b) Location: epigastric, left of midline, localized.
         (c) Occurrence: period pain, often 2 hours after eating.
         (d) Relief: antacids; may be aggravated, not relieved, by food.
      (2) Nausea.
      (3) History of risk factors as above.
   b. *Duodenal ulcers*
      (1) Pain
         (a) Type: gnawing, aching, burning, hungerlike, boring.
         (b) Location: right epigastric, localized; steady pain near midline of back may indicate perforation.
         (c) Occurrence: 1–3 hours after eating, worse at end of day or during the night; initial attack occurs spring or fall; history of remissions and exacerbations.
         (d) Relief: food and/or antacids.
      (2) Nausea.
      (3) History of risk factors as above.
   c. *Stress ulcers*
      (1) Pain: often painless until serious complication (hemorrhage, perforation) occurs.
      (2) History of risk factors as above.
2. Objective data
   a. *Gastric ulcer*
      (1) Vomiting.
      (2) Melena (tarry stools).
      (3) Weight loss.
      ▶ (4) X ray (upper GI series) confirms "crater" (punched out appearance, clean base).
      ▶ (5) Endoscopy confirms presence of ulcer; biopsy for cytology.
      (6) Monitor for blood loss: CBC, stool for occult blood.
   b. *Duodenal ulcer*
      (1) Eructation.
      (2) Vomiting.
      (3) Regurgitation of sour liquid into back of mouth.
      (4) Constipation.
      ▶ (5) X ray (upper GI series) confirms ulcer craters and niches as well as outlet deformities; round

or oval funnellike lesion extending into musculature.

(6) Common complications: hemorrhage or perforation.

c. *Stress ulcer*

(1) GI bleeding.

(2) Multiple, superficial erosions affecting large area of gastric mucosa.

D. Analysis/nursing diagnosis (all types):

1. *Pain* related to erosion of gastric lining.
2. *Ineffective individual coping* related to inability to change life-style.
3. *Altered nutrition, less than body requirements,* related to inadequate intake.
4. *Knowledge deficit* regarding preventive measures.
5. *Potential for injury* related to possible hemorrhage or perforation.

E. Nursing plan/implementation (all types):

1. Goal: *promote comfort.*

a. Medications as ordered to decrease pain (see 4. Goal: Health teaching below); sedatives to decrease anxiety.

▶ b. Prepare for diagnostic tests.

(1) X rays; upper GI series (barium swallow); lower GI (barium enema).

(2) Endoscopy.

(3) Gastric analysis, to determine amount of hydrochloric acid in GI tract.

2. Goal: *prevent/recognize signs of complications.*

a. Monitor vitals for shock.

b. Check stool for occult blood/hemorrhage.

c. Palpate abdomen for perforation (rigid, boardlike).

3. Goal: *provide emotional support.*

a. Stress-management techniques.

b. Restful environment.

c. Prepare for surgery, if necessary.

4. Goal: *health teaching.*

a. Medications:

(1) Antacids: *Give 1 to 3 hours after meals and at bedtime* to decrease pain by lowering acidity; monitor for:

(a) Diarrhea (seen most often with magnesium carbonate and magnesium oxide).

(b) Constipation (seen most often with calcium carbonate or aluminum hydroxide).

(c) Electrolyte imbalance (seen with systemic antacid, soda bicarbonate).

(d) Best 1–3 hours *after meals.*

(e) Liquids more effective than tablets; if taking tablets, chew slowly.

(2) Histamine antagonists: *Given with meals/bedtimes* to block the action of histamine-stimulated gastric secretions (basal and stimulated); inhibits pepsin secretion and reduces the volume of gastric secretion.

(a) Cimetidine (Tagamet) inhibits gastrin release, can be given PO, IV or IM; cannot be given within 1 hour of antacid therapy.

(b) Ranitidine (Zantac) has greater reduction of acid secretion, longer duration, less frequent administration (bid vs qid), and fewer side effects than cimetidine.

(3) Sucralfate (Carafate) *Given 1 hour before meals and at bedtime.*

(a) Locally active topical agent that forms a protective coat on mucosa, prevents further digestive action of both acid and pepsin.

(b) Must not be given within one half hour of antacids.

(4) Anticholinergic *when used, given before meals* to decrease gastric acid secretion and delay gastric emptying.

(5) Important: avoid aspirin (could increase bleeding possibility).

b. Diet:

(1) *Avoid*

(a) Stress at mealtimes.

(b) Milk (increases gastric acid production).

(c) Substances that cause pain.

(d) Coffee with or without caffeine.

(e) Foods or liquids containing caffeine.

(f) Alcohol.

(g) Tobacco.

(2) *Plan:*

(a) Small, frequent meals (to prevent exacerbation of symptoms related to an empty stomach).

(b) Weight control.

c. Complications: signs and symptoms

(1) Gastric ulcers may be premalignant.

(2) Perforation.

(3) Hemorrhage.

(4) Obstruction.

d. Life-style changes

(1) Decrease:

(a) Smoking.

(b) Noise.

(c) Rush.

(d) Confusion.

(2) Increase:

(a) Communications.

(b) Mental/physical rest.

(c) Compliance with medical regime.

F. Evaluation:

1. Remains on specified diet.
2. Takes prescribed medications.
3. Pain decreases.
4. No complications.
5. States signs and symptoms of complications.
6. Participates in stress-reduction activities.

IX. Gastric surgery: performed when ulcer medical regime is unsuccessful, ulcer is determined to be precancerous, or complications are present.

A. Types:

1. Subtotal gastrectomy: removal of a portion of the stomach.
2. Total gastrectomy: removal of the entire stomach.
3. Antrectomy: removal of entire antrum (lower) portion of the stomach.
4. Pyloroplasty: repair of the pyloric opening of the stomach.
5. Vagotomy: interruption of the impulses carried by the vagus nerve, which results in reduction of gastric secretions and decreased physical activity of the stomach.
6. Combination of vagotomy and gastrectomy.

B. Analysis/nursing diagnosis:

1. *Pain* related to surgical incision.
2. *Ineffective breathing pattern* related to high surgical incision.
3. *Potential for trauma* related to possible complications postgastrectomy.
4. *Knowledge deficit* related to inability to manage ulcer disease on medical regime.
5. *Fear* related to possible precancerous lesion.
5. *Ineffective individual coping* related to risk factors influencing peptic ulcer disease.

C. Nursing plan/implementation:

1. Goal: *promote comfort in the postoperative period.*
   a. Analgesics: to relieve pain and allow client to cough, deep breathe to prevent pulmonary complications.
   b. *Position:* semi-Fowler's to aid in breathing.
2. Goal: *promote wound healing.*
   a. Keep dressings dry.
   b. *NG tube* to low intermittent suction (Levine) or low continuous (Salem sump).
      (1) Check drainage from NG tube; normally bloody first 2–3 hours postsurgery, then brown to dark green.
      (2) Excessive bright red blood drainage: take vital signs; report: vital signs, color and volume of drainage to MD immediately.
      (3) Irrigate *gently* with saline in amount ordered; do **not** irrigate against resistance.
      (4) Tape securely to face, but prevent obstructed vision.
      (5) Frequent mouth and nostril care.
3. Goal: *promote adequate nutrition and hydration.*
   a. Administer parenteral fluids as ordered.
   b. Accurate I&O.
   c. Check bowel sounds, at least q4h; NPO 1–3 days; oral fluids as ordered when bowel sounds present—usually 30 mL, then small feedings, then bland liquids to soft diet.
   d. Observe for nausea and vomiting due to suture line edema, food intake (too much, too fast).
4. Goal: *prevent complications.*
   a. Check dressing q4h for bleeding.
   b. Vitamin B_{12} and iron replacement as ordered to avoid pernicious anemia or iron deficiency anemia.
   c. Avoid dumping syndrome.

D. Evaluation:

1. Hemorrhage, dumping syndrome avoided.
2. Healing begins.
3. Adjust life-style to prevent recurrence/marginal ulcer.

X. Dumping syndrome: hypoglycemic-type episode; occurs postoperatively after gastric resection (may also occur post vagotomy, antrectomy, or gastroenterostomy), when food and fluids that are more hyperosmolar than the jejunal secretions pass *quickly* into jejunum, producing fluid shifts from bloodstream to jejunum. This is a mild problem for about 20% of clients and will disappear in a few months to a year. Symptoms cause serious problem for about 7% of the clients. This discomfort may occur during a meal or up to 30 minutes after the meal and last from 20–60 minutes. The reaction is greatest after the ingestion of sugar.

A. Assessment:

1. Subjective data
   a. Feeling of fullness, weakness, faintness.
   b. Palpitations.
   c. Nausea.
   d. Discomfort during or after eating.
2. Objective data
   a. Diaphoresis.
   b. Diarrhea.
   c. Fainting.
   d. Symptoms of hypoglycemia.

B. Analysis/nursing diagnosis:

1. *Altered nutrition, more than body requirements,* related to body's inability to properly digest high-carbohydrate, high-sodium foods.
2. *Diarrhea* related to food passing into jejunum too quickly.
3. *Potential for injury* related to hypoglycemia.
4. *Knowledge deficit* related to dietary restrictions.

C. Nursing plan/implementation:

1. Goal: *health teaching.*
   a. *Include:*
      (1) Increased fat, protein to delay emptying.
      (2) Rest after meals.
      (3) Small, frequent meals.
      (4) Fluids *between* meals.
   b. *Avoid:*
      (1) Foods high in salt, carbohydrate.
      (2) Large meals.
      (3) Stress at mealtime.
      (4) Fluids at mealtime.

D. Evaluation:

1. No complications.
2. Client heals.

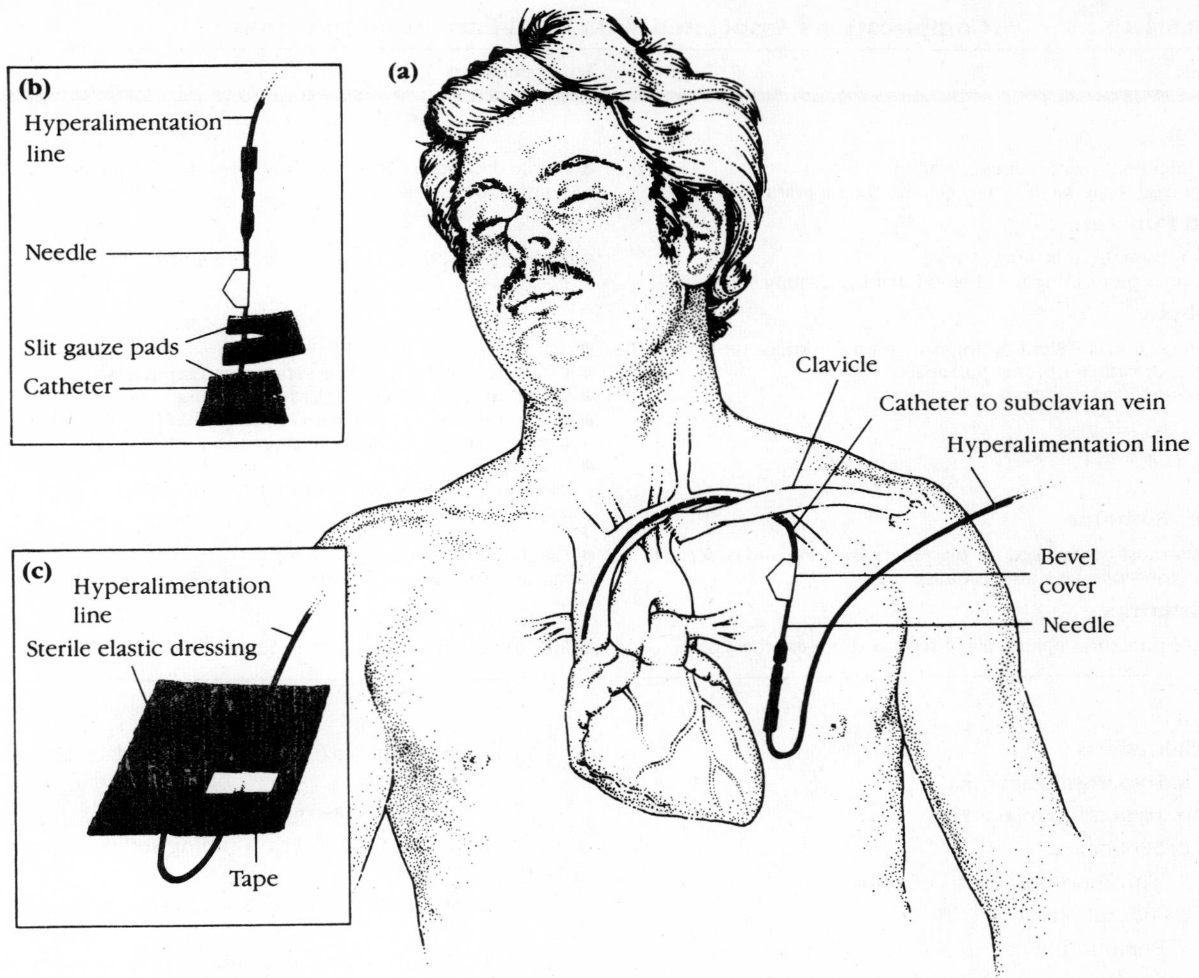

■ FIGURE 4.2
Hyperalimentation. (a) Client with subclavian hyperalimentation line. (b) Gauze dressing. (c) Taping hyperalimentation line. (From Saxton DF, et al.: *The Addison-Wesley Manual of Nursing Practice,* Addison-Wesley, Menlo Park, CA, 1983.)

3. No further ulcers.
4. Incorporates health teaching into life-style and prevents syndrome.

XI. Total parenteral nutrition: provide nutrition through a central venous line to clients who are in a catabolic state; are malnourished and cannot tolerate food by mouth; are in negative nitrogen balance; or have conditions that interfere with protein ingestion, digestion and absorption, e.g., Crohn's disease, major burns, and side effects of radiation therapy of abdomen.

A. Types of solutions:

1. Hydrolyzed proteins (Hyprotein, Amigen).
2. Synthetic amino acids (Freamine).
3. Usual components:
   a. 3–8% amino acid.
   b. 10% to 25% glucose.
   c. Multivitamins.
   d. Electrolytes.
4. Supplements that can be added:
   a. Fructose.
   b. Alcohol.
   c. Minerals: iron, copper, calcium.
   d. Trace elements: iodine, zinc, magnesium.
   e. Vitamins: A, B, C.
   f. Androgen hormone therapy.
   g. Insulin.

B. Administration:

1. Dosage varies with clinical condition; one liter q5–8h; rate of flow must be constant.
2. Solution prepared under laminar flow hood (usually in pharmacy); solution must be *refrigerated;* when refrigerated, expires in 24 h; once removed from refrigerator, expires in 12 h.
3. Incompatible with many antibiotics; check with pharmacy.
4. Route: catheter inserted in a large vein (e.g., subclavian) by physician; placement confirmed by X ray before beginning infusion (see Figure 4.2).

TABLE 4.19 Complications Associated With Total Parenteral Nutrition

Problem	Intervention
Infection	
■ Local infection (pain, redness, edema). ■ Generalized, systemic infection (elevated temperature, WBC).	■ Sterile dressings; administer antibiotics as ordered; general comfort measures.
Arterial Puncture	
■ Artery is punctured instead of vein. ■ Physician aspirates bright red blood that is pulsating strongly.	■ Needle is withdrawn and pressure is applied.
Air Embolus	
■ Air enters venous system during catheter insertion or tubing changes; or catheter/tubing pull apart. ■ Chest pain, dizziness, cyanosis, confusion.	■ Stat ABGs, chest X ray, ECG. ■ Connect catheter to sterile syringe, and aspirate air. ■ Clean catheter tip, connect to new tubing. ■ *Place client on left side with head lowered* (left Trendelenburg prevents air from going into pulmonary artery). ■ *Prevent: have client perform Valsalva maneuver or use plastic-coated clamp on catheter at insertion or tubing changes.*
Catheter Embolus	
■ Catheter must be checked for placement by X ray and observed when removed to be sure it is intact.	■ Careful observation of catheter. ■ Monitor for signs of distress.
Pneumothorax	
■ If needle punctures pleura, client reports dyspnea, chest pain.	■ May seal off or may need chest tubes.

5. Side effects:
   a. Hyperosmolar coma.
   b. Hyperglycemia >130.
   c. Septicemia.
   d. Thrombosis/sclerosis of vein.
   e. Air embolus.
   f. Pneumothorax.
6. Prolonged use: >10 days, fat needed; intralipids piggybacked close to insertion site; do not give through filter; observe for hypersensitivity (e.g., tachypnea, tachycardia, nausea, urticaria).

C. Analysis/nursing diagnosis:

1. *Fluid volume excess, potential,* related to inability to tolerate amount and consistency of solution.
2. *Fluid volume deficit* related to state of malnutrition.
3. *Potential for injury* related to possible complications.
4. *Altered nutrition, more or less than body requirements,* related to ability to tolerate parenteral nutrition.

D. Nursing plan/implementation:

1. Goal: *prevent infection.*
   a. Dressing change:
      (1) Strict aseptic technique.
      (2) Nurse and client wear mask during dressing change.
      (3) Cleanse skin with solution as ordered:
         (a) Acetone to defat the skin, destroy the bacterial wall.
         (b) Iodine 1% solution as antiseptic agent.
      (4) Dressing changed every 48–72 hours; transparent polyurethane dressings may be changed weekly.
      (5) Mark with nurse's initials, date and time of change.
      (6) Air occlusive dressing.
   b. Attach final filter on tubing setup, to prevent air embolism.
   c. Solution: change every 12 hours to prevent infection.
   d. Culture wound and catheter tip if signs of infection appear.
   e. Monitor temperature q4h.
   f. Use lumen line for feeding only (not for CVP or medications).
2. Goal: *prevent fluid and electrolyte imbalance.*
   a. Daily weights.
   b. I&O.
   c. Blood glucose q4h using glucometer; may need insulin coverage.
   d. Specific gravity q8h to determine hydration status.
   e. Infusion pump to maintain constant infusion rate.
3. Goal: *prevent complications.*
   a. Warm TPN solution to room temperature to prevent chills.
   b. Monitor for signs of complications (see Table 4.19).
      (1) Infiltration.
      (2) Thrombophlebitis.
      (3) Fever.
      (4) Hyperglycemia.
      (5) Fluid imbalance.
   c. Have client perform Valsalva's maneuver, or apply a plastic coated clamp when changing tubing to prevent air embolism.
   d. Tape tubings together to prevent accidental separation.

E. Evaluation:

1. No signs of infection.
2. Glycosuria between 1 + and 2 +.
3. Specific gravity between 1.010 and 1.020.
4. Wounds begin to heal.
5. Weight: no further loss, begins to gain.

XII. Diabetes: heterogeneous group of diseases involving the disruption of the metabolism of carbohydrates, fats, and protein. If uncontrolled, serious vascular and neurological changes occur.

A. Types:

1. *Type I: IDDM* (insulin dependent diabetes mellitus): formerly called "juvenile onset diabetes." Insulin needed to prevent ketosis; onset usually in youth but may occur in adulthood; prone to ketosis, unstable diabetes.
2. *Type II: NIDDM* (non-insulin dependent diabetes mellitus): formerly called "maturity onset or adult onset diabetes." May be controlled on diet and oral hypoglycemics or insulin; client less apt to have ketosis, except in presence of infection. May be further classified as *obese type* II or *non-obese type* II.
3. *Type III: GDM* (gestational diabetes mellitus): glucose intolerance during pregnancy in women who were not known diabetics prior to pregnancy; will be reclassified after delivery; may need to be treated or may return to prepregnancy state and need no treatment.
4. *Type IV:* diabetes secondary to another condition, such as pancreatic disease, other hormonal imbalances, or drug therapy such as involving glucocorticoids.

B. Pathophysiology:

1. IDDM—absolute deficiency of insulin due to destruction of pancreatic beta cells by the interaction of genetic, immunologic, hereditary or environmental factors.
2. NIDDM—relative deficiency of insulin due to:
   a. An islet cell defect resulting in a slowed or delayed response in the release of insulin to a glucose load; or
   b. Reduction in the number of insulin receptors from continuously elevated insulin levels; or
   c. A postreceptor defect; or
   d. A major peripheral resistance to insulin induced by hyperglycemia. These factors lead to deprivation of insulin-dependent cells → a marked decrease in the cellular rate of glucose uptake, and therefore elevated blood glucose.

C. Risk factors:

1. Obesity.
2. Family history of diabetes.
3. Elderly.
4. Women whose babies at birth weighed more than 9 pounds.
5. History of autoimmune disease.

D. Assessment:

1. Subjective data
   a. *Eyes:* blurry vision.
   b. *Skin:* pruritus vulvae.
   c. *Neuromuscular:* paresthesia, peripheral neuropathy, lethargy, weakness, fatigue, increased irritability.
   d. *GI:* polydipsia (increased thirst).
   e. *Reproductive:* impotence.
2. Objective data
   a. *Genitourinary:* polyuria, glycosuria, nocturia, (nocturnal enuresis in children).
   b. *Vital signs:*
      (1) Pulse and temperature normal or elevated.
      (2) BP normal or decreased, unless complications present.
      (3) Respirations, increased rate and depth (Kussmaul's respirations).
   c. *GI:*
      (1) Polyphagia, dehydration.
      (2) Weight loss, failure to gain weight.
      (3) Acetone breath.
   d. *Skin:* cuts heal slowly; frequent infections, foot ulcers, vaginitis.
   e. *Neuromuscular:* loss of strength, peripheral neuropathy.
   f. Lab data:
      (1) *Elevated:*
         (a) Blood sugar (above 130 mg/100 mL).
         (b) Glucose tolerance test.
         (c) Glycosuria (above 170 mg/100 mL).
         (d) Potassium (>5) and chloride (>145).
      (2) *Decreased:*
         (a) pH (<7.4).
         (b) P_{CO_2} (<32).
   g. Long-term pathological considerations:
      (1) *Cataract formation and retinopathy:* thickened capillary basement membrane, changes in vascularization and hemorrhage, due to chronic hyperglycemia.
      (2) *Nephropathy:* due to glomerulosclerosis, arteriosclerosis of renal artery and pyelonephritis, progressive uremia.
      (3) *Neuropathy:* due to reduced tissue perfusion; affecting motor, sensory, voluntary, and autonomic functions.
      (4) *Arteriosclerosis:* due to lesions of the intimal wall.
      (5) *Cardiac:* angina, coronary insufficiency, myocardial infarction.
      (6) *Vascular changes:* occlusions, intermittent claudication, loss of peripheral pulses, arteriosclerosis.

E. Analysis/nursing diagnosis:

1. ***Altered nutrition, less than body requirements,*** related to inability to metabolize nutrients and weight loss.
2. ***Altered nutrition, more than body requirements,*** related to excessive glucose intake.

3. *Potential for injury* related to complications of uncontrolled diabetes.
4. *Body image disturbance* related to long-term illness.
5. *Knowledge deficit* related to management of long-term illness.
6. *Ineffective individual coping* related to inability to follow diet/medication regime.
7. *Sexual dysfunction* related to impotence of diabetes and treatment.

F. Nursing plan/implementation:

1. Goal: *obtain and maintain normal sugar balance.*
   a. Monitor: vital signs; blood glucose before meals, at bedtime, and as symptoms demand (urine testing for glucose levels is *not* as accurate as capillary blood testing).
   b. Medications: oral hypoglycemics or insulin, as ordered.
   c. Diet, as ordered.
      (1) Carbohydrate, 50–60%; protein, 20%; fats, 30% (saturated fats limited to 10%, unsaturated fats, 90%).
      (2) Calorie reduction in obese adults; enough calories to promote normal growth and development for children or nonobese adults.
      (3) Limit refined sugars.
      (4) Add vitamins, minerals as needed for well-balanced diet.
   d. Monitor for signs of acute or chronic complications.
2. Goal: *health teaching.*
   a. Diet: foods allowed, restricted, substitutions.
   b. Medications: administration techniques, importance of utilizing room temperature insulin, and rotating injection sites to prevent tissue damage.
   c. Desired and side effects of prescribed insulin type; onset, peak, and duration of action of prescribed insulin.
   d. Urine and blood testing techniques.
   e. Signs of complications (see Table 4.20).
   f. Importance of health maintenance:
      (1) Infection prevention, especially foot and nail care.
      (2) Routine checkups.
      (3) Maintain stable balance of glucose by carefully monitoring glucose level and making necessary adjustments in diet and activity level; seeking medical attention when unable to maintain balance; regular exercise program.

G. Evaluation:

1. Optimal blood glucose levels achieved.
2. Ideal weight maintained.
3. Adequate hydration.
4. Carries out self-care activities; blood or urine testing, foot care, exchange diets, medication administration, exercise.
5. Recognizes and treats hyper- or hypoglycemic reactions.
6. Seeks medical assistance appropriately.

XIII. Hyperglycemic hyperosmolar nonketotic coma (HHNC): profound hyperglycemia and dehydration without ketosis or ketoacidosis; seen in non-insulin dependent diabetics; brought on by infection or illness. The client is *critically ill.*

A. Pathophysiology: hyperglycemia greater than 1000 mg/100 mL causes osmotic diuresis, depletion of extracellular fluid, and hyperosmolarity related to infection or another stressor as the precipitating factor. Client unable to replace fluid deficits with oral intake.

B. Risk factors:

1. Old age.
2. History of non-insulin dependent diabetes.
3. Infections: pneumonia, pyelonephritis, pancreatitis, gram-negative infections.
4. Kidney failure: uremia and peritoneal dialysis.
5. Shock:
   a. Lactic acidosis related to bicarbonate deficit.
   b. Myocardial infarction.
6. Hemorrhage:
   a. GI.
   b. Subdural.
   c. Arterial thrombosis.
7. Medications:
   a. Diuretics.
   b. Glucocorticoids.

C. Assessment:

1. Subjective data
   a. Confusion.
   b. Lethargy.
2. Objective data
   a. Nystagmus.
   b. Dehydration.
   c. Aphasia.
   d. Nuchal rigidity.
   e. Hyperreflexia.
   f. Lab data:
      (1) Blood glucose level 1000 mg/100 mL.
      (2) Serum sodium and chloride—normal to elevated.
      (3) BUN > than 60 mg/100 mL (higher than in ketoacidosis because of more severe gluconeogenesis and dehydration).
      (4) Arterial pH—slightly depressed.

D. Analysis/nursing diagnosis:

1. *Potential for injury* related to hyperglycemia.
2. *Altered renal peripheral tissue perfusion* related to vascular collapse.
3. *Ineffective airway clearance* related to coma.

E. Nursing plan/implementation:

1. Goal: *promote fluid and electrolyte balance.*
   a. IVs: fluids and electrolytes, saline solution used initially to combat dehydration. Lab values will determine fluid replacement.
   b. Monitor I&O because of the high volume of fluid replaced in the critical stage of this condition.

■ **TABLE 4.20** **Comparison of Diabetic Complications**

	Hypoglycemia	Ketoacidosis
Pathophysiology	Major metabolic complication when too little food or too large dose of insulin or hypoglycemic agents administered; interferes with oxygen consumption of nervous tissue.	Major metabolic complication in which there is insufficient insulin for metabolism of carbohydrates, fats, and proteins; seen most frequently with clients who are insulin-dependent. Precipitated in the known diabetic by stressors (such as infection, trauma, major illness) that increase insulin needs.
Risk Factors	Too little food. Emotional or added stress. Vomiting or diarrhea. Added exercise.	Insufficient insulin or oral hypoglycemics. Noncompliance with dietary instructions. Major illness/infections. Therapy with steroid administration. Trauma, surgery. Elevated blood sugar: >200 mg/100 mL.
Assessment	**Behavioral Change:** *Subjective data*—nervous, irritable, anxious, confused, disoriented. *Objective data*—abrupt mood changes, psychosis.	**Behavioral Change:** *Subjective data*—irritable, confused. *Objective data*—drowsy.
	Visual: *Subjective data*—blurred vision, diplopia.	**Visual:** *Objective data*—eyeballs: soft, sunken.
	Skin: *Objective data*—diaphoresis, **pale,** cool, clammy, goose bumps (piloerection).	**Skin:** *Objective data*—loss of turgor, **flushed face,** pruritus vulvae.
	Vitals: *Objective data*—tachycardia; palpitations.	**Vitals:** *Objective data*—respirations-Kussmaul's. Breath: fruity; BP: hypovolemic shock.
	Gastrointestinal: *Subjective data*— hunger, nausea. *Objective data*—diarrhea, vomiting.	**Gastrointestinal:** *Subjective data*—increased thirst, abdominal pain, anorexia, nausea. *Objective data*—vomiting, diarrhea, dry mucous membrane; lips, tongue: red, parched.
	Neurologic: *Subjective data*—headache; lips/tongue: tingling, numbness. *Objective data*—fainting, yawning; speech: incoherent; convulsions; coma.	**Neurologic:** *Subjective data*—headache; irritability; confusion; lethargy, weakness.
	Musculoskeletal: *Subjective data*—weak, fatigue. *Objective data*—trembling.	**Musculoskeletal:** *Subjective data*—fatigue; general malaise.
	Blood Sugar: <80 mg/100 mL.	**Blood Sugar:** >130 mg/100 mL.
Analysis/nursing diagnosis	■ *Potential for injury* related to deficit of needed glucose. ■ *Knowledge deficit* related to proper dietary intake or proper insulin dosage. ■ *Altered nutrition, less than body requirements,* related to glucose deficiency.	■ *Potential for injury* related to glucose imbalance. ■ *Knowledge deficit* related to proper balance of diet and insulin dosage.
Nursing plan/implementation	■ Goal: *provide adequate glucose to reverse hypoglycemia:* administer simple sugar stat, PO or IV, glucose paste absorbed in mucous membrane; monitor blood sugar levels: identify events leading to complication.	Goal: *promote normal balance of food and insulin:* **regular** insulin as ordered; IV saline, as ordered; bicarbonate and electrolyte replacements, as ordered; potassium replacements once therapy begins and urine output is adequate.
	■ Goal: *health teaching:* how to prevent further episodes (see Diabetes, Health teaching, p. 364); importance of careful monitoring of balance between glucose levels and insulin dosage.	Goal: *health teaching:* diet instructions; desired effects and side effects of prescribed insulin or hypoglycemic agent (onset, peak, and duration of action); importance of recognizing signs of imbalance.
Evaluation	■ Adheres to diet and correct insulin dosage. ■ Adjusts dosage when activity is increased. ■ Glucose level 80–120 mg/mL.	Serious complications avoided. Accepts prescribed diet. Takes medication (correct dose and time). Glucose level 80–120 mg/dL.

c. Administer nursing care for problem that precipitated this serious condition.

d. Food by mouth when client is able.

2. Goal: *prevent complications.*

a. Administer *regular* insulin (initial dose usually 5–15 U) and food, as ordered.

b. Uncontrolled condition leads to cardiovascular disease, renal failure, blindness, and diabetic gangrene.

F. Evaluation:

1. Blood sugar returns to normal level of 80–120 mg/100 mL.
2. Client is alert to time, place, and person.
3. Primary medical problem resolved.
4. Client recognizes and reports signs of imbalance.

XIV. Cholecystitis/cholelithiasis: inflammation of gallbladder due to bacterial infection, presence of cholelithiasis (stones, cholesterol, calcium, or bile in the gallbladder), or choledocholithiasis (stone in the common bile duct) and/or obstruction. Acute cholecystitis is abrupt in onset, but the client usually has a history of several attacks of fatty-food intolerance. Client with chronic cholecystitis has a history of several attacks of moderate severity and has usually learned to avoid fatty foods to decrease symptoms.

A. Pathophysiology: calculi from increased concentration of bile salts, pigments, or cholesterol due to metabolic or hemolytic disorders, biliary stasis → precipitation of salts into stones, or inflammation causing bile constituents to become altered.

B. Risk factors:

1. Women.
2. Obesity.
3. Pregnancy.
4. Cirrhosis of the liver.
5. Diabetes.

C. Assessment:

1. Subjective data

a. Pain:

(1) Type—severe colic, radiating to back under the scapula and to the right shoulder.

(2) Positive Murphy's sign—a sign of gallbladder disease consisting of pain on taking a deep breath when pressure is placed over the location of the gallbladder.

(3) Location—right upper quadrant, epigastric area, flank.

(4) Duration—spasm of duct attempting to dislodge stone lasts until dislodged or relieved by medication, or sometimes by vomiting.

b. GI—anorexia, nausea, feeling of fullness, indigestion, intolerance of fatty foods.

2. Objective data

a. GI—belching, vomiting, clay-colored stools.

b. Vital signs—increased pulse, fever.

c. Skin—chills, jaundice.

d. Urine—dark amber.

e. Lab data—*elevated:*

(1) WBC.

(2) Alkaline phosphatase.

(3) Serum amalyse, lipase.

(4) AST[SGOT].

(5) Bilirubin.

D. Analysis/nursing diagnosis:

1. *Pain* related to obstruction of bile duct due to cholelithiasis.
2. *Altered nutrition, more than body requirements,* related to fatty foods.
3. *Altered nutrition, less than body requirements,* related to hesitancy to eat due to anorexia and nausea.
4. *Potential fluid volume deficit* related to episodes of vomiting.
5. *Knowledge deficit* related to fat-free diet.

E. Nursing plan/implementation:

1. Nonsurgical interventions:

a. Goal: *promote comfort.*

(1) Medications as ordered: meperidine, antibiotics, antispasmodics, electrolytes.

(2) Avoid morphine due to spasmodic effect.

(3) NG tube to low suction.

(4) Diet: fat-free when able to tolerate food.

b. Goal: *health teaching.*

(1) Signs, symptoms, and complications of disease.

(2) Fat-free diet.

(3) Desired effects and side effects of prescribed medications.

(4) Prepare for possible removal of gallbladder (cholecystectomy) if conservative treatment unsuccessful.

2. Surgical interventions:

a. *Preoperative*—Goal: *prevent injury:* see I. Preoperative preparation, p. 342.

b. *Postoperative*—Goal: *promote comfort* (see also III. Postoperative experience, p. 345).

(1) Promote tube drainage.

(a) NG tube to low suction.

(b) *T tube* to closed-gravity drainage, to preserve patency of edematous common duct and ensure bile drainage; usual amount 500–1000 mL/24 h; dark brown drainage.

(c) Provide enough tubing to allow turning without tension.

(d) Empty and record bile drainage q8h.

(2) *Position:* low to semi-Fowler's to facilitate T-tube drainage.

(3) Dressing: dry to protect skin (as bile excoriates skin).

(4) Clamp T tube as ordered.

(a) Observe for abdominal distention, pain, nausea, chills, or fever.

(b) Unclamp tube and notify MD if symptoms appear.

c. Goal: *prevent complications.*
   (1) IV fluids with Berroca C.
   (2) Cough, turn, and deep breathe (prone to respiratory complication because of high incision).
   (3) Early ambulation to prevent vascular complications and aid in expelling flatus.
   (4) Monitor for jaundice: skin, sclera, urine, stools.
   (5) Monitor for signs of hemorrhage, infection.

d. Goal: *health teaching.*
   (1) Diet: fat-free for 6 weeks.
   (2) Signs of complications of food intolerance, pain, infection, hemorrhage.

F. Evaluation:
1. No complications.
2. Able to tolerate food.
3. Plans follow-up care.
4. Possible weight reduction.

■ ELIMINATION

CONDITIONS AFFECTING BOWEL ELIMINATION

I. Appendicitis: obstruction of appendiceal lumen and subsequent bacterial invasion of appendiceal wall.

A. Pathophysiology: when obstruction is partial or mild, inflammation begins in mucosa with slight appendiceal swelling, accompanied by periumbilical pain. As the inflammatory process escalates and/or obstruction becomes more complete, appendix becomes more swollen, lumen fills with pus, mucosal ulceration begins. When inflammation extends to peritoneal surface, pain is referred to right lower abdominal quadrant. *Danger:* rigidity over the entire abdomen is usually indicative of ruptured appendix; client then prone to peritonitis.

B. Risk factors:
1. Males more than females.
2. Most frequently seen between 10 and 30 years old.

C. Assessment:
1. Subjective data
   a. Pain: generalized, then right lower quadrant at McBurney's point, with rebound tenderness.
   b. Anorexia, nausea.
2. Objective data
   a. Vital signs: elevated temperature, shallow respirations.
   b. Either diarrhea or constipation.
   c. Vomiting, fetid breath odor.
   d. Splinting of abdominal muscles, flexion of knees onto abdomen.
   e. Lab data:
      (1) WBC elevated (above 10,000).
      (2) Neutrophil count elevated (above 75%).

D. Analysis/nursing diagnosis:
1. *Pain* related to inflammation of appendix.
2. *Potential for trauma* related to ruptured appendix.
3. *Knowledge deficit* related to possible surgery.

E. Nursing plan/implementation:
1. Goal: *promote comfort.*
   a. *Preoperative:*
      (1) Explain procedures.
      (2) Assist with diagnostic workup.
   b. *Postoperative:*
      (1) Relieve pain related to surgical incision.
      (2) Prevent infection: wound care, dressing technique.
      (3) Prevent dehydration: IVs, I&O, fluids to solids by mouth as tolerated.
      (4) Promote ambulation to prevent postoperative complications.

F. Evaluation:
1. No infection.
2. Tolerates fluid; bowel sounds return.
3. Heals with no complications.

II. Hernia: protrusion of the intestine through a weak portion of the abdominal wall.

A. Types:
1. *Reducible:* visceral contents return to their normal position, either spontaneously or by manipulation.
2. *Irreducible, or incarcerated:* contents cannot be returned to normal position.
3. *Strangulated:* blood supply to the structure within the hernia sac becomes occluded (usually a loop of bowel).
4. Most common hernias: umbilical, femoral, inguinal, incisional, and hiatus.

B. Pathophysiology: weakness in the wall may be either congenital or acquired. Herniation occurs when there is an increase in intra-abdominal pressure from coughing, lifting, crying, straining, obesity, or pregnancy.

C. Assessment:
1. Subjective data
   a. Pain, discomfort.
   b. History of feeling a lump.
2. Object data
   a. Soft lump, especially when straining or coughing.
   b. Sometimes alteration in normal bowel pattern.
   c. Swelling.

D. Analysis/nursing diagnosis:
1. *Activity intolerance* related to pain and discomfort.
2. *Potential for trauma* related to lack of circulation to affected area of bowel.
3. *Pain* related to protrusion of intestine into hernia sac.

E. Nursing plan/implementation:
1. Goal: *prevent postoperative complications.*
   a. Monitor bowel sounds.
   b. Prevent postoperative scrotal swelling with inguinal hernia by applying ice and support to scrotum.
2. Goal: *health teaching.*
   a. Prevent recurrence with correct body mechanics.
   b. Gradual increase in exercise.

F. Evaluation: healing occurs with no further hernia occurrence.

III. Diverticulosis: a *diverticulum* is a small pouch or sac composed of mucous membrane that has protruded through the muscular wall of the intestine. The presence of several of these is called *diverticulosis*. Inflammation of the diverticula is called *diverticulitis*.

A. Pathophysiology: weakening in a localized area of muscular wall of the colon, (especially the sigmoid colon), accompanied by increased intraluminal pressure.

B. Risk factors:

1. Diverticulosis
   a. Age: seldom before 35; 60% incidence in older adults.
   b. History of constipation.
   c. Diet history: low in vegetable fiber, high in carbohydrate.
2. Diverticulitis: highest incidence between ages 50 and 60.

C. Assessment:

1. Subjective data: pain: cramplike; left lower quadrant of abdomen.
2. Objective data
   a. Constipation or diarrhea, flatulence.
   b. Fever.
   c. Rectal bleeding.
   ▶ d. Diagnostic procedures:
      (1) Palpation reveals tender colonic mass.
      (2) Barium enema (done only in absence of inflammation) reveals presence of diverticula.
      (3) Sigmoidoscopy.

D. Analysis/nursing diagnosis:

1. *Constipation* related to dietary intake.
2. *Pain* related to inflammatory process of intestines.
3. *Potential fluid volume deficit,* related to episodes of diarrhea or bleeding.
4. *Potential for injury* related to bleeding.
5. *Knowledge deficit* related to prevention of constipation.

E. Nursing plan/implementation:

1. Goal: *bowel rest during acute episodes.*
   a. Diet: soft, liquid.
   b. Fluids, IVs if oral intake not adequate.
   c. Pain medications, as ordered.
   d. Monitor stools for signs of bleeding.
2. Goal: *promote normal bowel elimination.*
   a. Diet: bland, high in vegetable fiber
      (1) *Include:* fruits, vegetables, whole grain cereal, unprocessed bran.
      (2) *Avoid:* foods difficult to digest (corn, nuts).
   b. Bulk-forming agents as ordered: methylcellulose, psyllium.
   c. Monitor: abdominal distention, acute bowel symptoms.
3. Goal: *health teaching.*
   a. Methods to avoid constipation.
   b. Foods to include/avoid in diet.
   c. Relaxation techniques.
   d. Signs and symptoms of complications of chronic inflammation, abscess, obstruction, fistulas, perforation, or hemorrhage.

F. Evaluation:

1. Inflammation decreases.
2. Bowel movements return to normal.
3. Pain decreases.
4. No complications of perforation, fistulas, or abscesses noted.

IV. Ulcerative colitis: inflammation of mucosa and submucosa of the distal colorectal area. Inflammation leads to ulceration with bleeding. Involved areas are continuous. Disease is characterized by remissions and exacerbations.

A. Pathophysiology: specific physiological response to emotional trauma. Edema and hyperemia of colonic mucous membrane → superficial bleeding with increased peristalsis, shallow ulcerations, abscesses; bowel wall thins and shortens and becomes at risk for perforation. Increased rate of flow of liquid ileal contents → decreased water absorption and diarrhea.

B. Risk factors:

1. Highest occurrence in young adults (20-40 years of age).
2. Genetic predisposition: higher in Caucasians, Jews.
3. Autoimmune response.
4. Infections.
5. More common in urban areas (upper-middle incomes and higher educational levels).
6. May be influenced by smoking.
7. Exacerbations often related to stressful event.

C. Assessment:

1. Subjective data
   a. Urgency to defecate, particularly when standing (tenesmus).
   b. Loss of appetite, nausea.
   c. Coliclike stomach pain.
   d. History of intolerance to dairy products.
   e. Emotional depression.
2. Objective data
   a. *Diarrhea:* 10–20 stools per day; can be chronic or intermittent, episodic or continual; stools contain blood, mucus and pus.
   b. Weight loss and malnutrition, dehydration.
   c. Fever.
   d. Lab data: *decreased:* RBC, potassium, sodium, calcium, bicarbonate related to excessive diarrhea.
   e. Lymphadenitis.
   ▶ f. Diagnostic tests:
      (1) Sigmoidoscopy for visualization of lesions.
      (2) Barium enema.

D. Analysis/nursing diagnosis:

1. *Diarrhea* related to increased flow rate of ileal contents.

2. *Self-esteem disturbance* related to progression of disease and increased number and odor of stools.
3. *Pain* related to inflammatory process.
4. *Fluid volume deficit* related to frequent episodes of diarrhea.
5. *Knowledge deficit* related to methods to control symptoms.
6. *Social isolation* related to continual diarrhea episodes.

E. Nursing plan/implementation:

1. Goal: *reduce psychological stress.*
   a. Provide quiet environment.
   b. Encourage verbalization of concerns.
2. Goal: *relieve discomfort.*
   a. Administer medications as ordered.
      (1) Sedatives and tranquilizers to *promote rest and comfort.*
      (2) Absorbents, Kaopectate.
      (3) Anticholinergics and antispasmotics *to relieve cramping and diarrhea,* e.g., atropine sulfate, phenobarbital, Lomotil.
      (4) Antimicrobial agents *to relieve bacterial overgrowth* in bowel and *limit secondary infection.*
      (5) Steroids *to relieve inflammation and produce remission.*
      (6) Potassium supplements *to relieve deficiencies.*
3. Goal: *health teaching.*
   a. Diet:
      (1) *Avoid:* coarse-residue foods, e.g., raw fruits and vegetables, whole milk, cold beverages.
      (2) *Include:* bland, high-protein, high-vitamin, high-mineral, high-calorie foods.
      (3) Parenteral hyperalimentation for severely ill.
      (4) Force fluids by mouth.
4. Goal: *prepare for surgery if medical regime unsuccessful.*
   a. Possible surgical procedures:
      (1) Permanent ileostomy.
      (2) Continent ileostomy (Kock pouch).
      (3) Total colectomy, anastomosis with rectum.
      (4) Total colectomy, anastomosis with anal sphincter.

F. Evaluation:

1. Fluid balance is obtained and maintained.
2. Alterations in life-style managed.
3. Stress-management techniques successful.
4. Complications such as fistulas, obstruction, perforation, and peritonitis are avoided.
5. Client is prepared for surgery if medical regime is unsuccessful or complications develop.

V. Crohn's disease: a chronic, progressive inflammatory disease usually affecting the terminal ileum.

A. Pathophysiology: one of two conditions called "inflammatory bowel disease" (ulcerative colitis is the other) that affects all layers of the ileum and/or the colon, causing patchy shallow, longitudinal mucosal ulcers; possible correlation with autoimmune disease and adenocarcinoma of the bowel.

B. Risk factors:

1. Age: 15-20, 55-60.
2. Caucasian, especially Jewish.
3. Familial predisposition.
4. Possible virus involvement.
5. Possible psychosomatic involvement.
6. Possible hormonal or dietary influences.

C. Assessment (See IV. Ulcerative colitis for analysis/nursing diagnosis, nursing plan/implementation, and evaluation):

1. Subjective data
   a. Abdominal pain.
   b. Anorexia.
   c. Nausea.
   d. Malaise.
   e. History of isolated, intermittent, or recurrent attacks.
2. Objective data
   a. Diarrhea.
   b. Weight loss, vomiting.
   c. Fever, signs of infection.
   d. Fluid/electrolyte imbalances.
   e. Malnutrition, malabsorption.
   f. Occult blood in feces.

VI. Intestinal obstruction: blockage in movement of intestinal contents through small or large intestines.

A. Pathophysiology:

1. *Mechanical causes*—physical impediments to passage of intestinal contents, e.g., adhesions, hernias, neoplasms, inflammatory bowel diseases, foreign bodies, fecal impactions, congenital or radiational strictures, intussusception, or volvulus.
2. *Paralytic causes*—passageway remains open, but peristalsis ceases, e.g., after abdominal surgery, abdominal trauma, hypokalemia, myocardial infarction, pneumonia, spinal injuries, peritonitis, or vascular insufficiency.

B. Assessment:

1. Subjective data: pain related to
   a. *Proximal loop obstruction:* upper abdominal, sharp, cramping, intermittent pain.
   b. *Distal loop obstruction:* poorly localized, cramping pain.
2. Objective data
   a. Bowel sounds: initially loud, high pitched; then when smooth muscle atony occurs, bowel sound absent.
   b. Increased peristalsis above level of obstruction in attempt to move intestinal contents through the obstructed area.
   c. Obstipation (no passage of gas or stool through obstructed portion of bowel; no reabsorption of fluids).

d. Distension.

e. Vomiting:

(1) *Proximal loop obstruction:* profuse nonfecal vomiting.

(2) *Distal loop obstruction:* less frequent fecal-type vomiting.

f. Urinary output: decreased.

g. Temperature: elevated; tachycardia; hypotension → shock if untreated.

h. Dehydration, hemoconcentration, hypovolemia.

i. Lab data:

(1) Leukocytosis.

(2) *Decreased:* sodium (<138), potassium (<3.5).

(3) *Increased:* pH (>7.45), bicarbonates (>26 mm), BUN (>18 mg/dL).

C. Analysis/nursing diagnosis:

1. *Fluid volume deficit* related to vomiting.
2. *Pain* related to increased peristalsis above the level of obstruction.
3. *Altered nutrition, less than body requirements,* related to vomiting.
4. *Potential for trauma* related to potential perforation.

D. Nursing plan/implementation:

1. Goal: *obtain and maintain fluid balance.*

a. Nursing care of client with nasogastric tube (see Table 7.5):

(1) *Miller Abbott tube:* dual lumen, balloon inflated with air after insertion.

(2) *Cantor tube:* has mercury in distal sac, which helps move tube to point of obstruction.

Caution: do not tape either tube to face until tube reaches point of obstruction.

b. Nothing by mouth, IV therapy, strict I&O.

c. Take daily weights (early morning), monitor CVP for hydration status.

d. Monitor abdominal girth for signs of distention and urinary output for signs of retention or shock.

2. Goal: *relieve pain and nausea.*

a. Medications as ordered:

(1) Analgesics, antiemetics.

(2) If problem is paralytic: medical treatment includes neostigmine *to stimulate peristalsis.*

b. Observe for bowel sounds, flatus (tape intestinal tube to face once peristalsis begins).

c. Skin and frequent mouth care.

3. Goal: *prevent respiratory complications.*

a. Encourage coughing and deep breathing.

b. *Semi-Fowler's* or position of comfort.

4. Goal: *Postoperative nursing care* (if treated surgically): see III. Postoperative experience, p. 345.

E. Evaluation:

1. Fluid balance obtained and maintained.
2. Shock is prevented.
3. Obstruction is resolved.
4. Pain is decreased.
5. Fluids tolerated by mouth.
6. Complications such as perforation and peritonitis avoided.

VII. Fecal diversion—*stomas:* performed because of disease or trauma; may be temporary or permanent.

A. Types (See Table 4.21):

1. *Temporary*—fecal stream rerouted to allow GI tract to heal or to provide outlet for stool when obstructed.
2. *Permanent*—intestine cannot be reconnected. Rectum and anal sphincter removed (abdominal perineal resection). Often performed for cancer of the colon and/or rectum.

B. Analysis/nursing diagnosis:

1. *Bowel incontinence* related to lack of sphincter in newly formed stoma.
2. *Altered health maintenance* related to knowledge of ostomy care.
3. *Body image disturbance* related to stoma.
4. *Fluid volume deficit* related to increased output through stoma.

C. Nursing plan/implementation:

1. *Preoperative period*

a. Goal: *prepare bowel for surgery.*

(1) Administer neomycin as ordered to reduce colonic bacteria.

(2) Administer cathartics, enemas as ordered to cleanse the bowel of feces.

(3) Administer low-residue or liquid diet as ordered.

b. Goal: *relieve anxiety and assist in adjustment to surgery.*

(1) Provide accurate, brief, and reassuring explanations of procedures; allow time for questions.

(2) Have enterostomal nurse visit to discuss ostomy management and placement of stoma appliance.

(3) Offer opportunity for a visit with an Ostomy Association Visitor.

c. Goal: *health teaching.*

(1) Determine knowledge of surgery and potential impact.

(2) Begin teaching regarding ostomy.

2. *Postoperative period*

a. Goal: *maintain fluid balance.*

(1) Monitor I&O as large volume of fluid is lost through stoma.

(2) Administer IV fluids as ordered.

(3) Monitor losses through NG tube.

b. Goal: *prevent other postoperative complications.*

(1) Monitor for signs of intestinal obstruction.

(2) Maintain sterility when changing dressings; avoid fecal contamination of incision.

c. Goal: *initiate ostomy care.*

(1) Protect skin around stoma: use commercial preparation to toughen skin and use protective

TABLE 4.21 Comparison of Ileostomy and Colostomy

	Ileostomy	Colostomy
Procedure	Surgical formation of a fistula, or stoma, between the abdominal wall and *ileum*.	Surgical formation of an artificial opening between the surface of the abdominal wall and *colon*. *Single barrel*—only one loop of bowel is opened to the abdominal surface. *Double barrel*—two loops of bowel, a proximal and distal portion, are open to the abdominal wall. Feces will be expelled from the proximal loop, mucus will be expelled from the distal loop. Client may expel some excreta from rectum as well.
Reasons performed	Unresponsive ulcerative colitis: complications of ulcerative colitis, e.g., hemorrhage, carcinoma (suspected).	*Single barrel:* colon or rectal cancer. *Double barrel:* relieve obstruction.
Results	Permanent stoma.	*Single barrel:* permanent stoma. *Double barrel:* temporary stoma.
Discharge	Green liquid, nonodorous.	Consistency of feces dependent on diet and portion of the bowel used as the stoma; from brown odorous liquid to normal stool consistency.
Nursing care	See Table 7.6, 7.7; VII. Fecal diversion, p. 370.	See Table 7.6, 7.7, and VII. Fecal diversion, p. 370.

barrier wafer (Stomahesive) or paste (Karaya or substitute) to keep drainage (which can cause excoriation) off the skin.

(2) Keep skin around stoma clean and dry; empty appliance frequently. Check for drainage in appliance at least twice during each shift. If drainage present (diarrhea-type stool):

(a) Unclip the bottom of bag.

(b) Drain into bedpan.

(c) Use a squeeze-type bottle filled with warm water to rinse inside of appliance.

(d) Clean off clamp, if soiled.

(e) Put a few drops of deodorant in appliance if not odorproof.

(f) Fasten bottom of appliance securely (fold bag over clamp 2–3 times before closing).

(g) Check for leakage under appliance every 2–4 hours.

(3) Change appliance when drainage leaks around seal, or approximately every 2–3 days. Initially, size of stoma will be large due to edema. Pouch opening should be slightly larger than stoma so it will not constrict. Stoma will need to be measured for each change until swelling subsides to ensure appropriate fit.

(a) Gather equipment: gloves, skin prep packet, colostomy appliance measured to fit stoma properly (use stoma measuring guide), skin barrier, warm water and soap, face cloth/towel, plastic bag for disposal of old equipment.

(b) Remove old appliance carefully, pulling from area with least drainage to area with most drainage.

(c) Wash skin area (not stoma) with soap and water. Be careful not to: irritate skin, put soap on stoma, irritate stoma; do not put anything dry onto stoma. Remember: bowel is very fragile; working near bowel increases peristalsis so that feces and flatulence may be expelled.

(d) Observe skin area for potential breakdown.

(e) Use packet of skin prep on the skin around the stoma. Do not put this solution onto stoma, as it will cause irritation. Allow skin prep solution to dry on skin before applying colostomy appliance.

(f) Apply skin barrier you have measured and cut to size.

(g) Put appliance on so that bottom of appliance is easily accessible for emptying (e.g., if client is *out* of bed most of the time, put the bottom facing the feet; if client is *in* bed most of the time, have bottom face the side). Picture frame the adhesive portion of the appliance with 1-inch tape.

(h) Put a few drops of deodorant in appliance if not odorproof.

(i) Use clamp to fasten bottom of appliance.

(j) Talk to client (or communicate in best way possible during and after procedure). THIS IS A VERY DIFFICULT ALTERATION IN BODY IMAGE.

(k) Good handwashing technique.

(4) Use deodorizing drops in appliance and provide adequate room ventilation to decrease odors. *Caution:* deodorizing drops must be safe for mucous membranes. No pinholes in pouch.

d. Goal: *promote psychological comfort.*

(1) Support client and family—accept feelings and behavior.

(2) Recognize that such a procedure may initiate the grieving process.

e. Goal: *health teaching.*

(1) Self-management skills related to ostomy appliance and skin care.

(2) Diet: adjustments to control character of feces; avoid foods that increase flatulence.

(3) Signs of complications of infection, obstruction, or electrolyte imbalance.

(4) Community referral for follow-up care.

D. Evaluation:

1. Demonstrates self-care skill for independent living.
2. Makes dietary adjustments.
3. Ostomy functions well.
4. Adjusts to alteration in bowel elimination pattern.

VIII. Hemorrhoids: enlarged vein in mucous membrane of rectum.

A. Pathophysiology: venous congestion and interference with venous return from hemorrhoidal veins → increase in pelvic pressure, swelling, and distortion.

B. Risk factors:

1. Straining to expel constipated stool.
2. Pregnancy.
3. Intra-abdominal or pelvic masses.
4. Interference with portal circulation.
5. Prolonged standing or sitting.
6. History of low-fiber, high-carbohydrate diet, which contributes to constipation.
7. Family history of hemorrhoids.
8. Enlarged prostate.

C. Assessment:

1. Subjective data: discomfort, anal pruritus, pain.
2. Objective data

a. Bleeding, especially on defecation.

b. Narrowing of stool.

c. Grapelike clusters around anus (pink, red, or blue).

d. Diagnosis:

(1) Visualization for *external* hemorrhoids.

(2) Digital exam or proctoscopy for *internal* hemorrhoids.

D. Analysis/nursing diagnosis:

1. *Pain* related to defecation.
2. *Constipation* related to dietary habits and pain at time of defecation.
3. *Knowledge deficit* related to foods to prevent constipation.

E. Nursing plan/implementation:

1. Goal: *reduce anal discomfort.*

a. Sitz baths, as ordered; perineal care to prevent infection.

b. Hot or cold compresses as ordered to reduce inflammation and pruritus.

c. Topical medications as ordered:

(1) Anti-inflammatory: hydrocortisone cream.

(2) Astringents: witch-hazel-impregnated pads.

(3) Topical anesthetics: dibucaine (Nupercain).

2. Goal: *prevent complications related to surgery.*

a. Encourage postoperative ambulation.

b. Pain relief until packing removed.

c. Monitor for: bleeding, infection, pulmonary emboli, phlebitis.

d. Facilitate bowel evacuation: stool softeners, laxatives, suppositories, oil enemas as ordered.

e. Monitor for syncope/vertigo during first postoperative bowel movement.

f. Diet:

(1) Low-residue (postoperative)— until healing has begun.

(2) High-fiber to prevent constipation after healing.

g. Increase fluid intake.

3. Goal: *health teaching*—methods to avoid constipation.

F. Evaluation:

1. No complications.
2. Client has bowel movement.
3. Incorporates knowledge of correct foods into lifestyle.

CONDITIONS AFFECTING URINARY ELIMINATION

I. Pyelonephritis (PN): acute or chronic inflammation due to bacterial infection of the parenchyma and pelvis of the kidney; 95% of cases caused by gram-negative enteric bacilli (*Escherichia coli*); occurs more frequently in young women and older men.

A. Pathophysiology: inflammation of renal medulla or lining of the renal pelvis → nephron destruction; hypertrophy of nephrons needed to maintain urine output → impaired sodium reabsorption (salt-wasting); inability to concentrate urine; progressive renal failure; hypertension (two-thirds of all cases).

B. Risk factors:

1. Obstruction.
2. Hypertension.
3. Hypokalemia.
4. Diabetes mellitus.
5. Pregnancy.
6. Catheterization.

C. Assessment:

1. Subjective data

a. *Pain:* flank—one or both sides; back; dysuria; headache.

b. *Loss of appetite;* weight loss.

c. *Night sweats;* chills.

d. *Urination:* frequency, urgency.

2. Objective data

a. Fever.

b. Lab data:

(1) *Blood*—polymorphonuclear leukocytosis >11,000.

(2) *Urine*—leukocytosis, hematuria, white blood cell casts, proteinuria (<3 g in 24 h), positive cultures; specific gravity—normal or increased with acute PN, decreased with chronic PN; cloudy; foul-smelling.

c. Intravenous pyelogram (IVP)—may manifest structural changes.

D. Analysis/nursing diagnosis:

1. *Altered urinary elimination* related to kidney disease.
2. *Pain* related to dysuria and kidney damage.
3. *Altered nutrition, less than body requirements,* related to impaired sodium reabsorption and protein loss.
4. *Potential fluid volume excess* related to renal failure.

E. Nursing plan/implementation:

1. Goal: *combat infection, prevent recurrence, alleviate symptoms.*

a. Medications:

(1) *Antibiotics* and/or sulfonamides to support body defenses.

(2) *Analgesics* for pain—pentazocine lactate (Talwin), meperidine (Demerol) HCl.

(3) *Antipyretics* for fever—acetominophen (Tylenol).

b. Fluids: 1500-2000 mL/day to flush kidneys, relieve dysuria, reduce fever, prevent dehydration.

c. Observe hydration status: I&O (output minimum 1500 mL/24 h); daily weight; urine—check each voiding for protein, blood, specific gravity; vital signs q4h to monitor for hypertension, tachycardia; skin turgor.

d. Hygiene: meticulous perineal care; cleanse with soap and water; antimicrobial ointment may be used around urinary meatus with retention catheter.

e. Cooling measures: tepid sponging.

f. Diet: sufficient calories and protein to prevent malnutrition; sodium supplement as ordered.

2. Goal: *promote physical and emotional rest.*

a. Activity: bedrest or as tolerated—depends on whether anemia or fever is present; encourage activities of daily living as tolerated.

b. Emotional support: encourage expression of fears (possible renal failure, dialysis); provide diversional activities; include family in care; answer questions.

3. Goal: *health teaching.*

a. Medications: take regularly to maintain blood level; side effects.

b. Personal care: perineal hygiene; avoid urethral contamination; avoid tub baths.

c. Possible recurrence with pregnancy.

d. Monitoring daily weight.

F. Evaluation:

1. Normal renal function (minimum 1500 mL urine/24 h).
2. Blood pressure within normal range.
3. No recurrence of symptoms.

II. Acute glomerulonephritis: see Unit 3, p. 247.

III. Acute renal failure: broadly defined as rapid onset of oliguria accompanied by a rising BUN and serum creatinine; usually reversible.

A. Pathophysiology: acute renal ischemia → tubular necrosis → decreased urine output. *Oliguric phase* (<400 mL/24 h)—waste products are retained → metabolic acidosis → water and electrolyte imbalances → anemia. *Recovery phase*—diuresis → dilute urine → rapid depletion of sodium, chloride, and water → dehydration.

B. Types and risk factors:

1. *Prerenal*—due to factors outside of kidney; usually circulatory collapse—hemorrhage, severe dehydration, myocardial infarction, shock, vascular obstruction.
2. *Intrinsic renal*—parenchymal disease from ischemia or nephrotoxic damage; nephrotoxic agents—poisons, such as carbon tetrachloride; heavy metals (arsenic, mercury); antibiotics (kanamycin SO_4, neomycin SO_4); incompatible blood transfusion; alcohol myopathies; acute renal disease—acute glomerulonephritis, acute pyelonephritis.
3. *Postrenal*—obstruction in collecting system; renal or bladder calculi, tumors of bladder, prostate or renal pelvis, gynecologic or urologic surgery in which ureters are accidentally ligated.

C. Assessment:

1. Subjective data

a. Sudden decrease or cessation of urine output (<400 mL/24 h).

b. Anorexia, nausea, vomiting from azotemia.

c. Sudden weight gain from fluid accumulation.

d. Headache.

2. Objective data

a. Vital signs (vary according to cause and severity):

(1) *BP*—usually elevated.

(2) *Pulse*—tachycardia, irregularities.

(3) *Respirations*—increased rate, depth, rales, rhonchi.

b. Neurologic: decreasing mentation, unresponsive to verbal or painful stimuli, psychoses, convulsions.

c. Halitosis; cracked mucous membranes.

d. Skin: dry, rashes, purpura, itchy, pale.

e. Lab data:

(1) Blood: *increased*—potassium, BUN, creatinine, WBC; *decreased*—pH, bicarbonate, hematocrit, hemoglobin.

(2) Urine: *decreased*—volume, specific gravity (↓ 1.010); *increased*—protein, casts, red and white blood cells, sodium.

D. Analysis/nursing diagnosis:

1. *Altered urinary elimination* related to kidney malfunction.
2. *Fluid volume excess* related to decreased urine output.
3. *Altered nutrition, less than body requirements,* related to anorexia.
4. *Altered oral mucous membrane* related to stomatitis.
5. *Altered thought processes* related to uremia.

E. Nursing plan/implementation:

1. Goal: *maintain fluid and electrolyte balance and nutrition.*
   a. Monitor: daily weight (should not vary more than ± 1 lb); vital signs—include CVP; blood chemistries (BUN 6–20 mg/dL; creatinine 0.6–1.5 mg/dL).
   b. Fluids: IV as ordered; blood: plasma, packed cells, electrolyte solutions to replace losses; restricted to 400 mL/24 h if hypertension present or during oliguric phase to prevent fluid overload.
   c. Diet, as tolerated: high carbohydrate, low protein, may be low potassium and low sodium; hypertonic glucose (TPN) if oral feedings not tolerated; intravenous L-amino acids and glucose.
   d. Control hyperkalemia: infusions of hypertonic glucose and insulin to force potassium into cells; calcium gluconate (IV) to reduce myocardial irritability from K^+; sodium bicarbonate (IV) to correct acidosis; polystyrene sodium sulfonate (Kayexalate) or other exchange resins, orally or rectally (enema), to remove excess K^+; peritoneal or hemodialysis.
   e. Medications:
      (1) *Diuretics* (Edecrin, Lasix).
      (2) *Antacids* that bind phosphates (Amphogel, Alucaps).
      (3) *Anticonvulsants* (Valium, Dilantin).
2. Goal: *use assessment and comfort measures to reduce occurrence of complications.*
   a. Respiratory: monitor rate, depth, breath sounds, arterial blood gases; encourage deep breathing, coughing, turning; use incentive spirometer or nebulizer as indicated.
   b. Frequent oral care to prevent stomatitis.
   c. Observe for signs of:
      (1) *Infection*—elevated temperature, localized redness, swelling, heat, or drainage.
      (2) *Bleeding*—stools, gums, venipuncture sites.
3. Goal: *maintain continual emotional support.*
   a. Same caregivers, consistency in procedures.
   b. Give opportunities to express concerns, fears.
   c. Allow family interactions.
4. Goal: *health teaching.*
   a. Preparation for dialysis (indications: uremia, uncontrolled hyperkalemia, or acidosis).
   b. Dietary restrictions: low sodium, fluid restriction.
   c. Disease process; treatment regimen.

F. Evaluation:

1. Return of kidney function—normal creatinine level (< 1.5 mg/dL), urine output.
2. Resumes normal life pattern (about 3 months after onset).

IV. Chronic renal failure: as a result of progressive destruction of kidney tissue, the kidneys are no longer able to maintain their homeostatic functions; considered irreversible.

A. Pathophysiology: destruction of glomeruli → reduced glomerular filtration rate → retention of metabolic waste products; decreased urine output; severe fluid, electrolyte, acid-base imbalances → uremia. Clinical picture includes:

1. Ammonia in skin and alimentary tract by bacterial interaction with urea → inflammation of mucous membranes.
2. Retention of phosphate → decreased serum calcium → muscle spasms, tetany, and increased parathormone release → demineralization of bone.
3. Failure of tubular mechanisms to regulate blood bicarbonate → metabolic acidosis → hyperventilation.
4. Urea osmotic diuresis → flushing effect on tubules → decreased reabsorption of sodium → sodium depletion.
5. Waste product retention → depressed bone marrow function → decreased circulating RBCs → renal tissue hypoxia → decreased erythropoietin production → further depression of bone marrow → anemia.

B. Risk factors:

1. Polycystic kidney disease.
2. Chronic glomerulonephritis.
3. Chronic urinary obstruction, ureteral stricture, calculi, neoplasms.
4. Chronic pyelonephritis.
5. Severe hypertension.
6. Congenital or acquired renal artery stenosis.
7. Systemic lupus erythematosus.

C. Assessment:

1. Subjective data: excessive fatigue, weakness.
2. Objective data
   a. Skin: bronze-colored, uremic frost.
   b. Ammonia breath.
   c. Also see III. Acute renal failure; symptoms gradual in onset.

D. Analysis/nursing diagnosis:

1. In addition to the following, see III. Acute renal failure.
2. *Fatigue* related to severe anemia.
3. *Potential impaired skin integrity* related to pruritus.
4. *Ineffective individual coping* related to chronic illness.
5. *Body image disturbance* related to need for dialysis.
6. *Noncompliance* related to denial of illness.

E. Nursing plan/implementation:

1. Goal: *maintain fluid/electrolyte balance and nutrition.* (Also see III. Acute renal failure.)

TABLE 4.22 Comparison of Hemodialysis, Peritoneal Dialysis, and Continuous Ultrafiltration

	Hemodialysis	Peritoneal Dialysis	Continuous Ultrafiltration
Speed	Rapid—up to 8 hours per treatment.	Slow—up to 72 hours initially, up to 12 hours per treatment thereafter. Can be advantage in clients who cannot tolerate rapid fluid and electrolyte changes.	Slow—treatment is continuous during oliguric phase. Continuous slow removal of fluid and electrolytes is an advantage in patients who cannot tolerate rapid changes.
Cost	Expensive.	Manual—relatively inexpensive; automated—expensive.	Relatively inexpensive; one-to-one nursing care may be required.
Equipment	Complex.	Manual—simple and readily available; automated—complex.	Manual—simple and readily available.
Vascular access	Required.	Not necessary; therefore suitable for clients with vascular problems.	Arterial and venous access required.
Heparinization	Required; systemic or regional.	Little or no heparin necessary; therefore suitable for clients with bleeding problems.	Heparinization of filter/tubing required; minimal systemic heparinization.
Technical nursing skill necessary	High degree.	Manual—moderate degree; automated—high degree.	Moderate degree.
Complications (other than fluid and electrolyte imbalances, which are common to all)	Dialysis disequilibrium syndrome (preventable). Mechanical dysfunctions of dialyzer.	Peritonitis. Protein loss (0.5 g/L of dialysate). Bowel or bladder perforation.	Blood loss—filter rupture/ disconnection; system clotting.

Source: Holloway, N. *Nursing the Critically Ill Adult.* Menlo Park, CA: Addison-Wesley, 1988.

a. Diet: low sodium; foods high in calcium, vitamin B complex, vitamins C and D, and iron (to reduce edema, replace deficits, and promote absorption of nutrients).

b. Medications: calcium carbonate; supplemental vitamins if deficient.

c. I&O; intake should be no more than 600–800 mL more than previous day's output to prevent fluid retention.

2. Goal: *employ comfort measures that reduce distress and support physical function.*

a. Activity: bedrest; facilitate ventilation; turn, cough, deep breathe q2h; ROM—active and passive, to prevent thrombi.

b. Hygiene: mouth care to prevent stomatitis and reduce discomfort from mouth ulcers; perineal care.

c. Skin care: soothing lotions to reduce pruritus.

d. Encourage communication of concerns.

3. Goal: *health teaching.*

a. Dietary restrictions: no added salt when cooking; change cooking water in vegetables during process to decrease potassium; read food labels to avoid Na^+ and K^+.

b. Importance of daily weight: same scale, time, clothing.

c. Prepare for dialysis; transplantation.

F. Evaluation:

1. Acceptance of chronic illness (no indication of indiscretions, destructive behavior, suicidal tendency).

2. Compliance with dietary restriction—no signs of protein excess (e.g., nausea, vomiting) or fluid/sodium excess (e.g., edema, weight gain).

V. Dialysis: diffusion of solute through a semipermeable membrane that separates two solutions; direction of diffusion depends on concentration of solute in each solution; rate and efficiency depend on concentration gradient, temperature of solution, pore size of membrane, and molecular size; two methods available (see Table 4.22).

A. Indications: acute poisonings; acute or chronic renal failure; hepatic coma; metabolic acidosis; extensive burns with azotemia.

B. Goals

1. *Reduce level of nitrogenous waste.*

2. *Correct acidosis, reverse electrolyte imbalances, remove excess fluid.*

C. *Hemodialysis:* circulation of client's blood through a compartment formed of a semipermeable membrane (cellophane or cuprophane) surrounded by dialysate fluid.

1. Types of dialyzers

a. Coil type.

b. Parallel plate.

c. Capillary.

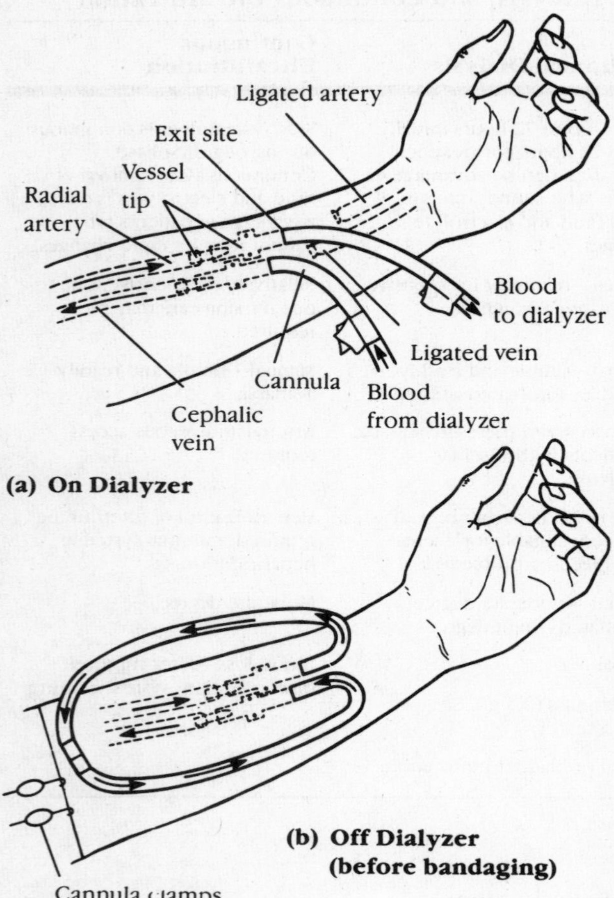

■ **FIGURE 4.3**
AV shunt (cannulae). Adapted and used by permission of Ann Holmes, RN, Head Nurse, West Contra Costa Dialysis Clinic, San Pablo, California.)

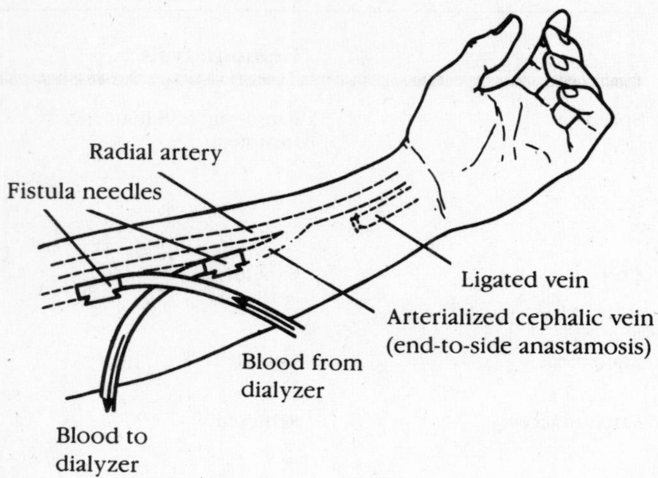

■ **FIGURE 4.4**
AV fistula. Adapted and used by permission of Ann Holmes, RN, Head Nurse, West Contra Costa Dialysis Clinic, San Pablo, California.)

2. Types of venous access for hemodialysis
   a. External shunt (Figure 4.3)
      (1) Cannula is placed in a large vein and a large artery that approximate each other.
      (2) External shunts, which provide easy and painless access to bloodstream, are prone to infection and clotting and cause erosion of the skin around the insertion area.
         (a) Daily cleansing and application of a sterile dressing.
         (b) Prevention of physical trauma and avoidance of some activities, such as swimming.
   b. Arteriovenous fistulas (Figure 4.4)
      (1) Large artery and vein are sewn together (anastomosed) below the surface of the skin.
      (2) Purpose is to create one blood vessel for withdrawing and returning blood.
      (3) *Advantages:* greater activity range than AV shunt and no protective asepsis.
      (4) *Disadvantage:* necessity of two venipunctures with each dialysis.
3. Complications during hemodialysis
   a. *Disequilibrium syndrome*—rapid removal of urea from blood → reverse osmosis, with water moving into brain cells → cerebral edema → possible headache, nausea, vomiting, confusion, and convulsions.
   b. *Hypotension*—results from excessive ultrafiltration or excessive antihypertensive medications.
   c. *Hypertension*—results from volume overload (water and/or sodium), causing disequilibrium syndrome or anxiety.
   d. *Transfusion reactions* (see Unit 7).
   e. *Arrhythmias*—due to hypotension, fluid overload, or rapid removal of potassium.
   f. *Psychologic problems*
      (1) Clients react in varying ways to dependence on hemodialysis.
      (2) Nurse needs to identify client reactions and defense mechanisms and to employ supportive behaviors, i.e., include client in care; continual repetition and reinforcement; do not interpret client's behavior—for example, do not say, "You're being hostile" or "You're acting like a child"; answer questions honestly regarding quality and length of life with dialysis and/or transplantation; encourage independence as much as possible.

D. *Peritoneal dialysis:* involves introduction of a dialysate solution into the abdomen, where the peritoneum acts as the semipermeable membrane between the solution and blood in abdominal vessels. *Procedures:*

1. Area around umbilicus is prepared, anesthetized with local anesthetic, and a catheter is inserted into the peritoneal cavity through a trocar; the catheter is then sutured into place to prevent displacement.
2. Warmed dialysate is then allowed to flow into the peritoneal cavity. Inflow time: 5–10 min; 2 liters of

ADULT NURSING

solution are used in each cycle in the adult; solutions contain: glucose, Na^+, Ca^{++}, Mg^{++}, K^+, Cl^-, and lactate or acetate.

3. When solution bottle is empty, dwell time (exchange time) begins. *Dwell time:* 20–30 min; processes of diffusion, osmosis, and filtration begin to move waste products from bloodstream into peritoneal cavity.
4. Draining of the dialysate begins with the unclamping of the outflow clamp. *Outflow time:* usually 20 min; returns <2 L usually result from incomplete peritoneal emptying; turn side to side to increase return; 30 cycles in 24 h is ideal.

E. *Continuous ambulatory peritoneal dialysis* (CAPD): functions on the same principles as peritoneal dialysis, yet allows greater freedom and independence for dialysis patients. *Procedure:*

1. Dialysis solution is infused into peritoneum three times daily and once prior to bedtime.
2. *Dwell time*—5 h for each daily exchange, and overnight for the fourth.
3. Indwelling peritoneal catheter is connected to solution bag at all times—serves to fill and drain peritoneum; concealed in cloth pouch, strapped to the body during dwell time; client can move about doing usual activities.

F. *Continuous ultrafiltration hemofiltration:* a method of controlling fluid and electrolyte balance in critically ill patients who cannot tolerate hemodialysis or peritoneal dialysis. Does not require hemodialysis machinery. Patient's own arterial blood pressure serves as the power source. *Procedures:*

1. Requires both arterial and venous access.
2. Patency maintained with a heparin infusion pump (hourly dose, 10–20 U/kg).
3. Assess hemodynamic function before beginning ultrafiltration (e.g., heart rate, blood pressure, cardiac output).
4. Monitor ultrafiltration rate for one minute after beginning (hourly rate varies from 150–800 mL/h).
5. Observe for: fluid depletion, clotting of the filter, and bleeding.

VI. Kidney transplantation: placement of a donor kidney (from sibling, parent, cadaver) into the iliac fossa of a recipient and the anastomosis of its ureter to the bladder of the recipient; indicated in end-stage renal disease.

A. Criteria for recipient: irreversible kidney function; under 55 years of age; patent and functional lower urinary tract; and good surgical risk, free of serious cardiovascular complications. *Contraindicated* in metastatic carcinoma and oxalosis (excessive oxalate in urine).

B. Donor selection

1. Sibling or parent—survival rate of kidney is greater; preferred for transplantation.
2. Cadaver—greater rate of rejection following transplantation, although majority of transplants are with cadaver kidneys.

C. Bilateral nephrectomy: necessary for clients with rapidly progressive glomerulonephritis, malignant hypertension, or chronic kidney infections; prevents complications in transplanted kidney (see VII. Nephrectomy for nursing care).

D. Analysis/nursing diagnosis:

1. *Altered urinary elimination* related to kidney failure.
2. *Fear* related to potential transplant rejection.
3. *Potential for infection* related to immunosuppression.
4. *Body image disturbance* related to immunosuppression.

E. Nursing plan/implementation:

1. *Preoperative*
   a. Goal: *promote physical and emotional adjustment.*
      (1) Informed consent.
      (2) Lab work completed—histocompatibility, CBC, urinalysis, blood type and crossmatch.
      (3) Skin preparation.
   b. Goal: *encourage expression of feelings:* origin of donor, fear of complications, rejection.
   c. Goal: *minimize risk of organ rejection:* Give medications: begin immunosuppression (Imuran, corticosteroids, cyclosporine); antiinfectives if ordered.
   d. Goal: *health teaching.*
      (1) Nature of surgery; placement of kidney.
      (2) Postoperative expectations: deep breathing, coughing, turning, early ambulation; reverse isolation.
      (3) Medications: immunosuppressive therapy: purpose, effect.
2. *Postoperative*
   a. Goal: *promote uncomplicated recovery of recipient.*
      (1) Vital signs; CVP; I&O—may see large amounts urine (3–20 L) in early postoperative period from sodium diuresis, or kidney may not work for a week or more and dialysis will be needed within 24–48 h.
      (2) *Isolation:* strict reverse isolation with immunosuppression; wear face mask when out of room.
      (3) *Position:* back to unoperative side; semi-Fowler's to promote gas exchange.
      (4) Indwelling catheter care: characteristics of urine—report gross hematuria, heavy sediment; clots; perineal care.
      (5) Activity: ambulate 24 h after surgery; avoid prolonged sitting.
      (6) *Weigh daily.*
      (7) Medications: immunosuppressives; analgesics as ordered.
      (8) Drains: irrigate *only* on physician order; *meticulous* catheter care.
      (9) Diet: regular; liberal amounts of protein; *restrict* fluids, sodium, potassium *only if* oliguric.
   b. Goal: *observe for signs of rejection*—most dangerous complication. Four classifications:
      (1) Hyperacute—occurs with 5–10 min after transplantation.

(2) Accelerated—within 24–36 h.

(3) Acute—occurs 1 week to 3 months.

(4) Chronic—occurs several months to years.

(5) **Assessment:**

(a) Subjective data

(i) Lethargy, anorexia.

(ii) Tenderness over graft site.

(b) Objective data

(i) Lab data: Urine: *decreased*—output, creatinine clearance, sodium; *increased*—protein. Blood: increased: BUN, creatinine.

(ii) Rapid weight gain.

(iii) Vital signs: BP, temperature—elevated.

c. Goal: *Maintain immunosuppressive therapy.*

(1) Azathioprine (Imuran)—an antimetabolite that interferes with cellular division. *Side effects:*

(a) Gastrointestinal bleeding (give PO form with food).

(b) Bone marrow depression; leukopenia; anemia.

(c) Development of malignant neoplasms.

(d) Infection.

(e) Liver damage.

(2) Glucocorticoids (Prednisone)—believed to affect lymphocyte production by inhibiting nucleic acid synthesis: anti-inflammatory action helps prevent tissue damage if rejection occurs. *Side effects:*

(a) Stress ulcer with bleeding (give with food).

(b) Decreased glucose tolerance (hyperglycemia).

(c) Muscle weakness.

(d) Osteoporosis.

(e) Moon facies.

(f) Acne and striae.

(g) Depression and hallucinations.

(3) Cyclosporine (Cyclosporin A)—a polypeptide antibiotic used to prevent rejection of kidney, liver, or heart allografts; PO dose given with room temperature chocolate milk or OJ in a glass dispenser. *Side effects:*

(a) Nephrotoxicity (increased BUN, creatinine).

(b) Hypertension.

(c) Tremor.

(d) Hirsutism, gingival hyperplasia.

(e) *GI*—nausea, vomiting, anorexia, diarrhea, abdominal pain.

(f) *Infections*—pneumonia, septicemia, abscesses, wound.

d. Goal: *health teaching.*

(1) Signs of rejection (see goal b. above).

(2) Drugs: side effects of immunosuppression (see goal c. above).

(3) Self-care activities: temperature, blood pressure, I&O, urine specimen collection.

(4) Avoidance of infection.

(5) See also goals of care, III. Postoperative experience, p. 346.

F. Evaluation:

1. No signs of rejection (e.g., weight gain, oliguria).
2. No depression.
3. Client resumes role responsibilities.

VII. Nephrectomy: removal of kidney through flank, retroperitoneal, abdominal, thoracic, or thoracic-abdominal approach; indicated with malignant tumors, severe trauma, or under certain conditions before renal transplantation (see VI. Kidney transplantation).

A. Analysis/nursing diagnosis:

1. *Pain* related to surgical incision.
2. *Potential for infection* related to wound contamination.
3. *Potential for aspiration* related to vomiting.
4. *Constipation* related to paralytic ileus.
5. *Anxiety* related to possible loss of function in remaining kidney.
6. *Dysfunctional grieving* related to perceived loss.

B. Nursing plan/implementation:

1. *Preoperative:* Goal: *optimize physical and psychologic functioning* (see I. Preoperative preparation, p. 342).
2. *Postoperative:* Goal: *promote comfort and prevent complications.*

a. Observe for signs of:

(1) *Paralytic ileus*—abdominal distention, absent bowel sounds, vomiting (common complication following renal surgery).

(2) *Hemorrhage.*

b. Fluid balance: daily weight—maintain within 2% of preoperative level.

C. Evaluation:

1. No complications (e.g., hemorrhage, paralytic ileus, wound infection).
2. Acceptance of loss of kidney.

VIII. Renal calculi (urolithiasis): formation of calculi (stones) in renal calyces or pelvis that pass to lower regions of urinary tract—ureters, bladder, or urethra; occurs after age 30, with greatest incidence in *men,* particularly over age 50.

A. Pathophysiology: organic crystals form (75% of stones contain calcium) → obstruction, infection; increased backward pressure in kidney → hydronephrosis → atrophy, fibrosis of renal tubules.

B. Risk factors:

1. Changes in urine pH and concentration from readily precipitable, crystalline materials—sulfonamides, uric acid, calcium salts.
2. Urinary tract infection.
3. Indwelling Foley catheter.
4. Vitamin A deficiency.

C. Assessment (depends on size, shape, location of stone):

1. Subjective data
   a. Pain: occasional, dull, in loin or back when stones are in calyces or renal pelvis; *excruciating* in flank area (renal colic), radiating to groin when stones are ureteral.
   b. Nausea associated with pain.
2. Objective data
   a. Pallor, sweating, syncope, shock, and vomiting due to pain.
   b. Palpable kidney mass with hydronephrosis.
   c. Fever and pyuria with infection.
   d. Lab data:
      (1) Urinalysis: abnormal—pH (acidic or alkaline); RBCs (injury); WBCs (infection); increased—specific gravity; casts; crystals; other organic substances, depending on type of stone (i.e., uric acid, calcium); positive culture.
      (2) Blood: *increased* calcium, phosphorus, total protein, alkaline phosphatase, creatinine, uric acid, BUN.
   ▶ e. Diagnostic tests:
      (1) IVP: reveals nonopaque stones, degree of obstruction.
      (2) X ray; radiopaque stones seen.
      (3) Ultrasound may also be used.

D. Analysis/nursing diagnosis:

1. *Pain* related to passage of stone.
2. *Altered urinary elimination* related to potential obstruction.
3. *Urinary retention* related to obstruction of urethra.

E. Nursing plan/implementation:

1. Goal: *reduce pain and prevent complications.*
   a. Medication: *narcotics, antiemetics, antibiotics.*
   b. Fluids: 3–4 L/day; IVs if nauseated, vomiting.
   c. Activity: ambulate to promote passage of stone, except bedrest during acute attack (colic).
   d. Reduce spasms: warm soaks to affected flank.
   e. Observe for signs of:
      (1) *Obstruction*—decreased urinary output, increased flank pain.
      (2) *Passage of stone*—cessation of pain; filter urine with gauze.
   f. Monitor: hydration status—I&O, daily weight; vital signs—particularly temperature for sign of infection; urine—color, odor.
2. Goal: *health teaching.*
   a. Importance of fluids: minimum 3000 mL/day; 2 glasses during night.
   b. Diet: modify according to stone type.
      (1) *Uric acid stones*—low purine.
      (2) *Calcium oxalate and calcium phosphate stones*—low calcium phosphorus, and oxalate (e.g., tea, cocoa, cola, beans, spinach, acidic fruits).
      (3) *Cystine stones*—low protein.
   c. *Acid-ash diet* with: calcium oxalate and calcium phosphate stones, magnesium and ammonium phosphate stones.
   d. *Alkaline-ash diet* with: calcium oxalate, uric acid, and cystine stones (see Common Therapeutic Diets in Unit 5, p. 473).
   e. Signs of urinary infection: dysuria, frequency, hematuria; seek immediate treatment.
   f. Prepare for removal if indicated; 60–80% of patients will have lithotripsy done; cystoscopy or ureterolithotomy may also be ordered; nephrectomy in *extreme cases.*

F. Evaluation:

1. Relief from pain.
2. No signs of urinary obstruction (e.g., increased flank pain, decreased urine output).
3. No recurrence of lithiasis (adheres to diet and fluid regimen).

IX. Extracorporeal lithotripsy: a noninvasive mechanical procedure used to break up renal calculi so they can pass spontaneously, in most cases. The trunk of the patient is submerged in water. In addition to being strapped to a frame, the patient may also be sedated, as the procedure takes 30–45 min, and remaining still is important. An underwater electrode generates shock waves that fragment the stone so it can be excreted in the urine a few days after the procedure. A degree of renal colic may occur requiring antispasmodics. Nursing measures should encourage ambulation and promote diuresis through forcing fluids.

X. Prostatic hypertrophy (prostatism): malfunction of the urinary tract resulting from a lesion (benign or malignant) of the prostate gland.

A. Pathophysiology: prostate enlarges, bulges upward, blocks flow of urine from bladder into urethra → obstruction → hydroureter, hydronephrosis.

B. Risk factors:

1. Benign
   a. Changes in estrogen and androgen levels.
   b. Men over 50.
2. Malignant
   a. Genetic tendency.
   b. Hormonal factors (e.g., late puberty, higher fertility).
   c. Diet (high fat).
   d. Chemical carcinogens (fertilizer, rubber, cadmium batteries).

C. Assessment:

1. Subjective data—*urination:*
   a. Difficulty starting stream.
   b. Smaller, less forceful.
   c. Dribbling.
   d. Frequency.
   e. Urgency.
   f. Nocturia.
   g. Retention (incomplete emptying).
   h. Inability to void after ingestion of alcohol or exposure to cold.
2. Objective data

a. Catheterization for residual urine: 25–50 mL after voiding.
b. Enlarged prostate on rectal exam.
c. Lab data:
(1) Urine—*increased* RBC, WBC.
(2) Blood—*increased* creatinine.

D. Analysis/nursing diagnosis:
1. *Urinary retention* related to incomplete emptying.
2. *Altered urinary elimination* related to obstruction.
3. *Urinary incontinence* related to urgency, pressure.
4. *Anxiety* related to potential surgery.
5. *Body image disturbance* related to threat to male identity.

E. Nursing plan/implementation:
1. Goal: *relieve urinary retention.*
a. Catheterization: release maximum of 1000 mL initially; *avoid* bladder decompression, which results in hypotension, bladder spasms, ruptured blood vessels in bladder; empty 200 mL every 5 min.
b. Patency: irrigate intermittently or continually, as ordered.
c. Fluids: minimum 2000 mL/24 h.
2. Goal: *health teaching.*
a. Preparation for surgery (cystostomy, prostatectomy):
(1) Expectations—indwelling catheter (will feel urge to void).
(2) *Avoid* pulling on catheter (this increases bleeding and clots).
(3) Bladder spasms common 24–48 h after surgery, particularly with TUR and suprapubic approaches.
(4) Threatening nature of procedure (possibility of impotence with perineal prostatectomy).
b. See also I. Preoperative preparation, p. 342.

XI. Prostatectomy: surgical procedure to relieve urinary retention and frequency caused by benign prostatic hypertrophy or cancer of the prostate.

A. Types
1. *Transurethral resection (TUR)*—removal of obstructive prostatic tissue surrounding urethra by an electric wire (resectoscope) introduced through the urethra; hypertrophy may recur, and TUR repeated.
2. *Suprapubic*—low midline incision is made directly over the bladder; bladder is opened and large mass of prostatic tissue is removed through incision in urethral mucosa.
3. *Retropubic*—removal of hypertrophied prostatic tissue high in pelvic area through a low abdominal incision; bladder is not opened.
4. *Perineal*—removal of prostatic tissue low in pelvic area is accomplished through an incision made between the scrotum and the rectum; usually results in impotency.

B. Nursing plan/implementation:
1. *Preoperative:* see X. Prostatic hypertrophy, above.
2. *Postoperative*
a. Goal: *promote optimal bladder function and comfort.*
(1) Urinary drainage: sterile closed-gravity system—maintain external traction as ordered.
(2) Reinforce purposes, sensations to expect.
(3) Bladder irrigation to control bleeding, keep clots from forming.
(4) Suprapubic catheter care (suprapubic prostatectomy)—closed-gravity drainage system; observe character, amount, flow of drainage.
(5) *After removal:*
(a) Observe for urinary drainage q4h for 24 hours.
(b) Skin care.
(c) Report excessive drainage to physician.
(6) Dressings: keep dry, clean; reinforce if necessary (may need to change suprapubic dressing if urinary drainage); notify physician of *excessive bleeding.*
(7) Observe for signs of:
(a) *Bladder distention*—distinct mound over pubis, slow drop in collecting bottle; irrigate catheter as ordered.
(b) *Increased bleeding*—bright red drainage and clots; cool, clammy, pale skin; and increased pulse rate.
b. Goal: *assist in rehabilitation.* Emotional support: *fears* of incontinence, loss of male identity, impotence.
c. Goal: *health teaching.*
(1) Expectations: mild incontinence, dribbling for a while (several months) after surgery; need to void as soon as urge is felt; push fluids.
(2) Exercises: perineal 1–2 days after surgery—buttocks are tightened for a count of ten, 20–50 times daily.
(3) *Avoid:*
(a) Long auto trips, vigorous exercise, heavy lifting, and sexual intercourse for about 3 weeks or until medical permission, as this may increase tendency to bleed.
(b) Alcoholic beverages for 1 month, as this may cause burning on urination.
(c) Tub baths, as this increases chance of infection.
(4) Medications: stool softeners or mild cathartics to decrease straining.

C. Evaluation:
1. Relief of symptoms.
2. No complications (e.g., hemorrhage, impotence).

XII. Urinary diversion (ileal conduit): implantation of ureters into a portion of the terminal ileum, with formation of a stoma; common method for urinary diversion; also known as Bricker's procedure.

A. Indications:
1. Congenital anomalies of bladder.
2. Neurogenic bladder.

3. Mechanical obstruction to urine flow (e.g., bladder cancer).
4. Severe cystitis.
5. Trauma to lower urinary tract.

B. Analysis/nursing diagnosis:

1. *Altered urinary elimination* related to surgical diversion.
2. *Potential impaired skin integrity* related to leakage of urine.
3. *Potential for infection* related to contamination of stoma.
4. *Constipation* related to absence of peristalsis.
5. *Body image disturbance* related to stoma.

C. Nursing plan/implementation:

1. *Preoperative:* optimal bowel and stoma-site preparation.
   a. Diet: nonresidue several days before surgery.
   b. Medications:
      (1) Neomycin (for bowel sterilization).
      (2) Cathartics, enemas.
   c. Site selection: appliance faceplate must bond securely; avoid areas of pressure from clothing (waistline); usual site is right or left lower abdominal quadrant.
   d. See also I. Preoperative preparation, p. 342.
2. *Postoperative*
   a. Goal: *present complications and promote comfort.*
      (1) Observe for signs of:
         (a) *Paralytic ileus* (common complication)—keep NG tube patent.
         (b) *Stoma necrosis*—dusky or cyanotic color (**emergency** situation).
      (2) Skin care: check for leakage around ostomy bag.
      (3) See III. Postoperative experience, p. 345.
   b. Goal: *health teaching.*
      (1) Self-care activities:
         (a) *Peristomal skin care*—prevent irritation, breakdown; proper cleansing—soap and water; adhesive remover, if needed.
         (b) *Appliance application and emptying;* do not remove each day; change appliance every 4–5 days or when leaking.
         (c) *Odor control*—dilute urine, acid-ash diet, hygiene, avoid asparagus, tomatoes; mucus normal.
         (d) *Use of night drainage system* if necessary for uninterrupted sleep.
      (2) Signs of *complications:* change in urine color, clarity, quantity, smell; stomal color change.

D. Evaluation:

1. Acceptance of new body image.
2. Regains independence.
3. Demonstrates confidence in management of self-care activities.

■ SENSORY-PERCEPTUAL FUNCTIONS

I. Laryngectomy (radical neck dissection): removal of entire larynx, lymph nodes, sternomastoid muscle, and jugular vein for cancer of the larynx that extends beyond the vocal cords. Permanent tracheostomy; new methods of speech will have to be learned.

Partial laryngectomy: removal of lesion on larynx. Client will be able to speak after operation, but quality of voice may be altered.

A. Assessment:

1. Subjective data
   a. Feeling of lump in throat.
   b. Pain: Adam's apple; may radiate to ear.
   c. Dysphagia.
2. Objective data
   a. Hoarseness: persistent, progressive.
   b. Lymphadenopathy: cervical.
   c. Breath odor: foul.

B. Analysis/nursing diagnosis:

1. *Impaired verbal communication* related to removal of larynx.
2. *Body image disturbance* related to radical neck dissection.
3. *Ineffective airway clearance* related to copious amounts of mucus.
4. *Fear* related to diagnosis of cancer.
5. *Impaired swallowing* related to edema.
6. *Impaired social interaction* related to altered speech.

C. Nursing plan/implementation:

1. *Preoperative*
   a. Goal: *provide emotional support and optimal physical preparation.*
      (1) Encourage verbalization of fears; answer all questions honestly, particularly about having no voice after surgery.
      (2) Visit from person with laryngectomy (contact International Association of Laryngectomees).
   b. Goal: *health teaching.*
      (1) Prepare for tracheostomy.
      (2) Other means to speak (esophageal "burp" speech).
2. *Postoperative*
   a. Goal: *maintain patent airway and prevent aspiration.*
      (1) *Position:* semi-Fowler's, preventing forward flexion of neck to reduce edema and keep airway open.
      (2) Observe for hypoxia:
         (a) *Early signs:* increased respiratory and pulse rates, apprehension, restlessness.
         (b) *Late signs:* dyspnea, cyanosis; swallowing difficulties—client should chew food well and swallow with water.

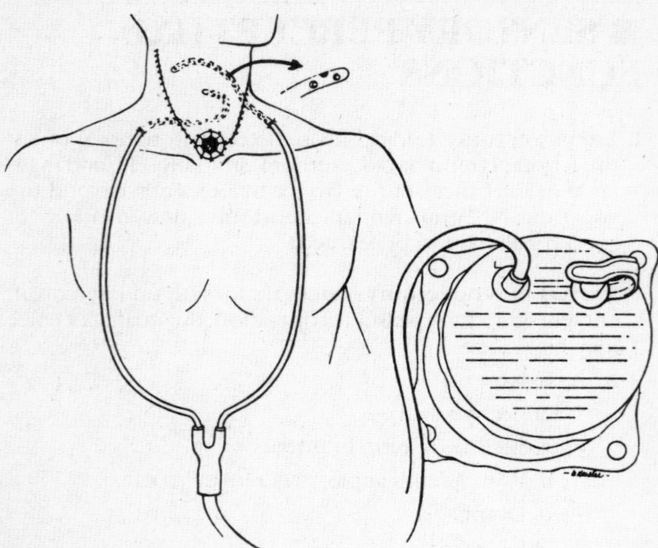

■ **FIGURE 4.5**
Hemovac apparatus for constant closed suction. In this system of wound drainage, suction is maintained by plastic container with spring inside that tries to force apart lids and thereby produces suction that is transmitted through plastic tubing. Neck skin is pulled down tight, and no external dressing is required. Container serves as both suction source and receptacle for blood. It is emptied as required, and drainage tubes are left in neck for three days. (From DeWeese DD, Saunders WH: *Textbook of Otolaryngology,* 6th ed., Mosby, St. Louis, 1987.)

(3) *Laryngectomy* tube care:

(a) Observe for stridor (coarse, high-pitched inspiratory sound)—**report immediately.**

(b) Have extra laryngectomy tube at bedside.

(c) Suction with sterile equipment; instill 2–3 mL sterile saline into stoma to loosen secretions.

b. Goal: *promote optimal physical and psychologic function.*

(1) Frequent mouth care.

(2) Dressings: may be pressure-type; note color and amount of drainage; reinforce as ordered.

(3) *Tubes:* Hemovac (Figure 4.5); expect 80–120 mL serosanguineous drainage first postoperative day; drainage should decrease daily; observe patency.

(4) Post-Hemovac removal—observe: skin flaps down, adherent to underlying tissue; may have to "roll" flaps to prevent drainage build-up.

(5) Use surgical asepsis.

(6) Answer call bell *immediately;* use preestablished means of communication.

(7) Reexplain all procedures while giving care.

(8) Support head when lifting.

c. Goal: *health teaching.*

(1) Speech rehabilitation as soon as esophageal suture is healed.

(a) Information on laryngeal speech (International Association of Laryngectomees, American Cancer Society, American Speech and Hearing Association).

(b) Esophageal speech best learned in speech clinic—learn to burp column of air needed for speech; new voice sounds are natural but hoarse.

(2) *Stoma* care:

(a) Cover with scarf or shirt of a porous material (material substitutes for nasal passage—warms and filters out particles).

(b) Use source of humidification ("mister" or commercial humidifier).

(c) Caution while bathing or showering, to decrease likelihood of aspiration.

(d) Swimming and boating permitted only with snorkel device.

(e) Procedure for suctioning if cough ineffective.

(3) Simple ROM of neck; how to support head.

(4) Possible contraindications: use of talcum powder, tissues.

D. Evaluation:

1. No surgical complications (e.g., airway obstruction, infection, hemorrhage).
2. Learns alternate speech 60–90 days after surgery.
3. Demonstrates proper stoma care.
4. Resumes productive life-style (work, family).
5. Normal response to change in body image (e.g., anger, grief, denial).

II. Aphasia: impaired ability to understand or use commonly accepted words or symbols; interferes with ability to speak, write, and/or read; usually occurs with right-sided hemiplegia with a cerebrovascular accident.

A. Types and pathophysiology:

1. *Receptive (sensory)*—lesion usually Wernicke's area of temporal lobe; difficulty understanding spoken word (auditory aphasia) or written word (visual aphasia).
2. *Expressive (motor)*—lesion usually in Broca's area of frontal lobe; difficulty expressing thoughts in speech or writing (motor aphasia).

B. Risk factors:

1. Vascular disease of the brain (cerebral vascular accident).
2. Alzheimer's disease.
3. Sickle cell anemia.

C. Analysis/nursing diagnosis:

1. *Impaired verbal communication* related to cerebral cortex disorder.
2. *Powerlessness* related to inability to express needs/concerns.
3. *Impaired social interaction* related to difficulty communicating.

D. Nursing plan/implementation: Goal: *assist with communication.*

1. Assess comprehension: use simple requests; write questions or use picture cards.

2. Stand on client's unaffected side (stay within client's visual field).
3. Talk slowly, clearly; do not shout or "talk down" (there is no intellectual impairment).
4. Use short, simple phrases, repeat words; ask questions needing one-word answers.
5. Use alternative ways to communicate; hand gestures, picture cards.
6. Avoid frustration for client: do not force client to repeat words; allow ample time to respond; anticipate needs.
7. Respond to client's speech; if not understood, tell client; encourage client to use other words.
8. Reinforce techniques taught by speech therapist.
9. Maintain one-way communication: receptive aphasia does not always accompany expressive aphasia.

E. Evaluation:

1. Communication reestablished.
2. Minimal frustration exhibited.
3. Participates in speech therapy.

III. Meniere's disease: chronic, recurrent disorder of inner ear; attacks of vertigo, tinnitus, and vestibular dysfunction; lasts 30 minutes to full day; usually no pain or loss of consciousness.

A. Pathophysiology: associated with excessive dilatation of cochlear duct (unilateral) from overproduction or decreased absorption of endolymph → progressive sensorineural loss.

B. Risk factors:

1. Emotional or endocrine disturbance (diabetes mellitus).
2. Spasms of internal auditory artery.
3. Head trauma.
4. Allergic reaction.
5. High salt intake.
6. Smoking.
7. Ear infections.

C. Assessment:

1. Subjective data
   a. Tinnitus.
   b. Headache.
   c. True vertigo; sudden attacks; room appears to spin.
   d. Depression; irritability; withdrawal.
   e. Nausea on sudden head motion.
2. Objective data
   a. Impaired hearing, especially *low* tones.
   b. Change in gait; lack of coordination.
   c. Vomiting with sudden head motion.
   d. Nystagmus—during attacks.
   ▶ e. Diagnostic test: caloric (cold water in ear canal)—may precipitate attack; audiometry—loss of hearing.

D. Analysis/nursing diagnosis:

1. *Potential for injury* related to vertigo, lack of coordination.
2. *Auditory sensory/perceptual alteration* related to progressive hearing loss.
3. *Anxiety* related to uncertainty of treatment.
4. *Potential activity intolerance* related to sudden onset of vertigo.
5. *Sleep pattern disturbance* related to tinnitus.
6. *Ineffective individual coping* related to chronic disorder.

E. Nursing plan/implementation:

1. Goal: *provide safety and comfort during attacks.*
   a. Activity: bedrest during attack; siderails up; lower to chair or floor if attack occurs while standing; assist with ambulation (sudden dizziness common).
   b. *Position:* recumbent; affected ear uppermost usually.
   c. Identify prodromal symptoms (aura, ear pressure, increased tinnitus).
   d. Call bell within reach.
2. Goal: *minimize occurrence of attacks.*
   a. Give medications as ordered:
      (1) *Diuretics* (Diuril, Diamox) to decrease endolymphatic fluids.
      (2) *Antihistamines* (Dramamine, Benadryl) to inhibit tissue edema.
      (3) *Vasodilators* (nicotinic acid) to control vasospasms.
      (4) *Antiemetics and antivertigo agents* (Valium, Antivert).
   b. Diet: low sodium; limited fluids to reduce endolymphatic pressure.
   c. Avoid precipitating stimuli: bright, glaring lights; noise; sudden jarring; turning head or eyes (stand in front of client when talking).
3. Goal: *health teaching.*
   a. No smoking (causes vasospasm) or alcoholic beverages (fluid retention, contraindicated with medications).
   b. Management of symptoms: play radio to mask tinnitus, particularly at night.
   c. Keep medication available at all times.
   d. Prepare for surgery if indicated (labyrinthectomy if hearing gone or endolymphatic sac decompression to preserve hearing).

F. Evaluation:

1. Decreased frequency of attacks.
2. Complies with treatment regimen and restrictions (e.g., low-sodium diet, no smoking).
3. Hearing preserved.

IV. Otosclerosis: insidious, progressive deafness; most common cause of conductive deafness; cause unknown.

A. Pathophysiology: formation of new spongy bone in labyrinth → fixation of stapes → prevention of sound transmission through ossicles to inner ear fluids.

B. Risk factors:

1. Heredity.
2. Females, puberty to 45 years.

C. Assessment:

1. Subjective data
   a. Tinnitus.
   b. Difficulty hearing—gradual loss in both ears.
2. Diagnostic tests:
   a. *Rinne* (tuning fork placed over mastoid bone)—reduced sound conduction by air and intensified by bone.
   b. *Weber* (tuning fork placed on top of head)—increased sound conduction to affected ear.
   c. *Audiometry*—diminished hearing ability.

D. Analysis/nursing diagnosis:

1. *Auditory sensory/perceptual alteration* related to hearing loss.
2. *Body image disturbance* related to aid.
3. *Ineffective individual coping* related to grief reaction to loss.
4. *Impaired social interaction* related to hearing loss.

E. Nursing plan/implementation/evaluation: see V. Stapedectomy, below.

V. Stapedectomy: removal of the stapes and replacing it with a prosthesis (steel wire, teflon piston, or polyethylene); treatment for deafness due to otosclerosis, which fixes the stapes, preventing it from oscillating and transmitting vibrations to the fluids in the inner ear.

A. Analysis/nursing diagnosis:

1. *Sensory/perceptual alteration* related to edema and ear packing.
2. See The Perioperative Experience, p. 342, for diagnoses relating to surgery.

B. Nursing plan/implementation:

1. *Preoperative:* health teaching.
   a. Important to keep head in position ordered by physician postoperatively.
   b. *Avoid:* sneezing, blowing nose, vomiting, coughing—all of which increase pressure in eustachian tubes.
   c. Breathing exercises.
2. *Postoperative*
   a. Goal: *promote physical and psychologic equilibrium.*
      (1) Position: as ordered by physician—varies according to preference; siderails up as vertigo is common.
      (2) Activity: assist with ambulation; avoid rapid turning, which might increase vertigo.
      (3) Dressings: check frequently; may change cotton pledget in outer ear.
      (4) Give medications as ordered:
         (a) *Antiemetics.*
         (b) *Analgesics.*
         (c) *Antibiotics.*
      (5) Reassurance: reduction in hearing is normal; hearing may *not* immediately improve after surgery.
   b. Goal: *health teaching.*
      (1) Ear care: keep covered outdoors; keep outer ear plug clean, dry, and changed.
      (2) *Avoid:*
         (a) Washing hair for 2 weeks.
         (b) Swimming for 6 weeks.
         (c) Air travel for 6 months.
         (d) Individuals with upper respiratory infections.
         (e) Heavy lifting or straining.

C. Evaluation:

1. Hearing improves—evaluate 1 month postoperatively (may require hearing aid).
2. Returns to work (usually 2 weeks after surgery).
3. Continues medical supervision.

VI. Deafness: (1) *Hard of hearing*—slight or moderate hearing loss that is serviceable for activities of daily living. (2) *Deaf*—hearing is nonfunctional for activities of daily living.

A. Risk factors:

1. *Conductive* hearing losses (transmission deafness):
   a. Impacted cerumen (wax).
   b. Foreign body in external auditory canal.
   c. Defects (thickening, scarring) of eardrum.
   d. Otosclerosis of ossicles.
2. *Sensory* hearing losses (perceptive or nerve deafness):
   a. Arteriosclerosis.
   b. Infectious diseases (mumps, measles, meningitis).
   c. Drug toxicities (quinine, streptomycin, neomycin SO_4).
   d. Tumors.
   e. Head traumas.
   f. High-intensity noises.

B. Assessment—objective data:

1. Inattentive or strained facial expression.
2. Excessive loudness or softness of speech.
3. Frequent need to clarify content of conversation or inappropriate responses.
4. Tilting of head while listening.
5. Lack of response when others speak.

C. Analysis/nursing diagnosis:

1. *Auditory sensory/perceptual alteration* related to loss of hearing.
2. *Impaired social interaction* related to deafness.

D. Nursing plan/implementation:

1. Goal: *maximize hearing ability and provide emotional support.*
   a. Gain person's attention before speaking; avoid startling.
   b. Provide adequate lighting so person can see you when you are speaking.
   c. Look at the person when speaking.
   d. Use nonverbal cues to enhance communication, e.g., writing, hand gestures, pointing.
   e. Speak slowly, distinctly; do not shout (excessive loudness distorts voice).
   f. If person doesn't understand, use different words; write it down.
   g. Use alternative communication system:
      (1) Speech (lip) reading.

(2) Sign language.

(3) Hearing aid.

(4) Paper and pencil.

(5) Flash cards.

h. Supportive, nonstressful environment.

2. Goal: *health teaching.*

▶ a. Prepare for evaluative studies—audiogram.

b. Appropriate community resources: National Association of Hearing and Speech Agencies for *counseling* services; National Association for the Deaf to assist with *employment, education, legislation;* Alexander Graham Bell Association for the Deaf, Inc., serves as *information* center for those working with the deaf; American Hearing Society provides educational information, employment services, *social clubs.*

c. Use of hearing aid: care; testing; carry spare battery at all times.

d. Safety precautions: when crossing street, driving.

E. Evaluation:

1. Method of communication established.

2. Achieves independence (use of Dogs for Deaf, special telephones, visual signals).

3. Copes with life-style changes (minimal depression, anger, hostility).

VII. Glaucoma (acute and chronic): increased intraocular pressure; affects 2% of population over 40 years of age.

A. Pathophysiology:

1. *Acute (closed-angle)*—impaired passage of aqueous humor into the circular canal of Schlemm due to closure of the angle between the cornea and the iris. *Medical emergency; requires surgery.*

2. *Chronic (open-angle)*—local obstruction of aqueous humor between the anterior chamber and the canal. *Most common; treated with medication* (miotics, carbonic anhydrase inhibitors).

3. Untreated: imbalance between rate of secretion of intraocular fluids and rate of absorption of aqueous humor → increased aqueous humor pressures → decreased peripheral vision → corneal edema → halos and blurring of vision → blindness.

B. Risk factors—unknown, but associated with:

1. Emotional disturbances.

2. Hereditary factors.

3. Allergies.

4. Vasomotor disturbances.

C. Assessment:

1. Subjective data

a. *Acute* (closed-angle):

(1) Pain: severe, in and around eyes.

(2) Headache.

(3) Halos around lights.

(4) Blurring of vision.

(5) Nausea, vomiting.

b. *Chronic* (open-angle):

(1) Eyes tire easily.

(2) Loss of peripheral vision.

2. Objective data

a. Corneal edema.

b. Decreased peripheral vision.

c. Increased cupping of optic disc.

d. Tonometry—pressures *over* 22 mm Hg.

e. Pupils: dilated.

f. Redness of eye.

D. Analysis/nursing diagnosis:

1. *Visual sensory/perceptual alterations* related to increased intraocular pressure.

2. *Pain* related to sudden increase in intraocular pressure.

3. *Potential for injury* related to blindness.

4. *Impaired physical mobility* related to impaired vision.

E. Nursing plan/implementation:

1. Goal: *reduce intraocular pressure.*

a. Activity: bedrest.

b. *Position:* semi-Fowler's.

c. Medications as ordered:

(1) *Miotics* (pilocarpine, carbachol).

(2) *Carbonic anhydrase inhibitors* (Diamox).

(3) *Anticholinesterase* (Humorsol) to facilitate outflow of aqueous humor.

2. Goal: *provide emotional support.*

a. Place personal objects within field of vision.

b. Assist with activities.

c. Encourage verbalization of concerns, fears of blindness, loss of independence.

3. Goal: *health teaching.*

a. *Prevent* increased intraocular pressure by avoiding:

(1) Anger, excitement, worry.

(2) Constrictive clothing.

(3) Heavy lifting.

(4) Excessive *fluid* intake.

(5) Atropine or other mydriatics.

(6) Straining at stool.

(7) Eye strain.

b. Relaxation techniques; stress-management if indicated.

c. Prepare for iridectomy (surgical removal of part of iris) if ordered; *each eye will be done 6 weeks apart; no patch; ambulate immediately following procedure.*

d. Medications: purpose, dosage, frequency; eyedrop installation; have extra bottle in case of breakage or loss.

e. Activity: moderate exercise—walking.

f. Safety measures: MedicAlert band or tag; avoid driving 1–2 h after instilling miotics.

g. Community resources as necessary.

F. Evaluation:

1. Eyesight preserved if possible.

2. Intraocular pressure lowered (*below 22* mm Hg).

3. Continues medical supervision for life—reports reappearance of symptoms immediately.

VIII. Cataract: developmental or degenerative opacification of the crystalline lens.

A. Risk factors:

1. Aging.
2. Trauma.
3. Toxins.
4. Congenital defect.

B. Assessment:

1. Subjective data—vision: blurring, loss of acuity; distortion; diplopia; photophobia.
2. Objective data
   a. Blindness: unilateral or bilateral (particularly in congenital cataracts).
   b. Loss of red reflex: gray opacity of lens.

C. Analysis/nursing diagnosis:

1. *Visual sensory/perceptual alterations* related to opacity of lens.
2. *Potential for injury* related to accidents.
3. *Social isolation* related to impaired vision.

IX. Cataract removal: removal of opacified lens because of loss of vision; extracapsular cataract extraction followed by intraocular lens (IOL) insertion is procedure of choice.

A. Nursing plan/implementation:

1. *Preoperative*
   a. Goal: *prepare for surgery.* Instill mydriatic eye drops as ordered; note dilation of pupils; avoid glaring lights; usually done under local anesthetic.
   b. Goal: *health teaching.* Postoperative expectations: do not rub, touch, or squeeze eyes shut after surgery; eye patches will be on; assistance will be given for needs; overnight hospitalization not required unless complications occur; mild iritis usually occurs.
2. *Postoperative*
   a. Goal: *reduce stress on the sutures and prevent hemorrhage.*
      (1) Activity: ambulate as ordered, usually soon after surgery; generally discharged 5–6 hours after surgery.
      (2) *Position:* flat or low Fowler's; on back or turn to *nonoperative* side, as turning to operative side increases pressure.
      (3) Avoid activities that increase intraocular pressure: vomiting, coughing, brushing teeth, brushing hair, shaving, *bending,* or *stooping.*
      (4) Provide: mouthwash, hair care, personal items within easy reach, "step-in" slippers.
   b. Goal: *promote psychologic well-being.* With elderly, frequent contacts to prevent sensory deprivation.
   c. Goal: *health teaching.*
      (1) Temporary (1–4 weeks) use of cataract spectacle lenses (aphakic glasses). Explain about magnification, perceptual distortion, blind areas in peripheral vision; guide through activities with glasses; need to look through central portion of lens and turn head to side when looking to the side to decrease distortion.
      (2) Eye care: instillation of eye drops (mydriatics and carbonic anhydrase inhibitors to prevent glaucoma and adhesions if IOL not inserted; with IOL steroid-antibiotic used); eye shield at night to prevent injury for one month.
      (3) Signs/symptoms of: infection (redness, pain, edema, drainage); iris prolapse (bulging or pear-shaped pupil); hemorrhage (sharp eye pain, half-moon of blood).
      (4) *Avoid:* heavy lifting; potential eye trauma.

B. Evaluation:

1. Vision restored.
2. No complications (e.g., severe eye pain, hemorrhage).
3. Performs self-care activities (e.g., instills eye drops).
4. Returns for follow-up ophthalmology care—recognizes symptoms requiring immediate attention.

X. Retinal detachment: separation of retina from choroid.

A. Risk factors:

1. Trauma.
2. Degeneration.

B. Assessment:

1. Subjective data
   a. Flashes of light before eyes.
   b. Vision: blurred, sooty (sudden onset); sensation of floating particles; blank areas of vision.
2. Objective data—ophthalmic exam: retina is grayish in area of tear; bright red, horseshoe-shaped tear.

C. Analysis/nursing diagnosis:

1. *Visual sensory/perceptual alteration* related to blurred vision.
2. *Anxiety* related to potential loss of vision.
3. *Potential for injury* related to blindness.

D. Nursing plan/implementation:

1. *Preoperative*
   a. Goal: *reduce anxiety and prevent further detachment.*
      (1) Encourage verbalization of feelings; answer all questions; reinforce physician's explanation of surgical procedures.
      (2) Activity: bedrest; eyes usually covered to promote rest and maintain normal position of retina; siderails up.
      (3) *Position:* according to location of retinal tear; involved area of eye should be in a dependent position.
      (4) Give medications as ordered: *cycloplegic* or *mydriatics* to dilate pupils widely and decrease intraocular movement.
      (5) Relaxing diversion: conversation, music.
   b. Goal: *health teaching.* Prepare for surgical intervention:
      (1) *Electrodiathermy*—electrode needle is passed through sclera, draining the subretinal fluid; retina will then adhere to the choroid.

(2) *Cryosurgery*—supercooled probe is applied to the sclera, causing a scar, which pulls the choroid and retina together.

(3) *Laser beam*—a beam of intense light from a carbon arc is directed through the dilated pupil onto the retina; effect is the same as in electrodiathermy.

(4) *Scleral buckling*—the sclera is resected or shortened to enhance the contact between the choroid and retina.

2. *Postoperative*

a. Goal: *reduce intraocular stress and prevent hemorrhage.*

(1) *Position:* flat or low Fowler's; sandbags may be used to position head; turn to nonoperative side if allowed.

(2) Activity: bedrest; decrease intraocular pressure by not stooping, bending, or prone positioning.

(3) Give medications as ordered:

(a) *Mydriatics.*

(b) *Antibiotics.*

(c) *Corticosteroids* to reduce eye movements, inflammation, and prevent infection.

(4) ROM—isometric, passive; elastic stockings to avoid thrombus related to immobility.

b. Goal: *support coping mechanisms.*

(1) Plan all care with client.

(2) Encourage verbalization of feelings, fears.

(3) Encourage family interaction.

(4) Diversional activities.

c. Goal: *health teaching.*

(1) Eye care: eye patch or shield at night to prevent touching of the eye while asleep; dark glasses; avoid rubbing, squeezing eyes.

(2) Limitations: no reading for 3 weeks, no physical exertion for 6 weeks.

(3) Medications: dosage, frequency, purpose, side effects: avoid nonprescription medications.

(4) Signs of redetachment: flashes of light, increase in "floaters," blurred vision.

E. Evaluation:

1. Vision restored.
2. No further detachment—recognizes signs and symptoms.
3. No injury occurs—accepts limitations.

XI. Blindness: legally defined as vision less than 20/200 with the use of corrective lenses, or a visual field of no greater than 20 degrees; greatest incidence after 65 years.

A. Risk factors:

1. Glaucoma.
2. Cataracts.
3. Diabetic retinopathy.
4. Atherosclerosis.
5. Trauma.

B. Analysis/nursing diagnosis:

1. *Visual sensory/perceptual alteration* related to blindness.
2. *Impaired social interaction* related to loss of sight.
3. *Potential for injury* related to visual impairment.
4. *Self-care deficit* related to visual loss.

C. Nursing plan/implementation:

1. Goal: *promote independence and provide emotional support.*

a. Familiarize with surroundings; encourage use of touch.

b. Establish communication lines; answer questions.

c. Deal with feelings of loss, overprotectiveness by family members.

d. Provide diversional activities: radio, records, talking books, tapes.

e. Encourage self-care activities; allow voicing of frustrations when activity is not done to satisfaction (spilling or misplacing something), to decrease anger and discouragement.

2. Goal: *facilitate activities of daily living.*

a. Eating:

(1) Establish routine placement for table pieces, e.g., plate, glass.

(2) Help person mentally visualize the plate as a clock or compass (e.g., "3 o'clock" or "east").

(3) Take person's hand and guide the fingertips to establish spatial relationship.

b. Walking:

(1) Have person hold your forearm: walk a half step in front.

(2) Tell the person when approaching stairs, curb, incline.

c. Talking:

(1) Speak when approaching person; tell them before you touch them.

(2) Tell them who you are and what you will be doing.

(3) Do not avoid words such as "see" or discussing the appearance of things.

3. Goal: *health teaching.*

a. Accident prevention in the home.

b. Community resources

(1) Voluntary agencies:

(a) American Foundation for the Blind—provides catalogs of devices for visually handicapped.

(b) National Society for the Prevention of Blindness—comprehensive educational programs and research.

(c) Recording for the Blind, Inc.—provides recorded educational books on free loan.

(d) Lion's Club.

(e) Catholic charities.

(f) Salvation Army.

(2) Government agencies;

(a) Social and Rehabilitation Service—counseling and placement services.

TABLE 4.23 Levels of Consciousness

Stage	Characteristics
Alertness	Aware of time and place.
Automatism	Aware of time and place but demonstrates abnormality of mood (euphoria to irritability).
Confusion	Inability to think and speak in coherent manner; responds to verbal requests but is unaware of time and place.
Delirium	Restlessness and violent activity; may not comply with verbal instructions.
Stupor	Quiet and uncommunicative; may appear conscious—sits or lies with glazed look; unable to respond to verbal instructions; bladder and rectal incontinence may occur.
Semicoma	Unresponsive to verbal instructions but responds to vigorous or painful stimuli.
Coma	Unresponsive to vigorous or painful stimuli.

(b) Veterans Administration—screening and pensions.

(c) State Welfare Department, Division for the Blind—vocational.

D. Evaluation:

1. Acceptance of disability—participates in self-care activities, remains socially involved.
2. Regains independence with rehabilitation.

XII. Traumatic injuries to the brain

A. Types:

1. *Concussion*—transient disorder due to injury in which there is brief loss of consciousness due to paralysis of neuronal function; recovery is usually total.
2. *Contusion*—structural alteration of brain tissue characterized by extravasation of blood cells (bruising); injury may occur on side of impact or on opposite side (when cranial contents shift forcibly within the skull with impact).
3. *Laceration*—tearing of brain tissue or blood vessels due to a sharp bone fragment or object or tearing force.
4. *Hematomas*
   a. *Subdural*—blood from ruptured or torn vein collects between arachnoid and dura; may be acute, subacute, or chronic.
   b. *Extradural* (epidural)—blood clot located between dura and inner surface of skull; most often from tearing of middle meningeal artery; **emergency** condition.

B. Pathophysiology of impaired CNS functioning:

1. Depressed neuronal activity in reticular activating system → depressed *consciousness* (Table 4.23).
2. Depressed neuronal functioning in lower brain stem and spinal cord → depression of reflex activity → decreased eye movements, unequal pupils → decreased response to light stimuli → widely dilated and fixed *pupils*.
3. Depression of respiratory center → altered respiratory pattern → decreased rate → *respiratory arrest*.

C. Risk factors: accidents—automobile, industrial and home, motorcycle, military.

D. Assessment:

1. Subjective data
   a. Headache.
   b. Dizziness, loss of balance.
   c. Double vision.
   d. Nausea.
2. Objective data
   a. Laceration or abrasion around face or head.
   b. Drainage from ears or nose.
   c. Projectile vomiting, hematemesis.
   d. Vital signs indicating increased intracranial pressure (see XIII. Increased intracranial pressure, below).
   e. Neurologic exam:
      (1) Altered level of consciousness; a numerical assessment, such as the Glasgow Coma Scale (see Table 4.24), may be used. The lower the score, the poorer the prognosis, generally.
      (2) Pupils—equal, round, react to light, *or* unequal, dilated, unresponsive to light.
      (3) Extremities—paresis or paralysis.

TABLE 4.24 Glasgow Coma Scale

Best eye-opening response	Purposeful and spontaneous	4
	To voice	3
	To pain	2
	No response	1
	Untestable	U
Best verbal response	Oriented	5
	Disoriented	4
	Inappropriate words	3
	Incomprehensible sounds	2
	No response	1
	Untestable	U
Best motor response	Obeys commands	6
	Localizes pain	5
	Withdraws to pain	4
	Flexion to pain	3
	Extension to pain	2
	No response	1
	Untestable	U

(4) Reflexes—hypo- or hypertonia; Babinski present (flaring of great toe when sole is stroked).

E. Analysis/nursing diagnosis:

1. *Altered thought processes* related to brain trauma.
2. *Sensory/perceptual alteration* related to depressed neuronal activity.
3. *Potential for injury* related to impaired CNS functioning.
4. *Potential for aspiration* related to respiratory depression.
5. *Self-care deficit* related to altered level of consciousness.
6. *Potential for disuse syndrome* related to paresis or paralysis.

F. Nursing plan/implementation:

1. Goal: *sustain vital functions and minimize or prevent complications.*
   a. Patent airway: endotracheal tube or tracheostomy may be ordered.
   b. Oxygen: as ordered (as hypoxia increases cerebral edema).
   c. *Position:* semiprone or prone with head level to prevent aspiration *(keep off back);* turn side to side to prevent stasis in lungs.
   d. Vital signs as ordered.
   e. Neurologic check: pupils, level of consciousness, muscle strength; report changes.
   f. Seizure precautions: padded siderails.
   g. Medications as ordered:
      (1) *Steroids.*
      (2) *Anticonvulsants* (Dilantin, phenobarbital).
      (3) *Analgesics* **(morphine contraindicated).**
   h. Cooling measures or hypothermia for elevated temperature.
   ▶ i. Assist with diagnostic tests:
      (1) Lumbar puncture (contraindicated with increased intracranial pressure).
      (2) Electroencephalogram (EEG).
   j. Diet: NPO for 24 hours, progressing to clear liquids if awake.
   k. Fluids: IVs; nasogastric tube feedings; I&O.
   l. Monitor blood chemistries: sodium imbalance common with head injuries.
2. Goal: *provide emotional support and use comfort measures.*
   a. Comfort: skin care, oral hygiene; sheepskins; wrinkle-free linen.
   b. Eyes: lubricate q4h with artificial tears if periocular edema present.
   c. ROM—passive, active; physical therapy as tolerated.
   d. Avoid restraints.
   e. Encourage verbalization of concerns about changes in body image, limitations.
   f. Encourage family communication.

G. Evaluation:

1. Alert, oriented—no residual effects (e.g., cognitive processes intact).
2. No signs of increased intracranial pressure (e.g., decreased respirations, increased systolic pressure with widening pulse pressure, bradycardia).
3. No paralysis—regains motor/sensory function.
4. Resumes self-care activities.

XIII. Increased intracranial pressure (ICP): intracranial hypertension associated with altered states of consciousness.

A. Pathophysiology: increases in intracranial blood volume, cerebrospinal fluid, and/or brain tissue mass → increased intracranial pressure → impaired neural impulse transmission → cellular anoxia, atrophy.

B. Risk factors:

1. Congenital anomalies (hydrocephalus).
2. Space-occupying lesions (abscesses or tumors).
3. Trauma (hematomas or skull fractures).
4. Circulatory problems (aneurysms, emboli).
5. Inflammation (meningitis, encephalitis).

C. Assessment:

1. Subjective data
   a. Headache.
   b. Nausea.
2. Objective data
   a. Changes in level of consciousness.
   b. Pupillary changes—unequal, dilated, and unresponsive to light.
   c. Vital signs—changes are variable.
      (1) Blood pressure—gradual or rapid elevation, widened pulse pressure.
      (2) Pulse—bradycardia, tachycardia; significant sign is *slowing of pulse* as *blood pressure rises.*
      (3) Respirations—pattern changes (Cheyne-Stokes, apneusis, Biot's), deep and sonorous.
      (4) Temperature—moderate elevation.
   d. Projectile vomiting.

D. Analysis/nursing diagnosis:

1. *Altered cerebral tissue perfusion* related to increased intracranial pressure.
2. *Altered thought processes* related to cerebral anoxia.
3. *Ineffective breathing pattern* related to compression of respiratory center.
4. *Potential for aspiration* related to unconsciousness.
5. *Self-care deficit* related to altered level of consciousness.
6. *Impaired physical mobility* related to abnormal motor responses.

E. Nursing plan/implementation: *promote adequate oxygenation and limit further impairment.*

1. Vital signs: report changes **at once.**
2. Patent airway: keep alkalotic, to prevent increased intracranial pressure from elevated CO_2; hyperventilate if necessary.
3. Give medications as ordered:
   a. *Hyperosmolar diuretics* (mannitol, urea) to reduce brain swelling.
   b. *Steroids* (Decadron) for antiinflammatory action.
   c. *Antacids* to prevent stress ulcer.

ADULT NURSING

d. *Anticholinergics*—prevent stress ulcer.

4. *Position:* head of bed elevated 30°.
5. Fluids: restrict; strict I&O.
6. Cooling measures to reduce temperature, as fever increases ICP.
7. Prepare for surgical intervention (see XIV. Craniotomy, below).

F. Evaluation:

1. No irreversible brain damage—regains consciousness.
2. Resumes self-care activities.

XIV. Craniotomy: excision of a part of the skull (burr hole to several centimeters) for exploratory purpose and biopsy; to remove neoplasms, evacuate hematomas or excess fluid, control hemorrhage, repair skull fractures, remove scar tissue, repair or excise aneurysms, and drain abscesses; produces minimal neurologic deficit.

A. Analysis/nursing diagnosis:

1. *Altered cerebral tissue perfusion* related to edema.
2. *Altered thought processes* related to disorientation.
3. *Self-care deficit* related to continued neurologic impairment.
4. Also see nursing diagnosis for XII. Traumatic injuries to the brain, XIII. Increased intracranial pressure, and The Perioperative Experience, p. 342.

B. Nursing plan/implementation:

1. *Preoperative*
   a. Goal: *obtain baseline measures.*
      (1) Vital signs.
      (2) Level of consciousness.
      (3) Mental, emotional status.
      (4) Pupillary reactions.
      (5) Motor strength and functioning.
   b. Goal: *provide psychologic support:* listen; give accurate, brief explanations.
   c. Goal: *prepare for surgery.*
      (1) Cut hair; shave scalp (may be done in surgery).
      (2) Cover scalp with clean towel.
      (3) Enema and/or cathartics as ordered.
      (4) Insert indwelling Foley catheter as ordered.
2. *Postoperative:*
   a. Goal: *prevent complications and limit further impairment.*
      (1) Vital signs (indications of complications):
         (a) Decreased blood pressure—*shock.*
         (b) Widened pulse pressure—*increased ICP.*
         (c) Respiratory failure—*compression* of medullary *respiratory* centers.
         (d) Hyperthermia—disturbance of heat-regulating mechanism; *infection.*
      (2) Neurologic:
         (a) Pupils—ipsilateral dilation (increased ICP), visual disturbances.
         (b) Altered level of consciousness.
         (c) Altered cognitive or emotional status—disorientation common.
         (d) Motor function and strength—hypertonia, hypotonia, seizures.
      (3) Blood gases, to monitor adequacy of ventilation.
      (4) Dressings: check frequently; aseptic technique; reinforce as necessary.
      (5) Observe for:
         (a) CSF leakage (glucose-positive drainage from nose, mouth, ears)—*report immediately.*
         (b) Periorbital edema—apply light ice compresses as necessary—remove crusts from eyelids.
      (6) Check integrity of seventh cranial nerve (facial)—incomplete closure of eyelids.
      (7) *Position:*
         (a) *Supratentorial* surgery (cerebrum)—semi-Fowler's (30° elevation); may *not* lie on operative side.
         (b) *Infratentorial* (brain stem, cerebellum)—*flat* in bed; may turn to either side but *not* onto back.
      (8) Fluids: NPO for 24–48 hours.
      (9) Medications as ordered:
         (a) *Osmotic diuretics* (mannitol).
         (b) *Corticosteroids* (Decadron).
         (c) *Mild analgesics* (do not mask neurologic or respiratory depression).
      (10) Orient frequently to person, time, place—to reduce restlessness, confusion.
      (11) Siderails up for safety.
      (12) Avoid restraints (may increase agitation and ICP).
      (13) Ice bags to head to reduce headache.
      (14) Activity: assist with ambulation.
   b. Goal: *provide optimal supportive care.*
      (1) Cover scalp once dressings are removed (scarves, wigs).
      (2) Deal realistically with neurologic deficits—facilitate acceptance, adjustment, independence.
   c. Goal: *health teaching.*
      (1) Prepare for physical, occupational, and/or speech therapy, as needed.
      (2) Activities of daily living.

C. Evaluation:

1. Regains consciousness—is alert, oriented.
2. Resumes self-care activities within limits of neurologic deficits.

XV. Epilepsy: seizure disorder characterized by sudden transient aberration of brain function; associated with motor, sensory, autonomic, or psychic disturbances.

A. Seizure: involuntary muscular contraction and disturbances of consciousness from abnormal electrical activity.

B. Risk factors:

1. Brain injury.

2. Infection (meningitis, encephalitis).
3. Water and electrolyte disturbances.
4. Hypoglycemia.
5. Tumors.
6. Vascular disorders (hypoxia or hypocapnia).

C. Generalized seizures:

1. *Tonic-clonic* (grand mal) seizures:
   a. **Pathophysiology:** increased excitability of a neuron → possible activation of adjacent neurons → synchronous discharge of impulses → vigorous involuntary sustained muscle spasms (*tonic* contractions). Onset of neuronal fatigue → intermittent muscle spasms (*clonic* contractions) → cessation of muscle spasms → fatigue.
   b. **Assessment:**
      (1) Subjective data—aura: flash of light; peculiar smell, sound; feelings of fear; euphoria.
      (2) Objective data
         (a) *Convulsive stage*—tonic and clonic muscle spasms, loss of consciousness, breath-holding, frothing at mouth, biting of tongue, urinary or fecal incontinence; lasts 2–5 minutes.
         (b) *Postconvulsion*—headache, fatigue (postictal sleep), malaise, nausea, vomiting, sore muscles, choking on secretions, aspiration.
2. *Absence* (petit mal) seizures:
   a. **Pathophysiology:** unknown etiology, momentary loss of consciousness (10–20 seconds); usually no recollection of seizure; resumes previously performed action.
   b. **Assessment**—objective data
      (1) Fixation of gaze; blank facial expression.
      (2) Flickering of eyelids.
      (3) Jerking of facial muscle or arm.
3. *Minor motor* seizures:
   a. *Myoclonic*—involuntary jerking contraction of major muscles; may throw person to the floor.
   b. *Akinetic*—momentary loss of muscle movement.
   c. *Atonic*—total loss of muscle tone; person falls to the floor.

D. Partial (focal) seizures:

1. *Partial motor:* arises from region in motor cortex (posterior frontal lobe); most commonly begins in upper extremities, spreading to face and lower extremity (Jacksonian march); noting progression is important in identifying area of cortex involved.
2. *Partial sensory:* sensory symptoms occur with partial seizure activity; varies with region in brain; transient.
3. *Partial complex* (psychomotor): arises out of anterior temporal lobe; frequently begins with an aura; characteristic feature is automatism (lip-smacking, chewing, patting body, picking at clothes); lasts from 2–3 min to 15 min; do not restrain.

E. Analysis/nursing diagnosis:

1. *Potential for injury* related to convulsive disorder.
2. *Anxiety* related to sudden loss of consciousness.
3. *Self-esteem disturbance* related to chronic illness.
4. *Impaired social interaction* related to self-consciousness.

F. Nursing plan/implementation (generalized seizures):

1. Goal: *prevent injury* during *seizure.*
   a. Do not force jaws open during convulsion.
   b. Do not restrict limbs—protect from injury; place something soft under head (towel, jacket, hands).
   c. Loosen constrictive clothing.
   d. Note time, level of consciousness, type and duration of seizure.
2. Goal: *postseizure care:*
   a. *Turn on side* to drain saliva and facilitate breathing.
   b. Suction as necessary.
   c. Orient to time and place.
   d. Oral hygiene if tongue or cheek injured.
   e. Check vital signs, pupils, level of consciousness.
3. Goal: *prevent or reduce recurrences of seizure activity.*
   a. Encourage client to identify precipitating factors.
   b. Moderation in diet and exercise.
   c. Medications as ordered: diphenylhydantoin (Dilantin); phenobarbital; carbamazepine (Tegretol); primidone (Mysoline); trimethadione (Tridione)—petit mal only.
4. Goal: *health teaching.*
   a. Medications:
      (1) Actions, side effects (apathy, ataxia, hyperplasia of gums).
      (2) Complications with sudden withdrawal (status epilepticus).
   b. Attitude toward life and treatment; adhere to medication program.
   c. Clarify misconceptions, fears—especially about insanity, bad genes.
   d. Maintain activities, interests—*except* no driving until seizure-free for period of time specified by state Department of Motor Vehicles.
   e. *Avoid:* stress; lack of sleep; emotional upset; alcohol.
   f. Relaxation techniques; stress management.
   g. Use MedicAlert band or tag.
   h. Appropriate community resources.

G. Evaluation:

1. Avoids precipitating stimuli—achieves seizure control.
2. Complies with medication regimen.
3. Retains independence.

XVI. Transient ischemic attacks (TIAs): temporary, complete, or relatively complete cessation of cerebral blood flow to a localized area of brain, producing symptoms ranging from weakness and numbness to monocular blindness; an important precursor to cerebral vascular accident (CVA). Surgical intervention includes *carotid endarterectomy;* most common postoperative cranial nerve damage

ADULT NURSING

causes vocal cord paralysis or difficulty managing saliva and tongue deviation (CN VII, X, XI, XII); usually temporary.

XVII. Cerebral vascular accident (CVA): brain lesions resulting from damage to blood vessels supplying brain.

A. Pathophysiology: reduced or interrupted blood flow → interruption of nerve impulses down corticospinal tract → decreased or absent voluntary movement on one side of the body (fine movements are more affected than coarse movements); later, autonomous reflex activity → spasticity and rigidity of muscles.

B. Risk factors:

1. Cerebral thrombosis (most common), embolism, hemorrhage.
2. Prior ischemic episodes (TIAs).
3. Hypertension.
4. Oral contraceptives.
5. Emotional stress.
6. Family history.
7. Age.
8. Diabetes mellitus.

C. Assessment:

1. Subjective data
   a. Weakness; sudden or gradual loss of movement of extremities on one side.
   b. Difficulty forming words.
   c. Difficulty swallowing (dysphagia).
   d. Nausea, vomiting.
   e. History of TIAs.
2. Objective data
   a. Vital signs:
      (1) BP—elevated; widened pulse pressure.
      (2) Temperature—elevated.
      (3) Pulse—normal, slow.
      (4) Respirations—tachypnea, altered pattern; deep; sonorous.
   b. Neurologic:
      (1) Altered level of consciousness.
      (2) Pupils—unequal; vision—homonymous hemianopia.
      (3) Ptosis of eyelid, drooping mouth.
      (4) Paresis or paralysis.
      (5) Loss of sensation and reflexes.
      (6) Incontinence of urine or feces.
      (7) Aphasia (see p. 382).

D. Analysis/nursing diagnosis:

1. *Impaired physical mobility* related to hemiplegia.
2. *Impaired swallowing* related to paralysis.
3. *Impaired verbal communication* related to aphasia.
4. *Potential for aspiration* related to unconsciousness.
5. *Sensory/perceptual alterations* related to altered cerebral blood flow.
6. *Altered thought processes* related to cerebral edema.
7. *Self-care deficit* related to paresis or paralysis.
8. *Body image disturbance* related to hemiplegia.
9. *Total incontinence* related to interruption of normal nerve transmission.
10. *Impaired social interaction* related to aphasia or neurologic deficit.
11. *Potential impaired skin integrity* related to immobility.

E. Nursing plan/implementation:

1. Goal: *reduce cerebral anoxia.*
   a. Patent airway:
      (1) Oxygen therapy as ordered; suctioning to prevent aspiration.
      (2) Turn, cough, deep breathe q2h due to high incidence of pneumonia.
   b. Activity: bedrest; progressing to out of bed as tolerated.
   c. *Position:*
      (1) Maximize ventilation.
      (2) Support with pillows when on side; use hand rolls and arm slings as ordered.
2. Goal: *promote cardiovascular function and maintain cerebral perfusion.*
   a. Vital signs; neurologic checks.
   b. Medications as ordered:
      (1) *Antihypertensives* to prevent rupture.
      (2) *Anticoagulants* to prevent thrombus.
   c. Fluids: IVs to prevent hemoconcentration; I&O; weigh daily.
   d. ROM exercises to prevent contractures, muscle atrophy, phlebitis.
   e. Skin care and position changes to prevent decubiti.
3. Goal: *provide for emotional relaxation.*
   a. Identify grief reaction to changes in body image.
   b. Encourage expression of feelings, concerns.
4. Goal: *health teaching.*
   a. Exercise routines.
   b. Diet: self-feeding, but assist as needed.
   c. Resumption of self-care activities.
   d. Use of supportive devices.

F. Evaluation:

1. No complications (e.g., pneumonia).
2. Regains functional independence—resumes self-care activities.
3. Return of control over body functions (e.g., bowel, bladder, speech).

XVIII. Bacterial meningitis (see Unit 3, p. 250).

XIX. Encephalitis: inflammation of the brain and its coverings, which usually results in a lengthy coma.

A. Pathophysiology: brain tissue injury → release of enzymes that increase vascular dilatation, capillary permeability → edema formation → increased intracranial pressure → depression of central nervous system function.

ADULT NURSING

B. Risk factors:

1. Syphilis.
2. Lead or arsenic poisoning.
3. Carbon monoxide.
4. Typhoid fever.
5. Measles; chickenpox.
6. Viruses.

C. Assessment:

1. Subjective data
   a. Headache—severe.
   b. Fever—sudden.
   c. Nausea, vomiting.
   d. Sensitivity to light (photophobia).
   e. Difficulty concentrating.
2. Objective data
   a. Altered level of consciousness.
   b. Nuchal rigidity.
   c. Tremors; facial weakness.
   d. Nystagmus.
   e. Elevated temperature.
   ▶ f. Diagnostic test: lumbar puncture—fluid cloudy; increased neutrophils, protein.
   g. Lab data: blood—slight to moderate leukocytosis (about 14,000).

D. Analysis/nursing diagnosis:

1. *Self-care deficit* related to altered level of consciousness.
2. *Potential for injury* related to coma.
3. *Sensory/perceptual alteration* related to brain tissue injury.
4. *Altered thought processes* related to increased intracranial pressure.

E. Nursing plan/implementation:

1. Goal: *support physical and emotional relaxation.*
   a. Vital signs; neurologic signs as ordered.
   b. Seizure precautions.
   c. *Position:* to maintain patent airway; prevent contractures; ROM.
   d. Medications as ordered:
      (1) Analgesics for pain.
      (2) Antipyretics for fever.
      (3) Sedatives for agitation.
      (4) Anticonvulsants for seizures.
      (5) Antibiotics for infection.
      (6) Osmotic diuretics (mannitol, urea) to reduce cerebral edema.
   e. No isolation.
2. Goal: *health teaching:* self-care activities with residual motor and speech deficits; physical therapy.

F. Evaluation:

1. Regains consciousness; is alert, oriented.
2. Performs self-care activities with minimal assistance.

■ COMFORT, REST, ACTIVITY, AND MOBILITY

I. Pain

A. *Types of pain:*

1. *Superficial somatic tissues*—skin, subcutaneous or fibrous tissue, and ligaments have pain receptors, and thus pain is localized.
2. *Deep somatic tissues and viscera*—may be diffuse and radiating pain because these do not have direct connection with sensory-discriminative system.
3. *Neurogenic pain*—results from damage to peripheral or central nervous system; any sensation may be perceived as pain due to abnormal processing of afferent impulses or paroxysmal activity.
4. *Psychogenic pain*—due to fantasies and psychologic need for injury or punishment (called conversion).

B. *Components of pain experience*—pain related to:

1. *Stimuli*—sources: chemical, ischemic, mechanical trauma, extremes of heat/cold.
2. *Perception*—viewed with fear by children, can be altered by level of consciousness, interpreted and influenced by previous and current experience, is more severe when alone at night or immobilized.
3. *Response*—variations in physiologic, cultural and learned responses; anxiety is created; pain seen as justified punishment; pain as means for attention-getting.

C. Assessment:

1. Subjective data
   a. *Site*—medial, lateral, proximal, distal.
   b. *Strength:*
      (1) Certain tissues are more sensitive.
      (2) Change in intensity.
      (3) Based on expectations.
      (4) Affected by distraction or concentration, state of consciousness.
      (5) Described as slight, medium, severe, excruciating.
   c. *Quality*—aching, burning, crushing, dull, piercing, shifting, throbbing, tingling.
   d. *Antecedent factors*—physical exertion, eating, extreme temperatures, physical and emotional stressors (fear, for example).
   e. *Previous experience*—influences reaction to pain.
   f. *Behavioral clues*—demanding, worried, irritable, restless, difficult to distract, sleepless.
2. Objective data
   a. *Verbal clues*—moaning, groaning, crying.
   b. *Nonverbal clues*—clenching teeth, grimacing, splinting of body parts, body position, knees drawn up, involuntary reflex movements, tossing/turning, rhythmic rubbing movements, voice pitch and speed, eyes shut.
   c. *Physical clues*—breathing irregularities, abdominal distention, skin color changes, skin temperature changes, excessive salivation, perspiration.

ADULT NURSING

d. *Time/duration*—onset, duration, recurrence, interval, last occurrence.

D. Analysis/nursing diagnosis:

1. *Pain,* acute or chronic, related to specific patient condition.
2. *Activity intolerance* related to discomfort.
3. *Sleep pattern disturbance* related to pain.
4. *Fatigue* related to state of discomfort or emotional stress.
5. *Ineffective individual coping* related to chronic pain.

E. Nursing plan/implementation:

1. Goal: *provide relief of pain.*
   a. Assess level of pain; ask patient to rate on scale of 0–10 (0 = no pain; 10 = worst pain).
   b. Determine cause and try nursing *comfort* measures *before* giving drugs:
      (1) *Environmental factors:* noise, light, odors, motion.
      (2) *Physiologic needs:* elimination, hunger, thirst, fatigue, circulatory impairment, muscle tension, ventilation, pressure on nerves.
      (3) *Emotional:* fear of unknown, helplessness, loneliness (especially at night).
   c. Determine pain reactions; explore meaning of "pain" (how much, when, how long, where, why, what it feels like).
   d. *Relieve:* anger, anxiety, boredom, loneliness.
   e. Report **sudden, severe, new** pain; pain **not** relieved by medications or comfort measures; pain associated with **casts or traction.**
   f. *Remove pain stimulus:*
      (1) Administer pain medication (e.g., analgesic, antispasmodic) at appropriate time intervals; do not withhold due to overestimated danger of addiction.
      (2) Avoid cold (to reduce immediate tissue reaction to trauma).
      (3) Apply heat (to relieve ischemia).
      (4) Change activity (e.g., restrict activity in cardiac pain).
      (5) Change, loosen dressing.
      (6) Comfort (e.g., smooth wrinkled sheets, change wet dressing).
      (7) Give food (e.g., for ulcer).
   g. *Reduce pain-receptor reaction.*
      (1) Ointment (use as coating).
      (2) Local anesthetics.
      (3) Padding (of bony prominences).
   h. Assist with medical/surgical interventions to *block pain-impulse transmission:*
      (1) Injection of local anesthetic into nerve (e.g., dental).
      (2) Chordotomy—sever anterolateral spinal cord nerve tracts.
      (3) Electrical stimulation—transcutaneous (skin surface), percutaneous (peripheral nerve).
      (4) Peripheral nerve implant—electrode to major sensory nerve.
      (5) Dorsal column stimulator—electrode to dorsal column.
   i. *Avoid causes of inadequate pain control:*
      (1) Incorrect assessment.
      (2) Insufficient knowledge of pharmacologic effects.
      (3) Personal attitudes, e.g., concern for addiction.
      (4) Fear of respiratory depression.
      (5) Reluctance to accept subjective data.
   j. *Document response to pain-relief measures.*
2. Goal: *alter pain perception* by raising pain threshold.
   a. *Distraction,* e.g., TV (cerebral cortical activity blocks impulses from thalamus).
   b. *Analgesics*—give *prior* to occurrence of severe pain; give routinely for chronic/terminal pain.
   c. *Hypnosis*—assess appropriateness for use for psychogenic pain and for anesthesia; needs to be open to suggestion.
   d. *Acupuncture*—assess emotional readiness and belief in it.
3. Goal: *alter interpretation and response to pain.*
   a. Administer narcotics—result: no longer sees pain as disturbing.
   b. Administer hypnotics—result: changes perception and decreases reaction.
   c. Help client obtain interpersonal satisfaction from ways other than attention received when in pain.
4. Goal: *promote patient control of pain and analgesia: Patient-controlled analgesia* (PCA), an analgesia administration system designed to maintain optimal serum analgesia levels, safely delivers intermittent bolus doses of a narcotic analgesic; preset to maximum hourly dose.
   a. *Advantages:* decreased patient anxiety; improved pulmonary function; fewer side effects.
   b. *Limitations:* requires an indwelling intravenous line; analgesia targets central pain, may not relieve peripheral discomfort; cost of PCA unit.
5. Goal: *health teaching.*
   a. Explain causes of pain and how to describe pain.
   b. Explain that it is acceptable to admit existence of pain.
   c. Relaxation exercises.
   d. Biofeedback methods of pain perception and control.
   e. Proper medication administration, when necessary, for self-care.

F. Evaluation:

1. Verbalizes comfort; awareness of pain decreased.
2. Knows source of pain; how to reduce stimulus and perception.
3. Uses alternative measures for pain relief.
4. Able to cope with pain, e.g., remains active, relaxed appearance; verbal and nonverbal clues of pain absent.

II. Immobility: impaired physical mobility or limitation of physical movement may be accompanied by a number of complications that can involve any or all of the major systems of the body. Regardless of the cause of immobilization, there are a number of conditions that arise primarily as a complication of immobility. These are discussed in Table 4.25.

A. Types of immobility:

1. *Physical*—physical restriction due to limitation in movement or physiologic processes (e.g., breathing).
2. *Intellectual*—lack of action due to lack of knowledge (e.g., mental retardation, brain damage).
3. *Emotional*—immobilized when highly stressed (e.g., after loss of loved person or diagnosis of terminal illness).
4. *Social*—decreased social interaction due to separation from family when hospitalized or when alone, as in old age.

B. Risk factors:

1. Pain, trauma, injury.
2. Loss of body function or body part.
3. Chronic disease.
4. Emotional, mental illness; neglect.
5. Malnutrition.
6. Bedrest, traction, surgery, medications.

C. Assessment:

1. Subjective data: *psychologic/social effects* of immobility:
   a. Decreased motivation to learn; decreased retention.
   b. Decreased problem-solving abilities.
   c. Diminished drives; decreased hunger.
   d. Changes in body image, self-concept.
   e. Exaggerated emotional reactions, inappropriate to situation or person; aggression, apathy, withdrawal.
   f. Deterioration of time perception.
   g. Fear, anxiety, worthlessness related to change in role activities, e.g., when no longer employed.
2. Objective data: *physical effects* of immobility:
   a. Cardiovascular
      (1) Orthostatic hypotension.
      (2) Increased cardiac load.
      (3) Thrombus formation.
   b. Gastrointestinal
      (1) Anorexia.
      (2) Diarrhea.
      (3) Constipation.
   c. Metabolic
      (1) Tissue atrophy and protein catabolism.
      (2) BMR reduced.
      (3) Fluid-electrolyte imbalances.
   d. Musculoskeletal
      (1) Demineralization (osteoporosis).
      (2) Contractures and atrophy.
      (3) Skin breakdown.
   e. Respiratory
      (1) Decreased respiratory movement.
      (2) Accumulation of secretions in respiratory tract.
      (3) O_2/CO_2 ratio imbalance.
   f. Urinary
      (1) Calculi.
      (2) Bladder distention, stasis.
      (3) Infection.
      (4) Frequency.

D. Analysis/nursing diagnosis:

1. *Impaired physical mobility* related to specific patient condition.
2. *Impaired skin integrity* related to physical immobilization.
3. *Urinary retention* related to incomplete emptying of bladder.
4. *Constipation* related to inactivity.
5. *Potential for disuse syndrome* related to lack of range of motion.
6. *Bathing/hygiene self-care deficit* related to musculoskeletal impairment.
7. *Sensory/perceptual alteration* related to complications of immobility.
8. *Body image disturbance* related to physical limitations.

E. Nursing plan/implementation:

1. Goal: *prevent physical, psychologic hazards.*
   a. Apply nursing measures to promote venous flow, muscle strength, endurance, joint mobility, skin integrity.
   b. Assess and counteract *psychologic* impact of immobility (e.g., feelings of helplessness, hopelessness, powerlessness).
   c. Help maintain accurate sensory processing to prevent and lessen *sensory disturbances.*
   d. Help adapt to *altered body image* due to increased dependency, sensory deprivation, and changes in status and power that accompany immobility.
   e. Offer counseling when sexual expression is impaired.
2. Goal: *health teaching:* how to prevent physical problems related to immobility (e.g., anticonstipation diet, range of motion, skin care); teach activities while immobile that encourage independence and provide sensory stimulation.

F. Evaluation:

1. Minimal contractures, skin breakdown, muscle atrophy or loss of strength.
2. Interest in self and environment; positive self-image.
3. Returns to optimal level of physical activity.

III. Fractures: disruptions in the continuity of bone as the result of trauma or various disease processes, such as Cushing's syndrome, that weaken the bone structure.

A. Types:

1. *Open or compound*—fractured bone extends *through skin* and mucous membranes; increased potential for infection.
2. *Closed or simple*—fractured bone *does not* protrude through skin.

■ TABLE 4.25 **Complications of Immobilization**

Disorder	Pathophysiology	Assessment	Analysis/Nursing Diagnosis
Orthostatic hypotension	A decrease in BP >30/15 caused by failure of vasomotor responses to compensate for change from a recumbent to an upright position.	*Subjective data:* weakness; dizziness. *Objective data:* decreased BP >30/15 measured 2 min after moving from a supine to a sitting or standing position; loss of muscle tone and strength; client may faint.	*Decreased cardiac output* related to orthostatic hypotension. *Potential for injury* related to vertigo. *Activity intolerance,* potential, related to dizziness.
Cardiac overload	When the body is recumbent, some of the total blood volume that would be in the legs due to gravity is redistributed to other parts of the body, thereby increasing the circulating volume and increasing the workload of the heart. Heart rate, which is decreased because blood is prevented from entering the thoracic vessels by pressure from the Valsalva maneuver, increases when normal breathing resumes.	*Subject data:* fear; apprehension. *Objective data:* Valsalva maneuver (pressure against the closed glottis when breath is held) 10–20 times/h, when trying to move in bed; tachycardia; decreased exercise tolerance.	*Potential for injury* related to increased workload of heart. *Activity intolerance* related to increased workload of heart. *Fear* related to tachycardia.

continued

3. *Complete*—fracture extends through *entire bone,* disrupting the periosteum on both sides of the bone, producing two or more fragments.
4. *Incomplete*—fracture extends *only part way* through bone; bone continuity is not totally interrupted.
5. *Greenstick or willow-hickory stick*—fracture of *one* side of bone; *other side merely bends;* usually seen only in children.
6. *Impacted or telescoped*—fracture in which bone fragments are *forcibly driven into* other or adjacent bone structures.
7. *Comminuted*—fracture having *more than one* fracture line and with bone fragment broken into *several pieces.*
8. *Depressed*—fracture in which bone or bone fragments are driven *inward,* as in skull or facial fractures.

B. Methods used to reduce/immobilize fractures: reduction or setting of the bone—restores bone alignment as nearly as possible.

1. *Closed reduction*—manual traction or manipulation. Usually done under general anesthesia to reduce pain and muscle spasm. Maintenance of reduction and immobilization is accomplished by casting (fiberglass or plaster of Paris).
2. *Open reduction*—operative procedure utilized to achieve bone alignment; pins, wire, nails, or rods may be used to secure bone fragments in position; prosthetic implants may also be used.
3. *Traction reduction*—force is applied in two directions, to obtain alignment and to reduce or eliminate muscle spasm. Used for fractures of long bones. May be:
   a. Continuous—used with fractures or dislocations of bones or joints.
   b. Intermittent—used to reduce flexion contractures or lessen pain and muscle spasm.
   c. Applied as follows:
      (1) *Skin*—traction applied to skin by using a commercial foam rubber Buck's traction splint or by using adhesive, plastic, or a moleskin strip bound to the extremity by elastic bandage; exerts indirect traction on bone or muscles (e.g., Buck's extension, Bryant's, Russell's, pelvic). See Figure 4.6, parts a–d, p. 408.
      (2) *Skeletal*—direct traction applied to bone using pins (Steinman), wires (Kirschner). Pin is inserted through the bone in or close to the involved area and usually protrudes through skin on both sides of the extremity. Skeletal traction for fractured vertebrae accomplished with tongs (Crutchfield tongs, Gardner-Wells tongs).
   d. Specific types of traction
      (1) *Cervical*—direct traction applied to cervical

■ **TABLE 4.25 *(Continued)***

Nursing Plan/ Implementation	Evaluation
Prevent trauma due to sudden decrease in BP. 1. Change position gradually. 2. Elastic stockings. 3. Leg exercises. 4. Dangle before getting up. 5. Tilt table. 6. Sitting and lying BP. 7. Monitoring side effects of drugs. *Health teaching.* 1. Explains signs and symptoms to client. 2. Encourage client to dangle before standing. 3. Encourage slow movement from sitting to standing. 4. Exercises to maintain muscle tone.	Client tolerates increased activity. No trauma occurs. BP remains within normal limits.
Prevent injury and further ischemic damage to cardiac tissue by decreasing workload of heart. 1. Out of bed in chair when possible. 2. Semirecumbent position when in bed; pillows between legs when side-lying. 3. Exercises: passive and active ROM, isometric. 4. Encourage participation in self-care. 5. Turn every 2 hours, dangle. 6. Avoid Valsalva, fatigue. 7. Minimize constipation. 8. Encourage slow, deep breathing when moving in bed. *Health teaching.* 1. Exhale while turning, don't hold breath. 2. Measures to conserve energy.	No complications noted. Client tolerates increased activity. Heart rate within normal limit.

continued

vertebrae using a head halter or Crutchfield, Gardner-Wells, or Vinke tongs that are inserted into the skull (see Figure 4.6, parts e and f). Traction is increased with weights until vertebrae move into position and alignment is regained. After reduction is obtained, weights are decreased to the amount needed to maintain reduction. *Weight amount is prescribed by physician.*

(2) *Balanced suspension*—countertraction produced by a force other than client's body weight; extremity is suspended in a traction apparatus that maintains the line of traction despite changes in the client's position (e.g., Russell's leg traction, Thomas' splint with Pearson's attachment). See Figure 4.6, parts c and g.

(3) *Running*—traction that exerts a pull in one plane; countertraction is supplied by the weight of the client's body or can be increased through use of weights and pulleys in the opposite direction (e.g., Buck's extension, Russell's traction). See Figure 4.6, parts a and c, p. 408.

(4) *Halo*—an apparatus that employs both a plastic and metal frame; molded frame extends from the axilla to iliac crest and houses a metal frame. The struts of the frame extend to skull and attach to round metal (halo) device. The halo is attached to skull by four pins—two located anterolaterally and two located posterolaterally. They are inserted into external cortex of the cranium (see Figure 4.6, part h). Used to: immobilize the cervical spine following spinal fusion, give some correction to scoliosis prior to spinal fusion, and immobilize nondisplaced fracture of spine.

4. *Immobilization*—maintains reduction and promotes healing of bone fragments. Achieved by:
   a. *External fixation*
      (1) Casts—types:
         (a) Spica—applied to immobilize hip or shoulder joints.
         (b) Body cast—applied to trunk.
         (c) Arm or leg cast—joints above and below site included in cast.
      (2) Splints, continuous traction.
      (3) External fixation devices (Charnley)—multiple pins/rods through limb above and below fracture site, attached to external metal supports. Client able to become ambulatory.
   b. *Internal fixation*—pins, wires, nails, rods. See VI. Total hip replacement, p. 405, and VII. Total knee replacement, p. 407.

C. Assessment:

1. Subjective data
   a. Pain, tenderness.
   b. Tingling, numbness.
   c. Nausea.
   d. History of traumatic event.
2. Objective data
   a. Function: abnormal or lost.
   b. Deformities.
   c. Ecchymosis, increased heat over injured part.
   d. Localized edema.
   e. Muscle spasm.
   f. Crepitation (grating sensations heard or felt as bone fragments rub against each other).
   g. Signs of shock.
   h. Indicators of anxiety.
   ▶ i. X ray: *fracture*—positive interruption of bone; *dislocation*—abnormal position of bone.

D. Analysis/nursing diagnosis:

1. *Pain* related to interruption in bone.
2. *Impaired physical mobility* related to fracture/treatment modality.
3. *Potential for injury* related to complications of fractures.

TABLE 4.25 *(Continued)* **Complications of Immobilization**

Disorder	Pathophysiology	Assessment	Analysis/Nursing Diagnosis
Thrombus formation	Mass of blood constituents formed in the heart or blood vessels due to pooling of blood from lack of activity; increased viscosity related to dehydration or possible external pressure.	*Subjective data:* discomfort over involved vessel. *Objective data:* increased RBC; venous stasis; hypercoagulability.	*Potential altered peripheral tissue perfusion* related to obstructed vessel. *Potential for injury* related to emboli.
Respiratory congestion related to decreased respiratory movements	Decreased thoracic movement due to restriction against bed or chair, lack of position change, restrictive clothing or binders/bandages, or abdominal distention.	*Subjective data:* dyspnea; pain. *Objective data:* trauma; immobilization of thorax or abdomen, due to position in bed; inability to cough or deep breathe; abdominal distention.	*Ineffective breathing pattern* related to splinting to reduce pain. *Ineffective airway clearance* related to retained secretions. *Impaired physical mobility* related to trauma.

continued

4. *Knowledge deficit* regarding cast care, crutch walking, traction.
5. *Constipation* related to immobilization.
6. *Potential impaired skin integrity* related to immobility or friction from materials used to immobilize the fracture during healing.

E. Nursing plan/implementation:

1. Goal: *promote healing and prevent complications of fractures* (see Table 4.26, pp. 409–411).
   a. Diet: high protein, iron, vitamins, to improve tissue repair; moderate carbohydrates to prevent weight gain; no increase in calcium, to prevent kidney stones (decalcification and demineralization occur when client is immobilized).
   b. Encourage increased fluid intake, to prevent kidney stones.
   c. Prevent or correct constipation through increasing bulk foods, fruits, and fruit juices, or utilizing prescribed stool softeners, laxatives, or cathartics as necessary.
   d. Provide activities to reduce perceptual deprivation—reading, handcrafts, music, special interests/hobbies that can be done while maintaining correct position for healing.
2. Goal: *prevent injury or trauma in relation to:*
   a. *Fracture care*
      (1) Maintain affected part in optimum alignment.
      (2) Maintain skin integrity; check all bony prominences for evidence of pressure q4h and p.r.n., depending on amount of pressure.
      (3) Monitor: circulation in, sensation of, and motion of (CSM) affected part q15min for first four hours; q1h until 24 h; q4h and p.r.n., depending on amount of edema.
      (4) Maintain mobility in unaffected limb and unaffected joints of affected limb by active and passive ROM; prevent foot drop by using ankle-top sneakers.
   b. *Skin traction*
      (1) Maintain correct alignment:
         (a) If tape or moleskin is used, shave extremity and apply benzoin to improve adherence of strip and reduce itching.
         (b) Check apparatus for slippage, bunching, and replace p.r.n.
      (2) Prevent tissue injury:
         (a) Check all bony prominences for evidence of pressure: q15min for first four hours; q1h

■ **TABLE 4.25 *(Continued)***

Nursing Plan/ Implementation	Evaluation
Prevent injury by reducing risk factors and venous stasis. 1. *Position:* change q12h. 2. Do not gatch bed (causes pressure against leg vessels). 3. Increase fluid intake. 4. Monitor coagulation lab values. 5. *Medications:* anticoagulation therapy, as prescribed for clients at risk (immobilized, trauma, low pelvic surgery.) 6. Ambulate as soon as possible. *Health teaching.* 1. How to recognize signs of thrombophlebitis/ thromboemboli. 2. Leg exercise program to strengthen muscles for improved tone, to prevent pooling of blood in vessels. 3. Precautions necessary when on anticoagulation therapy. 4. Side effects of anticoagulation therapy (bleeding from gums, body fluids, obvious bleeding).	No thromboemboli. *Note:* If Homans' sign present (discomfort behind knee on forced dorsiflexion of the foot), see nursing care for client with thromboemboli, p. 311.
Prevent complications related to respiratory status. 1. Maintain a clear airway, assist with ventilation p.r.n. 2. Remove or minimize causes of dyspnea. 3. Conserve client's energy (periods of rest and activity—client able to cough more effectively when rested). 4. Incentive spirometry. *Promote comfort.* 1. Maintain hydration and nutrition. 2. *Position:* change q2h; out of bed in chair when possible (chest expansion greater when sitting in chair). *Health teaching.* 1. Methods to allay anxieties precipitated by dyspnea. 2. Effective breathing and coughing exercises.	No respiratory complications or excess secretions noted.

continued

until 24 hrs, q4h and p.r.n., depending on amount of edema.

(b) Nonadhesive traction may be removed q8h to check skin (e.g., Bryant's).

c. *Skeletal traction*

(1) Maintain affected part in optimum alignment:

(a) Ropes on pulleys.

(b) Weights hang free.

(c) Elevate head of bed as prescribed.

(d) Check knots routinely.

(2) Maintain skin integrity:

(a) Frequent skin care.

(b) Keep bedlinens free of crumbs and wrinkles.

(3) Prevent infection: special skin care to pin insertion site tid. Keep area around pins clean and dry. Utilize prescribed solution for cleansing.

(4) Monitor: circulation, sensation, motion of affected part (see a. Fracture care, p. 398).

(5) Maintain mobility in unaffected limb and unaffected joints; prevent foot drop of affected limb.

d. *Running traction*

(1) Keep well centered in bed.

(2) *Elevate head of bed only* to point of countertraction.

(3) No turning from side to side—will cause rubbing of bony fragments.

(4) Check distal circulation frequently.

(5) Frequent back care to prevent skin breakdown.

(6) Fracture bed pan for toileting.

(7) Avoid excessive padding of splints in groin area to prevent tissue trauma.

e. *Balanced suspension traction:*

(1) Maintain alignment and countertraction:

(a) Ropes on pulleys.

(b) Weights hang free.

(c) Elevate head of bed as prescribed.

(d) Check knots routinely.

(2) May move client, but turn only slightly (no more than 30° to *unaffected* side).

(3) Heel of affected leg must remain free of the bed.

(4) 20° angle between thigh and bed.

(5) Check for pressure from sling to popliteal area.

(6) Provide foot support to prevent foot drop.

(7) Maintain *abduction* of extremity.

(8) Check for signs of infection at pin insertion sites; cleanse t.i.d. as ordered.

(9) If tape or moleskin is used, shave extremity and apply benzoin to improve adherence of strip and reduce itching.

f. *Cervical traction:*

(1) May be placed on specialized bed, e.g., Stryker frame.

(2) Position: maintain body alignment.

(3) Keep tongs free from bed, and keep weights hanging freely to allow traction to function properly.

g. *Halo traction:*

(1) Several times a day, check screws to the head and screws that hold the upper portion of the frame, to determine correct position.

(2) Pin sites cleansed t.i.d. with bacteriostatic solution to prevent infection.

(3) Monitor for signs of infection.

(4) Position as any other client in body cast, except no pressure to rest on halo—pillows may be

■ **TABLE 4.25 *(Continued)*** **Complications of Immobilization**

Disorder	Pathophysiology	Assessment	Analysis/Nursing Diagnosis
Respiratory congestion related to pooled secretions	Inability of cilia to move normal secretions out of bronchial tree due to ineffective coughing, lack of thoracic expansion, or effects of medications.	*Subjective data:* dyspnea; pain. *Objective data:* dehydration; drugs—anticholinergic, CNS depressants, anesthesia. Inadequate coughing. Stationary position.	*Ineffective airway clearance* related to pooled secretions. *Impaired gas exchange* related to ineffective coughing.
Oxygen-carbon dioxide imbalance	Imbalance in oxygen and carbon dioxide levels related to pulmonary congestion, ineffective breathing patterns, trauma, or effects of medications.	*Subjective data:* confusion, irritable, restless, dyspnea. *Objective data:* hypoxia, hypercapnia, cyanosis.	*Impaired gas exchange* related to immobilization.
Malnutrition of immobilized adult	Lack of adequate dietary intake to maintain healthy tissue related to: lack of food; lack of knowledge about food; problems with ingestion, digestion, or absorption; or psychosocial factors that influence client's motivation to eat.	*Subjective data:* anorexia, nausea; diet history validating lack of adequate nutritional intake; mental irritability. *Objective data:* 1. Recent weight loss of more than 10%. 2. Decreased: healing ability, GI motility, absorption, secretion of digestive enzymes. 3. Appearance: listlessness, muscle weakness; posture—sagging shoulders, sunken chest. 4. Anthropometric data (measurement of size, weight and body proportions) less than 85% of standard.	*Altered nutrition, less than body requirements,* related to decreased appetite. *Knowledge deficit* related to nutrition requirements.

continued

placed under abdomen and chest when client is prone.

(5) Institute ROM exercises to prevent contractures.

(6) Turn frequently to prevent development of pressure areas.

(7) Allow client to verbalize about having screws placed in skull.

(8) Post application nursing care same as pin insertion for other traction.

h. *External fixation devices:*

(1) Pin care same as for skeletal traction.

(2) Teach clothing adjustment.

(3) Teach to adjust for size of apparatus.

i. *Internal fixation devices:*

(1) Monitor for signs of infection/allergic reaction to materials used for maintenance of reduction (drainage, pain, increased temperature).

(2) Position as ordered to prevent dislocation.

j. *Casts:*

(1) Support drying cast on firm pillow; avoid finger imprints on cast.

(2) Elevate limb to reduce edema.

(3) Prevent complications of fractures as listed.

(4) Closely monitor: *circulation* (blanching, swelling, decreased temperature); *sensation* (absence of feeling or pain or burning); and *motion* (inability to move digits of affected limb).

TABLE 4.25 *(Continued)*

Nursing Plan/ Implementation	Evaluation
Prevent atalectasis, infection, stasis of air and secretions in lungs. 1. Maintain patent airway; cough; suction; change position. 2. See nursing plan for Respiratory congestions related to decreased respiratory movements, above. *Health teaching.* 1. Effective coughing techniques. 2. Importance of adequate hydration.	No respiratory complications. Client coughs and removes secretions.
Promote improved respirations. 1. Change position frequently. 2. Increase humidification. 3. Monitor side effects of administered medication, especially narcotics, barbiturates. 4. See nursing plan for Respiratory congestion related to decreased respiratory movements, above.	No respiratory complications. Respiratory rate and depth are adequate for maintaining balance of oxygen and carbon dioxide.
Improved nutritional intake to maintain basal metabolism requirements and replace losses from catabolism. 1. Provide balanced or prescribed diet, soft or ground food if cannot chew or is endentulous. 2. Increase fluid intake. 3. Attain/maintain normal weight. 4. Feed, assist with feeding, or place foods within client's reach. *Promote comfort.* 1. Mouth care: to facilitate mastication of food→ improved digestion and absorption. 2. Relieve constipation (see nursing plan for Constipation, below).	No complications. Client obtains/maintains normal weight. No tissue breakdown.

continued

(5) **Be prepared to notify MD or cut cast if circulatory impairment occurs.**

(6) Protect skin integrity: avoid pressure of edges of cast; petal p.r.n.

(7) Monitor for signs of infection if skin integrity impaired.

3. Goal: *provide care related to ambulation with crutches.*
   a. See Teaching Crutch Walking (Table 4.27, p. 412).
   b. Measure crutches correctly (see Table 4.28, p. 412).
      (1) Subtract 16 inches from total height; top of crutch should be 2 inches below the axilla.
      (2) Complete extension of the elbows should be possible without pressure of axilla bar into the axilla.
      (3) Handgrip should be adjusted so that complete wrist extension is possible.
      (4) Instruct in correct body alignment:
         (a) Head erect.
         (b) Back straight.
         (c) Chest forward.
         (d) Feet 6–8 inches apart, wide base for support.
4. Goal: *provide safety measures related to possible complications following fracture* (see Table 4.26).
5. Goal: *health teaching.*
   a. Explain and show apparatus before application, if possible.
   b. Pin care at least once daily to prevent granulation and cellulitis.
   c. Correct position for rest/sleep and prevention of injury with halo traction—no pressure on halo.
   d. Purpose of cast: to immobilize, to support body tissues, to prevent or correct deformities.
   e. Teach signs and symptoms of complications to report related to cast care (i.e., numbness, odor, crack/break in cast; extremity cold, bluish).
   f. Isometric exercises for use with affected joint.
   g. Safety measures with crutches:
      (1) Weight bearing on hands, not axilla.
      (2) Position crutches 4 inches to side and 4 inches to front.
      (3) Use short strides, looking ahead, not at feet.
      (4) Prevent injury: if client begins to fall, throw crutches to side to prevent falling on them; body should be relaxed.
      (5) Check for environmental hazards: rugs, water spills.

F. Evaluation:

1. No injury or complications related to apparatus or immobilization (e.g., infection, tissue injury, altered circulation/sensation, dislocation).
2. Bone remains in correct alignment and begins to heal.
3. Demonstrates elevated limb position to relieve edema with casted extremity.
4. Lists complications related to circulation and/or neurologic impairment and infection.
5. Begins to use affected part.
6. Demonstrates correct technique for ambulation with crutches—no pressure on axilla, utilizes strength of arms and wrists.
7. No falls while using crutches.

IV. Compartment syndrome: an accumulation of fluid in the muscle compartment, resulting in an increase in pressure that reduces blood flow to the tissues. Can lead to neuromuscular deficit, amputation, and death.

■ **TABLE 4.25 *(Continued)*** **Complications of Immobilization**

Disorder	Pathophysiology	Assessment	Analysis/Nursing Diagnosis
Malnutrition of immobilized adult (cont.)		5. Cardiovascular: tachycardia (over 100) on minimal exertion; bradycardia at rest. 6. Hair: brittle, dry, thin. 7. Skin: dry, scaly. 8. Lack of financial resources: sociocultural influences. 9. Decreased blood values: serum albumin, iron-binding capacity, lymphocyte levels, hemocrit, and hemoglobin.	
Constipation	Waste material in the bowel is too hard to pass easily; or bowel movements are so infrequent that client has discomfort.	*Subjective data:* discomfort, pain, distress, and pressure in the rectum; reported decrease in normal elimination pattern. *Objective data:* immobilization; hard-formed stool, possible palpable impaction; decreased bowel sounds; bowel elimination less frequent than usual.	*Constipation* related to decreased water and fiber intake. *Knowledge deficit* related to dietary and exercise requirements to prevent constipation.
Osteoporosis	Metabolic bone disorder in which there is a generalized loss of bone density due to an imbalance between formation and bone resorption. Immobilization can cause calcium losses of 200–300 mg/day.	*Subjective data:* backache. *Objective data:* demineralization of bone seen on X ray; kyphosis; spontaneous fracture of bone.	*Pain* related to bone fractures or body structural changes.

continued

A. Risk factors:
1. Fractures.
2. Burns.
3. Crushing injuries.
4. Restrictive bandages.
5. Cast.
6. Prolonged lithotomy positioning.

B. Pathophysiology: inability of the fascia surrounding the muscle group to expand to accommodate the increased volume of fluid → compartment pressure increases → venous flow impaired → arterial flow continues, increasing capillary pressure → fluid pushed into the extravascular space → intracompartment pressure further increased → prolonged or severe ischemia → muscle and nerve cells destroyed, contracture, loss of function, necrotic tissue, infection, release of potassium, hydrogen, and myoglobin into bloodstream.

C. Assessment:
1. Subjective data
   a. Severe, unrelenting pain, unrelieved by narcotics and associated with passive stretching of muscle.
   b. Paresthesias.
2. Objective data
   a. Edema; tense skin over limb.
   b. Paralysis.
   c. Decreased or absent pulses.
   d. Poor capillary refill.

■ **TABLE 4.25** ***(Continued)***

Nursing Plan/ Implementation	Evaluation
3. Observe for stomatitis, bleeding, changes in skin texture, color. 4. Medications: monitor nausea and vomiting side effects of prescribed medications; administer anti-emetics as ordered to control nausea and vomiting. 5. Ambulate to alleviate flatulence and distention. 6. Alleviate pain and discomfort by distractions, increased social interactions, pleasant environment, backrubs, and administration of p.r.n. pain medications, as ordered. *Health teaching.* 1. Diet and elimination. 2. See Unit 5 for foods high in protein and carbohydrate.	
Promote normal pattern of bowel elimination. 1. Administer: stool softeners or bulk cathartics as ordered; oil retention, soap suds enemas as ordered. 2. Encourage change of position and activity as tolerated. 3. Provide high-bulk diet. 4. Increase fluid intake. 5. Provide for privacy. 6. Encourage regular time for evacuation. *Health teaching.* 1. Dietary instructions regarding increased fiber. 2. Exercise program as tolerated. 3. Increase fluids.	Client has normal bowel elimination pattern. No impactions. Increases fluid and fiber in diet.
Prevent injury related to decreased bone strength. 1. Position: correct body alignment, firm mattress. 2. Encourages self-care activities: plan maximum activity allowed by physical condition; muscle exercises against resistance as tolerated.	No fractures. No renal calculi. Incorporates dietary improvements in daily menu selection. Participates in exercise program on a regular basis.

continued

e. Limb temperature change (colder).

▶ f. Ankle-arm pressure index (API) decreased; 0.4 indicates ischemia (see Unit 7, Doppler ultrasonography, p. 517).

g. Urine output—decreased (developing acute tubular necrosis); reddish-brown color.

D. Analysis/nursing diagnosis:

1. *Pain* related to tissue swelling and ischemia.
2. *Potential for injury* related to neuromuscular deficits.
3. *Impaired physical mobility* related to contracture and loss of function.
4. *Potential for infection* related to tissue necrosis.
5. *Altered urinary elimination* related to acute tubular necrosis from myoglobin accumulation.
6. *Body image disturbance* related to limb disfigurement.

E. Nursing plan/implementation:

1. Goal: *recognize early indications of ischemia.*
   a. Assess neurovascular status frequently (q1h): skin temperature, capillary refill, peripheral pulses, mobility, and sensation.
   b. Listen to patient complaints; report suspected complications.
   c. Report nonrelief of pain with narcotics.
   d. Recognize unrelenting pain with passive muscle stretching.
2. Goal: *prevent complications.*
   a. *Elevate* injured extremity initially; if ischemia suspected, keep extremity at heart level to prevent compensatory increase in blood flow.
   b. Avoid tight bandages, splints, or casts.
   c. Monitor intravenous infusion for signs of infiltation.
   d. Prepare patient for fasciotomy (incision of skin and fascia to release tight compartment).

F. Evaluation:

1. Relief from pain; normal perfusion restored.
2. Neurovascular status within normal limits.
3. Retains function of limb; no contractures or infection.
4. Compartment pressure returns to normal (less than 20 mm Hg.).
5. No systemic complications (e.g., normal cardiac and renal function, acid-base balance within normal limits).

V. Osteoarthritis: joint disorder characterized by degeneration of articular cartilage and formation of bony outgrowths at edges of weight-bearing joints.

A. Pathophysiology: excessive friction combined with risk factors → thinning of articular cartilage, narrowing of joint space, and loss of joint stability; cartilage erodes, producing shallow pits on articular surface and exposing bone in joint space. Bone responds by becoming denser and harder.

B. Risk factors:

1. Aging (over 50).
2. Rheumatoid arthritis.
3. Arteriosclerosis.
4. Obesity.
5. Trauma.
6. Family history.

C. Assessment:

1. Subjective data
   a. Pain; tender joints.
   b. Fatigability, malaise.
   c. Anorexia.

ADULT NURSING

■ **TABLE 4.25 *(Continued)*** **Complications of Immobilization**

Disorder	Pathophysiology	Assessment	Analysis/Nursing Diagnosis
Osteoporosis (cont.)			
Contractures	Abnormal shortening of muscle tissue, rendering the muscle highly resistant to stretching; related to lack of active or passive range of motion, or improper support and positioning of joints affected by arthritis or injury.	*Subjective data:* pain. *Objective data:* muscles—fixed, shortened, decreased tone; resistance of muscles to stretch; decreased ROM in affected limb.	*Impaired physical mobility* related to muscle weakness and contractures. *Pain* related to injury. *Self-care deficit* related to immobility.
Skin breakdown	Presence of risk factors that could lead to skin breakdown, such as immobility, inadequate nutrition, lack of position changes.	*Subjective data:* fatigue; pain; inability to turn on own. *Objective data:* interruption of skin integrity, especially over ears, occiput, heels, sacrum, scrotum, elbows, trochanter, ischium, scapular; immobilization; malnutrition.	*Impaired skin integrity* related to lack of frequent position change.

continued

d. Cold intolerance.

e. Extremities: numb, tingling.

2. Objective data

a. Joints

(1) Enlarged.

(2) Stiff, limited movement.

(3) Swelling, redness, and heat around affected joint.

(4) Shiny stretched skin over and around joint.

(5) Subcutaneous nodules.

b. Weight loss.

c. Fever.

d. Crepitation (creaking or grating of joints).

e. Deformities, contractures.

f. Cold, clammy extremities.

g. Lab data: decreased Hgb, elevated WBC.

▶ h. Diagnostic tests: X ray, thermography, arthroscopy.

D. Analysis/nursing diagnosis:

1. *Pain* related to friction of bones in joints.

2. *Bathing/hygiene self-care deficit* related to decreased mobility of involved joints.

3. *Potential for injury* related to fatigability.

4. *Impaired physical mobility* related to stiff, limited movement.

5. *Impaired home maintenance management* related to contractures.

E. Nursing plan/implementation:

1. Goal: *promote comfort: reduce pain, spasms, inflammation, swelling.*

a. Medications as prescribed:

(1) Anti-inflammatory agents: aspirin, Ecotrin, Motrin, Indocin, corticosteroids.

(2) Antimalarials: Aralen, Plaquenil, to relieve symptoms.

b. Heat to reduce muscle spasm.

c. Cold to reduce swelling and pain.

d. Prevent contractures:

(1) Exercise.

(2) Bedrest on firm mattress during attacks.

(3) Splints to maintain proper alignment.

■ **TABLE 4.25 *(Continued)***

Nursing Plan/ Implementation	Evaluation
3. Rest/activity pattern: encourage ROM exercise; *avoid* fatigue. 4. Weight-bearing positions, tilt table. 5. Diet: high protein, high vitamin C, calcium rich. 6. Increase fluids to prevent renal calculi (calcium from bones could cause kidney stones). *Health teaching.* 1. Dietary instructions, foods to include for high-protein, high-vitamin C, high-calcium diet. 2. Exercise program. 3. Signs and symptoms of renal calculi.	
Prevent deformities: 1. Active and/or passive ROM. 2. Positioning: functional, correct alignment. 3. Footboard to prevent footdrop. 4. Avoid knee gatch. *Health teaching.* 1. Importance of ROM exercises. 2. Correct anatomical positions.	ROM maintained. No deformities noted.
Prevent skin breakdown. 1. Change position q1–2h and p.r.n., out of bed when possible. 2. Protect from infection. 3. Increase dietary intake: protein, carbohydrates. 4. Increase fluids. *Assess for/reduce contributing factors known to cause decubitus ulcers:* incontinence, stationary position, malnutrition, obesity, sensory deficits, emotional disturbances, paralysis.	No skin breakdown.

continued

e. Elevate extremity to reduce swelling.

f. Rest.

g. Assistive devices to decrease weight bearing of affected joints (canes, walkers).

2. Goal: *health teaching to promote independence.*

a. Encourage self care with assistive devices for ADL.

b. Activity, as tolerated, with ambulation-assistive devices.

c. Scheduled rest periods.

d. Correct body posture and body mechanics.

3. Goal: *provide for emotional needs.*

a. Accept feelings of frustration regarding long-term debilitating disorder.

b. Provide diversional activities appropriate for age and physical condition to promote comfort and satisfaction.

F. Evaluation:

1. Remains independent as long as possible.
2. No contractures.
3. States comfort has improved.
4. Uses methods that are successful in pain control.

VI. Total hip replacement: femoral head and acetabulum are replaced by a prosthesis, which is cemented into the bone with plastic cement. Performed to replace a joint with limited and painful function due to bony alkalosis and deformity, caused by degenerative joint disease. Goal of the surgery: restore or improve mobilization of hip joint and prevent complications of extended immobilization.

A. Risk factors:

1. Rheumatoid arthritis.
2. Osteoarthritis.
3. Complications of femoral neck fractures (see Table 4.29, p. 413).
4. Congenital hip disease.

B. Analysis/nursing diagnosis:

1. *Potential for injury* related to implant surgery.
2. *Knowledge deficit* regarding joint replacement surgery.
3. *Impaired physical mobility* related to major hip surgery.
4. *Pain* related to surgical incision.
5. *Potential impaired skin integrity* related to immobility.

C. Nursing plan/implementation:

1. *Preoperative*

a. Goal: *prevent thrombophlebitis or pulmonary emboli.*

(1) Antiembolic stockings.

(2) Increase fluid intake.

b. Goal: *prevent infection:* antibiotics as ordered, given prophylactically.

c. Goal: *health teaching.*

(1) Isometric exercises—gluteal, abdominal, and quadricep setting, dorsiflexion and plantar flexion of the feet.

(2) Use of trapeze.

(3) Explain position of operative leg and hip postoperatively to prevent *adduction* and flexion.

(4) Transfer techniques—bed to chair and chair to crutches.

(5) Assist client with skin scrubs with antibacterial soap.

2. *Postoperative*

a. Goal: *prevent respiratory complications.*

(1) Turn, cough, and deep breathe.

(2) Incentive spirometry.

b. Goal: *prevent complications of shock or infection.*

(1) Check dressings for drainage q1h for first 4h; then q4h and p.r.n.; may have Hemovac or other drainage tubes inserted in wound to keep dressing dry.

(2) Monitor I&O and vital signs hourly for 4 hours, then q4h and p.r.n.

TABLE 4.25 *(Continued)* **Complications of Immobilization**

Disorder	Pathophysiology	Assessment	Analysis/Nursing Diagnosis
Skin breakdown (cont.)			
Urinary stasis	Immobility leads to inability to completely empty the bladder, which increases risk for urinary tract infection and renal calculi.	*Subjective data:* pain, due to infection or renal calculi. *Objective data:* difficulty in urinating due to position or lack of privacy; infection related to catheter insertion or stasis of urine; hematuria.	*Altered urinary elimination* related to inability to empty bladder.

continued

c. Goal: *prevent contractures, muscle atrophy:* initiate exercises as soon as allowed; isometric quadriceps, dorsiflexion and plantar flexion of foot, and flexion and extension of the ankle.

d. Goal: *promote early ambulation and movement.*
   (1) Use trapeze.
   (2) Transfer technique (pivot on unaffected leg); crutches/walker.
   (3) Initiate progressive ambulation as ordered.
   (4) Administer anticoagulation therapy as ordered prophylactically to prevent thromboemboli.
   (5) Recognize early side effects of medications and report appropriately.

e. Goal: *prevent constipation.*
   (1) Increase fluid intake.
   (2) Use fracture bed pan.

f. Goal: *prevent dislocation of prosthesis.*
   (1) Maintain *abduction* of the affected joint: elevate head of bed, turn according to physician's order. When turning to unaffected side, turn with abduction pillow between legs to maintain abduction.
   (2) Buck's extension or Russell's traction may be applied.
   (3) Plaster booties with an abduction bar may be used.
   (4) Wedge Charnley (triangle-shaped) pillow to maintain abduction between knees and lower legs.
   (5) Provide periods throughout day when client lies flat in bed to prevent hip flexion and strengthen hip muscles.
   (6) Report signs of dislocation: *anteriorly*—knee flexes, leg turns outward, leg looks longer than other, femur head may be felt in groin area; *posteriorly*—leg turns inward, appears shorter than other, greater trochanter elevated.

g. Goal: *promote comfort.*
   (1) Initiate skin care; monitor pressure points for redness; back care q2h.
   (2) Alternating pressure mattress; sheepskin when sitting in chair.

h. Goal: *health teaching.*
   (1) Exercise program with written list of activity restrictions.
   (2) Methods to prevent hip adduction.
   (3) Avoid sitting for more than 1 hour: stand, stretch, and walk frequently to prevent hip flexion contractures.
   (4) Advise not to exceed 90° of hip flexion (dislocation can occur, particularly with posterior incisions); avoid low chairs.

TABLE 4.25 *(Continued)*

Nursing Plan/ Implementation	Evaluation
Promote healing. 1. Wash gently, pat dry—to avoid skin abrasion. 2. Clean, dry, wrinkle-free bed linens and pads. 3. Massage skin with lotion that does not contain alcohol (alcohol dries skin). 4. Protect with wafer barrier, alternating mattress, sheepskin pads, protectors, floatation devices. 5. No "doughnuts" or rubber rings (interfere with circulation of tissue within center of ring).	
Prevent urinary infections, stasis, or renal calculi. 1. Increase activity as allowed. 2. Check for distended bladder. 3. Increase fluids, I&O. 4. Diet: acid ash to increase acidity, thereby preventing infection. 5. Avoid catheterization; use intermittent catheterization instead of Foley whenever possible or Crede maneuver to empty bladder (manual exertion of pressure on the bladder to force urine out). 6. Bladder training.	No urinary infections or evidence of renal calculi. Bladder emptied, no urinary stasis.

(5) Teach altered methods of usual self-care activities to prevent hip dislocation—e.g., *avoid:* bending from waist to tie shoes, sitting up straight in a low chair, using a low toilet seat.

(6) *Avoid* crossing legs, driving a car for 6 weeks.

(7) Wear support hose for 6 weeks to enhance venous return and avoid thrombus formation.

D. Evaluation:

1. Participates in postoperative nursing care plan to prevent complications.
2. Reports pain has decreased.
3. Ambulates with assistive devices.
4. Complications of immobility avoided.
5. Able to resume self-care activities.

VII. Total knee replacement: both sides of the joint are replaced by metal or plastic implants.

A. Analysis: see VI. Total hip replacement, p. 405.

B. Nursing plan/implementation:

1. See VI. Total hip replacement, p. 405.
2. Goal: *to achieve active flexion beyond 70°.*
   a. Immediately postop: may have continuous passive motion (CPM) device for flexion/extension of affected knee.
   b. Monitor drainage in Hemovac (q15min for first 4 hours, q1h until 24 hours; q4h and p.r.n. while Hemovac in place).
   c. Analgesics as ordered for pain.
   d. While dressings are still on: quadriceps setting exercises for approximately 5 days (consult with physical therapist for specific instructions).
   e. After dressings removed: active flexion exercises.
   f. Avoid pressure on heel.

C. Evaluation:

1. No complications of infection, hemorrhage noted.
2. ROM of knee increases with exercises.

VIII. Amputation: surgical removal of a limb due to trauma or circulatory impairment (gangrene). The amount of tissue amputated is determined by the severity of disease or trauma and the ability of the remaining tissue to heal.

A. Risk factors:

1. Artherosclerosis obliterans.
2. Uncontrolled diabetes mellitus.
3. Malignancy.
4. Extensive and intractable infection.
5. Result of severe trauma.

B. Assessment: *preoperative*

1. Subjective data: pain in affected part.
2. Objective data
   a. Soft tissue damage.
   b. Partial or complete severance of a body part.
   c. Lack of peripheral pulses.
   d. Skin color changes, pallor → cyanosis → gangrene.
   e. Infection, hemorrhage, or shock.

C. Analysis/nursing diagnosis:

1. *Impaired physical mobility* related to lower limb amputation.
2. *Body image disturbance* related to loss of body part.
3. *Pain* related to interruption of nerve pathways.
4. *Anxiety* related to potential change in life-style.
5. *Knowledge deficit* related to rehabilitation goals.

D. Nursing plan/implementation:

1. Goal: *prepare for surgery, physically and emotionally.*
   a. Validate that client and family are aware that amputation of body part is planned.
   b. Validate that informed consent is signed.
   c. Allow time for grieving.
   d. If time allows, prepare client for postoperative phase, e.g., teach arm-strengthening exercises if lower limb is to be amputated; teach altered methods of ambulation.
   e. Provide time to discuss feelings.
   f. Prepare surgical site to decrease possibility of infection (e.g., shave, scrub as ordered).
   g. Discuss postoperative expectations.
2. Goal: *promote healing postoperatively.*
   a. Monitor respiratory status q1–4h and p.r.n.: rate, depth of respiration; auscultate for signs of congestion; and question client about chest pain (pulmonary emboli common complication).

(*Continued on p. 412*)

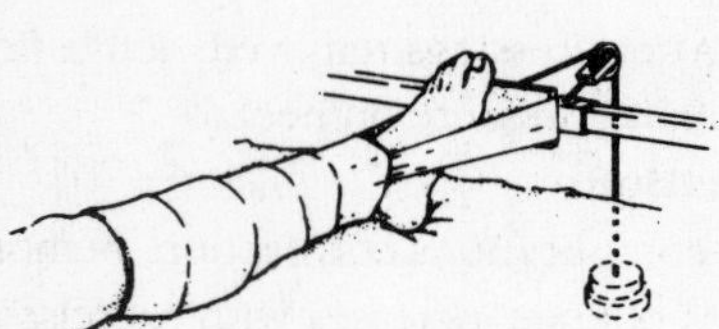

(a) Buck's extension. Skin traction applied to the medial and lateral aspects of an extremity with adhesive foam, moleskin, or use of "Buck's boot."

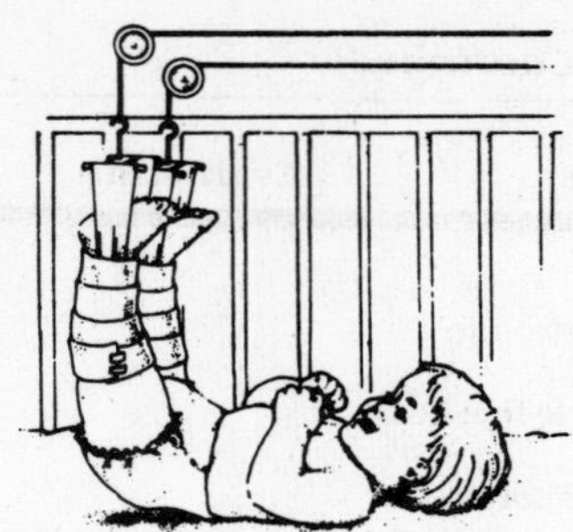

(b) Bryant's traction. Vertical suspension skin traction in which child's pelvis is elevated from the bed.

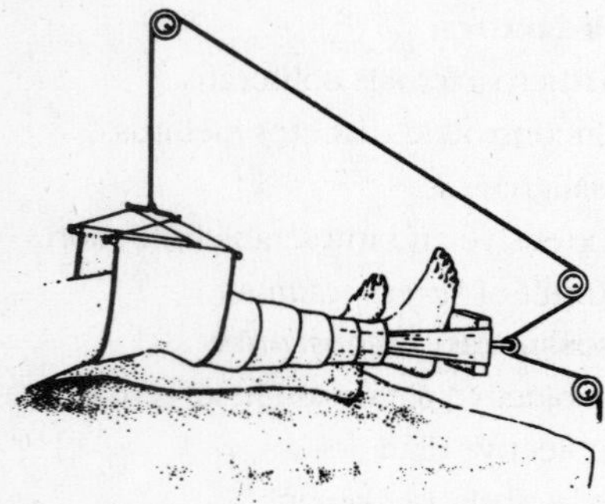

(c) Russell's traction. Skin traction composed of Buck's extension on the foreleg, three pulleys at the bottom, and a sling under the knee. Affords more freedom of movement than Buck's.

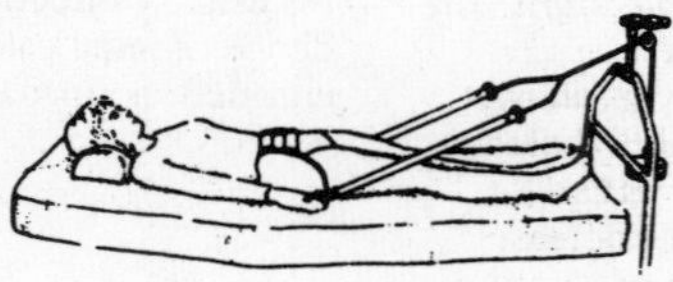

(d) Pelvic traction. Skin traction applied to the lumbosacral region by means of a pelvic belt.

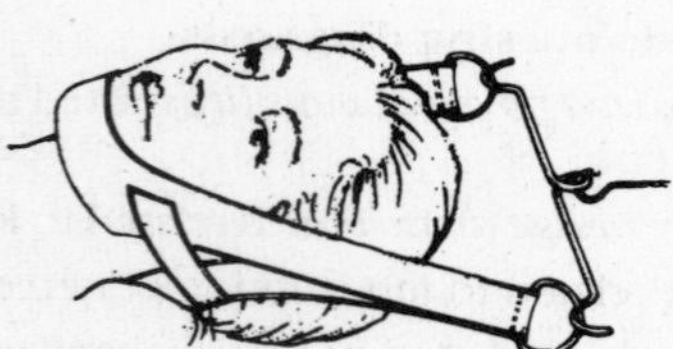

(e) Head halter. Cervical traction applied to the head by means of a halter under the chin.

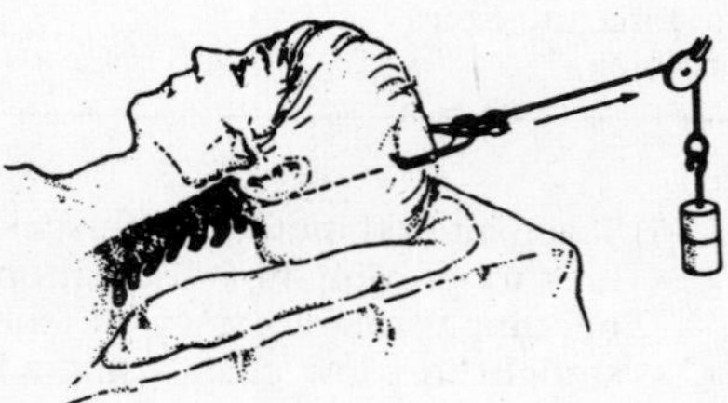

(f) Crutchfield tongs. Cervical traction using tongs into the skull.

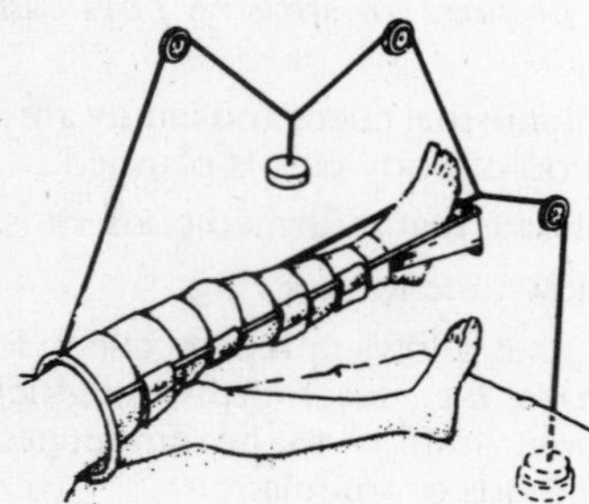

(g) Thomas' splint. Full-leg splint that keeps the leg fully extended and the long bones in alignment. Pressure is on the ischium and perineal area. May be used with skin or skeletal traction.

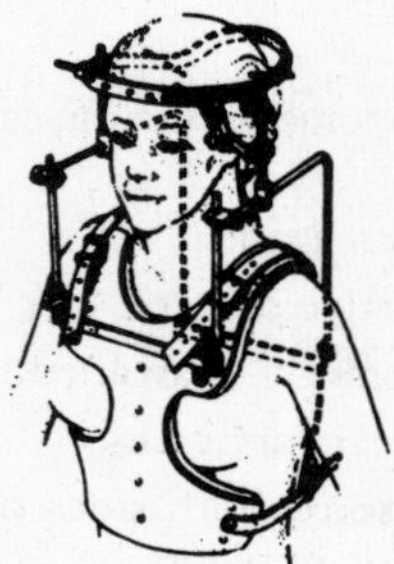

(h) Halo vest assembly. Applied in operating room. Patient will usually be ambulatory 24 hours after application.

■ **FIGURE 4.6**
Types of traction. (From Saxton DF, et al.: *The Addison-Wesley Manual of Nursing Practice,* Addison-Wesley, Menlo Park, CA, 1983.)

TABLE 4.26 **Complications of Fractures**

Complication	Assessment	Analysis/Nursing Diagnosis	Nursing Plan/Implementation	Evaluation
Shock (see p. 305)				
Thrombophlebitis (see p. 310)				
Fat emboli: serious, potentially life-threatening complication in which pressure changes in interior of fracture force molecules of fat from marrow into systemic circulation; may cause problems in respiratory or nervous system. Seen most frequently on third day after multiple fractures, fractures of long bones, or comminuted fracture.	*Subjective data:* dyspnea, severe chest pain; confusion, agitation; decrease in level of consciousness; numbness; feeling faint; history of diabetes, obesity. *Objective data:* cyanosis; pupillary changes; muscle twitching; petechiae—chest, buccal cavity, axilla, conjunctiva, soft palate; extremities—pallor, cold; shock; vomiting.	*Potential for injury* related to fat emboli. *Altered tissue perfusion* related to fat emboli.	1. *Position:* high Fowler's to relieve respiratory symptoms. 2. Administer oxygen stat, to relieve anoxia and reduce surface tension of fat globules. 3. Institute respiratory support measures, as ordered—IPPB, respiratory assistive devices. **Be prepared for CPR** in event of respiratory failure. 4. Monitor vital signs, cardiac monitor, q15min during acute episode and p.r.n. (shock/cardiac failure possible). 5. Obtain baseline data and monitor levei of consciousness, neurologic signs q15min during acute episode and p.r.n. (neurologic involvement possible). 6. Administer parenteral fluids, as ordered: IV alcohol, blood and fluid replacements. 7. Administer medications as ordered: corticosteroids; digitalis; aminophylline; heparin sodium. 8. **DO NOT RUB ANY LEG CRAMPS, BUT REPORT IMMEDIATELY.**	Client alert. Pain relieved. Respiratory, cardiac, and neurologic statuses have no permanent damage.
Nerve compression: pressure on nerve in affected area from edema, dislocation of bone, or immobilization apparatus. If pressure not relieved, permanent paralysis can result.	*Subjective data:* discomfort, pain, referred pain; burning, tingling, "stinging sensation"; numbness, altered sensation, inability to distinguish touch. *Objective data:* limited movement; muscle weakness; paralysis; reflexes—diminished, irritable, or absent; color changes related to impaired circulation.	*Pain* related to pressure on nerve. *Potential for physical injury* related to pressure on nerve. *Impaired tissue perfusion* related to impaired circulation. *Impaired physical mobility* related to joint contracture, numbness.	1. Monitor for potential signs q1h for first 48 h; neurovascular assessment q12h and p.r.n. as condition indicates (circulation, sensation, motion—CSM). 2. *Elevate* affected limb; flex hand or foot of affected extremity; passive and active ROM exercises. 3. **Be prepared to cut cast or remove constrictions if signs of impairment present.** 4. Begin active ROM exercises to unaffected extremities. 5. Use footboard to prevent footdrop. 6. Encourage use of trapeze if applicable. 7. Isometric exercises, as ordered. 8. Ambulation, weight-bearing as ordered, support casts.	Sensation, motor function are normal. No complications noted.

continued

TABLE 4.26 *(Continued)* **Complications of Fractures**

Complications	Assessment	Analysis/Nursing Diagnosis	Nursing Plan/ Implementation	Evaluation
Avascular necrosis/circulatory impairment: interference with normal circulation to affected area due to interruption of blood vessel, pressure on the vessel from dislocation, edema, or immobilization devices. Results of impaired circulation lead to discomfort and, if not corrected, necrosis of tissue and bone due to lack of oxygen supply.	*Subjective data:* tenderness; pain, especially on passive motion. *Objective data:* edema, swelling in affected area; decreased color, temperature, mobility; bleeding from wound.	*Potential altered peripheral tissue perfusion,* related to vessel damage.	1. Monitor for potential signs q1h for first 48 h; blanching, coolness, edema; palpate pulse above and below injury, report absent or major discrepancies stat. 2. *Elevate* affected limb to decrease edema. 3. Report to physician if signs persist. 4. Be prepared to assist with bivalving of casts, or cut cast to relieve pressue. 5. Monitor size of drainage stains on casts; measure accurately and report if size increases.	Circulation adequate to limb, to prevent tissue damage.
Infection	*Subjective data:* pain. *Objective data:* elevated temperature and pulse; erythema—discoloration of surrounding skin; edema—sudden, local induration; drainage—thin, watery, foul-smelling exudate; crepitus (may be indicative of gas gangrene); with cast—warm area, foul smell.	*Potential for injury* related to tissue destruction. *Altered peripheral tissue perfusion* related to swelling.	1. Monitor vital signs, drainage. 2. Ensure client has had prophylactic tetanus toxoid. 3. May have prophylactic antibiotics ordered if wound was contaminated at time of injury. 4. Instruct client not to touch open wound, pin sites or put anything inside cast (could interrupt skin interity and become potential source of infection).	No infection or heals with no serious complications.
Delayed union/non-union: failure of bone to heal within normal time related to lack of use, inadequate circulation, other complicating medical conditions such as diabetes or poor nutrition.	*Subjective data:* pain. *Objective data:* lack of callus formation on X ray; poor alignment.	*Potential for injury* related to poor healing of bone fracture. *Impaired physical mobility* related to lower limb fractures. *Dressing/grooming, bathing/hygiene, self-care deficit* related to upper-limb fracture.	1. Maintain immobilization and alignment of affected limb. 2. Maintain adequate nutrition. 3. Avoid trauma to affected limb. 4. Monitor for circulatory or infection complication. 5. Dietary instructions regarding foods containing calcium and protein necessary for bone healing.	Bone heals. No complications noted. Pain decreased. Ambulation and self-care return to preinjury status.

continued

■ **TABLE 4.26 *(Continued)***

Complications	Assessment	Analysis/Nursing Diagnosis	Nursing Plan/ Implementation	Evaluation
Skin breakdown (related to cast)	*Subjective data:* pain. *Objective data:* temperature and pulse elevated; erythema; edema—cast edges, exposed distal portion of limb, limb area within cast; drainage and foul odor from break in skin, may be under cast and stain through or exit at ends of cast; crepitus (crackling sound could indicate gas gangrene); hyperactive reflexes.	*Impaired skin integrity* related to cast trauma.	1. If open wound: verify tetanus administration; monitor site through cast window, change dressing daily and p.r.n. 2. Apply lotion or cornstarch to exposed skin (no powder). 3. Petal tape edges of cast to reduce irritation. 4. Inspect skin for irritation, edema, odor, drainage—q2h initially, then q3h. 5. Instruct client not to place any object under cast as skin abrasions may lead to decubitus ulcers. 6. Promote drying of cast by leaving it uncovered and exposed to air for 48 hours; use no plastic. 7. Prevent indenting casts with fingertips or hard surface: place on pillows; use palms of hands when positioning affected limb. 8. Avoid excessive padding of Thomas splint in groin area—padding traps moisture, skin breakdown.	No skin breakdown.
Duodenal distress (with spica cast): spica cast incorporates the trunk and affected limb and can cause respiratory or abdominal distress when edema is present under the cast or cast is too tight to allow for normal body functions.	*Subjective data:* anorexia, nausea, abdominal pain. *Objective data:* duodenal distress, vomiting, distention, cast too tight.	*Ineffective breathing pattern* related to pressure from cast. *Pain* related to abdominal distress from pressure. *Fear* related to cast constriction.	1. Place on firm mattress; use bed boards if necessary to reduce muscle spasm. 2. Maintain warmth by covering uncasted areas. 3. Avoid turning for first 8 hours. When turning: use enough personnel to log-roll; do not use bar between legs while turning device; support chest with pillows. 4. Monitor for signs of respiratory distress: increased respirations, apprehension. 5. Monitor for signs of duodenal distress: vomiting, distention. *If these signs occur:* place in prone position; have cast bivalved; may need NG tube; monitor for fluid imbalance. 6. Protect cast with nonabsorbent material during elimination.	Complications avoided or detected early enough to prevent serious damage.

■ TABLE 4.27 Teaching Crutch Walking

A. When only *one* leg can bear weight:
1. *Swing-to gait:* crutches forward; swing body to crutches.
   a. Move both crutches forward.
   b. Move both legs to meet the crutches.
   c. Continue pattern.
2. *Swing-through gait:* crutches forward; swing body through crutches.
   a. Move both crutches forward.
   b. Move both legs farther ahead than crutches.
   c. Continue pattern.
3. *Three-point gait:* crutches and affected extremity forward; swing forward, placing nonaffected foot ahead or between crutches.
   a. Both crutches and affected limb move at same time.
   b. Move both crutches and affected leg (e.g., left) ahead 6 inches.
   c. Move unaffected leg (e.g., right) to same place as left and crutches.
   d. Continue pattern.

B. When *both* legs can move separately and bear some weight:
1. *Four-point gait:* right crutch forward, left foot forward; swing weight to right side while bringing left crutch forward, then right foot forward; gait simulates normal walking.
   a. Move right crutch forward 4–6 inches.
   b. Move left foot forward same distance as right crutch.
   c. Move left crutch forward ahead of left foot.
   d. Move right foot forward to meet right crutch.
   e. Continue pattern.
2. *Two-point gait:* as four-point gait but faster; one crutch and opposite leg moving forward at same time.
   a. Opposite crutch and limb move together.
   b. Move right crutch and left leg ahead 6 inches.
   c. Move left crutch and right leg ahead.
   d. Continue pattern.

C. When client is *unable* to walk: *tripod gait:* crutches forward at a wide distance; drag legs to point just behind crutches, balance, and repeat.

■ TABLE 4.28 Measuring Crutches Correctly

1. Have client lie on a flat surface. Measure from anterior fold of axilla to 4 inches lateral to heel.
2. Have client stand. Measure from 1–2 inches below axilla to 2 inches in front of and 6 inches to the side of the foot.
3. Hand placement on bar of crutch: Have client stand upright, support body weight with hand on bar (not putting weight on axilla). Elbow flexion should be 30 degrees.
4. Slightly pad the shoulder rests of the crutches for general comfort.
5. Make sure there are nonskid rubber tips on the crutches.

(*Continued from p. 407*)

b. Monitor for hemorrhage; keep tourniquet at bedside.
c. Medicate for pain as ordered—client may have phantom pain.
d. Support stump on pillow for first 24 h; **remove pillow** after 24 h to prevent contracture.
e. *Position: turn client onto stomach* to prevent hip contracture.
f. ROM exercises for joint above amputation to prevent joint immobilization; strengthening exercises for arms, nonaffected limbs, abdominal muscles.
g. Stump care:
   (1) Early postoperative dressings changed p.r.n.
   (2) As incision heals, bandage is applied in cone shape to prepare stump for prosthesis.
   (3) Inspect for blisters, redness, abrasions.
   (4) Remove stump sock daily and p.r.n.
h. Assist in rehabilitation program.

E. Evaluation:
1. Begins rehabilitation program.
2. No hemorrhage, infection.
3. Adjusts to altered body image (see Body Image Disturbance, Unit 1, p. 19).

IX. Gout: disorder of purine metabolism; genetic disease believed to be transmitted by a dominant gene, characterized by recurrent attacks of acute pain and swelling of one joint (usually the great toe).

A. Pathophysiology: urate crystals and infiltrating leukocytes appear to damage the intracellular phagolysosomes, resulting in leakage of lysomal enzymes into the synovial fluid, causing tissue damage and joint inflammation.

B. Risk factors:
1. Men.
2. Age (over 50).
3. Genetic/familial tendency.
4. Prolonged hyperuricemia (elevated serum uric acid).

C. Assessment:
1. Subjective data
   a. Pain: excruciating.
   b. Fatigue.
   c. Anorexia.
2. Objective data
   a. Joint: erythema (redness), hot, swollen, difficult to move; skin stretched and shiny over joint.
   b. Subcutaneous nodules, trophi (deposits of non-sodium urate) on hands and feet.
   c. Weight loss.
   d. Fever.
   e. Sensory changes, with cold intolerance.

TABLE 4.29 Types of Hip Fractures

	Assessment	Treatment	Complications
Femoral neck	History of slight trauma. Pain in groin and hip. Pain with hip movement. Usually occurs in women over 60. Lateral rotation and shortening of leg with minimal deformity.	Femoral head replacement with prosthesis, threaded pins. Occasionally, primary total hip replacement.	Avascular necrosis of femoral head. Nonunion. Pin complications. Dislocation of prosthesis.
Intertrochanteric	History of direct trauma over trochanter. Severe pain. Tenderness over trochanter. Usually women 60 to 85 or younger women with osteoporosis. External rotation and shortening of leg with obvious deformity. Loss of hip motion.	Open reduction: internal fixation with nail, pin, compression plate with screw.	Shortening of the leg. Traumatic arthritis. Pin migration; bending or breaking of pin. Fracture impaction. Loss of reduction. Delayed union or nonunion of bone.
Subtrochanteric	History of direct trauma of great force. Proximal leg pain. Usually women over 60. External rotation and shortening of leg with some deformity. Large hematoma.	Open reduction: internal fixation with intra-medullary nail, sliding nail plates, and other fixed plates. Closed reduction with nail insertion.	Shortening of the leg; metal fatigue. Lateral displacement of proximal fragment.

Source: Dunajcik L: The Hip: Nursing Fracture Patients to Full Recovery. *RN* (April 1989):57.

f. Lab data:
   (1) Serum uric acid: increased significantly (6.5/100 mL in females, 7.5/100 mL in males) in chronic gout; only slightly increased in acute gout.
   (2) WBC: 12,000–15,000/mm.
   (3) Erythrocyte sedimentation rate: above 20 mm/h.
   (4) 24 h urinary uric acid: slightly elevated.
   (5) Proteinuria (chronic gout).
   (6) Axotemia (presence of nitrogen-containing compounds in blood) in chronic gout.

D. Analysis/nursing diagnosis:

1. *Pain* related to inflammation and swelling of affected joint.
2. *Impaired physical mobility* related to pain.
3. *Knowledge deficit* related to diet restrictions and increased fluid needs.
4. *Altered urinary elimination* related to kidney damage.

E. Nursing plan/implementation:

1. Goal: *decrease discomfort.*
   a. Administer anti-gout medications as ordered:
      (1) Treatment of acute attacks: Colchicine, Phenylbutazone (Butazolidin), Indomethacin (Indocin), Allopurinol (Zyloprim).
      (2) Preventive therapy: Probenecid (Benemid), Sulfinpyrazone (Anturane).
   b. Absolute rest of affected joint → gradual increase in activities, to prevent complications of immobilization; at the same time, rest for comfort.
2. Goal: *prevent kidney damage.*
   a. Increase fluid intake to 2,000–3,000 mL per day.
   b. Monitor urinary output.
3. Goal: *health teaching.*
   a. Need for low-purine diet during acute attack (see VII. Purine-restricted diet, Common Therapeutic Diets, Unit 5, p. 475).
   b. Importance of increased fluid in diet.
   c. Signs and symptoms of increased disease.
   d. Dosage and side effects of prescribed medications.

F. Evaluation:

1. Swelling decreased.
2. Discomfort alleviated.
3. Mobility returned to status prior to attack.
4. Lab values return to normal.

X. Herniated/ruptured disk (ruptured nucleus pulposus): strain or injury to a weakened cartilage between vertebrae can result in herniation of the nucleus, causing pressure on nerve roots in spinal canal, pain, and disability.

A. Pathophysiology: pulpy substance of disk interior (nucleus pulposus) bulges or ruptures through the outer annulus fibrosus → irritation and pressure on nerve endings in the spinal ligaments → muscle spasm and distortion of the joints of vertebral arches.

B. Risk factors:

1. Strain as result of poor body mechanics.
2. Trauma.
3. History of back injuries.

C. Assessment:

1. *Lumbar injuries* (90% of herniations):

a. Subjective data

(1) Pain: low back, radiating to buttocks, posterior thigh, and calf; relieved by recumbency; aggravated by sneezing, coughing, and flexion; sciatic pain continues even when back pain subsides.

(2) Numbness, tingling.

b. Objective data

(1) Muscle weakness—leg and foot.

(2) Inability to flex leg.

(3) Sensory loss, leg and foot.

(4) Alterations in posture: leans to side, unable to stand up straight.

(5) Edema: leg and foot.

(6) Positive Lasèque's sign: straight leg raising with hip flexed and knee extended will produce sciatic pain.

2. *Cervical injuries* (10% of herniations):

a. Subjective data

(1) Pain—upper extremities, radiating to hands and fingers; aggravated by coughing, sneezing, and straining.

(2) Tingling, burning sensation in upper extremities and back of neck.

b. Objective data

(1) Upper extremities: weakness and atrophy.

(2) Neck: restricted movement.

▶ (3) Diagnostic tests for both lumbar and cervical injuries.

(a) Spine X rays.

(b) CAT scan.

(c) MRI.

(d) Myelography (less preferred than CAT scan or MRI).

(e) Electromyography.

(f) Neurological exam: special attention to sensory status, including pain, touch, and temperature identification, and to motor status, including strength, gait, and reflexes.

D. Analysis/nursing diagnosis:

1. *Pain* related to pressure on nerve roots.
2. *Fear* related to disease progression and/or potential surgery.
3. *Knowledge deficit* related to correct body mechanics.
4. *Impaired physical mobility* related to continued pain.
5. *Sleep pattern disturbance* related to difficulty finding comfortable position.

E. Nursing plan/implementation:

1. Goal: *relieve pain and promote comfort.*

a. Bedrest with bedboard.

b. *Position*—avoid twisting.

(1) *Lumbar disk: William's* (head elevated 30 degrees, knee gatch elevated to flatten the lumbosacral curve).

(2) *Cervical:* low Fowler's.

c. Medications as ordered:

(1) Analgesics.

(2) Muscle relaxants.

(3) Anti-inflammatory.

(4) Stool softeners.

d. Moist heat.

e. Fracture bed pan.

f. Gradual increase in activity.

g. Brace application for support.

h. Traction application p.r.n. for comfort.

i. Prepare for surgery if medical regime unsuccessful.

2. Goal: *health teaching.*

a. Correct body mechanics, keep back straight.

b. Exercise program as symptoms decrease.

F. Evaluation:

1. Reports pain decreased.
2. Mobility increased, normal body posture attained.

XI. Laminectomy: excision of dorsal arch of vertebrae with or without spinal fusion of two or more vertebrae with a bone graft from iliac crest, to stabilize spine.

A. Analysis/nursing diagnosis:

1. *Pain* related to edema of surgical procedure.
2. *Impaired physical mobility* related to pain and discomfort resulting from surgery.

B. Nursing plan/implementation:

1. Goal: *relieve anxiety.*

a. Answer questions, explain routines.

b. See The Perioperative Experience, p. 342.

2. Goal: *prevent injury postoperatively.*

a. Monitor vital signs:

(1) Neurologic signs, e.g., check sensation and motor strength of limbs.

(2) Respiratory status (potential for respiratory depression with cervical laminectomy).

b. Monitor I&O (urinary retention common, especially with cervical laminectomy); may need catheterization. Encourage fluids.

c. Monitor bowel sounds (paralytic ileus common with lumbar laminectomy).

d. Monitor dressing for possible bleeding.

e. Bed *position* as ordered:

(1) *For lumbar laminectomy: head of bed flat;* supine with slight flexion of legs; with pillow between knees for turning and side-lying position.

(2) *For cervical laminectomy: head of bed elevated,* neck immobilized with collar or sand bags.

f. Encourage deep breathing to prevent respiratory complications.

3. Goal: *promote comfort.*

a. Administer analgesics as sciatic-type pain continues after lumbar surgery (arm pain after cervical surgery), due to edema from trauma of surgery.

4. Goal: *prepare for early discharge.*
   a. Clients having microsurgery for repair of herniated disk will usually be discharged from the hospital one day postoperative; teaching regarding allowed and restricted activities must be done early.
5. Goal: *health teaching.*
   a. How to turn and move from side to side in one motion, sit up, and get out of bed *without twisting spine;* to get out of bed: raise head of bed while in side-lying position, then put feet over edge of bed, and stand.
   b. Proper positioning and ambulation techniques.
   c. Correct posture, body mechanics, activities to prevent further injury; increase activities according to tolerance.
   d. Physiotherapy; encourage compliance for full rehabilitation.

C. Evaluation:

1. No respiratory, bowel, bladder complications noted.
   a. Lung sounds clear.
   b. Bowel sounds present; able to pass gas and feces.
   c. Urinary output adequate.
2. Regains mobility.
3. Comfort level increases: reports leg and back pain decreased.
4. Demonstrates protective positioning and ambulation techniques.

XII. Spinal cord injuries: trauma from hyperextension, hyperflexion, axial compression, lateral flexion, or shearing of the spine.

A. Types:

1. *C-1 and C-2 injury level*—resulting deficit:
   a. Phrenic nerve involvement.
   b. Diaphragmatic paralysis.
   c. Respiratory difficulties (require permanent ventilatory support).
   d. Possible quadriplegia.
   e. Possible death.
2. *C-4 through T-1 injury level*—resulting deficit: quadriplegia.
3. *Thoracic-lumbar injury level*—resulting deficit: paraplegia.

B. Pathophysiology: trauma → vertebral dislocation or fractures → cord trauma, compression or severance of the cord.

C. Risk factors:

1. Motor vehicle accidents.
2. Diving, surfing, contact sports.
3. Falls.
4. Gunshot wounds.

D. Assessment:

1. Subjective data
   a. Pain at the level of injury.
   b. Numbness/weakness, loss of sensation below level of injury.
   c. Psychological distress related to severity of injury and its effects.
2. Objective data
   a. Symptoms depend on extent of injury to spinal cord/spinal nerves.
   b. Paralysis: motor, sphincter.
      (1) Initially a period of *flaccid paralysis* and loss of reflexes, called spinal or neural shock.
      (2) *Incomplete injuries* may lead to loss of voluntary movement and sensory deficits below injury level (symptoms vary depending on injury).
      (3) *Complete injury* leads to loss of function and all voluntary movement below level of injury.
   c. Respiratory distress.
   d. Alterations in temperature control.
   e. Alterations in bowel and bladder function.
   f. Involved muscles become spastic and hyperreflexic within days or weeks.

E. Analysis/nursing diagnosis:

1. *Ineffective breathing patterns* related to high-level injury.
2. *Impaired physical mobility* related to injuries affecting lower limbs.
3. *Fear* related to uncertain future health status.
4. *Anxiety* related to loss of control over own activities of daily living.
5. *Bathing/hygiene self-care deficit* related to injuries above T-1.
6. *Impaired home maintenance management* related to quadriplegia and possibly paraplegia.
7. *Potential altered body temperature* related to absence of sweating below level of injury.
8. *Potential for injury* related to equipment necessary for daily activities.
9. *Tactile sensory/perceptual alterations* related to injury level.
10. *Body image disturbance* related to permanent change in physical status.

F. Nursing plan/implementation:

1. Goal: *maintain patent airway.*
   a. Suction, cough, tracheostomy care, p.r.n.
   b. Oxygen, ventilator care.
   c. Monitor blood gas levels.
2. Goal: *prevent further damage.*
   a. Immobilize spine.
   b. Firm mattress, Stryker frame, Foster frame, CircOelectric bed, traction, casts, braces, (see III. Fractures, p. 395).
   c. Skeletal traction via tongs: Crutchfield, Gardner Wells (see III. Fractures, p. 395).
   d. Halo traction (see III. Fractures, p. 395).
3. Goal: *relieve edema:* anti-inflammatory medications, corticosteroids.
4. Goal: *relieve discomfort:* analgesics, sedatives, muscle relaxants.

ADULT NURSING

5. Goal: *promote comfort:*
   a. Maintain fluid intake: PO/IV, I&O.
   b. Increase nutritional intake.
   c. Prevent contractures and decubiti.
   d. Assist client to deal with psychosocial issues, e.g., role changes.
   e. Begin rehabilitation plan.
6. Goal: *prevent complications.*
   a. Monitor for spinal shock during initial phase of injury (see XIII. Spinal shock, below).
   b. Monitor for hyperreflexia with severed spinal cord injuries (see XIV. Autonomic hyperreflexia, p. 417).
7. Goal: *health teaching.*
   a. Self-care techniques for highest level of independence; include significant others in teaching.
   b. How to use ambulation assistive devices (battery-operated wheel chair controlled by mouthpiece or hand controls, depending on level of paralysis).
   c. Identify community resources for follow-up care and career counseling.
   d. Signs and symptoms of autonomic hyperreflexia (see Section XIV, p. 417).
   e. Methods to prevent skin breakdown, infections of respiratory, urinary tract.
   f. Bowel, bladder program.

G. Evaluation:
1. Complications avoided.
2. Accomplishes self-care to greatest level for injury.
3. Participates in rehabilitation plan.
4. Grieves over loss and begins to integrate self into society.

XIII. Spinal shock: temporary flaccid paralysis and areflexia following a severe injury to the spinal cord.

A. Pathophysiology: squeezing or shearing of the spinal cord due to fractures or dislocation of vertebrae; interruption of sensory tracts; loss of conscious sensation; interruption of motor tracts; loss of voluntary movement; loss of facilitation; loss of reflex activity; loss of muscle tone; loss of stretch reflexes, leading to bowel and bladder retention. If injury between T-1 and L-2, leads to loss of sympathetic tone and decrease in blood pressure. Afferent impulses are unable to ascend from below the injured site to the brain, and efferent impulses are unable to descend to points below the site.

B. Risk factors:
1. Automobile/motorcycle accidents.
2. Athletic accidents, e.g., diving in shallow water.
3. Gunshot wounds.

C. Assessment:
1. Subjective data
   a. Loss of sensation below level of injury.
   b. Inability to move extremities.
   c. Pain at level of injury.
2. Objective data
   a. Neurologic exam:
      (1) *Absent:* pinprick, pressure, and vibratory sensations below level of injury; reflexes below level of injury.
      (2) Muscles: flaccid.
   b. Vital signs
      (1) BP decreased (loss of vasomotor tone below level of injury).
      (2) Bradycardia.
      (3) Elevated temperature.
      (4) Respirations: may be depressed; possible respiratory failure if diaphragm involved.
   c. Absence of sweating below level of injury.
   d. Urinary retention.
   e. Abdominal distention: retention of feces, paralytic ileus.
   f. Skin: cold, clammy.

D. Analysis/nursing diagnosis:
1. *Decreased cardiac output* related to loss of vasomotor tone below level of injury.
2. *Ineffective breathing pattern* related to injuries involving diaphragm.
3. *Impaired physical mobility* related to loss of voluntary movement of limbs.
4. *Urinary retention* related to loss of stretch reflexes.
5. *Fear* related to serious physical condition.
6. *Potential for injury* related to potential organ damage if shock continues.

E. Nursing plan/implementation:
1. Goal: *prevent injury related to shock.*
   a. Maintain patent airway: intubation and mechanical ventilation may be necessary with cervical spinal injuries due to involvement of diaphragm.
   b. Monitor vital signs; profound hypotension and bradycardia are most dangerous aspects of spinal shock.
   c. Administer blood/IV fluids as ordered.
   d. Nutrition and hydration:
      (1) NPO in acute stage: maintain nutrition by IV infusions as ordered.
      (2) When allowed to eat: high-protein, high-calorie, high-vitamin diet.
   e. Maintain proper *position* to prevent further injury.
      (1) Backboard is necessary to transport from place of injury.
      (2) Support head in neutral alignment and prevent flexion.
      (3) Skeletal traction will be applied once diagnosis is made.
   f. Monitor urinary output q1h; may have Foley catheter while in shock; later intermittent catheterization will be used as needed.
   g. Relieve bowel distention; use lubricant containing anesthetic, as necessary, when checking for or removing impaction.

F. Evaluation:
1. Complications are avoided.
2. Body functions are maintained.

XIV. Autonomic hyperreflexia (autonomic dysreflexia): a group of symptoms in which many spinal cord autonomic responses are activated simultaneously. This may occur when cord lesions are *above the sixth thoracic* vertebra; it is *most commonly* seen with cervical spinal cord injuries.

A. Pathophysiology: pathologic reflex condition, which is an acute **medical emergency** characterized by extreme hypertension and exaggerated autonomic responses to stimuli; primarily seen with cervical and high thoracic cord lesions.

B. Risk factors:

1. Distention of bladder or rectum.
2. Stimulation of skin, e.g., decubitus ulcers, wrinkled clothing.
3. Stimulation of pain receptors.

C. Assessment:

1. Subjective data
   a. Severe headache.
   b. Blurred vision.
   c. Nausea.
   d. Restlessness.
   e. Feels flushed.
2. Objective data
   a. Severe hypertension (may reach 300 mm Hg.).
   b. Bradycardia.
   c. Profuse diaphoresis.
   d. Flushing of skin above level of injury.
   e. Pale skin below level of injury.
   f. Pilomotor spasm (goose flesh).
   g. Nasal congestion.
   h. Distended bladder, bowel.
   i. Skin breakdown.

D. Analysis/nursing diagnosis:

1. *Dysreflexia* related to high spinal cord injury.
2. *Potential for injury* related to complications of hypertension, CVA.
3. *Visual sensory/perceptual alteration* related to blurred vision.
4. *Urinary retention* related to inability to empty bladder due to spinal injury.
5. *Constipation* related to inability to establish successful bowel training program.
6. *Impaired skin integrity* related to immobility.

E. Nursing plan/implementation:

1. Goal: *decrease symptoms to prevent serious side effects.*
   a. *Elevate head of bed;* this lowers BP in persons with high spinal cord injuries.
   b. Identify and correct source of stimulation if possible.
   c. Monitor vital signs (BP) q15min and p.r.n.; uncontrolled hypertension can lead to CVA, blindness, death.
   d. If hypertension persists, a ganglionic blocking agent, such as hexamethonium chloride or pentolinium (Ansolysen), or a vasodilator, such as nitroprusside (Nipride), will be given to prevent CVA.
2. Goal: *maintain patency of catheter.*
   a. Monitor output; palpate for distended bladder.
   b. Increase fluids.
   c. Check for tubing kinks; irrigate catheter p.r.n.
   d. Insert new catheter *immediately* if blocked.
   e. Culture if infection suspected.
3. Goal: *promote regular bowel elimination.*
   a. Bowel training program.
   b. Administer suppository/enemas/laxatives as ordered and p.r.n.
   c. When checking for and/or removing impaction, first use anesthetic ointment (e.g., dibucaine [Nupercainal] ointment) to decrease irritation.
4. Goal: *prevent decubitus ulcers.*
   a. Meticulous skin care.
   b. Position change q1–2h.
   c. Flotation pads, alternating pressure mattress on bed and wheelchair.
5. Goal: *health teaching.*
   a. How to recognize risk factors that could initiate this condition.
   b. Methods to prevent situations that increase risk, e.g., bowel program, bladder program, skin care, position change schedule.

F. Evaluation:

1. BP remains within normal limits.
2. No complications occur.

XV. Hyperthyroidism (also called Thyrotoxicosis; Graves' disease): spectrum of symptoms of accelerated metabolism caused by excessive amounts of circulating thyroid hormone.

A. Pathophysiology: diffuse hyperplasia of thyroid gland → overproduction of thyroid hormone and increased blood serum levels. Hormone stimulates mitochondria to increase energy for cellular activities and heat production. As metabolic rate increases, fat reserves are utilized, despite increased appetite and food intake. Cardiac output is increased to meet increased tissue metabolic needs, and peripheral vasodilation occurs in response to increased heat production. Neuromuscular hyperactivity → accentuation of reflexes, anxiety, and increased alimentary tract mobility. Graves' disease is caused by stimulation of the gland by immunoglobulins of the IgG class.

B. Risk factors:

1. Possible autoimmune response resulting in increase of a gamma globulin called *long-acting thyroid stimulator* (LATS).
2. Occurs in third and fourth decade.
3. Affects women more than men.
4. Emotional trauma, infection, increased stress.
5. Overdose of medications used to treat hypothyroidism.
6. Use of certain weight-loss products.

C. Assessment:

1. Subjective data
   a. Nervousness, mood swings.
   b. Palpitations.

c. Heat intolerance.
d. Dyspnea.
e. Weakness.

2. Objective data
   a. Eyes: exophthalmos, characteristic stare, lid lag.
   b. Skin:
      (1) Warm, moist, velvety.
      (2) Increased sweating, melanin pigmentation.
      (3) Pretibial edema with thickened skin and hyperpigmentation.
   c. Weight loss *despite* increased appetite.
   d. Muscle: weakness, tremors, hyperkinesia.
   e. Vital signs: BP—increased systolic pressure, widened pulse pressure; tachycardia.
   f. Goiter: thyroid gland noticeable and palpable.
   g. Abnormal menstruation.
   h. Frequent bowel movements.
   i. Activity pattern: overactivity leads to fatigue, which leads to depression, which stimulates client into overactivity, and pattern continues. *Danger:* total exhaustion.
   j. Lab data:
      (1) *Elevated:* serum T_4 (>11μg/100 mL), free T_4 or Free T_4 index, T_3 level (above 35%) and free T_3 level.
      (2) *Elevated:* Thyroid uptake of radioiodine (RAIU).
      (3) *Elevated:* Metabolic rate (BMR).
      (4) *Decreased:* WBC caused by decreased granulocytosis (<4,500).

D. Analysis/nursing diagnosis:

1. *Altered nutrition, less than body requirements,* related to elevated basal metabolic rate.
2. *Potential for injury* related to exophthalmos and tremors.
3. *Activity intolerance* related to fatigue from overactivity.
4. *Fatigue* related to overactivity.
5. *Anxiety* related to tachycardia.
6. *Sleep pattern disturbance* related to excessive amounts of circulating thyroid hormone.

E. Nursing plan/implementation:

1. Goal: *protect from stress:* private room, restrict visitors, quiet environment.
2. Goal: *promote physical and emotional equilibrium.*
   a. Environment: quiet, cool, well ventilated.
   b. Eye care:
      (1) Sunglasses to protect from photophobia, dust, wind.
      (2) Protective drops (methylcellulose) to soothe exposed cornea.
   c. Diet:
      (1) High: calorie, protein, vitamin B.
      (2) 6 meals/day, as needed.
      (3) Weigh daily.
      (4) Avoid stimulants (coffee, tea, colas, tobacco).
3. Goal: *prevent complications.*
   a. Medications as ordered:
      (1) Propylthiouracil to block thyroid synthesis.
      (2) Methimazole (Tapazole).
      (3) Iodine preparations: Used in combination with above medications when hyperthyroidism not well controlled; Saturated Solution of Potassium Iodide (SSKI) or Lugol's solution; more palatable if diluted with water, milk, or juice; give through a straw to prevent staining teeth. Takes 2–4 weeks before results are evident.
   b. Monitor for *thyroid storm (crisis)*—**medical emergency:** acute episode of thyroid overactivity caused when increased amounts of thyroid hormone are released into the bloodstream and metabolism is markedly increased.
      (1) **Risk factors** for thyroid storm: client with uncontrolled hyperthyroidism (usually Graves' disease) who undergoes severe sudden stress, such as:
         (a) Infection.
         (b) Surgery.
         (c) Pregnant woman begins labor.
         (d) Inadequate antithyroid medications before thyroidectomy.
      (2) Subjective data—thyroid storm:
         (a) Apprehension.
         (b) Restlessness.
      (3) Objective data—thyroid storm:
         (a) Vital signs: elevated temperature (106°F), hypotension, extreme tachycardia.
         (b) Marked respiratory distress, pulmonary edema.
         (c) Weakness and delirium.
         (d) **If untreated, client could die of heart failure.**
      (4) Medications—thyroid storm:
         (a) Propylthiouracil or methimazole (Tapazole) to decrease synthesis of thyroid hormone.
         (b) Sodium iodide IV; Lugol's solution orally.
         (c) Propranolol (Inderal) to slow heart rate.
         (d) Aspirin to decrease temperature.
         (e) Steroids to combat crisis.
         (f) Diuretics, digitalis to treat congestive heart failure.
4. Goal: *health teaching.*
   a. Stress-reduction techniques.
   b. Importance of medications, their desired and side effects.
   c. Methods to protect eyes from environmental damage.
   d. Signs and symptoms of thyroid storm (see above).
5. Goal: *prepare for additional treatment as needed.*
   a. Radioactive iodine therapy: ^{131}I, a radioactive isotope of iodine to decrease thyroid activity.
      (1) ^{131}I dissolved in water and given by mouth.

(2) Hospitalization necessary only when large dose is administered.

(3) Minimal precautions needed for usual dose.

(a) Sleep alone for several nights.

(b) Flush toilet several times after use.

(4) Effectiveness of therapy seen in 2–3 weeks.

(5) Monitor for signs of hypothyroidism.

b. Surgery: see XVI. Thyroidectomy.

F. Evaluation:

1. Complications avoided.
2. Compliance with medical regime.
3. No further weight loss.
4. Able to obtain adequate sleep.

XVI. Thyroidectomy: partial removal of thyroid gland (for hyperthyroidism) or total removal (for malignancy of thyroid).

A. Risk factor: unsuccessful medical treatment of hyperthyroidism.

B. Analysis/nursing diagnosis:

1. *Potential for injury* related to possible trauma to parathyroid gland during surgery.
2. *Ineffective breathing pattern* related to neck incision.
3. *Pain* related to surgical incision.
4. *Altered nutrition, less than body requirements,* related to difficulty in swallowing because of neck incision.
5. *Impaired verbal communication* related to possible trauma of nerve during surgery.
6. *Potential altered body temperature* related to thyroid storm.

C. Nursing plan/implementation: *prepare for surgery* (see I. Preoperative preparation, p. 342). *Postoperative:*

1. Goal: *promote physical and emotional equilibrium.*

a. *Position:* semi-Fowler's to reduce edema.

b. Immobilize head with pillows/sandbags.

c. Support head during position changes to avoid stress on sutures, prevent flexion or hyperextension of neck.

2. Goal: *prevent complications of hypocalcemia and tetany,* due to accidental trauma to parathyroid gland during surgery; signs of tetany indicate necessity of *calcium gluconate IV.*

a. Check *Chvostek's sign*—tapping face in front of ear produces spasm of facial muscles.

b. Check *Trousseau's* sign—compression of upper arm (usually with BP cuff) elicits carpal (wrist) spasm.

c. Monitor for respiratory distress (due to laryngeal nerve injury, edema, bleeding); keep tracheostomy set/suction equipment at bedside.

d. Monitor for elevated temperature, indicative of thyroid storm (see objective assessment data for thyroid storm, above).

e. Monitor vital signs, check dressing and beneath head, shoulders for bleeding q1h and p.r.n. for 24 h; *hemorrhage* is possible complication; if swallowing is difficult, loosen dressing. If client still complains of tightness when dressing is loosened, look for further signs of hemorrhage.

f. Check voice postoperatively as soon as responsive after anesthesia and every hour (assessing possible laryngeal nerve damage); crowing voice sound indicates laryngeal nerves on both sides have been injured, *respiratory distress possible.*

(1) Avoid unnecessary talking to lessen hoarseness.

(2) Provide alternate means of communication.

3. Goal: *promote comfort measures.*

a. Narcotics as ordered.

b. Offer iced fluids.

c. Ambulation and soft diet, as tolerated.

4. Goal: *health teaching.*

a. How to support neck to prevent pressure on suture line: place both hands behind neck when moving head or coughing.

b. Signs of hypothyroidism; needs supplemental thyroid hormone if total thyroidectomy.

c. Signs and symptoms of hemorrhage and respiratory distress.

d. Importance of adequate rest and nutritious diet.

e. Importance of voice rest in early recuperative period.

D. Evaluation:

1. No respiratory distress, hemorrhage, laryngeal damage, tetany.
2. Preoperative symptoms relieved.
3. Normal range of neck motion obtained.
4. States signs and symptoms of possible complications.

XVII. Hypothyroidism (myxedema): deficiency of circulating thyroid hormone; often associated with the end result of Hashimoto's thyroiditis and Graves' disease.

A. Pathophysiology: atrophy, destruction of gland by endogenous antibodies or inadequate pituitary thyrotropin production → insidious slowing of body processes, personality changes, and generalized, interstitial nonpitting (mucinous) edema—myxedema; pronounced involvement in systems with high protein turnover (e.g., cardiac, GI, reproductive, hematopoietic).

B. Risk factors:

1. Total thyroidectomy; inadequate replacement therapy.
2. Inherited autosomal recessive genes.
3. Hypophyseal failure.
4. Dietary iodine deficiencies.
5. Radiation of thyroid gland.
6. Overtreatment of hyperthyroidism.

C. Assessment:

1. Subjective data

a. Weakness, fatigue, lethargy.

b. Headache.

c. Slow memory, psychotic behavior.

d. Loss of interest in sexual activity.

2. Objective data

a. Depressed basal metabolism rate (BMR).
b. Cardiomegaly, bradycardia, hypotension, anemia.
c. Menorrhagia, amenorrhea, infertility.
d. Dry skin, brittle nails, coarse hair, hair loss.
e. Slow speech, hoarseness, thickened tongue.
f. Weight gain: edema, generalized interstitial; peripheral nonpitting; periorbital puffiness.
g. Intolerance to cold.
h. Hypersensitive to narcotics and barbiturates.

D. Analysis/nursing diagnosis:

1. *Potential for injury* related to hypersensitivity to drugs.
2. *Altered nutrition, more than body requirements,* related to decreased basal metabolic rate.
3. *Activity intolerance* related to fatigue.
4. *Constipation* related to decreased peristalsis.
5. *Decreased cardiac output* related to hypotension and bradycardia.
6. *Potential impaired skin integrity* related to dry skin and edema.
7. *Social isolation* related to lethargy.

E. Nursing plan/implementation:

1. Goal: *provide for comfort and safety.*
   a. Monitor for infection or trauma; may precipitate myxedema coma, which is manifested by unresponsiveness, bradycardia, hypoventilation, hypothermia, and hypotension.
   b. Provide warmth; prevent heat loss and vascular collapse.
   c. Administer thyroid medications as ordered: levothyroxine (Synthroid)—most common drug used; triiodothyronine (Cytomel); dosage adjusted according to symptoms.
2. Goal: *health teaching.*
   a. Diet: low-calorie, high-protein.
   b. Signs and symptoms of hypothyroidism and hyperthyroidism.
   c. Life-long medications, dosage, desired and side effects.
   d. Stress-management techniques.
   e. Exercise program.

F. Evaluation:

1. No complications noted. Most common complications: atherosclerotic coronary heart disease, acute organic psychosis, and myxedema coma.
2. Dietary instructions followed.
3. Medication regime followed.
4. Thyroid hormone balance obtained and maintained.

XVIII. Cushing's disease: overactivity of adrenal gland leading to prolonged elevated plasma concentration of adrenal steroids.

A. Pathophysiology:

1. Excess glucocorticoid production, leading to:
   a. *Increased* gluconeogenesis → raised serum glucose levels → glucose in urine, increased fat deposits in face and trunk.
   b. *Decreased* amino acids → protein deficiencies, muscle wasting, poor antibody response, and lack of collagen.

B. Risk factors:

1. Adrenal hyperplasia.
2. Excessive hypothalmic stimulation.
3. Tumors: adrenal, hypophyseal, pituitary, bronchogenic, or gallbladder.
4. Excessive steroid therapy.

C. Assessment:

1. Subjective data
   a. Headache, backache.
   b. Weakness, decreased work capacity.
   c. Mood swings.
2. Objective data
   a. Hypertension, weight gain, pitting edema.
   b. Characteristic fat deposits, supraclavicular (buffalo hump).
   c. Pendulous abdomen, purple striae, easy bruising.
   d. Moon face, acne.
   e. Hirsutism: face, arms, legs.
   f. Hyperpigmentation.
   g. Menstrual changes.
   h. Impotence.
   i. Lab data:
      (1) Urine: elevated 17 ketosteroids (>12 mg/24 h) and glucose (>120 mg/dL.)
      (2) Plasma: elevated 17 hydroxycorticosteroids, cortisol (>10μg/dL). Cortisol does not decrease during the day as it should.
      (3) Serum: *elevated*—glucose, RBC, WBC; *diminished*—potassium, chlorides, eosinophils, lymphocytes.
   ▶ j. X rays and scans to determine tumors/metastasis.

D. Analysis/nursing diagnosis:

1. *Body image disturbance* related to changes in physical appearance.
2. *Activity intolerance* related to backache and weakness.
3. *Potential for injury* related to infection and bleeding.
4. *Knowledge deficit* related to management of disease.
5. *Pain* related to headache.

E. Nursing plan/implementation.

1. Goal: *promote comfort.*
   a. Assist with preparation of diagnostic workup.
   b. Explain procedures.
   c. Protect from trauma.
2. Goal: *prevent complications;* monitor for:
   a. Fluid balance—I&O, daily weights.
   b. Glucose metabolism—blood, urine for sugar and acetone.
   c. Hypertension—vital signs.
   d. Infection—skin care, urinary tract; check temperature.

e. Mood swings—observe behavior.

3. Goal: *health teaching.*

a. Diet: *increased* protein, potassium; *decreased* calories, sodium.

b. Medications:

(1) Aminoglutethimide (Cytadren, Elipten), Metyrapone (Metopirone), Mitotane (Lysodren)—decrease cortisol production.

(2) Replacement hormones as needed.

c. Signs and symptoms of increased disease as noted in Assessment.

d. Preparation for adrenalectomy if medical regime unsuccessful.

F. Evaluation:

1. Symptoms controlled by medication.

2. No complications—adrenal steroids within normal limits.

3. If adrenalectomy necessary, see following section.

XIX. Adrenalectomy: surgical removal of adrenal glands because of tumors or uncontrolled overactivity; also bilateral adrenalectomy may be performed to control metastatic breast or prostate cancer.

A. Risk factors:

1. Pheochromocytoma.

2. Adrenal hyperplasia.

3. Cushing's syndrome.

4. Metastasis of prostate or breast cancer.

5. Adrenal cortex or medulla tumors.

B. Assessment:

1. Objective data: validated evidence of

a. Benign lesion (unilateral adrenalectomy) or malignant tumor (bilateral adrenalectomy).

b. Adrenal hyperfunction that cannot be managed medically.

c. Bilateral excision for metastasis of breast and sometimes metastasis of prostate carcinoma.

C. Analysis/nursing diagnosis:

1. *Knowledge deficit* related to planned surgery.

2. *Potential for physical injury* related to hormone imbalance.

3. *Decreased cardiac output* (potential) related to possible hypotensive state resulting from surgery.

4. *Potential for infection* related to decreased normal resistance.

5. *Altered health maintenance* related to need for self-administration of steroid medications, orally or by injection.

D. Nursing plan/implementation:

1. Goal: *preoperative: reduce risk of postoperative complications.*

a. Prescribed steroid therapy given 1 week before surgery, is gradually decreased; will be given again postoperatively.

b. Antihypertensive drugs are discontinued as surgery may result in severe hypotension.

c. Sedation as ordered.

d. General preoperative measures (see p. 342).

2. Goal: *postoperative: promote hormonal balance.*

a. Administer hydrocortisone parenteral therapy as ordered; rate indicated by: fluid and electrolyte balance, blood sugar, and blood pressure.

b. Monitor for signs of Addisonian crisis (see below).

3. Goal: *prevent postoperative complications.*

a. Monitor vital signs until stability is regained; if on *vasopressor* drugs such as metaraminol (Aramine):

(1) Maintain flow rate as ordered.

(2) Monitor BP q5–15min, notify physician of significant elevations in BP (dose needs to be decreased) or drop in BP (dose needs to be increased). *Note:* readings that are normotensive for some may be hypotensive for clients who have been hypertensive.

b. NPO—attach nasogastric tube to intermittent suction; abdominal distention is common side effect of this surgery.

c. Respiratory care:

(1) Turn, cough, and deep breathe.

(2) Splint flank incision when coughing.

(3) Administer narcotics to reduce pain and allow client to cough; flank incision is close to diaphragm, making coughing very painful.

(4) Auscultate breath sounds q2h; decreased or absent sounds could indicate pneumothorax.

(5) Sudden chest pain and dyspnea should be reported *immediately,* as spontaneous pneumothorax can occur.

d. *Position:* flat or semi-Fowler's.

e. Mouth care.

f. Monitor dressings for bleeding; reinforce p.r.n.

g. Ambulation, as ordered.

(1) Check BP q15min when ambulation is first attempted.

(2) Place elastic stockings on lower extremities to enhance stability of vascular system.

h. Diet—once NG tube removed, diet as tolerated.

4. Goal: *health teaching.*

a. Signs and symptoms of adrenal crisis:

(1) Pulse: rapid, weak, or thready.

(2) Temperature: elevated.

(3) Severe weakness and hypotension.

(4) Headache.

(5) Convulsions, coma.

b. Importance of maintaining steroid therapy schedule to ensure therapeutic serum level.

c. Weigh daily.

d. Monitor blood glucose levels daily.

e. Report undesirable side effects of steroid therapy or adrenal crisis to physician.

f. Avoid persons with infections, due to decreased resistance.

g. Daily schedule: include adequate rest, moderate exercise, good nutrition.

E. Evaluation:

1. Adrenal crisis avoided.
   a. Vitals within normal limits.
   b. No neurologic deficits noted.
2. Healing progresses: no signs of infection or wound complications.
3. Adjust to alterations in physical status.
   a. Complies with medication regime.
   b. Avoids infections.
   c. Incorporates good nutrition, periods of rest and activity into daily schedule.

XX. Addison's disease: chronic primary adrenal cortical insufficiency.

A. Pathophysiology:

1. Atrophy of adrenal gland is most common cause of adrenal insufficiency; manifested by *decreased* adrenal cortical secretions.
   a. Deficiency in mineralocorticoid secretion (*aldosterone*) → increased sodium excretion → dehydration → hypotension → decreased cardiac output and resulting decrease in heart size.
   b. Deficiency in glucocorticoid secretion (*cortisol*) → decrease in gluconeogenesis → hypoglycemia and liver glycogen deficiency, emotional disturbances, diminished resistance to stress. Cortisol deficiency → failure to inhibit anterior pituitary secretion of ACTH and melanocyte stimulating hormone → increased levels of ACTH and hyperpigmentation.
   c. Deficiency in androgen hormone → less axillary and pubic hair in women (testes supply adequate sex hormone in men, so no symptoms are produced).

B. Risk factors:

1. Autoimmune processes.
2. Infection.
3. Malignancy.
4. Vascular obstruction.
5. Bleeding.
6. Environmental hazards.
7. Congenital defects.
8. Bilateral adrenalectomy.

C. Assessment:

1. Subjective data
   a. Muscle weakness, fatigue, lethargy.
   b. Dizziness, fainting.
   c. Nausea, food idiosyncrasies, anorexia.
   d. Abdominal pain/cramps.
2. Objective data
   a. Vital signs: decreased BP, orthostatic hypotension, widened pulse pressure.
   b. Pulse—increased, collapsing, irregular.
   c. Temperature—subnormal.
   d. Vomiting and diarrhea.
   e. Tremors.
   f. Skin: poor turgor, excessive pigmentation (bronze tone).
   g. Lab data:
      (1) Blood:
         (a) *Decreased:* sodium (<135 mEq/L); glucose (<60 mg/dL), chloride (<98 mEq/L), bicarbonate (<23 mEq/L).
         (b) *Increased:* hematocrit, potassium (>5 mEq/L).
      (2) Urine: *decreased* (or absent) 17-ketosteroids, 17-hydroxycorticosteroids (<4 mg/24 h).

D. Analysis/nursing diagnosis:

1. *Fluid volume deficit* related to decreased sodium.
2. *Altered renal tissue perfusion* related to hypotension.
3. *Decreased cardiac output* related to aldosterone deficiency.
4. *Potential for infection* related to cortisol deficiency.
5. *Activity intolerance* related to muscle weakness and fatigue.
6. *Altered nutrition, less than body requirements,* related to nausea, anorexia, and vomiting.

E. Nursing plan/implementation:

1. Goal: *decrease stress.*
   a. Environment: quiet, nondemanding schedule.
   b. Anticipate events where extra resources will be necessary.
2. Goal: *promote adequate nutrition.*
   a. Diet: *acute phase*—high sodium, low potassium; *nonacute phase*—increase carbohydrates and protein.
   b. Fluids: force, to balance fluid losses; monitor I&O, daily weights.
   c. Administer life-long exogenous replacement therapy as ordered:
      (1) Glucocorticoids—cortisone, hydrocortisone.
      (2) Mineralcorticoids—fludrocortisone.
3. Goal: *health teaching.*
   a. Take medications *with* food or milk.
   b. May need antacid therapy to prevent GI disturbances.
   c. Side effects of steroid therapy.
   d. Avoid stress; may need adjustment in medication dosage when stress is increased.
   e. Signs and symptoms of *addisonian crisis:* very serious condition characterized by severe hypotension, shock, coma, and vasomotor collapse related to strenuous activity, infection, stress, omission of prescribed medications. **If untreated, could quickly lead to death.**
4. Goal: *prevent serious complications if addisonian crisis evident.*
   a. Complete bedrest; avoid stimuli.
   b. High dose of hydrocortisone IV or cortisone IM.
   c. Treat shock—IV saline.
   d. I&O, vital signs q15min to 1 h or p.r.n. until crisis passes.

F. Evaluation:

1. No complications occur.
2. Medication regimen followed, is adequate for client's needs.
3. Adequate nutrition and fluid balance obtained.

XXI. Multiple sclerosis: progressive neurologic disease, common in northern climates, characterized by demyelination of brain and spinal cord leading to degenerative neurologic function.

A. Pathophysiology: multiple foci (patches) of nerve degeneration throughout brain, spinal cord, optic nerve, and cerebrum cause nerve impulses to be interrupted (blocked) or distorted (slowed); chronic remitting and relapsing disease; cause unknown. Exacerbations aggravated by fatigue, chilling, and emotional distress.

B. Risk factors:

1. Northern climate.
2. Onset age: 20–40
3. Affects men and women equally.

C. Assessment:

1. Subjective data
   a. Extremities: weak, numb, decreased sensation.
   b. Emotional instability, apathy, irritability, mood swings, fatigue.
   c. Eyes: diplopia (double vision), spots before eyes (scotomas), potential blindness.
   d. Difficulty in swallowing.
2. Objective data
   a. Nystagmus (involuntary rhythmic movements of eyeball) and decreased visual acuity.
   b. Inappropriate outbursts of laughing or crying (sometimes related to ingestion of hot food).
   c. Disorders of speech.
   d. Susceptible to infections.
   e. Tremors to severe muscle spasms and contractures.
   f. Changes in muscular coordination; *gait:* ataxic, spastic.
   g. Changes in bowel habits, e.g., constipation.
   h. Urinary frequency and urgency.
   i. Incontinence, urine and feces.
   j. Lab tests: cerebrospinal fluid has presence of *y*-globulin, IgG.

D. Analysis/nursing diagnosis:

1. *Impaired physical mobility* related to changes in muscular coordination.
2. *Self-esteem disturbance* related to chronic, debilitating disease.
3. *Altered health maintenance* related to spasms and contractures.
4. *Potential impaired skin integrity* related to contractures.
5. *Constipation* related to immobility.
6. *Impaired swallowing* related to tremors.
7. *Visual sensory/perceptual alteration* related to nystagmus and decreased visual acuity.

E. Nursing plan/implementation:

1. Goal: *maintain normal routine as long as possible.*
   a. Maintain mobility—encourage walking as tolerated; active and passive ROM; splints to decrease spasticity.
   b. Avoid fatigue, infections.
   c. Frequent position changes to prevent skin breakdown and contractures; position at night: prone to minimize flexor spasms of knees and hips.
   d. Bowel/bladder training program to minimize incontinence.
   e. Avoid stressful situations.
2. Goal: *decrease symptoms*—medications as ordered:
   a. Baclofen (Lioresal) for alleviating spasticity: 5 mg 3 times daily increased by 5 mg every 3 days; not to exceed 80 mg/day (20 mg four times/day). Optimal effect between 40 and 80 mg; sudden withdrawal of medication may cause hallucinations and rebound spasticity.
   b. Steroids during exacerbations.
   c. Valium, Dantrolene (Dantrium) to relieve muscle spasm.
3. Goal: *health teaching to prevent complications.*
   a. Signs and symptoms of disease; measures to prevent exacerbations.
   b. Teach to monitor respiratory status to prevent infections.
   c. Importance of physical therapy to prevent contractures.
   d. Possible counseling or community support group for assistance in accepting long-term condition.
   e. Teach special skin care to prevent decubitus ulcers.
   f. Teach use of assistive devices to maintain independence.

F. Evaluation:

1. Establishes daily routine; adjusts to altered life-style.
2. Injuries prevented; no falls.
3. Urinary and bowel routines established; incontinence decreased.
4. Infections avoided.
5. Symptoms minimized by medications.

XXII. Myasthenia gravis: neuromuscular disease characterized by weakness and easy fatigability of facial, oculomotor, pharyngeal, and respiratory muscles.

A. Pathophysiology: inadequate acetylcholine or excessive or altered cholinesterase, leading to impaired transmission of nerve impulses to muscles at myoneural junction.

B. Risk factors:

1. Possible autoimmune reaction.
2. Thymus tumor.
3. Ages 20–40: affects women more than men.
4. Older age groups: affects men and women equally.

C. Assessment:

1. Subjective data
   a. Diplopia (double vision).

b. Severe generalized fatigue.

2. Objective data
   a. Muscle weakness: hands and arms affected first.
   b. Ptosis (drooping of eyelids), expressionless facies.
   c. Hypersensitivity to: narcotics, barbiturates, tranquilizers.
   d. Abnormal speech pattern, with high-pitched nasal voice.
   e. Difficulty chewing/swallowing food.
   f. Decreased: ability to cough and deep breathe, vital capacity.
   g. Positive Tensilon test (administration of Edrophonium chloride, 10 mg IV, produces relief of symptoms within 30 seconds).
   h. Positive Prostigmin test (1.5. mg subcutaneous Prostigmin produces relief of symptoms within 15 minutes, increased muscle strength within 30 minutes).

D. Analysis/nursing diagnosis:

1. *Ineffective breathing patterns* related to weakness.
2. *Potential for injury* related to muscle weakness.
3. *Activity intolerance* related to severe fatigue.
4. *Bathing/dressing self-care deficit* related to progressive disease.
5. *Impaired physical mobility* related to decrease in strength.
6. *Anxiety* related to physical symptoms and disease progression.
7. *Knowledge deficit* related to medication administration and expected effectiveness.

E. Nursing plan/implementation:

1. Goal: *promote comfort.*
   a. Passive and active ROM, as tolerated, to increase strength.
   b. Mouth care: before and after meals.
   c. Diet: as tolerated, soft, pureed, or tube feedings.
   d. Skin care to prevent decubiti.
   e. Eye care: remove crusts; patch affected eye p.r.n.
   f. Monitor respiratory status—suction airway p.r.n.
2. Goal: *decrease symptoms.*
   a. Administer medications as ordered:
      (1) Anticholinesterase (Prostigmin, Tensilon, Pyridostigmine) to elevate concentration of acetylcholine at myoneural junction.
      (2) Give *before* meals to aid in chewing, *with* milk or food to decrease GI symptoms; may be given parenterally.
3. Goal: *prevent complications.*
   a. Respiratory assistance if breathing pattern not adequate.
   b. Monitor for choking/increased oral secretion.
   c. **Avoid:** narcotics, barbiturates, tranquilizers.
4. Goal: *promote increased self-concept.*
   a. Encourage independence when appropriate.
   b. Encourage communications; provide alternate methods when speech pattern impaired.
5. Goal: *health teaching.*
   a. Medication information:
      (1) Adjust dosage to maintain muscle strength.
      (2) Medication must be taken at prescribed time to avoid:
         (a) Myasthenic crisis (too little medication).
         (b) Cholinergic crisis (too much medication).
   b. Signs and symptoms of crisis: dyspnea, severe muscle weakness, respiratory distress, difficulty in swallowing.
   c. Importance of avoiding upper respiratory infections.
   d. Determine methods to conserve energy, to maintain independence as long as possible, while avoiding overexertion.
   e. Refer to Myasthenia Gravis Foundation and other community agencies for assistance in reintegration into the community and plans for follow-up care.

F. Evaluation:

1. Independence maintained as long as possible.
2. Respiratory arrest avoided.
3. Infection avoided.
4. Medication regimen followed and crisis avoided.

XXIII. Parkinson's disease: progressive disease of the brain occurring in later life; characterized by stiffness of muscles and by tremors.

A. Pathophysiology: depigmentation of the substantia nigra of basal ganglia → decreased dopamine (neurotransmitter necessary for proper muscle movement) → decreased and slowed voluntary movement, wooden facies, and difficulty initiating ambulation. Decreased inhibitions of alphamotoneurons → increased muscle tone → rigidity of both flexor and extensor muscles and tremors at rest.

B. Risk factors:

1. Occurs in ages 50–60.
2. Affects men and women equally.
3. Cause unknown; possibly connected to arteriosclerosis or viral infection.
4. Drug-induced parkinsonian syndromes have been linked to:
   a. Phenothiazines.
   b. Reserpine (Serpasil).
   c. Butyrophenones (Haloperidol).

C. Assessment:

1. Subjective data
   a. Insomnia.
   b. Depression.
   c. Defects in judgment, emotional instability; intelligence not impaired.
2. Objective data
   a. Limbs, shoulders: stiff, offer resistance to passive ROM.
   b. Loss of coordination, muscular weakness with rigidity.
   c. Shuffling gait: difficulty in initiating, then propulsive, trunk bent forward.

d. Tremors: pill-rolling of fingers, to and fro head movements.

e. Loss of postural reflexes.

f. Weight loss, constipation.

g. Difficulty in maintaining social interactions because of impaired speech, lack of facial affect, drooling.

h. Facies: wide-eyed, eye blinking, decreased facial expression, akinesia (abnormal absence of movement).

i. Excessive salivation, drooling.

j. Speech: slowed, slurred; judgment defective; intelligence intact.

k. Heat intolerance.

D. Analysis/nursing diagnosis:

1. *Impaired physical mobility* related to loss of coordination.
2. *Altered health maintenance* related to defective judgment.
3. *Potential for injury* related to altered gait.
4. *Dressing/grooming self-care deficit* related to muscular rigidity.
5. *Sleep pattern disturbance* related to insomnia.
6. *Body image disturbance* related to tremors and drooling.
7. *Social isolation* related to altered physical appearance.
8. *Altered nutrition, less than body requirements,* related to lack of appetite.
9. *Impaired swallowing* related to excessive drooling.
10. *Constipation* related to dietary changes.

E. Nursing plan/implementation:

1. Goal: *promote maintenance of daily activities.*

a. ROM exercises, skin care, physical therapy.

b. Encourage ambulation; discourage sitting for long periods.

c. Assist with meals—high protein, high calorie; soft diet; small, frequent feedings; encourage increased fluids.

d. Encourage compliance with medication regimen:

(1) Levodopa: given in increasing doses until symptoms are relieved; given *with food* to decrease GI symptoms. *Side effects:* nausea, vomiting, anorexia, postural hypotension, mental changes, cardiac arrhythmias. Levodopa assists in restoring striated dopamine deficiency.

(2) Sinemet (Carbidopa and Levodopa): limits the metabolism of Levodopa peripherally and provides more levodopa for the brain.

(3) Anticholinergics: effective in lessening muscle rigidity.

(4) Antihistamines: exert mild central anticholinergic properties.

2. Goal: *protect from injury.*

a. Monitor BP, side effects of medications, e.g., orthostatic hypotension.

b. Monitor for GI disturbances.

c. Avoid pyridoxine (vitamin B_6): cancels effect of Levodopa.

d. Levodopa contraindicated with:

(1) Glaucoma (causes increased intraocular pressure).

(2) Monoamine oxidase (MAO) inhibitors (causes possible hypertensive crisis).

3. Goal: *health teaching.*

a. Teach client and family about medications: dosage range, side effects, not discontinuing medications abruptly.

b. Exercise program to maintain ROM and normal body posture; also to get adequate rest to prevent fatigue.

c. Dietary adjustment and precautions regarding cutting food in small pieces to prevent choking, taking fluid with food for easier swallowing.

d. Importance of adding roughage to diet to prevent constipation.

e. Assist client and family to adjust to this chronic debilitating illness.

F. Evaluation:

1. Activity level maintained.
2. Symptoms relieved by medications; no drug interactions.
3. Complications avoided.

XXIV. Amyotrophic lateral sclerosis (ALS; Lou Gehrig's disease): progressive degeneration of motor neurons within the brain and/or spinal cord, leading to death within 5–10 years, usually from respiratory or bulbar paralysis.

A. Pathophysiology: myelin sheaths destroyed, replaced by scar tissue; involves lateral tracts of spinal cord, eventually medulla and ventral tracts.

B. Risk factors:

1. Affects men more than women.
2. Usually in middle age.
3. Viral infection possible causal agent.
4. Possible familial or genetic component.

C. Assessment:

1. Subjective data

a. Early symptoms: fatigue, awkwardness.

b. Dysphagia, dysarthria.

c. Alert, no sensory loss.

2. Objective data

a. Symptoms depend on which motor neurons affected.

b. Decreased fine finger movement.

c. Progressive muscular weakness, atrophy.

d. Spasticity of flexor muscles; one side of body becomes more involved than other.

e. Progressive respiratory difficulties → diaphragmatic paralysis.

f. Progressive disability of upper and lower extremities.

g. Tongue fasciculations.

D. Analysis/nursing diagnosis:

1. *Ineffective airway clearance* related to difficulty in coughing.
2. *Ineffective breathing pattern* related to progressive respiratory difficulties and eventually respiratory paralysis.
3. *Altered health maintenance* related to inability to perform self-care activities.
4. *Impaired physical mobility* related to progressive muscular weakness.
5. *Bathing/hygiene and dressing/grooming self-care deficit* related to neuromuscular impairment.
6. *Powerlessness* related to life-style of progressive physical helplessness.
7. *Impaired swallowing* related to disease progression.

E. Nursing plan/implementation:

1. Goal: *maintain independence as long as possible.*
   a. Assistance with ADL; splints, prosthetic devices to support weak limbs and maintain mobility.
   b. Skin care to prevent decubiti.
   c. Soft/liquid diet to aid in swallowing, prevent choking; suction p.r.n.; head of bed elevated when eating.
   d. Respiratory assistance as needed; ventilator as disease progresses and diaphragm becomes involved.
   e. Arrange long-term care arrangements if home maintenance no longer feasible.
   f. Emotional support, when client is alert; continue involving client in decisions regarding care.
2. Goal: *health teaching.*
   a. Skin care to prevent decubitus ulcer.
   b. Explain ramifications of disease so client and family can make decisions regarding future care, whether client will remain at home as disease progresses or enter a long-term care facility.
   c. How to use suction apparatus to clear airway.
   d. Care of nasogastric or gastrostomy feeding tube.

F. Evaluation:

1. Obtains physical and emotional support.
2. Complications avoided in early stage of disease.
3. Remains in control of ADL as long as possible.
4. Skin breakdown avoided.
5. Peaceful death.

CANCER

I. The cancer client: Cancer is a multisystem stressor. Regardless of the specific type of cancer, certain aspects of the disease and of nursing care are the same. The following principles apply universally and should be referred to when studying individual kinds of cancer.

A. Pathophysiology: result of altered cellular mechanisms. Several theories about causation, but current thinking is multiple causation. Alterations result in a progressive, uncontrolled multiplication of cells, with selective ability to invade and metastasize.

B. Risk factors:

1. Heredity, e.g., retinoblastoma.
2. Familial susceptibility, e.g., breast.
3. Acquired diseases, e.g., ulcerative colitis.
4. Virus, e.g., Burkitt's tumor.
5. Environmental factors:
   a. Tobacco.
   b. Alcohol.
   c. Radiation.
   d. Occupational hazards.
   e. Drugs, e.g., immunosuppressive, cytotoxic.
6. Age.
7. Air pollution.
8. Diet, e.g., high animal protein.
9. Chronic irritation.
10. Precancerous lesions, e.g., gastric ulcers.
11. Stress.

C. Assessment:

1. Specific symptoms depend on the anatomical and functional characteristics of the organ or structure involved.
2. Mechanical effects:
   a. *Pressure*—tumors growing in confined areas such as bone produce pain early, whereas tumors growing in expandable areas such as the abdomen may be undetected for some time.
   b. *Obstruction*—tumors that compress tubular structures such as the esophagus, bronchi, or lymph channels may cause symptoms such as swallowing difficulties, shortness of breath, edema. Symptoms depend on location of tumor and on the particular organ or structure receiving pressure.
   c. *Interruptions of blood supply*—compression of blood vessels or diversion of blood supply may cause necrosis or ulceration or may precipitate hemorrhage.
3. Systemic effects:
   a. Anorexia, weakness, weight loss.
   b. Metabolic disturbances—malabsorption syndrome.
   c. Fluid and electrolyte imbalances.
   d. Hormonal imbalances—increased antidiuretic hormone (ADH), adrenocorticotropic hormone (ACTH), thyrotropin (TSH), or parathyroid hormone (PTH).
   ▶ e. Diagnostic tests:
      (1) *Biopsy*—excision of part of tumor mass.
      (2) *Needle biopsy*—aspiration of cells from subcutaneous masses or organs such as liver.
      (3) *Exfoliative cytology*—scraping of any endothelium (cervix, mucous membranes) and applying to slide.
      (4) *X rays*—detect tumor growth in GI, respiratory, and renal systems.
      (5) *Endoscopy*—visualization of body cavity through endoscope.

(6) *Computerized axial tomography*—visualization of a body part whereby layers of tissue can be seen utilizing the very narrow beams of this type of X ray equipment.

(7) *Magnetic resonance imaging (MRI) scan*—a scanning device using a magnetic field for visualization.

f. Lab data:

(1) *Blood and urine tests*—refer to Appendix G for normal values.

(2) *Alkaline phosphates*—greatly increased in osteogenic carcinoma (above 92 U/L).

(3) *Calcium*—elevated in multiple myeloma bone metastases (above 10.5 mg/dL).

(4) *Sodium*—decreased in bronchogenic carcinoma (below 135 mEq/L).

(5) *Potassium*—decreased in extensive liver carcinoma (below 3.5 mEq/L).

(6) *Serum gastrin*—measures gastric secretions. Decreased in gastric carcinoma. Normal value 40–150 pg/mL.

(7) *Neutrophilic leukocytosis*—tumors.

(8) *Eosinophilic leukocytosis*—brain tumors, Hodgkin's disease.

(9) *Lymphocytosis*—chronic lymphocytic anemia.

D. Analysis/nursing diagnosis:

1. *Pain* related to diagnostic procedures, pressure, obstruction, interruption of blood supply, or potential side effects of drugs.
2. *Anxiety* related to fear of diagnosis or disease progression, treatment, and its known or expected side effects.
3. *Altered nutrition, less than body requirements* related to anorexia.
4. *Potential for injury* related to radioactive contamination of excreta.
5. *Body image disturbance* related to loss of body parts, change in appearance as a result of therapy.
6. *Powerlessness* related to diagnosis and own perception of its meaning.
7. *Self-esteem disturbance* related to impact of cancer diagnosis.
8. *Potential for infection* related to immunosuppression from radiation and chemotherapy.
9. *Altered urinary elimination* related to dehydration.
10. *Potential for injury* related to normal tissue damage from radiation source.
11. *Fluid volume deficit* related to nausea and vomiting.
12. *Diarrhea* related to radiation of bowel.
13. *Constipation* related to dehydration.

E. Nursing plan/implementation—general care of the cancer client:

1. Goal: *promote psychosocial comfort.* (See also Unit 1.)

a. Assist with diagnostic work-up by providing psychologic support and information about diagnostic tests, diagnosis, and treatment options.

b. Reduce anxiety by listening, making referrals for special problems (peer support groups, self-help groups such as Reach to Recovery), supplying information, or correcting misinformation, as appropriate.

c. Stress-management techniques (see Orientation).

d. Nursing management related to depressed client (see Unit 1).

2. Goal: *minimize effects of complications.*

a. Anorexia/anemia:

(1) *Decrease anemia* by:

(a) Providing well-balanced, iron-rich, small, frequent meals.

(b) Administering supplemental vitamins and iron as ordered.

(c) Administering packed cells as ordered.

(d) Maintaining hyperalimentation as ordered.

(2) *Enhance nutrition* by providing nutritional supplements and a diet high in protein; necessary because of increased metabolism related to metastatic process. *Consult* with dietician for suggestions of best food for individual client.

b. Hemorrhage: monitor platelet count and maintain platelet infusions as ordered. Teach client to monitor for any signs of bleeding.

c. Infection: observe for signs of sepsis (changes in vital signs, temperature of skin, mentation, urinary output or pain); monitor laboratory values; administer antibiotics as ordered.

d. Pain and discomfort: alleviate by frequent position changes, diversions, conversations, imagery, relaxation, back rubs, and narcotics as ordered.

e. Assist in adjusting to altered body image by encouraging expression of fears and concerns. Don't ignore client's questions, and give honest answers: be available.

3. Goal: *general health teaching.*

a. Self-care skills to maintain independence; e.g., client who has a colostomy should know how to manage the colostomy before going home.

b. Importance of follow-up care and routine physical examinations to monitor for general health and possible signs of further disease.

c. Dietary instructions, adjustments necessary to maintain nutrition during and after treatment.

d. Health maintenance programs: teach hazards of the use of tobacco and alcohol. Avoid high-fat, low-roughage diet.

e. Risk factors: family history, stress, age, diet, occupation, environment.

F. General surgical intervention: surgery may be *curative* (when the lesion is localized or with minimal metastases to the lymph nodes) or *palliative* (to decrease symptomatology). (Also see The Perioperative Experience, p. 342, and specific types of cancer, following.)

ADULT NURSING

1. **Nursing plan/implementation**—*preoperative:*
   a. Goal: *prevent respiratory complications.*
      (1) Coughing and deep-breathing techniques.
      (2) No smoking for 1 week prior to surgery.
   b. Goal: *counteract nutritional deficiencies.*
      (1) Diet:
         (a) High protein, high carbohydrate for tissue repair.
         (b) Vitamin and mineral supplements.
         (c) Hyperalimentation as ordered.
      (2) Blood transfusions may be needed if counts are low.
   c. Goal: *reduce apprehension.*
      (1) Clarify postoperative expectations.
      (2) Explain care of ostomies or tubes.
      (3) Answer client's questions honestly.
2. *Postoperative*
   a. Goal: *prevent complications.*
      (1) Monitor respiratory status and hemodynamic status.
      (2) Wound care; active and passive exercises as allowed; respiratory hygiene; coughing, deep breathing, and turning; fluids See III. Postoperative experience, p. 345.
   b. Goal: *alleviate pain and discomfort.*
      (1) Encourage early ambulation, depending on surgical procedure.
      (2) Administer prescribed medications as needed.
      (3) Administer stool softeners and enemas as ordered.
   c. Goal: *health teaching.*
      (1) Involve client, significant others, and family members in rehabilitation program.
      (2) Prepare for further therapies, such as radiation or chemotherapy.
      (3) Support groups, as appropriate: Reach to Recovery, Ostomy Associates, Laryngectomy Association.
      (4) Develop skills to deal with disease progression if cure not realistic or metastasis evident (see J. Palliative care, p. 432).

G. Chemotherapy: used as single treatment or in combination with surgery and radiation, for early or advanced diseases. Antineoplastic agents' primary mode of action involves interfering with the supply and utilization of building blocks of nucleic acids as well as interfering with intact molecules of DNA or RNA, which are needed for replication and growth. Bone marrow, hair follicles, and the gastrointestinal tract are three areas of the body in which cells are actively dividing; this is why most side effects are related to these areas of the body.

1. *Types:* alkylating agents, antimetabolites, antitumor antibiotics, plant alkaloids, enzymes, hormones.
2. *Major problem:* lacks specificity, thus affecting normal as well as malignant cells.
3. *Major side effects:* bone marrow depression, stomatitis, nausea and vomiting, gastrointestinal ulcerations, diarrhea, and alopecia (see Table 4.30).
4. *Routes of administration:* oral, intramuscular, intravenous (Hickman catheter), subclavian lines, porta caths, peripheral, intra-arterial (may have infusion pump for continuous or intermittent flow rate), intracavity (e.g., bladder through cystoscopy). (See p. 522 for information about administration of IV chemotherapeutic agents.)
5. **Nursing plan/implementation:**
   a. Goal: *assist with treatment of specific side effects*
      (1) *Nausea and vomiting*—antiemetic drugs as ordered and scheduled; small, frequent, high-calorie, high-potassium, high-protein meals; include milk and milk products when tolerated for increased calcium; carbonated drinks; frequent mouth care; antacid therapy as ordered; rest after meals; avoid food odors during preparation of meals; pleasant environment during meals; appropriate distractions; IV therapy; nasogastric tube for control of severe nausea or as route for tube feeding if unable to take food by mouth; hyperalimentation.
      (2) *Diarrhea*—low-residue diet; increased potassium; increased fluids; Lomotil or Kaopectate as ordered; avoid hot or cold foods/liquids.
      (3) *Stomatitis* (painful mouth)—soft toothbrushes or sponges (toothettes); mouth care q2–4h; viscous Xylocaine as ordered before meals. Oral salt and soda mouth rinses; avoid commercial mouthwashes that contain high level of alcohol, which could be very irritating to mucous membranes. Avoid hot foods/liquids; bland foods; cool temperatures; remove dentures if sores are under dentures; moisten lips with petroleum jelly.
      (4) *Skin care*—monitor: wounds that do not heal, infections (client receives frequent sticks for blood tests and therapy); avoid sunlight; use sunblock, especially if receiving Adriamycin.
      (5) *Alopecia*—ice caps during therapy or tourniquet around forehead for 20 minutes before, during, and after infusion of a few drugs (as ordered by physician); be gentle when combing or lightly brushing hair; use wigs, night caps, scarves; provide frequent linen changes. Advise client to have hair cut short prior to treatment with drugs known to cause alopecia (Belomycin, Cuclophosphamide, Dactinomycin, Daunomycin hydrochloride, Doxorubicin hydrochloride, 5-Fluorouracil, ICRF-159, Hydroxyurea, Methotrexate, Mitomycin, VP 16-213, and Vincristine).
   b. Goal: *health teaching.*
      (1) Orient client and family to purpose of proposed drug regimen and anticipated side effects.
      (2) Advise that frequent checks on hematologic status will be necessary (client will receive frequent IV sticks, lab tests).
      (3) Advise client/family on increased risk for infection (avoid uncontrolled crowds and individuals with upper respiratory tract infections or childhood diseases).

■ TABLE 4.30 Common Side Effects of the Antineoplastic Agents*

	Myelo-suppression	Mucositis	Nausea and Vomiting	Alopecia and Skin Reactions	Other
L-Asparaginase					Anaphylaxis; CNS toxicity; hyperpyrexia.
Bleomycin	0	0	0	+	Anaphylaxis; hyperpyrexia; pulmonary toxicity.
Busulfan	+	–	0	–	Pulmonary toxicity.
Carmustine	+	+	+	–	Cardiac, hepatic, and pulmonary toxicity; skin necrosis.
Chlorambucil	+	–	0	–	
Cisplatin	+	–	+	–	Anaphylaxis; ototoxicity; renal toxicity; peripheral neuropathy.
Cyclophosphamide	+	–	+	+	Hemorrhagic cystitis.
Cytarabine	+	+	+	+	CNS and pulmonary toxicity with high doses.
Dacarbazine	+	–	+	–	Anaphylaxis; hypotension; skin necrosis.
Dactinomycin	+	+	+	+	Skin necrosis.
Daunorubicin	+	+	+	+	Cardiotoxicity; hepatic toxicity; skin necrosis.
Doxorubicin	+	+	+	+	Cardiotoxicity; hepatic toxicity; skin necrosis.
Etoposide	+	0	+	+	Anaphylaxis; hypotension.
Floxuridine	+	+	+	+	Diarrhea, gastritis; hepatic toxicity.
5-Fluorouracil	+	+	+	+	Diarrhea; cerebellar ataxia.
Hydroxyurea	+	0	+	0	
Lomustine	+	+	+	0	Hepatic and renal toxicity.
Mechlorethamine	+	–	+	+	Skin necrosis.
Melphalan	+	0	0	–	
6-Mercaptopurine	+	+	0	0	Hepatic toxicity.
Methotrexate	+	+	+	+	CNS toxicity (intrathecal); hepatic toxicity; pneumonitis; renal toxicity.
Mitomycin	+	+	+	+	Pulmonary and renal toxicity; skin necrosis.
Mitotane	–	+	+	0	Adrenal insufficiency; CNS toxicity.
Mitoxantrone	+	0	0	0	Cardiotoxicity.
Plicamycin	+	+	+	–	Hepatic and renal toxicity; skin necrosis.
Procarbazine	+	0	+	–	MAO inhibition.
Streptozocin	0	0	+	+	Diarrhea; abdominal cramps; renal toxicity.
6-Thioguanine	+	+	0	0	Hepatic toxicity.
Triethylene thiophosphoramide	+	–	+	–	
Vinblastine	+	+	0	+	Skin necrosis.
Vincristine	–	–	–	+	Skin necrosis; hepatic toxicity; neurotoxicity.

*Key: + = Common; 0 = occasional; – = uncommon.
Note: Long-term use of antineoplastic agents may lead to sterility and the development of secondary malignancies.
Source: Shlafer, M., Marieb, E: *The Nurse, Pharmacology, and Drug Therapy.* Menlo Park, CA: Addison-Wesley, 1989.

(4) Monitor injection site for signs of extravasation (infiltration) (site must be changed if leakage suspected, and guidelines to neutralize must be followed according to drug protocol).

6. *Nursing precautions with chemotherapy*
   a. Nurse should wear gloves and mask when preparing chemotheraphy drugs for administration.
   b. Drugs are toxic substance, and nurses must take every precaution to handle them with care.
   c. When expelling air bubbles from syringes, care must be taken that the drugs are not sprayed into the atmosphere.
   d. Contaminated needles and syringes should be disposed of intact (to prevent aerosol generation) in plastic-lined box and incinerated. Disposable equipment should be used whenever possible.
   e. If skin becomes contaminated with a drug, wash under running water.
   f. Nurses should know the half-life and excretion route of the drugs being administered and take the special precautions necessary. For example, while the drug is actively being excreted, use gloves when touching client, stool, urine, dressings, vomitus, etc.
   g. Nurses who are in the early phase of pregnancy should exercise caution when caring for the client receiving chemotherapeutic agents.

ADULT NURSING

H. Radiation therapy: used in high doses to kill cancer cells, or palliatively for pain relief. Side effects of radiation therapy depend on site of therapy (side effects are variable in each individual): nausea, vomiting, stomatitis, esophagitis, dry mouth, diarrhea, depression of bone marrow, suppression of immune response, decreased life span, and sterility.

1. **External radiation:** cobalt or linear accelerator machine.
   a. *Procedure:* daily treatments, Monday through Friday, for prescribed number of times according to size and location of tumor (length of treatment schedule is usually 4–6 weeks). Client remains alone in room during treatment. (Nurse, therapist, family members cannot stay in room with client due to radiation exposure during treatment.) Client instructed to lie still so exactly same area irradiated each treatment. Marks (tattoos or via permanent-ink markers) are made on skin to delineate area of treatment; marks must not be removed during entire treatment course.
   b. **Nursing plan/implementation:**
      (1) Goal: *prevent tissue breakdown.*
         (a) Do not wash off site-identification marks (tattoos cannot be removed); dosage area is carefully calculated and must be exact for each treatment.
         (b) Assess skin daily and teach client to do same (most radiation therapy is done on out-patient basis, so client needs skills to manage independently).
         (c) Keep skin dry; cornstarch usually the only topical application allowed:
         (d) *Contraindications:*
            (i) Talcum powders, due to potential radiation dosage alteration.
            (ii) Lotions, due to increased moistening of skin.
         (e) Reduce skin friction by avoiding constricting bedclothes or clothing and by using electric shaver.
         (f) Dress areas of skin breakdown with nonadherent dressing and paper tape.
      (2) Goal: *decrease side effects of therapy.*
         (a) Provide meticulous oral hygiene.
         (b) If diarrhea occurs, may need IV infusions, antidiarrheal medications; monitor bowel movements, possible adhesions from surgery and radiation treatments.
         (c) Monitor vital signs, particularly respiratory function, and BP (sloughing of tissues puts client at risk for hemorrhage).
         (d) Monitor hematologic status—bone marrow depression can cause fatal toxicosis and sepsis.
         (e) Institute reverse isolation as necessary to prevent infections (reverse isolation usually instituted if less than 50% neutrophils).
      (3) Goal: *health teaching.*
         (a) Instruct client to *avoid:*
            (i) Strong sunlight; must wear sunblock lotion, protective clothing over radiation site.
            (ii) Extremes in temperature to the area (hot-water bottles, ice caps).
            (iii) Synthetic, nonporous clothes or tight constrictive clothing over area.
            (iv) Eating 2–3 hours before treatment and 2 hours after, to decrease nausea; give small, frequent meals high in protein and carbohydrates and low in residue.
            (v) Strong alcohol-base mouthwash; use daily salt and soda mouthwash.
            (vi) Fatigue, an overwhelming problem. Need to pace themselves, nap; may need someone to drive them to therapy; can continue with usual activities as tolerated.
            (vii) Crowds and persons with upper respiratory infections or any other infections.
         (b) Provide appropriate birth control information for clients of childbearing age.

2. **Internal radiation: sealed** (radium, iridium, cesium)
   a. Used for localized masses, e.g., mouth, cervix, breast, testes. Due to exposure from radiation source, precautions must be taken while it is in place. Health care personnel and family must adhere to principles of time, distance, and shielding to decrease exposure (shortest amount of time possible, stay as far away from the source of radiation, and wear protective lead apron, gloves). If source of radiation accidentally falls out, it should be picked up only with *forceps.* Radiation officer should be notified immediately. Client should be in private room, and bed should be in the center

of the room, if possible, to protect others. Unless the walls are lead lined, radiation will penetrate them; placing the bed in center of room will decrease exposure. Once the source of radiation has been removed, there is no exposure from client, excretions, or linens.

b. **Nursing plan/implementation:**

(1) Goal: *assist with cervical radium implantation* (cervical radium is used here as the most common example of internal radiation source).

(a) *Prior to insertion*—give douche, enema, perineal prep; insert foley, as ordered.

(b) *After implantation*—check position of applicator q24h.

(i) Keep client on bedrest in flat position to avoid displacing applicator (may turn to side for eating).

(ii) Notify physician if: temperature elevates, nausea or/and vomiting occur (indicates radiation reaction or infection).

(iii) *After removal* of implant (48–144 hours)—bathe, douche, and remove catheter as ordered.

(2) Goal: *health teaching*.

(a) Explain that nursing care will be limited to essential activities in postinsertion period.

(b) Signs and symptoms of complications so client can notify staff if something unusual happens (bleeding, radiation source falls out, fever, etc.).

c. **Nursing precautions for sealed internal radiation**

(1) **Never handle radium directly**—if applicators should accidentally be removed, pick up applicator by strings with long-handled forceps and **notify radiation officer.**

(2) Linen must remain in client's room and not be sent to laundry until source of radiation has been accounted for and returned to its container.

(3) **Time, distance, and shielding** are factors that increase or decrease potential effects on personnel. Need to minimize exposure of nursing staff, client's family, and other health professionals. Nurses who may be pregnant should not care for clients with radiation because of possible damage to the unborn fetus due to radiation exposure.

3. **Internal radiation: unsealed** (radioisotope/radionuclide)

a. Source of radiation is given orally or intravenously or instilled into a cavity as a liquid.

b. **Nursing plan/implementation:** Goal: *reduce radiation exposure of others.*

(1) Isolate client and tag room with radioactivity symbol.

(2) Rotate personnel to avoid overexposure (principles of time, distance, and shielding). Staff should use good handwashing technique. Client should be in a room with running water. (Nurse who may be pregnant should not care for client while radiation source still active.)

(3) Encourage family to maintain telephone contact or use intercom, to decrease exposure to others.

(4) Plan independent diversional activities.

c. *Specific nursing precautions* (post in chart, on client's door)

(1) *Radioactive iodine* (^{131}I): half-life 8.1 days; excreted in urine, saliva, perspiration, vomitus, feces.

(a) Wear gloves and isolation gowns when handling client, excreta, or dressings directly.

(b) Collect paper plates, eating utensils, dressings, and linen in impermeable bags; label and dispose according to agency protocol.

(c) Collect excreta in shielded container and send to lab daily to monitor excretion rate and disposal.

(2) *Radioactive phosphorus* (^{32}P): half-life 14 days; injected into cavity or given IV or orally.

(a) If injected into cavity, turn client q10–15min for 2 hours to assure distribution.

(b) No radiation hazard unless leakage from instillation site or from client's excreta, which are collected in lead-lined containers and brought to the radioisotope laboratory for disposal. Linen is collected in container, marked *radioactive,* and brought to the radioisotope lab for special handling.

(c) Seepage will stain linens blue; wear gloves when handling contaminated linens, dressings. Excreta disposed of as in (b) above.

(3) *Radioactive gold* (^{198}Au): half-life 2.7 days; usually injected into pleural or abdominal cavity.

(a) May seep from instillation site or drainage tubes in cavity; stains purple.

(b) Turn client q15min for 2 hours, as in (2)(a) above.

(c) Same precautions regarding handling excreta as in (1)(a) and (2)(b) above.

4. **Precautions for nurses**

a. Use principles of time, distance and shielding when caring for clients who are having active radiation therapy treatments.

b. Nurses who may be pregnant should not accept an assignment caring for clients who have active radiation in place.

c. Always use gloves, gowns to protect skin and clothing.

d. Wear detection badge to determine exposure to energy source.

I. Immunotherapy: it has been hypothesized that clinical malignancy may occur as a result of failure of the immunologic surveillance system of the body to fight off cancer cells as they develop. The goal of immunotherapy is to immunize clients against their own tumors.

1. *Nonspecific* immunotherapy—encourages a host-immune response by use of an unrelated agent. BCG (Bacillus Calmette-Guerin) vaccine and *Corynebacterium parvum* are the two agents used for this type of immunotherapy.
2. *Specific* immunotherapy—uses substances that are antigenically related to the tumor that stimulate a specific host-immune response.
3. Side effects—malaise, chills, nausea, vomiting, diarrhea; local reaction at site of injection, such as pruritus, scabbing.
4. **Nursing plan/implementation:**
   a. Goal: *decrease discomfort associated with side effects of therapy.*
      (1) Identify measures to lessen symptoms of side effects (see D. Nursing plan/implementation—general care of the cancer client, previously).
      (2) Know type of immunotherapy being used, adverse and desirable effects of therapy.
      (3) Administer fluids, encourage rest.
      (4) Administer acetaminophen as ordered to decrease flulike symptoms.
      (5) Administer antiemetics as ordered for nausea.
      (6) Monitor for respiratory distress.
      (7) Administer analgesics as ordered for pain.
   b. Goal: *health teaching.*
      (1) Comfort measures to decrease side effects of therapy.
      (2) Expected and side effects of therapy.
      (3) Investigational nature of therapy.
      (4) Care of site of administration.
      (5) Answer questions honestly.

J. Palliative care: When treatment has been ineffective in control of the disease, the nurse must plan palliative, terminal care. Cure is not possible for such clients in an advanced phase of malignancy. Symptoms increase in severity; clients and family have many special problems.

1. General problems of terminal cancer client:
   a. *Cachexia:* progressive weakness, wasting, and weight loss.
   b. *Anemia:* leukopenia, thrombocytopenia, hemorrhage.
   c. *Gastrointestinal disturbances:* anorexia, constipation.
   d. *Tissue breakdown* leading to decubiti, seeping wounds.
   e. *Urine:* retention, incontinence, renal calculi, tumor obstruction of ureters.
   f. *Hypercalcemia* occurs in 10–30% of clients.
   g. *Pain* due to tumor growth, obstruction, vertebral compression, or secondarily to complications, e.g., decubiti, stiffened joints, stomatitis. Also neuropathy, due to prolonged use of neurotoxic chemotherapeutic agents such as vincristine.
   h. *Fatigue:* major and debilitating problem.
2. **Nursing plan/implementation:**
   a. Goal: *make client as comfortable as possible;* involve nursing staff, family, support personnel, clergy, volunteers, support groups, hospice, etc.
      (1) *Nutrition:* obtain nutritional consultation; high-calorie, high-protein diet; small, frequent meals; blenderized or strained commercial protein supplements (Vivonex, Sustagen).
      (2) Prevent tissue breakdown and vascular complications: frequent turning, massage, air mattress, active and passive ROM exercises.
      (3) GI tract disturbances: observe for toxic reactions to therapy, particularly vomiting and diarrhea; administer medications: anti-emetics, anti-diarrheal agents as ordered.
      (4) Relieve pain.
         (a) Use supportive measures such as massage, relaxation techniques, imagery, and drugs for pain relief; administer codeine, Percodan, Talwin, morphine, meperidine, methadone, and diamorphine as ordered.
         (b) Monitor for side effects of narcotics, depressed respiratory status, constipation, anorexia.
   b. Goal: *assist client to maintain self-esteem and identity.*
      (1) Encourage self-care.
      (2) Spend time with client; isolation is a great fear for the dying client.
   c. Goal: *assist client with psychologic adjustment*—see nursing care for clients with alterations in body image, grieving clients, dying clients (Unit 1).

K. Evaluation:

1. Tolerates treatment modality—complications of surgery are avoided; tolerates chemotherapy; completes radiation therapy.
2. Side effects of treatment are managed by effective nursing care and health teaching.
3. Maintains good nutritional status.
4. Uses effective coping mechanisms or seeks appropriate assistance to deal with psychosocial concerns.
5. Makes choices for follow-up care based on accurate information.
6. Finds methods to control pain and minimize discomfort.
7. Dignity maintained until and/or during death.

II. Lung cancer

A. Pathophysiology: *squamous cell carcinoma:* undifferentiated, pleomorphic in appearance; accounts for 45–60% of all lung cancer; *small cell (oat-cell) carcinoma:* small, dark cells located between cells of mucosal surfaces; characterized by early metastasis and poor prognosis; *large-cell (giant-cell) carcinoma:* located in the peripheral areas of the lung, has poor prognosis; *adenocarcinoma:* found in men and women; not necessarily related to smoking.

B. Risk factors:

1. Heavy cigarette smoking, 20-year smoking history.
2. Exposure to certain industrial substances, such as asbestos.
3. Increased incidence in women during the last decade of life.

C. Assessment:

1. Subjective data
   a. Dyspnea.
   b. Pain: on swallowing; dull and poorly localized chest pain, referred to shoulders.
   c. Anorexia.
   d. History of cigarette smoking over a period of years; recurrent respiratory infections with chills and fever, especially pneumonia or bronchitis.
2. Objective data
   a. Wheezing; dry to productive persistent cough; hemoptysis.
   b. Weight loss.
   c. Positive diagnosis: cytology report of cells from bronchoscopy.
   d. Chest pain.
   e. Signs of metastasis.

D. Annual incidence: 152,000 new cases; 139,000 estimated deaths.

E. Analysis/nursing diagnosis:

1. *Ineffective breathing pattern* related to pain.
2. *Impaired gas exchange* related to tumor growth.
3. *Pain* related to disease progressing.
4. *Fear* related to uncertain future.
5. *Powerlessness* related to inability to control symptoms.
6. *Knowledge deficit* related to disease and treatment.

F. Nursing plan/implementation:

1. Goal: *make client aware of diagnosis and treatment options.*
   a. Allow time to talk and to discuss diagnosis.
   b. Client makes informed decision regarding treatment.
2. Goal: *prevent complications related to surgery* for client who is diagnosed early and for whom surgery is an option: wedge or segmental resection, lobectomy, or pneumonectomy are usual procedures.
   a. See Nursing plan/implementation for the client having thoracic surgery, p. 333.
   b. Monitor vital signs, including accurate respiratory assessment for respiratory congestion, blood loss, infection.
   c. Assist client to deep breathe, cough, change position.
3. Goal: *assist client to cope with alternative therapies* when surgery is deemed not possible.
   a. *Radiation:* megavoltage X ray, cobalt—usual form of radiation. (See Nursing plan/implementation for the client having radiation therapy, p. 430.)
   b. *Chemotherapy*
      (1) Cytoxan, Adriamycin, CCNU, methotrexate, Oncovin are the usual drugs given for lung cancer.
      (2) See Nursing plan/implementation for the client having chemotherapy, p. 428.
4. Goal: *health teaching.*
   a. Encourage client to stop smoking to offer best possible air exchange.
   b. Encourage high-protein, high-calorie diet to counteract weight loss.
   c. Force fluids, to liquefy secretions so they can be expectorated.
   d. Encourage adequate rest and activity to prevent problems of immobility.
   e. Desired effects and side effects of medications prescribed for therapy and pain relief.
   f. Coping mechanisms for maximal comfort and advanced disease (see J. Palliative care, p. 432).

G. Evaluation:

1. Copes with disease and treatment.
2. Side effects of treatment are minimized by proper nursing management.
3. Acid–base balance is maintained by careful management of respiratory problems.
4. Client is aware of the seriousness of the disease.

III. Colon and rectal cancer

A. Risk factors:

1. Males, middle age, personal or family history of colon and rectal cancer, personal or family history of polyps in the rectum or colon, ulcerative colitis.
2. Diet high in beef and low in fiber.
3. Gardner's syndrome (multiple colonic adenomatous polyps, osteomas of the mandible or skull, multiple epidermoid cysts, or soft-tissue tumors of the skin).

B. Annual incidence: 147,000 new cases, 61,500 estimated deaths.

C. Assessment:

1. Subjective data
   a. Change in bowel habits.
   b. Anorexia.
   c. Weakness.
   d. Abdominal cramping or vague discomfort with or without pain.
2. Objective data
   a. Diarrhea (pencil-like or ribbon-shaped feces) or constipation.
   b. Weight loss.
   c. Rectal bleeding; anemia.
   d. Chills, fever.
   e. Digital exam reveals palpable mass if lesion is in ascending or descending colon.
   f. Signs of intestinal obstruction: obstipation, distention, pain, vomiting, fecal oozing.
   ▶ g. Diagnostic tests:
      (1) Digital examination.
      (2) Slides of stool specimen, for occult blood.
      (3) Proctoscopy.
      (4) Sigmoidoscopy.
      (5) Barium enema.
   h. Lab data: occult blood, blood serotonin increased, carcinoembryonic antigen (CEA); positive radioimmunoassay of serum or plasma indicates presence of carcinoma or adenocarcinoma of colon; positive results after resection indicates return of tumor.

ADULT NURSING

D. Analysis/nursing diagnosis:

1. *Constipation or diarrhea* related to presence of mass.
2. *Altered health maintenance* related to care of stoma.
3. *Sexual dysfunction* related to possible nerve damage during radical surgery.
4. *Body image disturbance* related to colostomy.

E. Nursing plan/implementation (see also E. Nursing plan/implementation—general care of the cancer client, p. 427).

1. *Radiation:* to reduce tumor or for palliation.
2. *Chemotherapy:* to reduce tumor mass and metastatic lesions.
   a. Antitumor antibiotics—Mitomycin C, doxorubicin hydrochloride (Adriamycin).
   b. Aklylating agents—methyl-CCNU.
   c. Antimetabolites—5-Fluorouracil (5-FU).
   d. Steroids and analgesics for symptomatic relief.
3. Prepare client for surgery (colostomy) if necessary.

F. Evaluation:

1. Return of peristalsis and formed stool following resection and anastamosis.
2. Adjusts to alteration in bowel elimination route following abdominoperineal resection (e.g., no depression, resumes life-style).
3. Demonstrates self-care skills with colostomy.
4. Makes dietary adjustments that affect elimination as indicated.
5. Identifies alternate methods of expressing sexuality, if needed.

IV. Breast cancer

A. Risk factors:

1. Women over age 50.
2. Family history of breast cancer.
3. Never bore children, or bore first child after age 30.
4. Had breast cancer in other breast.
5. Menarche before age 11.
6. Menopause after age 50.
7. Excessive animal fat in diet.
8. Exposure to endogenous estrogens.

B. Annual incidence: 135,900 new cases; 42,300 estimated deaths.

C. Assessment:

1. Subjective data
   a. Burning, itching of nipple.
   b. Reported painless lump.
2. Objective data
   a. Firm, nontender lump or mass.
   b. Asymmetry of breast.
   c. Nipple—retraction, discharge.
   d. Alteration in breast skin—redness, dimpling, ulceration.
   e. Palpation reveals lump.
   ▶ f. Diagnostic tests: mammography, needle biopsy, excisional biopsy—level of estrogen-receptor protein predicts response to hormonal manipulation of metastatic disease and may represent a prognostic indicator for primary cancer; carcinoembryonic antigen useful for client with metastatic disease of the breast.

D. Analysis/nursing diagnosis:

1. *Potential for injury* related to surgical intervention.
2. *Body image disturbance* related to effects of surgery, radiation, or chemotherapy.
3. *Altered sexuality patterns* related to loss of breast.

E. Nursing plan/implementation (see also E. Nursing plan/implementation—general care of the cancer client, p. 427):

1. Goal: *assist through treatment protocol.*
   a. Radiation—primary treatment modality; adjunctive, external, or implantation to primary lesion site or notes.
   b. *Chemotherapy*
      (1) Cytotoxic agents to destroy tumor and control metastasis.
      (2) Alkylating agents: cyclophosphamides (Cytoxan).
      (3) Antitumor antibiotics: doxorubicin (Adriamycin).
      (4) Antimetabolites: Fluorouracil (5-FU); methotrexate (Amethopterine, MTX).
      (5) Plant alkaloids: vincristine sulfate (Oncovin).
      (6) Hormones to control metastasis, provide palliation: androgens, fluoxymesterone (Halotestin), testosterone (Teslac).
      (7) Antiestrogens: Tamoxifen citrate (Nolvadex).
      (8) Cortisols: cortisone, prednisolone (Delta-Cortef), prednisolone acetate (Meticortelone), prednisone (Deltasone, Deltra).
      (9) Estrogens: diethylstilbesterol.
   c. *Surgery*
      (1) Preoperative
         (a) Goal: *prepare for surgery—types:*
            (i) *Lumpectomy* (with or without radiation)—used when lesion is small; section of breast is removed (often accompanied by radiation therapy and then radium interstitial implant).
            (ii) *Simple mastectomy*—breast removed, no alteration in nodes.
            (iii) *Modified radical mastectomy*—breast, some axillary nodes, subcutaneous tissue removed; pectoralis minor muscle removed.
            (iv) *Radical mastectomy*—breast, axillary nodes, and pectoralis major and minor muscles removed.
            (v) Reconstructive surgery—done at time of initial mastectomy or (most often) later, when other adjuvant therapy has been completed.
         (b) Goal: *promote comfort.*
            (i) Allow client and family to express fears, feelings.

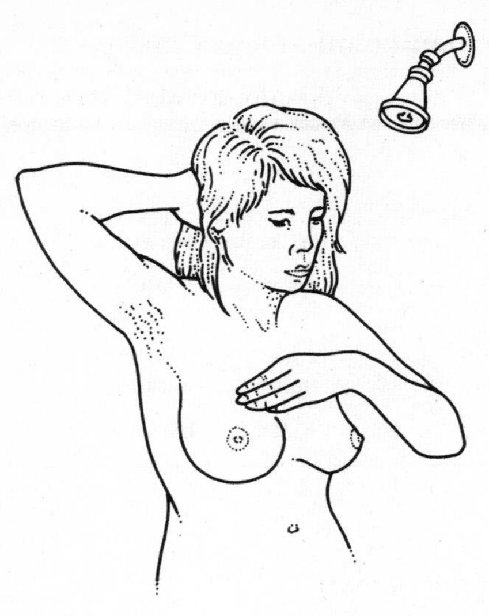

(a) Examine breasts during bath or shower since flat fingers glide easily over wet skin. Use right hand to examine left breast and vice versa.

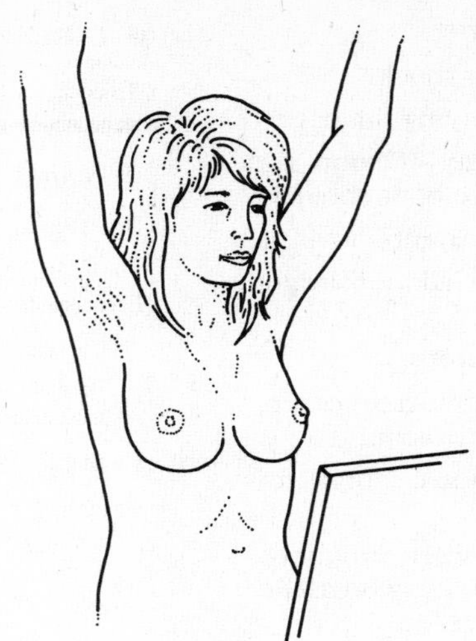

(b) Sit or stand before a mirror. Inspect breasts with hands at sides, then raised overhead. Look for changes in contour or dimpling of skin.

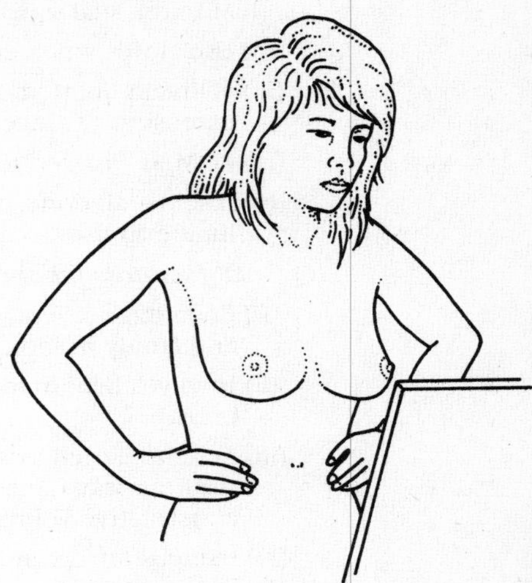

(c) Place hands on hips and press down firmly to flex chest muscles.

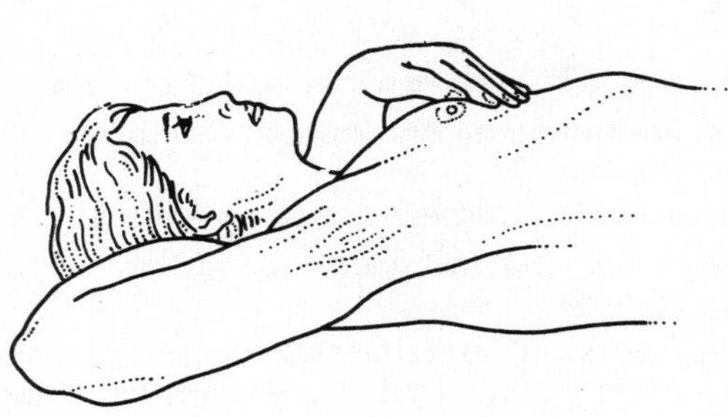

(d) Lie down with one hand under head and pillow or folded towel under that scapula.

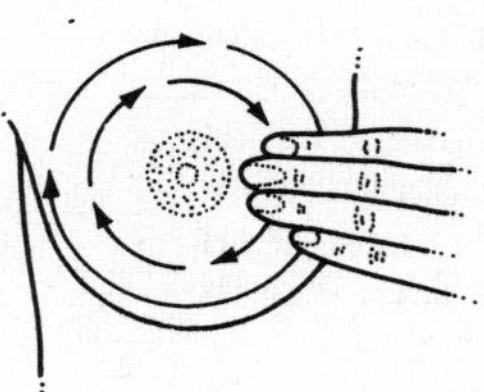

(e) Palpate that breast with the other hand using concentric circle method. It usually takes three circles to cover all breast tissue. Include the tail of the breast and the axilla. Repeat with other breast.

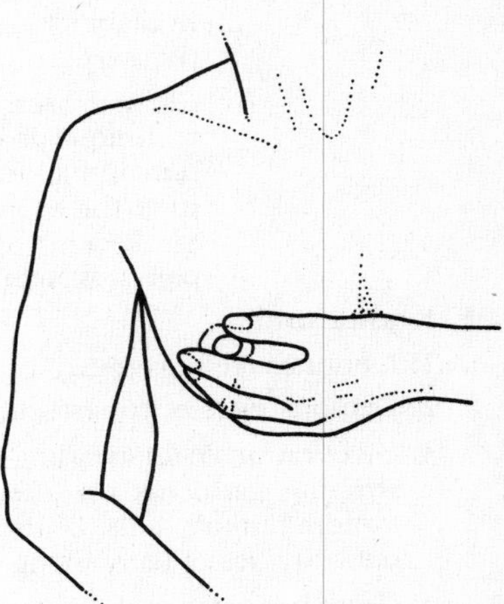

(f) End in a sitting position. Palpate the areola areas of both breasts, and inspect and squeeze nipples to check for discharge.

■ **FIGURE 4.7**
Breast self-examination. (From Phipps WJ, et al.: *Medical-Surgical Nursing,* Mosby, St. Louis, 1987.)

(ii) Provide correct information about diagnostic tests, operative procedure, postoperative expectations.

(2) Postoperative

(a) Goal: *facilitate healing.*

(i) Observe pressure dressings for bleeding; will appear under axilla and toward the back.

(ii) Report if dressing becomes saturated; reinforce dressing as needed; monitor drainage from Hemovac or suction pump.

(iii) *Position:* semi-Fowler's to facilitate venous and lymphatic drainage; use pillows to elevate affected arm above right atrium, to prevent edema if nodes removed.

(b) Goal: *prevent complications.*

(i) Monitor vital signs for shock.

(ii) Use gloves when emptying drainage.

(iii) Maintain joint mobility—flexion and extension of fingers, elbow, shoulder.

(iv) ROM as ordered to prevent ankylosis.

(v) If skin graft done, check donor site and limit exercises.

(c) Goal: *facilitate rehabilitation.*

(i) Encourage client, significant others, and family to look at incision.

(ii) Involve client in incisional care, as tolerated.

(iii) Refer to: Reach to Recovery program of the American Cancer Society Breast Reconstructive Volunteers.

(iv) Exercise program, hydrotherapy for postmastectomy clients, to reduce lymphedema.

(d) Goal: *health teaching.*

(i) How to avoid injury to affected area; how to prevent lymphedema.

(ii) Exercises to gain full ROM.

(iii) Availability of prosthesis, reconstructive surgery.

(iv) Correct breast self-examination (BSE) technique (is at risk for breast cancer in remaining breast). See Figure 4.7. Best time for exam: premenopausal women, seventh day of cycle, postmenopausal women, same day each month.

F. Evaluation:

1. Identifies feelings regarding loss.
2. Demonstrates postmastectomy exercises.
3. Gives rationale for avoiding fatigue and avoiding constricting garments on affected arm; necessity for avoiding injury (cuts, bruises, burns) while carrying out activities of daily living.
4. Describes signs and symptoms of infection.
5. Demonstrates correct BSE technique.

V. Uterine cancer (endometrial): originates from epithelial tissues of the endometrium; second only to cervical cancer as cause of pelvic cancer. Slow growing; metastizes late; responsive to therapy with early diagnosis; Pap test not as effective—more effective to have endometrial tissue sample. See Tables 4.31 and 4.32. Table 4.33 discusses cervical cancer.

A. Risk factors:

1. History of infertility (nulliparity).
2. Failure of ovulation.
3. Prolonged estrogen therapy.
4. Obesity.
5. Menopause after age 52.
6. Diabetes.

B. Annual incidence: 46,900 new cases; 10,000 estimated deaths.

C. Assessment:

1. Subjective data

a. History of risk factor(s).

b. Pain (late symptom).

2. Objective data

a. Obese.

b. Abnormal cells obtained from aspiration of endocervix or endometrial washings.

c. Postmenopausal uterine bleeding.

d. Abnormal menses; intermenstrual or unusual discharge.

D. Analysis/nursing diagnosis:

1. *Pain* related to surgery.
2. *Potential for injury* related to surgery.
3. *Body image disturbance* related to loss of uterus.

E. Nursing plan/implementation (see also care of the cancer client, p. 427):

1. Goal: *assist client through treatment protocol.*

a. *Radiation*—external and/or internal with poor surgical risk *clients.*

b. *Chemotherapy*—to reduce tumors and produce remission of metastasis. Antineoplastic drugs: dacarbazine (DTIC), Adriamycin, Provera, Megace.

TABLE 4.31 Papanicolau-Smear Classes

Class		Recommended Actions
I	Normal	
II	Atypical cells, nonmalignant	Treat vaginal infections; repeat Pap smears.
III	Suspicious cells	Biopsy; dilatation & curettage.
IV	Abnormal cells; suspicious of malignancy	Biopsy; dilatation & curettage; conization.
V	Malignant cells present	See Table 4.32.

TABLE 4.32 Uterine Cancer: Recommended Treatment, by Stage of Invasion

Stage of Invasion		Recommended Treatment
0	(In situ) Atypical hyperplasia.	Cryosurgery, conization.
I	Uterus is of normal size.	Hysterectomy.
II	Uterus slightly enlarged, but tumor is undifferentiated.	Radiation implant, X ray; hysterectomy 4–6 weeks postradiation.
III	Uterus enlarged, tumor extends outside uterus.	Radiation implant, total hysterectomy 4–6 weeks postradiation.
IV	Advanced metastatic disease.	Radiation, chemotherapy; progestin therapy to reduce pulmonary lesions.

2. Goal: *prepare client for surgery—types:*
   a. Subtotal hysterectomy: removal of the uterus; cervical stump remains.
   b. Total hysterectomy: removal of entire uterus, including cervix (abdominally—approximately 70%—or vaginally).
   c. Total hysterectomy with bilateral salpingo-oophorectomy: removal of entire uterus, fallopian tubes, and ovaries.
3. Goal: *reduce anxiety and depression:* allow for expression of feelings, concerns about femininity, role, relationships.
4. Goal: *prevent postoperative complications.*
   a. Catheter care—temporary bladder atony may be present as a result of edema or nerve trauma, especially when vaginal approach is used.
   b. Observe for abdominal distention and hemorrhage:
      (1) Auscultate for bowel sounds.
      (2) Measure abdominal girth.
      (3) Utilize rectal tube to decrease flatus.
   c. *Decrease pelvic congestion* and prevent venous stasis.
      (1) *Avoid* high Fowler's position.
      (2) Anti-embolic stockings as ordered.
      (3) Institute passive leg exercises.
      (4) Apply abdominal support as ordered.
      (5) Encourage early ambulation.
5. Goal: *support coping mechanisms* to prevent psychosocial response of depression: allow for verbalization of feelings.
6. Goal: *health teaching* to prevent complication of hemorrhage, infection, thromboemboli.
   a. Avoid:
      (1) Douching or coitus until advised by physician.
      (2) Strenuous activity and work, for 2 months.
      (3) Sitting for long time and wearing constrictive clothing, which tend to increase pelvic congestion.
   b. Explain hormonal replacement if applicable; correct dosage, desired and side effects of prescribed medications.
   c. Explain:
      (1) Menstruation will no longer occur.
      (2) Importance of reporting symptoms, e.g., fever, increased or bloody vaginal discharge, and hot flashes.

F. Evaluation:

1. Adjusts to altered body image.
2. No complications—hemorrhage, shock, infection, thrombophlebitis.

VI. Prostate cancer

A. Risk factors:

1. Men over age 50.
2. Familial history.
3. Geographic distribution, environmental (e.g., industrial exposure to cadmium).

■ TABLE 4.33 International System of Staging for Cervical Carcinoma

Stage	Location	Prognosis	Treatment
0	In situ.	Highly curable.	Conization.
I	Cervix.	Cure rate decreases as stage progresses.	Radiation.
II	Cervix to upper vagina.		Radiation.
III	Cervix to pelvic wall or lower third of vagina.		Surgeries: 1. Panhysterectomy, wide vaginal excision with removal of lymph nodes; ileal conduit.
IV	Cervix to true pelvis, bladder, or rectum.		2. Pelvic exenteration: a. Anterior: removal of vagina and bladder; ileal conduit. b. Posterior: removal of rectum and vagina; colostomy. c. Total: both anterior and posterior. 3. Chemotherapy.

B. Annual incidence: 99,000 new cases; 29,000 estimated deaths.

C. Assessment:

1. Subjective data
   a. Difficulty in starting urinary stream.
   b. Pain due to metastasis in lower back, hip.
   c. Symptoms of cystitis.
2. Objective data
   a. Urinary: smaller, less forceful stream; terminal dribbling; frequency, urgency, nocturia; *retention* (inability to void after ingestion of alcohol or exposure to cold).
   b. Cystoscopy, needle biopsy, or specimen reveals positive cancer cells.

D. Analysis/nursing diagnosis:

1. *Altered urinary elimination* related to incontinence.
2. *Altered sexuality pattern* related to nerve damage.
3. *Body image disturbance* related to surgery.

E. Nursing plan/implementation (see also care of the cancer client, p. 427).

1. Goal: *assist client through treatment protocol.*
   a. *Radiation*—alone or in conjunction with surgery.
   b. *Chemotherapy*—analgesics, antispasmodics, antibiotics, adrenocortical hormones, and cytotoxic drugs in conjunction with orchiectomy, to limit production of androgens.
   c. *Surgery*—see Prostatectomy, p. 380.

F. Evaluation: see Prostatectomy, p. 380.

ADULT NURSING

VII. Bladder cancer: The bladder is most common site of urinary tract cancer.

A. Risk factors:

1. Contact with certain dyes.
2. Cigarette smoking.
3. Excessive coffee intake.
4. Prolonged use of analgesics with phenacetin.
5. Three times more common in males.

B. Annual incidence: 46,000 new cases; 10,400 estimated deaths.

C. Assessment:

1. Subjective data
   a. Frequency, urgency.
   b. Pain: flank, pelvic; dysuria.
2. Objective data
   a. Painless hematuria (initially).
   ▶ b. Diagnostic tests:
      (1) Cytoscopy, intravenous pyelogram (IVP)—mass or obstruction.
      (2) Bladder biopsy, urine cytology—malignant cells.
   c. Lab data: urinalysis—increased RBC (>4.8/μL—men); (>4.3/μL—women); erythrocytes (>30 mg/dL).

D. Analysis/nursing diagnosis:

1. *Potential for injury* related to surgical intervention.
2. *Altered urinary elimination* related to surgery.

E. Nursing plan/implementation (see also care of the cancer client, p. 427):

1. Goal: *assist client through treatment protocol.*
   a. *Radiation*—cobalt, radioisotopes, radon seeds; often before surgery to slow tumor growth.
   b. *Chemotherapy*
      (1) Antitumor antibiotics: doxorubicin hydrochloride (Adriamycin).
      (2) Antimetabolites: 5-Fluorouracil (5-FU).
      (3) Alkylating agents: Thiotepa.
      (4) Sedatives, antispasmodics.
2. Goal: *prepare client for surgery*—types:
   a. Transurethral fulguration or excision: used for small tumors with minimal tissue involvement.
   b. Segmental resection: up to half the bladder may be resected.
   c. Cystectomy with urinary diversion: complete removal of the bladder; performed when disease appears curable.
3. Goal: *assist with acceptance of diagnosis and treatment.*
4. Goal: *prevent complication during postoperative period.*
   a. *Transurethral fulguration or excision:*
      (1) Monitor for clots, bleeding, spasms.
      (2) Maintain patency of Foley catheter.
   b. *Urinary diversion with stoma:*
      (1) Protect skin, ensure proper fit of appliance—because constantly wet with urine (see also Ileal conduit, p. 380, and ostomies and stoma care, pp. 370–371).
      (2) Prevent infection by increasing acidity of urine and increasing fluid intake.
      (3) Health teaching.
         (a) Self-care of stoma and appliance.
         (b) Expected and side effects of medications.
         (c) Importance of follow-up visits for early detection of metastasis.

F. Evaluation:

1. Accepts treatment plan.
2. Utilizes prescribed measures to decrease side effects of surgery, radiation, chemotherapy.
3. Plans follow-up visits for further evaluation.
4. Maintains dignity.

VIII. Laryngeal cancer

A. Risk factors:

1. Eight times more common in men.
2. Occurs most often after age 60.
3. Cigarette smoking.
4. Alcohol.
5. Chronic laryngitis, vocal abuse.
6. Family predisposition to cancer.

B. Annual incidence: 12,200 new cases; 3,800 estimated deaths.

C. Assessment:

1. Subjective data
   a. Dysphagia—pain in area of Adam's apple; radiates to ear.
   b. Dyspnea.
2. Objective data
   a. Persistent hoarseness.
   b. Cough and hemoptysis.
   c. Enlarged cervical nodes.
   d. General debility and weight loss.
   e. Foul breath.
   f. Diagnosis made by history, laryngoscopy with biopsy and microscopic study of cells.

D. Analysis/nursing diagnosis:

1. *Impaired verbal communication* related to removal of larynx.
2. *Body image disturbance* related to radical surgery.
3. *Ineffective airway clearance* related to increased secretions through tracheoctomy.

E. Nursing plan/implementation (see also care of the cancer client, p. 427): treatment primarily surgical (laryngectomy—see p. 381); radiation therapy may also be indicated.

F. Evaluation: see Laryngectomy, p. 382.

IX. Additional types of cancer—see Table 4.34

TABLE 4.34 Selected Cancer Problems

	Assessment				
	Subjective Data	Objective Data	Risk Factors	Annual Incidence	Specific Treatment
Gastrointestinal Tract					
Oral cancer	Difficulty chewing, swallowing, moving tongue or jaws; history of heavy smoking, drinking, or chewing tobacco.	Sore that bleeds and does not heal; persistent red or white patch; diagnosis by biopsy. Early detection: dental checks.	Heavy smoking and drinking, user of chewing tobacco, men over age 40 (affects twice as many men as women).	30,200 new cases; 9,050 estimated deaths.	*Surgery,* with reconstructive surgery useful for cure and palliatively (see care of cancer client having surgery, p. 427). *Radiation* using simulated computer localization to avoid destruction of normal tissue (see care of client having radiation therapy, p. 430).
Esophageal cancer	Dysphagia—difficulty in swallowing; discomfort described as lump in throat, pressure in chest, pain; fatigue, lethargy, apathy, depression; anorexia.	Weight loss; regurgitation, vomiting; diagnostic tests—barium swallow, esophagoscopy, biopsy.	Over age 50, alcoholism, use of tobacco; increasing risk in nonwhite females, in people with achalasia (inability to relax lower esophagus with swallowing) or hiatal hernias.	9,800 new cases, 9,200 estimated deaths.	*Surgery:* resection with anastomosis, or removal with gastrostomy. *Radiation:* best form of therapy. *Chemotherapy:* antineoplastic drugs ineffective; medications to reduce symptoms of pain, discomfort, and anxiety. See nursing plan/implementation for client: with cancer (p. 427); having radiation therapy (p. 430); having chemotherapy (p. 428); having surgery (p. 428).
Stomach cancer	Vague feeling of fullness, pressure, or epigastric pain following ingestion of food; anorexia, nausea, intolerance of meat; malaise.	Eructation, regurgitation, vomiting; melana, hematemesis, anemia; jaundice, diarrhea, ascites; big belly, upper gastric area; often palpable mass.	Men, lower socioeconomic classes, colder climates, early exposure to dietary carcinogens, blood group A, pernicious anemia, atrophic achlorhydric gastritis.	24,800 new cases; 14,400 estimated deaths.	*Surgery*—gastrectomy (see gastric surgery, p. 360 for nursing care). *Radiation*—not as useful because dosage needed would cause side effects unlikely to be tolerated by client. *Chemotherapy* alone or in conjunction with surgery: antitumor antibiotics, antimetabolites, nitrosureas, hematinics (see nursing plan for clients having chemotherapy, p. 428).
Pancreatic cancer	Anorexia, nausea; pain in upper abdomen, radiating to back; dyspnea.	Jaundice, vomiting, weight loss; determination of solid mass in area of pancreas by computed tomographic scanning and ultrasound; tissue identification by thin needle percutaneous biopsy.	Excessive use of alcohol; exposure to dry cleaning chemicals, gasoline; coffee and decaffeinated coffee; possibly diabetes and chronic pancreatitis.	27,000 new cases; 24,500 estimated deaths.	*Surgery*—removal (must then have supplemental pancreatic enzymes, so clients become insulin-dependent diabetics) or bypass to relieve obstruction (see nursing plan/implementation for client with diabetes, p. 364). *Chemotherapy*—pain relief, antiemetics, insulin, pancrelipase, 5-FU,

continued

■ **TABLE 4.34 *(Continued)*** **Selected Cancer Problems**

	Assessment				
	Subjective Data	**Objective Data**	**Risk Factors**	**Annual Incidence**	**Specific Treatment**
Gastrointestinal Tract (cont.)					
Pancreatic cancer (cont.)					cytoxan, methotrexate, vincristine, mitomycin-C (see nursing plan/implementation for client having chemotherapy, p. 428). *Radiation*—intraoperative high dose to pancreatic tumors with external high beam; palliative radiation therapy for pain (see nursing plan/implementation for client having radiation therapy, p. 430). See nursing plan/implementation for client with cancer, p. 427).
Skin					
Skin cancer: basal cell	Reported painless lesion.	Scaly plaques, papules that ulcerate; pale, waxy, pearly nodule or red, sharply outlined patch; unusual skin condition, change in size or color, or other darkly pigmented growth or mole.	Exposure to: sun, coal tar, pitch, arsenic compounds, creosote, radium; fair complexion.	500,000 new cases; 7,800 estimated deaths; 27,300 of these are malignant melonoma.	*Surgery*—electrodesiccation (dehydration of tissue by use of needle electrode); cryosurgery (destruction of tissue by application of extreme cold) (see care of cancer client, p. 427). *Radiation therapy* (see care of client having radiation therapy, p. 430). *Prevention*—avoid sun from 10–3; use protective clothing, sunblock lotion.
Nervous System					
Brain	*Headache:* steady, intermittent, severe (may be intensified by physical activity); nausea; lethargy, easy fatigability; forgetfulness, disorientation, impaired judgment; visual disturbances; blackouts.	Vomiting, may be projectile; sight loss, auditory changes; signs of increased intracranial pressure; seizures; *diagnostic studies*—CT scan, arteriography, cytology of cerebrospinal fluid; paraesthesia; behavior changes.	None known for primary tumors; brain is common site for metastasis.	14,700 new cases (brain and spinal cord); 10,900 estimated deaths.	*Surgery*—craniotomy with excision of lesion; ventricular shunt to allow for drainage of fluid (see nursing plan/implementation for craniotomy, p. 390; see nursing plan/implementation for client with cancer, p. 427). *Radiation*—cobalt (local or entire CNS); total brain radiation causes alopecia, which may be permanent (see nursing plan/implementation for client having radiation therapy, p. 430); could be used alone, with surgery, or with chemotherapy. *Chemotherapy:* antineoplastic

continued

■ **TABLE 4.34 *(Continued)***

	Assessment				
	Subjective Data	**Objective Data**	**Risk Factors**	**Annual Incidence**	**Specific Treatment**
Nervous System (cont.) Brain (cont.)					alkylating agents; nitrosureas (cross blood-brain barrier to reduce tumor)—carmustine (BCNU), lomustine (CCNU), semustine (Methyl-CCNU); cerebral diuretics to reduce edema; anticonvulsants; analgesics; sedatives (see nursing plan/implementation for client having chemotherapy, p. 428).
Endocrine					
Thyroid cancer	Painless nodule; dysphagia; difficulty breathing	Enlarged thyroid, thyroid nodule; palpable thyroid, lymph nodes; hoarseness; hypofunctional nodule seen on isotopic imaging scanning; needle biopsy for cytology studies.	Radiation in childhood.	11,000 new cases; 1,100 estimated deaths.	*Surgery*—total thyroidectomy, possible radical neck dissection (see Thyroidectomy, p. 419). *Radiation*—external, or with radioactive iodine (^{131}I) (see care of client having radiation therapy, p. 430). *Chemotherapy*—Leukeran, Adriamycin, Oncovin (see care of client having chemotherapy, p. 428).
Blood and Lymph Tissues					
Hodgkin's disease	Fatigue; generalized pruritis; anorexia.	Painless enlargement of lymph nodes, especially in cervical area; fever, night sweats; hepatosplenomegaly; anemia; peak age of incidence, 15–35; diagnostic tests—biopsy shows presence of Reed-Sternberg cells; X rays, scans, laparotomy.	For young adults from 15–35 years old, not clearly defined, some relationship to socioeconomic status; male/female ratio is 1.5/1; increased frequency among whites.	7,400 new cases; 1,500 estimated deaths.	*Staging and treatment:* *Stage I*—involvement of a single node or a single node region; excision of lesion, and total nodal radiation (see care of client having radiation therapy, p. 430). *Stage II*—involvement of two or more lymph node regions on same side of diaphragm; excision of lesion and radiation (see care of client having radiation therapy, p. 430). *Stage III*—involvement of lymph node regions on both sides of the diaphragm, which may include the spleen; combination of radiation and chemotherapy. *Stage IV*—involvement of one or more extralymphatic organs or tissues, with or without lymphatic involvement; treated with chemotherapy alone, radiation therapy alone, or both. Presence or absence of symptoms of night sweats, significant fever, and weight loss; treated with

continued

TABLE 4.34 *(Continued)* **Selected Cancer Problems**

	Assessment				
	Subjective Data	**Objective Data**	**Risk Factors**	**Annual Incidence**	**Specific Treatment**
Blood and Lymph Tissues (cont.)					
Hodgkin's disease (cont.)					*chemotherapy,* MOPP protocol—Mustargen (alkylating agent), Oncovin (plant alkaloid), procarbazine (antineoplastic); prednisone (corticosteroid) (see care of client having chemotherapy, p. 428).
Multiple myeloma	Weakness; history of frequent infections, especially pneumonias; severe bone pain on motion; neurologic symptoms, paralysis.	Fractures of long bones; deformity of—sternum, ribs, vertabrae, pelvis; hepatosplenomegaly; renal calculi, renal insufficiency; anemia and bleeding tendencies; elevated uric acid.	Exposure to ionizing irradiation; middle-aged or older females.	11,600 new cases; 8,200 estimated deaths.	*Radiation therapy*—for some lesions (see nursing plan/implementation for clients having radiation therapy, p. 430). *Surgery*—relieve spinal cord compression; orthopedic procedures to relieve or support bone problems (see nursing plan/implementation for: clients with internal fixation for fractures, p. 400; client with spinal cord injuries when paralysis occurs, p. 415). *Chemotherapy)*—alkylating agents; antitumor antibiotics; plant alkaloids; hormones—melphalan and prednisone (see nursing plan/implementation for clients having chemotherapy, p. 428).
Urinary Organs					
Kidney cancer	Anorexia, nausea; fatigue; abdominal or flank pain.	Painless, gross hematuria; firm, nontender, palpable kidney; vomiting and weight loss; *complications*—hypertension, nephrotic syndrome, lung metastasis; *lab and diagnostic tests:* IVP; urinalysis—presence of red cells and albumin; CBC—decrease in red cells and leukocytes, *reduction* in serum albumin, *elevation* of alpha globulin.	More common among men than women, whites than blacks; radiation exposure, possible familial influence; common site of metastasis from lung, breast.	22,500 new cases; 9,600 estimated deaths.	*Surgery*—nephrectomy (see pre/postoperative nursing care, p. 342). *Radiation*—local and irradiation of metastatic sites when tumor is radiosensitive (see nursing plan/implementation for client having radiation therapy, p. 430). *Chemotherapy:* plant alkaloids—vincristine (Oncovin); antitumor antibiotics—dactinomycin (Actinomycin D), doxorubicin (Adriamycin); alkylating agents—cyclophosphamide (Cytoxan) (see nursing plan/implementation for client having chemotherapy, p. 428).

continued

■ **TABLE 4.34 *(Continued)***

	Assessment				
	Subjective Data	**Objective Data**	**Risk Factors**	**Annual Incidence**	**Specific Treatment**
Genital Organs					
Testicular cancer	Aching or dragging sensation in groin, usually painless.	Gynecomastia; enlargement, swelling, lump, hardening of testes; young adult male. Early diagnosis—monthly testicular self-exam. See Figure 4.8, p. 453.	Second most common malignancy among men between 25 and 40; possibly exposure to chemical carcinogens; trauma, orchitis; gonadal dysgenesis; cryptorchidism (undescended testicles).	5,600 new cases; 350 estimated deaths; 95–100% 5-year survival rate for early-detected non-metastasized lesions.	*Surgery*—orchiectomy (see nursing plan/implementation for the pre- and postop client, p. 342). *Radiation*—see nursing plan/implementation for client having radiation therapy, p. 430. *Chemotherapy*—Leukeran, Methotrexate, steroids (see nursing plan/implementation for client having chemotherapy, p. 428).
Cervical cancer	Vague pelvic or low-back discomfort, pressure, or pain.	Intermenstrual, postcoital, or postmenopausal bleeding; vaginal discharge—serosanguineous and malodorous hypermenorrhea; abdominal distension with urinary frequency; abnormal Pap test (see Table 4.31). Recommended guidelines by American Cancer Society: Pap test annually; after 3 consecutive normal tests, MD may recommend less frequent testing. Pelvic/uterine exam every 3 years..	Early age at first intercourse; multiple sex partners; low socioeconomic status; exposure to herpes virus 2.	12,900 new cases; 7,000 estimated deaths.	*Staging:* (See Table 4.33, p. 437): *Stage 0*—carcinoma in situ; no distinct tumor observable; stage may last for 8–10 years; cure rate 100% following treatment of wedge or cone resection of cervix during childbearing years, or simple hysterectomy. *Stage I*—malignant cells infiltrate cervical mucosa; lesion bleeds easily; cure rate 80% with treatment of hysterectomy. *Stage II*—neoplasm spreads through cervical muscular layers, involves upper third of vaginal mucosa; cure rate 50% with treatment of radical hysterectomy. *Stage III*—neoplasm involves lower third of vagina; cure rate 25% with pelvic exoneration. *Stage IV*—involves metastasis to bladder, rectum, and surrounding tissues; considered incurable. *Radiation:* External and/or internal, in conjunction with surgery or alone, depending on stage of disease or condition of client (see nursing plan/implementation for client having radiation therapy, p. 430). *Chemotherapy:* progestin, antineoplastics, megestrol (Megace), Medroxyprogesterone (Curretab, Provera); alkylating agents—dacarbazine (DTIC).

■ EMERGENCY NURSING PROCEDURES

I. Purpose—to initiate assessment and intervention procedures that will speed total care of the client toward a successful outcome.

II. Emergency nursing procedures for adults are detailed in Table 4.35.

III. Legal issues in the emergency room—see Unit 8.

■ TABLE 4.35 Nursing Care of the Adult in Medical and Surgical Emergencies

Condition	Assessment: Signs and Symptoms	Prehospitalization Nursing Care	In-Hospital Nursing Care
Cardiovascular Emergencies			
Myocardial infarction—ischemia and necrosis of cardiac muscle secondary to insufficient or obstructed coronary blood flow.	*Prehospital:* *Chest pain:* vise-like choking, unrelieved by rest or nitroglycerin. *Skin:* ashen, cold, clammy. *Vital signs:* pulse—rapid, weak, thready; increased rate and depth of respirations; dyspnea. *Behavior:* restless, anxious. *In hospital:* *C/V:* blood pressure and pulse pressure decreased. *Heart sounds:* soft; S_3 may be present. *Respirations:* fine basilar rales. *Lab:* ECG consistent with tissue necrosis (Q waves) and injury (ST-segment elevation). Serum enzymes elevated.	1. If coronary suspected, call physician, paramedic service, or emergency ambulance. 2. Calm and reassure client that help is coming. 3. Place in semi-Fowler's position. 4. Keep client warm but not hot.	1. Rapidly assess hemodynamic and respiratory status. 2. Start IV as ordered—usually 5% D/W per microdrip to establish lifeline for emergency drug treatment. 3. Draw blood for electrolytes, enzymes, as ordered. 4. Place on cardiac monitor. 5. Relieve pain—morphine SO_4 IV as needed. 7. Take 12-lead ECG. Once client is stable, transfer to CCU.
Cardiac arrest—cardiac stenosis or ventricular fibrillation secondary to rapid administration or overdose of anesthetics or narcotic drugs, obstruction of the respiratory tract (mucus, vomitus, foreign body), acute anxiety, cardiac disease, dehydration, shock, electric shock, or emboli.	Cyanosis, gasping. *Respirations:* rapid, shallow, absent. *Pulse:* weak, thready, >120, absent. Muscle twitching. *Pupils:* dilated. *Skin:* cold, clammy. Loss of consciousness.	*CPR* 1. *Position:* flat on back. 2. Shake vigorously—establish unresponsiveness. 3. Call for help. 4. Tilt head back (chin lift). 5. Check for breathing—listen at mouth, look at chest, feel with cheek. *No breathing* 1. Kneel close to head. Place hand on forehead, bringing lower jaw forward and opening airway. 2. Pinch nostrils shut and blow two full breaths into client's mouth. 3. Lips must form airtight seal. 4. Watch chest for adequate expansion. Clear throat if indicated. 5. Check pulse—if present, breathe into mouth every 5 seconds.	1. If monitored, note rhythm. Call for help and note time. 2. Countershock if rhythm is ventricular fibrillation or ventricular tachycardia. 3. If countershock unsuccessful, begin CPR, as in prehospital care.

continued

■ **TABLE 4.35 *(Continued)***

Condition	Assessment: Signs and Symptoms	Prehospitalization Nursing Care	In-Hospital Nursing Care
Cardiovascular Emergencies (cont.)			
Cardiac arrest (cont.)		*No heartbeat* *Two-person CPR:* 80 chest compressions per minute, with one breath between every 5 compressions. *One-person CPR:* 80 chest compressions per minute, with two quick breaths between every 15 compressions. Check pulse at neck after 1 minute and every few minutes thereafter. Check pupils to determine effectiveness of CPR—should begin to constrict. *If heartbeat returns:* Assist respiration and monitor pulse. Continue CPR until help arrives.	*Two-person rescue* *First person:* begins CPR as described in prehospital care. *Second person:* 1. Pages arrest team. 2. Brings defibrillator to bedside and countershocks, if indicated by rhythm. 3. Brings emergency cart to bedside. 4. Suctions airway, if indicated due to vomitus or secretions. 5. Bags client with 100% O_2. 6. Assists with intubation when arrest team arrives. 7. Establishes intravenous line if one is not available.
Shock—cellular hypoxia and impairment of cellular function secondary to: trauma, hemorrhage, fright, dehydration, cardiac insufficiency, allergic reactions, septicemia, impairment of nervous system, poisons.	*Early shock* *Sensorium:* conscious, apprehensive, and restless; some slurring of speech. *Pupils:* dull but reactive to light. *Pulse:* rate <140/min; amplitude full to mildly decreased. *Blood pressure:* normal to slightly decreased. *Neck veins:* normal to slightly flat in supine position. May be full in septic shock or grossly distended in cardiogenic shock. *Skin:* cool, clammy, pale. *Respirations:* rapid, shallow. *GI:* nausea, vomiting, thirst. *Renal:* urine output 20–40 cc/hour.	1. Check breathing—clear airway if necessary. If no breathing, give artificial respirations. If breathing is irregular or labored, raise head and shoulders. 2. Control bleeding by placing pressure on the wound or at pressure points (proximal artery). 3. Make comfortable and reassure. 4. Cover lightly to prevent heat loss, but don't bundle up. 5. If you suspect neck or spine injury—do *not* move, unless victim in danger of more injury. If patient unconscious or has wounds of the lower face and jaw—place on *side* to promote drainage of fluids. Position client on *back* unless otherwise indicated.	1. Check vital signs rapidly—pulse, pupils, respirations. 2. Check airway; clear if necessary. Po_2 should be maintained above 60 mm Hg. Elevated Pco_2 indicates need for intubation and ventilatory assistance. 3. Control gross bleeding. 4. Prepare for insertion of intravenous line and central lines—if abdominal injuries present. 5. Peripheral line should be placed in upper extremity if fluids being lost in abdomen. 1. Draw blood for specimens: Hgb, Hct, CBC, glucose, CO_2, sodium amylase, BUN, K^+; type and cross-match, blood gases, enzymes, prothrombin times. 2. Prepare infusion of 5% D/NS *unless* hypernatremia suspected. Dextran if blood loss.

continued

ADULT NURSING

TABLE 4.35 *(Continued)* Nursing Care of the Adult in Medical and Surgical Emergencies

Condition	Assessment: Signs and Symptoms	Prehospitalization Nursing Care	In-Hospital Nursing Care
Cardiovascular Emergencies (cont.)			
Shock (cont.)	*Severe or late shock* *Sensorium:* confused, disoriented, apathetic, unresponsive; slow, slurred speech, often incoherent. *Pupils:* dilating, dilated, slow or nonreactive to light. *Pulse:* rate >150/min, thready, weak. *Blood pressure:* 80 mm Hg or unobtainable. *Neck veins:* flat in a supine position—no filling. Full to distended in septic or cardiogenic shock. *Skin:* cold, clammy, mottled; circumoral cyanosis, dusky, cyanotic. *Eyes:* sunken—vacant expression. *Renal:* urine output <20 cc/h.	1. *Raise* feet 6–8 inches unless client has head or chest injuries. If victim becomes less comfortable, lower feet. 2. If client complains of thirst, do *not* give fluids unless you are more than 6 hours away from professional medical help. Under *no* conditions give water to clients who are unconscious, having seizures or vomiting, appearing to need general anesthetic, or with a stomach, chest, or skull injury. 3. Be calm and confident; reassure client help is on the way.	1. Assess and intervene as above; then obtain information as to onset and past history. 2. Catheterize and monitor urine output as ordered. 3. Take 12-lead ECG. 4. Insert nasogastric tube and assess aspirate for volume, color, and blood. Save specimen if poison or drug overdose suspected. 5. *If CVP low*—infuse 200–300 mL over 5–10 min. *If CVP rises* sharply, fluid restriction necessary. If remains low, hypovolemia present. 6. If client febrile—blood cultures and wound cultures will be ordered. 7. If urine output scanty or absent—give mannitol as ordered.
Respiratory Emergencies			
Choking—obstruction of airway secondary to aspiration of a foreign object.	Gasping, wheezing. Looks panicky, but can still breathe, talk, cough. Cough: weak, ineffective; breathing sounds like high-pitched crowing; color—white, gray, blue. Difficulty speaking; clutches throat.	Do not interfere; watch closely; call for assistance. *Victim standing, sitting and conscious.* Perform *Heimlich maneuver:* stand behind victim, wrap arms around waist, place fist against abdomen, and with your other hand, press it into the victim's abdomen with a quick upward thrust until the obstruction is relieved or the victim becomes unconscious.	As in prehospital care. Do *not* slap on back.
		Victim lying down: Roll the victim onto his or her back. Straddle the victim's thighs. Place heel of hand in the middle of abdomen. Place other hand on top of the first; stiffen arms and deliver 6–10 abdominal thrusts.	As in prehospital care.
		Unconscious victim: Try to ventilate. If unsuccessful, deliver abdominal thrusts using technique described above. Probe mouth for foreign objects. Keep repeating above procedure until ventilation occurs. As victim becomes more deprived of air, muscles will relax and maneuvers that were previously unsuccessful will begin to work. When successful in removing obstruction, give two breaths. Check pulse. Start CPR if indicated. On obese or pregnant victims—use chest thrusts instead of abdominal thrusts.	As in prehospital care. When probing mouth for foreign object, turn head to side, unless client has neck injury. In event of neck injury, raise the arm opposite you and roll the head and shoulders as a unit, so that head ends up supported on the arm.

continued

■ TABLE 4.35 *(Continued)*

Condition	Assessment: Signs and Symptoms	Prehospitalization Nursing Care	In-Hospital Nursing Care
Respiratory Emergencies (cont.)			
Choking (cont.)		*You are victim and alone:* Place your two fists for abdominal thrusts. Bend over back of chair, sink, etc. and exert hard, repeated pressure on abdomen to force object up. Push fingers down your throat to encourage regurgitation.	
Acute respiratory failure—sudden onset of an abnormally low P_{O_2} (<60 mm Hg) and/or high P_{CO_2} (>60 mm Hg) secondary to lung disease or trauma, peripheral or central nervous system depression, cardiac failure, severe obesity, airway obstruction, environmental abnormality.	*Hypoxia* *Sensorium:* acute apprehension. *Respiration:* dyspnea; shallow, rapid respirations. *Skin:* circumoral cyanosis; pale, dusky skin and nailbeds. *C/V:* slight hypertension and tachycardia, or hypotension and bradycardia. *Hypercardia* *Sensorium:* decreasing mentation; headache. *Skin:* flushed, warm, moist. *C/V:* hypertension; tachycardia.	If you suspect respiratory distress, call physician. Calm and reassure client. Place in a chair or semi-sitting position. Keep warm but not hot. Phone for ambulance. If respirations cease or client becomes unconscious, clear airway and commence respiratory resuscitation. Check pulse: initiate CPR if necessary. Continue resuscitation until help arrives.	Check client's ability to speak. Maintain airway by placing in *high Fowler's* position. Check vital signs: BP, pulse rate and rhythm, temperature, skin color, rate and depth of respirations. Prepare for intubation if: 1. Client has flail chest. 2. Client is comatose without gag reflex. 3. Has respiratory arrest. Maintain mouth to mouth until intubation. 4. P_{CO_2}>55 mm Hg. 5. P_{O_2}<60 mm Hg. 6. F_1O_2>50% using nasal cannula, catheter, or mask. 7. Respiratory rate >36. *After intubation:* 1. Check bilateral lung sounds. 2. Observe for symmetrical lung expansion. 3. Maintain humidified oxygen at lowest F_1O_2 possible to achieve P_{O_2} of 60 mm Hg. *Improve ventilation (decreased P_{CO_2}) by:* 1. Liquefying secretions—oral and parenteral fluids. If intubated, frequent instillations of normal saline or sodium bicarbonate. 2. Frequent suctioning. 3. IPPB indicated if tidal volume ↓. 4. Chest physiotherapy. Administer *drugs* as ordered: sympathomimetics, xanthines, antibiotics, and steroids. Monitor: arterial blood gases, electrolytes, Hct, Hb, and WBC. *Do not:* 1. Administer sedatives. 2. Correct acid-base problems without monitoring electrolytes. 3. Overcorrect P_{CO_2}. 4. Leave client alone while oxygen therapy is initiated. Once client is stable, transfer to ICU.

continued

TABLE 4.35 *(Continued)* **Nursing Care of the Adult in Medical and Surgical Emergencies**

Condition	Assessment: Signs and Symptoms	Prehospitalization Nursing Care	In-Hospital Nursing Care
Respiratory Emergencies (cont.)			
Near-drowning—asphyxiation or partial asphyxiation due to immersion or submersion in a fluid or liquid medium.	*Conscious victim* Acute anxiety, panic. Increased rate of respirations. Pale, dusky skin. *Unconscious victim* Shallow or no respirationss. Weak or no pulse. If victim not breathing, as soon as you have firm support begin mouth-to-mouth resuscitation. Tilt head back, bring jaw forward, pinch nostril shut, give two quick breaths.	*Conscious victim* 1. Try to talk victim out of panic so can find footing and way to shore. 2. Utilize devices such as poles, rings, clothing to extend to victim. Do not let panicked victim grab you. Do not attempt swimming rescue unless specially trained. 3. If you suspect head or neck injury—handle carefully, floating victim back to shore with body and head as straight as possible. Do not turn head or bend back. *On shore:* 1. Check breathing. 2. Lay victim flat on back. Cover and keep warm. 3. Calm and reassure victim. 4. Do not give food or water. 5. Get to medical assistance as soon as possible. 6. *If unconscious and not breathing,* begin sequence for CPR. Compress water from abdomen *only* if interfering with ventilation attempts. 7. *If airway obstructed,* reposition head. Attempt to ventilate. Perform 6–10 abdominal thrusts. Sweep mouth deeply. Attempt to ventilate. Repeat until successful. 8. Once ventilation established, check pulse. If absent, begin chest compressions as in CPR, one-person or two-person rescue. 9. Continue CPR until victim revives or help arrives. 10. If victim revives, cover and keep warm. Reassure victim help is on the way. 11. Rescue personnel can further assist emergency room personnel by: a. Documenting prehospital resuscitation methods used. b. Immobilizing victims suspected of cervical spine injuries. c. Utilizing a sterile container to take a sample of immersion fluid. d. Taking on-scene arterial blood gas sample for later analysis.	*Nonsymptomatic near-drowning victim* 1. Draw blood for arterial blood gases with client breathing room air. 2. PA and lateral chest X ray. 3. Auscultate lungs. 4. Admit to hospital for further evaluation if: a. $Po_2 < 80$ mm Hg. b. pH$<$7.35. c. Pulmonary infiltrates present, or auscultation reveals rales. d. Victim inhaled fluids containing: chlorine, hydrocarbons, sewage, or hypotonic or fresh water. *Symptomatic near-drowning victim* 1. Provide basic or advanced cardiac life support. 2. Provide clear airway and adequate ventilation by: a. Suctioning airway. b. Inserting artificial airway and attaching it to ventilator as indicated. c. Inserting nasogastric tube to suction to minimize aspiration of vomitus. 3. Monitor ECG continuously. 4. Start IV infusion 5% D/W at keep-open rate for *fresh water near-drowning.* 5% D/NS in *salt water near-drowning.* 5. Assist with insertion of CVP and Swan-Ganz catheter to guide subsequent infusion rates. 6. Administer drugs as ordered: anticonvulsants; steroids, antibiotics, stimulants, antiarrhythmics. 7. Provide rewarming if hypothermia present. 8. Insert Foley to assess kidney output as fresh water near-drowning causes renal tubular necrosis due to RBC hemolysis. 9. Transfer to ICU when stabilized.

continued

ADULT NURSING

■ **TABLE 4.35 *(Continued)***

Condition	Assessment: Signs and Symptoms	Prehospitalization Nursing Care	In-Hospital Nursing Care
Systemic Injuries			
Multiple traumas	*Sensorium:* alert; disoriented, stuporous, comatose. *Respirations:* increased rate, depth; shallow; asymmetric; paradoxical breathing; mediastinal shift; gasping, blowing. *C/V:* signs of shock (see above). *Abdomen:* contusions; pain; abrasions; open wounds; rigidity; increasing distention. *Skeletal system:* pain; swelling; deformity; inappropriate or no movement. *Neurologic:* pupils round, equal, react to light; ipsilateral dilatation and unresponsive; fixed and dilated bilaterally. Bilateral movement and sensation in all extremities. Progressive contralateral weakness. Loss of voluntary motor function. See *Sensorium* above for level of consciousness.	1. *Don't* move client unless you must, to prevent further injury. Send for help. 2. Check breathing—give mouth-to-mouth resuscitation if indicated. 3. Check for bleeding. 4. Control bleeding by applying pressure on wound or on pressure points (artery proximal to wound). 5. Use tourniquet *only* if above pressure techniques fail to stop severe bleeding. 6. Check for shock (pulse, pupils, skin color) and other inujuries. 7. Fractures: keep open-fracture area clean. 8. Stop bleeding, observe for shock. 9. Do not try to set bone. 10. If client must be moved—splint broken bones with splints that extend past the limb joints. Tie splints on snugly but not so tight as to cut off circulation. 11. Check peripheral pulses. 12. If head or back injury suspected—keep body straight. Move only with help. 13. Reassure client that help is on the way.	1. Assess vital functions. 2. Establish airway; ventilate with ambu-bag, volume-cycled ventilator. 3. Draw arterial blood gases. 4. Control bleeding. 5. Support circulation by closed chest massage. 6. Prepare infusions of dextran, blood, crystalloids. 7. Assess for other injuries: head injuries—suspect cervical neck injury with all head injuries. 8. Place sandbags to immobilize head and neck. 9. Do *mini-neurologic exam:* level of consciousness, pupils, bilateral movement, and sensation. 10. Get history—time of injury; any loss of consciousness; any drug ingestion. 11. Stop bleeding on or about head. 12. Apply ice to contusions and hematomas. 13. Check for bleeding from nose, pharynx, ears. 14. Check for cerebrospinal fluid from ears or nose. 15. Assist with spinal tap if ordered. 16. Keep accurate I&O. 17. Protect from injury if restless; seizures: orient to time, place, person. 18. Administer steroids, diuretics, as ordered. 19. *Check for signs of increasing intracranial pressure:* slowing pulse and respiration, widened pulse pressure, decreasing mentation.
Spinal injuries			1. Assess and support vital functions as above. 2. Immobilize—no flexion or extension allowed. 3. If in respiratory distress—nasotracheal intubation or tracheostomy to avoid hyperextending neck. 4. *Check for level of injury and function,* asking client to: a. Lift elbow to shoulder height (C_5). b. Bend elbow (C_6). c. Straighten elbow (C_7). d. Grip your hand (C_8–T_1). e. Lift leg (L_3). f. Straighten knee (L_4, L_5). g. Wiggle toes (L_5). h. Push toes down (S_1).

continued

TABLE 4.35 *(Continued)* Nursing Care of the Adult in Medical and Surgical Emergencies

Condition	Assessment: Signs and Symptoms	Prehospitalization Nursing Care	In-Hospital Nursing Care
Systemic Injuries (cont.)			
Spinal injuries (cont.)			5. If client comatose: a. Rub sternum with knuckles. b. If all extremities move, severe injury unlikely. c. If one side moves and other does not, potential hemiplegia. d. If arms move and legs don't, lower spinal cord injury. 6. Administer steroids as ordered. 7. Assist with application of skull tongs—Vinke or Crutchfield. 8. Maintain IV infusions. 9. Insert Foley as indicated. 10. Assist with dressing of open wounds.
Chest injuries			1. Note color and pattern of respirations, position of trachea. 2. Auscultate lungs and palpate chest for: crepitus, pain, tenderness, and position of trachea. 3. Chest tubes if pneumothorax or hemothorax present. 4. Place gauze soaked in petroleum jelly over open pneumothorax (sucking chest wound) to seal hole and decrease respiratory distress. 5. Assist with tracheostomy if indicated.
Abdominal injuries			1. Observe for rigidity. 2. Check for hematuria. 3. Auscultate for bowel sounds. 4. Assist with paracentesis to confirm bleeding in abdominal cavity. 5. Prepare for exploratory laparotomy. 6. Insert nasogastric tube—to detect presence of UGI bleeding. 7. Monitor vital signs. *If organs protruding:* 1. Flex client's knees. 2. Cover intestines with sterile towel soaked in saline. 3. Do not attempt to replace organs.
Fractures			1. Administer tetanus toxoid as ordered. 2. Observe for: pain, peripheral pulses, pallor, loss of sensation and/or movement. 3. Assist with wound cleansing, casting, X rays, reduction. 4. Prepare for surgery if indicated. 5. Monitor vital signs.

continued

■ TABLE 4.35 *(Continued)*

Condition	Assessment: Signs and Symptoms	Prehospitalization Nursing Care	In-Hospital Nursing Care
Systemic Injuries (cont.)			
Burns—tissue trauma secondary to scalding fluid or flame, chemicals, or electricity.	*First degree:* Erythema and tenderness. Usually sunburn.	Relieve pain by applying cold, wet towel or cold water (not iced).	1. Cleanse thoroughly with mild detergent and water. 2. Apply gauze or sterile towel. 3. Administer sedatives and narcotics as ordered. 4. Arrange for follow-up care, or prepare for admission if burn ambulatory care impractical.
	Second degree: Swelling, blisters. Moisture due to escaping plasma.	1. Douse with cold water until pain relieved. 2. Blot skin dry and cover with clean towel. 3. Do *not* break blisters, remove pieces of skin, or apply antiseptic ointments. 4. If arm or leg burned, keep *elevated.* 5. Seek medical attention if *second degree* burns: a. Cover 15% of body surface in adult. b. Cover 10% of body surface in children. c. Involve hands, feet, or face.	1. Check tetanus immunization status. 2. Administer sedatives or narcotics as ordered. 3. Assess respiratory and hemodynamic status; oxygen or ventilatory assist as indicated, intravenous infusions as ordered to combat shock. 4. Remove all clothing from burn area. 5. Using aseptic technique, cleanse burns with antiseptic followed by soap and water, and irrigate with normal saline.
	Third degree: White, charred areas.	1. *Don't* remove charred clothing. 2. Cover burned area with clean towel, sheet. 3. *Elevate* burned extremities. 4. Apply cold pack to hand, face, or feet. 5. Sit up client with face or chest wound to assist respirations. 6. Maintain airway. 7. Observe for shock. 8. *Do not:* a. Put ice water on burns or immerse wounds in ice water—may increase shock. b. Apply ointments. 9. Calm and reassure victim. 10. Get medical help promptly. 11. *If* client conscious, not vomiting, and medical assistance is more than 6 hours away: may give sips of weak solution of salt, soda, and water.	1. Do not break blebs or attempt debridement. 2. Assist with application of dressings as ordered. 3. Maintain frequent checks of: vital signs, urine output. 4. Provide psychologic support—explain procedures, orient, etc. 5. Assist with application of splints as ordered. 6. Administer tetanus immune globulin or toxoid as ordered. 7. Assist with transfer to hospital unit.
	Chemical burns	1. Flush with copious amounts of water. 2. Get rid of clothing over burned area.	1. Flush with copious amounts of water. 2. Administer sedation or narcotics as ordered.
	Burns of the eye: Acid	1. Flush eye with water for at least 15 minutes. 2. Pour water from inside to outside of eye to avoid contaminating unaffected eye. 3. Cover—seek medical attention at once.	1. Irrigate with water. *Never* use neutralizing solution. 2. Instill 0.5% tetracaine as ordered. 3. Apply patch.

continued

ADULT NURSING

ADULT NURSING

■ **TABLE 4.35 *(Continued)*** **Nursing Care of the Adult in Medical and Surgical Emergencies**

Condition	Assessment: Signs and Symptoms	Prehospitalization Nursing Care	In-Hospital Nursing Care
Systemic Injuries (cont.)			
Burns (cont.)	Alkali (laundry detergent or cleaning solvent)	1. Don't allow client to rub eye. 2. Flush eye with water for at least 30 minutes. 3. Cover—seek medical attention at once.	As above for acid.
Abdominal Emergencies			
Aortic aneurysm—rupture or dissection.	Primarily males over age 60. Sudden onset of excruciating pain: abdominal, lumbosacral, groin, or rectal. Orthopnea, dyspnea. Fainting, hypotension. If dissecting, marked hypertension may be present. Palpable, tender, pulsating mass in umbilical area. Femoral pulse present. Dorsalis pedes—weak or absent.	1. Notify physician. 2. Lay client flat, or raise head if in respiratory distress. 3. Cover—keep warm but not hot. 4. Institute shock measures as above. 5. Calm; reassure that help is on the way.	1. Assess respiratory and hemodynamic status. 2. Institute shock measures as above if indicated. 3. Evaluate and compare peripheral pulses. 4. Assist with X rays. 5. Assist with emergency preoperative treatment.
Blunt injuries—Spleen	Left upper quadrant pain, tenderness and moderate rigidity. Left shoulder pain (*Kehr's sign*). Hypotension; weak, thready pulse; increased respirations (shock).	1. Lay client *flat*. 2. Institute shock measures as above.	1. Assess respiratory and hemodynamic status. a. Maintain airway and ventilation as indicated. b. Institute infusions of colloids and/or crystalloids as ordered. c. Insert both CVP and arterial monitoring lines. d. Insert Foley catheter. 2. Prepare for splenectomy.
Eye and Ear Emergencies			
Chemical burns	See *Burns*.	See *Burns*.	See *Burns*.
Blunt injuries secondary to flying missiles, e.g., balls, striking face against car dashboard.	Decreased visual acuity, diplopia, blood in anterior chamber. Pain, conjunctiva reddened, edema of eyelids.	1. Prevent victim from rubbing eye. 2. Cover with patch to protect eye. 3. Seek medical help immediately.	1. Test visual acuity of each eye using Snellen or Jaeger chart. 2. Assist with fluorescein administration—to facilitate identifying breaks in cornea.
Sharp ocular trauma—secondary to small or larger foreign bodies.	History of feeling as if something were hitting eye. Pain, tearing, reddened conjunctiva. Blurring of vision. Foreign object may be visible.	1. Keep victim from rubbing eye. 2. Cover very lightly—do not apply pressure.	1. Check visual acuity in both eyes. 2. Check pupils. 3. Instill 1% tetracaine HCl as ordered to relieve pain. 4. Administer antibiotic drops or ointment as ordered. 5. Apply eye patch. 6. Provide instructions for subsequent care and follow-up.
Foreign bodies in ears—beans, peas, candy, foxtails, insects.	Decreased hearing; pulling, poking at ear and ear canal; buzzing, discomfort.	1. Do *not* attempt to remove object. 2. Seek medical assistance.	1. Inspect ear canal. 2. Assist with sedating children—restraint may be necessary. 3. Assist with procedures to remove object: a. Forceps or curved probe for *foxtails, irregularly shaped* objects. b. #10 or #12 French catheter with tip cut squarely off and attached to suction to remove *round* object.

continued

■ **TABLE 4.35 *(Continued)***

Condition	Assessment: Signs and Symptoms	Prehospitalization Nursing Care	In-Hospital Nursing Care
Eye and Ear Emergencies (cont.)			
Foreign bodies in ears (cont.)			4. Irrigate external auditory canal to flush out *insects,* materials that do not absorb water. Do *not* irrigate if danger of perforation.

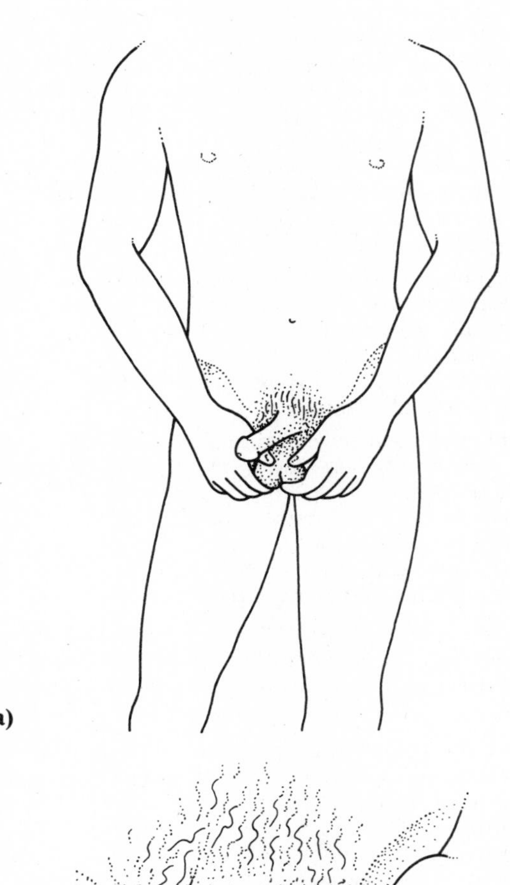

(a)

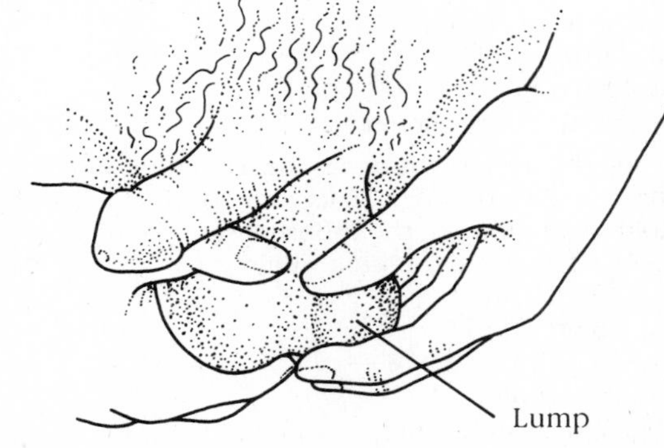

(b)

■ **FIGURE 4.8**
Testicular self-examination. (a) Grasp testis with both hands; palpate gently between thumb and fingers. (b) Abnormal lumps or irregularities are reported to physician. (From Fred Hutchinson Cancer Research Center, Cancer Control Program, Seattle, 1980, in Phipps WJ, et al.: *Medical-Surgical Nursing,* Mosby, St. Louis, 1987.)

■ QUESTIONS

Select the one best answer for each question, and fill in the answer circle beside the answer number.

Gladys Meeker is a 30-year-old advertising executive with a history of ulcerative colitis since age 22. Her chief complaint is severe abdominal cramping and 18–20 stools a day for 4 days. After 10 days of therapy, Ms. Meeker's physician decided to perform an ileostomy. For 3 days prior to surgery she was given neomycin. On the morning of surgery she was catheterized and a nasogastric tube was inserted.

1. Which of the following nursing interventions would be the most beneficial in preparing Ms. Meeker psychologically for this surgery?
○ 1. Include her family in preoperative teaching sessions. **PL 8**
○ 2. Encourage her to express her concerns and to ask questions regarding the management of the ileostomy. **PsI**
○ 3. Thorough, brief explanation of all preoperative and postoperative procedures.
○ 4. Have a member of an "ostomy club" visit her.

2. Two days postoperatively, Ms. Meeker begins to refuse care and repeatedly says to the staff, "Leave me alone, I just want to sleep." What would be your first nursing action?
○ 1. Provide accurate, brief, and reassuring explanations of all procedures. **IMP 8**
○ 2. Encourage ambulation in the hall with other clients. **PsI**
○ 3. Invite a member of an "ostomy club" to visit Ms. Meeker.
○ 4. Encourage Ms. Meeker to verbalize her feelings, fears, and questions.

Mrs. Dixon, a 35-year-old mother, was admitted with dysmenorrhea and excessive vaginal bleeding. A diagnostic D&C discovered uterine fibroid tumors. A hysterectomy was discussed and a decision to go home was made for child care arrangements. That night she experienced excessive vaginal bleeding and feelings of extreme weakness. She was readmitted at 2:00 A.M. after being examined by the ER physician. An emergency hysterectomy was performed. Her vital signs were: BP 94/60, apical pulse 126, respirations 28. Laboratory data: Hct 30%, Hgb 8.5.

3. On the morning of discharge, Mrs. Dixon is found sitting with her back to the door, staring out the window. She says that she no longer feels like a real woman. Your response should be to:
○ 1. Ask her if she would like her Valium. **IMP**

ADULT NURSING

○ 2. Notify the physician. **7**
○ 3. Ask, "Can you tell me what makes you feel that way?" **PsI**
○ 4. Reassure her that this is a common reaction.

Mr. Maestas, a 70-year-old Hispanic, sustained second-degree burns on his left leg and thigh when his pants caught fire while he was burning leaves. Vital signs were BP 96/70, pulse 116, respirations 26. Mr. Maestas was also restless and disoriented.

4. Burns are classified according to the depth of tissue destruction. You would recognize a second-degree burn because the burn:
○ 1. Involves the epidermis only. **AS**
○ 2. Extends to the dermis and is very painful. **1**
○ 3. Extends to subcutaneous tissues and is rarely painful. **PhI**
○ 4. Extends to muscle and bone and is very painful.

5. Equally important in determining severity of burns is the total body surface involved. The nurse would anticipate potential fluid and electrolyte problems when burns:
○ 1. Are first-degree and cover 20% of the body surface. **AN** **1**
○ 2. Are second-degree and cover 15% of the body surface. **PhI**
○ 3. Are third-degree and cover 10% of the body surface.
○ 4. Are fourth-degree and cover 5% of the body surface.

6. Besides assessing size and depth of the burn, which of the following physical parameters are also important baseline data for fluid replacement therapy?
○ 1. Age, sex, and vital signs. **AS**
○ 2. Age, weight, vital signs, and skin turgor. **6**
○ 3. Vital signs, level of mentation, and urine output. **PhI**
○ 4. Vital signs and quantity and specific gravity of urine.

7. The nurse knows that the physiologic response to the stress of extensive burns may result in the following complication in the postburn period:
○ 1. Curling's ulcer due to elevated serum cortisol. **AN**
○ 2. Positive nitrogen balance due to mobilization of body proteins. **1** **PhI**
○ 3. Decreased hematocrit due to red-blood-cell agglutination by epinephrine.
○ 4. Hypo- and hyperthermia due to failure of hypothalamic temperature regulators.

Admission ER lab values for Mr. Maestas were: hematocrit 50%, hemoglobin 17.2 g, serum sodium 140 mEq/L, serum potassium 7.6 mEq/L.

8. The nurse would expect the serum-sodium level to be within normal limits at the time of admission because:
○ 1. The pituitary has increased ADH release. **AN**
○ 2. Vascular fluid losses due to exudate and edema formation have resulted in hemoconcentration. **6** **PhI**
○ 3. Sodium has diffused from disrupted cells into the vascular compartment.
○ 4. Increased serum potassium depressed aldosterone secretion by the adrenal cortex.

9. During a client conference on Mr. Maestas, you discuss how the sodium and potassium levels are affected by severe burns. Hyponatremia may develop in burn clients due to:
○ 1. Displacement of sodium in edema fluids and loss through denuded areas of skin. **AN** **6**
○ 2. Increased aldosterone secretion. **PhI**
○ 3. Inadequate fluid replacement.
○ 4. Metabolic acidosis.

10. You can expect hyperkalemia to develop following burn damage because there is:
○ 1. Increased exudate formation at the burn site. **AN**
○ 2. Disruption of cell membrane integrity, allowing intracellular electrolytes to diffuse into the vascular compartment. **6** **PhI**
○ 3. Decreased aldosterone secretion, increasing sodium excretion, and retention of potassium.
○ 4. Hyperbilirubinemia secondary to red blood cell destruction.

11. In planning for Mr. Maestas, the nurse knows that the treatment of choice to reduce hyperkalemia is:
○ 1. Morphine sulfate. **PL**
○ 2. Kayexalate. **6**
○ 3. Insulin and 50% glucose solution. **SECE**
○ 4. Synthetic aldosterone.

12. During the initial stage of burns, a primary fluid imbalance occurs. The nurse knows that there has been a shift of fluids from:
○ 1. The cell to the interstitial space. **AN**
○ 2. The interstitial space into the cell. **6**
○ 3. The interstitial space to the plasma. **PhI**
○ 4. The plasma to the interstitial space.

Nursing care in the immediate 24 hours postburn is directed toward monitoring adequacy of fluid therapy. Initial intravenous therapy may include both colloidal and crystalloid solutions.

13. Which of the following replacement fluids will the nurse *least* often be expected to administer to a burn patient?
○ 1. Ringer's lactate. **PL**
○ 2. Whole blood. **6**
○ 3. Dextran. **SECE**
○ 4. Dextrose and water.

14. Fluid therapy postburn may necessitate as much as 7 L of fluid in 24 hours for a 70 kg individual. Using a 15-gtt/cc administration set, the drops per minute that you would set to deliver this volume would be:
○ 1. 48 gtt/min. **IMP**
○ 2. 75 gtt/min. **6**
○ 3. 60 gtt/min. **PhI**
○ 4. 90 gtt/min.

15. The adequacy of fluid volume replacement in the early postburn period is best reflected by:
○ 1. Blood pressure, pulse rates, and daily weights. **EV**

Key to codes following questions Nursing process: **AS**, Assessment; **AN**, Analysis; **PL**, Plan; **IMP**, Implementation; **EV**, Evaluation. Category of human function: **1**, Protective; **2**, Sensory-perceptual; **3**, Comfort, Rest, Activity, and Mobility; **4**, Nutrition; **5**, Growth and Development; **6**, Fluid-Gas Transport; **7**, Psycho-Social-Cultural; **8**, Elimination. Client need: **SECE**, Safe, Effective Care Environment; **PhI**, Physiological Integrity; **PsI**, Psychosocial Integrity; **HPM**, Health Promotion/Maintenance. See frontmatter for full explanation.

○ 2. Quantity of urinary output and vital signs. **6**
○ 3. Hemoglobin and hematocrit levels. **PhI**
○ 4. Serum-electrolyte levels and urinary output.

16. Fifty-four hours after Mr. Maestas sustained his burns, his urine output increased from 1000 mL/24 h to 2300 mL/24 h. Laboratory values were: serum sodium 136 mEq/L, serum potassium 4 mEq/L; hematocrit 34%. The nurse knows that the changes in Mr. Maestas' urinary output and lab studies indicate:
○ 1. Beginning of the interstitial-to-plasma fluid shift phase of burns. **AN 8**
○ 2. Kidney failure. **PhI**
○ 3. Circulatory overload due to rapid IV infusion rate.
○ 4. Hyponatremia.

17. The nurse knows that the hematocrit is reduced due to:
○ 1. Lack of erythropoietin factor. **AN**
○ 2. Hemodilution and volume overload. **6**
○ 3. Metabolic acidosis. **PhI**
○ 4. Hypoalbuminemia.

18. Mr. Maestas' burns were treated by the closed method. His left leg was cleaned and the left ankle debrided. Mafenide 1% (Sulfamylon) was applied, and his left leg was wrapped in fine mesh gauze. Nursing measures when this approach is used include:
○ 1. Cleansing of the wound daily and maintenance of strict isolation to prevent air contamination. **IMP 1**
○ 2. Cleansing of the wound daily, or more often if needed, and application of new dressings using clean technique. **PhI**
○ 3. Cleansing the wound one or more times each day and application of new dressing using sterile technique.
○ 4. Cleansing of the wound daily and utilization of heat lamps to help maintain normal body temperature.

19. The care plan includes observing for side effects of mafenide 1% (Sulfamylon), such as:
○ 1. Severe electrolyte disturbances. **PL**
○ 2. Metabolic acidosis. **1**
○ 3. Metabolic alkalosis. **PhI**
○ 4. Staining of linen.

20. Which of the following behaviors is *least* likely to be included in the nursing assessment of Mr. Maestas during his recovery period?
○ 1. Anxiety with mild confusion. **AS**
○ 2. Desperation and panic. **7**
○ 3. Withdrawal and depression. **PsI**
○ 4. Dependency and regression.

21. Mr. Maestas is withdrawn and depressed. The nurse can expect him to exhibit such psychologic reactions during the recuperative stage because of his:
○ 1. Pain and immobility. **AN**
○ 2. Changes in body image. **7**
○ 3. Financial concerns. **PsI**
○ 4. Anger.

Mr. Mangoni is a 51-year-old auto salesman admitted to your unit for recurrent complaints of burning epigastric pain, nausea and vomiting, and one episode of hemoptysis. He has been treated medically for gastric ulcer for the past year with antacids, antispasmodics, and an ulcer diet. He states he has had black stools two or three times in the past week, but he didn't really worry about it until he threw up blood this morning. A nasogastric tube was passed and attached to low intermittent suction. Gastric drainage resembles coffee grounds with a small amount of red blood.

22. The nurse's best explanation of the basic emotional issue underlying or contributing to the development of ulcers would be:
○ 1. Anxiety neurosis. **AN**
○ 2. Dependence-independence conflict. **7**
○ 3. Repressed anger and hostility. **PsI**
○ 4. Compulsive time orientation.

23. Forty-eight hours after admission, Mr. Mangoni is scheduled for an upper GI series. Nursing preparation for this procedure includes:
○ 1. Holding the client NPO for 24 hours before the procedure. **IMP 4**
○ 2. Administering an enema or cathartic to enhance visualization. **SECE**
○ 3. Discouraging the client from smoking the morning of the procedure because smoking can stimulate gastric motility.
○ 4. Instructing the client that the test involves insertion of a rubber gastroscopy tube.

24. Mr. Mangoni's barium X ray revealed a large cavitation in the antral portion of the stomach and scarring of the pyloric sphincter. The physician ordered a gastroscopy for the following day. Nursing preparations for this procedure include:
○ 1. Holding the client NPO for 24 hours before the procedure. **IMP 4**
○ 2. Having an operative or procedure permit signed. **PhI**
○ 3. Reassuring the client that gastroscopy is not an uncomfortable procedure, though he will need to lie quietly.
○ 4. Removing dentures and administering pain medication prior to the procedure.

Following these diagnostic tests, Mr. Mangoni's physician discussed possible therapies with him. It was decided that a partial gastrectomy, vagotomy, and gastrojejunostomy would be performed.

25. Mr. Mangoni asks why the vagotomy is being done. You explain that a vagotomy is done in conjunction with a subtotal gastrectomy because the vagus nerve:
○ 1. Stimulates increased gastric motility. **AN**
○ 2. Decreases gastric motility, thereby preventing the movement of HCl out of the stomach. **4 SECE**
○ 3. Stimulates both increased gastric secretion and gastric motility.
○ 4. Stimulates decreased gastric secretion, thereby increasing nausea and vomiting.

26. Which of the following nursing interventions would be included in the preoperative period for Mr. Mangoni?
○ 1. Insertion of a nasogastric tube on the morning of surgery. **PL 1**
○ 2. Administration of Valium 4 mg with 4 oz water 1 hour before surgery. **PhI**
○ 3. Detailed description of the possible complications that could happen postoperatively.
○ 4. Instructions to avoid taking pain medication too frequently in the first 2 postoperative days to avoid drug dependency.

27. Which of the following complications would you primarily anticipate in Mr. Mangoni's postoperative period?
○ 1. Thrombophlebitis from decreased mobility. **PL**

ADULT NURSING

○ 2. Abdominal distention due to air-swallowing. **1**
○ 3. Atelectasis due to shallow breathing. **PhI**
○ 4. Urinary retention due to prolonged use of anticholinergic medications.

28. The nurse would recognize drainage of blood from the nasogastric tube after surgery as abnormal if:
○ 1. It continued after 6 hours. **AN**
○ 2. It continued for a period greater than 12 hours. **1**
○ 3. It turned greenish yellow in less than 24 hours. **PhI**
○ 4. It was dark red in the immediate postoperative period.

29. Which of the following statements would the nurse include in teaching regarding nasogastric tubes?
○ 1. Nasogastric tubes should be irrigated with sterile water. **IMP** **4**
○ 2. Client should be in a sitting position with head slightly flexed for tube insertion. **SECE**
○ 3. When resistance is met while irrigating a nasogastric tube, pressure should be increased to complete that irrigation, and the physician should be notified at the completion.
○ 4. Ice chips can be taken as often as desired to promote comfort in the throat.

30. The nurse must observe for which of the following imbalances to occur with prolonged nasogastric suctioning?
○ 1. Hypernatremia. **AN**
○ 2. Hyperkalemia. **4**
○ 3. Metabolic alkalosis. **PhI**
○ 4. Hypoproteinemia.

31. Of the following mouth care measures by the nurse, which one should be used with caution when a client has a nasogastric tube?
○ 1. Regularly brushing teeth and tongue with soft brush. **PL** **1**
○ 2. Sucking on ice chips to relieve dryness. **PhI**
○ 3. Occasionally rinsing mouth with a nonastringent substance and massaging gums.
○ 4. Application of lemon juice and glycerine swabs to the lips.

32. The nurse tells Mr. Mangoni that the nasogastric tube will be removed:
○ 1. Standardly on the fourth postoperative day. **EV**
○ 2. When bowel sounds are established and the client has passed flatus or stool. **8** **SECE**
○ 3. Thirty-six hours after the cessation of bloody drainage.
○ 4. After 2 days of alternate clamping and unclamping of the tube.

33. Following surgery the nurse must observe for signs of pernicious anemia, which may be a problem after gastrectomy because:
○ 1. The extrinsic factor is produced in the stomach. **PL** **4**
○ 2. The extrinsic factor is absorbed in the antral portion of the stomach. **PhI**
○ 3. The intrinsic factor is produced in the stomach.
○ 4. Decreased hydrochloric acid production inhibits vitamin B_{12} reabsorption.

34. The nurse will usually ambulate the postgastrectomy patient beginning:
○ 1. The day after surgery. **PL**
○ 2. Three to four days after surgery. **3**
○ 3. After 4 days bedrest. **PhI**
○ 4. Immediately upon awakening.

35. The nurse tells Mr. Mangoni that dumping syndrome is a significant problem for:
○ 1. 70–80% of clients having gastrectomies. **AN**
○ 2. 50% of clients having gastrectomies. **4**
○ 3. 25% of clients having gastrectomies. **SECE**
○ 4. 5–10% of clients having gastrectomies.

36. Small, frequent feedings of which type of diet would the nurse recommend for clients experiencing dumping syndrome?
○ 1. Low-protein, high-fat, low-carbohydrate diet. **PL**
○ 2. High-protein, high-fat, high-carbohydrate diet. **4**
○ 3. High-protein, high-fat, low-carbohydrate diet. **PhI**
○ 4. Low-protein, low-fat, high-carbohydrate diet.

37. Clients suffering from dumping syndrome should be advised by the nurse to:
○ 1. Drink liquids between meals. **PL**
○ 2. Drink liquids only with meals. **4**
○ 3. Drink liquids any time they want. **PhI**
○ 4. Restrict fluid intake to 1200 cc per day.

38. Which of the following would the nurse expect to see with the dumping syndrome?
○ 1. Feeling of hunger. **AS**
○ 2. Constipation. **4**
○ 3. Increased strength. **PhI**
○ 4. Diaphoresis.

39. Before discharge Mr. Mangoni asks you pointedly, "How long will it be before I can eat three meals a day like the rest of my family?" You respond:
○ 1. "Eating six meals a day can be a bother, can't it?" **IMP** **4**
○ 2. "Some clients can tolerate three meals a day by the time they leave the hospital. It seems it will be a little longer for you." **PhI**
○ 3. "You will probably have to eat six meals a day for the rest of your life."
○ 4. "It varies from client to client, but generally in 6–12 months most clients can return to their previous meal patterns."

Mr. Victor Cloutier is a 34-year-old man admitted to your unit with a complaint of intermittent hematuria for about a month. Two days ago he developed a continual dull pain in his left side.

40. An angiogram was performed using a catheter inserted into the left femoral artery. Which of the following nursing actions is your *first* priority following this procedure?
○ 1. Monitoring vital signs until stable. **PL**
○ 2. Frequently checking the puncture site for fresh bleeding, swelling, or increasing tenderness. **6** **PhI**
○ 3. Measuring the quantity and specific gravity of urinary output.
○ 4. Checking the peripheral pulses distal to the femoral puncture site.

Following the angiogram, a diagnosis of probable carcinoma of the left kidney was made, and the client was scheduled for a left nephrectomy. Preoperative blood work indicated a mild polycythemia.

41. Postoperatively, Mr. Cloutier has a large flank incision. In order to facilitate deep breathing and coughing, you should:
○ 1. Have the client lie on the unaffected side. **PL**
○ 2. Coordinate breathing and coughing exercises with administration of analgesics. **6** **PhI**
○ 3. Maintain the client in high Fowler's position.

○ 4. Push fluid administration to loosen respiratory secretions.

42. Urinary output is closely assessed after nephrectomy. Which of the following assessment findings is an early indicator of fluid retention in the postoperative period?
○ 1. Increased specific gravity of urine. **AS**
○ 2. Daily weight gain of two or more pounds. **8**
○ 3. A urinary output of 50 mL/h. **PhI**
○ 4. Periorbital edema.

43. The postoperative nephrectomy client should also be closely observed by the nurse for:
○ 1. Hemorrhage. **AS**
○ 2. Hyperkalemia. **6**
○ 3. Respiratory alkalosis and tetany. **PhI**
○ 4. Polyuria.

44. Forty-eight hours after surgery, Mr. Cloutier complains of increasing nausea and abdominal pressure. Your *first* nursing action is to:
○ 1. Change the client's position to relieve abdominal pressure. **IMP 8**
○ 2. Auscultate bowel sounds. **PhI**
○ 3. Insert a rectal tube to relieve flatus.
○ 4. Administer morphine SO_4 6 mg as ordered for the relief of discomfort.

45. Mr. Cloutier has developed paralytic ileus. This dysfunction is described by the nurse as:
○ 1. Edema of the intestinal mucosa. **AS**
○ 2. Acute dilatation of the colon. **8**
○ 3. Absent, diminished, or uncoordinated autonomic stimulation of peristalsis. **PhI**
○ 4. High, tinkling bowel sounds over the area of obstruction.

46. Mr. Cloutier's physician decides to insert a Miller-Abbott tube to decompress the abdomen. Which of the following statements by the nurse accurately describes the Miller-Abbott tube?
○ 1. A double-lumen tube, with one lumen leading to the inflatable balloon and the other lumen used for aspiration. **IMP 8 PhI**
○ 2. A plastic or rubber tube with holes near its tip facilitating withdrawal of fluids from the stomach.
○ 3. A single-lumen, mercury-weighted tube approximately 6 feet long.
○ 4. A 10-foot-long rubber tube with a mercury bag at its end.

47. Before insertion of the Miller-Abbott tube, the balloon is tested for patency and capacity and then deflated. Which of the following nursing measures will ease the insertion of the nasoenteric tube?
○ 1. Chilling the tube before insertion. **PL**
○ 2. Administering a sedative to reduce anxiety. **8**
○ 3. Warming the tube before insertion. **PhI**
○ 4. Positioning the client in low Fowler's position.

48. What nursing action best facilitates the passage of the nasoenteric tube from the stomach through the pylorus and into the duodenum?
○ 1. Gently advancing the tube 1–4 inches at regular time intervals. **IMP 8**
○ 2. Positioning the client on his right side for 2 hours after insertion. **PhI**
○ 3. Maintaining strict bedrest and avoiding all unnecessary movement.
○ 4. Positioning the client in a flat supine position.

49. Two days before discharge, Mr. Cloutier expressed renewed concern over his ability to continue many of his activities with only one kidney. You respond:
○ 1. "You seem depressed. Actually you are very lucky, since the pathology reports indicate your tumor was encapsulated." **IMP 7 PsI**
○ 2. "Lots of people do quite well with only one kidney."
○ 3. "Would you like me to call the doctor so you can discuss it with him?"
○ 4. "I can understand your concern, but your remaining kidney is sufficient to maintain normal renal functions."

Mr. Robert Mackey, a 19-year-old college sophomore, sustained a transverse fracture of his right tibia and fibula when he tripped playing football. His fractures were reduced in the emergency room and his right leg immobilized in a long leg plaster of Paris cast, which extended from his groin to his toes, with the knee slightly flexed.

50. On his admission to the orthopedic unit, Mr. Mackey's cast is damp, and he is complaining that it feels very hot. The nurse should:
○ 1. Explain to Mr. Mackey that the cast will feel hot for several hours as the moisture evaporates and the cast hardens. **EV 3 PhI**
○ 2. Recognize that this is a sign of excessive pressure on the soft tissues and notify the physician.
○ 3. Tell Mr. Mackey not to worry, as this is a common complaint.
○ 4. Administer meperidine (Demerol) HCl 50 mg IM to relieve his discomfort.

51. After elevating Mr. Mackey's leg, you check his toes for circulation and motor activity. Which of the following indicates circulatory constriction?
○ 1. Tingling and numbness of toes. **AS**
○ 2. Inability to move toes. **3**
○ 3. Blanching or cyanosis of toes. **PhI**
○ 4. Complaints of pressure or tightness of the cast.

52. Several hours after Mr. Mackey is admitted, you notice his toes have become edematous. The physician decides to bivalve the cast. You explain to Mr. Mackey that this procedure:
○ 1. Requires recasting after 24 hours. **IMP**
○ 2. Includes splitting and spreading the cast down the middle to relieve constriction. **3 SECE**
○ 3. Includes splitting and spreading the cast on each side and cutting the underlying padding.
○ 4. Should be followed by placing the client's leg in a dependent position.

53. On entering Mr. Mackey's room 2 days later, the nurse observes him using a long pencil to scratch the skin under his cast. The nurse should:
○ 1. Ask the physician for a medication order to relieve itching. **IMP 2**
○ 2. Explain to the client that scratching under the cast should be avoided, as it may break the skin and cause an infection. **SECE**
○ 3. Assist Mr. Mackey by gently rolling the casted leg in the palmar surfaces of your hand.
○ 4. Take the pencil away from Mr. Mackey.

54. The doctor has ordered ambulation on crutches, with no weight-bearing on the affected limb. An appropriate crutch gait for the nurse to teach Mr. Mackey would be:

○ 1. Two-point gait. **PL**
○ 2. Three-point gait. **3**
○ 3. Four-point gait. **PhI**
○ 4. Tripod gait.

55. Which of the following instructions would be *inappropriate* when teaching a client to use crutches?
○ 1. Utilize axilla to help carry weight. **IMP**
○ 2. Use short strides to maintain maximum mobility. **3** **PhI**
○ 3. Keep feet 6–8 inches apart to provide a wide base for support.
○ 4. If he should begin to fall, throw crutches to the side to prevent falling on them.

Melissa Sue, a 29-year-old woman with a history of epilepsy since age 5, is admitted to the emergency room with repetitive seizures characterized by tonic and clonic contractions. Emergency measures for status epilepticus are started.

56. The nurse would explain that epileptic seizures or convulsions result from:
○ 1. Excessive exercise with lactic acid accumulation. **AN** **2**
○ 2. Excessive, simultaneous, disordered neuronal discharge. **PhI**
○ 3. Excessive cerebral metabolism, with local K^+ increased.
○ 4. Excessive circulating cerebrospinal fluid increasing cerebral pressures.

57. The nurse would recognize a generalized tonic-clonic seizure if which of the following occurred?
○ 1. Brief, abrupt loss of consciousness lasting 10–20 seconds. **AS** **2**
○ 2. Loss of consciousness for several minutes, with sustained and intermittent contractions of all motor muscle groups. **PhI**
○ 3. Sustained and intermittent contractions of selected motor groups in a somewhat confined area.
○ 4. Twitching of facial muscles.

58. You are to administer the drug of choice for long-term control of generalized tonic-clonic seizures. This drug is:
○ 1. Phenobarbital. **IMP**
○ 2. Diazepam (Valium). **2**
○ 3. Diphenylhydantoin (Dilantin) sodium. **PhI**
○ 4. Trimethadione (Tridione).

59. Which of the following nursing actions is your *first* priority during a generalized tonic-clonic seizure episode?
○ 1. Observe and record all events that occur prior to, during, and after the seizure. **PL** **2**
○ 2. Maintain a patent airway by turning the head to the side. **PhI**
○ 3. Protect the client from injury.
○ 4. Monitor vital signs, with special attention directed to respiratory status.

60. Emergency drug intervention for Melissa Sue included diazepam 10 mg intravenously and diphenylhydantoin 0.15 g IV in 0.05-g increments. Nursing implications with diphenylhydantoin include giving the intravenous injection slowly and in small increments to prevent:
○ 1. Respiratory depression and/or arrest. **IMP**
○ 2. Vasodepression and circulatory shock. **2**
○ 3. Irritation and/or necrosis of the vein and surrounding tissue. **PhI**
○ 4. Vasomotor stimulation, with a sudden, malignant increase in blood pressure.

Donald Lee, a 70-year-old retired businessman, went to his ophthalmologist with complaints of decreasing peripheral vision. Tonometry revealed increased intraocular pressures. Mr. Lee was admitted to the hospital with a diagnosis of open-angle glaucoma.

61. The signs and symptoms of open-angle glaucoma are related to:
○ 1. An imbalance between the rate of secretion of intraocular fluids and the rate of absorption of aqueous humor. **AN** **2** **PhI**
○ 2. A degenerative disease characterized by narrowing of the arterioles of the retina and areas of ischemia.
○ 3. An infectious process that causes clouding and scarring of the cornea.
○ 4. A dysfunction of aging in which the retina of the eye buckles from inadequate fluid pressures.

62. Assessment of the intraocular pressure as measured by tonometry would be normal if the value is in the range:
○ 1. 5–10 mm Hg. **AS**
○ 2. 12–22 mm Hg. **2**
○ 3. 10–20 cm H_2O. **PhI**
○ 4. 20–30 mm Hg.

63. While taking Mr. Lee's history, the nurse would be alerted to a sudden increase in intraocular pressure if he complained of:
○ 1. Generalized decrease in peripheral vision over the past year. **AS** **2**
○ 2. Difficulty with close vision. **PhI**
○ 3. Increasing discomfort in the left eye with radiation to his forehead and left temple.
○ 4. Halos around lights.

64. Client teaching about glaucoma should include a comparison of the two types. Open-angle, or chronic, glaucoma differs from closed-angle, or acute, glaucoma in that:
○ 1. Open-angle glaucoma occurs less frequently than closed-angle glaucoma. **AN** **2**
○ 2. Open-angle glaucoma's symptomatology includes pain, severe headache, nausea, and vomiting; whereas closed-angle glaucoma has a slow, silent, and generally painless onset. **SECE**
○ 3. The obstruction to aqueous flow in open-angle glaucoma generally occurs somewhere in Schlemm's canal or aqueous veins. It does not narrow or close the angle of the anterior chamber, as in closed-angle glaucoma.
○ 4. Open-angle glaucoma rarely occurs in families; however, there is a hereditary predisposition for closed-angle glaucoma.

65. Pilocarpine is the drug of choice in the treatment of open-angle glaucoma. The expected outcome following administration would be:
○ 1. Blocked action of cholinesterase at the cholinergic nerve endings, and therefore increased pupil size. **IMP** **2** **PhI**
○ 2. Constricted pupil and therefore widened outflow channels and increased flow of aqueous fluid.
○ 3. Impaired vision from decreased aqueous humor production.
○ 4. Constriction of aqueous veins and therefore decreased venous pooling in the eye.

66. Bedrest is ordered for Mr. Lee because activity tends to increase intraocular pressure. Which of the following activities of daily living should he be instructed to avoid?
- ○ 1. Watching television. **IMP**
- ○ 2. Brushing teeth and hair. **2**
- ○ 3. Self-feeding. **PsI**
- ○ 4. Passive range-of-motion exercises.

67. To correctly instill pilocarpine in Mr. Lee's eyes, the nurse should gently pull down the lower lid of the eye and instill the drops:
- ○ 1. Directly on the central surface of the cornea. **IMP**
- ○ 2. On the inner canthus of the eye. **2**
- ○ 3. Into the conjunctival sac. **PhI**
- ○ 4. Directly on the dilated pupil.

68. Which of the following aspects of open-angle glaucoma and its medical treatment is the *most frequent* cause of client noncompliance?
- ○ 1. Loss of mobility due to severe-driving restrictions. **EV** **2**
- ○ 2. The painful and insidious progression of this type of glaucoma. **PhI**
- ○ 3. Decreased light and near-vision accommodation due to miotic effects of pilocarpine.
- ○ 4. The frequent nausea and vomiting accompanying use of miotic drugs.

Ms. Ann Martin is a 23-year-old secretary readmitted to the hospital with pronounced weakness of the left facial muscles and difficulty swallowing. She was doing well until 2 weeks ago, when she developed some nausea and diarrhea and decided to discontinue her medications for myasthenia gravis.

69. The family of Ms. Martin asks about myasthenia gravis. The *best* explanation for the nurse to offer would be that myasthenia gravis is a:
- ○ 1. Degenerative dysfunction of the basal ganglia. **AN**
- ○ 2. Transmission dysfunction at the myoneural junction. **3** **PhI**
- ○ 3. Hypertrophic reaction in the anterior motor neurons of the spinal cord.
- ○ 4. Hereditary condition of cranial nerves VII, IX, and X.

70. Which of the following statements about myasthenia gravis is true?
- ○ 1. Thymectomies rarely produce remissions in myasthenia gravis. **PL** **3**
- ○ 2. Myasthenia gravis is an acute illness that progresses rapidly. **PhI**
- ○ 3. Myasthenia gravis has increased muscle strength as a major symptom.
- ○ 4. Myasthenia gravis may be an autoimmune disease.

71. Diagnosis of myasthenia gravis is frequently based on the client's response to an intravenous injection of edrophonium (Tensilon). If the client responds positively to this drug, the nurse should expect:
- ○ 1. Exacerbation of symptomatology. **EV**
- ○ 2. Relief of ptosis but not of weakness in other facial muscles. **3** **PhI**
- ○ 3. A prompt and dramatic increase in muscle strength.
- ○ 4. A slight increase in muscle strength that is countered by an increase in muscle fatigability.

The attending physician has ordered the following medical regimen for Ms. Martin:
- *Pyridostigmine bromide (Mestinon) 180 mg bid.*
- *Neostigmine bromide (Prostigmin) 0.05 mg sub q tid, ac.*
- *Ephedrine sulfate 25 mg tid.*
- *Potassium chloride tablets bid.*

72. The nurse anticipates that the backbone of treatment for clients with myasthenia gravis will be:
- ○ 1. Adrenergic drugs. **PL**
- ○ 2. Anticholinergic drugs. **3**
- ○ 3. Anticholinesterase drugs. **PhI**
- ○ 4. Cholinergic drugs.

73. The nursing care plan includes observing for the most common client problems arising from the use of Mestinon and Prostigmin, which include:
- ○ 1. Gastric distress—nausea, anorexia, diarrhea. **AN**
- ○ 2. Elimination problems—urinary retention. **3**
- ○ 3. Central nervous system excitation—flushing, irritability. **PhI**
- ○ 4. Cardiac arrhythmias—palpitations, PVCs.

74. Which of the following nursing interventions can aid in reducing the side effects of these drugs?
- ○ 1. Give oral medications along with milk, soda crackers, or antacids. **IMP** **3**
- ○ 2. Push fluids and encourage ambulation. **PhI**
- ○ 3. Keep room cool and discourage visitors.
- ○ 4. Encourage food high in potassium.

75. In order to take full advantage of the effects of pyridostigmine bromide and neostigmine bromide in reducing dysphagia, the nurse should plan to give the medications before meals. How long before?
- ○ 1. Two hours. **PL**
- ○ 2. 45–60 minutes. **3**
- ○ 3. 20–30 minutes. **PhI**
- ○ 4. 10–15 minutes.

76. Because Ms. Martin's medications have been increased, it is important that the nurse observe for signs of "cholinergic crisis." These include:
- ○ 1. Dilated pupils, profuse diaphoresis, and trembling. **AS** **2**
- ○ 2. Constricted pupils, hypersalivation, and hypotension. **PhI**
- ○ 3. Dilated pupils, nausea, and tachycardia.
- ○ 4. Constricted pupils, dry mucous membranes, and bradycardia.

77. If "cholinergic crisis" is established, all anticholinesterase drugs are withdrawn. To reduce symptoms, which of the following drugs should the nurse be prepared to give?
- ○ 1. Atropine. **PL**
- ○ 2. Ephedrine sulfate. **3**
- ○ 3. Potassium chloride. **PhI**
- ○ 4. Neostigmine bromide.

78. On evaluating Ms. Martin's dysfunction, the nurse recognizes that myasthena gravis is:
- ○ 1. An upper motor neuron lesion. **AN**
- ○ 2. A lower motor neuron lesion. **2**
- ○ 3. A combined upper and lower motor neuron lesion. **PhI**
- ○ 4. A genetic dysfunction.

Ms. Kim Landry, a 32-year-old teacher and mother of four school-age children, has just been diagnosed as having hypothyroidism.

79. Ms. Landry asks the nurse what causes hypothyroidism. The nurse would be correct in saying that two common causes of primary hypothyroidism are:
- ○ 1. Destruction of thyroid tissue by radioactive iodine during therapy for hyperthyroidism, and spontaneous atrophy due to autoimmune response. **AS 3 PhI**
- ○ 2. Spontaneous atrophy due to autoimmune response, and surgical removal of the thyroid gland.
- ○ 3. Surgical removal of the thyroid gland, and tumors of the pituitary gland that decrease the amount of circulating thyroxine.
- ○ 4. Tumors of the pituitary gland and/or large doses of antithyroid drugs.

80. The nursing assessment will likely reveal the most common clinical manifestations of hypothyroidism, which are:
- ○ 1. Increased body temperature, tachycardia, and fatigue. **AS 3 PhI**
- ○ 2. Decreased exercise tolerance and facial and pitting edema.
- ○ 3. Increased sluggishness, increased cold intolerance, and puffy eyelids, hands, and feet.
- ○ 4. Decreased facial expression, diarrhea, and weight gain.

81. If treatment with thyroid hormone is effective, the nurse should expect:
- ○ 1. Diuresis, a decrease in pulse rate, and an increase in blood pressure. **EV 3 PhI**
- ○ 2. Diuresis, a widening pulse pressure, and an increase in both temperature and respiratory rate.
- ○ 3. Increased pulse rate, decreased respiratory rate, and decreased puffiness.
- ○ 4. Weight loss, increased diastolic blood pressure, and decreased pulse rate.

82. In contrast to hypothyroidism, hyperthyroidism is due to excessive levels of thyroxine in the plasma. Clinical data gathered by the nurse indicating this endocrine dysfunction would include:
- ○ 1. Systolic hypertension and heat intolerance. **AS 3 PhI**
- ○ 2. Diastolic hypertension and widened pulse pressure.
- ○ 3. Heat intolerance and weight gain.
- ○ 4. Emotional hyperexcitabilty and anorexia.

83. The nurse knows that, in contrast to clients with hypothyroidism, clients with hyperthyroidism have:
- ○ 1. Increased serum cholesterol. **AN 3 PhI**
- ○ 2. Increased basal metabolic rate and Serum T_3 and T_4.
- ○ 3. Increased serum TSH (thyroid-stimulating hormone).
- ○ 4. Increased menstrual volume.

84. Of the following, which should the nurse recognize as the cardinal sign heralding the onset of thyroid storm?
- ○ 1. Fever. **AS 3 PhI**
- ○ 2. Tachycardia.
- ○ 3. Hypertension.
- ○ 4. Tremulousness.

85. Both Cushing's syndrome and Addison's disease are due to dysfunction of the adrenal cortex. In order to plan for the care of a client with Cushing's syndrome, the nurse should know that the primary pathology is:
- ○ 1. Increased cortisol secretion. **AS 3 PhI**
- ○ 2. Increased epinephrine secretion.
- ○ 3. Decreased aldosterone secretion.
- ○ 4. Decreased ACTH secretion.

86. Because cortisol is a glucocorticoid, the nurse should expect:
- ○ 1. Hypoglycemia due to increased insulin production. **EV 3 PhI**
- ○ 2. Skeletal-muscle wasting because glucocorticoids promote protein and fat mobilization.
- ○ 3. Dependent edema and severe hypokalemia due to abnormal aldosterone secretion.
- ○ 4. Discoloration or hyperpigmentation of the skin due to increased pituitary secretion of ACTH.

87. In Addison's disease, glucocorticoids, mineral corticoids, and androgenic hormones are all reduced. Therefore, in contrast to Cushing's syndrome, the nurse should expect to find:
- ○ 1. Hypotension, weight loss, and physical and mental exhaustion. **AS 3 PhI**
- ○ 2. Hypertension, moon facies, and masculinization in females.
- ○ 3. Hypotension, hyperglycemia, and weight gain.
- ○ 4. Hypertension, male impotency, and menstrual disturbances.

88. Since aldosterone is the major mineralocorticoid secreted by the adrenal cortex, which of the following fluid and electrolyte imbalances should the nurse anticipate with decreased secretion of this hormone?
- ○ 1. Hyperkalemia. **EV 6 PhI**
- ○ 2. Hypernatremia.
- ○ 3. Hypervolemia.
- ○ 4. Hypercalcemia.

89. Nursing actions for clients with Addison's disease will include:
- ○ 1. Providing a low-sodium diet. **IMP 3 PhI**
- ○ 2. Restriction of fluids to 1500 cc/day.
- ○ 3. Administering insulin-replacement therapy.
- ○ 4. Reducing physical and emotional stress.

90. Iron-deficiency anemia is best described as:
- ○ 1. Hypochromic microcytic. **AS 6 PhI**
- ○ 2. Hyperchromic macrocytic.
- ○ 3. Hyperchromic microcytic.
- ○ 4. Hypochromic macrocytic.

91. Mrs. Rhonda Sanchez is a 32-year-old flight attendant admitted to the hospital with acute rheumatoid arthritis. The nurse should expect that Mrs. Sanchez's emotional responses to her condition would primarily depend on:
- ○ 1. Her self-concept, body image, and usual affective coping strategies. **AN 7 PsI**
- ○ 2. Her relationship with her mother.
- ○ 3. Her usual affective or palliative coping strategies only.
- ○ 4. Economic status and work history.

Mr. Dunes was admitted to the hospital after an automobile accident. His major medical problems at the time of admission were multiple fractures of both lower legs. His medical treatment includes bedrest with skeletal traction.

92. Mr. Dunes complains that he has not had a bowel movement since he was admitted 2 days ago. Which of the following interventions would be the *most* appropriate nursing action?

○ 1. Administer an enema. IMP 8 PhI
○ 2. Put him on the bedpan every 2 hours.
○ 3. Ensure maximum fluid intake (3000 mL per day).
○ 4. Perform range of motion exercises to all extremities.

93. Understanding that prolonged immobilization could lead to decubitus ulcers, the nurse plans interventions to prevent alterations in skin integrity. Which would be the *least* appropriate intervention?
○ 1. Use of a bed cradle. PL 1 PhI
○ 2. Giving backrubs with alcohol.
○ 3. Encouraging a high-protein diet.
○ 4. Frequent assessment of the skin.

94. The nurse anticipates that osteoporosis may result from prolonged immobilization because of:
○ 1. Lack of weight-bearing, which decreases osteoblastic activity. AS 3 PhI
○ 2. Decreased dietary calcium intake.
○ 3. Deposition of excess calcium phosphate salts.
○ 4. Lack of weight-bearing, which increases bone formation.

95. Which of the following client problems relating to altered nutrition is a consequence of impaired physical mobility?
○ 1. Increased appetite. AN 3 PhI
○ 2. Decreased protein catabolism.
○ 3. Increased carbohydrate needs.
○ 4. Increased secretion of digestive enzymes.

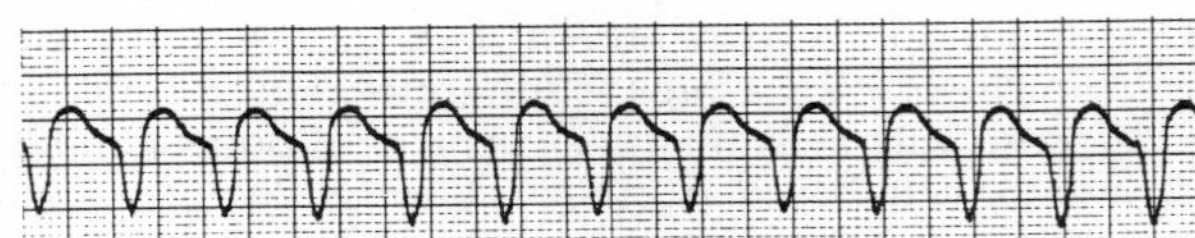

96. The nurse knows that the arrhythmia shown above, if untreated, is most likely to:
○ 1. Progress to ventricular fibrillation. AN 6 PhI
○ 2. Increase the blood pressure suddenly.
○ 3. Intensify chest pain from a myocardial infarction (MI).
○ 4. Cause no observable change in the client.

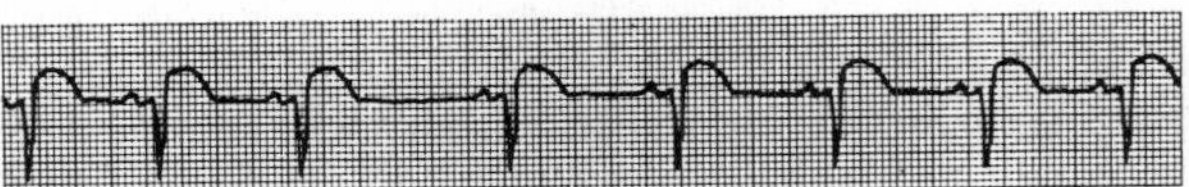

97. The appropriate nursing response to the above arrhythmia would be to:
○ 1. Administer a bolus of lidocaine 50 mg IV. IMP 6 PhI
○ 2. Limit client activity while the arrhythmia is present.
○ 3. Hold digoxin until atrioventricular node depression reverses.
○ 4. Do nothing, particularly with no symptoms.

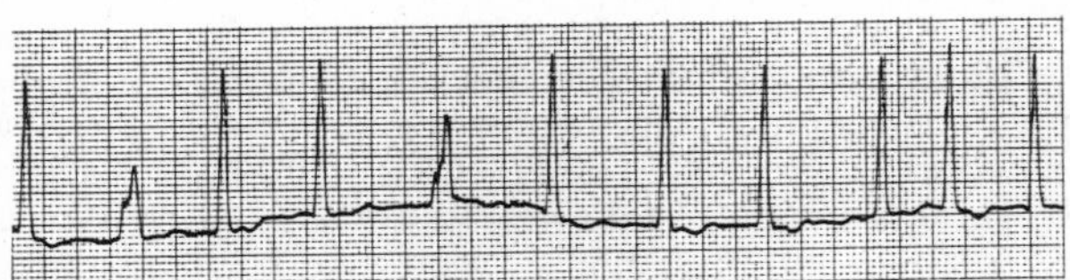

98. The correct interpretation of the above arrhythmia is:
○ 1. Sinus rhythm with multifocal premature ventricular contractions (PVCs). AN 6 PhI
○ 2. Atrial fibrillation with unifocal PVCs.
○ 3. Sinus tachycardia with unifocal PVCs.
○ 4. Second-degree atrioventricular block with unifocal PVCs.

■ ANSWERS/RATIONALE

1. (2) Although all of these interventions are appropriate in the preoperative period, research indicates that the *best* postoperative outcomes are related to the client's reduced preoperative anxiety levels. Clients who deny apprehension and refuse information, as well as those who are highly anxious and who are unable to ask and/or assimilate information, have the most difficult postsurgical course. Clients who are able to express their concerns and who are given emotional support as well as accurate, brief explanations tend to have less pain and fewer postoperative complications. Nos. 1, 3, and 4 do not address the client's need to verbalize concerns.

2. (4) It is important to recognize that the loss of anatomic integrity initiates a grieving process. Allowing the client to express feelings of depression, apathy, or disinterest indicates that such feelings are acceptable and not uncommon. No. 1 is always appropriate and should be consistently carried out; however, in the situation depicted it would *follow* the verbalization of feelings. Nos. 2 and 3 are also alternatives you may wish to employ *after* assessing the client's major concerns.

3. (3) It is not uncommon for a client to feel that she will no longer be able to fulfill her role and needs as a woman following a hysterectomy. Verbalization of feelings allows the nurse to assess the client's coping mechanisms and encourages the client to deal with her emotional response. No. 3 is an open-ended question that allows the client room to respond. Nos. 1 and 2 avoid the problem initially. No. 2 may be appropriate if, after talking to the client, you assess that the client's responses represent a more significant or deep-seated problem. No. 4 would be appropriate *after* the client has aired her feelings.

4. (2) Second-degree burns involve both the epidermis and some of the dermis. They have a pink-red appearance and are characterized by moisture or blisters. Second-degree burns are very painful, as nerve endings remain and may be exposed to the air. A *first*-degree burn involves only the epidermis (No. 1). An example is sunburn: the skin is usually red and dry. In *third*-degree burns, subcutaneous tissue, muscle, and even bone are also involved (Nos. 3 and 4). Typically, a *third*-degree burn is white, gray, or charred in color and is dry and leathery in appearance. Nerve endings have been destroyed, so the area is painless.

5. (3) Critical burns are classified as second degree over 30% of the body and/or third degree over 10% of the body. Extensive burns involving the face, hands, and feet or those associated with respiratory injuries are also considered critical. The most frequently used method of calculating the extent of a burn is called the "rule of nines." While this method is fairly simple to apply, it is somewhat inaccurate. This is particularly true when it is applied to children because allowances are not made for the proportional differences in head size and extremity size between children and adults. Hence first-degree

ADULT NURSING

burns (No. 1) are not serious unless large areas are involved and the client is very young or old. Second-degree burns (No. 2) are classified as a major burn if over 25% of the body is involved. The fourth-degree burn classification is not routinely used (No. 4).

6. (2) Age is important baseline data because IV infusion rates to maintain appropriate quantity and specific gravity of urinary output differ; for example, 10–20 mL/h for infants versus 50–70 mL/h for adults. Weight is significant if the Evans or Brooke formulas are used for fluid replacement therapy. Both these formulas utilize both the size of the burn and the weight of the client to calculate the amount of fluid to be replaced. Vital signs and skin turgor are both important measures of the degree or extent of hypovolemia. As dehydration develops, skin turgor becomes poor, mucous membranes dry, and the eyeballs feel soft. Likewise, the pulse may become thready and the blood pressure may decrease. Size (weight), as discussed, not sex, would determine therapy (No. 1). Level of mentation (No. 3) is less helpful in this particular situation because of the fear, pain, and acute anxiety experienced by some clients. Quantity and specific gravity of urine output (No. 4) are important in assessing the adequacy of fluid replacement rather than as part of the initial assessment.

7. (1) The hypovolemia and shock that accompany burns greatly increase the body's stress response. Increased serum levels of norepinephrine, epinephrine, and aldosterone facilitate venous return and thus assist in maintaining cardiac output and blood pressure. The pituitary is also stimulated in the stress response to increase circulating levels of ADH (decreases water output) and cortisol. Increased levels of the latter hormone are implicated in the development of Curling's ulcer (stress ulcer), which clients of all ages and with both minor and major burns may develop. Generally, H_2 antagonists and antacids are used to reduce its occurrence. No. 2 is incorrect because negative iron balance occurs due to protein mobilization for healing. Clients with burns are given high-protein, high-calorie meals as well as supplemental vitamins to promote wound-healing. No. 3 is incorrect because hemolysis of red blood cells and decreased hematocrit are primarily due to the injury itself rather than to epinephrine agglutination. In thermal burns, up to 40% of the red blood cell mass may be hemolyzed. Hypothermia is a problem in the postburn period but is the result of the loss of skin areas; hence No. 4 is incorrect. The client treated by the open or exposed method of burn therapy is particularly susceptible to chilling. Increased thermostat settings and radiant heat lamps may be employed to aid in maintaining normal body temperature.

8. (2) Aldosterone secretion by the adrenal cortex is stimulated by decreases in cardiac output. Aldosterone acts to conserve sodium in the kidney tubules, passively increasing water reabsorption and improving fluid volume balance. Normally, if Mr. Maestas had only a water loss, he would also be hypernatremic because of this mechanism. However, in burns the client's hypovolemia (hemoconcentration) is due to both fluid and electrolyte loss in edema fluids as well as through the denuded areas of skin. No. 1 is not the best answer because, although ADH is being released, its action has not at this time prevented hemoconcentration. No. 3 is incorrect because very little sodium is released due to cellular disruption. Sodium is the main cation of the extracellular fluid. No. 4 is incorrect because increased serum-potassium levels stimulate the release of aldosterone.

9. (1) Hyponatremia or decreased serum sodium may develop in burn clients because sodium tends to move with water into edema fluids as well as into denuded areas of skin. Nos. 2 and 4 are incorrect because both these mechanisms tend to increase sodium reabsorption by the kidney tubules. Inadequate fluid replacement (No. 3) would tend to mask hyponatremia because of hemoconcentration.

10. (2) Hyperkalemia (excesses in serum potassium) occurs in burns due to three separate mechanisms: (a) cellular injury resulting in the movement of potassium from the intracellular space into the extracellular space; (b) decreased glomerular filtration and urine output preventing excretion of increased serum potassium; and (c) inadequate tissue metabolism resulting in increased hydrogen ion formation (metabolic acidosis). In the kidney tubules, hydrogen and potassium ions are exchanged for sodium ions. In metabolic acidosis, more hydrogen ions are excreted than potassium ions. Exudate formation itself does not significantly affect serum-potassium levels (No. 1). During physical and emotional stress, aldosterone levels are increased, thereby lowering serum potassium (No. 3). Hyperbilirubinemia itself does not affect potassium concentration (No. 4), though red blood cell destruction probably increases the amount of circulating potassium, as potassium is the major intracellular cation.

11. (3) Potassium is transported back into the cells along with glucose; therefore the administration of insulin and glucose will facilitate the movement of potassium back into the cell. Kayexalate (No. 2) is a resin that attacks and binds potassium. It may be given either orally or as an enema; however, its use would not be indicated in this case unless more conservative means were unsuccessful. Morphine sulfate (No. 1) and synthetic aldosterone (No. 4) are not indicated for the management of hyperkalemia.

12. (4) The hypovolemia that occurs in the initial stage of burns is the result of fluid lost from denuded areas of skin and edema in and around the burned surface area. Edema formation is due to a shift of plasma fluids to the interstitial space. Nos. 1, 2, and 3 are incorrect because, when tissues are burned, a change in the permeability of both tissue and capillary membranes occurs. This change as well as increased vasodilation result in a shift of excessively large amounts of extracellular fluid (electrolytes and proteins) into the burned area. Most of this fluid loss occurs deep in the wound, where fluid moves into the deeper tissue. Burns of a highly vascular area (muscle, face) are believed to cause more severe fluid volume shifts than comparable burns to other areas of the body.

13. (2) With the exception of the Evans formula, whole blood is administered to burn clients only when the hematocrit begins to manifest red blood cell loss. Several fluid formulas have been developed to serve as a guideline for fluid replacement in the burn client. The Evans formula is the oldest and is based on both the size of the wound and the client's weight. Colloids (blood, dextran, plasma) and crystalloids (electrolyte solutions) are administered during the first 48 hours. The Brooke formula is quite similar, except that blood is not given until the hematocrit level has fallen and the need is demonstrated.

The Parkland formula, more recently developed, is based on the premise that volume expansion is dependent on the rate of infusion rather than the type of replacement. During the first 24 hours, fluid volume is replaced with electrolyte solutions (Ringer's lactate) only (No. 1). Colloids are used only if urine output is not maintained (No. 3). During the second 24 hours, dextrose and water (No. 4) are used to maintain fluid volume.

14. (2) Calculating the correct rate requires computation of the hourly volume (290 cc) and the minute volume (5 cc), and then multiplying the rate, in cc/min, by the drop factor (15 gtt/cc). (The hourly and minute volumes have been rounded to the nearest whole number.) Nos. 1 and 3 are not fast enough to deliver this large a volume in the prescribed period. No. 4 is too rapid. A quick method of computing the drip rate is to use the first two numbers in the 24-hour fluid volume, i.e., 7000 cc in 24 hours = 70 gtt/min. This shortcut may be useful when initially starting an infusion, before mathematically calculating the rate. Use only with 15 gtt/cc factor.

15. (2) Although each of the listed measures can be used to assess the adequacy of the fluid replacement, hourly urine outputs and vital signs provide significant information on fluid balance in the acute burn period. Decreased urine output, increased pulse rate, and restlessness are early signs of inadequate fluid replacement. Increases in blood pressure, pulse, respirations, and urine output are early signs of circulatory overload. Changes in daily weights provide accurate data over the long run and are extremely important in monitoring fluid volumes in clients on diuretic therapy, such as clients with congestive heart failure or cirrhosis. Nos. 1, 3, and 4 are *not* the *best* indicators.

16. (1) The diuretic stage of burns occurs 48–72 hours after injury. The fluid shift is just the opposite of that in the initial stage. Fluids, electrolytes, and proteins may move very rapidly from the interstitial space back into the vascular compartment. Unless renal damage has occurred and there is no indication (No. 2), diuresis ensues, due to the increased blood volume and renal blood flow. Serum eletrolytes and hematocrit are decreased due to hemodilution. If urine output is insufficient at this time, symptoms of circulatory overload and cardiac failure will occur. There are no data to support No. 3. The sodium value is within normal limits (No. 4).

17. (2) Hematocrit is reduced due to hemodilution and volume overload resulting from the interstitial-to-plasma fluid shift. Erythropoietin factor (No. 1) is produced by the kidneys and would only be reduced if there were kidney failure. Metabolic acidosis (No. 3) does increase red blood cell fragility, but it is not applicable in this situation. Hypoalbuminemia (No. 4) causes loss of oncotic pressures in the vascular compartment. The primary effect of this phenomenon is movement of fluid from the vascular compartment to the interstitial space, the outcome of which is hemoconcentration.

18. (3) Clients with burns limited to an extremity are generally treated by a closed method; that is, wounds are covered with a layer of sterile, fine mesh gauze impregnated with an antibacterial agent such as mafenide 1%. Wounds are cleansed one or more times per day, and dressings are reapplied using strict sterile technique. Clients treated by the closed or semi-open method do not have to be isolated (No. 1). Clients treated by the open method (wounds completely exposed to the air) require strict isolation to prevent infection. The open method is usually used for minor burns, areas difficult to dress (burns of trunk, perineum), or new skin grafts. No. 2 is incorrect because sterile technique must be used. Heat lamp (No. 4) is incorrect because the wound is covered in the closed method.

19. (2) Mafenide 1% (Sulfamylon) is a white antibacterial ointment applied once or twice daily. Besides causing pain on application, this medication is a carbonic anhydrase inhibitor that interferes with the kidney's ability to excrete hydrogen ions and thus may cause metabolic acidosis, not metabolic alkosis (No. 3). Clients who are treated with mafenide 1% need to have their acid–base balance monitored by blood-gas determinations. Clinical signs of metabolic acidosis are increased rate and depth of respirations. Silver nitrate causes black discoloration of linens, and its hypotonicity causes electrolyte imbalances (Nos. 1 and 4). Clients treated with silver nitrate will need supplemental sodium, potassium, and chloride.

20. (2) Desperation and panic may strike while the injury is occurring but rarely occur during the recovery period. During the acute stage of burn recovery, anxiety is common due to the stress and pain of injury and dressing changes. Anxiety decreases the individual's ability to perceive situations realistically, which may result in an altered mental state (No. 1). During the intermediate phase of burn recovery, clients may react to continued pain, changes in body image, and financial stress with various psychologic responses, ranging from withdrawal and depression (No. 3) to acting out anger by refusing to cooperate with the medical regimen and by dependency (No. 4).

21. (2) Body image changes are the most frequent basis for psychologic responses during the recuperative phase. This is particularly true if the client is young or has sustained facial or neck burns. Also, self-esteem is often lowered. The client needs to be encouraged to talk about the changes he perceives between what he was and what he is now. Sessions with a psychiatric nurse specialist may be helpful. Occasionally individual and/or group therapy is indicated. Pain and immobility (No. 1) create problems in the *acute* phase of burns. Financial concerns (No. 3) do affect responses during the recuperative phase, but they are not a significant concern for all clients. Anger (No. 4) may be a response during each phase as the client reacts to various real and imagined losses.

22. (2) Some authorities believe that the basic psychosomatic issue underlying the development of ulcers is an unresolved dependence-independence conflict. This conflict frequently prevents the client from accepting a dependent role, even on a temporary basis. However, the unresolved dependency wish that many of these people have frequently results in irritable, angry behavior when treatments aren't exactly on time. Other psychosomatic research has linked anxiety and neurotic behavior (No. 1) with the occurrence of angina pectoris; repressed anger and hostility (No. 3) with the development of rheumatoid arthritis; and compulsive time orientation (No. 4) (type A personality) with onset of myocardial infarction.

23. (3) Clients are NPO and encouraged not to smoke or take medications the morning of an upper GI series. Clients are NPO for 6–8 hours, not 24 hours (No. 1). Enemas and/or cathartics (No. 2) are *not* administered before an upper GI series; however, they are given *after* the series, to aid in the elimination of the barium. The test involves an X ray, using a barium swallow as contrast medium. Gastroscopy (No.4) is the direct visualization of the stomach.

24. (2) All permits must be signed before the procedure. Clients are NPO 6–8 hours, not 24 hours (No.1). Gastroscopy is an uncomfortable procedure; to mislead the client by telling him it isn't uncomfortable (No. 3) can only increase anxiety and discomfort during the procedure. This procedure involves the passage of a long tube into the stomach, with a lighted, mirrored lens that permits direct visualization of the stomach mucosa. The client must lie quietly during insertion of the tube to prevent perforation of the esophagus. Usually sedatives, not pain medications (No. 4), are given prior to the procedure.

25. (3) The vagus nerve stimulates both an increase in hydrochloric acid secretion and gastric motility. Vagotomy not only decreases hydrochloric acid secretion but also alters the motility of the stomach and intestines; this may result in a sensation of fullness after meals, eructation, and abdominal distention. No. 1 is incomplete. Nos. 2 and 4 are the reverse of effects of vagal action.

26. (1) A nasogastric tube will be inserted early on the surgical day. No. 2 is not correct because Mr. Mangoni will not be allowed anything by mouth; all medications will be administered by injection in the immediate preoperative period. No. 3 is not correct because, although it is important for the physician to explain possible complications when obtaining permission to perform the surgery, the timing is inappropriate for any lengthy descriptions of possible complications. No. 4 is not a good choice because Mr. Mangoni should be *encouraged,* not discouraged, to take an appropriate amount of pain medications so he will be able to cough, turn, and deep breathe to avoid respiratory complications.

27. (3) Clients with high abdominal incisions are prone to atelectasis following surgery because they tend to breathe shallowly to prevent incisional pain. However, the nurse must also institute measures to prevent thrombophlebitis (No. 1), wound infection, and dehiscence. Abdominal distention due to air-swallowing (No. 2) is unlikely because the client has a nasogastric tube in place. Urinary retention after surgery (No. 4) is generally due to the effects of anesthesia on the autonomic nervous system rather than to the residual effects of anticholinergic medications.

28. (2) Bloody drainage from the nasogastric tube more than 12 hours after surgery should be considered unusual and reported to the surgeon. Prolonged bleeding may be indicative of a slow bleeder, a blood dyscrasia, or problems with incisional closure. Any of these may increase blood loss and lead to shock. Nos. 1,3, and 4 are incorrect because they are normal findings in the early postgastrectomy period.

29. (2) The tube will be inserted with greater ease if the client is sitting up with head slightly flexed. The tube should be lubricated and will be passed into the stomach with greater accuracy if the client is given water to drink through a straw; at the same time that the client is swallowing, the tube is advanced. No. 1 is not correct because the tube should be irrigated with saline, *not* water, to prevent electrolyte imbalances. No. 3 is not correct because pressure must *not* be utilized during irrigation. If resistance is met, the physician should be notified immediately. Ice chips (No. 4) should be used *sparingly, not* as often as desired, to prevent electrolyte imbalances from excessive hypotonic water ingestion.

30. (3) Removal of gastric secretions incurs the loss of sodium, potassium, and hydrochloric acid ions. The loss of these ions may lead not only to metabolic alkalosis (↓ H^+) but also to hypokalemia. Nos. 1 and 2 are incorrect because hypernatremia and hyperkalemia indicate an excess in sodium and potassium ions. Hypoproteinemia (No. 4) occurs with liver dysfunctions and is not a side effect of nasogastric suctioning.

31. (2) The client should be cautioned to limit the number of ice cubes he sucks on because the nasogastric suction will remove not only the increased water ingested from the melted cubes but also essential electrolytes. Nos. 1, 3, and 4 are appropriate mouth care measures for a client who has a nasogastric tube.

32. (2) The nasogastric tube is removed after bowel sounds have been reestablished (generally around the third day) and after the client has passed flatus or stool. Nos. 1 and 3 are incorrect because they do not include the return of bowel sounds. Before removal, the tube is frequently clamped for a 2-to 4-hour period—not 2 days (No. 4)—to test the client's tolerance. Gastric residue is measured after this period. If it is more than 100 mL, the nasogastric tube is left in place. Likewise, if the client experiences any pain, nausea, vomiting, or distention during this period, the tube is left in. If no symptoms occur and there is a minimal amount of gastric residue, the tube is removed.

33. (3) Pernicious anemia may occur following subtotal gastrectomy (when large portions of the stomach are removed) due to the loss of tissue that produces the intrinsic factor. Loss of this factor necessitates the parenteral administration of vitamin B_{12}, the extrinsic factor. No. 1 is incorrect because the extrinsic factor is found in food. Nos. 2 and 4 are incorrect because it is the loss of intrinsic factor that results in the malabsorption of vitamin B_{12}.

34. (1) Clients are ambulated as soon as possible to prevent the complications of bedrest; generally ambulation can begin as soon as 24 hours after surgery. In some instances, as when the client is severely debilitated or has complications due to ulcer perforation, bedrest may be prolonged, as in Nos. 2 and 3. If this is the case, the nurse will need to observe closely for signs of complications (atelectasis, thrombophlebitis, etc.) and institute measures to prevent them. The client is rarely if ever gotten up immediately after awakening, as in No. 4.

35. (4) While 70–80% of clients having subtotal gastrectomies may experience some symptoms of dumping syndrome, it is a significant problem for only a small percentage (5–10%). The term *dumping* is used because the symptoms are believed to be due to the rapid emptying of the gastric contents into the small intestine. This produces gastric distention, and some authorities believe that large amounts of extracellular fluid then enter the intestines to dilute the hypertonic stomach contents. The subsequent lowering of the blood volume produces shocklike symptoms, such as weakness, diaphoresis, faintness, and palpitations. Nos. 1, 2, and 3 are incorrect percentages.

36. (3) The symptoms of dumping syndrome are most likely to occur following the ingestion of large amounts of sugars or carbohydrates. Therefore a diet that is high in protein and fats and low in carbohydrates is recommended, to reduce symptomatology and to provide the client with essential energy requirements. No. 1 is incorrect because it does not supply sufficient protein for energy and tissue repair. High protein intake is essential after surgery and most prolonged illnesses for rebuilding tissue. Nos. 2 and 4 are incorrect because they list high carbohydrates.

37. (1) Clients experiencing dumping syndrome should be advised to ingest liquids between meals rather than with meals (No. 2) or at any time they desire (No. 3). Taking fluids between meals allows for adequate hydration, reduces the amount of bulk ingested with meals, and aids in preventing rapid gastric emptying. Six small meals rather than three large meals, as well as resting after eating, are also measures used to prevent the occurrence of symptoms, which usually disappear over time. There is no need to restrict the quantity of fluids (No. 4), just the timing.

38. (4) Profuse perspiration, diaphoresis, is one of a group of symptoms that happens 5 to 30 minutes after a high-carbohydrate meal or when liquid is taken with the meal. This is caused by entrance of food into the jejunum before it has had a chance to begin the digestive process. Other symptoms include a feeling of fullness, *not* hunger (No. 1); diarrhea, *not* constipation (No. 2); and weakness, *not* increased strength (No. 3).

39. (4) In response to direct questioning by the client, the nurse needs to provide brief, accurate information. Some clients who have had gastrectomies are able to tolerate three meals a day before discharge from the hospital. However, for the majority of clients, it takes 6–12 months before their surgically reduced stomach has stretched enough to accommodate a larger meal. No. 1 is incorrect because it is an open-ended response designed to elicit additional information. No. 2 is correct as far as it goes, but still doesn't answer the client's question. If you don't know the answer to a question, admit that you do not know but will try to get the information. No. 3 is incorrect because it gives inaccurate information.

40. (2) After arterial punctures, your first nursing priority is to observe for bleeding or hematoma formation, particularly in the first 4 hours after the procedure. Vital signs (No. 1) are monitored. The specific gravity and urinary output (No. 3) are monitored, but this is not as significant as observing the puncture site. The peripheral pulse distal to the puncture site (No. 4) is also monitored. Because of the size of the vessel, bleeding can quickly cause volume depletion and shock.

41. (2) Because the flank incision in nephrectomy is directly below the diaphragm, deep breathing is painful. Additionally, there is a greater incisional pull each time the person moves than there is with abdominal surgery. Incisional pain following nephrectomy generally requires analgesic administration every 3–4 hours for 24–48 hours after surgery. Therefore turning, coughing, and deep breathing exercises should be planned to maximize the analgesic effects. Client may be on either side, as long as drainage tubes are not kinked and gravity flow is uninhibited (No. 1). A low Fowler's or semi-Fowler's position is generally more comfortable for the client and of sufficient height to encourage gravity flow from drainage tubes (No. 3). Fluid administration is directed toward maintaining blood volume and urinary output (No. 4).

42. (2) Daily weights are taken following nephrectomy. Daily increases of two or more pounds is indicative of fluid retention and should be reported to the physician. Intake and output records may also reflect this imbalance. Increased specific gravity of urine (No. 1) indicates that the client is underhydrated rather than overhydrated. A urinary output of 50 mL/h (No. 3) is the desired minimum following renal surgery. Periorbital edema (No. 4) is a later sign of excess fluid retention.

43. (1) Hemorrhage may follow nephrectomy because of the difficulty in securing ligatures in the short renal-artery stump. It may occur on the day of surgery or 8–12 days postoperatively, when normal tissue sloughing occurs with healing. Dressing and urine are observed for bright red bleeding, vital signs are monitored, and the client is continually observed for any other indications of shock. Hyperkalemia (No.2), tetany (No. 3), and polyuria (No. 4) are not common complications after nephrectomy.

44. (2) Though nausea may occur following the administration of narcotics, if it is accompanied by the absence of bowel sounds and upper abdominal distention, gastric or small-intestine dilatation should be suspected and your findings reported to the physician. Changing the client's position (No. 1) and insertion of a rectal tube (No. 3) are not helpful if peristalsis is not present (bowel sounds). Administering morphine (No. 4) is not indicated until the source of Mr. Cloutier's discomfort is diagnosed.

45. (3) Paralytic ileus is characterized by diminished, absent, or uncoordinated bowel sounds due to inappropriate or absent autonomic nervous system (vagal) stimulation of the intestinal tract. Paralytic ileus may occur due to anesthetic interruption of autonomic outflow or hypokalemia. Edema of the intestinal mucosa (No. 1) is usually found with inflammation or ulcerative colitis. Acute dilatation of the colon (No. 2) and high, tinkling bowel sounds (No. 4) are associated with large-bowel obstruction.

46. (1) The Miller-Abbott tube is a double-lumen tube, with one lumen leading to the inflatable balloon and the other lumen utilized for aspiration of intestinal contents. No. 2 is an example of a Levin tube, used for gastric suction. No. 3 is an example of a Harris tube, and No. 4, a Cantor tube, both utilized for intestinal decompression, like the Miller-Abbott.

47. (1) Chilling the tube before insertion assists in relieving some of the nasal discomfort. Water-soluble lubricants along with viscous xylocaine may also be used. However, since mercury is instilled into the balloon of the Miller-Abbott tube after insertion, it is usually only lightly lubricated before insertion. The client may be administered a sedative (No. 2) on physician's orders to reduce apprehension during insertion. Warming the tube (No. 3) has no advantages. The client is usually positioned (No. 4) in high Fowler's position during insertion to aid in swallowing the tube.

48. (2) After the tube has been inserted into the stomach, its movement into the duodenum is first facilitated by having the client lie on his right side for 2 hours, then on his back with head elevated for 2 hours, and finally on his left side for 2 hours. After the tube has passed the pylorus (this is usually checked by X ray), ambulating him will help move the tube to the point of obstruction. After positioning and ambulation, the physician or the nurse may advance the tube 1–4 inches at specified time intervals (No. 1) to provide slack for peristaltic action. Remaining quiet or flat in bed (Nos. 3 and 4) will not facilitate the advancement of the tube either through the pylorus or through the small intestine.

49. (4) Recognizing the client's concern is essential both in maintaining rapport and in keeping the lines of communication open. Having done this, you can then assure the client that one kidney is sufficient to handle renal functions. This statement can then be followed by other discharge instructions, such as the need for adequate fluid intake, avoiding infections, and untoward signs that the client needs to observe for. Nos. 1, 2, and 3 do not recognize the client's concern or facilitate open communication.

50. (1) A freshly applied cast generates heat as moisture evaporates and cast hardens. To facilitate drying, keep it exposed to the air. Do not use plastic covers or Chux on pillows to elevate the limb, as these tend to slow drying. No. 2 is incorrect; signs of increased pressure are numbness and tingling, pain, and loss of movement. No. 4 does not take into account that discomfort and apprehension can be reduced if the client understands what is to be expected. No. 3 is an inappropriate response to the question because it also fails to recognize the client's cognitive needs.

51. (3) Signs of circulatory constriction include blanching (delayed capillary refill) and cyanosis, swelling of the toes, pain that is out of proportion for the type of fracture, and temperature changes. Tingling and numbness (No. 1), loss of movement (No. 2), and constant pain (No. 4) are symptoms associated with constriction or pressure on a peripheral nerve.

52. (3) Bivalving the cast involves full-length splitting of the cast on each side. The underlying padding is also cut, as blood-soaked padding shrinks and can also cause circulatory constriction. After the cast is cut, it is spread sufficiently to relieve constriction. This procedure does not disturb reduction of the bone. The cast is then reapplied (No. 1) after the swelling has gone down. No. 2 is the technique used when the cast is removed. The client's limb should always be elevated (No. 4) following bivalving, as the underlying condition (edema and swelling) is best relieved by elevation of the limb, ice packs, and isometric exercises.

53. (2) It is not safe to insert any foreign object under a cast, as the skin may break and become infected. Scratching also disturbs the padded surface under the cast, causing it to become wrinkled, which may lead to skin irritation and breakdown. Itching under the cast can be relieved by directing air (from a blower) under the cast. Oral medication is not generally effective in relieving this type of skin irritation (No. 1). Rolling the cast (No. 3) while Mr. Mackey scratched would only increase the risk of skin damage. Taking the pencil from Mr. Mackey (No. 4) would deny his ability both to understand the rationale and to take responsibility for his actions.

54. (2) The three-point gait is appropriate when weight-bearing is not allowed on the affected limb. The swing-to and swing-through crutch gaits may also be used when only one leg can be used for weight-bearing. Nos. 1 and 3 are utilized when weight-bearing is allowed on both feet. No. 4, the tripod gait, is utilized when the client has little or no sensation or movement (paralysis) in the lower limbs.

55. (1) In the use of crutches, all weight-bearing should be on the hands. Constant pressure in the axilla from weight-bearing can lead to damage of the brachial plexus nerves and produce crutch paralysis. Nos. 2, 3, and 4 are appropriate instructions to give to the client preparing for crutch-walking.

56. (2) Epileptic seizures or convulsions are the result of excessive, simultaneous, disordered neuronal discharge in the brain. This dysrhythmic electrical discharge may be focal (Jacksonian seizure) or widely dispersed (grand mal seizures). Nos. 3 and 4 are incorrect because theories for the initiation of these convulsions vary from decreased intracellular K^+ to decreased cerebral spinal fluid to alteration in neuronal defenses due to trauma, toxins, or inflammation. Depending on existing potential in the individual, No. 1 may be a precipitating factor.

57. (2) Generalized tonic-clonic (grand mal) seizures are characterized by auras preceding the convulsive spasms of all muscle groups, loss of consciousness, and loss of sphincter control. Brief, abrupt loss of consciousness, with a characteristic "blank stare," is indicative of absence (petit mal) seizures (No. 1). Focal or partial seizures usually involve only a portion of the brain and reflect the area of the brain activated by abnormal discharge (such as tonic and clonic contractions of the large muscles in an arm or leg (No. 3). Localized twitching of facial muscles, especially of the angle of the mouth, or within a finger or toe, is characteristic of a Jacksonian seizure (No. 4).

58. (3) Dilantin (phenytoin, diphenylhydantoin) is consistently found to be effective against most types of seizures except absence seizures. Its precise action is unknown, but it appears to stabilize cell membranes by altering intracellular sodium concentrations. Plasma levels of the drug are checked frequently to avoid toxicity and to determine effective dosage. Side effects include gastritis and nervousness, and at toxic levels the drug may cause ataxia. Phenobarbital (No. 1) is also used in conjunction with Dilantin. Diazepam (No. 2) may be used as adjunct therapy in seizure disorders. Trimethadione (No. 4) is used in the control of absence seizures.

59. (3) The first priority is to protect the client from injury. Do not restrain the client's arms or legs, but make sure she does not hit anything. Protect the head with your hand, a towel, or jacket. During the initial tonic phase, the client usually stops breathing for up to a minute. There is no cause for alarm, as spontaneous breathing will, in most clients, return with no harm. In the absence of breathing, airway patency (No. 2) is *not* the *first* priority. Muscle contraction will prevent "positioning" of the head. The use of a padded tongue blade, once indicated during a seizure, is also no longer used. Nos. 1 and 4 are appropriate nursing actions after the seizure has ended.

60. (2) Dilantin must be injected IV slowly and in small increments to prevent vasodepression and circulatory collapse. Respiratory depression (No. 1) is generally associated with morphine sulfate. Adrenergic (alpha) drugs such as Levophed may cause vein and tissue necrosis (No. 3) and have only rarely caused sudden malignant increases in blood pressure (No. 4).

61. (1) Glaucoma is defined as an imbalance between the rate of secretion of intraocular fluids and the rate of their absorption. Glaucoma may be acute/closed-angle (obstruction of the angle between the cornea and iris) or chronic/open-angle (obstruction occurs proximal or distal to the angle). It is characterized by increased intraocular pressures. Narrowing of the arterioles and retinal ischemia (No. 2) are the result of prolonged hypertension. Clouding of the cornea (No. 3) is not seen in glaucoma. Buckling of the retina (No. 4) is associated with retinal detachment.

62. (2) The normal range of intraocular pressures is 12–22 mm Hg. No. 1 is below the range of normal pressures and may occur in hypovolemia (soft eyeballs) or dehydration. No. 3 is incorrect because ocular pressures are measured in millimeters of mercury. No. 4 is incorrect because pressures above 22 mm Hg are considered elevated.

63. (3) Generally the client with chronic, or open-angle, glaucoma has few complaints of intense symptomatology. The usual onset of this condition is slow, silent, and painless. However, some clients do experience prodromal symptoms, such as aching and discomfort around the eye, disturbed accommodation to darkness, and blurring of peripheral vision (No. 1). Any complaint of pain or increasing discomfort with radiation to the forehead and temporal area is a grave sign of a sudden increase in pressure. Difficulty with close vision (No. 2) is not characteristic of glaucoma. Halos around lights (No. 4) occur less commonly.

64. (3) In chronic, or open-angle glaucoma, the obstruction to aqueous outflow is due to degenerative changes in either the trabeculum, Schlemm's canal, or the aqueous veins. Closed-angle glaucoma is characterized by obstruction of aqueous outflow due to narrowing of the angle between the anterior chamber and the root of the iris. The other answers are incorrect because chronic, or open-angle, glaucoma occurs more frequently than closed-angle (No. 1), is characterized by slow, insidious, painless onset rather than the acute symptoms of closed-angle glaucoma (No. 2), and is certainly familial, if not hereditary (No. 4). Due to this latter characteristic, family members of clients with open-angle glaucoma should be encouraged to have their intraocular pressures assessed annually, particularly past age 40.

65. (2) Pilocarpine constricts the pupil by causing contraction of the ciliary muscles, thus widening the outflow channels and increasing aqueous flow. No. 1 is incorrect because pilocarpine is a parasympathomimetic; that is, it mimics the action of acetylcholine at cholinergic nerve endings, thus decreasing pupil size. No. 3 is incorrect, in that diuretics such as Diamox, which is a carbonic anhydrase inhibitor, are used to decrease aqueous production. No. 4 does not describe the actions of any medication utilized in glaucoma therapy.

66. (2) Vigorous activities such as brushing the teeth and brushing the hair are generally discouraged during periods of acute distress. These activities tend to increase aqueous production and therefore pressures because they activate sympathetic nervous system stimulation of the vasculature. Quiet activities such as watching TV (No. 1), moderate reading, self-feeding (No. 3), and passive range-of-motion exercises (No. 4) are encouraged.

67. (3) Eye drops should be instilled into the conjunctival sac to prevent medication from hitting the sensitive cornea. The client should then be instructed to close his eye, but not squeeze shut, so that the medication can be distributed evenly over the eye. Nos. 1 and 4 are incorrect because instillation on these structures would increase corneal irritation. No. 2 is incorrect because drops instilled into the inner canthus are likely to run down the outer aspects of the nose or be absorbed systemically through the tear duct.

68. (3) The most frequent cause of noncompliance to the medical treatment of chronic, or open-angle, glaucoma is the miotic effects of pilocarpine. Pupillary constriction impedes normal accommodation, making night driving difficult and hazardous, reducing the client's ability to read for extended periods, and making participation in games with fast-moving objects impossible. No. 1 is incorrect because daytime driving is not restricted. No. 2 is incorrect because this process is painless. The fact that the process is painless and insidious may in fact increase client's noncompliance because they do not usually experience any adverse reactions if they do not instill their eyedrops. Nausea and vomiting are rare toxic effects of pilocarpine and are usually very mild; hence No. 4 is incorrect.

69. (2) The primary dysfunction in myasthenia gravis occurs at the myoneural junction (the synapse between the end of a myelinated nerve fiber and a skeletal muscle fiber). Normally, acetylcholine is secreted by the nerve ending, which acts on the muscle fiber membrane by increasing its permeability to sodium. If sufficient sodium enters the muscle fiber membrane, an action potential is promulgated that causes the muscle fiber to contract. To enable the muscle fiber to repolarize, the acetylcholine in the synaptic junction is destroyed by cholinesterase. In myasthenia gravis, these normal impulses are blocked at the myoneural junction. No. 1 is incorrect because degeneration of the basal ganglia results in increased muscle tone, as occurs with Parkinson's disease. No. 3 is incorrect because increased stimulation of muscle fibers by anterior motor neurons would also increase muscle contractions. No. 4 is partially correct, in that there does seem to be a familial tendency toward the development of myasthenia; however, if myasthenia is generalized, it usually affects not only facial and mastication muscles but also ocular movement (diplopia and ptosis) as well as muscles of the neck, trunk (respirations), and limbs.

70. (4) Myasthenia gravis is a rare disease of unknown cause but is suspected to have autoimmune characteristics. No. 1 is not correct because thymectomy has *often* resulted in remission or improvement (in approximately 70% of clients), not rarely. No. 2 is not correct because myasthenia gravis runs a *chronic* and progressive, not acute and rapid course. One of the major symptoms is muscle weakness, *not* increased strength (No. 3).

71. (3) Edrophonium (Tensilon) is a short-acting anticholinesterase compound. A positive Tensilon test (a prompt and dramatic increase in muscle strength) is consistent with the diagnosis of myasthenia gravis. No. 1 is incorrect because an exacerbation of symptoms would indicate another cause for the muscle dysfunction. No. 2 is partially correct: ptosis is relieved, but so is sagging of the other facial muscles. No. 4 is incorrect because the increase in muscle strength is accompanied by decreased fatigability as long as the drug continues to circulate.

72. (3) The main treatment for clients with myasthenia gravis is anticholinesterase drugs. These drugs increase the response of muscles to nerve impulses and improve muscle strength by inhibiting the rapid removal of acetylcholine from the myoneural junction. No. 1 is partially correct, in that adrenergic drugs such as ephedrine sulfate are administered to improve muscle tone but these drugs do not inhibit cholinesterase at the myoneural junction. Likewise, anticholinergic drugs (No. 2) such as atropine are also utilized in the treatment of myasthenia, primarily to reduce the incidence of side effects of the anticholinesterase drugs and to reverse their effect if "cholinergic crisis" occurs. Cholinergic drugs (No. 4) are not indicated in the treatment of myasthenia gravis.

73. (1) The most common side effects of pyridostigmine (Mestinon) and neostigmine bromide (Prostigmin) include anorexia, nausea, diarrhea, and abdominal cramps. These symptoms are due to increased gastrointestinal secretions, smooth muscle contractions (peristalsis), and irritation of the gastric mucosa. No. 2 is incorrect because increased cholinergic discharge increases bladder tone and contraction, thus facilitating voiding. Nos. 3 and 4 are incorrect because the symptoms listed are consistent with increased adrenergic, not cholinergic, discharge or stimulation.

74. (1) The gastric distress that occurs with these medications can be reduced by administering the drugs along with milk, soda crackers, or antacids. Nos. 2, 3, and 4 are nursing actions consistent with Nos. 2, 3, and 4 in the previous question.

75. (3) In order to take full advantage of the effects of anticholinesterase drugs, they should generally be scheduled 20–30 minutes before eating. Nos. 1 and 2 are not totally incorrect, in that these drugs generally act over a 3-hour period; however, peak action occurs quickly, and clients with dysphagia need time to eat, chew, and swallow during meals. Rushing at meals causes unnecessary fatigue. No. 4 may not allow enough time for the drug to take effect.

76. (2) Signs of "cholinergic crisis" include pupils constricted to <2 mm, severe diarrhea, nausea, vomiting, hypersalivation, lacrimation, pallor, and hypotension. Bradycardia may occur but is uncommon. In severe cases, confusion progressing to coma may occur due to blockage of cerebral synapses. Nos. 1 and 3 are symptoms related to increased adrenergic discharge. No. 4 is only partially correct.

77. (1) In cholinergic crisis, all anticholinesterase drugs are withdrawn and atropine (an anticholinergic drug) is given in 2-mg doses IV every hour until signs of atropine toxicity develop (dry mouth, blurred vision, tachycardia, rash or flushing of the skin, and elevated temperature). Nos. 2, 3, and 4 are incorrect because they do not act to decrease cholinergic responses. Ephedrine (No. 2) is utilized in myasthenia gravis to increase muscle tone; potassium chloride (No. 3) is utilized to increase serum K^+ because it is believed that adequate serum-potassium levels potentiate the effects of cholinergic drugs; and neostigmine bromide (No. 4) is an anticholinesterase that acts to improve cholinergic transmission of impulses at the myoneural junction.

78. (2) Since the dysfunction in myasthenia gravis occurs at the myoneural junction, it is considered a lower motor neuron lesion. Upper motor neuron lesions (No. 1) involve cranial neurons and their axons in the spinal cord. Combined lesions (No. 3) generally occur with spinal injury when axons of cranial neurons are destroyed, resulting in hyperreflexia and increased muscle tone below the level of the lesion and destruction of motor neurons at the level of the injury, which in turn leads to hyporeflexia, decreased muscle tone, and muscle atrophy in those muscles normally innervated by these neurons. Myasthenia gravis is not an inherited disorder (No. 4). Recent evidence suggests an autoimmune basis.

79. (1) The most common cause of hypothyroidism today is excess thyroid tissue destruction due to radioactive iodine therapy for hyperthyroidism. Spontaneous hypothyroidism is believed due to an autoimmune response. Several studies have revealed a high incidence of antibodies for thyroid antigen in clients with spontaneous atrophy (No. 2). Other, less common causes include surgical removal (No. 3), Hashimoto's thyroiditis, overuse of antithyroid drugs (No. 4), and pituitary tumors or insufficiency that decrease the circulating levels of TSH (thyroid-stimulating hormone).

80. (3) A deficiency of thyroid hormone causes widespread metabolic changes. Alterations in fluid and electrolyte balance due to increased capillary permeability lead to fluid retention that results in edema, particularly of the eyelids, hands, and feet. No. 1 is incorrect because the lowered metabolic rate decreases cellular oxygen consumption; as a result, the heart rate, pulse pressure, and blood pressure are reduced. No. 2 is incorrect because there is eyelid edema, not facial edema. The basal metabolic rate is reduced, causing symptoms of anorexia, constipation, and intolerance to cold due to a lowered body temperature. No. 4 is incorrect because it includes diarrhea. Reduced cerebral blood flow affects both perception and coordination and results in symptoms of lethargy, generalized weakness, and slowing of both intellectual and motor functions.

81. (2) If treatment with thyroid hormone is effective, there should be an overall increase in metabolic rate and a decrease in fluid retention; that is, increased blood pressure, pulse rate, pulse pressure, temperature, and rate and depth of respirations. As a result of improved renal blood flow, glomerular filtration and urine output should also increase, thus reducing the weight gain due to fluid retention. Nos. 1, 3, and 4 are incorrect because each contains at least one outcome that is not consistent with improved status.

82. (1) The client with hyperthyroidism has an increased metabolic rate due to excess serum thyroxine leading to symptoms of systolic hypertension, heat intolerance, widened pulse pressure, and emotional excitability. No. 2 is incorrect because the diastolic blood pressure reduces due to decreased peripheral resistance. Weight loss (not gain, as in No. 3) occurs because of increased catabolism despite an increase in appetite. Anorexia in No. 4 is incorrect.

83. (2) Clients with hyperthyroidism have an increased BMR (basal metabolic rate) as well as increased T_3 and T_4. Increased serum cholesterol (No. 1), increased TSH (No. 3), and increased menstrual volume (No. 4) are findings consistent with hypothyroidism. Menstruation in hyperthyroidism characteristically is decreased in volume. Cycle lengths may be shortened or prolonged, but eventually amenorrhea develops.

84. (1) Thyroid storm may be precipitated by a number of stresses, such as infection, real or threatened loss of a loved one, or thyroid surgery undertaken before the client was prepared adequately with antithyroid drugs. A change heralding thyroid storm is a fever: the client's temperature may rise as high as 106 °F (41 °C). Nos. 2, 3, and 4 are symptoms of hyperthyroidism and become exaggerated during thyroid storm. Without treatment, the client progresses from delirium to coma; death ensues as the result of congestive heart failure.

85. (1) The primary pathology in Cushing's syndrome is increased serum cortisol, which acts to accelerate the rate of gluconeogenesis in the body, thus mobilizing stored fats and proteins. Serum glucose is increased, stimulating insulin secretion by the pancreas and resulting in abnormalities in fat metabolism and deposition. Weight gain is common; the torso enlarges and fat pads develop on the back of the neck and in the cheeks, giving the client the characteristic "buffalo hump" and "moon facies." Increased epinephrine secretion (No. 2) is associated with pheochromocytoma. Increased aldosterone (No. 3) is associated with primary aldosteronism. Decreased ACTH secretion (No. 4) is associated with dysfunctions of the pituitary gland.

86. (2) Lassitude and muscle weakness are early clinical signs of Cushing's syndrome. Catabolism from gluconeogenesis occasionally results in a marked decrease in skeletal mass and the client's extremities may appear wasted. No. 1 is incorrect because gluconeogenesis from excess cortisol secretion results in hyperglycemia. No. 3 is partially correct: hypersecretion of aldosterone in Cushing's disease is rare; however, large quantities of cortisol tend to increase sodium and water retention and potassium excretion. Edema and hypokalemia occur only in severe cases. Discoloration and hyperpigmentation (No. 4) occur with adrenal insufficiency.

87. (1) Signs and symptoms of Addison's disease include hypotension, hypoglycemia, muscular weakness, fatigue, weight loss, hyperkalemia, and depression. These symptoms are primarily due to disturbances in sodium, water, and potassium imbalances that cause severe dehydration. No. 2 includes symptoms of Cushing's syndrome. No. 3 is incorrect because hyperglycemia and weight gain are consistent also with Cushing's syndrome. No. 4 also includes symptoms of Cushing's syndrome.

88. (1) The primary fluid and electrolyte imbalances in Addison's disease are hyponatremia, hypovolemia, and hyperkalemia. These imbalances are caused by decreased aldosterone secretion. Nos. 2 and 3 are incorrect because they occur with excessive secretion of this hormone. Calcium levels are not affected by this condition (No. 4).

89. (4) Since the client's ability to react to stress is decreased, maintaining a quiet environment becomes a nursing priority. Dehydration is a common problem in Addison's disease, so close observation of the client's hydration level is crucial. To promote optimal hydration and sodium intake, fluid intake is increased, particularly fluids containing electrolytes, such as broths, carbonated beverages, and juices. No. 1 is incorrect because it limits sodium. No. 2 is incorrect because it limits fluids. Daily weights and intake and output records are essential for monitoring fluid balance. Drug therapy in Addison's disease is directed toward oral replacement of adrenocorticosteroids such as cortisone, prednisone, and fludrohydrocortisone (Florinef). Insulin (No. 3) is not required.

90. (1) Iron-deficiency anemia is characterized by a decrease in red blood cell color due to a decrease in iron (hypochromic) and an increase in immature red blood cells (microcytic). No. 2 describes the red blood cells in pernicious anemia. Nos. 3 and 4 describe no particular conditions.

91. (1) In assessing any client's emotional responses, you should first assess the client's ego strength, body image, and coping abilities for life situations in general. The manner in which the client views herself will greatly affect her attitudes toward her disease and her emotional response. If the client normally denies or represses threatening information or situations, desirable outcomes may be difficult to achieve. The evidence of recent research indicates that social supports are extremely important in maintaining health. The relationship between Mrs. Sanchez and her mother (No. 2) should be assessed. However, if Mrs. Sanchez has a strong self-image, the issues between mother and daughter should be resolvable either alone or with objective outside help. No. 3 is incomplete. Economic status and work history (No. 4), depending on their value to Mrs. Sanchez, may or may not be important determinants of her emotional response.

92. (3) The best early intervention would be to increase fluid intake because constipation is common when activity is decreased or usual routines have been interrupted. No. 1 is incorrect because this may not be necessary and also needs a doctor's order. No. 2 is incorrect because this is a great deal of exertion when the client is not expressing an urge to defecate. Although activity usually helps bowel evacuation, it would be impossible to exercise extremities that have unhealed fractures (No. 4).

93. (2) Alcohol is extremely drying and contributes to skin breakdown. An emollient lotion should be used. Bed cradles (No. 1) keep the pressure of bed clothing off pressure points. High-protein diet (No. 3) aids in the healing process. Assessment of skin (No. 4) is vital, to recognize any red areas.

94. (1) Osteoblastic activity (bone growth) needs the stress and strain of weight-bearing to be proportional to osteoclastic activity (bone breakdown). When the client is immobilized for an extended period of time, bone breakdown takes place. Although dietary intake is important, it is not recommended that there be an increase in calcium intake (No. 2) due to the potential for kidney stones as a result of immobilization. Osteoporosis is related to a *deficit* of calcium, not excess (No. 3). Bone growth is dependent on weight-bearing, not lack of it (No. 4).

95. (3) Increased carbohydrates are needed for healing and tissue repair. Anorexia, *not increased appetite* (No. 1), is a problem. Increased, *not decreased* protein catabolism is present (No. 2). Digestive enzyme secretion is decreased, *not increased* (No. 4).

96. (1) Ventricular tachycardia occurs most commonly in clients with acute MI and coronary artery disease. Of immediate significance to the client, if untreated, are the hemodynamic dysfunction, a drop in blood pressure rather than an increase (No. 2), and the possibility of progressing to ventricular fibrillation. No. 3 is incorrect because if pain does result it will be angina, not MI pain. No. 4 is incorrect because ventricular tachycardia is potentially life threatening and requires intervention.

97. (4) Sinus arrhythmia is the most frequent arrhythmia and occurs as a normal phenomenon, often related to the respiratory cycle. No. 1 is incorrect because lidocaine is used to treat life-threatening ventricular arrhythmias. No. 2 is incorrect because exercise, which increases the heart rate, will abolish the arrhythmia, so rest or limited activity is not indicated. No. 3 is incorrect because the arrhythmia originates in the sinoatrial node, not in the atrioventricular node, and digoxin is the treatment for atrial arrhythmias.

98. (2) The narrow QRS complexes are normal, within 0.12 sec, but there are no regular P waves for each QRS. The baseline appears "wavy" and the rhythm is "regularly irregular," which describes atrial fibrillation. The second and fifth QRS complexes are wide and bizarre but alike, indicating a unifocal origin. No. 1 is incorrect because there is not one P wave for every QRS, and the multifocal PVCs would look different in configuration. Even though the rate is 100, No. 3 is incorrect because the impulse is not originating from the SA node, which is necessary for a sinus rhythm. No 4 is incorrect because atrial tachycardia is more rapid and regular, and though the P waves are difficult to see, they are present. Also, the PVCs are unifocal, not multifocal, in origin.

UNIT

5 Review of Nutrition

NUTRITION DURING PREGNANCY AND LACTATION

See Table 5.1.

I. Milk group—important for calcium, protein of high biologic value, and other vitamins and minerals.

- **A.** *Pregnancy*—three to four servings.
- **B.** *Lactation*—four to five servings.
- **C.** *Count as one serving*—1 cup milk; ½ cup undiluted evaporated milk; ¼ cup dry milk; 1¼ cups cottage cheese; 2 cups low-fat cottage cheese; 1½ cups cheddar or Swiss cheese; or 1½ cups ice cream.

II. Meat group—important for protein, iron, and many B vitamins.

- **A.** *Pregnancy*—three servings.
- **B.** *Lactation*—two servings.
- **C.** *Count as one serving* (12–14 g protein)—6–8 oz lean meat, fish, or poultry; 2 eggs; 2 frankfurters; 4 tbsp peanut butter; or 1 cup cooked dry beans, dry peas, or lentils.

III. Vegetable and fruit group—vitamins and minerals (especially A and C) and roughage.

- **A.** *Pregnancy*—five to six servings.
- **B.** *Lactation*—five to six servings.
- **C.** *Count as one serving*—½ medium grapefruit; 1 medium apple, banana, or orange; ¾ cup fruit juice.
- **D.** *Good sources (vitamin C)*—citruses, cantaloupe, mango, papaya, strawberries, broccoli, and green and red bell peppers.
- **E.** *Fair sources (vitamin C)*—tomatoes, honeydew melon, asparagus tips, raw cabbage, collards, kale, mustard greens, potatoes (white and sweet), spinach, and turnip greens.
- **F.** *Good sources (vitamin A)*—dark green or deep yellow vegetables and a few fruits (apricots, broccoli, pumpkin, sweet potato, spinach, cantaloupe, carrots, and winter squash).
- **G.** *Good sources of folic acid*—dark green foliage-type vegetables.

IV. Bread and cereal group—good for thiamine, iron, niacin, and other vitamins and minerals.

- **A.** *Pregnancy*—ten servings.
- **B.** *Lactation*—ten servings.
- **C.** *Count as one serving*—1 slice bread, 1 oz ready-to-eat cereal, ½ to ¾ cup cooked cereal, cornmeal, grits, macaroni, noodles, rice, or spaghetti.

NUTRITIONAL NEEDS OF THE NEWBORN

I. Calories—115 Kcal/kg/day.

II. Protein—3.5 g/kg/day (1 g protein = 1 oz milk).

III. Fluids—3.5 oz/kg/24 hours.

IV. Vitamin D—400 IU daily for bottle-fed babies after week two.

V. Fluoride—0.25 mg daily regardless of content in local water supply.

■ **TABLE 5.1** **Nutrient Needs During Pregnancy**

Nutrient	Maternal Need	Fetal Need	Food Source
Protein	Maternal tissue growth: uterus, breasts, blood volume, storage.	Rapid fetal growth.	Milk and milk products; animal meats—muscle, organs; grains, legumes; eggs.
Calories	Increased BMR.	Primary energy source for growth of fetus.	Carbohydrates: 4 Kcal/g Proteins: 4 Kcal/g Fats: 9 Kcal/g
Minerals Calcium (and phosphorus)	Increase in maternal Ca^{2+} metabolism.	Skeleton and tooth formation.	Milk and milk products, especially Swiss cheese.*
Iron	Increase in RBC mass. Prevent anemia. Decrease infection risk.	Liver storage (especially in third trimester).	Organ meats—liver, animal meat; egg yolk, whole or enriched grains; green leafy vegetables; nuts.
Vitamins A	Tissue growth.	Cell development—tissue and bone growth and tooth bud formation.	Butter, cream, fortified margarine; green and yellow vegetables.
B's	Coenzyme in many metabolic processes.	Coenzyme in many metabolic processes.	Animal meats, organ meats; milk and cheese; beans, peas, nuts; enriched grains.
Folic acid	Meet increased metabolic demands in pregnancy. Production of blood products.	Meet increased metabolic demands, including production of cell nucleus material.	Liver; deep-green, leafy vegetables.
C	Tissue formation and integrity. Increase iron absorption.	Tissue formation and integrity.	Citrus fruit, berries, melons; peppers; green, leafy vegetables; broccoli; potatoes.
D	Absorption Ca^{2+}, phosphorus.	Mineralization of bone tissue and tooth buds.	Fortified milk and margarine.
E	Tissue growth; cell wall integrity; RBC integrity.	Tissue growth; cell integrity; RBC integrity.	Widely distributed: meat, milk, eggs, grains, leafy vegetables.

*Swiss cheese contains twice the amount of calcium as 8 oz of whole milk but only 0.09 as much lactose; therefore, it is a good source for those with lactose intolerance. Tofu (soybean cake) also is high in calcium, and contains *no* lactose.

■ PEDIATRIC NUTRITION

See Tables 5.2, 5.3, and 5.4.

■ **TABLE 5.2** **Recommended Energy Intake for Children of Various Ages**

	Age	Energy (Kcal/kg)
Infants	0–0.5	115
	0.5–1	105
Children	1–3	100
	4–6	85
	7–10	85
Males	11–14	60
	15–18	42
Females	11–14	48
	15–18	38

Source: Recommended Dietary Allowances, © 1989 by the National Academy of Sciences, National Academy Press.

■ ETHNIC FOOD PATTERNS

See Tables 5.5 and 5.6.

■ COMMON VITAMINS AND RELATED DEFICIENCIES

See Table 5.7.

■ NUTRITIONAL NEEDS OF THE ELDERLY

I. *Calories*—1500–2000 Kcal/day to maintain ideal weight; 15-20% of calories from protein sources.

II. *High fiber*—prevent or alleviate constipation and dependence on laxatives.

III. Sodium—3–4 g/day according to cardiac and renal status.

■ TABLE 5.3 Recommended Food-Group Intake and Serving Sizes

Food Group	Servings per Day	Average Size of Servings: 1 Year	2–3 Years	4–5 Years	6–9 Years	10–12 Years	13–15 Years
Milk and cheese (1.5 oz cheese = 1 c milk)	4	½ c*	½–¾ c	½–¾ c	½–1 c	½–1 c	½–1 c
Meat group (protein foods)	3 or more						
Eggs		1	1	1	1	1	1 or more
Lean meat, fish, poultry (liver once a week)		2 tbsp	2 tbsp	4 tbsp	2–3 oz (4–6 tbsp)	3–4 oz	4 oz or more
Peanut butter			1 tbsp	2 tbsp	2–3 tbsp	3 tbsp	3 tbsp
Fruits and vegetables	At least 4, including:						
Vitamin C source (citrus fruits, berries, tomato, cabbage, cantaloupe)	1 or more (twice as much tomato as citrus)	⅓ c (citrus)	½ c	½ c	1 medium orange	1 medium orange	1 medium orange
Vitamin A source (green or yellow fruits and vegetables)	1 or more	2 tbsp	3 tbsp	4 tbsp (¼ c)	¼ c	⅓ c	½ c
Other vegetables (potato and legumes, etc.) *or*	2	2 tbsp	3 tbsp	4 tbsp (¼ c)	⅓ c	½ c	¾ c
Other fruits (apple, banana, etc.)		¼ c	⅓ c	½ c	1 medium	1 medium	1 medium
Cereals (whole-grain or enriched)	At least 4						
Bread		½ slice	1 slice	1½ slices	1–2 slices	2 slices	2 slices
Ready-to-eat cereals		½ oz	¾ oz	1 oz	1 oz	1 oz	1 oz
Cooked cereal (including macaroni, spaghetti, rice, etc.)		¼ c	⅓ c	½ c	½ c	¾ c	1 c or more
Fats and carbohydrates	To meet caloric needs						
Butter, margarine, mayonnaise, oils: 1 tbsp—100 calories (Kcal)		1 tbsp	1 tbsp	1 tbsp	2 tbsp	2 tbsp	2–4 tbsp
Desserts and sweets: 100-calorie portions as follows: ⅓ c pudding or ice cream; 2 3″ cookies, 1 oz cake, 1⅓ oz pie, 2 tbsp jelly, jam, honey, sugar		1 portion	1½ portions	1½ portions	3 portions	3 portions	3–6 portions

*c = 1 cup or 8 oz or 240 mL.
†tbsp = tablespoon (1 tbsp = approx. 15 mL = approx. ½ oz).
Source: Marlow DR, Redding BA: *Textbook of Pediatric Nursing,* 6th ed. Philadelphia; Saunders, 1988.

IV. *Fluids*—6–8 glasses/daily.

V. Common deficiencies: calories, calcium, folic acid, thiamine, vitamins A and D, zinc.

VI. Factors contributing to food preferences:

A. Physical ability to prepare, shop for, and eat food.

B. Income.

C. Availability of food if dependent on others.

D. Food intolerances.

VII. See Table 5.8 for interventions for common eating problems in the elderly.

■ RELIGIOUS CONSIDERATIONS IN MEAL PLANNING

I. Orthodox Jews

A. Kosher meat and poultry.

B. No shellfish or pork products.

C. Milk and dairy products cannot be consumed with meat or poultry; requires separate utensils.

II. Conservative and Reform Jews: dietary practices may vary from religious laws.

III. Muslims: no pork or alcohol.

IV. Hindus: vegetarians (cows are sacred).

V. Seventh-day Adventists

A. Vegetarianism is common (lacto-ovo).

NUTRITION

■ **TABLE 5.4** **Fluid Maintenance Requirements for Infants and Children**

Age	Weight (kg)	Fluid Requirement (mL/24 hours)	Approximate Hourly Fluid Rate	Formula
Newborn (less than 72 h)	3.3	198–330	8–15	60–100 mL/kg body weight.
1 week	3.3	330	15	100mL/kg (can be increased if no renal or cardiac difficulties).
2 months	5.0	500	20	
6 months	8.0	800	35	
12 months	10.0	1000	40	
3 years	15.0	1250	50	1000 mL for the first 10 kg plus 50 mL/kg for each kg over 10 kg.
5 years	20.0	1500	60	
8 years	30.0	1750	70	1500 mL for the first 20 kg plus 25 mL/kg for each kg over 20 kg.
12 years	40.0	1850	80	1750 mL for the first 30 kg plus 10 mL/kg for each kg over 30 kg.

Source: James SR, Mott SR: *Child Health Nursing: Essential Care of Children and Families,* Menlo Park, CA: Addison-Wesley, 1988.

B. No shellfish or pork products.

C. Avoid stimulants (coffee, tea, other caffeine sources).

D. No alcohol.

VI. Mormons: no coffee, tea, or alcohol.

■ SPECIAL DIETS

I. Low-carbohydrate diet: epilepsy—ketogenic: low carbohydrate, high fat; dumping syndrome—low carbohydrate, high fat, high protein.

II. Gluten-free diet—elimination of all foods made from oats, barley, wheat and rye; used for celiac disease.

III. High-protein diet—lean meat, cheese, and green vegetables.

A. Nephrotic syndrome (may also be on low-sodium diet).

B. Acute leukemia (combined with high-calorie and soft-food diets).

C. Neoplastic disease.

IV. Low-protein diet

A. Usually accompanied by high-carbohydrate diet and normal fats and calories.

B. Renal failure; uremia; anuria; acute glomerulonephritis.

V. Low-sodium diet

A. Congestive heart failure.

B. Nephrotic syndrome.

C. Acute glomerulonephritis (varies with degree of oliguria).

■ COMMON THERAPEUTIC DIETS

I. Clear-liquid diet

A. *Purpose:* relieve thirst and help maintain fluid balance.

B. *Use:* postsurgically and following acute vomiting or diarrhea.

C. *Foods allowed:* carbonated beverages; coffee (caffeinated and decaffeinated); tea; fruit-flavored drinks; strained fruit juices; clear, flavored gelatins; broth, consommé; sugar; popsicles and hard candy.

D. *Foods avoided:* Milk and milk products, fruit juices with pulp, and fruit.

II. Full-liquid diet

A. *Purpose:* provide an adequately nutritious diet for clients who cannot chew or who are too ill to do so.

B. *Use:* acute infection with fever, gastrointestinal upsets, after surgery as a progression from *clear liquids.*

C. *Foods allowed:* clear liquids, milk drinks, cooked cereals, custards, ice cream, sherbets, eggnog, all strained fruit juices, vegetable juices, creamed vegetable soups, puddings, mashed potatoes, mild cheese sauce or puréed meat, and seasonings.

D. *Foods avoided:* nuts, seeds, coconut, fruit, jam, and marmalade.

III. Soft diet

A. *Purpose:* provide adequate nutrition for those who have trouble chewing.

B. *Use:* clients with no teeth or ill-fitting dentures; transition from full-liquid to general diet; and for those who cannot tolerate highly seasoned, fried, or raw foods following acute infections or gastrointestinal disturbances, such as gastric ulcer or cholelithiasis.

TABLE 5.5 Ethnic Food Patterns

Ethnic Group	Cultural Food Patterns	Dietary Excesses or Omissions
Mexican (native)	Basic sources of protein—dry beans, flan, cheese, many meats, fish, eggs. Chili peppers and many deep-green and yellow vegetables. Fruits include: zapote, guava, papaya, mango, citrus. Tortillas (corn, flour); sweet bread; fideo; tacos, burritos, enchiladas.	*Limited* meats, milk, and milk products. Some are using flour tortillas more than the more nutritious corn tortillas. *Excessive* use of lard (manteca), sugar. Tendency to boil vegetables for long periods of time.
Filipino (Spanish-Chinese influence)	Most meats, eggs, nuts, legumes. Many different kinds of vegetables. Large amounts of rice and cereals.	May *limit* meat, milk, and milk products (the latter may be due to lactose intolerance). Tend to prewash rice. Tend to fry many foods.
Chinese (mostly Cantonese)	Cheese, soybean curd (tofu), many meats, chicken and pigeon eggs; nuts; legumes. Many different vegetables, leaves, bamboo sprouts. Rice and rice-flour products; wheat, corn, millet seed; green tea. Mixtures of fish, pork, and chicken with vegetables—bamboo shoots, broccoli, cabbage, onions, mushrooms, pea pods.	Tendency among some immigrants to use *excess* grease in cooking. May be *low* in protein, milk, and milk products (the latter may be due to lactose intolerance). Often wash rice before cooking. Large amounts of soy and oyster sauces, both of which are *high in salt*.
Puerto Rican	Milk with coffee. Pork, poultry, eggs, dried fish; beans (habichuelas). Viandas (starchy vegetables; starchy ripe fruits). Avocados, okra, eggplant, sweet yams. Rice, cornmeal.	Utilize *large* amounts of lard for cooking. *Limited* use of milk and milk products. *Limited* amounts of pork and poultry.
Black American	Milk with coffee. Pork, poultry, eggs, dried fish; beans (habichuelas). Viandas (starchy vegetables; starchy ripe fruits). Avocados, okra, eggplant, sweet yams. Rice, cornmeal. Cereals (including grits, hominy, hot breads). Molasses (dark molasses is especially good source of calcium, iron, vitamins B_1 and B_2, and niacin).	*Limited* use of milk group (lactose intolerance). Extensive use of frying, "smothering," simmering for cooking. *Large* amounts of fat: salt pork, bacon drippings, lard, gravies. May have *limited* use of citrus and enriched breads.
Middle Eastern (Greek, Syrian, Armenian)	Yogurt. Predominantly lamb, nuts, dried peas, beans, lentils. Deep-green leaves and vegetables; dried fruits. Dark breads and cracked wheat.	Tend to use *excessive* sweeteners, lamb fat, olive oil. Tend to fry meats and vegetables. *Insufficient* milk and milk products (almost no butter—use olive oil, which has no nutritive value except for calories); deficiency in fresh fruits.
Middle European (Polish)	Many milk products. Pork, chicken. Root vegetables (potatoes); cabbage; fruits. Wheat products. Sausages, smoked and cured meats; noodles, dumplings; bread; cream with coffee.	Tend to use *excessive* sweets and to overcook vegetables. *Limited* amounts of fruits (citrus), raw vegetables, and meats.
Native American (American Indian—much variation)	If "Americanized," use milk and milk products. Variety of meats: game, fowl, fish; nuts, seeds, legumes. Variety of vegetables, some wild; variety of fruits, some wild, rose hips; roots. Variety of breads, including tortillas, cornmeal, rice.	*Nutrition-related problems:* obestiy, diabetes, dental problems, iron-deficiency anemia; alcoholism. *Limited* quantities of high-protein foods depending on availability (flocks) and economic situation. *Excessive* use of sugar.
Italian	Staples are pasta with sauces; bread; eggs; cheese; tomatoes and vegetables such as artichokes, eggplant, greens, and zucchini. Only small amount of meat is used.	*Limited* use of whole grains; *insufficient* servings from milk group; tendency to overcook vegetables; enjoy sweets.

C. *Foods allowed:* very tender minced, ground, baked, broiled, roasted, stewed, or creamed beef, lamb, veal, liver, poultry, or fish; crisp bacon or sweetbreads; cooked vegetables; pasta; all fruit juices; soft raw fruits; soft breads and cereals; all desserts that are soft; and cheeses.

D. *Foods avoided:* coarse whole-grain cereals and breads; nuts; raisins; coconut; fruits with small seeds; fried foods; high-fat gravies or sauces; spicy salad dressings; pickled meat, fish, or poultry; strong cheeses; brown or wild rice; raw vegetables as well as lima beans and corn; spices such as horseradish, mustard, and catsup; and popcorn.

IV. Sodium-restricted diet

A. *Purpose:* reduce sodium content in the tissues and promote excretion of water.

B. *Use:* congestive heart failure, hypertension, renal disease, cirrhosis, toxemia of pregnancy, and cortisone therapy.

C. *Modifications:* mildly restrictive 2-g sodium diet to extremely restricted 200-mg-sodium diet.

D. *Foods avoided:* table salt; all commercial soups, including bouillon; gravy, catsup, mustard, meat sauces, soy sauce, buttermilk, ice cream, sherbet, sodas, beet greens, carrots, celery, chard, sauerkraut, spinach, *all canned* vegetables, frozen peas, all baked products containing salt, baking powder or baking soda, potato chips, popcorn, fresh or canned shellfish, all cheeses, smoked or commercially prepared meats, salted butter or margarine, bacon, olives, and commercially prepared salad dressings.

TABLE 5.6 Hot-Cold Theory of Disease Treatment*

Hot Diseases or Conditions	Cold Diseases or Conditions	Hot Foods	Cold Foods	Hot Medicines and Herbs	Cold Medicines and Herbs
Infections	Cancer	Chocolate	Fresh vegetables	Penicillin	Bicarbonate of soda
Kidney diseases	Earache	Cheese	Tropical fruits	Aspirin	Milk of magnesia
Diarrhea	Rheumatism	Temperate-zone fruits	Dairy products	Castor oil	Sage
Rashes and other skin eruptions	Tuberculosis	Chili peppers	Low-prestige meats (goat, fish, chicken)	Cod liver oil	Linden
Sore throat	Common cold	Cereal grains	Honey	Iron preparations	Orange flower water
Warts	Headache	Goat milk	Raisins	Vitamins	
Constipation	Paralysis	High-prestige meats (beef, water fowl, mutton)	Bottled milk	Anise	
Ulcers	Stomach cramps	Oils	Barley water	Cinnamon	
Liver complaints	Teething	Hard liquor	Cod	Garlic	
	Menstrual period	Aromatic beverages		Mint	
	Joint pain	Coffee		Ginger root	
	Malaria	Onions		Tobacco	
	Pneumonia	Peas			
		Eggs			

*A Latin American, particularly Puerto Rican, approach to treating diseases. A "hot" disease is treated with "cold" treatments (foods, medicines) and vice versa.
Source: Reprinted with permission from Wilson HS, Kneisl CR: *Psychiatric Nursing,* 2nd ed. Menlo Park, CA: Addison-Wesley, 1983, p. 774.

V. Renal diet

A. *Purpose:* control protein, potassium, sodium, and fluid levels in body.

B. *Use:* acute and chronic renal failure, hemodialysis.

C. *Foods allowed:* high-biologic proteins such as meat, fowl, fish, cheese, and dairy products—range between 20 and 60 mg per day. Potassium is usually limited to 40 mEq per day. Vegetables such as cabbage, cucumber, and peas are lowest in potassium. Sodium is restricted to 500 mg per day. See Sodium-restricted diet. Fluid intake is restricted to the daily urine volume plus 500 mL, which represents insensible water loss. Fluid intake measures water in fruit, vegetables, milk, and meat.

D. *Foods avoided:* cereals, bread, macaroni, noodles, spaghetti, avocados, kidney beans, potato chips, raw fruit, yams, soybeans, nuts, gingerbread, apricots, bananas, figs, grapefruit, oranges, percolated coffee, Coca-Cola, Orange Crush, Gatorade, and breakfast drinks such as Tang or Awake.

VI. High-protein, high-carbohydrate diet

A. *Purpose:* corrects large protein losses and raises the level of blood albumin. May be modified to include low-fat, low-sodium, and low-cholesterol diets.

B. *Use:* burns, hepatitis, cirrhosis, pregnancy, hyperthyroidism, mononucleosis, protein deficiency due to poor eating habits, geriatric clients with poor food intake, nephritis, nephrosis, and liver and gallbladder disorders.

C. *Foods allowed:* general diet with added protein. In adults, high-protein diets usually contain 135–150 g protein.

D. *Foods avoided:* restrictions depend on modifications added to the diet. These modifications are determined by the client's condition.

VII. Purine-restricted diet

A. *Purpose:* designed to reduce the amount of consumed uric-acid-producing foods.

B. *Use:* high uric acid retention, uric acid renal stones, and gout.

C. *Foods allowed:* general diet plus 2–3 quarts of liquid daily.

D. *Foods avoided:* cheese containing spices or nuts, fried eggs, meat, liver, seafood, lentils, dried peas and beans, broth, bouillon, gravies, oatmeal and whole wheats, pasta, noodles, and alcoholic beverages. *Limited* quantities meat, fish, and seafood allowed.

VIII. Bland diet

A. *Purpose:* provision of a diet low in fiber, roughage, mechanical irritants, and chemical stimulants.

B. *Use:* ulcers (gastric and duodenal), gastritis, hyperchlorhydria, functional GI disorders, gastric atony, diarrhea, spastic constipation, biliary indigestion, and hiatus hernia.

C. *Foods allowed:* varied to meet individual needs and food tolerances.

D. *Foods avoided:* fried foods, including eggs, meat, fish, and seafood; cheese with added nuts or spices; commercially prepared luncheon meats; cured meats such as ham; gravies and sauces; raw vegetables; potato skins; fruit juices with pulp; figs; raisins; fresh fruits; whole wheats; rye bread; bran cereals; rich pastries; pies; chocolate; jams with seeds; nuts; seasoned dressings; regular coffee; strong tea; cocoa; alcoholic and carbonated beverages; and pepper.

IX. Low-fat, cholesterol-restricted diet

A. *Purpose:* reduce hyperlipemia, provide dietary treatment for malabsorption syndromes and clients having acute intolerance for fats.

■ TABLE 5.7 Physiologic Functions and Deficiency Syndromes of Common Vitamins

Nutrient	Functions	Signs of Deficiency
Fat-Soluble Vitamins		
Vitamin A	Essential for formation and maintenance of epithelial cells; essential for normal function of the retina and the synthesis of rhodopsin (visual purple).	Night blindness; xerosis and softening of the cornea; dry, bumpy skin.
Vitamin D	Necessary for absorption and metabolism of calcium and phosphorus; important for the formation of normal teeth and bones.	Rickets in children; osteomalacia in adults.
Vitamin E	Anti-oxidant that protects red blood cells from hemolysis; utilized in epithelial tissue maintenance and prostaglandin synthesis.	Increased hemolysis of red blood cells, macrocytic anemia, increased capillary fragility.
Vitamin K	Essential for the formation of prothrombin and other clotting factors by the liver.	Hypoprothrombinemia; hemorrhagic disease in newborns.
Water-Soluble Vitamins		
Vitamin C	Essential for the formation of collagen; promotes healing of wounds and fractures; reduces susceptibility to infections; promotes the absorption of iron; necessary for the conversion of folic acid to folinic acid, tryptophan to serotonin, and cholesterol to bile salts. May play a role in resistance to certain types of cancer.	Scurvy—petechiae and ecchymoses, joint pain, delayed wound healing, gingivitis, bleeding gums, loss of teeth.
Vitamin B_1 (thiamine)	Coenzyme in carbohydrate metabolism; essential for normal nerve function.	Beri beri—peripheral neuropathy, muscle cramping, paresthesias, muscle degeneration, and heart failure.
Vitamin B_2 (riboflavin)	Coenzyme in cellular metabolism and respiration; essential for healthy eyes.	Red conjunctivae; fissures at corners of mouth, around nose and ears, and on tongue; magenta tongue.
Vitamin B_3 (niacin)	Coenzyme in the metabolism of carbohydrates and amino acids; essential for the synthesis of fatty acids and cholesterol and the conversion of phenylalanine to tyrosine.	Pellagra—cracks in skin and lips; red lesions of hands, feet, face,, and neck; dementia.
Vitamin B_6 (pyridoxine)	Coenzyme in protein metabolism and several other enzymatic reactions; necessary for the formation of norepinephrine, epinephrine, tyramine, dopamine, and serotonin.	Seborrheic dermatitis, cheilosis, peripheral neuritis, and convulsions.
Vitamin B_9 (folic acid)	Essential for DNA synthesis and normal maturation of red blood cells.	Megaloblastic and macrocytic anemia; reduced platelet levels.
Vitamin B_{12} (cyanocobalamin)	Coenzyme in protein metabolism; essential for red blood cell formation and maintenance of myelin sheaths of nerves.	Pernicious anemia, progressive neuropathy owing to demyelination.

Source: Shlafer M, Marieb E: *The Nurse, Pharmacology and Drug Therapy.* Menlo Park, CA: Addison-Wesley, 1989.

B. *Use:* hyperlipidemia, atherosclerosis, pancreatitis, cystic fibrosis, sprue, gastrectomy, massive resection of the small intestine, and cholecystitis.

C. *Foods allowed:* nonfat milk; low-carbohydrate, low-fat vegetables; most fruits; breads; pastas; cornmeal; lean meats; unsaturated fats such as corn oil; desserts made without whole milk; and unsweetened carbonated beverages.

D. *Foods avoided:* whole milk and whole-milk or cream products, avocados, olives, commercially prepared baked goods such as donuts and muffins, poultry skin, highly marbled meats, shellfish, fish canned in oil, nuts, coconut, commercially prepared meats, butter, ordinary margarines, olive oil, lard, pudding made with whole milk, ice cream, candies with chocolate, cream, sauces, gravies, and commercially fried foods.

X. Diabetic diet

A. *Purpose:* maintain blood glucose as near normal as possible; prevent or delay onset of diabetic complications.

B. *Use:* diabetes mellitus.

C. *Foods allowed:* comprised of 50–60% carbohydrates, 30–38% fats, and 12–20% protein. Foods are divided into groups from which exchanges can be made. Coffee, tea, broth, bouillon, spices, and flavorings can be used as desired. Vegetable A exchanges, one cup, contain mostly green vegetables; vegetable B exchanges, one-half cup, contain the remaining vegetables. The amounts of the remaining exchanges depend on the food selected. Fruit exchanges are fruits without sugar or syrup. Meat, fat, and milk exchanges. The number of exchanges allowed from each group is dependent on the total number of calories allowed. Non-nutritive sweeteners (aspartame) if desired. Nutritive sweeteners (sorbitol) in moderation with controlled, normal weight diabetics.

D. *Foods avoided:* concentrated sweets or regular soft drinks.

XI. Acid and alkaline ash diet

A. *Purpose:* furnish a well-balanced diet in which the total acid ash is greater than the total alkaline ash each day.

■ **TABLE 5.8** **Dietary Interventions for Eating Problems of the Elderly**

Problem	Rationale	Dietary Interventions
Difficulty chewing.	Missing or ill-fitting dentures.	Provide liquid, semisolid, mashed, or chopped foods as tolerated.
Difficulty swallowing.	Paralysis related to stroke.	Thickened and gelled liquids are usually better tolerated than thin liquids. Baby food can be used as a nutritious thickener. Avoid overuse of purèed foods because of the negative connotations associated with it.
Lack of appetite.	Depression. Acute or chronic disease. Loss of sense of smell and taste. Side effect of medication. Loneliness. Early satiety.	Offer small, frequent meals. Solicit food preferences. Allow plenty of time to eat. Because appetite is usually greatest in the morning, emphasize a nutritious breakfast. Encourage group eating.
Impaired ability to feed self.	Poor vision. Arthritis of the hands; stroke.	Describe the meal and how it is arranged on the plate. Assist the client by opening packages of bread and crackers, buttering bread and vegetables; cutting meat, and opening milk cartons. Assess the client's ability to grasp utensils and guide food to the mouth. Refer the client to an occupational therapist to evaluate the need for assistive devices or retraining.

Source: Dudek S: *Nutrition Handbook for Nursing Practice.* Philadelphia: Lippincott, 1987, p. 308. Reprinted by permission of J.B. Lippincott Company.

NUTRITION

B. *Use:* retard the formation of renal calculi. The type of diet chosen depends on laboratory analysis of the stones.

C. *Acid and alkaline ash food groups:*

1. *Acid ash:* meat, whole grains, eggs, cheese, cranberries, prunes, plums.
2. *Alkaline ash:* milk, vegetables, fruit (except cranberries, prunes, and plums).
3. *Neutral:* sugars, fats, beverages (coffee and tea).

D. *Foods allowed:* all you want of the following.

1. Breads: any, preferably whole grain; crackers, rolls.
2. Cereals: any, preferably whole grain.
3. Desserts: angel food or sunshine cake; cookies made without baking powder or soda; cornstarch pudding, cranberry desserts, custards, gelatin desserts, ice cream, sherbet, plum or prune desserts; rice or tapioca pudding.
4. Fats: any, such as butter, margarine, salad dressings, Crisco, Spry, lard, salad oils, olive oil, etc.
5. Fruits: cranberries, plums, prunes.
6. Meat, eggs, cheese: any meat, fish or fowl, two servings daily; at least one egg daily.
7. Potato substitutes: corn, hominy, lentils, macaroni, noodles, rice, spaghetti, vermicelli.
8. Soup: broth as desired; other soups from foods allowed.
9. Sweets: cranberry or plum jelly; sugar, plain sugar candy.
10. Miscellaneous: cream sauce, gravy, peanut butter, peanuts, popcorn, salt, spices, vinegar, walnuts.

E. *Restricted foods:* no more than the amount allowed each day.

1. Milk: 1 pint daily (may be used in other ways than as beverage).
2. Cream: 1/3 cup or less daily.
3. Fruits: one serving of fruit daily (in addition to the prunes, plums, and cranberries); certain fruits listed under *Foods avoided* below are not allowed at any time.
4. Vegetables, including potatoes: two servings daily; certain vegetables listed under *Foods avoided* below are *not allowed at any time.*

F. *Foods avoided:*

1. Carbonated beverages, such as ginger ale, cola, root beer.
2. Cakes or cookies made with baking powder or soda.
3. Fruits: dried apricots, bananas, dates, figs, raisins, rhubarb.
4. Vegetables: dried beans, beet greens, dandelion greens, carrots, chard, lima beans.
5. Sweets; chocolate or candies other than those listed under *Foods allowed* above; syrups.
6. Miscellaneous: other nuts, olives, pickles.

XII. High-fiber diet

A. *Purpose:* soften stool; exercise digestive tract muscles; speed passage of food through digestive tract to prevent exposure to cancer-causing agents in food; lower blood lipids; prevent sharp rise in blood glucose after eating.

B. *Use:* diabetes, hyperlipidemia, constipation, diverticulosis, anticarcinogenic (colon).

C. *Foods allowed*—recommended intake about 6 g crude fiber daily: all bran cereals; watermelon, prunes, dried peaches, apple with skin; parsnips, peas, brussels sprouts; sunflower seeds.

XIII. Low-residue (low-fiber) diet

A. *Purpose:* reduce stool bulk and slow transit time.

B. *Use:* bowel inflammation during acute diverticulitis or ulcerative colitis, preparation for bowel surgery, esophageal and intestinal stenosis.

C. *Foods allowed:* eggs; ground or well-cooked tender meat, fish, poultry; milk; mild cheeses; strained fruit juice (except prune); cooked or canned apples, apricots, peaches, pears; ripe bananas; strained vegetable juice; canned, cooked, or strained asparagus, beets, green beans, pumpkin, acorn squash, spinach; white bread; refined cereals (Cream of Wheat).

■ FOOD LIST FOR READY REFERENCE IN MENU PLANNING

I. High-cholesterol foods—over 50 mg/100-g portion: beef, butter, cheese, egg yolks, fish, kidney, liver, pork, veal.

II. High-sodium foods—over 500 mg/100-g portion: bacon—cured, Canadian; baking powder; beef—corned, cooked, canned, dried, creamed; biscuits, baking powder; bouillon cubes; bran, added sugar and malt; bran flakes with thiamine; raisins; breads—wheat, french, rye, white, whole wheat; butter, cheese—cheddar, parmesan, Swiss, pasteurized American; cocoa; cookies, gingersnaps; corn flakes; cornbread; crackers—graham, saltines; margarine; milk—dry, skim; mustard; oat products; olives—green, ripe; peanut butter; pickles, dill; popcorn with oil and salt; salad dressing—blue, roquefort, French, thousand island; sausages—bologna, frankfurters; soy sauce; tomato catsup; tuna in oil.

NUTRITION

III. High-potassium foods—more than 400 mg/100-g portion: almonds; bacon, Canadian; baking powder, low-sodium; beans—white, lima; beef, hamburger; bran with sugar and malt; cake—fruitcake, gingerbread; cashew nuts; chicken, light meat; cocoa; coffee, instant; cookies, gingersnaps; dates; garlic; milk—dry, skim, powdered; peanuts, roasted; peanut butter; peas; pecans; potatoes, boiled in skin; scallops; tea, instant; tomato puree; turkey, light meat; veal; walnuts, black; yeast, brewers.

IV. Foods high in B vitamins

A. *Thiamine:* pork, dried beans, dried peas, liver, lamb, veal, nuts, peas.

B. *Riboflavin:* liver, poultry, beef, oysters, tongue, fish, cottage cheese, veal.

C. *Niacin:* liver, fish, poultry, peanut butter, lamb, veal, beef, pork.

V. Foods high in vitamin C: orange, strawberries, dark-green leafy vegetables, potatoes, grapefruit, tomato, cabbage, broccoli, melon, liver.

VI. Foods high in iron, calcium, and residue

A. *Iron:* breads—brown, corn, ginger; fish, tuna; poultry; organ meats; whole-grain cereals; shellfish; egg yolk; fruits—apples, berries; dried fruits—dates, prunes, apricots, peaches, raisins; vegetables—dark-green leafy, potatoes, tomatoes, rhubarb, squash; molasses; dried beans and peas; peanut butter; brown sugar; noodles; rice.

B. *Calcium:* milk—dry, skim, whole, evaporated, buttermilk; cheese—American, Swiss, hard; kale; turnip greens; mustard greens; collards.

C. *Residue:* whole-grain cereals—oatmeal, bran, shredded wheat; breads—whole wheat, cracked wheat, rye, bran muffins; vegetables—lettuce, spinach, Swiss chard, raw carrots, raw celery, corn, cauliflower, eggplant, sauerkraut, cabbage; fruits—bananas, figs, apricots, oranges.

VII. Foods to be used in low-protein and low-carbohydrate diets

A. *Low-protein*:* milk—buttermilk, reconstituted evaporated, low-sodium, skim and dry; meat—chicken, lamb, turkey, beef (lean), veal; fish—sole, flounder, haddock, perch; cheese—cheddar, American, Swiss, cottage; eggs; fruits—apples, grapes, pears, pineapple; vegetables—cabbage, cucumbers, lettuce, tomatoes; cereals—cornflakes, puffed rice, puffed wheat, farina, rolled oats.

B. *Low-carbohydrate:* all meats; cheese—hard, soft, cottage; eggs; shellfish—oysters, shrimp; fats—bacon, butter, French dressing, salad oil, mayonnaise, margarine; vegetables—asparagus, green beans, beet greens, broccoli, brussels sprouts, cabbage, celery, cauliflower, cucumber, lettuce, green pepper, spinach, squash, tomatoes; fruits—avocados, strawberries, cantaloupe, lemons, rhubarb.

■ QUESTIONS

Select the one best answer for each question, and fill in the answer circle beside the answer number.

Diet and weight control are the foundation of diabetic management. In discussing Ms. Marble's diet with her before her discharge, you go over possible food exchanges. She has been placed on an 1800-calorie diet. A typical lunch includes two meat exchanges, two bread exchanges, one vegetable exchange, one fruit exchange, one fat exchange, and one milk exchange. (Refers to questions 1 and 2.)

1. Ms. Marble states she is a "peanut butter" freak. Which of the following exchanges would be equivalent to 2 tbsp peanut butter?
○ 1. Eight ounces of whole milk. **IMP**
○ 2. Two tbsp of butter. **4**
○ 3. One-quarter cup cottage cheese. **PhI**
○ 4. Two tbsp cream cheese.

2. Given her allowances, which of the following would be inappropriate for Ms. Marble to eat at her birthday luncheon?
○ 1. A piece of plain sponge cake. **PL**
○ 2. Eight-ounce glass of Coca-Cola. **4**
○ 3. A taco (tortilla, meat, cheddar cheese, lettuce). **PhI**
○ 4. Avocado and orange salad.

3. A client has been placed on a high-protein diet. Which one of the following foods would you suggest he select for his diet?
○ 1. Rice (1 cup). **IMP**
○ 2. Eggnog (8 oz). **4**
○ 3. Cheddar cheese (1 oz). **PhI**
○ 4. Broccoli (1 cup).

4. Which of the following foods would you recommend be *avoided* by the client experiencing dumping syndrome?
○ 1. Liver and bacon. **PL**

* These proteins are allowed in various amounts in controlled-protein diets for renal decompensation.

○ 2. Orange and avocado salad.
○ 3. Creamed chicken.
○ 4. Glazed donuts and coffee.

4
PhI

5. Dietary restriction of protein in chronic renal failure is used to prevent the accumulation of nitrogenous wastes and resulting azotemia. Which of the following foods containing amino acids would be allowed in a diet for a client with chronic renal failure?
   ○ 1. Roast beef.
   ○ 2. Milk and eggs.
   ○ 3. Chicken and turkey.
   ○ 4. Shellfish.

   PL
   4
   PhI

6. Of the following foods, which one may be more likely to cause discomfort in a patient with cholecystitis?
   ○ 1. Whole milk.
   ○ 2. Cottage cheese.
   ○ 3. Whole-grain breads.
   ○ 4. Eggs.

   IMP
   4
   PhI

7. Which of the following foods should you advise the colostomy client to *avoid*?
   ○ 1. Carbonated drinks.
   ○ 2. Fresh-cooked green beans.
   ○ 3. Liver and bacon.
   ○ 4. Cooked cereals.

   PL
   4
   PhI

8. Mary Lane is a 30-year-old gravida 3 para 2 who is 4 weeks pregnant. She has been a vegetarian for 8 years. She eats no eggs or dairy products (vegan vegetarian). When assessing the adequacy of Mary's diet, to which of the following food groups would the nurse pay particular attention?
   ○ 1. Grains.
   ○ 2. Protein foods.
   ○ 3. Vitamin-C-rich foods.
   ○ 4. Fruits and vegetables.

   AS
   4
   PhI

9. Ann Miller is a 17-year-old primigravida. At 30 weeks gestation she is diagnosed with an iron deficiency anemia. Ann takes her iron and vitamin supplements sporadically due to unacceptable GI side effects but eats many foods high in iron. In planning diet teaching, which of the following nutrients will the nurse emphasize to promote heme production?
   ○ 1. Niacin.
   ○ 2. Vitamin A.
   ○ 3. Vitamin D.
   ○ 4. Folic acid.

   PL
   4
   PhI

■ ANSWERS/RATIONALE

1. (3) A diabetic's diet is most often based on an exchange system. Foodstuffs in this system are divided into six types. Foods from within each list can be substituted for another in the same list because they have approximately the same food value. Peanut butter is in the meat exchange list, as is cottage cheese, and therefore these can be substituted for one another. Whole milk (No. 1) is on the milk exchange list. Butter and cream cheese (Nos. 2 and 4) are considered to be fats.
2. (2) Given Ms. Marble's food allowances, all these foods (Nos. 1, 3, and 4) would be allowed except for the Coca-Cola. All concentrated sweets and regular soft drinks are contraindicated on a diabetic diet.
3. (2) Eggs and milk are two sources of protein with the highest biologic values (high-quality proteins). Eggnog (8 oz) contains 15 g protein. Rice (No. 1) contains 4 g, cheddar cheese (No. 3) 7 g, and broccoli (No 4) 5 g. Meat, fish, and legumes contain more protein than does eggnog, but their percent of protein utilization is lower, making them almost equal in value to eggnog.
4. (4) Concentrated sugars and carbohydrates should be avoided by these clients. Likewise, fluid ingestion with meals or snacks should also be avoided to prevent rapid emptying of the stomach. Nos. 1, 2, and 3 are examples of high-protein, high-fat, low-carbohydrate foods, which are appropriate.
5. (2) The diet for clients with chronic renal failure is restricted in total amount of protein and amino acid content. Eggs and milk are generally included in the diet because they contain all the essential amino acids. Meats from animals (No. 1), fowl (No. 3), and fish (No. 4) are restricted due to their sulfur-containing, nonessential amino acids.
6. (1) Whole milk has a high fat content, so a client with cholecystitis is generally advised to switch to low-fat or skim milk. Cottage cheese (No. 2), whole-grain breads (No. 3), and eggs (No. 4), are allowed in a low-fat diet, though eggs may be limited to four per week.
7. (1) Carbonated drinks, cabbage, sauerkraut, and nuts tend to increase flatulence, and most clients feel uncomfortable passing flatus into the colostomy bag, as it causes it to inflate. Onions, cheese, and fish may cause odorous drainage. Generally the initial diet following a colostomy is a low-fiber diet for several weeks. As the diet is increased, the individual client can determine more accurately which foods cause constipation, diarrhea, flatus, or dyspepsia. Nos. 2, 3, and 4 are not troublesome to most such clients.
8. (2) Vegetarians who omit dairy foods may be unable to meet the requirement for an additional 30 g of protein per day over their nonpregnant needs. No. 1 is incorrect because individuals who have been vegetarians for some time usually have evolved diets adequate in grain intake. Nos. 3 and 4 are incorrect because individuals who are vegan vegetarians usually ingest a wide variety of fruits and vegetables to meet pregnancy requirements for vitamin C, fiber, and other nutrients.
9. (4) Folic acid (folacin) is essential for increased heme production for hemoglobin and prevention of megaloblastic anemia. No. 1 is incorrect because niacin has no direct or indirect role in erythropoeisis or heme production. No. 2 is incorrect because vitamin A is essential for fetal bone growth and tooth development. No. 3 is incorrect because vitamin D is essential for mineralization of bone tissue and calcium and phosphorus absorption.

Key to codes following questions Nursing process: **AS**, Assessment; **AN**, Analysis; **PL**, Plan; **IMP**, Implementation; **EV**, Evaluation. Category of human function: **1**, Protective; **2**, Sensory-perceptual; **3**, Comfort, Rest, Activity, and Mobility; **4**, Nutrition; **5**, Growth and Development; **6**, Fluid-Gas Transport; **7**, Psycho-Social-Cultural; **8**, Elimination. Client need: **SECE**, Safe, Effective Care Environment; **PhI**, Physiological Integrity; **PsI**, Psychosocial Integrity; **HPM**, Health Promotion/Maintenance. See frontmatter for full explanation.

UNIT

6 Review of Pharmacology

PHARMACOLOGY

GUIDELINES FOR ADMINISTERING MEDICATIONS TO INFANTS AND CHILDREN

I. Developmental considerations*

A. Be honest. Do not bribe or threaten child to obtain cooperation.

B. Describe any sensations child may expect to experience, e.g., "pinch" of needle during IM.

C. Explain how child can "help" nurse, e.g., "Lie as still as you can."

D. Tell child that it's OK to cry; provide privacy.

E. Offer support, praise, and encouragement during and after giving medication.

F. Allow child opportunity for age-appropriate therapeutic play to work through feelings and experiences, to clarify any misconceptions, and to teach child more effective coping strategies.

II. Safety considerations

A. Be absolutely sure dose you are giving is both safe (check recommended mg/kg) and accurate (have another nurse check your calculations). Remember: total volume of dose should be much smaller than adult dose.

B. Check identification band or ask parent or another nurse for child's first and last name.

C. Restrain child to avoid injury while giving medication; a second person is often required to help hold child.

III. Oral medications

A. Use syringe without needle to draw up medication.

B. Position: upright or semi-upright.

C. Place tip of syringe midway back at side of child's mouth and give medication. **Never** pinch infant or child's nostrils to force him or her to open mouth.

D. When infant will suck from nipple, place nipple in infant's mouth; as infant begins to suck, the liquid medication can be placed in nipple.

E. When giving tablets or capsules (that are **not** enteric coated), crush and mix into smallest possible amount of food or liquid to ensure that child takes entire dose. Do not mix with essential food or liquid (e.g., milk); select an "optional" food, such as applesauce.

IV. Ophthalmic installations

A. Position: lying down or sitting so that head is tilted back.

B. For eye drops: hold dropper 1–2 cm above middle of conjunctival sac.

C. For eye ointment: squeeze 2 cm of ointment from tube onto conjunctival sac.

D. After giving drops or ointment, encourage child to keep eyes closed briefly, to maximize contact with eyes.

V. Otic installations

A. Position: head to side so that affected ear is uppermost.

---

*Adapted from James, S. R., and Mott, S. R., *Child Health Nursing: Essential Care of Children and Families.* Menlo Park, CA: Addison-Wesley, 1988, pp. 613–620.

B. For child **under** 3 years of age: pull pinna gently **down** and back.

C. For child **over** 3 years of age: pull pinna gently **up** and back.

D. After administering ear drops, encourage child to remain with head to side with affected ear uppermost, to maximize contact with entire external canal to reach eardrum.

VI. Dermatologic installations

A. Remember: young child's skin is more permeable, therefore there is increased risk for medication absorption and resultant systemic effects; monitor for systemic effects.

B. Apply thin layer of cream or ointment, and confine it to portions of skin where it is essential.

VII. Rectal medication

A. Prepare child emotionally and physically; rectal route is invasive and embarrassing, particularly for children.

B. Position: side-lying with upper leg flexed.

C. Lubricate rounded end of suppository and insert past anal sphincter with gloved fingertip (wear gloves when inserting rectal medication).

D. Remove fingertip but hold child's buttocks gently together until child no longer strains or indicates urge to expel medication.

VIII. Intramuscular medication

A. Because the infant or child is much smaller physically than an adult, the nurse should select a shorter needle, generally 5/8″ (infant) to 1″ (child).

B. Preferred injection sites are on the thigh: vastus lateralis—lateral aspect; rectus femoris—anterior aspect. The deltoid muscle, though small, provides easy access and can be used in children with adequate muscle mass.

C. **Avoid** posterior gluteal muscle in children under age 4.

D. Because of vast differences in size, muscle mass, and subcutaneous tissue, it is especially important to note bony prominences as landmarks for intramuscular injections.

■ PSYCHOPHARMACOLOGY: COMMON PSYCHOTROPIC DRUGS

I. Antipsychotics

A. Phenothiazines (Compazine, Sparine, Thorazine, Mellaril, Stelazine, Trilafon, Vesprin, Prolixin Enanthate).

B. Butyrophenones (Haldol, Innovar, Serenace).

C. Thioxanthenes (Taractan, Navane)—chemically related to phenothiazines, with similar therapeutic effects.

1. *Use*—acute and chronic psychoses; most useful in cases of disorganization of thought or behavior; to decrease panic, fear, hostility, restlessness, aggression, and withdrawal.
2. **Assessment**—*side effects:*
   a. *Hypersensitivity* effects
      (1) *Blood dyscrasia*—agranulocytosis, leukopenia, granulocytopenia.
      (2) *Skin reactions*—photosensitivity, dermatitis, flushing, blue-gray skin.
      (3) Obstructive *jaundice.*
   b. *Extrapyramidal symptoms (EPS)* affecting voluntary movement and skeletal muscles
      (1) *Parkinsonism*—tremors, cogwheel rigidity, shuffling gait, pill-rolling, masklike facies, salivation, and difficulty starting muscular movement (dyskinesia).
      (2) *Dystonia*—limb and neck spasms (torticollis), extensive rigidity of back muscles (opisthotonus), oculogyric crisis, speech and swallowing difficulties, and protrusion of tongue.
      (3) *Akathisia*—motor restlessness, pacing, foot-tapping, inner tremulousness, and agitation.
      (4) *Tardive dyskinesia (TD)*—excessive blinking; vermiform tongue movement; stereotyped, abnormal, involuntary sucking, chewing, licking, and pursing movements of tongue and mouth; grimacing, blinking, frowning, rocking.
         (a) *Cause*—long-term use of high doses of antipsychotic drugs.
         (b) *Predisposing factors*—age, women, OBS; history of ECT or use of tricyclics or anti-Parkinson drugs.
   c. *Potentiates* central nervous system depressants.
   d. *Orthostatic hypotension* (less with butyrophenones).
   e. *Anticholinergic effects* (atropinelike)—dry mouth, stuffy nose, blurred vision, urinary retention, and constipation.
   f. Ocular changes (lens and corneal opacity).
3. **Nursing plan/implementation:**
   a. Goal: *anticipate, observe for, and check for side effects.*
      (1) Protect the person's skin from sunburn when outside.
      (2) For hypotension: take BP and have person lie down for 30 minutes, especially after an injection.
      (3) Watch for signs of blood dyscrasia: sore throat, fever, malaise.
      (4) Observe for symptoms of *hypo-* or *hyperthermic* reaction due to effect on heat-regulating mechanism.
      (5) Observe for, withhold drug for, and report early symptoms of *jaundice* and bile tract obstruction, high fever, upper abdominal pain, nausea, diarrhea, rash; monitor liver function tests.
      (6) Relieve excessive *mouth dryness:* mouth rinse, increased fluid intake.
      (7) Relieve gastric irritation, *constipation:* take with and increase fluids and roughage in diet.
      (8) Observe for and report changes in carbohydrate metabolism (glycosuria, weight gain, polyphagia): change diet.
   b. Goal: *health teaching.*
      (1) Dangers of drug potentiation with alcohol or sleeping pills.

(2) Advise about driving or occupations where blurred vision may be a problem.

(3) Caution against abrupt cessation at high doses.

(4) Warn regarding dark urine.

(5) Have client with respiratory disorder breathe deeply and cough as drug is a cough depressant.

(6) Need for continuous use of drug and follow-up care.

(7) Prompt reporting of hypersensitivity symptoms: fever, laryngeal edema; abdominal distention (constipation, urinary retention); jaundice; blood dyscrasia.

4. **Evaluation:**

a. Behavior is less agitated.

b. Knows side effects to observe for, lessen, and/or prevent.

c. Continues to use drug.

II. Antidepressants

A. Tricyclic (Tofranil, Norpramin, Pamelor, Surmontil, Elavil, Triavil, Aventyl, Vivactil, Sinequan)—effective in 1–3 weeks.

1. *Use*—elevate mood in depression, increase physical activity and mental alertness; may bring relief of symptoms of depression so that client can attend individual or group therapy; bipolar disorder, depressed; dysthmic disorder.

2. **Assessment**—*side effects:*

a. *Behavioral*—activation of latent schizophrenia; hypomania; suicide attempts; mental confusion. Withhold drug if observed.

b. *Central nervous system* (CNS)—tremors, ataxia, jitteriness.

c. *Autonomic nervous system* (ANS)—dry mouth, nasal congestion, aggravation of glaucoma, constipation, urinary retention, edema, paralysis, ECG changes (flattened T waves; arrhythmia severe in overdose).

3. **Nursing plan/implementation:**

a. Goal: *assess risk of suicide during initial improvement:* careful, close observation.

b. Goal: *prevent risk of cardiac arrhythmias and hypotension:* use caution with client with hyperthyroidism, having ECT or surgery (gradually discontinue 2–3 days *prior* to surgery). Monitor BP, pulse ×2 per day; ECGs, 2–3 per week until dose adjusted.

c. Goal: *observe for signs of urinary retention, constipation:* monitor I&O and weight gain.

d. Goal: *cautious drug use with glaucoma or history of seizures.* Observe seizure precautions due to lowered seizure threshold.

e. Goal: *health teaching:*

(1) Advise against driving car or participating in activities requiring mental alertness, due to *sedative* effects.

(2) Encourage increased fluid intake and frequent mouth rinsing to combat dry mouth.

(3) Avoid smoking, which decreases drug effects.

(4) Avoid use of alcohol and other drugs, due to adverse interactions, especially O.T.C. (e.g., antihistamines).

(5) Advise of delay in desired effect (2–4 weeks).

(6) Instruct gradual discontinuance to avoid withdrawal symptoms.

4. **Evaluation:** diminished symptoms of agitated depression and anxiety.

B. Monoamine-oxidase inhibitors (MAOI)—Nardil, Marplan, Parnate, Marsilid, Eutonyl, Niamid.

1. **Assessment**—*side effects:*

a. *Behavioral*—may activate latent schizophrenia, mania, excitement.

b. *CNS*—tremors; *hypertensive crisis* (avoid cheese, Coca-Cola, caffeine, wine, beer, yeast, chocolate, chicken liver, or other substances high in tyramine or pressor amine; for example, amphetamines and cold and hay fever medication); *intracerebral hemorrhage; hyperpyrexia.*

c. *ANS*—dry mouth, aggravation of glaucoma, bowel and bladder control problems; edema, paralysis, ECG changes (arrhythmia severe in overdose).

d. *Allergic* hepatocellular jaundice.

2. **Nursing plan/implementation:**

a. Goal: *reduce risk of hypertensive crisis:* diet restrictions of foods high in *tyramine* content.

b. Goal: *observe for urinary retention:* measure I&O.

c. Goal: *health teaching.*

(1) Therapeutic response takes 2–3 weeks.

(2) Food and alcohol restrictions: avocado, bananas, raisins, licorice, chocolate, cheese, yogurt, sour cream, liver, herring, soy sauce, meat tenderizers, wine, beer, caffeine.

(3) Change position gradually to prevent postural hypotension.

(4) Report any stiff neck, palpitations, chest pain, headaches because of possible hypertensive crises (can be fatal).

(5) Take *no nonprescribed* drugs.

3. **Evaluation:**

a. Improvement in: sleep, appetite, activity, interest in self and surroundings.

b. Lessening of anxiety and complaints.

III. Antianxiety

A. Chlordiazepoxide (Librium)

1. *Use*—alcoholism, tension, and irrational fears; has muscle relaxant and anticonvulsant properties.

2. **Assessment**—*side effects:* hypotension, drowsiness, motor uncoordination, confusion, skin eruptions, edema, menstrual irregularities, constipation, extrapyramidal symptoms, blurred vision, lethargy; ↑ or ↓ libido.

3. **Nursing plan/implementation:**

a. Goal: *administer cautiously, as drug may:*

(1) Be habituating (causing withdrawal convulsions; therefore gradual withdrawal necessary).

(2) Potentiate CNS depressants.

(3) Have adverse effect on pregnancy.

(4) Be dangerous for those with suicidal tendencies or severe psychoses.

(5) Reduce GI effects: crush tablet or take with meals or milk; give antacids 1 hour before.

(6) Check chart for results of periodic liver function tests and blood counts, especially with upper respiratory infection.

b. Goal: *health teaching.*

(1) Advise against suddenly stopping drug (withdrawal symptoms begin in 5–7 days).

(2) Talk with physician if plans to be or is pregnant.

(3) Drink fluids.

(4) Avoid alcohol, over-the-counter drugs, and heavy smoking.

4. **Evaluation:** decreased alcohol withdrawal symptoms or preoperative anxiety.

B. Diazepam (Valium)

1. *Use*—muscle relaxant; *not* used for psychotics.

2. **Assessment**—*side effects:* same as for Librium, plus double or blurred vision, difficult speech, headache, hypotension, incontinence, tremor, and urinary retention, liver damage.

3. **Nursing plan/implementation:**

a. Goal: *anticipate, observe for, and check for side effects,* especially depression, suicidal risk, and constipation.

b. Goal: *reduce risk of hypotension, respiratory depression, phlebitis, venous thrombosis.* Give: IM, in large muscles, slowly, and rotate sites, have client lie down; IV: over 1-minute period.

c. Goal: *observe for psychologic and physical dependence:* avoid abrupt discontinuation.

d. Goal: *health teaching:* sedative effects, potentiation of other CNS-depressant drugs and alcohol, and problem of habituation.

4. **Evaluation:** relief of tension, anxiety, skeletal muscle spasm.

IV. Antimanic

A. Lithium—effect occurs 1–3 weeks after first dose.

1. *Use*—acute manic attack and prevention of recurrence of cyclic manic-depressive episodes of bipolar disorders.

2. **Assessment**—*side effects:* levels from 1.6–2.0 mEq/L may cause tremors, nausea and vomiting, diarrhea, polyuria, polydipsia; levels *above* 2 mEq/L may cause motor weakness, headache, edema, and lethargy; *signs of severe toxicity:* neurologic, for example, twitching, marked drowsiness, slurred speech, dysarthria, athetotic movements, convulsions, delirium, stupor, coma.

a. *Precautions*—cautious use with clients: on *diuretics;* with disturbed *electrolytes* (sweating, dehydrated, and postoperative clients); with *thyroid* problems, on *low-salt diets;* with congestive *heart failure,* and with impaired *renal function.* Risk of suicide.

b. *Dosage—therapeutic* level 0.8–1.6 mEq/L; dose for maintenance 300–1500 mEq/day; *toxic* level >2.0 mEq/L; blood sample drawn in acute phase 10–14 hours after last dose, taken tid.

3. **Nursing plan/implementation:**

a. Goal: *anticipate, observe for, and check for signs and symptoms of toxicity.*

(1) Reduce GI symptoms: take with meals.

(2) Check for edema: daily weight.

(3) Monitor blood levels (1.6–2.0 mEq/L) for signs of toxicity: nausea, vomiting, diarrhea, anorexia, ataxia, weakness, drowsiness, fine tremor or muscle-twitching, slurred speech.

(4) Monitor results from repeat thyroid and kidney function tests.

b. Goal: *report fever right away.*

c. Goal: *monitor effect:* (therapeutic and toxic) through blood samples taken:

(1) 10–14 hours after last dose.

(2) Every 2–3 days until 1.6 mEq/L is reached.

(3) Once a week while in hospital.

(4) Every 2–3 months to maintain blood levels under 1 mEq/L.

d. Goal: *health teaching.*

(1) Advise client of 7–10-day lag time for effect.

(2) Urge to drink adequate liquids (2–3 L/day).

(3) Report: polyuria and polydypsia.

(4) Diet: avoid caffeine, crash diets, diet pills, self-prescribed low-salt diet, antacids, high-sodium foods (which increase lithium excretion and reduce drug effect); take with meals.

(5) Caution against driving, operating machinery that requires mental alertness until drug is effective.

(6) Warn *not* to change or omit dose.

4. **Evaluation:**

a. Changed facial affect.

b. Improved: posture, ability to concentrate, sleep patterns.

c. Assumption of self-care.

V. Antiparkinson agents

A. Trihexyphenidyl HCl (Artane).

B. Benztropine mesylate (Cogentin).

1. *Use*—counteract extrapyramidal reactions.

2. **Assessment:**

a. Artane

(1) *Side effects*—dry mouth, blurred vision, dizziness, nausea, constipation, drowsiness, urinary hesitancy or retention, pupil dilation, headache, and weakness.

(2) *Precautions*—cautious use with cardiac, liver, or kidney disease or obstructive gastrointestinal-genitourinary disease. Do not give if glaucoma present.

b. Cogentin—*side effects:* same as for Artane, plus:

(1) Effect on *body temperature* may result in life-threatening state.

(2) *Gastrointestinal distress.*

(3) *Inability to concentrate,* memory difficulties, and mild confusion (often mistaken for senility).

TABLE 6.1 **Major Substances Used for Mind Alteration**

Official Name	Slang Name	Usual Single Adult Dose/Duration	Legitimate Medical Uses (Present and Projected)	Short-Term Effects	Long-Term Effects
Alcohol—whisky, gin, beer, wine	Booze, hooch, suds	1½ oz gin or whisky, 12 oz beer/2–4 h	Rare: sometimes used as a sedative (for tension).	CNS depressant; relaxation (sedation); euphoria; drowsiness; impaired judgment, reaction time, coordination, and emotional control; frequent aggressive behavior and driving accidents.	Diversion of energy and money from more creative and productive pursuits; habituation; possible obesity with chronic excessive use; irreversible damage to brain and liver; addiction with severe withdrawal illness (DTs) with heavy use; many deaths.
Caffeine—coffee, tea, Coca-Cola, No-Doz, APC	Java	1–2 cups, 1 bottle, 5 mg/2–4 h	Mild stimulant; treatment of some forms of coma.	CNS stimulant; increased alertness; reduction of fatigue.	Sometimes insomnia, restlessness, or gastric irritation; habituation.
Nicotine (and coal tar)—cigarettes, cigars	Fags, nails	1–2 cigarettes/1–2 h	None (used as an insecticide).	CNS stimulant; relaxation or distraction.	Lung (and other) cancer, heart and blood vessel disease, cough, etc; higher infant mortality; many deaths; habituation; diversion of energy and money; air pollution; fire.
Sedatives	Downers				
Alcohol—see above					
Barbiturates—Amytal, Nembutal, Seconal, Phenobarbital	Barbs, blue devils, yellow jackets, dolls, red devils, phennies, goofers	50–100 mg	Treatment of insomnia and tension. Induction of anesthesia	CNS depressants; sleep induction; relaxation (sedation); sometimes euphoria; drowsiness; impaired judgment, reaction time, coordination, and emotional control; relief of anxiety/tension; muscle relaxation.	Irritability, weight loss, addiction with severe withdrawal illness (like DTs); diversion of energy and money; habituation, addiction.
Doriden (Glutethimides)		500 mg			
Chloral hydrate		500 mg			
Miltown, Equanil (Meprobamate)		400 mg/4 h*			
Stimulants	Uppers				
Caffeine—see above					
Nicotine—see above					
Amphetamines Benzedrine Methedrine Dexedrine	Pep pills, wake-ups, Bennies, cartwheels, Crystal, speed, meth, Dexies or Xmas trees (spansules)	2.5–15.0 mg	Treatment of obesity, narcolepsy, fatigue, depression.	CNS stimulants; increased alertness; reduction of fatigue; loss of appetite; insomnia; often euphoria.	Restlessness, weight loss, toxic psychosis (mainly paranoid); diversion of energy and money; habituation; extreme irritability, toxic psychosis.
Preludin		25 mg			
Cocaine	Coke, snow	Variable/4 h*	Anesthesia of the eye and throat.		

Tranquilizers				
Librium (chlordiazepoxide) Phenothiazines Thorazine Compazine Stelazine		5–25 mg 10–50 mg 5–10 mg 2–5 mg	Treatment of anxiety, tension, alcoholism, neurosis, psychosis, psychosomatic disorders, and vomiting.	Selective CNS depressants; relaxation, relief of anxiety/tension; suppression of hallucinations or delusions, improved functioning.	Sometimes drowsiness, dryness of mouth, blurring of vision, skin rash, tremor; occasionally jaundice, agranulocytosis, or death.
Reserpine (Rauwolfia)		0.1–0.25 mg/4–6 h*			
Marijuana or Cannabis†	Pot, grass, tea, weed, stuff, hash, joint, reefers	Variable—1 cigarette or pipe, or 1 drink or cake (India)/4 h*	Treatment of depression, tension, loss of appetite and high blood pressure.	Relaxation, euphoria, increased appetite, some alteration of time perception, possible impairment of judgment and coordination; mixed CNS depressant-stimulant.	Usually none; possible diversion of energy and money; habituation; occasional acute panic reactions.
Antidepressants					
Ritalin Dibenzazepine (Tofranil, Elavil) MAO inhibitors (Nardil, Parnate)		5–10 mg 25 mg, 10 mg 10 mg, 15 mg/4–6 h*	Treatment of moderate to severe depression.	Relief of depression (elevation of mood), stimulation.	Basically the same as tranquilizers above.
Narcotics (Opiates, Analgesics)					
Opium Heroin Morphine Codeine Percodan Demerol Methadone Cough syrups (Cheracol, Hycodan, Romilar, etc.)	Op Horse, H, smack, shit, junk	10–12 "pipes" (Asia)/4 h* Variable—bag or paper with 5–10% heroin. 10–15 mg 15–30 mg 1 tablet 50–100 mg 2.5–40 mg 2–4 oz (for euphoria)/4–6 h*	Treatment of severe pain, diarrhea, and cough.	CNS depressants; sedation, euphoria, relief of pain, impaired intellectual functioning and coordination.	Constipation, loss of appetite and weight, temporary impotency or sterility; habituation, addiction with unpleasant and painful withdrawal illness.
Hallucinogens					
LSD Psilocybin STP DMT Mescaline (peyote)	Acid, sugar cubes, trip Mushrooms Cactus	150 μg/10–12 h 25 mg 6 mg 350 mg/12–14 h	Experimental study of mind and brain function; enhancement of creativity and problem solving; treatment of alcoholism, mental illness, and the dying person; chemical warfare.	Production of visual imagery, increased sensory awareness, anxiety, nausea, impaired coordination; sometimes consciousness expansion.	Usually none; sometimes precipitates or intensifies an already existing psychosis; more commonly can produce a panic reaction.
Miscellaneous					
Glue, gasoline, and solvents Amyl nitrite Antihistamines Nutmeg Nonprescription "sedatives" (Compoze) Catnip Nitrous oxide		Variable 1–2 ampules 25–50 mg Variable/2 h	None except for antihistamines used for allergy and amyl nitrite for fainting.	When used for mind-alteration generally produces a "high" (euphoria) with impaired coordination and judgment.	Variable—some of the substances can seriously damage the liver or kidney, and some produce hallucinations.

*Time given pertains to all drugs listed.

†Hashish or charas is a more concentrated form of the active ingredient THC (tetrahydrocannabinol) and is consumed in smaller doses, analogous to vodka–beer ratios.

TABLE 6.2 Regional Analgesia-Anesthesia in Labor and Delivery

Types	Characteristics	Nursing Implications
Common Agents in 0.5–1.0% Solution		
Lidocaine (Xylocaine) Bupivacaine (Marcaine) HCl Tetracaine (Pontocaine) HCl Mepivacaine HCl (Carbocaine) Chloroprocaine HCl (Nesacaine)	Used with epinephrine (or other vasoconstrictor drug) to delay absorption, prolong anesthetic effect, and decrease chance of hypotension.	Note any history of allergy; note response: allergic reaction, hypotension, and lack of wearing off of anesthetic effect; observe for hypertensive crisis if agent combined with epinephrine and Pitocin is also being given.
Peripheral Nerve Block		
Pudendal (5–10 mL each side) anesthetizes lower two-thirds of vagina and perineum.	Perineal anesthesia of short duration (30 minutes); local anesthesia; simple and safe; does not depress neonate; may inhibit bearing-down reflex.	To get cooperation, give explanation during procedure.
Paracervical (uterosacral) block (5–10 mL given into each side) anesthetizes cervix and upper two-thirds of vagina.	May be given between 3 and 8 cm by physician when woman is having at least three contractions in ten minutes; lasts 45–90 minutes; can be repeated; can be followed by local, epidural, or other; may cause temporary fetal bradycardia.	Explain: especially length and type of needle; take maternal vital signs and FHR; have her void; help position; monitor FHR continuously; monitor contractions; and watch for return of pain.
Local infiltration	Useful for perineal repairs.	No special nursing care.
Peridural (epidural) block		
Caudal	Useful during first and second stages; can be given "one-shot" or continuously; given in peridural space through sacral hiatus.	Hypotension (with resultant fetal bradycardia): (a) turn from supine to lateral, or elevate legs, (b) administer humidified oxygen by mask at 8–10 liters/minute, (c) increase rate of IV fluids (use infusate *without* Pitocin). Will need coaching to push and low forceps with be required.
Continuous lumbar	T10 to S5 for vaginal delivery; T8 to S1 for abdominal delivery. Complete anesthesia for labor and delivery.	See Caudal.
Intrathecal morphine	0.5 mg MS produces marked analgesia for 12–24 h. Onset in 20–30 min.	Considerable side effects: respiratory depression, pruritis, nausea, vomiting, sleepiness, urinary retention. Keep Naloxone 0.4 mg at bedside and respiratory support equipment readily available.
Subarachnoid spinal (continous)	Useful during first or second stage of labor or for abdominal surgery.	Instruct when to bear down. Keep flat minimum of 8 h.
Low spinal ("saddle," "one shot") block	Same as subarachnoid spinal.	Same as subarachnoid spinal.

(4) May lead to toxic psychotic reactions.

(5) *Subjective sensations*—light or heavy feelings in legs, numbness and tingling of extremities, light-headedness or tightness of head, and giddiness.

3. **Nursing plan/implementation:**

a. Goal: *relieve GI distress* by giving after or with meals or at bedtime.

b. Goal: *monitor adverse effects:*

(1) Hypotension, tachycardia: check pulse, blood pressure.

(2) Constipation and fecal impaction: add roughage to diet.

(3) Dry mouth: increase fluid intake; encourage frequent mouth rinsing.

(4) Blurred vision, dizziness: assist with ambulation; use siderail.

c. *Health teaching.*

(1) Avoid driving, and limit activities requiring alertness.

(2) Delayed drug effect (2–3 days).

(3) Potential abuse due to hallucinogenic effects.

(4) Avoid alcohol and other CNS depressants.

4. **Evaluation:**

a. Less rigidity, drooling, and oculogyric crisis.

b. Improved: gait, balance, posture.

MIND-ALTERING SUBSTANCES

Major substances used by the public to alter mental states are compared in Table 6.1.

REGIONAL ANALGESIA-ANESTHESIA IN LABOR AND DELIVERY

See Table 6.2.

COMMON DRUGS

See Table 6.3.

FOOD AND DRUG CONSIDERATIONS

See Table 6.4.

■ TABLE 6.3

Common Drugs

Drug and Dosage	Use	Action	Assessment: Side Effects	Nursing Implications
Adrenergics				
Alpha and beta agonists				
Epinephrine (Adrenalin)—subcutaneous or IM 0.2–1 mg in 1:1000 solution; IV—intracardiac 1:10,000 solution; ophthalmic 1:1000–1:50,000 solution.	Asystole, bronchospasm, anaphylaxis, glaucoma.	Stimulates pacemaker cells; inhibits histamine and mediates bronchial relaxation; ↓ intraocular pressure.	Ventricular arrhythmias, fear, anxiety, anginal pain, decreased renal blood flow, burning of eyes, headache.	Use TB syringe for greater accuracy; massaging injection site hastens action; repeated injections may cause tissue necrosis; *avoid* injection in buttocks because bacteria in area may lead to gas gangrene; may make mucous plugs in lungs more difficult to dislodge.
Norepinephrine (Levophed)—IV 2–4 μg/min titrated to desired response.	Acute hypertension, cardiogenic shock.	Increases rate and strength of heart beat; increases vasoconstriction.	Palpitations, pallor, headache, hypertension, anxiety, insomnia, dilated pupils, nausea, vomiting, glycosuria, tissue sloughing.	Observe vital signs, mentation, skin temperature, and color (earlobes, lips, nailbeds); tissue necrosis occurs with infiltration; antidote is phentolamine 5–10 mg in 10–15 mL normal saline.
Metaraminol (Aramine)—IM 2–10 mg; IV 15–100 mg in 500 mL D_5W titrated to desired response.	Hypotension, shock.	Vasoconstriction; ↑ myocardial contractility; ↓ pulse rate.	Reflex bradycardia, ventricular arrhythmias, tissue sloughing.	Injury to local tissue may occur with infiltration; continuous monitoring of vital signs.
Beta agonists				
Isoproterenol (Isuprel)—10–15 mg sublingually; IV 0.5–4.0 μg/min in solution.	Cardiogenic shock, heart block, brochospasm—asthma, emphysema.	↑ Cardiac contractility: facilitates AV conduction and pacemaker automaticity.	Tachyarrhythmias, hypotension, headache, flushing of skin, nausea, tremor, dizziness.	Monitor vital signs, ECG: oral inhalation solutions must *not* be injected.
Dopamine (Intropin)—IV 2–5 μg/kg/min titrated to desired response.	Acute heart failure.	↑ Cardiac contractility; ↑ renal blood flow.	Ectopic beats, nausea, vomiting, tachycardia, anginal pain, dyspnea, hypotension.	Monitor vital signs, urine output, and signs of peripheral ischemia; will cause tissue sloughing if infiltration occurs.
Ritodrine (Premar)—PO 10–20 mg q2–6h; IV 0.15–0.35 mg/min.	Manage premature labor in selected clients.	Stimulates $beta_2$ receptors in uterine smooth muscle to reduce intensity and frequency of contractions.	Altered maternal and fetal heart rates, temporary hyperglycemia, arrhythmias, vomiting, restlessness.	Requires hospitalization; need to hydrate prior to infusion; monitor fetal heart rate and uterine activity; place in left lateral recumbent position to reduce risk of hypotension.
Dobutamine (Dobutrex)—IV 2.5–10 μg/kg/min.	Acute heart failure.	Stimulates cardiac contractile force (positive inotropy); fewer changes in heart rate than dopamine or isoproterenol.	Tachycardia, arrhythmias.	Mix with 5% dextrose. Do not dilute until ready to use. Protect from light. Administer with infusion pump. Check vital signs constantly. Extravasation can produce tissue necrosis. See norepinephrine.
Adrenocortical Steroids				
Cortisone acetate—PO or IM 20–100 mg qd in single or divided doses.	ACTH insufficiency; rheumatoid arthritis; allergies; ulcerative colitis; nephrosis.	Antiinflammatory effect of unknown action.	Moon facies, hirsutism, thinning of skin, striae, hypertension, menstrual irregularities, delayed healing, psychoses.	Give oral form pc, with snack at bedtime; give deep IM (*never* deltoid); monitor vital signs; observe for behavior changes; skin care and activity to tolerance; diet—salt-restricted, high-protein, KCl supplement; protect from injury.

continued

TABLE 6.3 *(Continued)* **Common Drugs**

Drug and Dosage	Use	Action	Assessment: Side Effects	Nursing Implications
Desoxycorticosterone acetate (hydrocortisone)—IM 1–5 mg.	Addison's disease; burns; surgical shock; adrenal surgery.	Promotes reabsorption of sodium, and restores plasma volume, BP, and electrolyte balance.	Edema, hypertension, pulmonary congestion, hypokalemia.	Salt restriction according to blood pressure readings; monitor vital signs; weigh daily.
Dexamethasone (Decadron)—PO 0.5–5 mg qd; IM or IV 4–20 mg qd.	Addison's disease; allergic reactions; leukemia; Hodgkin's disease; iritis; dermatitis; rheumatoid arthritis.	Antiinflammatory effect.	See Cortisone acetate.	*Contraindicated* in tuberculosis; see Cortisone acetate for nursing care.
Prednisone—PO 2.5–15 mg qd.	Rheumatoid arthritis; cancer therapy.	Antiinflammatory effect of unknown action.	Insomnia and gastric distress.	See Cortisone acetate.
Methylprednisolone sodium (Solu-Medrol)—IV, IM 10–40 mg, slowly.	Glucocorticoid, corticosteroid.	See Dexamethasone.	See Dexamethasone.	See Dexamathasone.
Analgesics				
Aspirin (acetylsalicylic acid)—PO or rectal 0.3–0.6 g.	Minor aches and pains; fever of colds and influenza; rheumatoid arthritis; anticoagulant therapy.	Selectively depresses subcortical levels of CNS.	Erosive gastritis with bleeding, coryza, urticaria, nausea, vomiting, tinnitus, impaired hearing, and respiratory alkalosis.	Administer with food or after meals; observe for nasal, oral, or subcutaneous bleeding; push fluids; check Hct, Hgb, prothrombin times frequently. Avoid use in children with flu.
Ecotrin (enteric coated aspirin).	See Aspirin.	See Aspirin.	See Aspirin.	See Aspirin.
Ibuprofen (Motrin)—300–800 mg oral 3–4/day not to exceed 3200 mg/day.	Nonsteroid antiinflammatory, antirheumatic used in chronic arthritis pain.	Inhibition of prostaglandin synthesis or release.	GI upset; leukopenia; sodium/water retention.	Give on empty stomach for best result; may mix with food if GI upset severe; teach caution when using other medications.
Acetaminophen (Tylenol, Datril, Panadol)—PO 325–650 mg q4h.	Simple fever or pain.	Analgesic and antipyretic actions. No antiinflammatory or anticoagulant effects.	No remarkable side effects when taken for a short period.	Consult with physician if no relief after 4 days of therapy.
Indomethacin (Indocin)—25 mg 3–4/day; increase to max 200 mg daily in divided doses.	Rheumatoid arthritis; bursitis; gouty arthritis.	Antipyretic/antiinflammatory action; inhibits prostaglandin biosynthesis.	GI distress; GI bleeding; rash; headache; blood dyscrasias; corneal changes.	Monitor GI side effects; administer after meals for best effect or with food, milk, or antacids if GI symptoms severe.
Meperidine HCl (Demerol)—PO or IM 50–100 mg q3–4h.	Pain due to trauma or surgery; allay apprehension prior to surgery.	Acts on CNS to produce analgesia, sedation, euphoria, and respiratory depression.	Palpitations, bradycardia, hypotension nausea, vomiting, syncope, sweating, tremors, and convulsions.	Check respiratory rate and depth before giving drug; give IM, as subcutaneous administration is painful and can cause local irritation.
	Obstetric use: maternal relaxation may either slow labor or speed up labor.	Depresses CNS, maternal and fetal; allays apprehension; PO peak action—1–2 h; IM peak action first hour.	As above; also can depress fetus.	Monitor maternal vital signs, contractions, progress of labor, and response to drug; fetal heart rate; if delivery occurs during peak action, prepare to give narcotic antagonist to mother and/or neonate.
Morphine SO_4—PO 10–30 mg (Roxanol, MS Contin); subcutaneous 8–15 mg; IV 4–10 mg. Rectal 10–20 mg.	Control pain and relieve fear, apprehension, restlessness, as in pulmonary edema.	Depresses CNS reception of pain and ability to interpret stimuli; depresses respiratory center in medulla.	Nausea, vomiting, flushing, confusion, urticaria, depressed rate and depth of respirations, and decreased blood pressure.	Check rate and depth of respirations before administering drug; observe for gas pains and abdominal distention; smaller doses for aged; monitor vital signs; observe for postural hypotension.

	Obstetric use: preeclampsia-eclampsia; uterine dysfunction; pain relief.	Increases cerebral blood flow; provides antihypertensive action; CNS depressant.	Respiratory and circulatory depression in mother and neonate; may depress contractions.	Observe for level of sedation, respirations, arousability, and deep tendon reflex; give narcotic antagonist as necessary; check I&O (urinary retention possible).
Alphaprodine HCl (Nisentil)—subcutaneous 40–60 mg.	*Obstetric use:* control pain, especially during labor.	Synthetic narcotic similar to meperidine HCl; subcutaneous peak action 1–2h; IV peak action first hour.	Addictive; may depress fetus, especially if used with barbiturate; respiratory depression; dizziness; sweating, nausea, vomiting, and restlessness.	See Meperidine HCl.
Codeine—PO IM or subcutaneous 15–60 mg (gr ¼ to 1).	Control pain; may be used during the puerperium.	Nonsynthetic narcotic analgesic.	Of little use during labor; allergic response; constipation; GI upset.	Note client's response to the medication. Less respiratory depression; preferred for head injury client.
Oxycodone HCl (Percodan, Tylox)—PO 3–20 mg; subcutaneous 5 mg.	*Postpartum use:* control pain; may be used during puerperium; 5–6 times more potent than codeine.	Less potent and addicting than morphine; for moderate pain—episiotomy and "after pains"; peak action 1 hour.	See Morphine SO_4.	Administer per order and observe for effect.
Pentazocine (Talwin)—PO 50–100 mg; IM 30–60 mg q3–4h.	Relief of moderate to severe pain.	Narcotic agonist, opioid antagonist properties, equivalent to codeine.	Respiratory depression, nausea, vomiting, dizziness, light-headedness, seizures.	Monitor respirations, BP; *caution* with clients with MI, head injuries, COPD.
Antacids				
Aluminum hydroxide gel (Amphojel)—PO 5–10 mL q2–4h or 1h pc.	Gastric acidity; peptic ulcer; phosphatic urinary calculi; ↓ phosphorus level in chronic renal failure.	Buffers HCl in gastric juices without interfering with electrolyte balance.	Constipation and fecal impaction.	Shake well before administering; encourage fluids to prevent impaction and milk-alkali syndrome.
Calcium carbonate (Titralac, Ducon)—PO 1–2 g taken with H_2O after meals and at bedtime.	Peptic ulcer and chronic gastritis.	Reduces hyperacidity.	Constipation or laxative effect.	See Aluminum hydroxide gel.
Aluminum hydroxide and magnesium trisilicate (Gelusil)—PO 5–30 mL pc and hs.	Peptic acid gastritis; heartburn; esophagitis.	Neutralizes and absorbs excess acid.	Diarrhea and hypermagnesemia.	*Avoid* prolonged administration to clients with renal insufficiency.
Magnesium and aluminum hydroxides (Maalox suspension)—PO 5–30 mL pc and hs.	Gastric hyperacidity; peptic ulcer; heartburn.	Neutralizes and binds acids.	Constipation and fecal impaction.	Encourage fluid intake; *contraindicated* for debilitated clients or those with renal insufficiency.
Antiarrhythmics				
Quinidine SO_4—PO 0.2–0.6 g q2h loading dose. Maintenance: 400–1000 mg tid, qid. IV 5–10 mg/kg over 30–60 min.	Atrial fibrillation; PAT; ventricular tachycardia; PVCs.	Lengthens conduction time in atria and ventricles; blocks vagal stimulation of heart.	Nausea, vomiting, diarrhea, vertigo, tremor, headache, abdominal cramps, AV block, and cardiac arrest.	Count pulse before giving; report changes in rate, quality, or rhythm; give drug with food; monitor BP daily. Supine during IV administration.
Procainamide HCl (Pronestyl)—PO, IM 500–1000 mg 4–6 times qd; IV 1 g.	Atrial and ventricular arrhythmias; PVCs; overdose of digitalis; general anesthesia.	Depresses myocardium, and lengthens conduction time between atria and ventricles.	Polyarthralgia, fever, chills, urticaria, nausea, vomiting, psychoses, and rapid decrease in BP.	Check pulse rate *before* giving; monitor heart action during IV administration.
Lidocaine HCl—IV 50–100 mg; bolus; 1–4 mg/min IV drip.	Ventricular tachycardia; PVCs.	Depresses myocardial response to abnormally generated impulses.	Drowsiness, dizziness, nervousness, confusion, and paresthesias.	Check apical and radial pulses for deficits; observe for signs of CNS toxicity; monitor ECG for prolonged PR interval.

continued

■ **TABLE 6.3 *(Continued)*** **Common Drugs**

Drug and Dosage	Use	Action	Assessment: Side Effects	Nursing Implications
Diphenylhydantoin (Dilantin)—PO 100–200 mg 3–4 times daily; IV loading dose 10–15 mg/kg (not to exceed 50 mg/min), 50–100 mg over 5–10 min.	Digitalis toxicity; ventricular ectopy.	Depresses pacemaker activity in SA node and Purkinje tissue without slowing conduction velocity.	Severe pain if administered in small vein. Ataxia, vertigo, nystagmus, seizures, confusion, skin eruptions, hypotension if administered too fast.	With IV use monitor vital signs; observe for CNS side effects; have O_2 on hand; seizure precautions (padded siderails, nonmetal airway, suction, mouth gag). Also see anticonvulsants.
Propranolol HCl (Inderal)—0.5–1 mg IV push (up to 3 mg); 20–60 mg orally 3 to 4 times daily.	Ventricular ectopy; angina unresponsive to nitrites, paroxysmal atrial tachycardia; hypertension.	Beta adrenergic blocker. ↓ Cardiac contractility, ↓ heart rate, ↓ myocardial oxygen requirements.	Bradycardia, hypotension, vertigo, paresthesia of hands.	Instruct client to take pulse *before* each dose; do *not* give to clients with history of asthma or obstructive pulmonary disease; no smoking, as hypertension may occur.
Bretylium (Bretylol)—IV 0.5–10 mg/kg q6h; IM 5–10 mg/kg (max 250 mg in one site).	Ventricular fibrillation; ventricular tachycardia.	Inhibits norepinephrine release from sympathetic nerve endings; increased fibrillation threshold.	Worsening of arrhythmia; tachycardia, and increased BP initially; nausea, vomiting; hypotension later.	Monitor BP and cardiac status closely. Rotate IM injection sites; no more than 5 mL/site.
Antiasthmatics				
Cromolyn sodium—inhale, 1 cap 4 times qd.	Perennial bronchial asthma (not acute asthma or status asthmaticus).	Inhibits release of bronchoconstrictors—histamine and SRS-A; suppresses allergic response.	Cough, hoarseness, wheezing, dry mouth, bitter aftertaste, urticaria, urinary frequency.	Instruct on use of inhaler—exhale; tilt head back; inhale rapidly, deeply, steadily; remove inhaler; exhale—repeat until dose is taken; gargle or drink water after treatment.
Antibiotics				
Sulfisoxazole (Gantrisin), sulfamethizole (Thiosulfil), and sulfisomidine (Elkosin).	Acute, chronic, and recurrent urinary tract infections.	Bacteriostatic and bactericidal.	Nausea, vomiting, oliguria, anuria, anemia, leukopenia, dizziness, jaundice, skin rashes, and photosensitivity.	Maintenance of blood levels very important; encourage fluids to prevent crystal formation in kidney tubules—push up to 3000 mL/day.
Penicillin—penicillin G, penicillin G potassium, penicillin G procaine, ampicillin.	*Streptococcus; Staphylococcus; Pneumococcus; Gonococcus; Treponema pallidum.*	Primarily bactericidal.	Dermatitis and delayed or immediate anaphylaxis.	Outpatients should be observed for 20 minutes postinjection; hospitalized clients should be observed at frequent intervals for 20 minutes postinjection.
Erythromycin—adults, PO 250 mg q6h; children, PO 30–50 mg/kg qd.	Pneumonia; pelvic inflammatory disease; intestinal amebiasis; ocular infections; used if allergic to penicillin.	Inhibits protein synthesis of microorganism; more effective against gram-positive.	Abdominal cramping, distention, diarrhea.	Be sure culture and sensitivity done before treatment; give on empty stomach 1 h before or 3 h after meals; do *not* crush or chew tabs; do *not* give with fruit juice.
Tetracyclines—chlortetracycline (Aureomycin), doxycycline (Vibramycin hyclate), oxytetracycline (Terramycin), and tetracycline HCl (Sumycin).	Wide-spectrum antibiotic.	Primarily bacteriostatic.	GI upsets such as diarrhea, nausea, and vomiting; sore throat; black, hairy tongue; glossitis; and inflammatory lesions in anogenital region.	Phototoxic reactions have been reported; clients should be advised to stay out of direct sunlight, and medication should *not* be given with milk or snacks, as food interferes with absorption of tetracyclines. Do not give to pregnant women and children under 8 yrs.

Cephalexin (Keflex)—PO 1–4 g daily in 2–4 equally divided doses.	Infections caused by gram-positive cocci; infections; respiratory, biliary, urinary, bone, septicemia, abdominal; surgical prophylaxis.	Bacteriocidal effects on susceptible organisms; inhibition of bacterial cell wall synthesis.	Nausea, vomiting; urticaria; toxic paranoid reactions; dizziness; increased alkaline phosphatase; nephrotoxicity; bone marrow supression.	Peak blood levels delayed when given with food; report nausea, flushing, tachycardia, headache; monitor for nephrotoxicity and for bleeding.
Cephalothin (Keflin, Seffin)—IM, IV 2–12 g/day in 4–6 equally divided doses.	Same as Cephalexin except not recommended for biliary tract infections.	Same as Cephalexin.	Same as Cephalexin.	Same as Cephalexin; pain at site of IM; given in large muscle; rotate sites.
Cefazolin (Ancef, Kefzol)—IM or IV 250 mg–1.5 g q6–12h.	*Staphylococcus aureus; E. coli; Klebsiella;* Group A and B *Streptococcus; Pneumococcus.*	Bactericidal.	Allergic reaction: urticaria, rash; abnormal bleeding.	See Penicillin. May cause false positive lab tests (Coombs', urine glucose). Oral probenecid may be taken concurrently to prolong effects of drug.
Co-trimoxazole (Bactrim, Septra)—PO 160 mg twice daily or 20 mg/kg/day for *P. carinii* pneumonia.	Acute otitis media; urinary tract infection; shigellosis; *P. carinii* pneumonia; prostatitis.	Bacteriostatic; antiinfective; antagonizes folic acid production; combination of sulfamethoxazole and trimethoprim.	Hypersensitivity. See Sulfisoxazole.	IV administration can cause phlebitis and tissue damage with extravasation.
Gentamicin (Garamycin, Jenamicin)—IM, IV 3–5 mg/kg/day in 3–4 divided doses; topical. Skin, eye.	Serious gram-negative bacillary infections; possible *Staph. aureus,* uncomplicated urinary infections.	Bacteriocidal effects on susceptible gram-positive and gram-negative organisms and mycobacteria.	Serious toxic effects: kidneys, ear; causes muscle weakness/paralysis.	Monitor plasma levels (peak is 4–10 μg/mL); patients with burns, cystic fibrosis may need higher doses.
Anticholinergics				
Atropi[illegible]—0.3–1.2 mg PO, subcutaneous, IM, or IV; ophthalmic 0.5–1% up to 6 times qd.	Peptic ulcer; spasms of GI tract; Stokes-Adams syndrome; control excessive secretions during surgery.	Blocks parasympathomimetic effects of acetylcholine on effector organs.	Dry mouth, dysphasia, skin rash, face and upper trunk, skin flushing, urinary retention. *Contraindications:* glaucoma and paralytic ileus.	Observe for postural hypotension in ambulating clients; administer cautiously in aged; and monitor vital signs for pulse and respiratory rate changes.
Tincture of belladonna—0.3–0.6 mL tid.	Hypermotility of stomach; bowel, biliary and renal colic; prostatitis.	Blocks parasympathomimetic effects of acetylcholine.	Dry mouth, thirst, dilated pupils, skin flushing, elevated temperature, and delirium.	Administer 30–60 min before meals; observe for side effects; physostigmine salicylate is antidote.
Propantheline bromide (Probanthine)—PO 15 mg qid; IM or IV 30 mg.	Decreases hypertonicity and hypersecretion of GI tract; ulcerative colitis; peptic ulcer.	Blocks neural transmission at ganglia of autonomic nervous system and at parasympathetic effector organs.	Nausea, gastric fullness, constipation, and mydriasis.	Give before meals; observe urinary output to avoid retention, particularly in elderly; mouth care pc will relieve dryness. Contraindicated with glaucoma.
Anticoagulants				
Heparin—initial dose: SC 10,000–20,000 units; IV 20,000–40,000 units.	Acute thromboembolic emergencies.	Prevents thrombin formation.	Hematuria, bleeding gums, and ecchymosis.	Observe clotting times—should be 20–30 min; antagonist is protamine sulfate.
Warfarin sodium (Coumadin)—initial dose: PO 10–15 mg; maintenance dose—PO 2–10 mg qd.	Venous thrombosis; atrial fibrillation with embolization; pulmonary emboli; myocardial infarction.	Depresses liver synthesis of prothrombin and factors VII, IX, and X.	Minor or major hemorrhage, alopecia, fever, nausea, diarrhea, and dermatitis.	Drug effects last 3–4 days; antagonist is vitamin K. Avoid foods high in vitamin K. No aspirin.
Anticoagulant Antidotes				
Protamine sulfate 1%—IV 10 mg/mL slowly; 1 mg per 100 U heparin.	Overdose of heparin.	Positive electrostatic charge inactivates negatively charged heparin molecules.	Excessive coagulation; hypotension; bradycardia; dyspnea.	Slow IV; no more than 50 mg in 10 minute period; monitor VS continuously. Check APTT for effectiveness.

continued

■ **TABLE 6.3 *(Continued)*** **Common Drugs**

Drug and Dosage	Use	Action	Assessment: Side Effects	Nursing Implications
Vitamin K_1 (Aquamephyton, Konakion)—PO, IM, SC 2.5–25 mg; 0.5–1.0 mg in newborns.	Warfarin (Coumadin) hypoprothrombinemia; hemorrhagic disease in newborns.	Counteracts the inhibitory effects of oral anticoagulants on hepatic synthesis of vitamin K-dependent clotting factors.	Flushing; hypotension; allergic reactions; reappearance of clotting problems (high doses).	Give IV only if absolutely necessary; dilute with preservative-free 0.9% NaCl, D_5W, or D_5NaCl. Protect solution from light; repeated injection may cause redness and pain. Check PT for drug effect.
Anticonvulsants				
Phenytoin or diphenylhydantoin (Dilantin) SO_4—PO 30–100 mg 3–4 times qd; IM 100-200 mg 3–4 times qd; IV 150–250 mg.	Psychomotor epilepsy; convulsive seizures; ventricular arrhythmias.	Depresses motor cortex by preventing spread of abnormal electrical impulses.	Nervousness, ataxia, gastric distress, nystagmus, slurred speech, hallucinations, and gingival hyperplasia.	Give with meals or pc; frequent and diligent mouth care; advise client that urine may turn pink to red-brown; teach client signs of adverse reactions. Mix IV with normal saline (precipitates with 5% D/W).
Ethosuximide (Zarontin)—PO 500 mg/day, increase by 250 mg/day until effective.	Absence seizures.	Depresses motor cortex and reduces CNS sensitivity to convulsive nerve stimuli.	GI distress: nausea, vomiting, cramps; diarrhea; anorexia; blood dyscrasias.	Administer with meals; regular CBC; precautions to avoid injury from drowsiness.
Valporic acid (Depakene)—PO 15 mg/kg/day, increase up to 60 mg/kg/day.	Absence, tonic-clonic, myoclonic, focal, or local seizures.	Inhibits spread of abnormal discharges through brain.	Nausea, vomiting, diarrhea (disappear over time); drowsiness or sedation if taken in combination with other anticonvulsants.	Assess responses; monitor blood levels; precautions against excessive sedation; discourage alcohol use.
Trimethadione (Tridione)—PO 900 mg/day up to 2400 mg/day, taken 3–4 times/day.	Refractory absence seizures.	Exact mechanism unknown. May increase seizure threshold in cortex and thalamus.	Hepatic impairment; nephrosis; blood dyscrasias; SLE; drowsiness; photophobia; nausea/vomiting; weight loss.	Not used as a first-line drug. Monitor closely for adverse effects. If pregnant, notify MD at once.
Primidone (Mysoline)—PO 100–250 mg, increase over 10 days.	Tonic-clonic, focal, or local seizures.	Inhibits abnormal brain electrical activity; dose-dependent CNS depression.	Excessive sedation or ataxia; vertigo.	Careful neurologic, cardiovascular, and respiratory assessment; have resuscitation equipment available.
Diazepam (Valium)—PO 2–10 mg bid–qid; IM or IV 5–10 mg.	All types of seizures.	Induces calming effect on limbic system, thalamus, and hypothalamus.	Drowsiness, ataxia, and paradoxical increase in excitability of CNS.	IV may cause phlebitis; give IV injection slowly, as respiratory arrest can occur; inject IM deeply into tissue.
Magnesium sulfate—PO 1–5 g/ IM or IV 1–4 g at rate of 1.5 mL/min.	Control seizures in pregnancy, epilepsy; relief of acute constipation; reduces edema, inflammation, and itching of skin; may inhibit preterm contractions.	Depresses CNS as well as smooth, cardiac, and skeletal muscle; promotes osmotic retention of fluid.	Flushing, sweating, extreme thirst, complete heart block, dehydration, depressed or absent reflexes, ↓ respirations.	If given IV, monitor vital signs contінously; I&O; do *not* give during the 2 hours preceding delivery; observe mother and newborn for signs of toxicity if given near delivery.
Antidiarrheals				
Paregoric or camphorated opium tincture—5–10 mL q2h, not more than qid.	Diarrhea.	Acts directly on intestinal smooth muscle to increase tone and decrease propulsive peristalsis.	Occasional nausea; prolonged use may produce dependence.	Contains approximately 1.6 mg morphine or 16 mg opium and is subject to federal narcotic regulations; administer with partial glass of water to facilitate passage into stomach; observe number and consistency of stools—discontinue drug as soon as diarrhea is controlled; keep in tight light-resistant bottles.

Kaolin with pectin (Kaopectate)—adults, PO 60–120 mL after each bowel movement (BM); children over 12, PO 60 mL; 6–12 yr, PO 30–60 mL; 3–6 yr, PO 15–30 mL after each BM.	Diarrhea.	Reported to absorb irritants and soothe.	Granuloma of the stomach.	Do not administer for more than 2 days, in presence of fever, or to children younger than 3 years.
Diphenoxylate HCl with atropine sulfate (Lomotil)—PO 5–10 mg tid–qid.	Diarrhea.	Increases intestinal tone and decreases propulsive peristalsis.	Rash, drowsiness, dizziness, depression, abdominal distention, headache, blurred vision, and nausea.	May potentiate action of barbiturates, opiates, and other depressants; closely observe clients receiving these drugs, and administer narcotic antagonists such as levallorphan (Lorfan) tartrate, naloxone HCl (Narcan), and nalorphine HCl (Nalline) as ordered; administer cautiously to clients with hepatic dysfunction—may precipitate hepatic coma.
Antiemetics				
Trimethobenzamide HCl (Tigan)—250 mg qid, PO, IM, rectal.	Nausea; vomiting.	Suppresses chemoreceptors in the trigger zone located in the medulla oblongata.	Drowsiness, vertigo, diarrhea, headache, hypotension, jaundice, blurred vision, and rigid muscles.	Give deep IM to prevent escape of solution; can cause edema, pain, and burning.
Prochlorperazine dimaleate (Compazine)—5–30 mg qid PO, IM, rectal.	Nausea, vomiting, and retching.	See Trimethobenzamide HCl.	Drowsiness, orthostatic hypotension, palpitations, blurred vision, diplopia, and headache.	Use cautiously in children, pregnant women, and clients with liver disease.
Antifungal				
Nystatin (Nilstat)—PO, rectal, vaginal 100,000–1,000,000 U 3–4 times qd.	Skin, mucous membrane infections *(Candida albicans)*; oral thrush, vaginitis; intestinal candidiasis.	Fungiastatic and fungicidal; binds to sterols in fungal cell membrane.	Nausea, vomiting, GI distress, diarrhea.	Oral use—clear mouth of food; keep medication in mouth several minutes before swallowing; vaginal—usually requires 2-week therapy; continue use during menses; consult physician before using antiinfective douches; determine predisposing factors to infection (diabetes, pregnancy, antibiotics, tight-fitting nylon pantyhose).
Amphotericin B (Fungizone)—IV 5 mg/250 mL dextrose over 4–6h (to 1 mg/kg body weight).	Severe fungal infections; histoplasmosis.	Fungistatic or fungicidal; binds to sterols in cell membrane, altering cell permeability.	Febrile reactions; chills, N/V, muscle/joint pain; renal damage; hypotension, tachycardia arrhythmias; hypokalemia.	Monitor for side effects; thrombophlebitis at IV site; BUN >40; creatinine 3 or >; stop drug because of nephrotoxicity.
Ketoconaszole (Nizoral)—oral 200–400 mg daily.	Histoplasmosis, systemic fungal infections.	Antifungal.	Headache, fatigue, dizziness; N/V; decreased libido, impotence; gynecomastia, esp. in males.	Administer with food; avoid concomitant use of antacids, H_2 blockers; advise to report side-effect symptoms.
Antigout				
Allopurinol (Lopurin, Zyloprim)—PO 100 mg initially, 300 mg daily with meals or pc.	Primary hyperuricemia, secondary hyperuricemia with cancer therapy.	Lowers plasma and urinary uric acid levels; no analgesic, antiinflammatory, or uricosuric actions.	Rash, itching, nausea, vomiting, anemia, drowsiness.	Report side effects, particularly rash, as drug must be stopped; avoid driving or other complex tasks until drug effects known; give at least 3000 mL fluid daily; minimum urine output of 2000 mL/day; keep urine neutral or alkaline with sodium bicarbonate or potassium citrate; use cautiously with liver disease, impaired renal function, history of peptic ulcers, lower GI disease, or bone marrow depression.

continued

■ TABLE 6.3 *(Continued)* **Common Drugs**

Drug and Dosage	Use	Action	Assessment: Side Effects	Nursing Implications
Colchicine—PO 1–1.2 mg acute phase; 0.5–2 mg nightly with milk or food; IV 1–2 mg initially.	Gouty arthritis, acute gout.	Inhibits leukocyte migration and phagocytosis in gouty joints; nonanalgesic, nonuricosuric.	Nausea, vomiting, diarrhea, abdominal pain, peripheral neuritis, bone marrow depression (sore throat, bleeding gums, sore mouth), tissue and nerve necrosis with IV use.	Do *not* dilute IV form with normal saline or 5% dextrose—use sterile water to prevent precipitation; infuse over 3–5 min IV; potentiate drug action with alkaline ash foods (milk, most fruits and vegetables).
Probenecid (Benemid)—PO 0.25–0.5 g twice daily pc.	Chronic gouty arthritis, no value in acute; adjuvant therapy with penicillin to increase plasma levels.	Inhibits renal tubular reabsorption of uric acid; no analgesic or anti-inflammatory activity. Competively inhibits renal tubular secretion of penicillin and many weak organic acids.	Headache, nausea, vomiting, anorexia, sore gums, urinary frequency, flushing.	Give with food, milk, or prescribed antacid; 3000 mL/day fluids; avoid alcohol, which increases serum urates; do *not* take with aspirin—inhibits action of drug; renal function and hematology should be evaluated frequently; during acute gout, give with colchicine (Colbenemid).
Antihistamines				
Diphenhydramine HCl (Benadryl)—PO 25–50 mg tid–qid; IM or IV 10–20 mg.	Allergic and pyrogenic reactions; motion sickness; radiation sickness; hay fever; Parkinson's disease.	Inhibits action of histamine on receptor cells, and decreases action of acetylcholine.	Sedation, dizziness, inability to concentrate, headache, anorexia, dermatitis, nausea, diplopia, and insomnia.	Avoid use in newborn or premature infants and clients with glaucoma; supervise ambulation; caution against driving or operating mechanical devices. Excitation or hallucinations may occur in children.
Chlorpheniramine maleate (Chlor-Trimeton)—PO 2–4 mg tid–qid; subcutaneous, IM or IV 10–20 mg.	Asthma; hay fever; serum reactions; anaphylaxis.	Inhibits action of histamine.	Nausea, gastritis, diarrhea, headache, dryness of mouth and nose, nervousness and irritability.	IV may drop blood pressure; give slowly; caution client about drowsiness.
Tripelennamine HCl (Pyribenzamine)—PO 25–50 mg bid–qid; IV or IM 25 mg.	Asthma; hay fever, pruritus; motion sickness.	Inhibits histamine and promotes sedation.	Dry mouth, vertigo, headache, nervousness, frequency, blood dyscrasia, blurred vision and drowsiness.	Caution against driving or handling mechanical equipment.
Antihyperglycemics				
Sulfonylureas				
Acetohexamide (Dymelor)—200–1500 mg qd; 1–2 per day; duration 12–24 h.	Oral hypoglycemic; antidiabetic.	Lowers blood glucose by stimulating insulin release from beta cells; effective only if pancreas has ability to produce insulin.	Hypoglycemia (profuse sweating, hunger, headache, nausea, confusion, ataxia, coma), skin rashes, bone marrow depression, liver toxicity.	Drug therapy must be combined with diet therapy, weight control, and planned, graded exercise; alcohol intolerance may occur (disulfiram reaction—flushing, pounding headache, sweating, nausea, vomiting); should not be taken at bedtime unless specifically ordered (nocturnal hypoglycemia more likely); take at same time each day; *contraindicated* in liver disease, renal disease, pregnancy.
Chlorpropamide (Diabinese)—100–500 mg; 1 per day; duration 30–60 h.	See Acetohexamide.	See Acetohexamide.	See Acetohexamide.	See Acetohexamide.
Tolazamide (Tolinase)—100–500 mg; 1 per day; duration 10–14 h.	See Acetohexamide.	See Acetohexamide.	See Acetohexamide.	See Acetohexamide.

Tolbutamide (Orinase)—500–2000 mg; 2–3 per day; duration 6–12 h.	See Acetohexamide.	See Acetohexamide.	See Acetohexamide.	See Acetohexamide.
Insulin—rapid acting Crystalline zinc (Regular) (Humulin R) (clear)—onset 0.5–1 h; peak 2–4 h; duration 6–8 h.	Poorly controlled diabetes; trauma; surgery, coma.	Enhances transmembrane passage of glucose into cells; promotes CHO, fat, and protein metabolism.	Hypoglycemia (profuse sweating, nausea, hunger, headache, confusion, ataxia, coma), allergic reaction at injection site.	Monitor blood and urine for glucose and acetone levels; insulin currently being used can be kept at room temperature for 1 month; refrigerate stock insulin only; rotate injection sites; cold insulin leads to lipodystrophy, reduced absorption, and local reaction; only form of insulin that is given IV.
Prompt insulin zinc suspension (Semilente) purified pork (cloudy)—onset 1–2 h; peak 4–10 h; duration 12–16 h.	Clients allergic to Regular; used in combination with longer-lasting insulin.	See Crystalline zinc (Regular).	See Crystalline zinc (Regular).	See Crystalline zinc (Regular). Compatible with all Lente preparations.
Insulin—intermediate acting NPH insulin (isophane insulin suspension) purified pork (Humulin N+) (cloudy)—onset 1–2 h; peak 5–12 h; duration 18–24 h.	Clients who can be controlled by one dose per day.	See Crystalline zinc (Regular).	See Crystalline zinc (Regular).	Gently rotate vial between palms, invert several times to mix; do not shake; See Crystalline zinc (Regular).
Insulin zinc suspension (Lente insulin) (cloudy)—onset 1–3 h; peak 6–12 h; duration 18–24 h.	Clients allergic to NPH.	See Crystalline zinc (Regular).	See Crystalline zinc (Regular).	See Crystalline zinc (Regular).
Insulin—slow acting PZI (Protamine zinc insulin suspension) (cloudy)—onset 4–8 h; peak 14–24 h; duration 24–36 h.	Rarely used, only if uncontrolled by other types.	See Crystalline zinc (Regular).	See Crystalline zinc (Regular).	Between-meal snacks may be necessary; bedtime snacks are essential; See Crystalline zinc (Regular).
Extended insulin zinc suspension (Ultralente) purified beef (cloudy)—onset 4–8 h; peak 12–24 h; duration 36 h.	Often mixed with Semilente for 24-hour curve.	See Crystalline zinc (Regular).	See Crystalline zinc (Regular).	See Crystalline zinc (Regular).
Antihypertensives				
Reserpine (Serpasil)—PO 0.25 mg qd.	Mild and moderate hypertension.	Depletes catecholamines and decreases peripheral vasoconstriction, heart rate, and BP.	Depression, nasal stuffiness, increased gastric secretions, rash, and pruritus.	Watch for signs of mental depression; closely monitor pulse rates of clients also receiving digitalis; avoid alcohol.
	Obstetric use: preeclampsia-eclampsia.	CNS depressant, tranquilizer; sedation is major effect; decreases neural transmission to nerves; decreases tone in in blood vessels.	Low level of toxicity; nasal stuffiness; weight gain; diarrhea; allergic reactions—dry mouth, itching, skin eruptions.	Siderails up; must not stand up without assistance; observe carefully; monitor BP.
Guanethidine SO_4 (Ismelin)—PO 10–50 mg qd in divided doses.	Severe to moderately severe hypertension.	Blocks norepinephrine at postganglionic synapses.	Orthostatic hypotension, diarrhea, and inhibition of ejaculation.	Postural hypotension is marked in the morning and accentuated by hot weather, alcohol, and exercise; teach to rise slowly, with assistance.
Methyldopa (Aldomet)—PO 500 mg–2 g in divided doses.	Severe to moderately severe hypertension.	Inhibits formation of dopamine, a precursor of norepinephrine.	Initial drowsiness, depression with feelings of unreality, edema, jaundice, and dry mouth.	Contraindicated in acute and chronic liver disease; encourage not to drive car if drowsy.

continued

■ **TABLE 6.3 *(Continued)*** **Common Drugs**

Drug and Dosage	Use	Action	Assessment: Side Effects	Nursing Implications
Hydralazine HCl (Apresoline)—PO 10–50 mg qid.	Moderate hypertension.	Dilates peripheral blood vessels, increases renal blood flow.	Palpitations, tachycardia, angina pectoris, tremors, and depression.	Encourage moderation in exercise and identification of stressful stimuli.
	Obstetric use: preeclampsia-eclampsia.	Relaxes peripheral blood vessels (opens vascular bed—physiologic dehydration).	Headache, heart palpitation, gastric irritation, coronary insufficiency, edema, chills, fever, and severe depression.	Siderails up; must not stand without assistance; may be given with diuretics; observe carefully; IM route only; monitor BP.
Guanfacine hydrochloride (Tenex)—PO 1 mg daily to maximum dose of 3 mg/day.	Hypertension, in combination with thiazidelike diuretics.	Centrally-acting alpha2-adrenergic receptor agonist.	Drowsiness; weakness; dizziness; dry mouth; constipation; impotence.	Warn patient not to drive or perform activities requiring alertness. Take at bedtime to minimize sedation. Monitor BP and pulse.
Pentolinium (Ansolysen) tartrate—PO 60–600 mg qd in divided doses.	Malignant hypertension; hypertensive crisis.	Blocks sympathetic stimulation at ganglion; dilates peripheral vasculature; very potent.	Orthostatic hypotension, diarrhea, and inhibition of ejaculation.	Teach to rise slowly.
Phentolamine hydrochloride (Regitine)—PO 50 mg 4–6 doses daily; IV, IM, or local 5–10 mg, diluted in minimum 10 mL normal saline.	Prevents dermal necrosis; hypertensive crisis; diagnosis pheochromocytoma.	Blocks alpha adrenergic receptors.	Weakness, dizziness, orthostatic hypotension, nausea, vomiting, abdominal pain.	When giving parenterally, client should be supine; monitor for overdosage (preciptous drop in BP); do *not* give with epinephrine.
Antilactogenics				
Deladumone (testosterone enanthate and estradiol valerate)—IM 200 mg once.	*Postpartum use:* suppresses lactation; prevents breast engorgement when given immediately prior to 3rd stage labor.	Depresses production of lactogenic hormone by anterior pituitary.	Rare, following one dose; masculinization and electrolyte imbalance with long-term therapy.	Observe for hypercalcemia, edema; *contraindicated* in pregnant women.
Testosterone cypionate—IM 100 mg.	*Postpartum use:* suppresses lactation; controls breast engorgement; palliative therapy for breast cancer and menopausal symptoms.	See Deladumone.	See Deladumone.	See Deladumone.
Bromocriptine mesylate (Parlodel)—PO 2.5 mg bid for 14 days.	Prevents lactation; also used for Parkinson's.	Inhibits prolactin secretion.	Fatigue; ovulation returns; hypertension; postural hypotension; nausea/vomiting; dizziness.	Contraceptive counseling; monitor VS; take with meals to ↓ GI upset.
Antilipemics				
Cholestyramine resin (Questran)—PO 4-g packet tid before meals.	Reduction of blood cholesterol.	Binds bile acids in the intestine and prevents their reabsorption, thus reducing serum cholesterol 10–20%.	Mild nausea, constipation; epigastric distress and diarrhea.	Watch for deficiencies of vitamins A, D, and K (fat-soluble vitamins); give all other drugs 1 h before or 4 h after Questran to avoid blocking absorption.
Clofibrate (Atromid-S)—PO 500 mg qid.	Endogenous hyperlipemias.	Inhibits hepatic synthesis of triglycerides, phospholipids, and cholesterol.	Urticaria, stomatitis, pruritus, leukopenia, nausea, elevation of SGOT and SGPT activity, and weight gain.	*Contraindicated* in pregnancy, lactation, renal and hepatic impairment, and in children.
Niacin (vitamin B_3, nicotinic acid)—PO 1.5–6 g.	Hypercholesterolemia.	Decreases liver's production of low-density lipoproteins (LDL) and synthesis of triglycerides.	GI upset, flushing, pruritus, hyperuricemia, hyperglycemia.	Take the drug with meals; prevent flushing by taking an aspirin 30 min before; monitor closely during first year of therapy.

Lovastatin (Mevacor)—PO 20–80 mg.	Primary hypercholesterolemia.	Blocks the liver's production of cholesterol; decreases synthesis of LDL.	Adverse reactions are rare; cataracts and liver damage with prolonged use; muscle pain and weakness.	Take with evening meal; report muscle pain and weakness immediately.
Gemfibrozil (Lopid)—1200 mg/day.	Hypercholesterolemia.	May inhibit peripheral lipolysis and reduce triglyceride synthesis in liver.	GI upset (abdominal pain, epigastric pain, diarrhea, nausea, vomiting), rash, headache, dizziness, blurred vision.	Use caution when driving or doing tasks requiring alertness; take before meals.
Antimycobacterials				
First-line drugs Isoniazid—5–10 mg/kg up to 300 mg PO or IM.	Tuberculosis	Suppresses or interferes with biosynthesis; bacteriostatic.	Peripheral neuritis, hepatitis, hypersensitivity.	Give pyridoxine (B_6) 10 mg as prophylaxis for neuritis; 50–100 mg as treatment.
Ethambutol—15–25 mg/kg PO.			Optic neuritis (reversible with discontinuation of drug; very rare at 15 mg/kg), skin rash.	Use with caution with renal disease or when eye testing is not feasible; used in combination with other drug.
Rifampin—10–20 mg/kg up to 600 mg PO.			Hepatitis, febrile reaction, purpura (rare).	Orange urine color; negates effect of birth control pills.
Streptomycin—15–20 mg/kg up to 1 g IM.			Eighth cranial nerve damage, nephrotoxicity.	Use with caution in older clients or those with renal disease.
Second-line drugs Viomycin—15–30 mg/kg up to 1 g IM.			Auditory toxicity, nephrotoxicity, vestibular toxicity (rare).	Use with caution in older clients; rarely used with renal disease.
Capreomycin—15–30 mg/kg up to 1 g IM.			Eighth cranial nerve damage, nephrotoxicity.	Use with caution in older clients; rarely used with renal disease.
Kanamycin—15–30 mg/kg up to 1 g IM.			Auditory toxicity, nephrotoxicity, vestibular toxicity (rare).	Use with caution in older clients; rarely used with renal disease.
Ethionamide—15–30 mg/kg up to 1 g PO.			GI disturbance, hepatotoxicity, hypersensitivity.	Divided dose may help GI side effects.
Pyrazinamide—15–30 mg/kg up to 3 g PO.			Hyperuricemia, hepatotoxicity.	Combination with an aminoglycoside is bactericidal.
Paraaminosalicylic acid (aminosalicylic acid)—150 mg/kg up to 12 g PO.			GI disturbance, hypersensitivity, hepatoxicity, sodium load.	GI side effects very frequent, making cooperation difficult.
Cycloserine—10–20 mg/kg up to 1 g PO.			Psychosis, personality changes, convulsions, rash.	Very difficult drug to use; side effects may be blocked by pyridoxine, ataractic agents, or anticonvulsant drugs.

Note: To minimize resistant strains, combination therapy is used long term.

Antiviral				
Zidovudine (Retrovir)—PO 200 mg q4h.	AIDS and related disorders.	Inhibits replication of human immunodeficiency virus (HIV).	Blood disorders, especially anemia and granulocytopenia; headache; nausea; insomnia; myalgia.	Monitor for signs of opportunistic infection and adverse drug effects; drug must be taken around the clock; regular blood tests (q 2 weeks).

continued

■ **TABLE 6.3 *(Continued)***

Common Drugs

Drug and Dosage	Use	Action	Assessment: Side Effects	Nursing Implications
Acyclovir (Zovirax)—PO 200 mg, 3–5 times/day; IV 5 mg/kg q8h over 1 h. Topical 6 times daily for 1 week.	Herpes simplex 1, 2; genital herpes.	Converts to an active cytotoxic metabolite that inhibits viral DNA replication.	Headache; nausea and vomiting; diarrhea; increased serum BUN and creatinine.	Measure I&O q8h; ensure adequate hydration; assess for common side effects; apply topical with finger cot or rubber glove; refer for counseling.
Pentamidine (Pentam 300)—IM or IV 4 mg/kg/day; give IV diluted in dextrose solution over 60 min.	*P. carinii* pneumonia.	Antiprotozoal.	Severe hypotension; nephrotoxicity; hyper- and hypoglycemia.	Injections are painful and may cause sterile abscesses; rotate sites and observe for inflammation.
Bronchodilators				
Aminophylline—PO 250 mg bid–qid; rectal 250–500 mg; IV 250–500 mg over 10–20 min.	Rapid relief of bronchospasm; asthma; pulmonary edema.	Relaxes smooth muscles and increases cardiac contractility; interferes with reabsorption of Na^+ and Cl^- in proximal tubules.	Nausea, vomiting, cardiac arrhythmias, intestinal bleeding, insomnia, restlessness, and rectal irritation from suppository.	Give oral with or after meals; monitor vital signs for changes in BP and pulse; weigh daily; IM injections are painful.
Ephedrine SO_4—PO, subcutaneous, or IM 25 mg tid–qid.	Asthma; allergies; bradycardia; nasal decongestant.	Relaxes hypertonic muscles in bronchioles and GI tract.	Wakefulness, nervousness, dizziness, palpitations, and hypertension.	Monitor vital signs; avoid giving dose near bedtime; check urine output in older adults.
Isoproterenol HCl (Isuprel)—inhalation of 1:100 or 1:200 solution.	Mild to moderately severe asthma attack; bronchitis; pulmonary emphysema.	Relaxes hypertonic bronchioles.	Nervousness, tachycardia, hypertension, and insomnia.	Monitor vital signs before and after treatment; teach client how to use nebulizer.
Theophylline—PO 400 mg/daily in divided doses; max adult dose: 900 mg divided dose.	Treatment/prevention of emphysema, asthma (bronchoconstriction); chronic bronchitis.	Bronchodilation.	Restlessness; increased respiration/heart rate; palpitations, arrhythmias; N/V; increased urine output → dehydration.	Monitor theophylline levels: 10–20 μg/mL; monitor signs of toxicity; take with 8 oz water or with meals to decrease GI symptoms.
Isoetharine (Bronkosol) Inhalant.	Bronchial asthma, reversible spasm of bronchitis; emphysema.	Smooth muscle relaxant; beta-adrenergic agonist; bronchodilator.	Tachycardia, palpitations; BP changes; dizziness; paradoxical airway; resistance with repeated doses.	Increase fluids; teach proper use/dose inhalation therapy.
Terbutaline (Brethine)—PO 2.5–5 mg q6h (not to exceed 20 mg/24 h); SC 0.25 mg, repeat 15–30 min (not to exceed 0.5 mg/h); inhalation—2 puffs (0.2 mg each) q4–6h.	Bronchospasm.	See Isoproterenol.	See Isoproterenol.	See Isoproterenol.
Calcium Channel Blocker				
Verapamil (Calan, Isopten)—PO 240–480 mg, 3–4 times/day; IV 75–150 μg/kg over 2 min.	Angina; supraventricular arrhythmias; essential hypertension.	Inhibits calcium movement into smooth muscle cells; lowers pressure by reducing cardiac contractility.	Constipation; AV block; hepatotoxicity.	Monitor VS and ECG for bradycardia and arrhythmias; observe for jaundice, abdominal pain; encourage fluids and bulk-forming foods.
Cardiac Glycosides				
Digitoxin—digitalizing dose: PO 200 μg twice/day; IM or IV 200–400 μg; maintenance dose: PO 50–300 μg qd.	Congestive heart failure; atrial fibrillation and flutter; supraventricular tachycardia.	Increases force of cardiac contractility, slows heart rate, decreases right atrial pressures, promotes diuresis.	Arrhythmias; nausea; vomiting; anorexia, malaise, color vision, yellow or blue.	Hold medication if pulse rate less than 60 or over 120; encourage foods high in potassium (e.g., bananas, orange juice); observe for signs of electrolyte depletion, apathy, disorientation, and anorexia.

Digoxin (Lanoxin)—digitalizing dose: PO up to 750 μg; IM or IV up to 600 μg; maintenance dose: PO 200 μg qd.	See Digitoxin.	See Digitoxin.	See Digitoxin.	See Digitoxin.
Chemotherapy				
Antimetabolites Cytosine arabinoside; 6-mercaptopurine; methotrexate; 5 FU.	Acute leukemia; bladder, breast, colorectal, stomach, testicular tumors.	Inhibits DNA synthesis; metabolized by liver and kidneys.	Nausea, vomiting, diarrhea, GI ulcers, stomatitis, photosensitivity, and alopecia.	Antiemetics; good oral hygiene; bland diet; methods to cope with alopecia.
Corticosteroids Prednisone; cortisone acetate; hydrocortisone.	Leukemia; hypercalcemia; anemia; reduction of CNS edema; Hodgkin's disease.	See Adrenocortical steroids.	No acute toxicity; increased appetite, fluid retention; long-term effects include moon face, striae, trunk obesity, purpura, osteoporosis, muscle weakness, psychosis, and possible hypertension, infection due to immunosuppression, gastric bleeding, and ulcers.	Prepare client and family for body changes and possible effects on behavior; avoid exposure to infection; avoid aspirin; give medication with food or beverage to minimize gastric irritation.
Alkalating agents Chlorambucil; cyclophosphamide (Cytoxan); Thiotepa; BCNU; CCNU; methyl-CCNU.	Chronic leukemia; Hodgkin's disease; lymphomas—bladder, brain, breast, cervical, colorectal, kidney.	Alter property of DNAs, nucleic acid, preventing mitosis.	Nausea, vomiting, dermatitis, leukopenia, thrombocytopenia, fever, and hemorrhagic cystitis.	Watch for signs and symptoms of infection; administer antiemetic.
Natural products Doxorubicin (Adriamycin), dactinomycin (Actinomycin D) (antibiotic); vinblastine SO_4; vincristine SO_4 (Oncovin); daunomycin (Daunorubicin) (antibiotic).	Sarcomas; Wilm's tumors; acute leukemia; lymphomas; neuroblastoma; rhabdomyosarcoma (bladder, breast, cervical, thyroid, colorectal, kidney, stomach, uterus); Hodgkin's disease.	Proposed mechanism for action—inhibition of RNA and DNA.	Nausea, vomiting, fever, stomatitis, anorexia, acne, alopecia, bone marrow depression, malaise, and diarrhea or neurotoxia with constipation and urinary retention.	Good oral hygiene; bland diet; attractive meals in social atmosphere; antiemetic; prepare client (and parents or SOs) for resulting hair loss.
Miscellaneous agents Hydroxyurea; procarbazine HCl.	Chronic leukemia; Hodgkin's disease; sarcomas.	Inhibits DNA synthesis, crosses blood-brain barrier, metabolized by liver, and excreted by kidneys.	Nausea, vomiting, bone marrow depression, alopecia, rash, pruritus, GI toxicity.	Antiemetic; bland diet; observe for infection; prepare client for loss of hair.
Cholinergic Drugs				
Bethanechol Cl (Urecholine)—PO, 5–30 mg; subcutaneous, 2.5–5 mg; Neostigmine bromide (Prostigmin)—PO, 10–30 mg; IM or subcutaneous 0.25–1 mg.	Postoperative abdominal atony and distention; bladder atony with retention; postsurgical or postpartum urinary retention; myasthenia gravis.	Increases GI and bladder tone; decreases sphincter tone.	Belching, abdominal cramps, diarrhea, nausea, vomiting, incontinence, profuse sweating, salivation, and respiratory depression.	Check respirations; have urinal or bedpan close at hand and answer calls quickly; atropine SO_4 is the antidote for cholinergic drugs.
Cholinergic Miotics				
Pilocarpine HCl—1–2 gtts 1%–2% solution up to 6 times/day. Physostigmine salicylate (Eserine)—0.1 mL of 0.25–10% solution; not more than qid.	Chronic open-angle and acute angle-closure glaucoma.	Contraction of the sphincter muscle of iris, resulting in miosis.	Brow ache, headache, ocular pain, blurring and dimness of vision, allergic conjunctivitis, nausea, vomiting, and profuse sweating; bronchoconstriction in patients with bronchial asthma.	Initially the medication may be irritating; teach proper sterile technique for instilling drops—wipe excess solution to prevent systemic symptoms; discard cloudy solutions.

continued

TABLE 6.3 *(Continued)* **Common Drugs**

Drug and Dosage	Use	Action	Assessment: Side Effects	Nursing Implications
CNS Stimulants				
Amphetamine SO_4—PO 5–60 mg qd in divided doses.	Mild depressive states; narcolepsy; postencephalitic parkinsonism; obesity control; minimal brain dysfunction in children (attention deficit disorder).	Raises blood pressure, decreases sense of fatigue, elevates mood.	Restlessness, dizziness, tremors, insomnia; increases libido; suicidal and homicidal tendencies; palpitations; angina pain.	Give before 4 P.M. to avoid sleep disturbance; dependence on drug may develop; *contraindicated* with MAO inhibitors, hyperthyroidism, and psychotic states.
Methylphenidate hydrochloride (Ritalin)—PO 0.3 mg/kg/d or adults 20–60 mg in divided doses.	Childhood hyperactivity; narcolepsy; MBD (attention deficit disorder) in children.	Mild CNS and respiratory stimulation.	Anorexia, dizziness, drowsiness, insomnia, nervousness, BP and pulse changes.	To avoid insomnia take last dose 4–5 h before bedtime; monitor vital signs; check weight 2–3 times weekly and report losses.
Diuretics				
Hydrochlorothiazide (Hydrodiuril and Esidrix 25–100 mg tid)—PO Diuril 0.5–1 g qd.	Edema; congestive heart failure; Na^+ retention in steroid therapy; hypertension.	Inhibits sodium chloride and water reabsorption in the distal ascending loop and the distal convoluted tubule of the kidneys.	Hypokalemia, nausea, vomiting, diarrhea, dizziness, and paresthesias; may accentuate diabetes.	Watch for muscle weakness; give well-diluted potassium chloride supplement; monitor urine for changes in sugar and acetone.
Spironolactone (Aldactone)—PO 25 mg bid–qid.	Cirrhosis of liver; when other diuretics are ineffective.	Inhibits effects of aldosterone in distal tubules of kidney.	Headache, lethargy, diarrhea, ataxia, skin rash, gynecomastia.	Potassium-sparing drug; do *not* give supplemental KCl; monitor for signs of electrolyte imbalance.
Furosemide (Lasix)—PO 40–80 mg qd in divided doses.	Edema and associated heart failure; cirrhosis; renal disease; nephrotic syndrome; hypertension.	Inhibits Na^+ and Cl^- reabsorption in the Loop of Henle.	Dermatitis pruritis, paresthesia, blurring of vision, postural hypotension, nausea, vomiting, diarrhea, dehydration, electrolyte depletion, and hearing loss (usually reversible).	Assess for weakness, lethargy, leg cramps, anorexia; peak action in 1–2 h; duration 6–8 h; do not give at bedtime; supplementary KCl indicated; may induce digitalis toxicity.
Ethacrynic acid (Edecrin)—PO 50–200 mg qd in divided doses.	Pulmonary edema; ascites; edema of congestive heart failure.	Inhibits the reabsorption of Na^+ in the ascending Loop of Henle.	Nausea, vomiting, diarrhea, hypokalemia, hypotension, gout, dehydration, deafness, and metabolic acidosis.	Assess for dehydration—skin turgor, neck veins; hypotension; KCl supplement.
Osmotic diuretic 30% urea, 10% invert sugar, 20% mannitol.	Cerebral edema.	Hypertonic solution that kidney tubules cannot reabsorb, thereby causing obligatory water loss.	↑ Extracellular fluid volume.	Usually Foley catheter required; monitor cardiac and respiratory status.
Acetazolamide (Diamox)—PO 250–1000 mg/d; IV, 500 mg.	Glaucoma; congestive heart failure; convulsive disorders.	Weak diuretic; produces acidosis; self-limiting effect; increases bicarbonate excretion.	Electrolyte depletion symptomatology—lassitude, apathy, decreased urinary output, and mental confusion.	Weigh daily; I&O; assess edema; give early in day to allow sleep at night; observe for side effects; replace electrolytes as ordered.
Enzymes				
Chymotrypsin (Chymar)—PO 50,000–100,000 U qid; IM 0.5–1.0 mL qd.	Inflammatory edema; hematomas from traumatic injuries.	Accelerates healing by removing fibrinlike material that blocks capillaries and lymphatics.	Pain, local edema, urticaria, allergic reactions.	Institute hypersensitivity test before administration.
Pancreatin (Viokase)—adults, PO 325 mg–1 g qd, during meals; children, PO 300–600 mg tid.	Chronic pancreatitis; cystic fibrosis; gastrectomy; pancreatectomy; sprue.	Assists in digestion of starch, protein, and fats; decreases nitrogen and fat content of stool.	Anorexia, nausea, vomiting, diarrhea, buccal/anal soreness (infants), sneezing, skin rashes, diabetes.	May be taken with antacid or cimetidine; do *not* crush or chew tabs; monitor I&O, weight; be alert for signs of diabetes; children may use sprinkles.

Expectorants				
Ammonium Cl—PO 300 mg.	Stimulates secretory activity of respiratory tract; diuretic.	NH_4 ions cause gastric irritation, which reflexly stimulates respiratory tract secretions.	Nausea, vomiting, and bradycardia.	Monitor respirations; keep IV record to avoid dehydration and metabolic acidosis.
Ipecac syrup—PO 15–30 mL for emesis, followed by 1–2 glasses H_2O (adults and children >1 yrs); 5–10 mL followed by ½–1 glass H_2O (children <1 yr).	Emergency emetic for poison ingestion.	See Ammonium Cl.	Violent emesis, tachycardia, decreased BP, and dyspnea.	*Contraindicated* in liver and renal disease; if given for emesis, follow dose with as much water as client will drink.
Potassium iodide—PO 300 mg tid–qid.	Bronchial asthma; bronchitis; actinomycosis; blastomycosis; sporotrichosis.	Reduces viscosity of bronchial secretions by stimulating flow of respiratory tract fluids.	Sore mouth, sore throat, conjunctivitis, headache, mental depression, ataxia, fever, and sexual impotence.	Give diluted in milk or juice to decrease gastric irritation; observe for side effects and teach client signs.
Terpin hydrate—PO 5–10 mL q3–4h.	Bronchitis; emphysema.	Liquefies bronchial secretions.	Nausea, vomiting, and gastric irritation.	Give undiluted; push fluids.
Guaifenesin (Robitussin) 100–400 mg q4h.	Respiratory congestion.	Increases expectoration by causing irritation of gastric mucosa; reduces adhesiveness/surface tension of respiratory tract fluid.	Low incidence of GI upset; drowsiness.	Encourage to stop smoking; increase fluid intake; respiratory hygiene.
Fibrinolytic Agents				
Alteplase, recombinant (Activase, tPA)—IV bolus, 6–10 mg over 1–2 min; IV infusion, 60 mg first h, 20 mg second h, 20 mg third h.	Acute MI; under investigation for pulmonary emboli, deep vein thrombosis, and peripheral artery thrombosis.	Promotes conversion of plasminogen to plasmin, which is fibrinolytic.	Internal or local bleeding; urticaria; dysrhythmias related to reperfusion; hypotension, nausea, and vomiting.	Assess for signs of reperfusion (relief of chest pain, no ST segment elevation). Observe for bleeding; avoid IM injection; do not mix other meds in line.
Streptokinase IV—250,000 IU over 30 min; 100,000 IU/h.	Lysis of pulmonary or systemic emboli or thrombi; acute MI.	Reacts with plasminogen, dissolves fibrin clots.	Prolonged coagulation; allergic reactions; mild fever.	Monitor for signs of excessive bleeding, particularly at injection sites; avoid nonessential handling of client.
Fibrinolytic Antidote				
Aminocaproic acid (Amicar)—PO, IV 5 g loading dose; 1 g/h to 30 g in 24 h.	Management of streptokinase or urokinase overdose.	Inhibits plasminogen activator and antagonizes plasmin.	Hypotension; bradycardia; cardiac arrhythmias.	Give slowly IV to prevent side effects; not recommended for DIC.
Hematinics				
Ferrous sulfate (Feosol, Fer-in-Sol)—adults, PO 300 mg–1.2 g qd; children under 6 yr, PO 75–225 mg qd; 6–12 yr, PO 120–600 mg qd.	Iron deficiency anemia; prophylactically during infancy, childhood, pregnancy.	Corrects nutritional Fe deficiency anemia.	Nausea, vomiting, anorexia, constipation, diarrhea, yellow-brown discoloration of eyes, teeth.	To minimize GI distress, give with meals; do *not* give with antacids or tea; liquid form should be taken through straw to prevent staining of teeth; causes dark green/black stool.

continued

TABLE 6.3 *(Continued)* **Common Drugs**

Drug and Dosage	Use	Action	Assessment: Side Effects	Nursing Implications
Hormones				
Testosterone—PO 5–10 mg qd; IM 25–50 mg 2–3 times/week; 200–400 mg IM q 2–4 weeks for breast cancer.	Hypogonadism; eunuchism; impotence; advanced cancer of breast.	Growth of sex organs and appearance of secondary male sex characteristics; counteracts excessive amounts of estrogen.	Nausea, dyspepsia, masculinization, hypercalcemia, menstrual irregularities, renal calculi, and Na^+, K^+, and H_2O retention.	Observe for edema; weigh daily; I&O; push fluids for bed-ridden clients, to prevent renal calculi.
Progesterone—subcutaneous or IM 5–10 mg qd; sublingual 5–10 mg.	Amenorrhea; dysmenorrhea; endometriosis; habitual abortion.	Converts endometrium into secreting structure; prevents ovulation; stimulates growth of mammary tissue.	Nausea, vomiting, dizziness, edema, headache, protein metabolism.	Give deep IM and rotate sites; weigh daily to ascertain fluid retention.
Estradiol—PO 1–2 mg up to 10 mg for CA qd–tid; cyclic (on 3 weeks, off 1 week).	Menopausal symptoms; osteoporosis; hypogenitalism; sexual infantilism; postpartum breast engorgement; breast and prostatic carcinoma.	Inhibits release of pituitary gonadotropins; promotes growth of female genital tissues.	Anorexia, nausea, vomiting, diarrhea, fluid retention, mental depression, headache, thromboembolism and feminization in males.	Baseline VS; weigh daily; encourage frequent physical check-ups to check serum lipids; teach BSE.
Chlorotrianisene (TACE), estrogen—PO 12–50 mg.	Suppresses lactation; prostatic cancer; menopause.	Nonsteroidal synthetic estrogen.	Rare after one course of treatment; thromboembolism; impotence and gynecomastia in males.	Rebound engorgement may occur. Supply client with package insert; *contraindicated* in blood coagulation disorders.
Diethylstilbestrol (DES)—PO or IM 0.2–5.0 mg qd; vaginal suppository 0.1–0.5 mg at bedtime.	Prostate carcinoma; menopausal symptoms; osteoporosis; pain; mammary carcinoma; atrophic vaginitis.	Synthetic nonsteroidal compound with estrogenic effects on pituitary, ovaries, myometrium, endometrium, and other tissues.	Anorexia, nausea, vomiting, headache, diarrhea, dizziness, and fainting—many side effects with long-term use.	*Never* give if woman is pregnant—predisposes to vaginal cancer in female offspring at puberty.
Medroxyprogesterone (Provera)—PO 2.5–10 mg; IM 400–1000 mg weekly.	Amenorrhea; functional uterine bleeding; threatened abortion; dysmenorrhea; adjunctive and palliation with renal cancer and endometriosis; PMS.	Similar to progesterone, but can be taken orally; thickens uterine decidua.	Drowsiness: cyclic menstrual withdrawal bleeding; GI upset; headache; edema; breast congestion.	Teach client regarding self-administration; breast self-exam for possible breast changes.
Hydroxyprogesterone caproate (Delalutin)—IM 250 mg/2 mL q4wk.	Menstrual disorders; ovarian and uterine dysfunction.	Synthetic derivative of progesterone; long-acting.	GI symptoms, headache, and allergy.	Requires test for endogenous estrogen production; tell patient onset of menstrual cycle may take 2–3 months after treatment; BSE.
Menotropins (Pergonal)—IM 1 amp (FSH + LH)/day for 9–12 days (followed by 5000–10,000 U HCG, if ovulation does not occur, repeat with 2 ampules).	*Infertility use:* treatment of secondary anovulation; stimulation of spermatogenesis.	Human gonadotropic responses; induces ovulation; sperm stimulation.	Abortions occur in 25%; failure rate 55–80% of clients; possible multiple births; ovarian enlargement; gynecomastia in males.	Assist in collection of urine to assess estrogen levels; counsel regarding couple's need to have daily intercourse from day of HCG injection until ovulation.
Mucolytic Agents				
Entex—PO 1 cap qid, or adult 2 tsp qid.	Bronchitis; bronchial asthma; sinusitis.	Decongests swollen mucous membranes, enhances flow of respiratory tract fluid, promotes ciliary action.	CNS stimulation with overdose.	Monitor vital signs, particularly in clients with hypertension, heart disease, diabetes. *Contraindicated* in clients receiving MAO inhibitors.
Acetylcysteine (Mucomyst)—1–10 mL of 20% solution per nebulizer tid.	Emphysema; pneumonia; tracheostomy care; atelectasis; cystic fibrosis.	Lowers viscosity of respiratory secretions by opening disulfide linkages in mucus.	Stomatitis, nausea, rhinorrhea, bronchospasm.	Observe respiratory rate; maintain open airway with suctioning as necessary. Observe asthmatics carefully for increased bronchospasm. Discontinue treatment immediately if this occurs. Odor disagreeable initially.

Muscle Relaxants				
Baclofen (Lioresal)—5 mg tid up to 10–20 mg 4/day maintenance dose.	Relief of spasticity of multiple sclerosis, spinal cord injury.	Centrally acting skeletal muscle relaxant; depresses polysynaptic afferent reflex activity at spinal cord level.	Pruritis, tinnitus; N/V, diarrhea or constipation; drowsiness.	Administer with food if GI symptoms; monitor for safety when ambulating; do not discontinue abruptly.
Dantrolene sodium (Dantrium)—25 mg/day to 25 mg bid–qid to 100 mg qid max.	See Baclofen.	See Baclofen.	See Baclofen.	See Baclofen.
Narcotic Antagonists				
Naloxone (Narcan) HCl—IV 0.1–0.2 mg repeated.	Reverses respiratory depression due to narcotics.	Reverses respiratory depression of morphine SO_4, meperidine HCl, and methadone HCl; does not itself cause respiratory depression, sedation, or analgesia.	No known side effects.	Note time, type of narcotic, dosage received; not useful with CNS depression from other drugs. Respiratory depression may return. Monitor closely.
Naltrexone (Trexan).	Treatment of narcotic addiction, refer to a pharmacology text.	See Naloxone.	See Naloxone.	See Naloxone.
Sedatives and Hypnotics				
Chloral hydrate—PO 250 mg tid; hypnotic: PO 0.5–1.0 g; rectal supplement 0.3–0.9 g.	Sedation for elderly; delirium tremens; pruritus; mania; barbiturate and alcohol withdrawal.	Depresses sensorimotor areas of cerebral cortex.	Nausea, vomiting, gastritis; pinpoint pupils; delirium; rash; decreased BP, pulse, respirations, and temperature; hepatic damage.	*Caution*—should not be taken in combination with alcohol; dependency is possible.
Diazepam (Valium)—PO 2–10 mg tid–qid; IM or IV 2–10 mg q3–4h.	Anxiety disorders; alcohol withdrawal; adjunctive therapy in seizure disorders; status epilepticus; tetanus; preoperative or preprocedural sedation (also see Midazolam).	Induces calming effect on limbic system, thalamus, and hypothalamus.	CNS depression—sedation or ataxia (dose-related); dry mouth; blurred vision; mydriasis; constipation; urinary retention.	Do not mix with other drugs; IM injection painful; observe for phlebitis; monitor response; measures to ensure patient safety (e.g., falls); high potential for abuse; *contraindicated* in acute angle closure glaucoma and porphyria.
Flurazepam (Dalmane)—PO >15 yrs, 30 mg hs; elderly or debilitated, 15 mg hs.	Hypnotic.	Fastest acting. See Diazepam.	See Diazepam.	See Diazepam.
Lorazepam (Ativan)—PO 1–2 mg bid–tid (up to 10 mg); 2–4 mg hs; IM 4 mg max; IV 2 mg max.	Anxiety disorders; insomnia; alternative to diazepam for status epilepticus; preanesthesia.	See Diazepam.	See Diazepam.	See Diazepam.
Phenobarbital Na—sedative, PO 20–30 mg tid; hypnotic, PO 50–100 mg; IV or IM 100–300 mg. Butabarbital Na (Butisol), pentobarbital Na (Nembutal), secobarbital Na (Seconal).	Preoperative sedation; emergency control of convulsions; absence seizures.	Depresses CNS, promoting drowsiness.	Cough, hiccups, restlessness, pain, hangover, and CNS and circulatory depression.	Observe for hypotension during IV administration; put up siderails on bed of older clients; observe for increased tolerance.
Chlordiazepoxide (Librium) HCl—PO 5–10 mg; IM or IV 50–100 mg.	Psychoneuroses; preoperative apprehension; chronic alcoholism; anxiety.	CNS depressant resulting in mild sedation; appetite stimulant; and anticonvulsant.	Ataxia, fatigue, blurred vision, diplopia, lethargy, nightmares, and confusion.	Ensure anxiety relief by allowing client to verbalize feelings; advise client to avoid driving and alcoholic beverages.

continued

■ **TABLE 6.3 *(Continued)*** **Common Drugs**

Drug and Dosage	Use	Action	Assessment: Side Effects	Nursing Implications
Hydroxyzine pamoate (Vistaril)—PO 25–100 mg qid.	See Chlordiazepoxide (Librium); antiemetic in postoperative conditions; adjunctive therapy.	CNS relaxant with sedative effect on limbic system and thalamus.	Drowsiness, headache, itching, dry mouth, and tremor.	Give deep IM only; potentiates action of warfarin (Coumadin), narcotics, and barbiturates.
Meprobamate (Equanil, Miltown)—PO 400 mg tid–qid.	Anxiety; stress; absence seizures.	See Hydroxyzine pamoate (Vistaril).	Voracious appetite, dryness of mouth, and ataxia.	Older clients prone to drowsiness and hypotension; observe for jaundice.
Midazolam (Versed)—IM 0.05–0.08 mg/kg; IV 0.1–0.15 mg/kg.	Preanesthesia; prediagnostic procedures; induction of general anesthesia.	Penetrates blood-brain barrier to produce sedation and amnesia.	Respiratory depression; apnea; disorientation and behavioral excitement.	Monitor ventilatory status and oxygenation; prevent injuries from CNS depression; nonirritating to vein.
Promethazine (Phenergan) 25–50 mg IV, IM, PO.	Preoperative sedation; postoperative sedation.	Antihistaminic; sedative, antiemetic, anti-motion sickness.	Drowsiness, coma, hypo/hypertension; leukopenia; photosensitivity; irregular respirations; blurred vision; urinary retention; dry mouth, nose, throat.	Administer oral med with food, milk; IM deep into large muscles, rotate sites; verify compatability with other drugs; safety concerns due to sedative effect.
Thyroid Hormone Inhibitor				
Propylthiouracil—PO 300–400 mg/day, divided initial dose; 100–150 mg/day maintenance dose; Methimazole (Tapazole) 15–60 mg/day initial dose; 5–15 mg/day maintenance dose.	Hyperthyroidism; return patient to euthyroid state; also used preoperatively.	Inhibits functional thyroid hormone synthesis by blocking reactions; responsible for iodide conversion to iodine; inhibition of T4 conversion to T3.	Blood dyscrasias; hepatotoxity; hypothyroidism.	Teach importance of compliance with med protocol; avoid iodine-rich foods (seafood, iodized salt); caution when using other drugs.
Lugol's solution—PO 2–6 drops tid 10 days prior to thyroidectomy.	To reduce size, vascularity of thyroid before thyroid surgery; emergency treatment of thyroid storm; or control of hyperthyroid symptoms after radioiodine (^{131} Iodine) therapy.	Inhibits thyroid hormone secretion, synthesis.	GI distress; stains teeth; increased respiratory secretions; rashes, acne.	Dilute in juice, give through straw; bloody diarrhea/vomiting indicates acute poisoning.
Saturated potassium iodide (SSKI)—300 mg tid–qid.	Same as Lugol's solution.	Same as Lugol's solution.	Same as Lugol's solution.	Same as Lugol's solution.
Thyroid Hormone Replacement				
Levothyroxine (Levothroid, Synthroid)—PO 0.05–0.1 mg/day oral.	Hypothyroidism.	Replacement therapy to alleviate symptoms.	Symptoms of hyperthyroidism.	Teach signs and symptoms of hyper/hypothyroidism; monitor bowel activity; teach diet to combat constipation; keep meds in tight light-proof containers; avoid foods that inhibit thyroid secretion (turnips, cabbage, carrots, peaches, peas, strawberries, spinach, radishes).
200–500 μg IV	Myxedema coma.	Emergency replacement therapy.		
Liothyronine (Cytomel)—25 μg/day to maintenance dose 25–75 μg.	Mild hypothyroidism in adults.	Replacement therapy.	See Levothyroxine.	See Levothyroxine.

Uterine Contractants				
Oxytocin (Pitocin, Syntocinon)—IM 0.3–1 mL; IV 1 mL (10 U) in 1000 mL solution.	Stimulates rhythmic contractions of uterus.	Induces labor; augments contractions; prevents or controls postpartum atony; antidiuretic effect.	Tetanic contractions, uterine rupture, cardiac arrhythmias, FHR deceleration.	*Contraindicated* if cervix is unripe, in CPD, abruptio placentae, and cardiovascular disease; monitor FHR, contractions, maternal BP, pulse, I&O, watch for signs of water intoxication with prolonged IV use; drug of choice in presence of hypertension. Never use undiluted; DC if tetanic contractions occur.
Methylergonovine maleate (Methergine)—PO 0.2 mg; IM, IV 0.2 mg (gr 1/320).	Postpartum hemorrhage, after delivery of placenta.	Stimulates stronger and longer contractions than ergonovine maleate (Ergotrate).	Nausea, vomiting, transient hypertension, dizziness, tachycardia; cramping.	Do *not* give if mother is hypertensive; do *not* use if solution is discolored; *do not use in labor.*
Ergonovine maleate (Ergotrate)—PO, IM, IV 0.2 mg (gr 1/320).	Postabortal or postpartum hemorrhage; promotes involution after delivery of placenta.	Stimulates uterine contractions for 3 or more hours.	Nausea, vomiting, occasional transient hypertension, especially if given IV; cramping.	Store in cool place; monitor maternal BP and pulse; *do not use in labor.*
Vasodilators				
Nitroglycerin—sublingual 0.15–0.3 mg p.r.n.; transdermal (patch) 2.5–15 mg/day; topical 2–3 in. q8h; IV 10–20 μg/min.	Angina pectoris; adjunctive treatment in MI, heart failure, hypertension (IV form).	Directly relaxes smooth muscle, dilating blood vessels; lowers peripheral vascular resistance; increases blood flow.	Faintness, throbbing headache, vomiting, flushing, hypotension, visual disturbances.	Instruct client to sit or lie down when taking drug, to reduce hypotensive effect; onset 1–3 min; may take 1–3 doses at 5-min intervals to relieve pain; up to 10 per day may be allowed; if headache occurs, tell client to expel tab as soon as pain relief occurs; keep drug at bedside or on person; watch expiration dates—tabs lose potency with exposure to air and humidity; alcohol ingestion soon after taking may produce shocklike syndrome from drop in BP; smoking causes vasoconstricting effect; causes burning under tongue; may crush between teeth to ↑ absorption.
Cyclandelate (Cyclospasmol)—PO 100–200 mg qid with meals and hs.	Thrombophlebitis; intermittent claudication; frostbite; Raynaud's disease; peripheral arteriosclerosis.	Acts directly on vascular smooth muscle to relax it and enhance blood flow.	Faintness, flushing, and hypotension.	Give with meals to reduce GI symptoms, or give with antacid; *contraindicated* in pregnancy, glaucoma, obliterative coronary artery disease, CVA, and clients with bleeding tendencies.
Erythrityl tetranitrate (Cardilate)—PO 10 mg tid.	Long-term treatment of angina pectoris.	Acts directly to relax smooth muscle of coronary musculature; slow onset; long duration.	Faintness, dizziness, headache, hypotension, and skin flushing.	Protect drug from light and exposure, as this reduces potency; see Nitroglycerin.

TABLE 6.4 Guide to Important Food and Drug Considerations

Key to Nursing Implications (with codes for medication administration records):

1. Take with food or milk (F-M).
2. Take on empty stomach (1 hour a.c. or 2 to 3 hours p.c.).
3. Don't drink milk or eat other dairy products (M-D).
4. Take with full glass of water (+ H_2O).
5. Take before meals (½ hour a.c.).
6. May take without regard to meals (OK c̄ meals).

A

acebutolol 6
Achromycin V 2, 3
allopurinol 1
Amcill 2
aminophylline 1
amiodarone 1
amoxicillin 6
amoxicillin/clavulanate 6
Amoxil 6
ampicillin 2
aspirin 1
Augmentin 6
Azo Gantrisin 4, 6
Azolid 1

B

Bactrim 4, 6
Benemid 4
bisacodyl 3
Butazolidin 1

C

Capoten 2
captopril 2
Carafate 2
Carprofen 1
Ceclor 6
cefaclor 6
Ceftin 6
cefuroxime axetil 6
cephalexin 6
chlorothiazide 1
cimetidine 1
Cipro 6
ciprofloxacin 6
Cleocin 4, 6
clindamycin 4, 6
cloxacillin sodium 2
Cloxapen 2
ColBENEMID 1, 4
Cordarone 1
co-trimoxazole 4, 6
Cuprimine 2

D

Declomycin 2, 3
Deltasone 1
demeclocycline 2, 3
Depen 2
Desyrel 1
dicloxacillin sodium 2
diflunisal 1
Diuril 1
Dolobid 1
Donnatal 5
Dopar 1
doxycycline hyclate 3, 6
Dulcolax 3
Dynapen 2

E

Ecotrin 3
E.E.S. 2
E-Mycin 6
enalapril 6
ERYC 2
Ery-Tab 6
Erythrocin 2
erythromycin estolate 6
erythromycin ethylsuccinate 6
erythromycin stearate 2
etretinate 1

F

famotidine 6
Feldene 1
ferrous sulfate 3
Flagyl 1
flecainide 6
fluoxetine 6
Fulvicin 1
Furadantin 1

G

Gantrisin 4, 6
glycopyrrolate 5
Grifulvin V 1
Grisactin 1
griseofulvin 1

H

Hydropres 1
Hytrin 6

I

Ilosone 6
Indocin 1
indomethacin 1
INH 2
isoniazid 2

K

Kaon 1
Kay Ciel 1
Keflex 6
ketoconazole 1
ketoprofen 1
K-Lor 1
K-Lyte 1

L

Larodopa 1
Larotid 6
levodopa 1
Lincocin 2
lincomycin 2
lisinopril 6
Lorelco 1
lovastatin 1

M

Macrodantin 1
Marax 1
methysergide maleate 1
metronidazole 1
Mevacor 1
mexiletine 1
Mexitil 1
Minocin 3, 6
Minocyline 3, 6

N

nafcillin 2
nitrofurantoin 1
nitrofurantoin macrocrystals 1
Nizoral 1
norfloxacin 2, 4
Noroxin 2, 4

O

Omnipen 2
Orazinc 3
Orudis 1
oxacillin sodium 2
oxytetracycline 2, 3

P

penicillamine 2
penicillin G (oral) 2
penicillin V 6
Pen-Vee K 6
Pepcid 6
phenylbutazone 1
pindolol 6
piroxicam 1
Polycillin 2
potassium chloride 1
prednisone 1
Prinivil 6
Pro-Banthine 5
probenecid 4
probucol 1
procainamide 6
Pronestyl 6
propantheline bromide 5
Prostaphlin 2
Prozac 6

R

ranitidine 6
Raudixin 1
rauwolfia serpentina 1
Regroton 1
reserpine 1
Rifadin 2
rifampin 2
Rimactane 2
rimadyl 1
Robinul 5

S

Sansert 1
Sectral 6
Septra 4, 6
Ser-Ap-Es 1
Serpasil 1
Sinemet 1
Slow-K 1
Somophyllin 1
sucralfate 2
sulfisoxazole 4, 6
Sumycin 2, 3

T

Tagamet 1
Tambocor 6
Tedral 1
Tegison 1
terazosin 6
Terramycin 2, 3
tetracycline HCl 2, 3
Theobid 6
Theo-Dur 6

U

Unipen 2

V

Vasotec 6
V-Cillin K 6
Vibramycin 3, 6
Visken 6

Z

Zantac 6
Zestril 6
zinc sulfate 3
Zyloprim 1

Source: McGavin K: 10 Golden Rules for Administering Drugs Safely, *Nursing 88, 18* (8).

PHARMACOLOGY

■ QUESTIONS

Select the one best answer for each question, and fill in the answer circle beside the answer number.

1. A client has meperidine 75 mg every 3–4 hours p.r.n. ordered for postoperative pain. Prior to administering this narcotic, the nurse should:
○ 1. Position in a semi-Fowler's position to minimize respiratory effects. **AS**
○ 2. Assess the type, location, and intensity of discomfort. **3**
○ 3. Evaluate whether the pain is real. **PhI**
○ 4. Try other measures to relieve discomfort, such as position change.

2. Prostigmin 0.5 mg subcutaneously stat is ordered by a client's physician to relieve urinary retention. The nurse knows that this drug is classified as:
○ 1. A cholinergic. **PL**
○ 2. An anticholinesterase. **8**
○ 3. An anticholinergic. **PhI**
○ 4. A beta blocker.

3. You explain to a client that although salicylates are given to relieve pain in rheumatoid arthritis, they also function as an:
○ 1. Analgesic. **IMP**
○ 2. Antiinflammatory. **3**
○ 3. Anticholinergic. **PhI**
○ 4. Antiadrenergic.

4. Drug therapy goals for a client included strengthening cardiac contraction and increasing glomerular filtration rate. Which of the following medications would you prepare to accomplish both goals?
○ 1. Epinephrine. **PL**
○ 2. Digoxin. **6**
○ 3. Lasix. **PhI**
○ 4. Hydralazine.

5. Which of the following outcomes is the best indicator that the drug has been effective?
○ 1. Increased systolic and diastolic pressures. **EV**
○ 2. Unlabored respirations and increased urinary output. **6**
○ 3. Decreased pulse rate and increased urinary output. **PhI**
○ 4. Increased blood pressure and decreased pulse rate.

6. Your client teaching includes the side effects of theophylline administration, which are:
○ 1. Tachycardia and palpitations. **IMP**
○ 2. Anorexia, nausea, and gastritis. **6**
○ 3. Restlessness and tremors. **PhI**
○ 4. Headache and nausea.

7. Based on the peak action of furosemide (Lasix) PO, you will evaluate the drug's effects in:
○ 1. 30–60 minutes. **EV**
○ 2. 1–2 hours. **8**
○ 3. 3–4 hours. **PhI**
○ 4. 6–8 hours.

8. You administer Kayexalate knowing that the drug reduces hyperkalemia by:
○ 1. Exchanging sodium ions for potassium ions in the GI tract, thereby increasing potassium excretion in the feces. **IMP 8 PhI**
○ 2. Inhibiting potassium absorption sites in the GI tract.
○ 3. Promoting diarrhea, thereby decreasing potassium absorption from the gut.
○ 4. Altering the effects of aldosterone in the kidney tubules.

9. The nurse knows that the best time to give oral iron preparations is:
○ 1. With meals, to decrease gastric upset. **PL**
○ 2. One hour before eating, to enhance absorption. **4 PhI**
○ 3. One hour after eating, to slow absorption.
○ 4. At bedtime.

10. The client is instructed to report the following side effect of neomycin administration:
○ 1. Deafness. **EV**
○ 2. Nausea. **2**
○ 3. Diarrhea. **PhI**
○ 4. Anaphylaxis.

11. Before administering morphine sulfate, the nurse should check:
○ 1. Apical and radial pulse. **AS**
○ 2. Respiratory rate. **6**
○ 3. Urinary output. **PhI**
○ 4. Skin color and turgor.

12. The nurse administers spironolactone (Aldactone) knowing that it is classified as:
○ 1. An aldosterone antagonist. **IMP**
○ 2. A carbonic anhydrase inhibitor. **6**
○ 3. A thiazide. **PhI**
○ 4. An osmotic diuretic.

13. Which of the following supplements would the nurse not ordinarily administer to the client receiving spironolactone?
○ 1. Vitamin B_6. **PL**
○ 2. Potassium chloride. **4**
○ 3. Ascorbic acid. **PhI**
○ 4. Calcium carbonate.

14. The primary objective in giving prednisone along with aspirin for acute rheumatoid arthritis is:
○ 1. To inhibit the autoimmune factors associated with rheumatoid arthritis. **AN 3**
○ 2. To prevent further joint destruction. **PhI**
○ 3. To decrease inflammation and suppress symptomatology.
○ 4. To increase glucose levels for tissue repair.

15. The nurse would recognize prednisone toxicity if which of the following occurred?
○ 1. Tinnitus. **EV**
○ 2. Exfoliative dermatitis. **8**
○ 3. Glucosuria. **PhI**
○ 4. Nausea and vomiting.

PHARMACOLOGY

Key to codes following questions Nursing process: **AS**, Assessment; **AN**, Analysis; **PL**, Plan; **IMP**, Implementation; **EV**, Evaluation. Category of human function: **1**, Protective; **2**, Sensory-perceptual; **3**, Comfort, Rest, Activity, and Mobility; **4**, Nutrition; **5**, Growth and Development; **6**, Fluid-Gas Transport; **7**, Psycho-Social-Cultural; **8**, Elimination. Client need: **SECE**, Safe, Effective Care Environment; **PhI**, Physiological Integrity; **PsI**, Psychosocial Integrity; **HPM**, Health Promotion/Maintenance. See frontmatter for full explanation.

16. Probanthine bromide is given to clients with cholelithiasis and cholecystitis because it:
- ○ 1. Reduces gastric secretions and intestinal hypermobility. **IMP 4 PhI**
- ○ 2. Decreases bile secretion by the liver and gallbladder.
- ○ 3. Slows the emptying of the stomach, thereby reducing chyme in the duodenum.
- ○ 4. Inhibits contraction of the gallbladder and the bile duct.

17. The nurse would most likely give papaverine HCl for relief of gallbladder pain rather than morphine SO_4 because:
- ○ 1. Morphine depresses gallbladder contractions, thereby decreasing bile secretions. **EV 3 PhI**
- ○ 2. Opiates tend to mask symptoms in clients with acute abdomens.
- ○ 3. Morphine tends to increase contractions of the sphincter of Oddi, thereby increasing intraductal pressures.
- ○ 4. Morphine relaxes smooth muscles, thereby increasing bile production.

18. The nurse can anticipate side effects of hydrochlorothiazide because it is classified as:
- ○ 1. An aldosterone inhibitor. **EV 8 PhI**
- ○ 2. A carbonic anhydrase inhibitor.
- ○ 3. A potassium-sparing drug.
- ○ 4. A potassium-wasting drug.

PHARMACOLOGY

19. The nurse knows that hydrochlorothiazide exerts its primary effect on:
- ○ 1. The proximal and distal tubules of the kidney. **AN 8 PhI**
- ○ 2. The distal convoluted tubule of the kidney only.
- ○ 3. The ascending loop of Henle and the distal tubule of the kidney.
- ○ 4. The descending loop of Henle and the proximal tubule of the kidney.

20. Assessment for the side effects of hydrochlorothiazide includes signs of:
- ○ 1. Hypernatremia. **AS 8 PhI**
- ○ 2. Hyperkalemia.
- ○ 3. Hypochloremia.
- ○ 4. Hypouricemia.

21. Two-year-old Kelly (diagnosis: meningitis) is to be sedated with phenobarbital 18 mg PO q6h. The label reads "20 mg per 5 cc." How much phenobarbital should the nurse administer to Kelly?
- ○ 1. 4 cc. **IMP 2 SECE**
- ○ 2. 4.3 cc.
- ○ 3. 4.5 cc.
- ○ 4. 4.8 cc.

22. Kelly's CSF culture is positive for *Hemophilus influenzae* meningitis. To protect other members of Kelly's family who have been exposed to meningitis, the nurse should explain that they may be given:
- ○ 1. Augmentin. **IMP 1 HPM**
- ○ 2. Sulfisoxazole.
- ○ 3. Rifampin.
- ○ 4. Immune serum globulin.

23. The nurse is to administer pancreatin to Shariff Black, a five-year-old with cystic fibrosis. To evaluate the effect of this medication, the nurse should know that the primary purpose of this medication is to increase the absorption of:
- ○ 1. Glucose. **AN 4 SECE**
- ○ 2. Vitamin C.
- ○ 3. Sodium chloride.
- ○ 4. Fats.

24. The nurse about to administer medication to 5-year-old Shariff notes that the child has no ID bracelet. The best way for the nurse to identify Shariff would be to ask:
- ○ 1. The child, "Is your name Shariff?" **IMP 1 SECE**
- ○ 2. The adult visiting, "Her name is Shariff?"
- ○ 3. The other children in the room what her name is.
- ○ 4. Another staff nurse to identify her.

25. Elixir of Lanoxin is available with 0.05 mg of the drug in 1 cc of solution. How much of this elixir should the nurse administer if the physician's order reads "0.125 mg PO bid."
- ○ 1. 2 cc. **IMP 6 SECE**
- ○ 2. 2.25 cc.
- ○ 3. 2.5 cc.
- ○ 4. 2.75 cc.

26. In teaching a parent how to administer cortisporin eye drops to an infant, the nurse would be most correct in advising the parent to place the drops:
- ○ 1. Directly onto the infant's sclera. **IMP 2 HPM**
- ○ 2. In the inner canthus of the infant's eye.
- ○ 3. In the outer canthus of the infant's eye.
- ○ 4. In the middle of the lower conjunctival sac of the infant's eye.

27. Two-year-old Paco Ruiz has iron deficiency anemia. The doctor orders Fer-in-Sol 0.6 cc PO tid. For maximum absorption, the nurse plans to administer this medication:
- ○ 1. Between meals. **PL 4 SECE**
- ○ 2. Before meals.
- ○ 3. During meals.
- ○ 4. After meals.

28. Two weeks after starting the oral iron supplement, Paco's mother tells the nurse that the child's stools are black in color. The nurse should tell her:
- ○ 1. "This is a normal side effect and means the medication is working." **EV 8 SECE**
- ○ 2. "I will notify the doctor, who will probably decrease the dosage slightly."
- ○ 3. "I will need a specimen to check the stool for possible bleeding."
- ○ 4. "You sound quite concerned. Would you like to talk about this further?"

Mona Ames, age 18, is seen in clinic for her first prenatal visit at 12 weeks gestation. She complains of severe pruritus, dysuria, and thick, creamy vaginal discharge for the past 3 days. Microscopic analysis establishes a diagnosis of monilial vaginitis.

29. Which of the following assessment factors from Mona's history is considered predisposing to the development of yeast vaginitis?
- ○ 1. Pregnancy. **AS 5 PhI**
- ○ 2. Late adolescence.
- ○ 3. High-carbohydrate diet.
- ○ 4. Sickle cell anemia.

30. Health teaching for Mona should be planned and implemented to ensure her consistent and appropriate use of the prescribed medication. Which of the following medications is effective in the treatment of monilial (yeast) vaginitis?

○ 1. Metronidazole (Flagyl) oral tablets. **IMP**
○ 2. Nystatin (Mycostatin) vaginal suppositories. **1**
○ 3. Local applications of podophyllin. **PhI**
○ 4. Antibiotic (bacitracin) ointment.

31. Reviewing the results of Mona's routine prenatal lab work, the nurse notes that her VDRL is positive. To protect the fetus from congenital syphilis, Mona must receive treatment before weeks 18–20. History suggests possible allergy to penicillin. Which of the following drugs would be ordered to treat venereal disease in the penicillin-allergic client?
○ 1. Streptomycin. **PL**
○ 2. Sulfasoxizole (Gantrisin). **1**
○ 3. Chloramphenicol (Chloromycetin). **PhI**
○ 4. Erythromycin.

32. Health teaching regarding uncomfortable signs and symptoms of side effects of oral antibiotic therapy includes:
○ 1. Tinnitus (ringing in the ears). **IMP**
○ 2. Nausea, vomiting, and abdominal pain. **1**
○ 3. Nausea and glossitis. **PhI**
○ 4. Nausea, diarrhea, and vaginal yeast infections.

Paula Paris has been admitted at 32 weeks gestation with threatened premature labor. She exhibits intermittent, irregular, mild to moderate contractions; cervical dilatation is 1–2 cm.

33. Which of the following medications is ordered most commonly to attempt to inhibit premature labor?
○ 1. Magnesium sulfate. **PL**
○ 2. Betamethasone. **5**
○ 3. Ritodrine (Yutopar) **PhI**
○ 4. Bromocryptine mesolate (Parlodel).

34. In evaluating Paula's response to betamimetic therapy used to inhibit premature labor, for which of the following signs of side effects must the nurse be alert?
○ 1. Maternal hypertension. **EV**
○ 2. Fetal bradycardia. **5**
○ 3. Maternal and fetal tachycardia. **PhI**
○ 4. Uterine hypertonia.

35. When a parturient is given a paracervical block, the nurse can expect:
○ 1. Low forceps delivery. **AN**
○ 2. Depression of contractions, maternal hypotension, fetal bradycardia, postnatal uterine atony. **5** **PhI**
○ 3. Depression of contractions and fetal bradycardia.
○ 4. Loss of bearing-down reflex, low forceps delivery.

36. When a parturient is given an epidural (or caudal) anesthesia, the nurse could expect:
○ 1. Maternal hypotension, low forceps delivery, need to remain flat in bed for some hours after delivery. **AN** **5** **PhI**
○ 2. Loss of bearing-down reflex, depression of contractions, maternal hypotension, fetal bradycardia, low forceps delivery.
○ 3. Loss of bearing-down reflex, depression of contractions, maternal hypotension, fetal bradycardia, low forceps delivery, postnatal bladder atony, postnatal uterine atony.
○ 4. Depression of contractions, maternal hypotension.

37. When a parturient is given a saddle block (low spinal) anesthesia, the nurse can expect:
○ 1. Loss of bearing-down reflex, maternal hypotension, low forceps delivery, need to remain flat in bed for some hours after delivery. **AN** **1** **PhI**
○ 2. Fetal bradycardia, low forceps delivery, postnatal uterine atony, need to remain flat in bed for some hours after delivery.
○ 3. Loss of bearing-down reflex, low forceps delivery, postnatal bladder atony, postnatal uterine atony.
○ 4. Loss of bearing-down reflex, maternal hypotension, low forceps delivery, need to remain flat in bed for some hours after delivery, fetal bradycardia, postnatal uterine atony, postnatal bladder atony.

38. A client is receiving tetracycline preoperatively in preparation for bowel surgery. Which common side effect should the nurse instruct the patient to expect with tetracycline?
○ 1. Urticaria. **IMP**
○ 2. Urinary retention. **1**
○ 3. Jaundice. **PhI**
○ 4. Deafness.

39. The following activities have been planned for Ms. Carson, a client who is mute and autistic. In which of the following activities will it be important for the nursing staff to take precautionary measures for a common side effect of Thorazine (chlorpromazine), which has been prescribed for this client?
○ 1. Shopping in an enclosed mall after lunch. **PL**
○ 2. Attending the symphony on Wednesday evening. **3** **PhI**
○ 3. A day at the beach, if the weather permits.
○ 4. A morning at the art museum.

40. Some clients who are on phenothiazines are also given Cogentin. The nurse administers this medication in order to:
○ 1. Prevent skin reactions. **PL**
○ 2. Increase the effectiveness of the phenothiazines. **7** **PhI**
○ 3. Decrease motor restlessness.
○ 4. Reduce extrapyramidal side effects.

41. A client has been on Prolixin IM for 3 years now. He has recently complained of frequent sore throats and malaise. What potentially serious side effect might these symptoms indicate to the nurse?
○ 1. Agranulocytosis. **AN**
○ 2. Akathisia. **7**
○ 3. Dystonia. **PhI**
○ 4. Dyskinesia.

42. When nialamide (Niamid) or isocarboxazid (Marplan) are administered, what must the nurse know about the effects of these drugs?
○ 1. They lower the threshold for seizures. **EV**
○ 2. They potentiate the effects of many other drugs and common foods. **7** **PhI**
○ 3. They decrease muscular contractions.
○ 4. They commonly cause obstructive jaundice.

43. Lithium salts are frequently used to treat manic disorders. What side effect is the nurse *least* likely to observe?
○ 1. Slurred speech. **EV**
○ 2. Twitching and athetotic movements. **7**
○ 3. Motor weakness. **PhI**
○ 4. Tardive dyskinesia.

44. Mike Wu, 9 months old, has been diagnosed with Hirschsprung's disease. At this time, he is admitted to the hospi-

tal for a temporary colostomy; preoperatively, the doctor orders Kanamycin. The nurse caring for Mike should know that Kanamycin is being given to:
- ○ 1. Increase peristalsis. **AN**
- ○ 2. Decrease amount of GI secretions. **1**
- ○ 3. Promote passage of stool and flatus. **SECE**
- ○ 4. Decrease number of intestinal flora.

45. Amy Sutter, age 22 months, is admitted to the pediatrics unit for observation following accidental ingestion of 17 children's Tylenol caplets. In the first 2–3 days following Amy's admission, it is essential that the nurse plan to observe her closely for signs of:
- ○ 1. Hepatic failure. **PL**
- ○ 2. Renal failure. **1**
- ○ 3. Hyperthermia. **PhI**
- ○ 4. Hemorrhage.

46. Amy's nurse should also have on hand the antidote to acetaminophen, which is:
- ○ 1. Mucomyst. **IMP**
- ○ 2. Potassium chloride. **1**
- ○ 3. Aspirin. **SECE/PhI**
- ○ 4. Heparin.

47. Bruce Minor, 9 years old, has an acute asthmatic attack. The doctor orders aminophylline 100 mg via IV. The nurse should know that the main reason the doctor ordered aminophylline for Bruce is because it is a(n):
- ○ 1. Bronchodilator. **AN**
- ○ 2. Anticholinergic. **6**
- ○ 3. Expectorant. **SECE/PhI**
- ○ 4. Mucolytic agent.

48. The nurse is to administer 100 mg of aminophylline IV to Bruce. The ampule contains 500 mg (gr 7½) of aminophylline in 10 cc of solution. How much solution should the nurse withdraw from the ampule?
- ○ 1. 2 cc. **IMP**
- ○ 2. 4 cc. **6**
- ○ 3. 6 cc. **SECE**
- ○ 4. 8 cc.

49. While Bruce's aminophylline is infusing, the nurse should plan to closely monitor his:
- ○ 1. Level of consciousness. **PL**
- ○ 2. Blood pressure. **6**
- ○ 3. Cardiac rhythm. **SECE**
- ○ 4. Temperature.

50. The nurse should know that, to prevent future asthmatic attacks, Bruce will most likely receive:
- ○ 1. Theophylline. **AN**
- ○ 2. Cromolyn sodium. **6**
- ○ 3. Prednisone. **SECE**
- ○ 4. Dipenhydramine.

51. Franco Jimenez, 15 years old, is admitted to the hospital with a diagnosis of infectious hepatitis (type A). To protect other members of Franco's family who have been exposed to infectious hepatitis, the nurse should explain that they may be given:
- ○ 1. Augmentin. **IMP**
- ○ 2. Sulfisoxazole. **1**
- ○ 3. Rifampin. **HPM**
- ○ 4. Immune serum globulin.

52. Yu Chang, 17 months old, has retropharyngeal abscess. She is to receive ampicillin four times a day; she weighs 15 kg (33 lb). The nurse's reference indicates that the correct dosage is 75 mg/kg/day. Which dose should the nurse give to Yu at 10 A.M.?
- ○ 1. 11 mg. **IMP**
- ○ 2. 28 mg. **1**
- ○ 3. 280 mg. **SECE**
- ○ 4. 1125 mg.

53. Four-year-old Marco Dane is scheduled for repair of left undescended testicle. To administer a nembutal suppository preoperatively to Marco, in which position should the nurse place him?
- ○ 1. Prone with legs abducted. **IMP**
- ○ 2. Sitting on a potty seat. **1**
- ○ 3. Supine with foot of bed elevated. **SECE**
- ○ 4. Side lying with upper leg flexed.

54. Marco appears very anxious and frightened prior to receiving his medication. Which statement by the nurse would be most appropriate in helping Marco take his medication?
- ○ 1. "Be a big boy! Everyone's waiting for you." **IMP**
- ○ 2. "You look so scared, Marco. Want to know a secret? This won't hurt a bit!" **5** **PsI**
- ○ 3. "Lie still now and I'll let you have one of your presents before you even have your operation."
- ○ 4. "Take a nice, big, deep breath and then let me hear you count to five."

55. Ten-year-old Laurel John is scheduled for an appendectomy. In preparing her preop injections, which size needle should the nurse select to administer Laurel's IM?
- ○ 1. 25 G, 5/8 in. **IMP**
- ○ 2. 22 G, 1 in. **1**
- ○ 3. 20 G, 1½ in. **SECE**
- ○ 4. 18 G, 1½ in.

■ ANSWERS/RATIONALE

1. (2) Prior to administering any narcotic, the nurse should assess the type, location, and intensity of pain, as well as factors that seem to precipitate or relieve it. Meperidine, like morphine, has hypotensive and respiratory depressant effects. Positioning in anticipation of respiratory changes is not indicated (No. 1). Pain and discomfort are subjective symptoms that are always real to the client (No. 3). Based on the information gained in No. 2, it is then possible to decide whether the client needs supportive measures (such as back rub or position change as in No. 4), the bedpan, and/or the administration of a narcotic.

2. (2) Prostigmin is an anticholinesterase. It enhances bladder tone and contraction, enabling complete emptying of the bladder. It is also used in the treatment of myasthenia gravis. Urecholine is an example of a cholinergic drug (No. 1), also used to treat postoperative urinary retention. Atropine is an example of an anticholinergic drug (No. 3), which would act to inhibit initiation of urination. Beta blockers (No. 4) such as propranolol do not affect the bladder.

3. (2) Salicylates, particularly acetylsalicylic acid (aspirin), are given in divided doses after each meal and at bedtime for their analgesic (reduced pain), antiinflammatory (reduced swelling), and antipyretic (reduced fever) effects. No. 1 is incorrect because relief of pain was already described in the question. Nos. 3 and 4 are incorrect because salicylates neither inhibit nor stimulate the autonomic nervous system synapses.

4. (2) Digoxin increases the force and velocity of cardiac contraction and slows the heart rate by delaying conduction through the atrioventricular node. The hemodynamic effects of its action include increased cardiac output, decreased right atrial and venous pressures, decreased left ventricular filling pressure, and increased excretion of sodium and water. Epinephrine (No. 1) increases the force of cardiac contractions but also increases heart rate, which in this case would increase cardiac embarrassment. Furosemide (Lasix) (No. 3) is a rapidly acting diuretic that enhances excretion of sodium and water. However, although its use is indicated to reduce fluid volume during the acute phase of pulmonary edema, it has no known direct effects on the cardiac musculature. Hydralazine (No. 4) is a peripheral vasodilator used in hypertensive therapy. It is not indicated in this situation.

5. (3) The best indicator that digoxin has been effective in strengthening cardiac contraction and increasing glomerular filtration is a decrease in heart rate (vagal effect) and increased urinary output. As a result of these drug effects, cardiac output is improved, raising blood pressure and decreasing pulmonary congestion. Nos. 1, 2, and 4 are only partially correct.

6. (2) Theophylline relaxes bronchial smooth muscles, which helps to relieve the wheezing and coughing associated with bronchospasm. Side effects are rare, but the earliest signs of overdose are usually anorexia, nausea, and vomiting. Tachycardia (No. 1), restlessness and tremors (No. 3), headache (No. 4), and insomnia are side effects associated with catecholamine bronchodilators, such as ephedrine and isoproterenol.

7. (2) Furosemide is a rapidly acting diuretic with a peak action in 1–2 hours and a duration of 6–8 hours.

8. (1) Kayexalate (sodium polystyrene sulfonate) is a cation-exchange resin. As it passes along the intestine or is retained in the colon after enema administration, sodium ions are partially released and replaced by potassium ions, allowing for fecal excretion of potassium ions. Kayexalate is extremely unpalatable and may be administered in syrup, chilled, or mixed in the diet, and if necessary, administered directly into the stomach per nasogastric tube. Side effects of Kayexalate administration include anorexia, nausea, vomiting constipation, hypokalemia, hypocalcemia, and sodium retention. Nos. 2, 3, and 4 are not actions of Kayexalate.

9. (1) Ideally, oral iron preparations should be taken on an empty stomach (No. 2). However, they tend to irritate the gastric mucosa, so they should be administered with or immediately after meals to ensure client compliance. Thus Nos. 2, 3, and 4 are not the best answers. Clients may complain of constipation or loose stools. Stools will change color (dark green to black). Ferrous sulfate is apt to deposit on teeth and gums, so frequent oral hygiene is necessary, and therapy will need to continue even after hemoglobin levels return to normal, in order to ensure adequate iron stores in the body.

10. (1) Toxic doses of neomycin may result in eighth cranial nerve damage much like that produced by streptomycin. Kidney damage may also occur, extending from milk albuminuria to elevation in blood urea nitrogen. Nausea (No. 2) is common with ingestion of antibiotics, though not specific to neomycin. Erythromycin most commonly causes nausea, vomiting, and diarrhea (No. 3). Anaphylactic reactions (No. 4) are associated most commonly with penicillin administration.

11. (2) Morphine strongly depresses the medullary respiratory centers. Therefore, before administering the narcotic, the nurse should assess the client's respiratory rate and depth to prevent severe respiratory depression. Nos. 1, 3, and 4 are not affected by morphine.

12. (1) Spironolactone (Aldactone) is an aldosterone inhibitor, inhibiting the effects of hyperaldosteronemia, which is common in cirrhosis. This drug safely increases sodium and water excretion but does not cause concomitant losses of potassium as do other diuretics. For this reason, potassium supplements are not generally given to the client. An example of a carbonic anhydrase inhibitor (No. 2) is Diamox; of a thiazide (No. 3) is Diuril or Hydrodiuril; and of an osmotic diuretic (No. 4) is mannitol.

13. (2) Potassium chloride—see preceding rationale. Spironolactone would not contraindicate the administration of vitamin B_6 (No. 1), ascorbic acid (No. 3), or calcium gluconate (No. 4).

14. (3) The primary objective in giving corticosteroids is to lessen the symptoms of the disease process. Most clients initially respond well to these drugs; however, as the disease progresses, higher and higher doses are required to relieve symptoms. Nos. 1 and 2 are incorrect because corticosteroids have no curative effects, only palliative. Many of the side effects of corticosteroid administration are due to the effects of these drugs on glucose metabolism (No. 4), such as Cushing's-like syndrome.

15. (3) Side effects of prednisone therapy mimic the manifestations of Cushing's syndrome (moon facies, abnormal fat deposits, purple striae, hyperglycemia with glucosuria, hypertension, obesity, and emotional disturbances). Side effects of other drugs utilized in the management of rheumatoid arthritis include tinnitus (No. 1), nausea, vomiting (No. 4), headaches, and vertigo with indomethacin (Indocin) administration, and dermatitis ranging from erythema to exfoliative dermatitis (No. 2) with gold salts therapy.

16. (4) Although the primary use of probantheline bromide in many clinical situations involving the gastrointestinal tract is to reduce gastric secretions and intestinal hypermobility, it is used in gallbladder disease because of its antispasmodic effects on the gallbladder and bile duct. No. 1 is therefore correct, but not the best choice. Nos. 2 and 3 are incorrect because probantheline bromide does not reduce bile secretions, and its calming effect on gastric motility does not reduce the amount of chyme entering the duodenum.

17. (3) Morphine sulfate causes spasms of the sphincter of Oddi, thereby increasing intraductal pressures and abdominal pain. Papaverine and meperidine, both synthetic opiates, as well as nitroglycerin may be administered to relieve pain associated with gallbladder disease. No. 1 is incorrect because the effect of morphine is to increase spasms in the gallbladder. No. 2, through correct, is not the *best* answer. Opiates are withheld when a client has an acute abdomen and the diagnosis is unknown or tentative. In this case, the client has an established history of gallbladder disease and rather specific symptomatology. No. 4 is incorrect, in that, although morphine does relax vascular smooth muscle, this effect does not increase bile synthesis in the liver.

18. (4) Hydrochlorothiazide is a thiazide diuretic that promotes the excretion of water, sodium, and chloride by inhibiting the reabsorption of sodium ions in the distal ascending limb of the loop of Henle and in the distal convoluted tubule of the nephron. Natriuresis promotes the secondary loss of potassium, so this drug is classified as potassium-wasting. Spironclactone is an example of an aldosterone inhibitor and is a potassium-sparing diuretic (Nos. 1 and 3). Diamox is the most frequently employed carbonic anhydrase inhibitor (No. 2).

19. (3) See answer 18 for the site of hydrochlorothiazide action in the kidney. No. 1 describes the effect of the carbonic anhydrase inhibitors, e.g., Diamox. No. 2 would be the effect of the potassium-sparing diuretics such as Aldactone. Finally, No. 4 is the site for the osmotic diuretics, e.g., mannitol, urea.

20. (3) Thiazide diuretics promote the excretion of sodium, chloride, bicarbonate, and potassium. However, chloride excretion tends to be proportionately greater than bicarbonate excretion, so therapy may result in hypochloremic alkalosis. Hyponatremia, not hypernatremia (No. 1) occurs. Hypokalemia, not hyperkalemia (No. 2), may develop, especially with brisk diuresis. Supplemental KCl therapy and/or increased dietary intake of potassium is indicated with thiazide therapy. No. 4 is incorrect because it says hypouricemia and hyperuricemia results, which may precipitate frank gout.

21. (3) The formula for finding the correct answer is:

dose desired/dose on hand = x/amount on hand.

$$18/20 = x/5$$
$$20x = 18(5)$$
$$x = \frac{18(5)}{20}$$
$$x = 4.5 \text{ cc}$$

22. (3) Rifampin is the drug of choice for the prophylactic treatment of *Hemophilus influenzae* meningitis. The usual dose is 20 mg/kg/day in a single dose for four days. Augmentin (No. 1), sulfisoxazole (No. 2), and immune serum globulin (No. 3) are not the drugs of choice to prevent *Hemophilus influenzae* meningitis.

23. (4) Pancreatin (Viokase) is an exocrine pancreatic supplement used as a digestive aid in cystic fibrosis; its primary use is to promote the absorption of fats. Pancreatin has no effect on the absorption of glucose (No. 1), vitamin C (No. 2), or sodium chloride (No. 3).

24. (4) The only acceptable way to identify a 5-year-old client is to have a parent or another staff member identify the client. No. 1 is incorrect because most 5-year-old children, under the age of reason, cannot legally be held accountable for self-identification. No. 2 is incorrect unless the nurse is sure this adult is Shariff's parent. Also, it would be better to ask, "What is the child's name?" No. 3 is also incorrect; children cannot legally be held accountable for identifying other children.

25. (3) The correct answer is found using the following formula:

dose desired/dose on hand = x/amount on hand.

$$0.125/0.05 = x/1$$
$$0.05x = 0.125(1)$$
$$x = \frac{0.125(1)}{0.05}$$
$$x = 2.5 \text{ cc}$$

26. (4) The recommended procedure for administering eye drops to any client calls for the drops to be placed in the middle of the lower conjunctival sac. Placing drops directly onto the sclera (No. 1) is irritating and less effective. Placing drops in the inner canthus of the eye (No. 2) may lead to systemic effects from absorption via tear ducts. Placing drops in the outer canthus of the eye (No. 3) results in loss of medication and may also cause infection.

27. (1) Maximum absorption of Fer-in-Sol occurs between meals, when hydrochloric acid is freely available in the stomach. When given before meals (No. 2), it may cause GI upset, which will interfere with eating. When given during meals (No. 3) or after meals (No. 4), there is slowed absorption of the drug; however, GI upset is minimized.

28. (1) When oral iron preparations are given correctly, the stools normally turn dark green/black in color. Parents of children receiving this medication should be advised that this side effect indicates the medication is being absorbed and is working well. Nos. 2, 3, and 4 would only increase the parent's anxiety and lead them to believe that the stool color was abnormal.

29. (1) Normal pregnancy alters vaginal pH and favors the growth of yeast organisms *(monilia)*. No. 2 is wrong because age is not a factor in the development of yeast vaginitis. No. 3 is wrong because ingestion of large amounts of carbohydrates does not alter vaginal pH. No. 4 is wrong because sickle cell anemia is not a predisposing factor in yeast vaginitis.

30. (2) Nystatin is the drug of choice for treatment of vaginal infections caused by *Candida albicans*. No. 1 is wrong because metronidazole is used in treatment of trichomonal vaginitis. No. 3 is wrong because podophyllin is used in treating venereal warts. No. 4 is wrong because bacitracin ointment is used in treating skin infections.

31. (4) Erythromycin or tetracycline is commonly used in treating penicillin-allergic clients with venereal disease. No. 1 is wrong because streptomycin is used in treating tuberculosis. No. 2 is wrong because Gantrisin is most commonly used to treat urinary tract infections. Further, its use is contraindicated in pregnancy. No. 3 is wrong because Chloromycetin is used in treating *salmonella* infections and is also contraindicated during pregnancy.

32. (4) Prolonged, heavy doses of oral antibiotics are irritating to the GI tract and result in nausea and diarrhea; yeast infections are common sequelae of antibiotic therapy. No. 1 is wrong; tinnitus is a symptom of streptomycin toxicity. No. 2 is wrong because abdominal pain is more commonly associated with Gantrisin therapy. No. 3 is wrong because glossitis and stomatitis are associated with Chloromycetin therapy.

33. (3) Ritodrine is the drug of choice when attempting to inhibit labor. No. 1 is wrong because magnesium sulfate is used most commonly in treating preeclampsia/eclampsia. No. 2 is wrong because betamethasone is used to stimulate production of fetal pulmonary surfactant. No. 4 is wrong because Parlodel is used to inhibit lactation in nonbreastfeeding mothers.

34. (3) Persistent maternal tachycardia (over 140 bpm) is a sign of impending pulmonary edema in clients receiving betamimetic drugs; fetal tachycardia is a common result of ritodrine therapy. No. 1 is wrong because ritodrine commonly results in maternal hypotension. No. 2 is wrong because the common fetal reaction to betamimetics is tachycardia. No. 4 is wrong because ritodrine is given to reduce uterine hyperirritability and threatened premature labor.

35. (3) Depression of contractions and fetal bradycardia are expected effects of paracervical block. No. 1 is incorrect because the bearing-down reflex is not affected by this anesthesia. No. 2 is incorrect because maternal blood pressure and postnatal uterine contractility are not affected by paracervical block. No. 4 is incorrect because the bearing-down reflex is not affected, and therefore forceps delivery is usually not needed.

36. (3) The medication never mixes with cerebral spinal fluid, and therefore there is no need for the woman to lie flat for several hours after receiving this form of anesthesia (No. 1). Nos. 2 and 4 are incorrect because their lists are incomplete.

37. (4) All of the listed effects are to be expected following spinal anesthesia: loss of bearing-down reflex, depression of contractions, maternal hypotension, fetal bradycardia, low forceps delivery, postnatal bladder atony, need to remain flat in bed for some hours after delivery, and postnatal uterine atony. Nos. 1, 2, and 3 are incorrect because their lists are incomplete.

38. (1) Hypersensitivity reactions (urticaria and hives) are common drug reactions. Photosensitization (exaggerated sunburn) in certain hypersensitive persons may also occur with exposure to direct or artificial sunlight during tetracycline use. Urinary retention (No. 2) is a side effect of anticholinergic and antihistamine drugs. Jaundice (No. 3) from drug toxicity is more common with isoniazid (INH), acetaminophen, phenothiazines (Thorazine), sulfonamides, and antidiabetic drugs (e.g., Orinase). Hepatotoxicity may occur with tetracycline, but it is less common. No. 4, deafness (ototoxicity), is a major side effect of the aminoglycoside antibiotics (e.g., gentamycin, neomycin, streptomycin, tobramycin) and diuretics, such as furosemide and ethacrynic acid.

39. (3) The client needs to be protected against photosensitivity and dermatitis when exposed to the sun; a sunscreen preparation should be applied to exposed parts of the skin, and the client should wear long sleeves and cover-up clothing. Nos. 1, 2, and 4 refer to *indoor* activities, where there is no danger of sunburn.

40. (4) This is the best choice as it *encompasses* No. 3. Nos. 1 and 2 are definitely incorrect.

41. (1) Blood dyscrasias often are overlooked when first symptoms of possible adverse drug effects appear in the form of a minor cold. Nos. 2, 3, and 4 refer to extrapyramidal tract symptoms that are *not* life-threatening.

42. (2) Hypertensive crisis can be precipitated by combining this drug with common cold medications and foods high in tyramine or pressor amines (yogurt, Chianti wine, cheese, Coca-Cola, and coffee, for example). All other options are incorrect.

43. (4) This effect is seen in clients taking a *major tranquilizer.* All of the other options are likely side effects of lithium salts.

44. (4) Kanamycin is an antibiotic that, although poorly absorbed in the GI tract, is often used as part of bowel prep prior to abdominal surgery. It acts as a bacteriocidal agent, thus significantly decreasing the number of intestinal flora and reducing risk of peritonitis in the postop period. Kanamycin does not increase peristalsis (No. 1), promote passage of stool or flatus (No. 3), or decrease amount of GI secretions (No. 2).

45. (1) The major toxic effect of an overdose of acetaminophen (Tylenol) is liver failure; Amy's liver function should be closely monitored during the first 2–3 days following her ingestion of Tylenol. Renal failure (No. 2) may occur as a **late** complication of acetaminophen toxicity, as may bleeding and hemorrhage (No. 4). Hyperthermia (No. 3) is not a major symptom of this type of ingestion; it is more common in salicylate ingestions.

46. (1) Mucomyst is the antidote for acetaminophen poisoning; it serves to protect the liver. It is usually given orally in a carbonated beverage (e.g., cola), but it can also be given via nasogastric tube. A loading dose is followed by q4h doses until a total of 18 doses have been given. KCl (No. 2), aspirin (No. 3), and heparin (No. 4) are not antidotes for acetaminophen and do not serve to protect the child's liver.

47. (1) Aminophylline, a bronchodilator that acts as a smooth muscle relaxant, is used to prevent and relieve symptoms of bronchial asthma. Anticholinergics (No. 2) are used to treat muscle spasms along the GI tract. Aminophylline is neither an expectorant (No. 3), which would assist in the removal of mucus from the respiratory tract, nor a mucolytic agent (No. 4), which would help thin out viscid secretions.

48. (1) The formula for finding the correct answer is:

dose desired/dose on hand = x/amount on hand.

$$100/500 = x/10$$
$$500x = 100(10)$$
$$x = \frac{100(10)}{500}$$
$$x = 2 \text{ cc}$$

49. (3) A transient side effect of IV aminophylline is an increase in heart rate; toxic effects include a prolonged increase in heart rate and abnormalities in cardiac rhythm. While he is receiving IV aminophylline, Bruce should be on a cardiac monitor, and both his rate and rhythm should be closely monitored and documented by the nurse. Aminophylline may also cause a transient change in the blood pressure (No. 2), but this is not as much a concern as Bruce's cardiac rhythm. Aminophylline should not affect Bruce's level of consciousness (No. 1) or his temperature (No. 4); thus, there is no particular need for the nurse to monitor these specifically at this time.

50. (2) Cromolyn sodium, an uncategorized drug used as an adjunct in the treatment of asthma, is used only after the acute attack is relieved; its primary intent is prophylaxis, i.e., to prevent future attacks. Cromolyn is used in an inhaler. It is absorbed into the systemic circulation after its inhalation into the lungs. It acts on the mast cells and also inhibits the release of histamine. Theophylline (No. 1), prednisone (No. 3), and dipenhydramine (No. 4) do not prevent future asthmatic attacks and have no prophylactic value.

51. (4) Immune serum globulin (ISG) offers the family members some protection against type A infectious hepatitis. It contains antibodies against the organism and will aid the family members in resisting this infectious disease. Augmentin (No. 1) and sulfisoxazole (No. 2) are antibiotics used for a variety of infections, but they would not prevent hepatitis. Rifampin (No. 3) is used prophylactically for *Hemophilus influenzae* meningitis and to treat Tb but, again, would not prevent hepatitis.

52. (3) The nurse should give Yu 280 mg at 10 A.M. Using the formula of 75 mg/kg/day, 75 mg × 15 kg = 1125 mg per day, to be divided into four doses. 1125 mg divided by 4 doses = 280 mg per dose.

53. (4) The recommended position to administer rectal medications to children is side lying with the upper leg flexed. This position allows the nurse to safely and effectively administer the medication while promoting comfort for the child. If Marco were to lie prone (No. 1), the nurse could not administer the medication as safely or effectively, even if his legs were abducted; further, this position would most likely cause Marco some discomfort. If Marco were sitting on a potty seat (No. 2), the nurse could not reach his rectum to insert the suppository, and it is very likely the suppository would be immediately expelled. If Marco were to lie supine (No. 3), again the nurse could not administer the medication comfortably for the child.

54. (4) Preschool children commonly experience fears and fantasies regarding invasive procedures. The nurse should attempt to momentarily distract Marco with a simple task that he can easily accomplish while remaining in the side-lying position. The suppository can be slipped into place while Marco is counting, and then the nurse can praise him for his cooperation while gently holding his buttocks together to prevent him from expelling the suppository. The nurse should not pressure him into acting like a "big boy" (No. 1) in such a frightening situation. The nurse should not lie to him, breaking a trust by telling him something "won't hurt a bit" (No. 2). Finally, the nurse should never "bribe" (No. 3) a child with gifts to ensure his cooperation.

55. (2) In selecting the correct needle to administer an IM injection to a school-age child, the nurse should always look at the child and use her judgment in evaluating muscle mass and amount of subcutaneous fat. In Laurel's case, in the absence of further data, the nurse would be most correct in selecting a needle gauge and length appropriate for the "average" school-age child. A medium gauge needle (22 G) that is 1 in. long would be most appropriate. A 5/8 in. needle (No. 1) would be too small, and a 1½ in. (18–20 G) needle would be too long and unnecessarily large (Nos. 3 and 4). A 23 or 25 G needle would be too thin to use on most school-age children (No. 1) and would be better suited for use with a newborn or an infant.

PHARMACOLOGY

UNIT

7 Common Nursing Treatments

COMMON DIAGNOSTIC PROCEDURES

I. Noninvasive diagnostic procedures are those procedures that provide an indirect assessment of organ size, shape, and/or function; these procedures are considered safe, are easily reproducible, need less complex equipment for recording, and generally do not require the written consent of client and/or guardian.

A. General nursing responsibilities:

1. Reduce client's anxieties and provide emotional support by
   a. Explaining purpose and procedure of test.
   b. Answering questions regarding safety of the procedure, as indicated.
   c. Remaining with client during procedure when possible.
2. Utilize procedures in the collection of specimens that avoid contamination and facilitate diagnosis—clean-catch urine and sputum specimens after deep breathing and coughing, for example.

B. Graphic studies of heart and brain

1. *Electrocardiogram (ECG)*—graphic record of electrical activity generated by the heart during depolarization and repolarization; *used to:* diagnose abnormal cardiac rhythms and coronary heart disease.
2. *Echocardiography* (ultrasound cardiography)—graphic record of motions produced by cardiac structures as high-frequency sound vibrations are echoed through chest wall into the heart; transesophageal echocardiography produces a clearer image, particularly in obese, barrel chested, or COPD patients; *used to:* demonstrate valvular or other structural deformities, detect pericardial effusion, diagnose tumors and cardiomegaly, or evaluate prosthetic valve function.
3. *Phonocardiogram*—graphic record of heart sounds; *used to:* keep a permanent record of client's heart sounds before and after cardiac surgery.
4. *Electroencephalogram (EEG)*—graphic record of the electrical potentials generated by the physiologic activity of the brain; *used to detect:* surface lesions or tumors of the brain and presence of epilepsy.
5. *Echoencephalogram*—beam of pulsed ultrasound is passed through the head, and returning echoes are graphically recorded; *used to:* detect shifts in cerebral midline structures caused by subdural hematomas, intracerebral hemorrhage, or tumors.

C. Roentgenologic studies (X ray)

1. *Chest—used to determine:* size, contour, and position of the heart; size, location, and nature of pulmonary lesions; disorders of thoracic bones or soft tissue; diaphragmatic contour and excursion; pleural thickening or effusions; and gross changes in the caliber or distribution of pulmonary vasculature.
2. *Kidney, ureter, and bladder (KUB)—used to:* determine size, shape, and position of kidneys, ureters, and bladder.
3. *Mammography*—examination of the breast with or without the injection of radiopaque dye into the ducts of the mammary gland; *used to:* determine the pres-

ence of tumors or cysts. *Patient preparation:* no deodorant, perfume, powders or ointment in underarm area on day of X ray. May be uncomfortable.

4. *Skull*—outline configuration and density of brain tissues and vascular markings; *used to:* determine the size and location of intracranial calcifications, tumors, abscesses, or vascular lesions.

D. Roentgenologic studies (fluoroscopy)—require the ingestion or injection of a radiopaque substance to visualize the target organ.

1. *Additional nursing responsibilities* may include:
   a. Administration of *enemas or cathartics* prior to the procedure and a laxative after.
   b. Keeping the client *NPO* 6–12 hours prior to examination; check with MD regarding oral medications.
   c. Ascertaining client's history of allergies or allergic reactions (e.g., iodine, seafood).
   d. Observing for *allergic* reactions to contrast medium following procedure.
   e. Providing fluid and food following procedure, to counteract dehydration.
   f. Observing stool for color and consistency until barium passes.
2. Common fluoroscopic examinations:
   a. *Upper GI*—ingestion of barium sulfate or Gastrografin (a white, chalky, radiopaque substance), followed by fluoroscopic and X-ray examination; *used to determine:*
      (1) Patency and caliber of *esophagus;* may also detect esophageal varices.
      (2) Mobility and thickness of *gastric* walls, presence of ulcer craters, filling defects due to tumors, pressures from outside the stomach, and patency of pyloric valve.
      (3) Rate of passage in small bowel and presence of structural abnormalities.
   b. *Lower GI*—rectal instillation of barium sulfate followed by fluoroscopic and X-ray examination; *used to determine:* contour and mobility of colon and presence of any space-occupying tumors; perform before upper GI. *Patient preparation:* explain purpose; *no food after evening meal* the evening before test; *stool softeners, laxatives, enemas, and suppositories* to cleanse the bowel before the test; *NPO after midnight* prior to test; oral medications *not* permitted day of test. *After completion of exam:* food, *increased liquid* intake and rest; *laxatives for at least two days* or until stools are normal in color and consistency.
   c. *Cholecystogram*—ingestion of organic iodine contrast substance Telepaque (iopanoic acid), or Oragrafin followed in 12 hours by X-ray visualization; gallbladder disease is indicated with *poor* or no visualization of the bladder; accurate only if gastrointestinal and liver function is intact; perform before barium enema or upper GI. *Patient preparation:* explain purpose; administer large amount of *water* with contrast capsules; *low-fat meal* evening *before* X ray; *oral laxative or stool softener after meal; no food* allowed after contrast capsules; water, tea, or coffee, with no cream or sugar, usually allowed. *After completion of exam:* fluids, food, and rest; observe for any signs of allergy to contrast capsules.
   d. *Cholangiogram*—intravenous injection of a radiopaque contrast substance, followed by fluoroscopic and X-ray examination of the bile ducts; failure of the contrast substance to pass certain points in the bile duct pinpoints *obstruction.*
   e. *Intravenous urography (IVU) or pyelography (IVP)*—injection of a radiopaque contrast substance, followed by fluoroscopic and X-ray films of kidneys and urinary tract; *used to:* identify lesions in kidneys and ureters and provide a rough estimate of kidney function.
   f. *Cystogram*—instillation of radiopaque medium through a catheter into the bladder; *used to:* visualize bladder wall and evaluate ureterovesical valves for reflux.
   g. *Phlebography* (lower limb venography)—determines patency of the tibial-popliteal, superficial femoral-common femoral, and saphenous veins. A contrast medium is injected into the superficial and/or deep veins of the involved extremity, followed by X rays, while the leg is placed in a variety of positions; *used to:* detect deep vein thrombosis and to select a vein for use in arterial bypass grafting; localized clotting may result.

E. Computerized axial tomography (CAT or CT scan)—an X-ray beam sweeps around the body, allowing measurement of various tissue densities; provides clear radiographic definition of structures that are not visible by other techniques, permitting earlier diagnosis and treatment and more effective and efficient follow-up. Initial scan may be followed by "contrast enhancement" using an injection of an intravenous contrast (iodine), followed by a repeat scan. *Patient preparation:* instructions for eating before test vary. Clear liquids up to 2 hours before are usually permitted.

F. Magnetic resonance imaging (MRI): noninvasive, nonionic technique produces cross-sectional images by exposure to magnetic energy sources. Provides superior contrast of soft tissue, including healthy, benign, and malignant tissue, along with veins and arteries; utilizes no contrast medium; takes 30–90 minutes to complete; client must stay still for periods of 5–20 minutes at a time. *Patient preparation:* client can take food and medications except for low abdominal and pelvic studies (food/fluids withheld 4–6 hours to decrease peristalsis). *Restrictions:* clients who have metal implants, permanent pacemakers, implanted medication pumps such as insulin, pregnant, or on life support systems. Obese clients may not be able to have full body MRI because they may not fit in the scanner tunnel.

G. Multiple-gated acquisition scan (MUGA)—also known as blood pool imaging. Red blood cells are tagged with a radioactive isotope. A computer-operated camera takes sequential pictures of actual heart wall motion; complement to cardiac catheterization; *used to:* determine valvular effectiveness, follow progress of heart disease, diagnose cardiac aneurysms, detect coronary artery disease, determine effects of cardiovascular drug therapy. No special preparation. Painless, except for injections. Wear gloves if contact with patient urine occurs within 24 hours after scan.

H. Ultrasound (sonogram)—scanning by ultrasound is used to diagnose disorders of the thyroid, kidney, liver, uterus, gallbladder, fetus and the intracranial structures in the neonate. It is not useful when visualization through air or bone is required (lung studies). In some hospitals the sonogram has taken the place of the oral cholecystogram in diagnosing gallbladder distention, bile duct distention, and calculi. *Patient preparation* for the client is minimal, i.e., NPO for at least 8 hours for gallbladder studies. No X-radiation. Thirty-two ounces of water PO 30 min prior to studies of lower abdomen or uterus.

I. Pulmonary function studies

1. Ventilatory studies—utilization of a spirometer to determine how well the lung is ventilating.
   a. *Vital capacity (VC)*—largest amount of air that can be expelled after maximal inspiration.
      (1) *Normally* 4000–5000 mL.
      (2) Decreased in restrictive lung disease.
      (3) May be normal, slightly increased, or decreased in chronic obstructive lung disease.
   b. *Forced expiratory volume (FEV_T)*—percentage of vital capacity that can be forcibly expired in 1, 2, or 3 seconds.
      (1) *Normally* 81–83% in 1 second, 90–94% in 2 seconds, and 95–97% in 3 seconds.
      (2) *Decreased* values indicate expiratory airway obstruction.
   c. *Maximum breathing capacity (MBC)*—maximum amount of air that can be breathed in and out in 1 minute with maximal rates and depths of respiration.
      (1) Best overall measurement of ventilatory ability.
      (2) *Reduced* in restrictive and chronic obstructive lung disease.
2. Diffusion studies—measure the rate of exchange of gases across alveolar membrane. Carbon monoxide single-breath, rebreathing, and steady-state techniques—utilized because of special affinity of hemoglobin for carbon monoxide; *decreased* when fluid is present in alveoli or when alveolar membranes are thick or fibrosed.

J. Sputum studies

1. Gross sputum evaluations—collection of sputum samples to ascertain quantity, consistency, color, and odor.
2. *Sputum smear*—sputum is smeared thinly on a slide so that it can be studied microscopically; *used to determine:* cytologic changes (malignant cell) or presence of pathogenic bacteria, e.g., tubercle bacilli.
3. *Sputum culture*—sputum samples are implanted or inoculated into special media; *used to:* diagnose pulmonary infections.
4. *Gastric lavage or analysis*—insertion of a nasogastric tube into the stomach to siphon out swallowed pulmonary secretions; *used to:* detect organisms causing pulmonary infections; especially useful for detecting tubercle bacilli in children.

K. Examination of gastric contents

1. Gastric analysis—aspiration of the contents of the fasting stomach for analysis of free and total acid.
   a. Gastric acidity is generally *increased* in presence of duodenal ulcer.
   b. Gastric acidity is usually *decreased* in pernicious anemia, cancer of the stomach.
2. Stool specimens—*examined for:* amount, consistency, color, character, and melena; *used to:* determine presence of urobilinogen, fat, nitrogen, parasites, and other substances.

L. Thermography—a picture of the surface temperature of the skin using infrared photography (not ionizing radiation) detects the circulation pattern of areas in the breasts. Tumors produce more heat than normal breast tissue. Useful with large tumors, but may not detect small or deep lesions. Requires expensive equipment and is difficult to interpret accurately.

M. Doppler ultrasonography—*used to:* measure blood flow in the major veins and arteries. The transducer of the test instrument is placed on the skin, sending out bursts of ultra-high-frequency sound. The ratio of ankle to brachial systolic pressure (API ≥ 1) provides information about vascular insufficiency. Sound varies with respiration and Valsalva's maneuver. No discomfort to the patient.

N. Caloric stimulation test—*used to:* evaluate the vestibular portion of the eighth cranial nerve, identify the impairment or loss of thermally induced nystagmus. Reflex eye movements (nystagmus) result in response to cold or warm irrigations of the external auditory canal if the nerve is intact. A diminished or absent response occurs with Meniere's or acoustic neuroma. Nausea, vomiting, or dizziness can be precipitated by the test.

II. Invasive diagnostic procedures—procedures that directly record the size, shape, or function of an organ and that are often complex or expensive or require utilization of highly trained personnel; these procedures may result in morbidity and occasionally mortality of the client and therefore require the written consent of the client or guardian.

A. General nursing responsibilities:

1. *Prior to procedure:* institute measures to provide for client's safety and emotional comfort.
   a. Have client sign permit for procedure.
   b. Ascertain and report any client history of allergy or allergic reactions.
   c. Explain procedure briefly, and accurately advise client of any possible sensations, such as flushing or a warm feeling, as when a contrast medium is injected.
   d. Keep client NPO 6–12 hours before procedure if anesthesia is to be used.
   e. Allow client to verbalize concerns, and note attitude toward procedure.
   f. Administer preprocedure sedative, as ordered.
   g. If procedure done at bedside:
      (1) Remain with client, offering frequent reassurance.
      (2) Assist with optional positioning of client.
      (3) Observe for indications of complications—shock, pain, or dyspnea.
2. *Following procedure:* institute measures to avoid complications and promote physical and emotional comfort.

a. Observe and record vital signs.

b. Check injection cut-down or biopsy sites for bleeding, infection, tenderness, or thrombosis.

(1) Report untoward reactions to physician.

(2) Apply warm compresses to ease discomfort, as ordered.

c. Encourage relaxation by allowing client to discuss experience and verbalize feelings.

B. Procedures to evaluate the cardiovascular system:

1. *Angiocardiography*—intravenous injection of a radiopaque solution or dye for the purpose of studying its circulation through the client's heart, lungs, and great vessels; *used to:* check the competency of heart valves, diagnose congenital septal defects, detect occlusions or coronary arteries, confirm suspected diagnoses, and study heart function and structure prior to cardiac surgery.

2. *Cardiac catheterization*—insertion of a radiopaque catheter into a vein to study the heart and great vessels.

a. *Right-heart catheterization*—catheter is inserted through a cut-down in the antecubital vein into the superior vena cava and through the right atrium, ventricle, and into the pulmonary artery.

b. *Left-heart catheterization*—catheter may be passed retrograde to the left ventricle through the brachial or femoral artery; it can be passed into the left atrium after right-heart catheterization by means of a special needle that punctures the septa; or it may be passed directly into the left ventricle by means of a posterior or anterior chest puncture.

c. Cardiac catheterizations are *used to:*

(1) Confirm diagnosis of heart disease and determine the extent of disease.

(2) Determine existence and extent of congenital abnormalities.

(3) Measure pressures in the heart chambers and great vessels.

(4) Obtain estimate of cardiac output.

(5) Obtain blood samples to measure oxygen content and determine presence of cardiac shunts.

d. *Specific nursing interventions*

(1) *Preprocedure client teaching:*

(a) Fatigue due to lying still for 3 or more hours is a common complaint.

(b) Some fluttery sensations may be felt—occurs as catheter is passed backward into the left ventricle.

(c) Flushed, warm feeling may occur when contrast medium is injected.

(2) *Postprocedure observations:*

(a) Monitor ECG pattern for arrhythmias.

(b) Check: extremities for color and temperature; peripheral pulses (femoral and dorsalis pedis) for quality.

3. *Angiography (arteriography)*—injection of a contrast medium into the arteries to study the vascular tree; *used to:* determine obstructions or narrowing of peripheral arteries.

4. *Pericardiocentesis (pericardial aspiration)*—puncture of the pericardial sac is performed to remove fluid accumulating with pericardial effusion. The goal is to prevent cardiac tamponade (compression of the heart). *Nursing responsibilities:* Monitor ECG and CVP during the procedure; have resuscitative equipment ready. HOB elevated to 45° to 60°. Maintain peripheral IV with saline or glucose. Following the procedure, monitor BP, CVP, and heart sounds for recurrence of tamponade (pulsus paradoxus).

C. Procedures to evaluate the respiratory system:

1. *Pulmonary circulation studies—used to:* determine regional distribution of pulmonary blood flow.

a. *Lung scan*—injection of radioactive isotope into the body, followed by lung scintiscan, which produces a graphic record of gamma rays emitted by the isotope in lung tissues; *used to:* determine lung perfusion when space-occupying lesions or pulmonary emboli and infarction are suspected.

b. *Pulmonary angiography*—X-ray visualization of the pulmonary vasculature after the injection of a radiopaque contrast medium; *used to:* evaluate pulmonary disorders, e.g., pulmonary embolism, lung tumors, aneurysms, and changes in the pulmonary vasculature due to such conditions as emphysema or congenital defects.

2. *Bronchoscopy*—introduction of a special lighted instrument (bronchoscope) into the trachea and bronchi; *used to:* inspect tracheobronchial tree for pathologic changes, remove tissue for cytologic and bacteriologic studies, remove foreign bodies or mucus plugs causing airway obstruction, assess functional residual capacity of diseased lung, and apply chemotherapeutic agents.

a. *Prebronchoscopy nursing actions*

(1) Oral hygiene.

(2) Postural drainage is indicated.

b. *Postbronchoscopy nursing actions*

(1) Instruct client not to swallow oral secretions but to let saliva run from side of mouth.

(2) Save expectorated sputum for laboratory analysis, and observe for frank bleeding.

(3) NPO until gag reflex returns.

(4) Observe for subcutaneous emphysema and dyspnea.

(5) Apply ice collar to reduce throat discomfort.

3. *Thoracentesis*—needle puncture through the chest wall and into the pleura; *used to:* remove fluid and, occasionally, air from the pleural space. *Nursing responsibilities prior* to thoracentesis:

a. Position: high Fowler's position or sitting up on edge of bed, with feet supported on chair to facilitate accumulation of fluid in the base of the chest.

b. If client is unable to sit up—turn on unaffected side.

c. Evaluate continually for signs of shock, pain, cyanosis, increased respiratory rate, and pallor.

D. Procedures to evaluate the renal system:

1. *Renal angiogram*—small catheter is inserted into the femoral artery and passed into the aorta or renal artery, radiopaque fluid is instilled, and serial films are taken.

a. *Used to:* diagnose renal hypertension and pheochromocytoma and differentiate renal cysts from renal tumors.

b. *Postangiogram nursing actions:* check pedal pulse for signs of decreased circulation.

2. *Cystoscopy*—visualization of bladder, urethra, and prostatic urethra by insertion of a tubular, lighted, telescopic lens (cytoscope) through the urinary meatus.

a. *Used to:* directly inspect the bladder, collect urine from the renal pelvis, obtain biopsies from bladder and urethra, remove calculi, and treat lesions in the bladder, urethra, and prostate.

b. *Nursing actions following* procedure

(1) Observe for urinary retention.

(2) Warm Sitz baths to relieve discomfort.

3. *Renal biopsy*—needle aspiration of tissue from the kidney for the purpose of microscopic examination.

E. Procedures to evaluate the digestive system:

1. *Celiac angiography, hepatoportography, splenoportography, and umbilical venography*—injection of a contrast medium into the portal vein or related vessel; *used to:* determine patency of vessels supplying target organ or detect lesions in the organs that distort the vasculature.

2. *Esophagoscopy and gastroscopy*—visualization of the esophagus, the stomach, and sometimes the duodenum by means of a lighted tube inserted through the mouth.

3. *Proctoscopy*—visualization of rectum and colon by means of a lighted tube inserted through the anus.

4. *Peritoneoscopy*—direct visualization of the liver and peritoneum by means of a peritoneoscope inserted through an abdominal stab wound.

5. *Liver biopsy*—needle aspiration of tissue for the purpose of microscopic examination; *used to:* determine tissue changes, facilitate diagnosis, and provide information regarding a disease course. *Nursing action:* place client on right side and position pillow for pressure, to prevent bleeding.

6. *Paracentesis*—needle aspiration of fluid from the peritoneal cavity; *used to:* relieve excess fluid accumulation or for diagnostic studies.

a. *Specific nursing actions prior to paracentesis*

(1) Have client void—to prevent possible injury to bladder during procedure.

(2) Position—sitting up on side of bed, with feet supported by chair.

(3) Check vital signs and peripheral circulation frequently throughout procedure.

(4) Observe for signs of hypovolemic shock—may occur due to fluid shift from vascular compartment following removal of protein-rich ascitic fluid.

b. *Specific nursing actions following paracentesis*

(1) Apply pressure to injection site and cover with sterile dressing.

(2) Measure and record amount and color of ascitic fluid; send specimens to lab for diagnostic studies.

7. *Small bowel biopsy*—a specimen is obtained by passing a tube through the oral cavity and is microscopically examined for changes in cellular morphology. *Nursing responsibilities:* no food or fluids 8 hours prior to procedure. Obtain written consent. Remove dentures if present. Monitor vital signs prior to, during, and after procedure for indications of hemorrhage. Procedure takes about an hour.

F. Procedures to evaluate the reproductive system in women:

1. *Culdoscopy*—operative procedure in which a culdoscope is inserted into the posterior vaginal cul-de-sac; *used to:* visualize uterus, fallopian tubes, broad ligaments, and peritoneal contents.

2. *Hysterosalpingography*—X-ray examination of uterus and fallopian tubes following insertion of a radiopaque dye into the uterine cavity; *used to:* determine patency of fallopian tubes and detect pathology in uterine cavity.

3. *Breast biopsy*—needle aspiration or incisional removal of breast tissue for microscopic examination; *used to:* differentiate among benign tumors, cysts, and malignant tumors in the breast tissue.

4. *Cervical biopsy and cauterization*—removal of cervical tissue for microscopic examination and cautery; *used to:* control bleeding or obtain additional tissue samples.

5. *Uterotubal insufflation (Rubin's test)*—injection of carbon dioxide into the cervical canal; *used to:* determine fallopian tube patency.

G. Procedures to evaluate the neuroendocrine system:

1. *Radioactive iodine uptake test (iodine 131 uptake)*—ingestion of a tracer dose of ^{131}I, followed in 24 hours by a scan of the thyroid for amount of radioactivity emitted.

a. *High* uptake indicates hyperthyroidism.

b. *Low* uptake indicates hypothyroidism.

2. *Eight-hour intravenous ACTH test*—administration of 25 units of ACTH in 500 mL of saline over an 8-hour period.

a. *Used to:* determine function of adrenal cortex.

b. 24-hour urine specimens are collected, before and after administration, for measurement of 17-ketosteroids and 17-hydroxycorticosteroids.

c. In Addison's disease, urinary output of steroids does *not increase* following administration of ACTH; *normally* steroid excretion *increases three- to fivefold* following ACTH stimulation.

d. In Cushing's syndrome, hyperactivity of the adrenal cortex *increases* the urine output of steroids in the second urine specimen tenfold.

3. *Cerebral angiography*—fluoroscopic visualization of the brain vasculature after injection of a contrast medium into the carotid or vertebral arteries; *used to:* localize lesions (tumors, abscesses, intracranial hemorrhages, and occlusions) that are large enough to distort cerebral vascular blood flow.

4. *Myelogram*—through a lumbar-puncture needle, a contrast medium is injected into the subarachnoid space of the spinal column to visualize the spinal

cord; *used to:* detect herniated or ruptured intervertebral disks, tumors, or cysts that compress or distort spinal cord. *Nursing responsibilities:* elevate HOB with water-soluble contrast; flat with oil contrast; check for bladder distention with metrizamide (water-soluble); vital signs every 4 hours for 24 hours.

5. *Brain scan*—intravenous injection of a radioactive substance, followed by a scan for emission of radioactivity.
   a. *Increased* radioactivity at site of pathology.
   b. *Used to:* detect brain tumors, abscesses, hematomas, and arteriovenous malformations.
6. *Lumbar puncture*—puncture of the lumbar subarachnoid space of the spinal cord with a needle to withdraw samples of cerebrospinal fluid (CSF); *used to:* evaluate CSF for infections and determine presence of hemorrhage. Not done if ↑ ICP suspected.

H. Procedures to evaluate the skeletal system: *Arthroscopy*—examination of a joint through a fiberoptic endoscope called an athroscope. Usually done in the OR (same day surgery) under aseptic conditions using a local anesthetic, although a general anesthetic may be used. A tourniquet is used to reduce blood flow to the area while the scope is introduced through a cannula. Saline is used as the viewing medium. Biopsy or removal of loose bodies from the joint may be done. A compression dressing (e.g., Ace bandage) is applied. Restrictions vary according to surgeon preference and nature of procedure. Weight-bearing may be immediate or restricted for 24 hours. Teach patient to observe for signs of infection.

■ INTRAVENOUS THERAPY

I. Infusion systems

A. Plastic bag

1. Contains no vacuum—needs no air to replace fluid as it flows from container.
2. Medication can be added with syringe and needle through a resealable latex port.
   a. During infusion, administration set should be completely clamped before medications are added.
   b. Prevents undiluted, and perhaps toxic, dose from entering administration set.

B. Closed system

1. Requires partial vacuum—however, only filtered air enters container.
2. Medication may be added during infusion through air vent in administration set.

C. Administration sets

1. *Standard*—deliver 10–15 drops/mL.
2. *Pediatric or mini-drop sets*—deliver 60 drops/mL.
3. *Controlled-volume sets*—permit accurate infusion of measured volumes of fluids.
   a. Particularly valuable when piggybacked into primary infusion.
   b. Solutions containing drugs can then be administered intermittently.
4. *Y-type administration sets*—allow for simultaneous or alternate infusion of two fluids.
   a. May contain filter and pressure unit for blood transfusions.
   b. Air embolism significant hazard with this type of administration set.
5. *Positive-pressure sets*—designed for rapid infusion of replacement fluids.
   a. In emergency, built-in pressure chamber increases rate of blood administration.
   b. Pump chamber *must* be filled at all times to avoid air embolism.
   c. Application of positive pressure to infusion fluids is responsibility of *physician.*
6. *Infusion pumps*—utilized to deliver small volumes of fluid or doses of high-potency drugs.
   a. Used primarily in neonatal, pediatric, and adult intensive-care units.
   b. Have increased the safety of parenteral therapy and reduced nursing time.

II. Fluid administration

A. Factors influencing rate:

1. Client's size.
2. Client's physical condition.
3. Age of client.
4. Type of fluid.
5. Client's tolerance to fluid.

B. Flow rates for parenteral infusions can be computed using the following formula:

$$\frac{\text{gtt/mL of given set}}{\text{60 min/h}} \times \text{total volume/h} = \text{gtt/minute}$$

If 1000 mL are to be infused in an 8-hour (125 mL/h) period and the administration set delivers 15 gtt/mL, the rate is 31.2 gtt/minute:

$$\frac{15}{60} \times 125 = \frac{1}{4} \times 125 = 31.2 \text{ gtt/minute}$$

C. Generally the type of fluid administration set determines its rate of flow.

1. Fluid administration sets—approximately 15 gtt/minute.
2. Blood administration sets—approximately 10 gtt/minute.
3. Pediatric administration sets—approximately 60 gtt/minute.
4. Always check information on the administration set box to determine the number of gtt/mL before calculating; varies with manufacturer.

D. Factors influencing flow rates:

1. *Gravity*—a change in the height of the infusion bottle will increase or decrease the rate of flow; for example, raising the bottle higher will increase the rate of flow, and vice versa.
2. *Blood clot* in needle—stopping the infusion for any reason or an increase in venous pressure may result in partial or total obstruction of needle by clot.
   a. Delay in changing infusion bottle.
   b. Blood pressure cuff on, or restraints on or above infusion needle.
   c. Client lying on arm in which infusion is being made.

3. Change in *needle position*—against or away from vein wall.
4. *Venous spasm*—due to cold blood or irritating solution.
5. *Plugged vent*—causes infusion to stop.

III. Fluid and electrolyte therapy

A. Types of therapy

1. Maintenance therapy—provides water, electrolytes, glucose, vitamins, and, in some instances, protein to meet daily requirements.
2. Restoration of deficits—in addition to maintenance therapy, fluid and electrolytes are added to replace previous losses.
3. Replacement therapy—infusions to replace current losses in fluid and electrolytes.

B. Types of intravenous fluids

1. *Isotonic solutions*—fluids that approximate the osmolarity (290 mOsm/L) of normal blood plasma.
   a. Sodium chloride (0.9%)—normal saline.
      (1) *Indications*
         (a) Extracellular fluid replacement when Cl^- loss is equal to or greater than Na^+ loss.
         (b) Treatment of metabolic alkalosis.
         (c) Na^+ depletion.
         (d) Initiating and terminating blood transfusions.
      (2) Possible *side effects*
         (a) Hypernatremia.
         (b) Acidosis.
         (c) Hypokalemia.
         (d) Circulatory overload.
   b. 5% dextrose in water (5% D/W).
      (1) Provides calories for energy, sparing body protein and development of ketosis from fat breakdown.
         (a) 3.75 calories are provided per gram of glucose.
         (b) USP standards require use of monohydrated glucose, so only 91% is actually glucose.
         (c) 5% D/W yields 170.6 calories; 5% D/W means 5 g glucose/L.

$$50 \times 3.75 = 187.5 \text{ calories}$$
$$0.91 \times 187.5 = 170.6 \text{ calories}$$

      (2) *Indications*
         (a) Dehydration.
         (b) Hypernatremia.
         (c) Drug administration.
      (3) Possible *side effects*
         (a) Hypokalemia.
         (b) Osmotic diuresis—dehydration.
         (c) Transient hyperinsulinism.
         (d) Water intoxication.
   c. 5% dextrose in normal saline.
      (1) Prevents ketone formation and loss of potassium and intracellular water.
      (2) *Indications*
         (a) Hypovolemic shock—temporary measure.
         (b) Burns.
         (c) Acute adrenocortical insufficiency.
      (3) Same *side effects* as normal saline.
   d. Isotonic multiple-electrolyte fluids—utilized for replacement therapy; ionic composition approximates blood plasma.
      (1) Types—Plasmanate, Polysol, and lactated Ringer's.
      (2) *Indicated in:* vomiting, diarrhea, excessive diuresis, and burns.
      (3) Possible *side effect*—circulatory overload.
      (4) Lactated Ringer's is *contraindicated* in severe metabolic acidosis and/or alkalosis and liver disease.
      (5) Same *side effects* as normal saline.
2. *Hypertonic solutions*—fluids with an osmolarity much higher than 290 mOsm (+50 mOsm); increase osmotic pressure of blood plasma, thereby drawing fluid from the cells.
   a. 10% dextrose in normal saline.
      (1) Administered in large vein to dilute and prevent venous trauma.
      (2) *Used for:* nutrition and to replenish Na^+ and Cl^+.
      (3) Possible *side effects*
         (a) Hypernatremia (excess Na^+).
         (b) Acidosis (excess Cl^-).
         (c) Circulatory overload.
   b. 3% and 5% sodium chloride solutions.
      (1) Slow administration essential to prevent overload (100 mL/h).
      (2) *Indicated in:* water intoxication and severe sodium depletion.
3. *Hypotonic solution*—fluids whose osmolarity is significantly less than that of blood plasma (−50 mOsm); these fluids lower plasma osmotic pressures, causing fluid to enter cells.
   a. 0.45% sodium chloride—utilized for replacement when requirement for Na^+ use is questionable.
   b. 2.5% dextrose in 0.45% saline, 5% dextrose in 0.45% saline, and 5% dextrose in 0.2% saline—these are all hydrating fluids.
      (1) *Indications*
         (a) Fluid replacement when some Na^+ replacement is also necessary.
         (b) Encourage diuresis in clients who are dehydrated.
         (c) Evaluate kidney status before instituting electrolyte infusions.
      (2) Possible *side effects*
         (a) Hypernatremia.
         (b) Circulatory overload.
         (c) Use with *caution* in edematous clients with cardiac, renal, or hepatic disease.
         (d) After adequate renal function is established, appropriate electrolytes should be given to avoid hypokalemia.

4. *Alkalizing agents*—fluids used in the treatment of *metabolic acidosis:*
   a. 1/6 M lactate
      (1) Administration—rate usually not more than 300 mL/h.
      (2) *Side effects*—observe carefully for signs of alkalosis.
   b. Sodium bicarbonate
      (1) *Indications*
         (a) Replace excessive loss of bicarbonate ion.
         (b) Emergency treatment of life-threatening acidosis.
      (2) Administration
         (a) Depends on client's weight, condition, and carbon dioxide level.
         (b) Usual dose is 500 mL of a 1.5% solution (89 mEq).
      (3) *Side effects*
         (a) Alkalosis.
         (b) Hypocalcemic tetany.
         (c) Rapid infusion may induce cellular acidity and death.
5. *Acidifying solutions*—fluids used in treatment of *metabolic alkalosis.*
   a. Types
      (1) Normal saline (see B.1. *Isotonic solutions,* p. 521).
      (2) Ammonium chloride.
   b. Administration—dosage depends on client's condition and serum lab values.
   c. *Side effects*
      (1) Hepatic encephalopathy in presence of decreased liver function since ammonia is metabolized by liver.
      (2) Toxic effects of irregular respirations, twitching, and bradycardia.
      (3) *Contraindicated* with renal failure.
6. *Blood and blood products* (see Table 7.1).
   a. *Indications*
      (1) Maintenance of blood volume.
      (2) Supply red blood cells to maintain oxygen-carrying capacity.
      (3) Supply clotting factors to maintain coagulation properties.
      (4) Exchange transfusion.

IV. Intravenous cancer chemotherapy

A. Usual sites: forearm, dorsum of hand, wrist, antecubital fossa.

B. Procedure:

1. Normal saline infusion usually started first, to verify vein patency, position of needle. Chemotherapy "piggy-backed" into IV that is running.
2. Rate: usually 1 mL/min. Running slowly decreases nausea, vomiting, and the degree of vein damage.
3. Check vein patency ever 3–5 minutes.
4. If more than one drug is to be infused, normal saline should be infused between drugs.
5. Never infuse against resistance.
6. Stop treatment if client reports pain at needle site. Extravasation (infiltration of toxic drugs into tissue surrounding vessel) may be present.
7. If extravasation present: begin protocol appropriate to drug administered (e.g., flushing of line with saline, applying ice or heat, local injection of site with antidote drugs, topical application of steroid creams).
8. Once treatment is completed: remove needle, apply Bandaid, exert pressure to prevent hematoma formation.

V. Complications of IV therapy: see Table. 7.2.

NURSING TREATMENTS

TABLE 7.1 **Transfusion With Blood or Blood Products**

Blood or Blood Product	Indications	Assessment: Side Effects	Nursing Plan/ Implementation
Whole blood	1. Acute hemmorhage. 2. Hypovolemic shock.	1. Hemolytic reaction. 2. Fluid overload. 3. Febrile reaction. 4. Pyogenic reaction. 5. Allergic reaction.	1. See Table 4.16, Postoperative Complications, p. 347, for complete discussion of nursing responsibilities. 2. Protocol for checking blood before transfusion is begun varies with each institution; however, at least *two* people must verify that the unit of blood has been cross-matched for a specific client.
Red blood cells, packed	1. Acute anemia with hypoxia. 2. Aplastic anemia. 3. Bone marrow failure due to malignancy. 4. Clients who need red blood cells but not volume.	See Whole blood.	See Whole blood.

continued

■ **TABLE 7.1** ***(Continued)*** **Transfusion With Blood or Blood Products**

Blood or Blood Product	Indications	Assessment: Side Effects	Nursing Plan/ Implementation
Red blood cells, frozen	1. See Red blood cells, packed. 2. Clients sensitized by previous transfusions.	1. Less likely to cause antigen reaction. 2. Decreased possibility of transmitting hepatitis.	See Whole blood.
White blood cells (leukocytes)	Currently being used in severe leukopenia with infection (research still being done).	1. Elevated temperature. 2. Graft versus host disease.	1. Careful monitoring of temperature. 2. *Must* be given as soon as collected.
Platelet concentrate	1. Severe deficiency. 2. Bleeding thrombocytopenic clients with platelet counts *below* 10,000.	1. Fever, chills. 2. Hives. 3. Development of antibodies that will destroy platelets in future transfusions. *Contraindications:* 1. Idiopathic thrombocytopenic purpura. 2. Disseminated intravascular coagulopathy.	Monitor temperature.
Single-donor fresh plasma	1. Clotting deficiency or concentrates not available or deficiency not fully diagnosed. 2. Shock.	1. Side effects rare. 2. Congestive heart failure. 3. Possible hepatitis.	Use sterile, pyrogen-free filters.
Plasma removed from whole blood (up to 5 days after expiration date, which is 21 days)	1. Shock due to loss of plasma. 2. Burns. 3. Peritoneal injury. 4. Hemorrhage. 5. While awaiting blood cross-match.	See Single-donor fresh plasma.	See Single-donor fresh plasma.
Freeze-dried plasma	See Plasma removed from whole blood	See Single-donor fresh plasma.	Must be reconstituted with sterile water before use.
Single-donor fresh-frozen plasma.	1. See Single-donor fresh plasma. 2. Inherited or acquired disorders of coagulation. 3. Presurgical hemophiliac.	See Single-donor fresh plasma.	1. Notify blood bank to thaw about 30 minutes before administration. 2. Give *immediately.*
Cryoprecipitate concentrate (factor VIII—antihemophilic factor)	For hemophilia: 1. Prevention. 2. Preoperatively. 3. During bleeding episodes.	Rare.	0.55 mL cryoprecipitate concentrate has same effect on serum level as 1600 mL of fresh frozen plasma.
Factor II, VII, IX, and X compiled.	Specific deficiencies.	Hepatitis.	Commercially prepared.
Fibrinogen (factor I).	Fibrinogen deficiency.	Increased risk of hepatitis since the hepatitis virus combines with fibrinogen during fractionation.	1. Reconstitute with sterile water. 2. Do *not* warm fibrinogen or use hot water to reconstitute. 3. Do *not* shake. 4. Must be given with a filter.
Albumin or salt-poor albumin.	1. Shock due to: hemmorrhage, trauma, infection, surgery, or burns. 2. Treatment of cerebral edema. 3. Low serum-protein levels.	None; these are heat-treated products.	Commercially prepared.
Dextran	Hypovolemic shock.	1. Rare allergic reaction. 2. Clients with heart or kidney disease susceptible to heart failure or pulmonary edema.	Commercially prepared.

■ **TABLE 7.2** **Complications of IV Therapy**

Complication	Assessment: Subjective Data	Assessment: Objective Data	Nursing Plan/ Implementation
Infiltration—fluid infusing into surrounding tissue rather than into vessel	Pain around needle insertion.	1. Infusion rate slow. 2. Swelling, hardness, coolness, blanching of tissue at site of needle. 3. Blood does not return into tubing when bag/bottle lowered. 4. Puffiness under surface of arm.	1. Stop IV. 2. Apply warm towel to area. 3. Restart at another site. 4. Record.
Thrombophlebitis—inflammatory changes in vessel; *Thromboemboli*—the development of venous clots within the inflamed vessel	Pain along the vein.	Redness, swelling around affected area (red line).	1. Stop IV. 2. Notify physician. 3. Cold compresses or warm towel, as ordered. 4. Restart in another site. 5. *Rest affected limb; do not rub.* 6. See nursing care of Thrombophlebitis, Unit 4.
Pyrogenic reaction—contaminated equipment/solution	1. Headache. 2. Backache. 3. Nausea. 4. Anxiety.	1. ↑ Temperature. 2. Chills. 3. Face flushed. 4. Vomiting. 5. ↓ BP. 6. Cyanosis.	1. Discontinue IV. 2. Vital signs. 3. Send equipment for culture/analysis. 4. Antibiotic ointment, as ordered, at injection site. 5. *Prevention:* change tubing q24–48h; meticulous sterile technique; check: for precipitation, expiration dates, damage to containers, tubings etc.; refrigerate hyperalimentation fluids; discard hyperalimentation fluids that have been at room temperature from 8–12 h and use new bag regardless of amount left in first bag (change, to prevent infection—excellent medium for bacterial growth).
Fluid overload—excessive amount of fluid infused; infants/elderly at risk.	1. Headache. 2. Shortness of breath. 3. Syncope. 4. Dyspnea.	1. ↑ pulse, venous pressure. 2. Venous distention. 3. Flushed skin. 4. Coughing. 5. ↑ respirations. 6. Cyanosis, pulmonary edema. 7. Shock.	1. Stop IV. 2. Semi-Fowler's position. 3. Notify physician. 4. Be prepared for diuretic therapy. 5. *Preventive measures:* monitor flow rate and client's response to IV therapy (see Fluid volume excess, p. 316, for subjective and objective data).
Air emboli—air in circulatory system.	Loss of consciousness.	1. Hypotension, cyanosis. 2. Tachycardia. 3. ↑ venous pressure. 4. Tachypnea.	1. Turn on left side, with head down. 2. Administer oxygen therapy. 3. **Medical emergency—call physician.**
Nerve damage—improper position of limb during infusion or *tying* limb down too tight during infusion → damage to nerve.	Numbness: fingers, hands.	Unusual position for limb.	1. Untie. 2. Passive ROM exercises. 3. Monitor closely for return of function. 4. Record limb status.
Pulmonary embolism—blood clot enters pulmonary circulation and obstructs pulmonary artery	Dyspnea.	1. Orthopnea. 2. Signs of circulatory and cardiac collapse.	1. Slow IV to keep vein open (rate: 5–6 drops/min). 2. Notify physician. 3. **Medical emergency.** 4. Be prepared for life-saving measures and anticoagulation therapy.

■ OXYGEN THERAPY

I. Purpose—to relieve hypoxia and provide adequate tissue oxygenation.

II. Clinical indications

A. Shock.

B. Cardiac disorders—myocardial infarction and congestive heart failure.

C. Respiratory depression, insufficiency, or failure.

D. Anemia.

E. Supportive therapy for unconscious clients.

F. Fetal decelerations during labor.

III. Precautions

A. Clients with chronic obstructive pulmonary disease should receive *low* flow rates of oxygen, to prevent inhibition of hypoxic respiratory drive.

B. *Excessive* amounts of oxygen for prolonged periods of time will cause retrolental fibroplasia and blindness in premature infants.

C. Oxygen delivered *without* humidification will result in drying and irritation of respiratory mucosa, decreased ciliary action, and thickening of respiratory secretions.

D. Oxygen supports combustion, and *fire* is a potential hazard during its administration.

1. Ground electrical administration.
2. Prohibit smoking.
3. Institute measures to decrease static electricity.

E. *High* flow rates of oxygen per ventilator or cuffed tracheostomy and endotracheal tubes can produce signs of oxygen toxicity in 24–48 hours.

1. Cough, sore throat, decreased vital capacity, and substernal discomfort.
2. Pulmonary manifestations due to:
   a. Atelectasis.
   b. Exudation of protein fluids into alveoli.
   c. Damage to pulmonary capillaries.
   d. Interstitial hemorrhage.

IV. Oxygen administration

A. Oxygen is dispensed from cylinder or piped-in system.

B. Methods of delivering oxygen:

1. Nasal catheter
   a. Effective and comfortable.
   b. Delivers 30–40% oxygen at flow rates of 6–8 L/min.
   c. Can produce excoriation of nares.
2. Nasal prongs.
   a. Comfortable and simple, and allows client to move about in bed.
   b. Delivers 30–40% oxygen at flow rates of 6–8 L/min.
   c. Difficult to keep in position unless client is alert and cooperative.
3. Face tent
   a. Well tolerated and provides means for supplying extra humidity.
   b. Delivers 30–55% oxygen at flow rates of 4–8 L/min.
4. Venturi mask
   a. Allows for accurate delivery of prescribed concentration of oxygen.
   b. Delivers 25–35% oxygen at flow rates of 4–8 L/min.
5. Face mask
   a. Poorly tolerated—utilized for short periods of time.
   b. Delivers 35–65% oxygen at flow rates of 6–12 L/min.
   c. Significant rebreathing of carbon dioxide at low oxygen flow rates.
   d. Hot—may produce pressure sores around nose and mouth.
6. T-tube
   a. Provides humidification and enriched oxygen mixtures to tracheostomy or ET tube.
   b. Delivers 40–60% oxygen at flow rates of 4–12 L/min.

V. Ventilators

A. *Indications*

1. Hypoventilation.
2. Hypoxia.
3. Counteract pulmonary edema by changing pressure gradient.
4. Decrease work of breathing.

B. *Contraindications*

1. Tuberculosis—may rupture tubercular bleb.
2. Hypovolemia—increased intrathoracic pressures decrease venous return.
3. Air trapping—increased because adequate exhalation is not allowed.

C. *Complications* (see Table 7.3):

1. Decreased blood pressure.
2. Atelectasis.
3. Infection.
4. Oxygen toxicity.
5. Difficulties weaning.
6. Gastric dilatation.
7. Pneumothorax.

D. *Types of ventilators*

1. Oscillating or rocking bed.
   a. Indirectly aids respirations by using weight and gravity of abdominal contents to change position of diaphragm.
   b. *Used with:* paralytic disease, as an aid in weaning.
2. Iron lung and chest respirators.
   a. Driven by motors that create negative pressure within tank or shell and thus allow air to enter client's lungs.
   b. *Used for:* neuromuscular disease.
3. Intermittent positive-pressure breathing.
   a. Produces greater-than-atmospheric pressures, intermittently.
   b. Improves tidal volume and minute volume and aids in overcoming respiratory insufficiency.

■ TABLE 7.3 Recognizing Complications of Mechanical Ventilation

Complication	Assessment Findings
Hyperventilation	1. ↑ respiratory rate (>20). 2. ↑ depth of respirations. 3. ↑ pH (>7.45, indicating alkalosis). 4. ↓ $Paco_2$ (<40 mm Hg). 5. Numbness. 6. Tingling of fingers and toes. 7. Lightheadedness.
Hypoventilation	1. ↓ respiratory rate (<10). 2. ↓ depth of respirations. 3. Diminished breath sounds. 4. ↓ pH (< 7.35, indicating acidosis). 5. ↑ $Paco_2$ (>40 mm Hg)*. 6. ↓ Pao_2 (below normal for patient). 7. ↑ pulse. 8. Dysrhythmias. 9. Anxiety.
Tracheal injury	1. Inspiratory stridor after extubation. 2. Blood-tinged sputum.
Pneumothorax	1. Dyspnea. 2. Diminished breath sounds. 3. Decreased chest movement on affected side. 4. Restlessness. 5. Deviated trachea.
Impaired venous return	1. Weak, rapid pulse. 2. ↓ urine output. 3. ↓ blood pressure.

*May be normal in patients with chronic obstructive pulmonary disease.
Source: Winters C: Monitoring Ventilator Patients for Complications. *Nursing 88, 18* (6), 40.

c. Produces more uniform distribution of alveolar aeration and reduces work of breathing.

d. *Used to:* deliver both oxygen and medications during treatment and rehabilitative pulmonary therapy, particularly if patient has decreased tidal volume.

e. *Contraindicated in:* pneumothorax, active tuberculosis, and history of recent hemoptysis.

4. Pressure-constant ventilators.
   a. *Bird*—Mark VII.
      (1) Pressure-cycled, pneumatic-powered.
      (2) When preset pressure is reached, valve closes, terminating inspiration.
      (3) Flow rate, sensitivity, and pressure limit are all adjustable.
      (4) Adjustable flow rate allows for increasing tidal volume.
      (5) Disadvantage—changes in compliance or airway resistance can affect oxygen concentration and tidal volume.
   b. *Bennett*—PR II.
      (1) Positive-pressure-cycled, time-cycled, flow-sensitive.
      (2) May be triggered by client's inspiration or controlled by pressure or time setting.
      (3) Oxygen delivery variable, so frequent monitoring is *essential.*
5. Volume-constant ventilators.
   a. Bennett—MA 1.
      (1) Delivers preset tidal volume.
      (2) Oxygen concentration adjusted by lighter flow being fed into machine.
      (3) Sophisticated alarms.
      (4) Has a sigh mechanism and positive end-expiration pressure (PEEP), which maintains lung inflation.
      (5) *Used for:* decreased compliance (stiff lungs).
      (6) Excellent humidification system.
6. Minute volume ventilators—Servo 990 C.
   a. Delivers preset inspiratory minute volume.
   b. Has PEEP, continuous positive airway pressure (CPAP), spontaneous intermittent mandatory ventilation (SIMV), and inverse ratio ventilation (IRV) capabilities.
   c. *Used for:* clients with ARDS who have not responded to conventional treatment (PEEP, IMV) and need the advantage of IRV and prolonged inspiratory ventilation.

■ POSITIONING THE CLIENT

See Table 7.4.

■ COMMONLY USED TUBES

See Table 7.5.

■ COLOSTOMY CARE

See Tables 7.6 and 7.7.

■ BASIC PROSTHETIC CARE

See Tables 7.8 and 7.9.

■ UNIVERSAL PRECAUTIONS

See Table 7.10.

■ **TABLE 7.4** **Positioning the Client for Specific Surgical Conditions**

Surgical Condition	Key Points	Rationale
Amputation: lower extremity	*No* pillows under stump after first 24 hours. Turn client prone several times a day.	Prevents flexion deformity of the limb.
Appendicitis: ruptured	Keep in Fowler's position—not flat in bed.	Keeps infection from spreading upward in the peritoneal cavity.
Burns (extensive)	Usually *flat* for first 24 hours.	Potential problem is hypovolemia, which will be more symptomatic in a sitting position.
Cast, extremity	Keep extremity elevated.	Prevents edema.
Coronary surgery	May be ordered flat on back for 24 hours.	Important to prevent possible hypotension, which may occur if head of bed raised.
Craniotomy	Head *elevated* with supratentorial incision; flat with cerebellar or brainstem incision.	Prevents collection of fluid in surgical area, which might contribute to increased intracranial pressure.
Flail chest	Position on *affected* side.	Reduces the instability of the chest wall that is causing the paradoxical respiratory movements.
Gastric resection	Lie down after meals.	May be useful in preventing dumping syndrome.
Hiatal hernia (*before* repaired)	Head of bed elevated on shock blocks.	Prevents esophageal irritation from gastric regurgitation.
Hip prosthesis	1. Keep affected leg in *abduction* (splint or pillow between legs). 2. Avoid adduction and flexion of the hip. 3. Use trochanter roll along outside of femur anterior joint capsule incision to keep affected leg turned slightly *inward*. No trochanter roll with posterior joint capsule incision as leg is turned slightly *outward*.	If affected leg is flexed and allowed to adduct and internally rotate, the head of the femur may be displaced from the socket.
Laminectomy; fusion	Avoid twisting motion when getting out of bed, ambulating.	Prevents any bending of the spine.
Liver biopsy	Place on right side, and position pillow for pressure.	Prevents bleeding.
Lobectomy	Do *not* put in Trendelenburg position. Position of comfort—sides, back.	Pushes abdominal contents against diaphragm. May cause respiratory embarrassment.
Mastectomy	1. Do *not* abduct arm first few days. 2. Elevate hand and arm *higher* than shoulder if lymph glands removed.	Puts tension on suture line. Prevents lymphedema.
Pneumonectomy	Turn only toward operative side for short periods; no extreme lateral positioning.	1. Gives unaffected lung room for full expansion. 2. Prevents mediastinal shift. 3. In case of bleeding there will be no drainage into the unaffected bronchi.
Radium implantation in cervix	Bedrest—usually may elevate head to 30°.	Must keep radium insert positioned correctly.
Respiratory distress	Orthopnea position usually desirable.	Allows for maximum expansion of lungs.
Retinal detachment	1. Affected area toward bed—complete bedrest. 2. *No sudden* movements of head—may use sand bags to prevent turning.	1. Gravity may help retina fall in place. 2. Any sudden increase in intraocular pressure may further dislodge retina. 3. Necessary to cover both eyes to reduce ocular movements.

continued

■ TABLE 7.4 *(Continued)* Positioning the Client for Specific Surgical Conditions

Surgical Condition	Key Points	Rationale
Traction		
Straight traction	Check specific orders about how much head may be elevated.	Body is used as the countertraction—this must not be less than the pull of the traction.
Balanced suspension	May give client more freedom to move about than in straight traction.	In balanced suspension additional weights supply countertraction.
Unconscious client	Turn on side with head slightly *lowered*—"coma" position.	1. Important to let secretions drain out by gravity. 2. Must prevent aspiration.
Vascular		
Ileo-femoral bypass; arterial insufficiency	1. Do *not* elevate legs. 2. *Avoid* hip flexion—walk or stand, but do *not* sit.	1. Arterial flow is helped by gravity. 2. Flexion of the hip compresses the vessels of the extremity.
Vein strippings; vein ligations	1. Keep legs elevated. 2. Do *not* stand or sit for long periods.	1. Prevents venous stasis. 2. Prevents venous pooling.

Source: Jane Vincent Corbett, RN, MS, Ed.D., Associate Professor, School of Nursing, University of San Francisco. Used with permission.

■ TABLE 7.5 Review of the Use of Common Tubes

Tube or Apparatus	Purpose	Examples of Use	Key Points
Chest tubes	1. *Anterior tube* drains mostly air from pleural space. 2. *Posterior tube* drains mostly fluid from pleural space. 3. Removal of fluid and air from pleural space is necessary to reestablish negative intrapleural pressure.	1. *Thoracotomy.* 2. *Open heart surgery.* 3. *Spontaneous pneumothorax.* 4. *Traumatic pneumothorax.*	1. See Key Points for each of the three entries under Drainage System, below. 2. Sterile technique is used when changing dressings around the tube insertions. 3. Fowler's position to facilitate air and fluid removal. 4. Cough, deep breathe q1h; splint chest; medicate for pain. 5. Manage pain carefully in order *not* to depress respirations. 6. Prepare for removal when: there is little or no drainage, air leak disappears, or fluctuations stop in water seal; have suture set, petrolatum gauze (or other ointment), 4x4s, and sturdy elastic tape ready; medicate for pain before removal; monitor breathing after removal (breath sounds, rate, chest pain).
Drainage System (see Figure 7.1, p. 531)			
#1: drainage bottle or compartment	Collects drainage.		1. Mark level in bottle each shift to keep accurate record—*not* routinely emptied; replaced when full. 2. *Never* raise glass bottle above the level of the chest, otherwise back flow will occur.
#2: water-seal bottle or chamber	Water seal prevents flow of atmospheric air into pleural space. Essential to prevent recollapse of the lung.		1. Air bubbles from postoperative residual air *will* continue for 24–48 hours. 2. *Persistent* large amounts of air bubbles in this compartment indicate an *air leak* between the alveoli and the pleural space. 3. Clamp tube(s) only to: verify a leak, replace a broken, cracked, or full drainage unit, or verify readiness of patient for tube removal. Not necessary to clamp when ambulating if water seal intact. 4. If tube becomes disconnected, clean off tubing ends and reconnect; if dislodged from chest, seal insertion site immediately on expiration if possible; use sterile petrolatum gauze and adhesive tape to form air-occlusive dressing. 5. If air leak is present, clamping the tube for very long may cause a tension pneumothorax. 6. Fluctuation of the fluid level in this bottle is *expected* (when the suction is turned off) because respiration changes the pleural pressure. If there is *no fluctuation* of the fluid in the tube of this bottle (when the suction is turned off), then either the lung is fully expanded or the tube is blocked by kinking or by a clot.

continued

■ **TABLE 7.5 *(Continued)*** **Review of the Use of Common Tubes**

Tube or Apparatus	Purpose	Examples of Use	Key Points
Drainage System (cont.)			7. Although not routinely used, milking (gently squeezing) the tubes, if ordered, will prevent blockage from clots or debris. Otherwise gravity drainage is sufficient to maintain patency. 8. Drainage of >100 mL in 1 hour should be reported to physician.
#3: suction control or breaker bottle—connected to wall suction	Level of the column of water (i.e., 15–20 cm) is used to control the amount of suction applied to the chest tube—if the water evaporates to only *10 cm* depth, then this will be the *maximum* suction generated by the wall suction.		1. Air ***should continuously bubble*** through this compartment when the suction is on. The bubbles are from the atmosphere—not the client. When the wall suction is turned higher, the bubbling will increase, but the increased pulling of air is from the atmosphere and ***not*** from the pleural space. 2. Since the level of H_2O determines the maximum negative pressure that can be obtained, make sure the water does *not* evaporate—keep filling the bottle to keep the ordered level. If there is ***no*** bubbling of air through this bottle, the wall suction is *too low.*
Heimlich flutter valve	1. Has a one-way valve so fluids and air can drain out of the pleural space but cannot flow back. 2. Eliminates the need for a water seal—no danger when tube is unclamped below the valve.	Same as for other chest tubes.	1. Can be connected to suction if ordered. 2. Sometimes can just drain into portable bag so client is more mobile.
Tracheostomy tube	1. Maintains patent airway and promotes better O_2–CO_2 exchange. 2. Makes removal of secretions by suctioning easier. 3. Cuff on trach is necessary if need airtight fit for an assisted ventilation.	1. *Acute respiratory distress* due to poor ventilation. 2. ***Severe burns of head and neck.*** 3. *Laryngectomy* (trach is permanent).	1. Use oxygen *before* and *after* each suctioning. 2. Humidify oxygen. 3. Sterile technique in suctioning. 4. Cleanse inner cannula as needed—only leave out 5–10 minutes. 5. Hemostat handy if outer cannula is expelled—have obturator taped to bed and another trach set handy. 6. Cuff must be deflated periodically to prevent necrosis of mucosa, unless low-pressure cuff used.
Penrose drain	Soft collapsible latex rubber drain inserted to drain serosanguineous fluid from a surgical site. Usually brought out to the skin via a stab wound.	Bowel resection.	1. Expect drainage to progress from serosanguineous to more serous. 2. Sterile technique when changing dressing—do often. 3. Physician will advance tube a little each day.
Nasogastric (NG) tubes Levin tube and small bore feeding tubes	1. Inserted into stomach to decompress by removing gastric contents and air—prevents any buildup of gastric secretions, which are continous. 2. Used when stomach needs to be washed out (lavaged). 3. Used for feedings when client is unable to swallow.	1. Any abdominal or other ***surgery where peristalsis is absent*** for a few days. 2. *Overdoses.* 3. *Gastrointestinal hemorrhage.* 4. *Cancer of the esophagus.* 5. *Early postoperative laryngectomy client* or ***radical neck dissection.***	1. Connect to *low* intermittent suction. 2. Irrigate p.r.n. with normal saline. 3. Clean, but *not* sterile, procedure. 4. Mouth care needed. 5. Report *"coffee ground"* material (digested blood). 6. For overdose, stomach is pumped out as *rapidly* as possible. 7. For hemorrhage, normal saline is usually used to lavage. 8. Critical to make sure tube still in stomach *before* beginning feeding; aspirate stomach contents, listen for air passing into stomach, and if possible aspirate gastric contents. Small bore tubes need placement check by X ray. 9. Follow feeding with some water to rinse out the tube. 10. Clamp tube when ambulating. 11. With larger bore tubes, determine residuals and withhold feeding if large residuals obtained.

continued

TABLE 7.5 *(Continued)* **Review of the Use of Common Tubes**

Tube or Apparatus	Purpose	Examples of Use	Key Points
Nasogastric Tubes (cont.)			
Miller-Abbott tube Cantor tube	Longer than Levin tube—has mercury or air in bags so tube can be used to *decompress the lower intestinal tract.*	1. *Small bowel obstructions.* 2. *Intussusception.* 3. *Volvulus.*	1. Care similar to that for Levin NG tube—irrigated. 2. Connected to suction, not sterile technique. 3. Orders will be written on how to advance the tube, gently pushing tube a few inches each hour; client position may affect advancement of tube. 4. X rays determine the desired location of tube.
Salem sump	Double-lumen tube with vent to protect gastric mucosa from trauma of suctioning.	Same as Levin tube.	1. Irrigate vent (blue tubing) with air only. 2. See Levin tube.
Gastrostomy tube	1. Inserted into stomach via abdominal wall. 2. May be used for decompression. 3. Used *long term for feedings.*	Conditions affecting *esophagus* where it is impossible to insert a nasogastric tube.	1. Principles of tube feedings same as with Levin nasogastric tube, *except* no danger that tube may be near trachea. 2. If permanent, tube may be replaceable.
T-tube	To drain bile from the common bile duct *until* edema has subsided.	*Cholecystectomy* when a CDE (common duct exploration) or choledochostomy was also done.	1. Bile drainage is controlled by the *height* of the drainage bag. 2. Clamp tube as ordered to see if bile will flow into duodenum normally.
Hemovac	A type of closed-wound drainage connected to suction—used to *drain* a *large amount* of serosanguineous drainage from under an incision.	1. *Mastectomy.* 2. *Total hip procedures.* 3. *Total knee procedures.*	1. May compress unit, and have portable vacuum or connect to wall suction. 2. Small drainage tubes may get clogged—physician may irrigate these at times.
Jackson-Pratt	1. A method of closed-wound suction drainage—indicated when tissue displacement and tissue trauma may occur with rigid drain tubes (i.e., Hemovac). 2. See Hemovac.	1. *Neurosurgery.* 2. *Neck surgery.* 3. *Mastectomy.* 4. *Total knee and hip replacement.* 5. *Abdominal surgery.* 6. *Urologic procedures.*	1. Empty reservoir when full, to prevent loss of wound drainage and back-contamination. 2. See Hemovac.
Three-way Foley	To provide avenues for *constant irrigation* and *constant drainage* of the urinary bladder.	1. Transurethral resection (TUR). 2. *Bladder* infections.	1. Watch for blocking by clots—causes bladder spasms. 2. Irrigant solution often has antibiotic added to the normal saline.
Suprapubic catheter	To *drain bladder* via an opening through the abdominal wall above the pubic bone.	*Suprapubic* prostatectomy.	May have orders to irrigate p.r.n. or continuously.
Ureteral catheter	To *drain urine* from the pelvis of one kidney, or for *splinting* ureter.	1. *Cystoscopy* for diagnostic work-ups. 2. *Ureteral surgery.* 3. *Pyelotomy.*	1. *Never* clamp the tube—pelvis of kidney only holds 4–8 cc. 2. Use *only* 5 cc sterile normal saline if ordered to irrigate.

Note: This review focuses on care of the tubes, not on total client care.
Source: Jane Vincent Corbett, RN, MS, Ed.D., Associate Professor, School of Nursing, University of San Francisco. Used with permission.

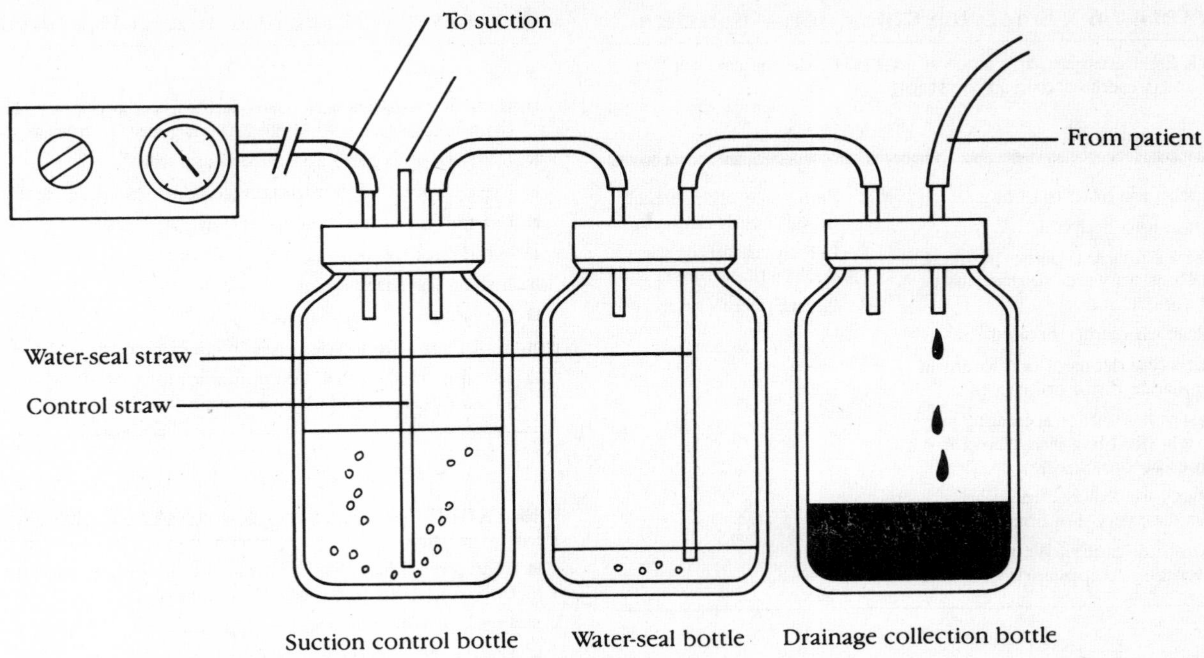

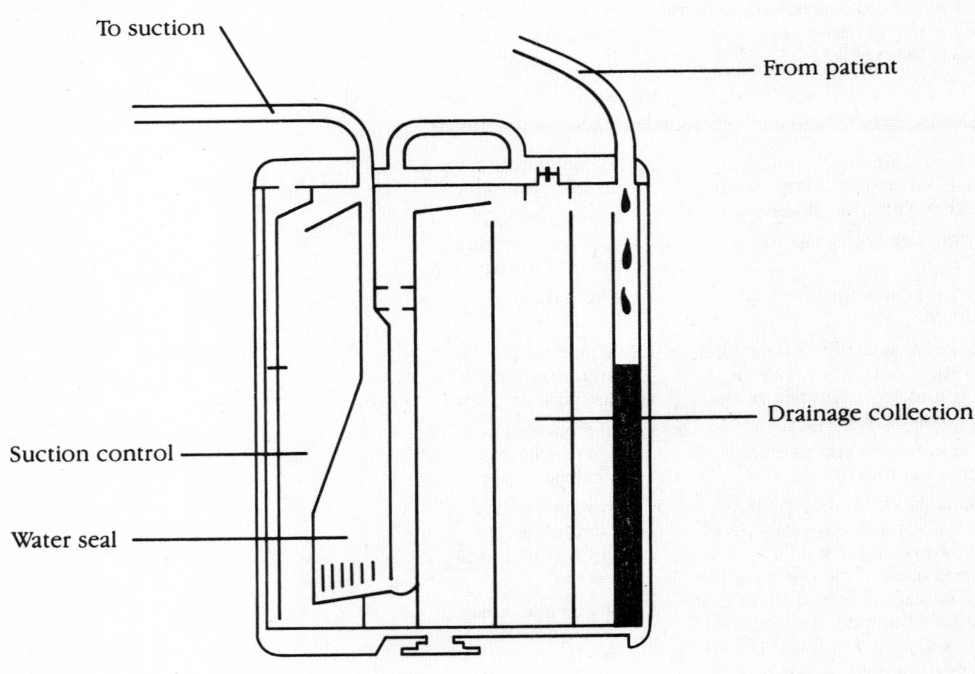

■ FIGURE 7.1
Comparison of (a) chest bottles and (b) the Pleurovac. (Reprinted with permission from the May issue of *Nursingyear.* Copyright © 1990. Springhouse Corporation, 1111 Bethlehem Pike, Springhouse, PA 19477. All rights reserved.)

TABLE 7.6 Emptying Colostomy Appliance

Check for drainage in appliance at least twice during each shift If drainage present (diarrhea type stool):

Do	Do Not
1. Unclip the bottom of bag.	1. Remove appliance each time it needs emptying.
2. Drain into bedpan.	2. Use any materials that could irritate bowel.
3. Use a squeeze type bottle filled with warm water to rinse inside of appliance.	3. Ignore client's needs.
4. Clean off clamp if soiled.	
5. Put a few drops of deodorant in appliance if not odorproof.	
6. Fasten bottom of appliance securely (fold bag over clamp 2–3 times before closing).	
7. Check for leakage under appliance every 2–4 hours.	
8. Communicate with client while attending to appliance.	

TABLE 7.7 Changing Colostomy Appliance

Gather equipment: gloves, skin prep packet, colostomy appliance measured to fit stoma properly (if new surgical stoma, it will continue to shrink with the healing process; use stoma measuring guide), skin barrier, warm water and soap, face cloth/towel, plastic bag for disposal of old equipment. Remember that bowel is very fragile; also, working near bowel increases peristalsis, and feces and flatulence may be expelled.

Do	Do Not
1. Remove old appliance carefully, pulling from area with least drainage to area with most drainage.	1. Tear appliance quickly from skin.
2. Wash skin area with soap and water.	2. Wash stoma with soap; put anything dry onto stoma.
3. Observe skin area for potential breakdown.	3. Irritate skin or stoma.
4. Use packet of skin prep on the skin around the stoma. Allow skin prep solution to dry on skin before applying colostomy appliance.	4. Put skin prep solution onto stoma; it will cause irritation.
5. Apply skin barrier you have measured and cut to size.	5. Make opening too large (increases risk of leakage).
6. Put appliance on so that the bottom of the appliance is easily accessible for emptying (e.g., if client is out of bed most of the time, put the bottom facing the feet; if client is in bed most of the time, have bottom face the side). Picture-frame the adhesive portion of the appliance with 1-inch tape.	6. Have appliance attached so client can't be involved in own care.
7. Put a few drops of deodorant in appliance if not odorproof.	7. Use any materials that would irritate bowel.
8. Use clamp to fasten bottom of appliance.	8. Avoid conversation/eye contact.
9. Talk to client (or communicate in best way possible for client) during and after procedure.	9. Contaminate other incisions.
10. Use good handwashing technique.	

TABLE 7.8 Care of Artificial Dentures

- Wear gloves.
- If client cannot remove own dentures, grasp upper plate at the front teeth and move up and down gently to release suction.
- Lift the upper plate up one side at a time.
- Use extreme care not to damage dentures while cleaning.
- Use tepid, not hot, water to clean.
- Avoid soaking for long periods of time.
- Inspect for sharp edges.
- Do oral cavity assessment.
- Replace moistened dentures in client's mouth.
- Use appropriately labeled container for storage when dentures are to remain out of client's mouth.

TABLE 7.9 Caring for an Artificial Eye

- With gloved hand pull lower eyelid down over the infraorbital bone and exert pressure below the eyelid.
- Pressure will make the eye pop out.
- Handle eye prosthesis carefully.
- Using aseptic techniques, cleanse socket with saline-moistened gauze, stroking from the inner to outer canthus.
- Wash the prosthesis in warm normal saline.
- To reinsert, gently pull the client's lower lid down, raise the upper lid if necessary, slip the saline-moistened eye prosthesis gently into the socket, and release the lids.

NURSING TREATMENTS

■ TABLE 7.10 Universal Blood and Body Fluid Precautions

The Centers for Disease Control recommend universal blood and body fluid precautions (also referred to as *universal precautions*) in the care of *all* clients, especially those in emergency care settings, in which the risk of blood exposure is increased and the infection status of the client is unknown. In other words, the nurse should treat all body substances or fluids of all cients as if they are potentially infectious.

The CDC (1988) recommend that these precautions apply to blood and to body fluids containing visible **blood,** as well as to **semen** and **vaginal** secretions; to tissues, and to the following fluids: **cerebrospinal fluid, synovial fluid, pleural fluid, peritoneal fluid, pericardial fluid,** and **amniotic fluid.** Universal precautions do *not* apply to *nasal secretions, sputum, saliva, sweat, tears, urine, feces,* and *vomitus unless* they contain visible blood. Blood is the single most important source of HIV, HBV, and other bloodborne pathogens in the health care setting.

Protective barriers—gloves, gowns, masks, and protective eyewear—reduce the risk of exposure to potentially infective materials. The following specific precautions are recommended.

- Wash your hands thoroughly and immediately after accidental contact with body substances containing blood, between clients, and immediately after gloves are removed.
- Wear gloves when touching blood and body fluids containing blood as well as when handling items or surfaces soiled with blood or body fluids.
- Change gloves between client contacts.
- Use sterile gloves for procedures involving contact with normally sterile areas of the body.
- Use examination gloves for procedures involving contact with mucuous membranes, unless otherwise indicated, and for other client care or diagnostic procedures that do not require the use of sterile gloves.
- Do not wash or disinfect surgical or examination gloves for reuse. Washing with surfactants may cause *wicking,* i.e., the enhanced penetration of liquids through undetected holes in the glove. Disinfecting agents may cause deterioration.
- Use general-purpose utility gloves (e.g., rubber household gloves) for housekeeping chores involving potential blood contact and for instrument cleaning and decontamination procedures. Utility gloves may be decontaminated and reused but should be discarded if they are peeling, cracked, or discolored or if they have punctures, tears, or other evidence of deterioration.
- Wear gloves when performing phlebotomy (venipuncture):
  - if the nurse has cuts, scratches, or other breaks in the skin.
  - in situations where hand contamination with blood may occur, e.g., with an uncooperative client.
  - when the nurse is learning phlebotomy techniques.
- Wear gloves when performing finger and/or heel sticks on infants and children.
- Wear masks and protective eyewear (glasses, goggles) or face shields to protect the mucous membranes of your mouth, nose, and eyes during procedures that are likely to generate droplets of blood or other body fluids to which universal precautions apply.
- Wear a disposable plastic apron or gown during procedures that are likely to generate splatters of blood or other body fluid (e.g., peritoneal fluid) and soil your clothing.
- To prevent injuries, place used disposable needle-syringe units, scalpel blades, and other sharp items in puncture-resistant containers for disposal. Discard used needle-syringe units *uncapped* and *unbroken.* Puncture-resistant containers should be located as close as practicable to use areas.
- Place mouthpieces, resuscitation bags, or other ventilation devices in areas where the need for emergency mouth-to-mouth resuscitation is predictable—even though saliva has *not* been implicated in HIV transmission.
- If a nurse has exudative lesions or weeping dermatitis, it is necessary to refrain from all direct client care and from handling client-care equipment until the condition is resolved.
- Handle soiled linen as little as possible and with minimum agitation to prevent gross microbial contamination of the air and of persons handling the linen. Place and transport linen soiled with blood or body fluids in leakage-resistant bags.
- Put all specimens of blood and listed body fluids in well-constructed containers with secure lids to prevent leakage during transport. When collecting specimens, take care to avoid contaminating the outside of the container.
- Use a chemical germicide that is approved for use as a hospital disinfectant to decontaminate work surfaces after there is a spill of blood or other body fluids. In the absence of a commercial germicide, a solution of sodium hypochlorite (household bleach) in a 1:10 dilution is effective. Before decontaminating areas, first remove visible material. Wear gloves during cleaning and decontaminating procedures.
- Follow agency policies for disposal of infective waste both when disposing of and when decontaminating contaminated materials.
- Carefully pour bulk blood, suctioned fluids, and excretions containing blood and secretions down drains that are connected to a sanitary sewer.

Source: U.S. Department of Health and Human Services. Public Health Service. Update: Universal precautions for prevention of transmission of Human Immunodeficiency Virus, Hepatitis B Virus, and other bloodborne pathogens in health care settings, *MMWR,* June 24, 1988; 37:107. Centers for Disease Control. Recommendations for prevention of HIV transmission in health care settings. *MMWR Supplement.* August 21, 1987; 36:25–185.

NURSING TREATMENTS

■ QUESTIONS

Select the one best answer for each question, and fill in the answer circle beside the answer number.

1. A client's laboratory values indicate hemoconcentration secondary to fluid loss. Which of the following intravenous solutions should the nurse anticipate will be ordered as the most appropriate during initial fluid replacement therapy?

○ 1. 10% dextrose and saline. **AN**
○ 2. 5% dextrose and water with 60 mEq KCl. **8**
○ 3. 5% dextrose and water only. **PhI**
○ 4. Distilled water.

2. Prior to surgery, Mr. Chen was instructed in the use of an incentive spirometer. The *primary* purpose of this activity is:

○ 1. To encourage coughing. **AN**
○ 2. To arouse and stimulate the client. **6**
○ 3. To encourage deep breathing. **PhI**
○ 4. To measure tidal volume and expiratory reserve volume.

3. The nurse explains to Mr. Chen's family that humidification is given with oxygen administration because:

○ 1. Oxygen is highly permeable in water, thereby increasing gaseous diffusion. **AN 6**
○ 2. Oxygen is very drying to the mucous membranes. **PhI**

○ 3. The partial pressures of oxygen are increased by water dilution, allowing more oxygen to reach the alveoli.
○ 4. Water acts as a carrier substance facilitating movement of oxygen across the respiratory membrane.

4. To correctly administer 1000 mL of 5% dextrose/water in 10 hours using a standard 15-drop administration set, you would adjust Mr. Chen's infusion rate to:
○ 1. 32 drops per minute. **IMP**
○ 2. 25 drops per minute. **6**
○ 3. 20 drops per minute. **PhI**
○ 4. 15 drops per minute.

5. The nurse would conclude that a client's fasting serum-glucose levels are normal if the results are:
○ 1. 30–60 mg/100 mL of blood. **AN**
○ 2. 80–120 mg/100 mL of blood. **4**
○ 3. 120–140 mg/100 mL of blood. **PhI**
○ 4. 140–200 mg/100 mL of blood.

6. A laboratory test to measure serum- and urine-glucose levels before and after ingestion of a glucose load has been ordered. The nurse knows that the test to be done is called:
○ 1. Fasting blood sugar. **AN**
○ 2. Glucose tolerance test. **4**
○ 3. Postprandial blood glucose. **PhI**
○ 4. Tolbutamide response test.

7. After a glucose tolerance test, the nurse would look for the blood-glucose levels to return to normal in about how many hours?
○ 1. One. **EV**
○ 2. Two. **4**
○ 3. Three. **PhI**
○ 4. Four

8. Following a gastroscopy, the nurse will plan to offer the client food or fluid:
○ 1. As soon as he returns to the room. **PL**
○ 2. One hour later, or after he is fully alert. **4**
○ 3. Three to 4 hours later, or when the gag reflex returns. **PhI**
○ 4. Six to 8 hours later to prevent the electrolyte imbalance that may occur with this procedure.

9. The nurse knows that a 24-hour urine-for-creatinine clearance measures which of the following kidney functions?
○ 1. Filtration fraction. **AS**
○ 2. Glomerular filtration rate. **8**
○ 3. Renal blood flow. **PhI**
○ 4. Quantity and specific gravity of urinary output.

10. A client asks why the intravenous pyelogram (IVP) is being done. You tell him the purpose is to:
○ 1. Determine the size, shape, and placement of the kidneys. **IMP**
○ 2. Test renal tubular function and the patency of the urinary tract. **8** **SECE**
○ 3. Measure renal blood flow.
○ 4. Outline the kidney vasculature.

11. Your care of a client before an IVP includes:
○ 1. Warning the client that the contrast medium may produce a warm, flushed feeling in the face and a salty taste in the mouth. **IMP** **8** **PhI**
○ 2. Administering radiopaque capsules 6 hours before the test.
○ 3. Ascertaining whether or not the client has any allergies to mercury.
○ 4. Pushing fluids until 2 hours before the test, to prevent dehydration.

12. The nurse's preparation of the client undergoing IV cholangiogram includes:
○ 1. Administering radiopaque tablets the evening before the examination. **PL** **4**
○ 2. A fatty meal the evening before examination. **SECE**
○ 3. Forcing fluids for 6–8 hours before examination.
○ 4. Informing the client he/she may experience a feeling of warmth, flushing of face, and/or a salty taste when the contrast medium is injected.

13. The nurse knows that the most important effect of intermittent positive-pressure breathing (IPPB) is:
○ 1. Mobilization of bronchial secretions. **EV**
○ 2. Increased alveolar ventilation. **6**
○ 3. Prevention of atelectasis. **PhI**
○ 4. Decreased airway resistance.

■ ANSWERS/RATIONALE

1. (3) Initial fluid therapy is directed toward increasing fluid volume and urine output. No. 1, being a hypertonic solution that would act to increase intracellular dehydration, is therefore contraindicated. Once adequate urinary output has been established, potassium salts are added (No. 2) to relieve hypokalemia. The amount of added potassium chloride depends on the extent of hypokalemia. No. 4, distilled water, is a hypotonic solution; that is, it does not contain any additional electrolytes. Hypotonic solutions, such as 0.45% sodium chloride, are frequently given to relieve hypertonic syndromes. However, distilled water is never given in fluid replacement therapy.

2. (3) The purpose of the incentive spirometer is to encourage deep breathing. The client is able to directly visualize his progress by the number and height of balls he is able to raise. *After-effects* of this activity may indeed be coughing up of sputum (No. 1) and arousal (No. 2) as the client competes with himself. Incentive spirometry can be used as a rough measure of tidal volume and expiratory reserve volume (No. 4) since the client breathes in deeply and exhales completely into the incentive spirometer.

3. (2) Humidification of oxygen is extremely important in reducing its drying effects on the mucous membranes of

NURSING TREATMENTS

Key to codes following questions Nursing process: **AS**, Assessment; **AN**, Analysis; **PL**, Plan; **IMP**, Implementation; **EV**, Evaluation. Category of human function: **1**, Protective; **2**, Sensory-perceptual; **3**, Comfort, Rest, Activity, and Mobility; **4**, Nutrition; **5**, Growth and Development; **6**, Fluid-Gas Transport; **7**, Psycho-Social-Cultural; **8**, Elimination. Client need: **SECE**, Safe, Effective Care Environment; **PhI**, Physiological Integrity; **PsI**, Psychosocial Integrity; **HPM**, Health Promotion/Maintenance. See frontmatter for full explanation.

the bronchial tree. Humidification of oxygen is generally provided by a water nebulizer. Nos. 1, 3, and 4 are incorrect because oxygen is not highly permeable in water; thus water tends to inhibit rather than facilitate oxygen diffusion across the respiratory membrane. Humidification expands the volume of the inhaled gas, but by doing so it decreases the partial pressure of the gas in the alveoli. Normal alveolar partial pressures of oxygen are approximately 100 mm Hg, whereas the partial pressures of oxygen in the atmosphere are approximately 135 mm Hg.

4. (3) Maintenance of infusion rates as ordered is extremely important. In this example, you can use the following equation:

$$\frac{\text{gtts/mL of given set}}{\text{60 min/h}} \times \text{total volume/h} = \text{gtts/minute}$$

Thus,

$$\frac{15}{60} \times 100 = \frac{1}{4} \times 100 = 25 \text{ gtts/min}$$

5. (2) Normal fasting serum-glucose levels are 80–120 mg/100 mL of blood. Levels below 60 (No. 1) indicate hypoglycemia; levels about 120 mg/100 (Nos. 3 and 4) indicate hyperglycemia.

6. (2) Procedurally, the client to receive the glucose tolerance test consumes a high-carbohydrate diet for 3 days before the test. All drugs that may influence the test are discontinued during this period (oral contraceptives, aspirin, steroids). On the day of the test, a fasting blood sugar (No. 1) and urine are collected before the test, as controls. After ingestion of a glucose load, specimens of blood and urine are collected at hourly intervals for 3 hours. In diabetes mellitus, glucose levels are elevated. The postprandial blood glucose (No. 3) is determined by giving the client an oral glucose load only. Blood-glucose levels are then evaluated in 2 hours. Usually glucose levels will return to normal during this period of time. The tolbutamide response test (No. 4) may also be utilized to confirm diabetes. After the client fasts overnight, a baseline FBS is drawn. Intravenous tolbutamide is then given, and blood samples drawn in 20–30 minutes. After this test the client should be given orange juice and instructed to eat breakfast.

7. (3) Within 3 hours the client's serum-glucose levels should not only have returned to normal, but some hypoglycemia should be expected. Nos. 1, 2, and 4 are incorrect.

8. (3) Following gastroscopy, food and fluids are withheld until the gag reflex returns (generally 2–3 hours) in order to prevent aspiration. The gag reflex is inactivated by either an anesthetic spray or an oral preparation gargled by the client prior to insertion of the gastroscopy tube. Inhibition of the gag reflex facilitates insertion. Nos. 1 and 2 are incorrect because the period of time is too brief. No. 4 is incorrect not only because it is generally unnecessary to wait 6–8 hours for the gag reflex to return, but because this procedure does not precipitate an electrolyte imbalance.

9. (2) Decreased amounts of creatinine in the urine are a reflection of the glomerular filtration rate, indicating the ability of the kidney to clear the renal blood of this substance. The filtration fraction is simply the amount of glomerular filtrate entering the tubules (No. 1). Renal blood flow is estimated by measuring renal excretion of PAH (para-aminohippuric acid) (No. 3). Though the amount and specific gravity of urine may be determined, it is not the primary function of this laboratory test (No. 4).

10. (2) Intravenous pyelogram tests both the function and patency of the kidneys. After the intravenous injection of a radiopaque dye, the size, location, and patency of the kidneys can be observed by roentgenogram, as well as the patency of the urethra and bladder as the kidneys function to excrete the dye. No. 1 is an example of a KUB, or flat plate of the abdomen, which can reveal gross structural changes in the kidneys and urethra. Renal blood flow (No. 3) is determined by the injection of PAH (para-aminohippuric acid) and measurement of its excretion in the urine. No. 4 is an example of renal angiogram.

11. (1) Client teaching includes telling the client that a warm, flushed sensation and salty taste may occur from the contrast medium. The contrast medium is given by IV injection during the procedure, not in capsule form (No. 2). No. 3 is incorrect because allergies to iodine, not to mercury, are the concern. Fluids are not pushed prior to this procedure; they are withheld for up to 8 hours prior to testing, to produce a slight dehydration that aids in concentrating the contrast medium in the kidneys and urinary system (No. 4).

12. (4) The client is informed of possible reaction to injection of the contrast medium, which is administered by an IV injection at the time of the test, not by tablets the evening before (No. 1). No. 2 is incorrect because clients given anything by mouth are given a low-fat meal the evening before IV cholangiogram or oral cholecystogram. Since the client is quite ill at this time, she may or may not be able to tolerate oral intake. However, in order to have a clear visualization of the gallbladder, the bowel is cleansed, food and fluids are withheld, not forced (No. 3), for 6–8 hours.

13. (2) The most important effect of intermittent positive-pressure breathing (IPPB) is increased alveolar ventilation. It also helps to mobilize secretions (No. 1), decrease the occurrence of atelectasis (No. 3), and decrease airway resistance (No. 4) through mechanical bronchodilation.

■ UNIT

8

Ethical and Legal Aspects in Nursing

ETHICS/LAW

■ NURSING ETHICS

Nursing ethics involves rules and principles to guide right conduct in terms of moral duties and obligations to protect the rights of human beings. In nursing, ethical codes provide professional standards and formal guidelines for nursing activities to protect both the nurse and the client.

I. Code of ethics—serves as a frame of reference when judging priorities or possible courses of action. *Purposes:*

A. To provide a basis for regulating relationships between nurse, client, co-workers, society, and profession.

B. To provide a standard for excluding unscrupulous nursing practitioners and for defending nurses unjustly accused.

C. To serve as a basis for nursing curricula.

D. To orient new nurses and the public to ethical professional conduct.

ANA CODE FOR NURSES*

1. The nurse provides services with respect for human dignity and the uniqueness of the client unrestricted by considerations of social or economic status, personal attributes, or the nature of health problems.
2. The nurse safeguards the client's right to privacy by judiciously protecting information of a confidential nature.
3. The nurse acts to safeguard the client and the public when health care and safety are affected by the incompetent, unethical, or illegal practice of any person.
4. The nurse assumes responsibility and accountability for individual nursing judgments and actions.
5. The nurse maintains competence in nursing.
6. The nurse exercises informed judgment and uses individual competence and qualifications as criteria in seeking consultation, accepting responsibilities, and delegating nursing activities to others.
7. The nurse participates in activities that contribute to the ongoing development of the profession's body of knowledge.
8. The nurse participates in the profession's efforts to implement and improve standards of nursing.
9. The nurse participates in the profession's efforts to establish and maintain conditions of employment conducive to high-quality nursing care.

*American Nurses Association. *1985 Code for Nurses, with Interpretive Statements.* Kansas City, Missouri: American Nurses Association. Reprinted with permission. (Interpretive statements for each portion of the above Code for Nurses are available from ANA.)

10. The nurse participates in the profession's effort to protect the public from misinformation and misrepresentation and to maintain the integrity of nursing.

11. The nurse collaborates with members of the health professions and other citizens in promoting community and national efforts to meet the health needs of the public.

II. Bioethics—a philosophical field that applies ethical reasoning process for achieving clear and convincing reasons to issues and dilemmas (conflicts between two obligations) in health care.*

A. Purpose of applying ethical reflection to nursing concerns:

1. Improve quality of professional nursing decisions.
2. Increase sensitivity to others.
3. Offer a sense of moral clarity and enlightenment.

B. Framework for analyzing an ethical issue:

1. Who are the relevant participants in the situation?
2. What is the required action?
3. What are the probable and possible consequences of the action?
4. What is the range of alternative actions or choices?
5. What is the intent or purpose of the action?
6. What is the context of the action?

C. Principles of bioethics:

1. *Autonomy*—the right to make one's own decisions.
2. *Nonmaleficence*—the intention to do no wrong.
3. *Beneficence*—the principle of attempting to do things that benefit others.
4. *Justice*—the distribution, as fairly as possible, of benefits and burdens.
5. *Veracity*—the intention to tell the truth.
6. *Confidentiality*—the social contract guaranteeing another's privacy.

III. Client rights*

A. Right to appropriate treatment.

B. Right to individualized treatment plan, subject to review and reassessment.

C. Right to active participation in treatment, with the risk, side effects, and benefits of all medication and treatment (and alternatives) to be discussed.

D. Right to give and withhold consent (exceptions: emergencies and when under conservatorship).

E. Right to be free of experimentation unless following recommendations of the National Commission on Protection of Human Subjects.

F. Right to be free of restraints except in an emergency.

G. Right to human environment.

H. Right to confidentiality.

I. Right of access to personal treatment record.

J. Right to as much freedom as possible to exercise constitutional rights of association (e.g., having visitors) and expression.

K. Right to information about these rights in both written and oral form, presented in an understandable manner at outset and periodically thereafter.

L. Right to assert grievances through a grievance mechanism that includes the power to go to court.

M. Right to obtain advocacy assistance.

N. Right to criticize or complain about conditions or services without fear of retaliatory punishment or other reprisals.

O. Right to referral to complement the discharge plan.

IV. Conflicts and problems

A. *Personal values versus professional duty*—nurses have the right to refuse to participate in those areas of nursing practice that are against their personal values, as long as a client's welfare is not jeopardized. Example: therapeutic abortions.

B. *Nurse versus agency*—conflict may arise regarding whether or not to give out needed information to a client or to follow agency policy, which does not allow it. Example: an emotionally upset teenager asks a nurse about how to get an abortion, a discussion which is against agency policy.

C. *Nurse versus colleagues*—conflict may arise when determining whether to ignore or report others' behavior. Examples: you see another nurse steal medications; you know that a peer is giving a false reason when requesting time off; or you observe an intoxicated colleague.

D. *Nurse versus client/family*—conflict may stem from knowledge of confidential information. Should you tell? Example: client or family member relates a vital secret to the nurse.

E. *Conflicting responsibilities*—to whom is the nurse primarily responsible when needs of the agency and the client differ? Example: an MD asks a nurse not to list all supplies used for client care, as the client cannot afford to pay the bill.

F. *Ethical dilemmas*—stigma of diagnostic label (e.g., AIDS, schizophrenic, addict); involuntary psychiatric confinement; right to control individual freedom; right to suicide; right to privacy and confidentiality.

V. Trends in nursing practice

A. Overall characteristics:

1. Some trends are subtle and slow to emerge; others are obvious and quickly emerge.
2. Trends may conflict; some will prevail, others get modified by social forces.

B. General trends:

1. *Broadened focus of care*—from care of ill to care of sick and healthy, from care of individual to care of family. Focus on prevention of illness, promotion of optimum level of health, holism.
2. *Increasing scientific base*—in bio-social-physical sciences, not mere reliance on intuition, experience, and observation.
3. *Increasingly complex technical skills* and use of *technologically advanced equipment,* such as monitors and computers.

* Davis AJ: Ethical Dilemmas in Nursing. Recorded at JONA and Nurse Educator's 1981 Joint Leadership Conference. Available from Teach 'Em, Inc., 160 E. Illinois St., Chicago, IL 60611.

4. *Increased independence* in use of judgment, such as teaching nutrition in pregnancy and providing primary prenatal care.
5. *New roles,* such as *nurse-clinician,* require advanced skills in a particular area of practice. Examples: psychiatric nurse consults with staff about problems; *primary care* nurse takes medical histories and does physical assessment; one nurse coordinates 24-hour care during hospital stay; *independent nurse practitioner* has her or his own office in community where clients come for care; case management.
6. *Community nursing services* rather than hospital-based; needs of the healthy are served as well as those of the ill.
7. *Development of nursing standards* to reflect specific nursing functions and activities.
   a. Assure *safe* standard of care to clients and families.
   b. Provide criteria to measure *excellence* and *effectiveness* of care.

C. Trends in care of childbearing family

1. *Consumerism*
   a. Consumer push for humanization and individualization of health care during the childbearing cycle to reflect client's role in decision making, preferences, and cultural diversity.
   b. Emphasis on family-centered care (including father, siblings, grandparents).
   c. Increase in options available for conduct of birth experience and setting for birth: birthing homes, alternative birth center (ABC) in hospitals; birthing chairs; side-lying position for birth; family-centered cesarean delivery; health care provider (MD, RN, lay midwife); length of postpartum stay.
   d. Increased consumer awareness of legal issues, clients' rights.
   e. Major nursing role: client advocate.
2. *Social trends*
   a. Alternative life-styles of families—single parenthood, communal living, surrogate motherhood, marriages without children.
   b. Earlier sexual experimentation—availability of assistance to emancipated minors.
   c. Increase in number of older (over 38) primiparas.
   d. Legalization of abortion; availability to emancipated minors.
   e. Smaller families.
   f. Rising divorce rates.
3. *Technologies*
   a. Development of genetic and bioengineering techniques.
   b. Development of prenatal diagnostic techniques, with options for management of each pregnancy.
   c. In-vitro fertilization and embryo transplantation.

D. Trends in community mental health (1960s–1980s):

1. Shift from institutional to community-based care.
2. Preventive services.
3. Consumer participation in planning and delivery of services.
4. Original 12 essential services (1975) reduced to 5(*) (1981).
   *a. 24-hour in-patient care.
   *b. Outpatient care.
   *c. Partial hospitalization (day or night).
   d. Emergency care.
   *e. Consultation and education.
   f. Follow-up care.
   g. Transitional services.
   h. Services for children and adolescents.
   i. Services for elderly.
   *j. Screening services (courts).
   k. Alcohol abuse services.
   l. Drug abuse services.
5. Protecting human rights of persons in need of mental health care.
6. Developing an advocacy program for chronically mentally ill.
7. Improving delivery of services to underserved and high risk populations (e.g., minorities).

E. ANA Standards of Nursing Practice:

STANDARDS OF NURSING PRACTICE*

1. The collection of data about the health status of the client/patient is systematic and continual. The data are accessible, communicated, and recorded.
2. Nursing diagnoses are derived from health status data.
3. The plan of nursing care includes goals derived from the nursing diagnoses.
4. The plan of nursing care includes priorities and the prescribed nursing approaches or measures to achieve the goals derived from the nursing diagnoses.
5. Nursing actions provide for client/patient participation in health promotion, maintenance, and restoration.
6. The nursing actions assist the client/patient to maximize his health capabilities.
7. The client/patient's progress or lack of progress toward goal achievement is determined by the client/patient and the nurse.
8. The client/patient's progress or lack of progress toward goal achievement directs reassessment, reordering of priorities, new goal setting, and revision of the plan of nursing care.

*American Nurses Association. *1973 Standards of Nursing Practice.* Kansas City, Missouri. Reprinted with permission. (Rationale and assessment factors for the above Standards of Nursing Practice are available from the ANA.)

ETHICS/LAW

F. *Four levels* of nursing practice:
 1. *Promotion of health* to increase level of wellness. Example: provide dietary information to reduce risks of coronary artery diseases.
 2. *Prevention of illness or injury.* Example: immunizations.
 3. *Restoration of health.* Example: teach how to change dressing, care for wound.
 4. *Consolation of dying*—assist person to attain peaceful death.

G. *Five components* of nursing care:
 1. *Nursing care activities*—assist with basic needs, give medications and treatments; observe response and adaptation to illness and treatments; teach self-care; guide rehabilitation activities for daily living.
 2. *Coordination of total client care*—all health team members should work together toward common goals.
 3. *Continuity of care*—when the location of care is transferred.
 4. *Evaluation of care*—flexibility and responsiveness to changing needs: clients' reactions and perceptions of their needs.
 5. *Delegate responsibility and direct nursing care provided by others*—based on particular client/family needs and on skills of other nursing personnel.

H. *Three main nursing roles* in relation to care of clients and their families. The emphasis of each role varies with the situation, with adaptation of skills and modes of care as necessary.
 1. *Therapeutic role* (instrumental). Function: work toward "cure" in acute setting.
 2. *Caring role* (expressive). Function: provide support through human relations, show concern, demonstrate acceptance of differences.
 3. *Socializing role.* Function: offer distractions and respite from focus on illness.

■ NURSING ORGANIZATIONS

I. International Council of Nurses (ICN)

A. *Purpose:* to provide a medium through which national nursing associations can work together, share common interests. Formed in 1899.

B. *Functions:*
 1. Serves as representatives of and spokespersons for nurses at international level.
 2. Promotes organization of national nurses' associations.
 3. Assists national organizations to develop and improve services for public health practice of nursing and social/economic welfare of nurses.

II. World Health Organization (WHO)—special intergovernmental agency of the UN, formed in 1948.

A. *Purpose:* to bring all people to the highest possible level of health.

B. *Functions:* provides assistance in the form of education, training, improving health standards, fighting disease, and reducing water pollution in member countries.

III. American Nurses Association (ANA)—national professional association in the US, composed of the nurses' associations of the 50 states, Guam, Virgin Islands, Puerto Rico, and Washington, D.C.

A. *Purpose:* to foster high standards of nursing practice and promote the education and welfare of nurses.

B. *Functions:* officially represents professional nurses in this country and internationally; defines practice of nursing; lobbies and promotes legislation affecting nurses' welfare and practice.

IV. National League for Nursing (NLN)—composed of both individuals and agencies.

A. *Purpose:* to foster the development and improvement of all nursing services and nursing education.

B. *Functions*
 1. Provides educational workshops.
 2. Assists in recruitment for nursing programs.
 3. Provides testing services for both RN and LPN (LVN) nursing programs.

■ LEGAL ASPECTS OF NURSING

I. Definition of terms

A. *Common law:* accumulation of law as a result of judicial court decisions.

B. *Civil law* (private law): law that derives from legislative codes and deals with relations between private parties.

C. *Public law:* concerns relationships between an individual and the state. The thrust of public law is to attain what are deemed valid public goals, such as reporting child abuse.

D. *Criminal law:* concerns actions against the safety and welfare of the public, such as robbery. It is part of the public law.

E. *Informed consent*—implies that significant benefits and risks of any procedure, as well as alternative methods of treatment, have been explained; person has had time to ask questions and have these answered; person has agreed to the treatment voluntarily and is legally competent to give consent; and communication is in a language known to the client.

F. *Reasonably prudent nurse*—nurse must react as a reasonably prudent nurse trained in that specialty area would react. For example, if a nurse works with fetal monitors, she must know how to use the monitors, know how to read the strips, and know what actions to take based on the findings.

II. Nursing licensure—mandatory licensure required in order to practice nursing.

A. *Nurse Practice Act:* each state has one to protect nurses' professional capacity, to legally control nursing through licensing, and to define standards of professional nursing.

B. *American Nurses Association (1980):* "The practice of nursing means the performance for compensation of professional services requiring substantial specialized knowledge of the biological, physical, behavioral, psychological, and sociological sciences and of nursing theory as the basis for assessment, diagnosis, planning, intervention, and evaluation in the promotion and maintenance of health; the casefinding and management of illness, injury, or infirmity; the restoration of optimum function; or the achievement of a dignified death. Nursing practice includes but is not limited to administration, teaching, counseling, supervision, delegation, and evaluation of practice and execution of the medical regimen, including the administration of medications and treatments prescribed by any person authorized by state law to prescribe. Each registered nurse is directly accountable and responsible to the consumer for the quality of nursing care rendered."*

C. *Revoking a license:* Board of Examiners in each state in the US and each province in Canada has the power to revoke licenses for just cause, such as incompetence in nursing practice, conviction of crime, drug addiction, obtaining license through fraud, or hiding criminal history.

III. Crimes and torts

A. *Crime:* an act committed in violation of societal law and punishable by fine or imprisonment. A crime does not have to be intended (as in giving a client an accidental overdose that proves to be lethal).

1. *Felonies:* crimes of a serious nature (such as murder) punishable by imprisonment of greater than six months.
2. *Misdemeanors:* crimes of a less serious nature (such as shoplifting), usually punishable by fines or short prison term or both.

B. *Tort:* a wrong committed by one individual against another or another's property. Fraud, negligence, and malpractice are torts (such as losing a client's hearing aid or bathing him in water that burns him).

1. *Fraud:* misrepresentation of fact with intentions for it to be acted upon by another person (such as falsifying college transcripts when applying for a graduate nursing program).
2. *Negligence:* "Omission to do something that a reasonable person, guided by those *ordinary* considerations which ordinarily regulate human affairs would *do,* or doing something which a reasonable and prudent person would *not* do" (Creighton, 1975, p. 119). Types of negligent acts related to:
   a. Sponge counts: incorrect counts or failure to count.
   b. Burns: heating pads, solutions, steam vaporizers.
   c. Falls: siderails left down, baby left unattended.
   d. Failure to observe and take appropriate action—forgetting to take vital signs and check dressing in a newly postoperative client.
   e. Wrong medicine, wrong dose and concentration, wrong route, wrong client.
   f. Mistaken identity—wrong client for surgery.
   g. Failure to communicate—ignore, forget, fail to report complaints of client or family.
   h. Loss of or damage to client's property—dentures, jewelry, money.
3. *Malpractice:* part of the law of negligence as applied to the *professional* person; any professional misconduct, unreasonable lack of skill, or lack of fidelity in professional duties, such as accidentally giving wrong medication or forgetting to give correct medication or instilling wrong strength of eyedrops into the client's eyes. Proof of intent to do harm is not required in acts of commission or omission.

IV. Invasion of privacy—compromising a person's right to withhold self and own life from public scrutiny. Implications for nursing—avoid unnecessary discussion of client's medical condition; client has a right to refuse to participate in clinical teaching; obtain consent prior to teaching conference.

V. Libel and slander—wrongful action of communication that damages person's reputation by print, writing, or pictures (libel), or by spoken word using false words (slander). Implications for nursing—make comments about client only to another health team member caring for that client.

VI. Privileged communications—information relating to condition and treatment of client requires confidentiality and protection against invasion of privacy. This applies only to court proceedings. Selected person does not have to reveal in court a client's communication to him or her. The purpose of privileged communication is to encourage the client to communicate honestly with the treating practitioner. It is the client's privilege at any time to permit the professional to release information.

Therefore, if the client asks the nurse to testify, the nurse must truthfully give all information. However, if the nurse is a witness against the client, without the client's permission to release information, the nurse must keep the information confidential by invoking the privileged communication rule if the state law recognizes it and if it applies to the nurse.

VII. Assault and battery—violating a person's right to refuse physical contact with another.

A. Definitions

1. *Assault*—the attempt to touch another or the threat to do so.
2. *Battery*—physical harm through willful touching of person or clothing.

B. Implications for nursing—need to obtain consent to treat, with special provisions when clients are under age, unconscious, or mentally ill.

VIII. Good Samaritan Act—protects health practitioners against malpractice claims resulting from assistance provided at scene of an emergency (unless there was willful wrongdoing) as long as the level of care provided is the same as any other reasonably prudent person would give under similar circumstances.

IX. Nurses' responsibilities to the law

A. A nurse is liable for nursing acts, even if directed to do something by an MD.

B. A nurse is not responsible for the negligence of the employer (hospital).

C. A nurse is responsible for refusing to carry out an order for an activity believed to be injurious to the client.

D. A nurse cannot legally diagnose illness or prescribe treatment for a client. (This is the MD's responsibility.)

E. A nurse is legally responsible when participating in a criminal act (such as assisting with criminal abortions or taking medications for own use from client's supply).

ETHICS/LAW

*American Nurses Association. 1980. *The Nursing Practice Act; Suggested State Legislation,* p. 6. Kansas City, Missouri. American Nurses Association. Reprinted with permission.

F. A nurse should reveal client's confidential information only to appropriate health care team members.

G. A nurse is responsible for explaining nursing activities but not for commenting on medical activities in a way that may distress the client or the MD.

H. A nurse is responsible for recognizing and protecting the rights of clients to refuse treatment or medication, and for reporting their concerns and refusals to the MD or appropriate agency people.

I. A nurse needs to respect the dignity of each client and family.

QUESTIONS MOST FREQUENTLY ASKED BY NURSES ABOUT NURSING AND THE LAW

I. Taking orders

A. *Should I accept verbal phone orders from an MD?* Generally, no. Specifically, follow your hospital's bylaws, regulations, and policies regarding this. Failure to follow the hospital's rules could be considered negligence.

B. *Should I follow an MD's orders if (a) I know it is wrong, or (b) I disagree with his judgment?* Regarding (a)—No, if you think a reasonable, prudent nurse would not follow it; but first inform the MD and record your decision. Report it to your supervisor. Regarding (b)—Yes, because the law does not allow you to substitute your nursing judgment for a doctor's medical judgment. Do record that you questioned the order and that the doctor confirmed it before you carried it out.

C. *What can I do if the MD delegates a task to me for which I am not prepared?* Inform the MD of your lack of education and experience in performing the task. Refuse to do it. If you inform him or her and still carry out the task, both you and the MD could be considered negligent if the client is harmed by it. If you do not tell the MD and carry out the task, you are solely liable.

II. Obtaining client's consent for medical and surgical procedures: *Is a nurse responsible for getting a consent for medical/surgical treatment?* Obtaining consent requires explaining the procedure and risks involved, which is the MD's responsibility. A nurse may accept responsibility for *witnessing* a consent. This carries with it little legal liability other than obtaining the correct signature and describing the client's condition at time of signing.

III. Client's records

A. *What should be written in the nurse's notes?* All facts and information regarding a person's condition, treatment, care, progress, and response to illness and treatment. Purpose of record: factual documentation of care given to meet legal standards; used to refute unwarranted claims of negligence or malpractice.

B. *How should data be recorded?* Entries should:

1. State time given.
2. Be written and signed by caregiver or supervisor who observed action.
3. Follow chronologic sequence.
4. Be accurate, precise, and clear.
5. Be legible.
6. Use universal abbreviations.

IV. Confidential information

A. *If called on the witness stand in court, do I have to reveal confidential information?* It depends on your state, as each state has its own laws pertaining to this. Consult a lawyer. Inform the judge and ask for specific directions before relating in court information that was given to you within a confidential, professional relationship.

B. *Am I justified in refusing (on the basis of "invasion of privacy") to give information about the client to another health agency to which a client is being transferred?* No. You are responsible for providing continuity of care when the client is moved from one facility to another. Necessary and adequate information should be transferred between professional health care workers. The client's consent for this exchange of information should be obtained. Circumstances under which confidential information can be released include:

1. By authorization and consent of the client.
2. By order of the court.
3. By statutory mandate, as in reporting cases of child abuse or communicable diseases.

V. Liability for mistakes—yours and others.

A. *Is the hospital or the nurse liable for mistakes made by the nurse while following orders?* Both the hospital and the nurse can be sued for damage if a mistake made by the nurse injures the client. The nurse is responsible for her own actions. The hospital would be liable, based on the doctrine of *respondeat superior.*

B. *Who is responsible if a nursing student or another staff nurse makes a mistake. The supervisor? The instructor?* Ordinarily the instructor and/or supervisor would not be responsible unless the court thought the instructor and/or supervisor was negligent in supervising or in assigning a task beyond the capability of the person in question. No one is responsible for another's negligence unless he or she contributed to or participated in that negligence. Each person is personally liable for his or her own negligent actions and failure to act as a reasonably prudent nurse.

C. *Am I responsible for injury to a client by a staff member who was observed (but not reported) by me to be intoxicated while giving care?* Yes, you may be responsible. You have a duty to take reasonable action to prevent a client's injury.

VI. Good Samaritan Act: *For what would I be liable if I voluntarily stopped to give care at the scene of an accident?* You would be protected under the Good Samaritan Act and required to live up to reasonable and prudent nursing standards in those specific circumstances. You would not be treated by the law as if you were performing under professional standards of properly sterile conditions, with proper technical equipment.

VII. Leaving against medical advice (AMA): *Would I or the hospital be liable if a client left "AMA," refusing to sign the appropriate hospital forms?* None of the involved parties would ordinarily be liable in this case as long as (a) the medical risks were explained, recorded, and witnessed, and (b) the client is a competent adult. The law permits clients to make decisions that may not be in their own best health interest. You cannot interfere with the right and exercise of the decision to accept or reject treatment.

VIII. Restraints: *Can I put restraints on a client who is combative even if there is no order for this?* Only in an emergency, for a limited time, for the limited purpose of protecting the client from injury, not for convenience of personnel. Notify attending MD immediately. Consult with another staff member, obtain client's consent if possible, document facts and reasons, get co-worker to witness the record. Apply restraints properly, check frequently to ensure they do not impair circulation, cause pressure sores, or other injury. Remove restraints at the first opportunity, and use them only as a last resort after other reasonable means have not been effective. Restraints of any degree may constitute false imprisonment. Freedom from unlawful restraint is a basic human right protected by law.

IX. Wills: *What do I do when a client asks me to be a witness to her or his will?* There is no legal obligation to participate as a witness, but there is a moral and ethical obligation to do so. You should not, however, help draw up a will as this could be considered practicing law without a license. You would be witnessing that (a) the client is signing the document as her or his last will and testament; (b) at that time, to the best of your knowledge, the client (testator) was of sound mind, was lucid, and understood what she or he was doing (that is, she or he must not be under the influence of drugs or alcohol or otherwise unable to know what she or he is doing); and (c) the testator was under no overt coercion, as far as you could tell, but was acting freely, willingly, and under her or his own impetus.

X. Disciplinary action

A. *For what reasons may the RN license be suspended or revoked?*

1. Obtaining license by fraud (omission of information, false information).
2. Negligence and incompetence.
3. Substance abuse.
4. Conviction of crime (state or federal).
5. Practicing medicine without a license.
6. Practicing nursing without a license (expired, suspended).
7. Allowing unlicensed person to practice nursing or medicine.
8. Giving client care while under the influence of alcohol or other drugs.
9. Habitually using drugs.
10. Discriminatory and prejudicial practices in giving client care (pertaining to race, color, sex, age, or ethnic origin).

B. *What could happen to me if I am proven guilty of professional misconduct?*

1. License may be revoked.
2. License may be suspended.
3. Behavior may be censured and reprimanded.
4. You may be placed on probation.

C. *Who has the authority to carry out any of the above penalties?* The State Board of Registered Nursing that granted your license.

D. *I am the head nurse. One of my nurses aides has a history of failing to appear to work and not giving notice of or reason for absence. How should I handle this?* An employee has the right to know hospital policies, what is expected of an employee, and what will happen if an employee does not meet the expectations stated in his or her job description or in hospital policies and procedures. As a head nurse, you need to document behavior factually, clearly, and concisely, as well as any discussion and decision about future course of action. The employee needs the chance to read and sign it. The head nurse then sends a copy to her or his supervisor.

XI. Floating: *Is a nurse hired to work in psychiatry obligated to cover in ICU when the latter is understaffed?* The issue is the hiring contract (implied or expressed). The contract is a composite of the mutual understanding by involved parties of rights and responsibilities, any written documents, and hospital policies. If the nurse was hired as a psychiatric nurse, he or she could legally refuse to go to the ICU. If the hospital intends to float personnel, such a policy should be clearly stated during the hiring process. Also at this time the employer should determine the employee's education, skills, and experience. On the other hand, if emergency staffing problems exist, a nurse should go to the ICU regardless of personal preference.

XII. Dispensing medication: *Can a nurse legally remove a drug from a pharmacy when the pharmacy is closed (during the night) if the MD insists that the nurse go to the pharmacy to get the specifically prescribed medication immediately?* Within the legal boundaries of the Pharmacy Act, a nurse may remove one dose of a particular drug from the pharmacy for a particular client during an unanticipated emergency within a limited time and availability of resources. However, the hospital should have a written policy for the nurse to follow and should authorize a specific person to use the services of the pharmacy under certain circumstances.

XIII. Illegible orders: *What should I do if I cannot decipher the MD's handwriting when she or he persists in leaving illegible orders?* Talk to the MD regarding the dangers of your giving the wrong amount of the wrong medication via the wrong route at the wrong time. If that does not help, follow appropriate channels. Do not follow an order you cannot read. You will be liable for following orders you thought were written.

XIV. Heroic measures: *The wife of a terminally ill client approaches me with the request that heroic measures not be used on her husband. She has not discussed this with him but knows that he feels the same way. Can I act on this request?* No. The client is the only one who can legally make the decision as long as he or she is mentally competent.

XV. Medication: *An MD orders pain medication p.r.n. for a client. The client asks for the medication, but when I question her she says the pain "isn't so bad." If in my judgment the client's pain is not severe, am I legally covered if I give half of the pain medication dosage ordered by the MD?* A nurse cannot substitute his or her judgment for the MD's. If you alter the amount of medication prescribed by the MD without a specific order to do so, you may be liable for practicing medicine without a license.

XVI. Malfunctioning equipment: *At the end-of-shift report the nurse going off duty tells me that the tracheal suctioning machine is malfunctioning and describes how she got it to work. Should I plan to use the machine in the evening shift and follow her suggestions about how to make it work?* Do not plan to use equipment that you know is not functioning properly. You could be held liable since you could reasonably foresee that proper functioning of equipment would be needed for your client. You have been put on notice that there are defects. Report this to the supervisor or person responsible for maintaining equipment in proper working order.

ETHICAL AND LEGAL CONSIDERATIONS IN INTENSIVE CARE OF THE ACUTELY ILL NEONATE

I. Responsibilities of the health agency

A. Provide an NICU or transfer to another hospital.

B. *Personnel—adequate number trained in neonate diseases, special treatment, and equipment.*

C. Equipment—adequate supply on hand, functioning properly (especially temperature regulator in incubator, oxygen analyzer, blood-gas machine).

II. Dying infants

A. Decision regarding resuscitation in cardiac arrest, with brain damage from cerebral anoxia. It is difficult to predict the effect of anoxia in infancy on the child's later life.

B. Decision to continue supportive measures.

C. Issue of euthanasia, such as in severe myelomeningocele at birth.

1. Active euthanasia (giving overdose).
2. Passive euthanasia (not placing on respirator).

III. Extended role of nurse in NICU—may raise issues of nursing practice versus medical practice, as when a nurse draws blood samples for blood-gas determinations without prior order. To be legally covered:

A. The nurse must be trained to perform specialized functions.

B. The functions must be written into the nurse's job description.

IV. Issue of negligence—such as cross-contamination in nursery.

V. Issue of malpractice—such as assigning care of critically il infant on respirator to untrained student or aide.

A. May be liable for inaccurate bilirubin studies for neonatal jaundice; may be legally responsible if brain damage occurs in absence of accurate laboratory tests.

B. May be liable for brain damage in infant due to respiratory or cardiac distress. Nurse needs to make sure that there are frequent blood-gas determinations to ensure adequate oxygen to prevent brain damage. Nurse also needs to make sure that the infant is not receiving too high a concentration of oxygen, which may lead to retrolental fibroplasia.

LEGAL ASPECTS OF PSYCHIATRIC CARE

I. Four sets of criteria to determine criminal responsibility at time of alleged offense

A. *M'Naghten Rule* (1832)—a person is not guilty if:

1. Person did not know the *nature and quality* of the act.
2. Person could not distinguish right from wrong—if person did not know what he or she was doing, person did not know it was wrong.

B. *The Irresistible Impulse Test* (used together with M'Naghten Rule)—person knows right from wrong, but:

1. Driven by *impulse* to commit criminal acts regardless of consequences.
2. Lacked premeditation in sudden violent behavior.

C. *American Law Institute's Model Penal Code (1955) Test*

1. Not responsible for criminal act if person lacks capacity to "appreciate" the wrongfulness of it or to "conform" conduct to requirements of law.
2. Excludes "an abnormality manifested only by repeated criminal or antisocial conduct"—namely, psychopathology.
3. Includes "knowledge" and "control" criteria.

D. *Durham Test* (Product Rule—1954): accused not criminally responsible if act was a "product of mental disease." Discarded in 1972.

II. Types of admissions

A. *Voluntary:* person, parent, or legal guardian applies for admission; person agrees to receive treatment and to follow hospital rules; civil rights are retained.

B. *Involuntary:* process and criteria vary among states (Figure 8.1).

III. Legal and civil rights of hospitalized clients—the right to:

A. Wear own clothes, keep and use personal possessions and reasonable sum of money for small purchases.

B. Have individual storage space for private use.

C. See visitors daily.

D. Have reasonable access to confidential phone conversations.

E. Receive unopened correspondence and have access to stationery, stamps, and a mailbox.

F. Refuse: shock treatments, lobotomy.

IV. Concepts central to community mental health (Community Mental Health Act, 1980)

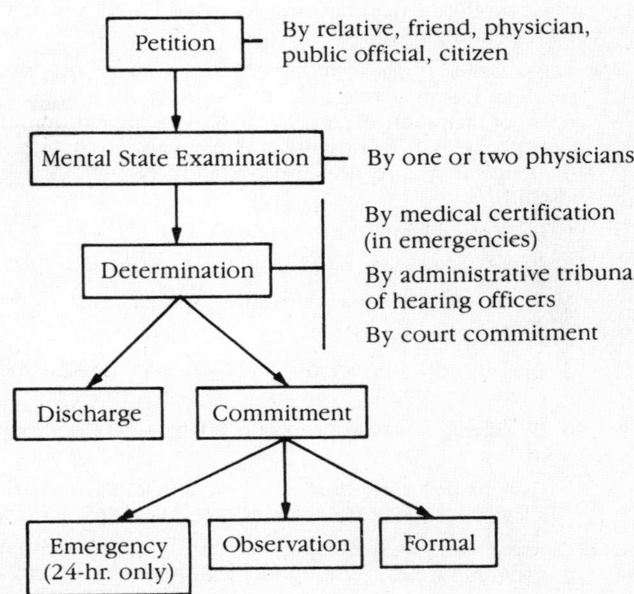

■ **FIGURE 8.1**
Typical procedure for involuntary commitment.

ETHICS/LAW

A. *Systems* perspective: scope of care moves beyond the individual to the community, with influences from biologic, psychologic, and sociocultural forces.

B. Emphasis on *prevention: primary* (reduce incidents by preventing harmful social conditions); *secondary* (early identification and treatment of disorders to reduce duration); *tertiary* (early rehabilitation to reduce impairment from disorders).

C. *Interdisciplinary collaboration:* flexible roles based on unique areas of expertise.

D. *Consumer participation and control.*

E. *Comprehensive services:* outpatient care, partial hospitalization, 24-hour hospitalization and emergency care; consultation and education; screening services.

F. *Continuity of care.*

LEGAL ASPECTS OF PREPARING A CLIENT FOR SURGERY

I. No surgical procedure, however minor, can proceed without the voluntary, informed, and written consent of the client.

A. Surgical permits are witnessed by the physician, nurse, or other authorized person.

B. Surgical permits protect the client against unsanctioned surgery and also protect the surgeon and hospital staff against claims of unauthorized operations.

C. Informed consent means that the operation has been fully explained to the client, including possible complications and disfigurements, as well as whether any organ or parts of the body are to be removed.

D. Adults and emancipated minors may sign their own operative permits if they are mentally competent; permission for surgery of minor children and incompetent or unconscious adults must be obtained from a responsible family member or guardian.

E. The signed operative permit is placed in a prominent place on the client's chart and accompanies the client to the operating room.

F. *Legal issues in the emergency room: record keeping* plays an essential role in both the prevention and defense of malpractice suits. Detailed documentation not only provides for continuity of care but also perpetuates evidence that care was appropriately given. Records should:

1. Be written legibly.
2. Clearly note events and time of occurrence.
3. Contain all lab slips and results of other tests.
4. Describe events and clients objectively.
5. Clearly note physician's parting instructions to the client.
6. Be signed where appropriate, such as with doctor's orders.
7. Contain descriptions of every event that might lead to a lawsuit, such as fights, injuries, equipment failures.

G. *Consent*—although there is no law requiring written consent before performing medical treatment, all elective procedures can only be performed if the client has been fully informed and voluntarily consents to the procedure.

1. If informed consent cannot be obtained because of the client's condition and immediate treatment is necessary to save life or safeguard health, the emergency rule can be applied. This rule implies consent. However, if time allows, it is advisable to obtain either oral or written informed consent from someone who has authority to act for the client.
2. Verbal consents should be recorded in detail, witnessed and signed by *two* individuals.
3. Written or verbal consent can be given by alert, coherent, or otherwise competent adults, by parents, legal guardian, or person in loco parentis (one standing in for the parent with the parent's rights, duties, and responsibilities) of minors or incompetent adults.
4. If the minor is 14 years old or older, consent must be acquired from the minor as well as from the parent or legal guardian. Emancipated minors can consent for themselves.

■ QUESTIONS

Select the one best answer for each question, and fill in the answer circle beside the answer number.

1. An ambiguous order was written by a physician. The nurse, familiar only with the injectible form of the medication and unaware of the elixir form, believed the order incorrect. The nurse should:

○ 1. Ask the two physicians who are currently on the unit whether she should give the medication as she understood the order. **IMP 7 SECE**
○ 2. Ask her head nurse if the order is correct.
○ 3. Call the physician who ordered the medication.
○ 4. Contact the nursing supervisor about the problem.

2. A female client had been receiving a drug by injection over a number of weeks. As the client's clinical symptoms changed, the physician wrote an order on the client's order sheet changing the mode of administration from injection to oral. When the nurse on the unit, who had been off duty for several days, was preparing to give the medication to the client by injection, the client objected and referred the nurse to the physician's new orders. The nurse should:

○ 1. Go back to the order sheet and check for the order. **IMP 7**
○ 2. Talk with the nurse who had taken care of this particular client while she had been off duty. **SECE**
○ 3. Talk with the head nurse about the advisability of using oral rather than injectible medications.
○ 4. Check the order sheet for the changed order and then speak with the attending physician concerning the changed order.

3. A nurse had been caring for a female client whose vital signs had previously been unstable. The nurse had not had a coffee break or a lunch break all day. By 2 P.M. the client had been stable for a number of hours. The physician in charge had seen the client and had told the nurse that the client appeared "much improved." The nurse should:

○ 1. Leave for lunch break. **IMP**
○ 2. Forego lunch break because of the client's previous unstable condition. **7 SECE**

○ 3. Arrange to eat lunch in the client's room.
○ 4. Discuss the situation with the nurse in charge of the unit and determine who should cover the client while the staff nurse is at lunch.

4. In a certain hospital, whenever there are clients in the recovery room, two nurses are usually present. The hospital policy expects the nurses to take their breaks before clients arrive from surgery. On this particular day, there are two nurses on duty and two clients in the recovery room who have had minor surgeries performed that morning. Nurse A had not had a coffee break that morning. Nurse A should:
○ 1. Stay because hospital policy expects there to be two nurses in attendance while there are clients in the recovery room. **IMP** 7 **SECE**
○ 2. Leave for coffee break because there are only two clients in the recovery room and one nurse can handle two clients quite easily.
○ 3. Talk with the nursing supervisor and secure permission from him or her.
○ 4. Leave to get coffee and come right back.

5. While driving down a freeway, a nurse spots an overturned car with the driver lying next to the car. Which of the following best describes what the nurse can do without being held liable?
○ 1. She or he may drive on without stopping, or stop and render emergency first aid. **PL** 7
○ 2. She or he may stop, start to render aid, and then leave. **SECE**
○ 3. She or he must stop at the scene of an accident and render first aid.
○ 4. She or he may stop and render aid, but if he or she performs a medical act, he or she may be charged with illegal practice of medicine.

6. Your client is terminally ill and has asked you to witness his will. Which of the following statements is true?
○ 1. As a nurse, you have a legal obligation to act as a witness to a will. **EV** 7
○ 2. As a nurse, you should help the client draw up a will. **SECE**
○ 3. As a nurse, you should make sure that the client is of sound mind, is lucid (not under the influence of drugs or alcohol), and understands what he or she is doing.
○ 4. Only lawyers or family members can act as a witness to a will. If the nurse acts as a witness, the will may automatically be declared invalid.

7. Your client has just returned from the recovery room. He is complaining of pain that is not "too severe" and has requested pain medication. You noted that the client had been given pain medication in the recovery room. Which of the following statements indicates the best action to take?
○ 1. Administer the dosage the physician had ordered on a p.r.n. basis. **IMP** 7
○ 2. Consult the physician and let him know that the client is requesting medication for pain that is "not too severe." **SECE**
○ 3. Give half of the pain medication dosage ordered as p.r.n. by the physician.
○ 4. Chart that the client was complaining of pain but that it was "not too severe."

8. As a nurse, if I am being sued for malpractice, which of the following will occur?
○ 1. My license will be revoked or suspended *automatically.* **EV** 7
○ 2. I will automatically be put on probation until the matter is cleared up. **SECE**
○ 3. I will automatically be charged with a crime.
○ 4. The State Board of Registered Nurses would be notified of the suit, and, depending on the offense and outcome of the suit, it might hold a hearing to determine the status of the license.

9. A nurse's license will be revoked or she or he will be put on probation for which of the following?
○ 1. The nurse lost a malpractice suit. **EV**
○ 2. The nurse was found guilty of practicing while under the influence of drugs or alcohol. 7 **SECE**
○ 3. The nurse was accused of negligence.
○ 4. The nurse gave a wrong medication.

10. If a nurse applies restraints on her client, she *may* be held liable by the client for restraint of freedom of movement (false imprisonment) if:
○ 1. She does not immediately obtain an order from the physician. **EV** 7
○ 2. She does so after other means to subdue the client have failed. **SECE**
○ 3. She tries but fails to obtain the client's consent.
○ 4. She applies restraints for the convenience of the personnel.

11. The nurse has been working with a terminally ill male client for weeks. The client is lucid. His wife pleads with the nurse not to use heroic measures on her husband but to let him die "with dignity." The nurse should:
○ 1. Tell the wife that she needs to talk with the attending physician, client (if possible), and other significant people about her concerns. **IMP** 7 **HPM**
○ 2. Act on the wife's request.
○ 3. Ignore the wife's request and proceed with the client's care.
○ 4. Tell the wife that to do as she had requested would be equivalent to murdering the client.

12. The surgical unit has not been busy all day. The head nurse and a few of the senior staff nurses are talking near the desk. You, as a new nurse, answer the telephone so that the other nurses may continue their conversation. Dr. D is on the line and would like you to take a telephone order. He states that the order is important. You do not know Dr. D or the client to whom he is referring very well. As a new nurse, your best response would be:
○ 1. To take the telephone order. **IMP**
○ 2. To refuse to take the order. 7
○ 3. To ask the head nurse or one of the other senior staff nurses to take the order. **SECE**
○ 4. To ask the physician to call back so you can take the telephone order *after* you have read the hospital policy manual.

Key to codes following questions Nursing process: **AS**, Assessment; **AN**, Analysis; **PL**, Plan; **IMP**, Implementation; **EV**, Evaluation. Category of human function: **1**, Protective; **2**, Sensory-perceptual; **3**, Comfort, Rest, Activity, and Mobility; **4**, Nutrition; **5**, Growth and Development; **6**, Fluid-Gas Transport; **7**, Psycho-Social-Cultural; **8**, Elimination. Client need: **SECE**, Safe, Effective Care Environment; **PhI**, Physiological Integrity; **PsI**, Psychosocial Integrity; **HPM**, Health Promotion/Maintenance. See frontmatter for full explanation.

13. Which of the following statements concerning consent is *false?*
- ○ 1. If an informed consent is not obtained from the client, then the nurse, doctor, and/or hospital may be liable for assault. **EV 7 SECE**
- ○ 2. One need only obtain a general consent to treatment.
- ○ 3. In an emergency a nurse may do what she or he can do to save life and limb, even in cases in which she or he has no consent.
- ○ 4. Consent may be given by conduct as well as expressed words.

14. A nurse gave a client the wrong medication. The client was seriously injured. The client sued. Who will most likely be held liable?
- ○ 1. The nurse. **EV**
- ○ 2. No one, because it was just an accident. **7**
- ○ 3. The hospital. **SECE**
- ○ 4. The nurse and the hospital.

15. The supervisor of a cardiovascular unit was responsible for checking staffing patterns. She assigned Nurse B to work on the unit because Nurse B had had numerous years of experience on that particular unit. That evening, Nurse B made a treatment error and a client was injured. Who is liable?
- ○ 1. Nurse B. **AN**
- ○ 2. Nurse B and the supervisor. **7**
- ○ 3. Nurse B and the hospital. **SECE**
- ○ 4. Nurse B, the supervisor, and the hospital.

16. Nurse A noticed that Nurse B was intoxicated while giving care. However, Nurse A did not report this fact to her supervisor. That same day, Nurse B made a medication error and a client was injured. Who *may* be held responsible?
- ○ 1. Nurse B (the one intoxicated). **AN**
- ○ 2. Nurse A, nurse B, and the hospital. **7**
- ○ 3. Nurse A (the one who did not report nurse B). **SECE**
- ○ 4. Nurse B (the one intoxicated) and the hospital.

17. A graduate nurse who was new to a unit was caring for an elderly gentleman. The physician on call ordered a treatment that the nurse had not heard of. She should:
- ○ 1. Inform the physician of her lack of education and experience and refuse to do the treatment without supervision. **IMP 7 SECE**
- ○ 2. Inform the physician of her lack of education and experience and then proceed to perform the treatment.
- ○ 3. Refuse to perform the treatment.
- ○ 4. Carry out the treatment as best she can.

18. Which of the following is *not* true about informed consent?
- ○ 1. Obtaining consent is the responsibility of the physician. **AN 7**
- ○ 2. A nurse may accept responsibility for witnessing a consent form. **SECE**
- ○ 3. A physician subjects himself or herself to liability if he or she withholds any facts that are necessary to form the basis of an intelligent consent.
- ○ 4. If a nurse witnesses a consent for surgery, the nurse is, in effect, indicating that the client is "informed."

19. You are a staff nurse coming on shift. The *day* nurse has just told you that the suction equipment in Mr. Clay's room is not working properly. Since you will be working with Mr. Clay, you should do which of the following?
- ○ 1. Follow the *day* nurse's suggestions on how to get the malfunctioning equipment to work. **IMP 7**
- ○ 2. Continue to use the malfunctioning machine, hoping that it will function for your shift. **SECE**
- ○ 3. Ask your supervisor to show you how to work with the malfunctioning equipment.
- ○ 4. Replace the equipment or report it to whomever is responsible for maintaining equipment in proper working condition.

20. Duncan Green is a competent adult who has refused treatment and wishes to leave AMA (against medical advice). Mr. Green has also refused to sign any of the appropriate AMA forms. All of the following statements are true except:
- ○ 1. The physician and/or hospital is always liable for any injury that might occur as a result of the client's decision to leave AMA. **EV 7 SECE**
- ○ 2. The law usually permits competent adult clients to make decisions that may not be in their own best health interest.
- ○ 3. Even if the client is a competent adult, the law may interfere with the client's decision to refuse medical treatment if the client has small children that need care.
- ○ 4. The physician might be held liable if it can be proven that the client did not receive sufficient information about risks involved with leaving AMA.

21. Nurse A, the only Spanish-speaking emergency room nurse, admitted a 6-year-old child. The child's mother explained in Spanish that she had removed two ticks from the child the previous day. The child was now running a very high temperature and had a rash on his abdomen. Nurse A reported her information to the emergency room physician, who did not speak Spanish. The nurse failed to tell the doctor about the ticks. The physician diagnosed the child as having measles. Over the course of the day, the child's health deteriorated until he died. Who is liable?
- ○ 1. Nurse A. **EV**
- ○ 2. Nurse A and the physician. **7**
- ○ 3. Nurse A and the hospital. **SECE**
- ○ 4. Physician.

22. Nurse B was on weekend call for the operating room. Late Saturday night, the nursing supervisor called nurse B to tell her that they were expecting an emergency appendectomy within the hour. While gowning the surgeon, nurse B smelled alcohol on the doctor's breath. Nurse B mentioned this to the anesthesiologist, who also admitted smelling alcohol on the surgeon. Both the nurse and the anesthesiologist felt the surgeon was somewhat unstable on his feet. However, neither the nurse nor the other doctor said anything. If the client had been injured during the surgery, who would have been liable?
- ○ 1. Nurse B, anesthesiologist, surgeon, and hospital. **AN 7**
- ○ 2. Nurse B and surgeon. **SECE**
- ○ 3. Surgeon and hospital.
- ○ 4. Hospital, surgeon, and anesthesiologist.

23. A child about 11 months old was brought by her mother to a hospital for examination, diagnosis, and treatment. The child was seen by a nurse and physician. At the time, the child was suffering from a comminuted spiral fracture of the right tibia and fibula that gave the appearance of having been caused by twisting. The child also had numerous bruises and burns on her body. In addition, she had a nondepressed linear fracture of the skull in the process of healing. When approached, the child demonstrated fear and apprehension. The mother had no explanation for the child's wounds. No further X rays were taken, and the child was released to the mother without report to concerned agencies. One month later the child was brought in again by the mother and was seen by a different physician. The second physician correctly diagnosed the battered-child syndrome and filed the proper reports. The child was placed in a foster home, and the foster home filed suit. Who may be liable?

- ○ 1. First nurse, first doctor, and hospital. **AN**
- ○ 2. First doctor. **7**
- ○ 3. No one. **SECE**
- ○ 4. First nurse.

24. While getting a client ready for surgery, Nurse A removed the client's dentures. The nurse wrapped the dentures in a towel so as not to break them and left them on the bedside stand. While the nurse was out of the room, two nurses' aides stripped the bed and threw all the linen, including the towel, in the laundry hamper. Upon returning from surgery, the client requested her dentures. However, the nurse and nursing aides were unable to find them. Who is liable?

- ○ 1. The nurse. **AN**
- ○ 2. The nurse and the hospital. **7**
- ○ 3. The nurse and nursing aides. **SECE**
- ○ 4. The nurse, nursing aides, and hospital.

25. A teenage girl who had complained of dizziness the previous day wanted to take a shower. The physician gave his permission for the client to shower with assistance. The nurse started to get the girl out of bed and over to the shower. The nurse questioned the client about her dizziness. The girl replied that she was not dizzy. The mother then said that she would watch her daughter in the shower and help her back to bed. The nurse then left the room. While the nurse was out, the client fainted getting back into bed. The client injured her head. Who is liable?

- ○ 1. The nurse. **EV**
- ○ 2. The doctor, nurse, and hospital. **7**
- ○ 3. The nurse and the hospital. **SECE**
- ○ 4. No one.

26. What does the Durham Test state about the accused?

- ○ 1. It states the same thing as the M'Naghten rule. *
- ○ 2. Accused is not criminally responsible if the act was the product of mental disease. **7** **SECE**
- ○ 3. Accused is not criminally responsible if the act was a result of impulsiveness.
- ○ 4. Accused is not criminally responsible if he or she does not appreciate the wrongfulness of the act.

27. What does voluntary admission require of the individual?

- ○ 1. The individual must ask to be admitted to a psychiatric hospital and must agree to abide by its rules. **EV** **7** **SECE**
- ○ 2. The request for hospitalization needs to originate with the individual to be admitted.
- ○ 3. The individual needs to make written application to a hospital, agree to treatment, and agree to abide by the rules.
- ○ 4. The individual needs to be responsible for the hospital bill.

28. Standards of practice for psychiatric mental health nursing have been developed by:

- ○ 1. A joint commission of psychiatric nurses and psychiatrists. * **7**
- ○ 2. Psychiatric nurses who are members of the American Nurses' Association. **SECE**
- ○ 3. A panel of representative psychiatric nurses in the United States.
- ○ 4. The Division on Psychiatric and Mental Health Nursing Practice of the American Nurses' Association.

29. The standards of practice for psychiatric mental health nursing are organized around:

- ○ 1. Different models of treatment. *
- ○ 2. Rights of the clients. **7**
- ○ 3. The nursing process. **SECE**
- ○ 4. Legal aspects of treatment.

30. The Community Mental Health Centers Amendments of 1975, Title III of Public Law 94–63:

- ○ 1. Cut the flow of funds to community mental health centers and set forth general guidelines for service. * **7** **SECE**
- ○ 2. Extended the flow of funds to community mental health centers and set forth specific guidelines for service.
- ○ 3. Cut the flow of funds to community mental health centers and set forth specific guidelines for service.
- ○ 4. Extended the flow of funds to community mental health centers and set forth general guidelines for service.

31. Congress, in the Mental Health Centers Act of 1974, also stated that it wanted to:

- ○ 1. Increase federal operation funds to centers and have centers under federal support. * **7**
- ○ 2. Provide funding on a declining basis at the federal level and encourage the goal of independence from federal support. *
- ○ 3. Provide funding on a declining basis at the federal level but maintain federal control.
- ○ 4. Get out of the community mental health business.

32. The principal recommendation of the Report of the President's Commission on Mental Health, 1978, was:

- ○ 1. The federal government should get out of mental health. * **7**
- ○ 2. The government should upgrade the old federal grant program for community mental health to encourage the creation of necessary services where they are inadequate and to increase the flexibility of communities planning a comprehensive network of services. *
- ○ 3. Community mental health programs should strictly adhere to the provision of specific services to all communities.
- ○ 4. A new federal grant program should be established for community mental health to encourage the creation of necessary services where they are inadequate and to increase the flexibility of communities planning a comprehensive network of services.

ETHICS/LAW

* Nursing process step or client need not applicable.

33. In order for nurses to control their own profession, they need to demonstrate:
- ○ 1. Expertise in implementing client care levels already determined by law. **EV 7**
- ○ 2. The ability to participate in the drafting of health care laws that directly reflect client care levels. **SECE**
- ○ 3. The ability to participate in the drafting of laws at all levels and in all areas of health care.
- ○ 4. Neutrality by ignoring political power, thus being free from political influence in giving health care.

34. The ICN's Code for Nurses, "Ethical Concepts Applied to Nursing," approved by the Council of Nurse Representatives in 1973, states that:
- ○ 1. The professional body of nurses of a particular country carries the responsibility for nursing practice and for maintaining competence. *** 7 SECE**
- ○ 2. The hospital employing the nurse carries the responsibility for nursing practice and for maintaining competence.
- ○ 3. The laws of the country in which the nurse works carry the responsibility for nursing practice and for maintaining competence.
- ○ 4. The individual nurse carries personal responsibility for nursing practice and for maintaining competence by continual learning.

35. The National Health Planning and Resource Development Act of 1974 allows:
- ○ 1. Physicians the largest representation on local and state health care boards that make decisions about health care. *** 7 ***
- ○ 2. Hospital administrators the largest representation on local and state health care boards that make decisions about health care.
- ○ 3. The consumer the largest representation on local and state health care boards that make health care decisions.
- ○ 4. Health professionals as a group the largest representation on local and state health care boards that make health care decisions.

ETHICS/LAW

■ ANSWERS/RATIONALE

1. (3) The nurse would be negligent for any untoward effects of the drug if she or he failed to contact the physician who ordered the drug before the nurse administered it. In *Norton* v. *Argonaut Insurance Co.* [144 So. 2nd 249 (La. Ct. App. 1962)], the court stated that it was the responsibility of the nurse to clarify the order with the physician *involved,* not with other nurses (Nos. 2 and 4). No. 1 is incorrect because the doctors on the unit are not the ones who wrote the order.

2. (4) Although No. 1 is a correct answer, No. 4 is the *best* answer because the nurse would validate the changed order and learn the physician's rationale for the change. In *Larrimore* v. *Homeopathic Hospital Association* [54 Del. 449, 181 A. 2d 573 (1962)], the court found that the nurse who went ahead and gave the medication was negligent. The courts went on to say that the jury could find the nurse negligent by applying ordinary common sense to establish the applicable standard of care. Nos. 2 and 3 are incorrect because talking with nurses is not the direct way to clarify and validate an order.

3. (4) The nurse would come back to the client revitalized after having a lunch break, and the client would be covered the whole time the nurse is away. In deciding that the nurse would not be negligent to leave such a client, the court would emphasize that the question of liability should be determined in light of the circumstances as they existed at the time. When the nurse left the client, it was not foreseeable that an increased risk to the client would result. On the contrary, the client would be looked after, and the nurse could take care of her own needs, too. *Child* v. *Vancouver General Hospital* [71 W.W.R. 656 (1979)]. No. 1 does not provide for client's care. Nos. 2 and 3 are not necessary actions, for the client's condition at the time did not warrant the nurse's foregoing lunch or eating in the client's room.

4. (1) In a court of law, hospital policy may be used to set the standard of care by which the nurses' actions are judged. Since the hospital policy states that two nurses must be in attendance while clients are in the recovery room, both the nurse who left (Nos. 2 and 4) and the supervisor who authorized the nurse's absence (No. 3) would be held liable for any untoward effect on the client. *Laidlaw* v. *Lions Gate Hospital* [70 W.W.R. 727 (1969)].

5. (1) The court has stated that no one is obliged by law to assist a stranger, even if he or she can do so by a word and without the slightest danger to himself or herself. Hence, No. 3 is incorrect. But once one has undertaken to give assistance, the law imposes on him or her a duty of care toward the person assisted. Hence No. 2 is incorrect. The court also states that, under emergency circumstances, a nurse, like any other person, may perform a medical act to preserve life and limb. Either law or custom exempts such actions from coming within the medical practice acts. This, then, would rule out No. 4.

6. (3) Anyone can act as a witness. No. 1 is incorrect because a nurse has no legal obligation to participate as a witness, only a moral and ethical obligation. No. 2 would also be incorrect because only a lawyer or the client can draw up a will. If the nurse draws up the will, she or he could be charged with practicing law without a license. If a nurse does act as a witness, he or she should determine that the client is of sound mind or the will could be declared invalid—not because the nurse acted as a witness (No. 4) but because the client was not of sound mind.

7. (2) The physician should be notified of the client's complaints, and the new orders should be established. This is what the courts would consider prudent under the circumstances and what a reasonable nurse should do. No. 1 would not be the best choice because the client had already been given pain medication in the recovery room, and another full dose might be too much. Without further information, this is a very dangerous choice, and the nurse would be held liable for any untoward effects. No. 3 would also be incorrect because a nurse cannot substitute her judgment for the physician's without consulting the physician first. If a nurse alters the amount prescribed without an order from the physician, the nurse could be charged with practicing medicine without a license. No. 4 is incomplete. A nurse must chart the client's complaints but must also indicate what was done about them.

8. (4) Only the State Board of Registered Nurses has the authority to revoke or suspend a license. This can occur only after the nurse has been given a fair hearing before an impartial hearing body. Hence, Nos. 1, 2, and 3 are incorrect because they assume a penalty should be applied before the State Board is notified.

9. (2) All State Practice Acts list "guilty of practicing while under the influence of drugs or alcohol" as a reason for revocation of a license or for putting a nurse on probation. Nos. 1, 3, and 4 may cause the nurse to lose her license; however, other circumstances would have to be considered first, such as the frequency with which these had occurred.

10. (4) Freedom from unlawful restraint is a basic human right. Restraints of any type may constitute false imprisonment. False imprisonment is an actionable tort for which a nurse may be held liable by a client. The client may have an actionable case of false imprisonment if the restraints were applied for staff convenience only. Most likely the nurse would not be held liable for false imprisonment even if she does not immediately obtain an order from the physician for the restraints. However, No. 1 is not the *best* choice. Restraints should be used only in emergency situations, for a limited time, for the limited purpose of protecting the client, and not for the convenience of the staff. Even though the client's consent (No. 3) is not usually obtainable under the circumstances, the nurse should try in order to avoid being held liable for false imprisonment. However, these restraints should only be applied as a last resort (No. 2).

11. (1) This type of case is an example of the most difficult medical ethical and legal questions today. The answers are ambiguous at best. However, in this case No. 1 would be best since neither the nurse (No. 3), the wife (No. 2), nor the doctor can make that decision as long as the client is a competent adult. No. 4 is incorrect because the nurse's values should not supersede the wife's concerns for her husband's welfare.

12. (3) Get a senior nurse who knows the policies, the client, and the doctor. Generally speaking, a nurse should not accept telephone orders. However, if it is necessary to take one, follow the hospital's policy regarding telephone orders. Failure to follow hospital policy could be considered negligence. In this case, the nurse was new and did not know the hospital's policy concerning telephone orders. The nurse was also unfamiliar with the doctor and the client. Therefore the nurse should not take the order unless (a) no one else is available and (b) it is an emergency situation. Nos. 1 and 2 are both incomplete, as they do not take into account the mitigating circumstances described above. Since the doctor has said that the order is important, the nurse should not delay the doctor while she or he reads the manual; hence, No. 4 is incorrect.

13. (2) *Assault* is the unjustifiable attempt to touch another person or the threat to do so in such circumstances as to cause the other reasonably to believe that it will be carried out. The lack of informed consent is an important part of the meaning of assault. Consent is a defense to an action for assault. However, if the treatment or procedure goes beyond the client's consent (as it probably would if consent was only to "general" treatment, as in No. 2), the nurse, the doctor, and/or the hospital may be liable. Hence, No. 1 is a true statement. In an emergency situation in which the nurse is trying to save the client's life, if the client does not or cannot consent to treatment, the nurse usually will not be held to have assaulted the client. Hence, No. 3 is also a true statement. Consent may be given by conduct as well as by expressed words, as in No. 4. For example, in a case in which a person held up his arm to be vaccinated, the court said he had consented. However, it is best to get the consent in writing, specifically outlining the treatment or procedure to be performed. The consent will most likely be deemed invalid, however, if the client is a child, is mentally incompetent, or is intoxicated.

14. (4) *Both* the nurse and the hospital can be sued for damages if a mistake the nurse makes injures the client. The nurse is always responsible for his or her own actions. The hospital, as the employer, will be vicariously liable under the *respondeat superior doctrine*—the employer is liable for the negligent conduct of its nurses when the act was committed within the scope of employment. Nos. 1 and 3 are incomplete; No. 2 is incorrect.

15. (3) The hospital is *always* initially held liable under the theory of *respondeat superior*—vicarious liability of the employer. Nos. 2 and 4 are incorrect because the supervisor would *not* be responsible unless the court thought that the supervisor was negligent in supervising or assigning a task beyond the capabilities of another. In this case, Nurse B had had numerous years of experience on the cardiovascular unit. Without further data, the supervisor would not be considered negligent for assigning Nurse B to the cardiovascular unit. No. 1 is incomplete.

16. (2) This answer includes all parties: the hospital, Nurse A, and Nurse B. The hospital, as the employer, might be held liable under the theory of *respondeat superior*—vicarious liability. Nurse B would be held responsible since each nurse is personally liable for his or her own negligent actions. Nurse A might also be held responsible since every nurse is obligated to act so that clients are safe from injury. In this case, Nurse A knew of B's intoxicated state. Nurse A did not act as a *reasonably prudent nurse* when she failed to inform a supervisor. Nos. 1, 3, and 4 are incomplete.

17. (1) If the nurse informs the physician and still carries out the treatment (No. 2), both the nurse and the physician could be held liable if the client is negligently harmed. The nurse would be liable for not acting as a reasonably prudent nurse, and the physician would be liable because he knew of the nurse's lack of knowledge and did not step in to protect the patient. If the nurse does not tell the physician and still carries out the treatment (No. 4), the nurse would be solely liable. The nurse should not refuse to perform the treatment (No. 3) unless she or he has no supervision.

18. (4) The nurse who witnesses a consent for surgery or other procedure is witnessing only that the signature is that of the purported person and that the person's condition is as indicated at the time of signing. The nurse is not witnessing that the client is "informed." Nos. 1, 2, and 3 are all true statements.

19. (4) As a nurse, you should *not* plan to use equipment that you know is malfunctioning. You could be held liable since you were on notice and could reasonably foresee that properly functioning equipment would be needed by your client. Hence, Nos. 1, 2, and 3 are incorrect.

20. (1) This is the *only clearly false* option. Neither the physician nor the hospital would ordinarily be liable if (a) the medical risk is explained and a full report concerning the incident is documented and (b) the client is a competent adult. The court does not usually interfere with one's right to refuse treatment, as in No. 2. However, the court will closely scrutinize a situation in which the client's refusal to accept treatment results in death or in the client's inability to care for children. If the children might be left as wards of the court, the court may force the client to accept treatment, as in No. 3. Hence, Nos. 2, 3, and 4 do not apply, as they are true.

21. (3) The court in *John Ramsey, Jr. et al.* v. *Physicians Memorial Hospital, Inc. et al.* stated: ". . . evidence supported finding that the failure of nurse to notify physician of client history involving removal of ticks from one of the children constituted a violation of her duties as a nurse, and failure to relate the information to the physician was the contributing proximate cause of death of the child." The hospital is *also* held liable under the doctrine of *respondeat superior* for the negligent conduct of its nurses when committed within the scope of their employment. Hence, No. 1 is incomplete because it doesn't include the hospital. The physician would most likely *not* be held liable because of the language barrier and the nurse's clear failure to communicate. Hence, Nos. 2 and 4 are incorrect.

22. (1) Both nurses and doctors are under a duty to protect the safety of their clients. In this case, the client's safety was potentially jeopardized, yet neither the anesthesiologist nor the nurse reported the situation. Therefore, if something had happened to the client during surgery, the court could have made a good argument that all were negligent. Hence, Nos. 2, 3, and 4 are incomplete. When a nurse encounters a situation as described here, what can she do? First, for her own safety, the nurse should prepare a summary of the incidents. The nurse might also consult with nurse colleagues who have worked with the physician, as they could confirm or deny the problem and possibly offer support. Second, the nurse should report the incident to her supervisor and director of nursing, who have a liaison with the surgical/medical staff. If the action is not pursued successfully, the nurse can bring the problem to the attention of the hospital administrator. Again, if no action is forthcoming, the nurse may seek out a board member who might be sensitive to the situation. In any case, these are difficult situations a nurse may find himself in. There is no easy solution.

23. (1) Most state statutes provide that every hospital to which any person is brought who is suffering from any injuries inflicted by another must report the fact immediately to the local law enforcement authorities. Most state statutes also impose the same duty on other health care professionals, school officials and teachers, child care supervisors, and social workers. Hence Nos. 2 and 4 are incomplete; No. 3 is incorrect. From *Landeros* v. *Flood* as well as other cases, it seems clear that the responsibility of professional people—doctors, nurses, and others who must deal with injured children—includes the duty to report suspicious evidence to the proper authorities.

24. (2) However, it could be argued that No. 1 is correct. The nurse's liability for the negligent loss of or damage to a client's property is based on her duty as a person, trained or untrained, to act as a reasonable and ordinary, prudent person. In this case, the nurse put the dentures in a towel without a label. She might reasonably expect that aides would be stripping the linen after the client left for surgery. Therefore, her act was not that of an ordinary prudent person. The nurse would be liable. Since the nurse is liable, the hospital, as her employer, *might* also be held liable. This would be for court determination. Since the aides had no knowledge of the dentures, and they were acting reasonably, they would not be liable for the lost dentures. Hence, Nos. 3 and 4 are incorrect.

25. (4) Although No. 4 is best, this is a very close case. When family members help with a hospitalized client, liability becomes complicated. Where members of the nursing team offer to assist clients in bathing, feeding, etc., and an apparently capable family member prefers to assist the client, this is usually acceptable and neither the hospital nor the health care team is liable. Thus, Nos. 1, 2, and 3 can be eliminated as correct choices. However, the nurse should never assume that the presence of a family member obviates her helping the client.

26. (2) The Durham Test says that a person is not criminally responsible if the act was a product of mental disease. No. 1 is incorrect because the M'Naghten rule states that a person is insane if he or she cannot determine right from wrong. No. 3 is wrong because it is *not* what the Durham Test states. No. 4 is wrong because it is an interpretation of the M'Naghten rule.

27. (3) The request must be in writing. Nos. 1 and 2 are true but incomplete. No. 4 has nothing to do with voluntary admission.

28. (4) This division of the ANA sets the standards; therefore, No. 1 cannot be correct. Nos. 2 and 3 are also incorrect, although they may be part of No. 4.

29. (3) Nos. 1, 2, and 4 may be referred to in the standards, but the standards were organized around the nursing process.

30. (2) The Amendments extended the flow of funds and set forth specific guidelines for service. No. 1 is incorrect because it did not cut funds or set general guidelines. No. 3 is incorrect because it did not cut funds. No. 4 is incorrect because it did not set general guidelines.

31. (2) Congress intended to provide funding on a declining basis and to encourage independence from federal support. No. 1 is incorrect because Congress does not want centers under continual federal support. No. 3 is incorrect because it did not want to maintain federal control. No. 4 is incorrect because, although Congress wanted declining funding and control, it remains interested in community mental health centers.

32. (4) This was the principal recommendation. No 1 is incorrect. No. 3 is incorrect because the commission wanted flexibility in services. No. 2 is incorrect because the commission did not want to upgrade the old grant; it wanted to provide a new one.

33. (3) Nurses, for control and better health care, should be active at all levels and in all areas of health care. No. 1 passively carries out others' ideas. No. 2 is too limited in scope. No. 4 is also passive, with an additional loss of control.

34. (4) This is what the document states. *Other* choices do not give the individual nurse primary responsibility.

35. (3) The Act states that the boards must be comprised of 60% *consumers* who are not affiliated with any health professional group; hence, Nos. 1, 2, and 4 are incorrect.

Pre Test

INTRODUCTION

The **Pre Test** is an *initial assessment* tool intended to help you to assess your strengths and weaknesses in your ability to apply the material you have learned in specific clinical areas to any nursing situation. By taking the **Pre Test**, you can focus your subsequent review of content, based on your own analysis of your results.

We suggest that you take the **Pre Test** before you read any of the content units in this book. After taking the **Pre Test**, you should:

1. Score your answers.
2. Take another look at the questions where your answer was wrong.
3. Identify the clinical areas where you need further review, i.e., Childhood and Adolescence, Behavioral and Emotional, etc.
4. Go back and read those specific content units in detail.
5. Then test yourself again on the **Post Test**.

QUESTIONS

David, a 16-year-old white Jewish male, attends a private school and was doing exceptionally well until 6 months ago, when he was arrested for drunk driving and his license was temporarily suspended. His parents placed him on house restriction for several months. When David's mother was cleaning his room she found some pills and some things that looked like joints. David accused his mother of being "nosy" and of "invading his privacy," and he stormed out of the house. Later David's mother received a call from University Hospital's emergency room informing her that her son had just been brought there by the police after he was found on school property running around in the nude with several other students. He appeared to be hallucinating. He was admitted and sent to the adult medical/surgical unit because the adolescent unit was full.

1. After a few days in the hospital, the nurse finds a marijuana joint under David's pillow. After being confronted, David promises not to smoke marijuana again if the nurse will not report the incident. The nurse fears that David is manipulating her. The *most* therapeutic nursing intervention when working with manipulative clients is to:

○ 1. Make decisions for them. **PL**
○ 2. Reinforce use of alternative behaviors. **7**
○ 3. Set rigid limits. **PsI**
○ 4. Confront them in front of others.

2. David asks the nurse whether marijuana is addictive. The most appropriate response would be:

○ 1. "It is addictive." **IMP**
○ 2. "It causes a psychologic dependence." **7**
○ 3. "It is not addictive." **PsI**
○ 4. "It is physiologically addictive."

3. David feels very isolated from his peer group because he has been placed on an adult medical floor. In planning care for David, which of the following would be most effective?

○ 1. Assisting him to develop a working relationship with his 51-year-old roommate. **PL** **7**
○ 2. Encouraging his friends to visit frequently. **PsI**

PRE TEST

○ 3. Asking him what he enjoys doing.
○ 4. Establishing a one-to-one relationship with him.

4. Which recreational activity would be most appropriate for the nurse to support?
○ 1. A television to watch in his room. **PL**
○ 2. Schoolwork that can be brought to the hospital. **5** **HPM**
○ 3. A board game such as checkers or backgammon.
○ 4. Various novels David says he wants to read.

After David has been hospitalized 8 days, his father discusses his condition with the physician. The physician indicates that an in-patient, short-term drug treatment program would probably be best for David at this time. David's father becomes very hostile and states, "My son is no addict and he isn't going to be put away in any crazy house."

5. To assess David's father's reaction to the physician's recommendation, the nurse should realize that David's father is:
○ 1. Expressing anger about the incompetent treatment he thinks David is receiving. **AN** **7**
○ 2. Denying that David is a drug abuser. **PsI**
○ 3. Projecting the blame onto someone else.
○ 4. Looking for the best possible treatment for his son.

Mr. and Mrs. Franco arrive in the emergency room at 4:00 A.M. with their son José, a 3-month old born at 8 months gestation. Mrs. Franco tells the nurse that she had just finished nursing Carlos, the twin brother, when she noticed he was not moving and not breathing. Mr. Franco grabbed José and shook him to try to make him breathe. José did not respond. He never regained consciousness and was pronounced dead at 5:00 A.M.

6. Mrs. Franco becomes hysterical. She begins to cry uncontrollably. Mr. Franco asks the nurse to "do something." The most appropriate intervention would include:
○ 1. Providing the Francos with privacy. **PL**
○ 2. Obtaining an order for a tranquilizer. **7**
○ 3. Sitting quietly with the couple. **PsI**
○ 4. Asking Mrs. Franco to calm down.

7. The most appropriate plan for immediate follow-up care for the Franco family would include:
○ 1. Referring the family to a psychotherapist. **PL**
○ 2. Arranging for the social worker to visit the family. **7** **PsI**
○ 3. Asking the family to identify their needs.
○ 4. Assessing the family's need for follow-up care.

8. The nurse working with a SIDS (Sudden Infant Death Syndrome) family should:
○ 1. Be knowledgeable about various theories of psychotherapy. **PL** **7**
○ 2. Have extensive experience working with dying clients. **PsI**
○ 3. Be able to identify personal feelings about death.
○ 4. Be able to suppress personal feelings about death.

Henry Miller, 8 weeks old, is diagnosed as being susceptible to extended periods of apnea. The physician suggests placing Henry on an apnea monitor at home.

9. Mrs. Miller tells the nurse that Henry looks so frail and sick on the apnea monitor. The best response for the nurse to make is:
○ 1. "Henry does have a life-threatening illness." **IMP**
○ 2. "Have you seen many infants Henry's age?" **7**
○ 3. "Try not to think of him like that. Think positive!" **PsI**
○ 4. "I know how you must feel. It can be very scary to see your baby looking like this."

Ten days after admission of Mr. Smith for a myocardial infarction, his physician decides that he has stabilized sufficiently to be transferred to floor care. Mrs. Smith has stopped by the nurses' station on her way out after visiting hours. She states, "Keep an eye on Mr. Smith, will you? He doesn't seem himself tonight." You decide to check Mr. Smith immediately, and you find him slumped on the siderails of his bed. He does not respond when you shake his shoulder or loudly call his name. You initiate CPR, and he resuscitates.

10. Three days after successful resuscitation, Mr. Smith states to you, "I'm all washed up. I don't think I'll ever be the same man again." Your best response would be:
○ 1. "Most clients who have been as ill as you have feel that way, Mr. Smith." **IMP** **7**
○ 2. "How do you feel you have changed from before your illness?" **PsI**
○ 3. "Getting depressed won't help you get better."
○ 4. "Tell me more."

Gladys Meeker is a 30-year-old advertising executive with a history of ulcerative colitis since age 22. Her chief complaint is severe abdominal cramping and 18–20 stools per day for 4 days.

11. Blood and fluid loss from frequent diarrhea may cause hypovolemia. You can quickly assess volume depletion in Ms. Meeker by:
○ 1. Measuring the quantity and specific gravity of her urine output. **AS** **8**
○ 2. Taking her blood pressure first supine, then sitting, noting any changes. **PhI**
○ 3. Comparing the client's present weight with her weight on her last admission.
○ 4. Administering the oral water test.

12. The nurse would recognize other signs of hypovolemia, which include:
○ 1. Dry mucous membranes and soft eyeballs. **AS**
○ 2. Decreased hematocrit and hemoglobin. **8**
○ 3. Decreased pulse rate and widened pulse pressure. **PhI**
○ 4. Dyspnea and crackles.

13. With severe diarrhea, electrolytes as well as fluids are lost. The nurse would conclude that the client is experiencing hypokalemia if which of the following were observed?
○ 1. Spasms, diarrhea, irregular pulse. **AS**
○ 2. Kussmaul breathing, thirst, furrowed tongue. **8**
○ 3. Apathy, weakness, GI disturbance. **PhI**
○ 4. Pitting edema, confusion, bounding pulse.

Key to codes following questions Nursing process: **AS**, Assessment; **AN**, Analysis; **PL**, Plan; **IMP**, Implementation; **EV**, Evaluation. Category of human function: **1**, Protective; **2**, Sensory-perceptual; **3**, Comfort, Rest, Activity, and Mobility; **4**, Nutrition; **5**, Growth and Development; **6**, Fluid-Gas Transport; **7**, Psycho-Social-Cultural; **8**, Elimination. Client need: **SECE**, Safe, Effective Care Environment; **PhI**, Physiological Integrity; **PsI**, Psychosocial Integrity; **HPM**, Health Promotion/Maintenance. See frontmatter for full explanation.

14. Three days after admission Ms. Meeker continued to have frequent stools. Her oral intake of both fluids and solids was poor. Her physician ordered parenteral hyperalimentation. While administering the ordered solution, it is important to remember that hyperalimentation solutions are:

○ 1. Hypotonic solutions used primarily for hydration when hemoconcentration is present. **IMP 8 SECE**
○ 2. Hypertonic solutions used primarily to increase osmotic pressure of blood plasma.
○ 3. Alkalyzing solutions used to treat metabolic acidosis, thus reducing cellular swelling.
○ 4. Hyperosmolar solutions used primarily to reverse negative nitrogen balance.

15. Maintaining the infusion rate of hyperalimentation solutions is a nursing responsibility. What side effects from too rapid an infusion rate would the nurse expect Ms. Meeker to demonstrate?

○ 1. Cellular dehydration and potassium depletion. **EV 6 PhI**
○ 2. Circulatory overload and hypoglycemia.
○ 3. Hypoglycemia and hypovolemia.
○ 4. Potassium excess and congestive heart failure.

16. Which of the following statements is correct regarding nursing care of Ms. Meeker while she is receiving hyperalimentation?

○ 1. The client's urine should be tested for glucose-acetone every 8–12 hours. **IMP 6 SECE**
○ 2. The hyperalimentation subclavian line may be utilized for CVP readings and/or blood withdrawal.
○ 3. Occlusive dressings at the catheter insertion site are changed every 48 hours using the clean technique.
○ 4. Records of intake and output and daily weights should be kept.

After 10 days of therapy, Ms. Meeker's physician decided to perform an ileostomy. For 3 days prior to surgery she was given neomycin. On the morning of surgery she was catheterized and a nasogastric tube was inserted.

17. Neomycin was administered by the nurse prior to surgery:

○ 1. To decrease the incidence of postoperative atelectasis due to decreased depth of respirations. **AN 8 PhI**
○ 2. To increase the effectiveness of the body's immunologic response following surgical trauma.
○ 3. To reduce the incidence of wound infections by decreasing the number of intestinal organisms.
○ 4. To prevent postoperative bladder atony due to catheterization.

18. Following ileostomy, the nurse would expect the drainage appliance to be applied to the stoma:

○ 1. 24 hours later, when edema has subsided. **IMP 8 SECE**
○ 2. In the operating room.
○ 3. After the ileostomy begins to function.
○ 4. When the client is able to begin self-care procedures.

19. Which of the following goals would be described to Ms. Meeker as the highest postoperative nursing priority?

○ 1. Relief of pain to promote rest and relaxation. **PL 8 SECE**
○ 2. Assisting the client with self-care activities.
○ 3. Maintenance of fluid, electrolyte, and nutritional balances.
○ 4. Skin care and control of odors.

20. During the early postoperative period, the nurse initiates ileostomy teaching with Ms. Meeker. The primary objective of this procedure is:

○ 1. To facilitate maintenance of intake and output records. **PL 8 SECE**
○ 2. To control unpleasant odors.
○ 3. To prevent excoriation of the skin around the stoma.
○ 4. To reduce the risk of postoperative wound infection.

21. After discharge, Ms. Meeker calls you at the hospital to report the sudden onset of abdominal cramps, vomiting, and watery discharge from her ileostomy. What would you advise?

○ 1. Call the physician if symptoms persist for 24 hours. **IMP 4 PhI**
○ 2. Take 30 cc of m.o.m. (milk of magnesia).
○ 3. NPO until vomiting stops.
○ 4. Call the physician immediately.

Mr. Pook Loo is a 63-year-old electrician admitted to the hospital for bronchoscopy. He has a smoking history of two packs per day for 30 years, although he has not smoked for the last 6 months. Ten days ago he developed an upper respiratory infection with mild fever. Six days ago, his fever increased and his cough was productive of greenish sputum. He went to the neighborhood health clinic, where he had a chest X ray taken. The chest X ray was positive for pneumonia, but the physician also noted an abnormality in the left lower lobe.

22. Physical assessment of Mr. Loo revealed a thin, muscular man with rhonchi and wheezes in the left lung and some wheezes in the right lower lobe. Rhonchi and wheezes are due to:

○ 1. Total obstruction of small bronchioles. **AN 6 PhI**
○ 2. Partial obstruction of bronchi and bronchioles.
○ 3. Fluid in the alveoli.
○ 4. Inflammation of the pleura.

23. The nurse explains to Mr. Loo that a bronchoscopy is:

○ 1. An X-ray procedure that allows for multiple views of the lungs. **EV 6 SECE**
○ 2. A procedure utilizing a lighted mirror lens to observe the walls of the trachea, mainstem bronchus, and major bronchial tubes.
○ 3. A diagnostic test during which a radiopaque substance is inserted into the tracheobronchial tree for clear visualization.
○ 4. A needle puncture of the lung mass, identified on an X ray with aspiration of cells for microscopic examination.

24. Following bronchoscopy, what is your most important nursing observation?

○ 1. Blood pressure, pulse, and temperature. **PL 6 PhI**
○ 2. Color and consistency of sputum.
○ 3. Function of the tenth cranial nerve.
○ 4. Presence of urticaria.

25. The nurse recognizes dyspnea as:

○ 1. Increased awareness of respiratory effort. **AN 6 PhI**
○ 2. Decreased alveolar ventilation.
○ 3. Increased rate and depth of respiration.
○ 4. Decreased oxygen saturation of venous blood.

26. Bronchoscopy revealed a squamous cell carcinoma. The lesion appeared fairly localized, and Mr. Loo's surgeon decided to do a lower left lobectomy. Preoperative teaching for Mr. Loo includes coughing, deep breathing, and arm exercises. The most important postoperative activity the thoracic client performs is:
- ○ 1. Arm exercises to prevent shoulder ankylosis. **IMP**
- ○ 2. Deep breathing and coughing up of sputum to prevent airway obstruction. **6** **SECE**
- ○ 3. Leg exercises to prevent thrombophlebitis due to prolonged bedrest.
- ○ 4. Deep breathing only to prevent undue suture stress while maintaining ventilation.

27. Which of the following instructions would be *inappropriate psychologic* instruction for Mr. Loo regarding his surgery and postoperative care?
- ○ 1. Explain to him that he will be surrounded by equipment, such as chest tubes, oxygen, and IV infusions, and that these are routine. **PL** **6** **SECE**
- ○ 2. Tell him he will have periods of rest but will be awakened approximately every 2 hours for turning, coughing, and deep breathing.
- ○ 3. Assure him he will receive medication that will assist in relieving his discomfort.
- ○ 4. Assure him that anesthesia will not have any untoward effects on his respiratory status.

28. Prior to surgery, pulmonary function tests are done and arterial blood gases are drawn to establish baseline data. Given Mr. Loo's respiratory symptomatology, the nurse would expect which of the following outcomes?
- ○ 1. Increased vital capacity and respiratory acidosis. **AN** **6**
- ○ 2. Decreased vital capacity and respiratory alkalosis. **PhI**
- ○ 3. Increased total lung capacity and metabolic acidosis.
- ○ 4. Decreased FEV_1 and respiratory acidosis.

On returning from the recovery room, Mr. Loo has a chest tube to a two-bottle, water-sealed drainage system and oxygen per nasal cannula. Postoperative orders included:
- *Meperidine 100 mg IM every 3–4 hours p.r.n. for pain.*
- *1000 mL 5% dextrose/water every 10 hours.*
- *Ampicillin 500 mg IM every 6 hours.*
- *Tigan 200 mg IM every 3–4 hours p.r.n. nausea and vomiting.*
- *IPPB with normal saline qid.*
- *Incentive spirometer qid.*

29. The essential purpose of the water-sealed drainage system is to:
- ○ 1. Prevent early precipitous reinflation of the lung. **AN** **6**
- ○ 2. Drain off excess fluid and air, thereby promoting reestablishment of negative intrapleural pressures. **SECE**
- ○ 3. Drain off excess fluid and air, thereby promoting reestablishment of positive intrapleural pressures.
- ○ 4. Decrease atelectasis in unaffected lung tissue and to monitor blood loss.

30. In a two-bottle, water-sealed drainage system, the nurse knows that:
- ○ 1. The first bottle establishes the suction pressure and the second bottle collects the drainage. **PL** **1** **SECE**
- ○ 2. The first bottle establishes the suction pressure and the second bottle is attached to motor suction.
- ○ 3. The first bottle collects the drainage and the second bottle provides easy access for removing drainage specimens.
- ○ 4. The first bottle collects the drainage and the second bottle establishes the suction pressure.

31. After making Mr. Loo comfortable in bed, your first nursing measure concerning the water-sealed drainage is:
- ○ 1. Milking the tubing to prevent accumulation of fibrin and clots. **IMP** **6**
- ○ 2. Raising the bottle to bed height to accurately assess the meniscus level. **SECE**
- ○ 3. Attaching the chest tubes to the bed linen to assure that airflow and drainage are unhindered by kinks.
- ○ 4. Marking the time and the amount of drainage in the collection bottle.

32. On the second postoperative day, the fluid in the suction bottle's glass tube ceases to fluctuate. The nurse knows that this most likely indicates:
- ○ 1. The chest tube is plugged by fibrin or a clot. **EV**
- ○ 2. There is an air leak in the system. **6**
- ○ 3. Pulmonary edema has occurred due to increased blood volume in remaining lung tissue. **SECE**
- ○ 4. The client's position needs to change to facilitate drainage.

33. The nurse explains to Mr. Loo that the purpose of intermittent positive-pressure breathing (IPPB) with normal saline is to maintain patent airways and to mobilize secretions. To accomplish this, IPPB exerts:
- ○ 1. Positive pressures on inspiration. **AN**
- ○ 2. Negative pressures on inspiration. **6**
- ○ 3. Positive pressures on expiration. **PhI**
- ○ 4. Negative pressures on expiration.

34. Passive arm exercises are instituted on Mr. Loo's left arm 4 hours after surgery. The nurse does these exercises to prevent which of the following dysfunctions?
- ○ 1. Hyperflexion of the wrist. **EV**
- ○ 2. Ankylosis of the shoulder. **3**
- ○ 3. Flexion of the elbow. **PhI**
- ○ 4. Spasticity of the intercostal muscles.

35. On the fifth postoperative day, fluctuation in the water-sealed bottle again ceased. Auscultation of Mr. Loo's upper left chest indicated the lung had reexpanded. The physician ordered a chest X ray to assess the degree of reexpansion. To safely transport Mr. Loo to X ray, the nurse would:
- ○ 1. Remove the chest tubes, immediately covering the incision site with a sterile petrolatum gauze to prevent air from entering the chest. **PL** **6** **SECE**
- ○ 2. Disconnect the drainage bottles from the chest tubes, covering the catheter tip with a sterile dressing to prevent contamination.
- ○ 3. Send Mr. Loo to X ray with his chest tube clamped but still attached to the drainage system to prevent air from entering the chest wall if the bottles are accidentally broken.
- ○ 4. Send Mr. Loo to X ray with his chest tube attached to the drainage system, taking precautions to prevent breakage.

Ms. Geraldine Phillips is a 21-year-old woman admitted to the hospital for an arthrotomy. She has had diabetes mellitus for 2 years. She is on NPH insulin, 40 units, which she administers to herself every A.M. This dose was ordered for the day of surgery, as well as rainbow coverage with regular insulin, on the following scale:

0 none
1+ none
2+ 6 units
3+ 10 units
4+ 14 units

On the morning of surgery her urine sample tested 1+ for sugar and acetone.

36. The nurse knows that acetonuria develops in diabetes due to:
- ○ 1. Excessive oxidation of fatty acids for energy, which increases ketones in glomerular filtrate. **AS 6 PhI**
- ○ 2. Osmotic diuresis, accompanying elevation in serum-glucose levels, which decreases exchange of electrolytes in renal tubules.
- ○ 3. Failure of sodium-hydrogen ion exchange mechanism in the renal tubules to secrete excess hydrogen ions.
- ○ 4. Increased volatile H^+ ions and decreased nonvolatile H^- ions in the glomerular filtrate.

On the evening of her first postop day, Ms. Phillips began to complain of increasing nausea. Her face was flushed, she appeared lethargic, and her vital signs were BP 108/78, pulse 100, respirations 24 and deep. Intake 2100 cc/IV. Urine output 2000 cc.

37. What is your first nursing action?
- ○ 1. Call the attending physician. **AN 4 PhI**
- ○ 2. Check her blood glucose and her urine for sugar and acetone.
- ○ 3. Administer an antiemetic.
- ○ 4. Decrease her IV infusion rate.

38. The nurse recognizes that Ms. Phillips' vital signs and urine output reflect:
- ○ 1. Increased ADH release in response to physiologic stress of surgery. **AN 4 PhI**
- ○ 2. Decreased ECF (Extracellular Fluid) volume due to osmotic diuresis.
- ○ 3. A hypo-osmolar fluid imbalance.
- ○ 4. Circulatory overload.

39. You explain to your client that regular or crystalline insulin is utilized as an adjunct to NPH therapy because:
- ○ 1. There is increased tissue metabolism with surgery. **AN 4 PhI**
- ○ 2. Insulin production is decreased even further with the stress of surgery.
- ○ 3. Physiologic and psychologic stress increases serum-glucose levels via sympathetic nervous system stimulation.
- ○ 4. An increased insulin load is necessary to prevent hyperkalemia.

40. The nurse knows that NPH insulin reaches its peak action:
- ○ 1. 4 hours after injection. **IMP 4 PhI**
- ○ 2. 6–12 hours after injection.
- ○ 3. 12–14 hours after injection.
- ○ 4. 15–18 hours after injection.

41. When can you expect the client who is receiving NPH insulin to *most* likely have a hypoglycemic reaction?
- ○ 1. Before lunch (10–11 A.M.). **PL 4 SECE**
- ○ 2. Early afternoon (1–3 P.M.).
- ○ 3. Late afternoon (4–7 P.M.).
- ○ 4. After supper (8–10 P.M.).

42. Objective data seen with hypoglycemic reactions include:
- ○ 1. Irritability, confusion, and lethargy. **AS 4 PhI**
- ○ 2. Increased temperature and flushing of skin.
- ○ 3. Muscle tremors and hyperreflexia.
- ○ 4. Decreased blood pressure and fatigue.

43. Which of the following statements would the nurse make to differentiate ketoacidosis from insulin shock?
- ○ 1. Deep and rapid respirations are characteristic of ketoacidosis, whereas slow, shallow respirations are characteristic of insulin shock. **AS 4 PhI**
- ○ 2. Acetone breath characterizes ketoacidosis, whereas the breath of the client in insulin shock is frequently fetid.
- ○ 3. Warm, dry, flushed skin and loss of turgor characterize the client with ketoacidosis, whereas the skin of the client with insulin shock is usually pale, cool, and diaphoretic.
- ○ 4. Apprehension, irritability, and combative behavior occur with ketoacidosis, whereas the client in insulin shock is more likely to be confused, lethargic, or comatose.

Mrs. Dixon, a 35-year-old mother, was admitted with dysmenorrhea and excessive vaginal bleeding. A diagnostic D&C discovered uterine fibroid tumors. A hysterectomy was discussed and a decision was made to go home for child care arrangements. That night she experienced excessive vaginal bleeding and feelings of extreme weakness. She was readmitted at 2:00 A.M. after being examined by the ER physician. An emergency hysterectomy was performed. Her vital signs were: BP 94/60, apical pulse 126, respirations 28. Laboratory data: Hct 30%, Hgb 8.5.

44. The nurse explains to Mrs. Dixon and her family that her surgery was an emergency because it had to be performed:
- ○ 1. Upon completion of the necessary surgical preparation. **PL 1 SECE**
- ○ 2. Immediately.
- ○ 3. Within 24 hours.
- ○ 4. At the start of the next surgical day.

45. The nurse explains to Mrs. Dixon's family that the surgical treatment *most* often implemented for excessive vaginal bleeding due to uterine fibroids is:
- ○ 1. Panabdominal hysterectomy. **IMP 5 SECE**
- ○ 2. Vaginal hysterectomy.
- ○ 3. Dilatation and curettage.
- ○ 4. Abdominal hysterectomy.

46. The nurse knows that such emergency procedures increase the surgical risk to the client because:
- ○ 1. The surgery is performed immediately. **AN 1 PhI**
- ○ 2. There is little time for psychologic/physical preparation.
- ○ 3. There is decreased physiologic stress.
- ○ 4. The anesthesia of choice is different for emergency surgery.

47. The nurse must assess past medical history and use of medications for any surgical candidate. Which of the following drugs can negatively interfere with anesthesia or contribute to postoperative complications?
- ○ 1. Anticoagulants and antihypertensives. **EV 1 PhI**
- ○ 2. Anticoagulants and insulin.
- ○ 3. Digoxin and thiazide diuretics.
- ○ 4. Vitamins and mineral replacements.

48. The laboratory data recorded an Hgb of 8.5. What is your *first* nursing responsibility?
○ 1. To attach the lab report to the chart. **AN**
○ 2. To hang a unit of blood. **6**
○ 3. To notify the physician immediately. **PhI**
○ 4. To chart the report in the nurses' notes.

49. One potential complication of an abdominal hysterectomy is abdominal distention. Postoperative nursing measures designed to *avoid* abdominal distention are:
○ 1. Auscultation of the abdomen for bowel sounds. **PL** **1**
○ 2. Abdominal massage and bedrest. **SECE**
○ 3. Insertion of nasogastric and rectal tubes and ambulation, as ordered.
○ 4. Progression of postoperative diet.

50. During discharge teaching, the nurse should include the following instructions:
○ 1. Avoid sitting for long periods of time. **IMP**
○ 2. Evacuate bowels daily. **1**
○ 3. Restrict sexual activity for 6 months after hysterectomy. **SECE**
○ 4. Avoid all household chores for 2 months.

51. Which of the following postoperative instructions includes *inaccurate* information?
○ 1. Monitor vaginal drainage and report any color changes. **IMP** **5**
○ 2. Expect that vaginal discharge will diminish and cease gradually. **PhI**
○ 3. Plan on contraception, considering her ovaries are still intact.
○ 4. Expect that menses will no longer occur.

Mr. Will Chuska, a Native American, is admitted to the hospital with complaints of increasing dyspepsia, intermittent bouts of diarrhea, increasing fatigue, and weight loss. Laboratory results: decreased bromsulphalein (BSP) excretion, increased serum alkaline phosphatase, increased ALT[SGOT] and AST[SGPT], serum sodium 135 mEq/L, serum potassium 3.6 mEq/L, total serum proteins 4.8 g/100, A/G ratio—albumin 3.0, globulin 5.2, Hct 32%, Hgb 9.4 g. Following a liver biopsy, diagnosis was postnecrotic cirrhosis.

52. Which of the following best describes the metabolic functions of the liver?
○ 1. Detoxification of endogenous and exogenous substances. **AN** **4**
○ 2. Fluid volume control and acid-base balance. **PhI**
○ 3. Erythrocyte and leukocyte breakdown.
○ 4. Concentration and storage of bile.

53. The nurse must be alert to the development of spontaneous bleeding (ecchymoses) in cirrhosis due to:
○ 1. Rupture of esophageal varices. **AN**
○ 2. Decreased synthesis of blood-clotting factors by the liver. **6** **PhI**
○ 3. Failure of the gut to absorb water-soluble vitamins needed to promote coagulation.
○ 4. Decreased venous pressures and slow blood flow.

54. Which of the following contributes to the development of ascites in cirrhosis of the liver?
○ 1. Portal hypertension, venous dilatation, and stasis. **AN** **4**
○ 2. Increased hepatic synthesis of albumin. **PhI**
○ 3. Decreased serum levels of aldosterone and ADH.
○ 4. Increased blood volume causing increased blood hydrostatic pressure in the capillary bed.

55. You explain to Mr. Chuska that his anemia is the result of:
○ 1. Increased RBC fragility due to folic acid deficiencies from inadequate dietary intake. **AN** **6**
○ 2. Decreased efficiency of Kupffer cells in the liver. **SECE**
○ 3. Increased blood-ammonia levels.
○ 4. Decreased amino acid breakdown and synthesis.

Mr. Chuska was placed on a moderate-protein, high-carbohydrate, high-calorie, low-salt diet. Medications included water- and fat-soluble vitamin supplements and the diuretic spironolactone (Aldactone).

56. Which statement would the nurse select as the *best* rationale for Mr. Chuska's diet?
○ 1. Since the liver may not be able to detoxify proteins, carbohydrates are substituted to meet his metabolic and nutritional needs. **PL** **4** **PhI**
○ 2. Proteins are given in sufficient amount to facilitate tissue repair. High-carbohydrate diet prevents further weight loss and spares proteins from energy metabolism. Sodium restriction facilitates management of fluid imbalances.
○ 3. High-protein foods are harder to digest and also have a high sodium content. Carbohydrates are more palatable and will more quickly correct Mr. Chuska's weight loss.
○ 4. High-carbohydrate diets, particularly if they contain adequate fiber, are more likely to decrease dyspepsia and diarrhea. Sodium is always restricted when the client is edematous.

57. One nursing measure that might increase Mr. Chuska's compliance with his diet is to:
○ 1. Sit with him until he has eaten everything. **IMP**
○ 2. Give his wife the responsibility of seeing that he eats. **4** **PhI**
○ 3. Feed him yourself.
○ 4. Offer frequent, small feedings instead of three large ones.

58. Paracentesis is a minor surgical procedure done at the bedside; its purpose is to remove ascitic fluid. After explaining the procedure to Mr. Chuska, your *next* nursing action would be to:
○ 1. Position the client in a chair or in high Fowler's position. **IMP** **6**
○ 2. Instruct the client to void. **PhI**
○ 3. Take vital signs.
○ 4. Drape the abdomen with sterile towels.

59. Since ascitic fluids are rich in serum proteins, the nurse would observe for which of the following complications following this procedure?
○ 1. Disequilibrium. **AN**
○ 2. Hypotension. **4**
○ 3. Hypoalbuminuria. **PhI**
○ 4. Paralytic ileus.

60. The nurse can anticipate that the amount of ascitic fluid removed will generally be:
○ 1. 500 mL. **AN**
○ 2. 1000 mL. **6**
○ 3. 2000 mL. **PhI**
○ 4. 3000 mL.

61. Four days after admission Mr. Chuska began to bleed from an esophageal varix. The earliest indications of bleeding noted by the nurse would include:
- ○ 1. Tachycardia, restlessness, and pallor. **AS**
- ○ 2. Tachycardia, lethargy, and flushing. **6**
- ○ 3. Sudden drop in blood pressure of 10 mm Hg or more. **PhI**
- ○ 4. Increasing combativeness and widening pulse pressure.

62. Initially Mr. Chuska's bleeding was controlled by the insertion of a Sengstaken-Blakemore tube. The nurse knows that this tube is used to:
- ○ 1. Prevent bleeding by applying pressure to the esophageal varices. **AN** **1**
- ○ 2. Prevent accumulation of blood in the GI tract, which could precipitate hepatic coma. **PhI**
- ○ 3. Stop bleeding by applying pressure to the cardiac portion of the stomach and against the esophageal varices.
- ○ 4. Reduce transfusion requirements.

63. The physician has left orders to deflate the tubes for 5 minutes every 12 hours to prevent esophageal erosion. Two hours following the second reinflation, Mr. Chuska suddenly became severely dyspneic and dusky. You should:
- ○ 1. Call a code blue (cardiac arrest). **IMP**
- ○ 2. Deflate the balloons. **6**
- ○ 3. Decrease the traction on the tube where it enters the nose. **PhI**
- ○ 4. Irrigate the tube with ice-cold saline to facilitate movement of the balloons into the stomach.

64. Twenty-four hours after the above incident, Mr. Chuska became increasingly confused and disoriented. The physician diagnosed hepatic coma. Which of the following nursing actions is designed to reduce ammonia intoxication in this client?
- ○ 1. Active and passive range-of-motion exercises to prevent venous stasis. **IMP** **4**
- ○ 2. Tap-water enemas to remove blood that may still be in the gut from the bleeding esophageal varices. **PhI**
- ○ 3. Administration of insulin and glucagon to reduce serum-potassium levels.
- ○ 4. Holding all antibiotic medications so that the action of the intestinal bacteria on protein is enhanced.

65. Mr. Chuska's prognosis is guarded. The nurse can anticipate a marked improvement in his prognosis if his hepatic coma lasts no longer than:
- ○ 1. 24 hours. **AN**
- ○ 2. 36 hours. **4**
- ○ 3. 48 hours. **PhI**
- ○ 4. 72 hours.

Both Sue Hoyt and her sister-in-law Judi Hill are pregnant with their first babies. Both are Rh negative. Sue is a 25-year-old diabetic who has been well controlled on insulin for the past 10 years. Judi is 20 years old, with a history of rheumatic fever at age 8. For both women, close observation and ongoing assessment are important to detect early signs of problems and assure prompt, appropriate management. Their estimated dates of confinement are 2 weeks apart. They come to their prenatal visits together.

66. Appropriate prenatal assessments are based on the nurse's understanding of the normal physiology of pregnancy and the interactive effects of coexisting disorders during pregnancy. For which of the following complications of pregnancy are Sue and Judi at equal risk?
- ○ 1. Spontaneous abortion. **AN**
- ○ 2. Preeclampsia. **6**
- ○ 3. Dystocia. **PhI**
- ○ 4. Erythroblastosis fetalis.

67. To enhance the pregnancy experience for both Sue and Judi, health teaching could be planned and implemented to meet both shared and individual needs. When discussing common complaints arising from normal maternal adaptations to pregnancy, which of the following normal physiologic changes has greater implications for Sue and requires more teaching about danger signs requiring prompt medical evaluation?
- ○ 1. Increased venous pressure in lower extremities. **IMP** **4**
- ○ 2. Placental production of HPL. **PhI**
- ○ 3. Increased cardiac output.
- ○ 4. Relaxation of the cardiac sphincter.

68. Which of these normal physiologic changes has greater implications for Judi and requires more teaching about danger signs requiring prompt medical evaluation?
- ○ 1. Increased venous pressure in lower extremities. **IMP** **6**
- ○ 2. Placental production of HPL. **PhI**
- ○ 3. Increased cardiac output.
- ○ 4. Relaxation of the cardiac sphincter.

69. The physician has told Sue she may require hospitalization during the pregnancy for treatment of any problems associated with her pregnancy and/or for diagnostic tests. When asked to verbalize her understanding of the discussion, which of Sue's responses indicates a need for further health teaching?
- ○ 1. "Pregnancy may change the amount of insulin I need for regulation of my diabetes." **EV** **4**
- ○ 2. "I may need to be hospitalized to evaluate how well my placenta is functioning." **PhI**
- ○ 3. "If this awful morning sickness keeps up, the doctor may put me in to control it."
- ○ 4. "The doctor said he might take a sample of my water (amniocentesis) to see if the baby has the gene for diabetes."

70. Individualizing Judi's health teaching requires discussing and explaining actions that will reduce the risk of further heart compromise during pregnancy. Which of the following should be emphasized as the most important factor in safeguarding Judi's heart during her pregnancy?
- ○ 1. Adequate exercise. **IMP**
- ○ 2. Adequate rest. **5**
- ○ 3. Low-salt diet. **PhI**
- ○ 4. Ferrous sulfate.

71. Judi is admitted for evaluation of her cardiac status at 24-weeks gestation. During the evening, she complains of dyspnea and shortness of breath while ambulating. She has a moist cough. Her physician orders her placed on complete bedrest. Which of the following nursing interventions is most appropriate to prevent further deterioration of Judi's condition?
- ○ 1. Place Judi in Trendelenberg position to encourage venous return to the heart. **IMP** **3**

PRE TEST

○ 2. Assist Judi with activities of daily living to reduce energy expenditures. **PhI**
○ 3. Encourage frequent coughing and deep breathing to prevent pulmonary complications of immobility.
○ 4. Initiate a regimen of lower limb exercises to prevent venous stasis and leg thrombosis.

72. Sue delivers an 8-pound 11-ounce boy at 38 weeks. On her first postpartum day, she is eating a full diet and her insulin has been cut to one-third of the dosage during pregnancy. The night nurse is making rounds and wants to assess the sleeping woman for signs indicating her response to the lowered insulin dosage. Which of the following indicates Sue is hyperglycemic?
○ 1. A flash of light in her face does not elicit a squint or turn of the head. **AN 4**
○ 2. Sue seems restless, her face is flushed, her pulse is rapid and her respirations deep. **HPM**
○ 3. Sue is perspiring profusely.
○ 4. She awakens with a headache.

73. Anticipatory guidance planned for Sue includes health teaching regarding self-care health maintenance actions in the postpartum. Sue wants to breastfeed her baby. Which of the following should be emphasized as part of her postpartum instructions?
○ 1. Breastfeeding is contraindicated because it stimulates gluconeogenesis. **IMP 5**
○ 2. Her caloric needs will decrease during the postpartum, so she must be alert for signs of hyperglycemia. **HPM**
○ 3. She should breastfeed the baby before feeding herself so that she can relax; stress inhibits the flow of breast milk.
○ 4. She must prevent hypoglycemia because it can inhibit the let-down reflex and decrease her milk supply.

74. On the third postpartum day, Sue prepares to return home with her new infant. Which of the following is the priority information to be discussed with Sue before she leaves the hospital?
○ 1. The statistical probability of her infant developing diabetes. **PL 1**
○ 2. The type of medical and obstetric problems that may occur in subsequent pregnancies. **HPM**
○ 3. Coping strategies with her new baby and her disease in the immediate postpartum period.
○ 4. Follow-up medical visits for both the infant and herself in the next 6 weeks.

75. Judi is admitted in labor 4 days before her EDD. If implemented during labor and delivery, which of the following would *increase* the stress on her heart?
○ 1. Helping her maintain a semi-recumbent position. **AN 4**
○ 2. Monitoring her pulse more frequently than her other vital signs. **HPM**
○ 3. Preparing her for regional anesthesia (epidural or caudal).
○ 4. After complete dilatation, coaching her to bear down only once per contraction.

Dian and Ben Kind have been married for 5 years. For the past 2 years, they have expected Dian to get pregnant and have used no contraception. However, Dian has not achieved pregnancy, and she asks the nurse what tests can be done to find out why. An infertility assessment begins with a thorough health history.

76. Which of the following factors is likely to be implicated in female infertility?
○ 1. Moderate alcohol intake. **AS 5**
○ 2. Menstrual cycle of 26 to 28 days.
○ 3. History of pelvic inflammatory disease. **PhI**
○ 4. Past use of diaphragm and spermicide for contraception.

Mr. Lawson is a 38-year-old, married business executive who is admitted for increasing fatigue and nocturia from glomerulonephritis.

77. Mr. Lawson states that he doesn't understand what caused his condition. You explain that acute glomerulonephritis is the result of:
○ 1. Acute infection of the kidney by gram-negative bacteria. **IMP 8**
○ 2. An immune response of the glomerular membrane to protein of the beta-hemolytic streptococcus. **PhI**
○ 3. Destruction of the glomerular membrane by gram-positive streptococci.
○ 4. Ischemia of glomerular capillary and vasa recta.

78. Several tests were ordered by the physician to evaluate Mr. Lawson's present kidney function. You know a decreased hematocrit occurs in chronic renal failure because:
○ 1. Secretion of erythropoietin factor by the diseased kidney is decreased. **AN 8**
○ 2. Chronic hypertension tends to suppress bone marrow centers. **PhI**
○ 3. Metabolic alkalosis tends to increase red blood cell fragility.
○ 4. Excretion of red blood cells in the urine is increased.

79. The nurse expects hyperkalemia on assessment to occur in chronic renal dysfunction because:
○ 1. As metabolic acidosis increases, the kidneys selectively secrete more H^+ than K^+ in exchange for Na^+. **AN 8 PhI**
○ 2. As edema forms, sodium diffuses into the interstitial space and is balanced by increased serum potassium.
○ 3. Respiratory compensation for metabolic acidosis tends to increase K^+ reabsorption by the kidneys.
○ 4. The nausea and vomiting that occur with metabolic acidosis tend to increase serum potassium to compensate for chloride losses.

80. Mr. Lawson has been NPO for the last 21 hours in preparation for an IVP (intravenous pyelogram). He has been complaining of thirst. The specific gravity of his urine has been averaging 1.008. Your explanation for these signs and symptoms is:
○ 1. The hypothalamus is stimulating increased secretion of ADH. **IMP 6**
○ 2. Extracellular fluid has become hypo-osmolar. **PhI**
○ 3. The kidneys are no longer able to concentrate urine, making the extracellular fluid hyperosmolar.
○ 4. Most clients complain of thirst after fluid restriction.

81. Besides omission of food and fluids by mouth, your preparation of Mr. Lawson for IVP would include:
○ 1. Ingestion of contrast medium the night before the procedure. **PL 8**
○ 2. Administration of cathartics or enemas to improve visualization of contrast medium in renal structures. **PhI**

○ 3. A low-protein and low-salt diet the evening before to increase hyperosmolarity of ECF.
○ 4. Institution of an intravenous line to maintain fluid and electrolyte balance.

82. In assessing Mr. Lawson's acid-base status, you would be alert to the following signs of metabolic acidosis:
○ 1. Hyperreflexia, paresthesias, and tetany. **AS**
○ 2. Giddiness, irregular respiratory pattern, and moist, cool skin. **6** **PhI**
○ 3. Muscle weakness, and numbness and tingling in the extremities.
○ 4. Lethargy, disorientation, and increased rate and depth of respirations.

Mr. Lawson's physician ordered: bedrest with commode privileges, methyldopa (Aldomet) 250 mg every 6 hours, and diazepam (Valium) 5 mg tid and a 40-g-protein diet.

83. You explain to Mr. Lawson's nursing student that methyldopa acts to decrease hypertension by:
○ 1. Dilating peripheral blood vessels and increasing renal flow. **IMP** **6**
○ 2. Depleting norepinephrine at postganglionic synapses. **PhI**
○ 3. Inhibiting formation of dopamine, a precursor of norepinephrine.
○ 4. Depressing reticular activating system activity.

84. The following is the best single measure of Mr. Lawson's fluid volume status:
○ 1. Skin turgor. **EV**
○ 2. Vital signs. **8**
○ 3. Daily weights. **PhI**
○ 4. Intake and output.

Mr. Lawson was discharged on a low-protein, low-salt diet and the above medication. Four weeks later he was readmitted to the hospital with complaints of joint pain, weight gain (15 lb), oliguria, muscle cramps, and lethargy.

85. The best explanation the nurse could give for Mr. Lawson's signs and symptoms would be:
○ 1. Renal ischemia due to increase in circulating toxins and chronic hypertension. **AN** **8**
○ 2. A decrease in the number of functioning nephrons, which further decreases glomerular filtration. **PhI**
○ 3. Increased water and salt loss due to flushing effect in the diseased kidney tubules.
○ 4. Water and salt retention due to insufficient renal blood flow.

86. Nursing measures to eliminate the cause of Mr. Lawson's joint pain would include:
○ 1. Amphogel to lower the elevated blood phosphate that occurs with renal failure. **AN** **3**
○ 2. Preparing for dialysis to decrease serum-creatinine levels. **PhI**
○ 3. Increasing his activity level.
○ 4. A low-purine diet to decrease uric-acid level.

87. What ECG changes would you anticipate Mr. Lawson to demonstrate on assessment, given his potassium level of 6.5 mEq/L?
○ 1. Peaked T waves. **AS**
○ 2. Flattened T waves. **6**
○ 3. ST-segment depression. **PhI**
○ 4. ST-segment elevation.

88. Your interpretation of Mr. Lawson's blood gases (pH 7.36; PO_2 90; PCO_2 34; serum bicarbonate 20 mEq/L) would be:
○ 1. Metabolic acidosis. **AN**
○ 2. Compensated metabolic acidosis. **6**
○ 3. Respiratory alkalosis with metabolic compensation. **SECE**
○ 4. Metabolic acidosis with minimal respiratory compensation.

89. Objective assessment data indicating circulatory overload in this client would include:
○ 1. Neck vein distention, apprehension, soft eyeballs. **AS** **6**
○ 2. Periorbital edema, distended neck veins, moist crackles. **PhI**
○ 3. Increased blood pressure, flattened neck veins, shock.
○ 4. Decreased pulse pressure, cool, dry skin, decreased skin turgor.

Mr. Lawson's physician ordered complete bedrest, Kayexalate 15 g tid, furosemide 40 mg bid, and Aldomet 500 mg qid.

90. After 3 days of the above therapy, Mr. Lawson's physician decides to institute peritoneal dialysis to decrease Mr. Lawson's increasing symptoms of azotemia. After explaining the procedures to Mr. Lawson and his wife and obtaining a signed operative permit, your next nursing action is to:
○ 1. Have the client empty his bladder. **IMP**
○ 2. Position the client in a comfortable supine position. **8** **PhI**
○ 3. Weigh the client and record vital signs.
○ 4. Cleanse and drape the abdomen.

91. Following the insertion of the catheter into the abdominal cavity, the warmed dialyzing solution is allowed to run rapidly (10–20 minutes) into the abdominal cavity. The nurse warmed the solution to body temperature to prevent abdominal pain and to:
○ 1. Expand the molecules and increase the osmotic gradient. **PL** **8**
○ 2. Increase dilation of the peritoneal vessels, thereby increasing urea clearance. **SECE**
○ 3. Decrease the likelihood of peritonitis due to constriction of peritoneal vessels.
○ 4. Expedite the movement of the dialyzing solute into the abdomen.

92. Care of the client on peritoneal dialysis must allow a dwell time, or equilibration period, of the dialyzing fluid, which is normally:
○ 1. 10–15 minutes. **IMP**
○ 2. 20–30 minutes. **8**
○ 3. 50–60 minutes. **PhI**
○ 4. More than one hour.

93. The drainage period generally takes 20 minutes, though this may vary from client to client. If fluid is not draining properly, you can facilitate return by:
○ 1. Turning the client to a prone position. **IMP**
○ 2. Manipulating the indwelling catheter. **3**
○ 3. Elevating the head of the bed, thereby increasing intraabdominal pressures. **SECE**
○ 4. Elevating the foot of the bed, thereby increasing abdominal pressures and gravity flow.

94. Which of the following signs and symptoms are *least* likely to occur if fluid drainage is inadequate?
○ 1. A negative balance between the amount drained and the amount instilled. **EV** **8**
○ 2. Confusion, lethargy, and coma. **PhI**
○ 3. Moist crackles and rhonchi.
○ 4. Flattened neck veins in a supine position.

95. The effectiveness of Mr. Lawson's treatment would be measured by:
- ○ 1. Serum potassium less than 3.5 mEq/L and serum sodium greater than 148 mEq/L. **EV 8 SECE**
- ○ 2. Quantity and specific gravity of urine unchanged.
- ○ 3. BUN less than 20 mg%, serum creatinine less than 1.2 mg%.
- ○ 4. Abdomen moderately soft and percussion note dull.

96. Ms. Bell has second-degree burns of the left leg and thigh. You plan to help prevent contractures in the burned leg by:
- ○ 1. Maintaining abduction of the left leg, extension of the left knee, and flexion of the left ankle. **PL 3 HPM**
- ○ 2. Maintaining adduction of the left leg and extension of the left knee and ankle.
- ○ 3. Maintaining abduction of the left leg and flexion of the left knee and ankle.
- ○ 4. Maintaining adduction of the left leg, flexion of the left knee, and extension of the left ankle.

Mr. Robert Mackey, a 19-year-old college sophomore, sustained a transverse fracture of his right tibia and fibula when he tripped playing football. His fractures were reduced in the emergency room and his right leg immobilized in a long leg plaster of paris cast, which extended from his groin to his toes, with the knee slightly flexed.

97. Which of the following is an appropriate exercise for Mr. Mackey to engage in to prevent complications of immobility?
- ○ 1. Quadriceps setting. **PL 3 HPM**
- ○ 2. Extension of the right knee.
- ○ 3. Passive range of motion of hip.
- ○ 4. Flexion of right knee.

Ms. Martin, a 23-year-old secretary, has been diagnosed as having myasthenia gravis.

98. In order to assess accurately her functional and vocational rehabilitation potential with myasthenia gravis, the nurse must *first* ascertain:
- ○ 1. The degree of physical and emotional stress in Ms. Martin's present occupation. **AS 3 HPM**
- ○ 2. The activities of daily living that cause the greatest degree of muscle weakness and fatigue.
- ○ 3. Ms. Martin's understanding of and attitude toward myasthenia gravis, as well as her ability to cope with activity restrictions.
- ○ 4. Whether or not Ms. Martin will be allowed to sit down and rest when necessary in her current occupation.

Mr. Dunes was admitted to the hospital after an automobile accident. His major medical problems at the time of admission were multiple fractures of both lower legs. His medical treatment includes bedrest with skeletal traction.

99. The nursing intervention that would be *most* effective in prevention of footdrop would be use of:
- ○ 1. A bed cradle. **PL 3 HPM**
- ○ 2. A footboard.
- ○ 3. Passive range of motion every shift.
- ○ 4. A trochanter roll.

Mr. Kealey is a moderately overweight 58-year-old retired policeman admitted to your unit for repair of bilateral indirect inguinal hernias. He reports to you that he has worn a truss for several years. Mr. Kealey also reveals that he had the right hernia repaired 5 years ago, but that it returned after he helped a fellow officer move into his new home. He has smoked for 25 years and has a smoker's cough.

100. You identify the *most* likely cause for herniation in Mr. Kealey as:
- ○ 1. Intestinal obstruction. **AN 8 PhI**
- ○ 2. Failure of resected muscles in previous operations to heal properly.
- ○ 3. Chronic cough and vigorous exercise.
- ○ 4. Obesity.

101. A truss is a pad of firm material that is placed over the hernial opening and held in place with a belt. A truss should be applied by the nurse:
- ○ 1. After getting out of bed but before engaging in strenuous activity. **AN 3 PhI**
- ○ 2. After the hernia has been reduced, by lying down with the feet elevated.
- ○ 3. Whether or not the hernia has been reduced to prevent further extrusion of the bowel.
- ○ 4. Not at all, for physicians no longer recommend the use of a truss because athletic supporters are sufficient in preventing further herniation.

102. Given Mr. Kealey's medical history and the surgery he is about to have, which of the following preoperative nursing actions will be *a priority?*
- ○ 1. Explanation of the surgical procedure. **PL 6 SECE**
- ○ 2. Respiratory hygiene measures and instructions in deep breathing.
- ○ 3. Discussion of postoperative nursing-care measures.
- ○ 4. Assurance that pain medication will be available whenever he needs it.

103. Again considering the above nursing history data, which type of surgical anesthesia may be most appropriate for this situation?
- ○ 1. General. **PL 1 PhI**
- ○ 2. Intravenous.
- ○ 3. Spinal.
- ○ 4. Local infiltration.

The following preoperative orders were written by Mr. Kealey's physician:
- *NPO after midnight.*
- *Abdominal surgical prep.*
- *CBC and UA.*
- *Chest X ray.*
- *Pulmonary ventilation testing this P.M.*

104. Pulmonary function testing revealed a vital capacity within normal limits but a reduced forced expiratory volume (FEV_1). The nurse explains to the family that this means Mr. Kealey:
- ○ 1. Has difficulty moving air in and out of his lungs. **AN 6 SECE**
- ○ 2. May have some airway obstruction.
- ○ 3. Has weakened expiratory muscles of respirations.
- ○ 4. May have some areas of atelectasis in his lungs.

105. The nurse explains that the surgical preparation for Mr. Kealey would include cleansing and shaving of:
- ○ 1. The entire abdomen from just below the nipple line to the mid-thigh. **IMP 1 PhI**
- ○ 2. The entire abdomen from the axilla to the pubis.
- ○ 3. From the waistline of the abdomen to below both knees.
- ○ 4. Lower abdomen, the pubic area, perineum, and inner sides of thighs and buttocks.

106. Mr. Kealey has a spinal anesthetic. In the recovery room, it will be important that the nurse immediately position him:
- ○ 1. On his side to prevent obstruction of airway by tongue. **IMP 1 SECE**
- ○ 2. Flat on his back.
- ○ 3. On his back, with knees flexed 15°.
- ○ 4. Flat on his stomach, with head turned to side.

107. After positioning the client, the recovery room nurse initially should make which of the following observations?
- ○ 1. Status of reflexes. **AS 1 PhI**
- ○ 2. Vital signs.
- ○ 3. Client's level of consciousness.
- ○ 4. Integrity of airway.

Postoperative orders include:
- *Flat in bed for 8 hours.*
- *Vital signs until stable and then every hour for 4 hours and every 2 hours for 4 hours.*
- *Meperidine 100 mg IM every 3–4 hours p.r.n. pain.*
- *Diet as tolerated.*

108. Shortly after Mr. Kealey returns to the surgical unit, the nurse observes that his scrotum is quite swollen. The *first* nursing action is to:
- ○ 1. Notify the surgeon stat. **IMP 3 SECE**
- ○ 2. Elevate the scrotum on a rolled towel and apply ice bags.
- ○ 3. Administer p.r.n. pain medication.
- ○ 4. Encourage vigorous deep breathing and coughing.

109. Mr. Kealey became extremely lethargic following administration of meperidine HCl 100 mg IM for pain. What is the most appropriate nursing action?
- ○ 1. Give only 50 mg of meperidine next time pain medication is required. **IMP 2 PhI**
- ○ 2. Administer an oral preparation of meperidine instead of intramuscular preparation.
- ○ 3. Consult with physician about decreasing the amount of pain medication ordered.
- ○ 4. Endeavor to prolong the time between medication dosages by employing alternate pain relief strategies.

110. Ten hours after surgery, and despite repeated efforts, Mr. Kealey has still not been able to void. He states he feels like he could void but just can't seem to get his stream started. You should:
- ○ 1. Try getting him up in a standing position once again. **IMP 8 SECE**
- ○ 2. Insert a Foley catheter stat.
- ○ 3. Run water while he attempts to use the urinal.
- ○ 4. Consult with his physician to obtain either a medication or catheterization order.

111. The nurse explains to Mr. Kealey that urinary retention may be a problem after spinal anesthesia because:
- ○ 1. Conduction of autonomic nervous system impulses as well as central nervous system impulses is inhibited. **AN 8 SECE**
- ○ 2. Sensation and motor responses are decreased.
- ○ 3. Clients tend to secrete less ADH with spinal anesthesia than they do with general anesthesia.
- ○ 4. Vasomotor depression, which occurs with spinal anesthesia, reduces the glomerular filtration rate.

112. On the fifth postoperative day, Mr. Kealey complains of a "giving" sensation around his wound when he is walking about. After assisting him back in bed, you note that the dressing covering the right incision is saturated with clear, pink drainage. You should suspect:
- ○ 1. Late hemorrhage. **AN 1 PhI**
- ○ 2. Dehiscence.
- ○ 3. Infection.
- ○ 4. Evisceration.

113. On lifting the edges of Mr. Kealey's dressings, you note the wound edges are entirely separated. What is your *next* nursing action?
- ○ 1. Tell the client to remain quiet and not to cough. **IMP 1 PhI**
- ○ 2. Offer the client a warm drink to relax him.
- ○ 3. Position the client in a chair with his feet elevated.
- ○ 4. Apply a Scultetus bandage.

114. Of the following activities of daily living, which should you recommend that Mr. Kealey avoid after discharge?
- ○ 1. Driving to and from work. **PL 3 PhI**
- ○ 2. Walking 3 miles a day.
- ○ 3. Washing and polishing his car.
- ○ 4. Carrying out the garbage cans.

Mrs. Jane LaChance is a 41-year-old administrative assistant. She relates a history of increasing gastric discomfort and heartburn after meals. Approximately 2 hours after a business luncheon today, she experienced an abrupt stabbing pain in her upper abdomen that tended to radiate to her right shoulder. Physician's orders were:
- *NPO.*
- *ProBanthine 30 mg IM every 6 hours.*
- *Papaverine HCl 30 mg IM every 3–4 hours p.r.n. for pain.*
- *Tetracycline.*
- *Schedule for IV cholangiogram in A.M.*

115. The nurse knows that the function of the gallbladder is to:
- ○ 1. Synthesize and manufacture bile. **AS 4 SECE**
- ○ 2. Collect, concentrate, and store bile.
- ○ 3. Collect and dilute bile.
- ○ 4. Regulate bile flow into the duodenum.

116. If bile flow into the duodenum is obstructed, absorption of fat-soluble vitamins is reduced. Which of the following complications would you therefore observe for?
- ○ 1. Peripheral neuritis. **AN 4 SECE**
- ○ 2. Scurvy.
- ○ 3. Increased bleeding tendencies.
- ○ 4. Macrocytic anemia.

117. Besides jaundice of the sclera and skin, what other clinical parameters might indicate biliary obstruction in the client?
- ○ 1. Increased systolic and diastolic pressures. **AS 4 PhI**
- ○ 2. Frequent eructation between meals.
- ○ 3. Darkened urine and clay-colored stools.
- ○ 4. Longitudinal ridging of the fingernails.

118. In preparing Mrs. LaChance for her IV cholangiogram, it is important for the nurse to ascertain:
- ○ 1. If she has ever had the procedure before. **PL 4 PhI**
- ○ 2. If she has any known allergies, particularly to fish or other iodine-containing substances.
- ○ 3. If her epigastric discomfort occurs only with fatty-food ingestion.
- ○ 4. If there is a family history of gallstones.

119. Which of the following nursing actions is inappropriate in the preparation of a client for *oral* cholecystography?
- ○ 1. Administering a fat-free diet the evening before the test. **PL** **4**
- ○ 2. Administering Telepaque tablets in 5-minute intervals 1 hour after supper. **SECE**
- ○ 3. Administering at least 6 oz of water with each Telepaque tablet.
- ○ 4. Allowing the client, after she has ingested the tablets, to drink water until midnight, then NPO.

Following Mrs. LaChance's cholecystogram, a diagnosis of cholelithiasis and cholecystitis is made, and arrangements are made for surgery in 3 days.

120. Preoperative nursing measures for Mrs. LaChance include:
- ○ 1. Observing for bruising or easy bleeding due to potential prothrombin deficiency. **IMP** **1**
- ○ 2. Informing Mrs. LaChance of the purpose of the postoperative Hemovac. **PhI**
- ○ 3. Providing relief for abdominal discomfort by placing a heating pad on the upper abdomen.
- ○ 4. Providing a low-carbohydrate diet to stimulate release of glycogen stores in the liver.

121. Postoperative coughing and deep breathing may become a nursing problem following cholecystectomy because:
- ○ 1. Clients having abdominal surgery are prone to pulmonary complications. **PL** **6**
- ○ 2. Clients with biliary surgery tend to breathe shallowly to prevent pain and discomfort. **PhI**
- ○ 3. Women tend to be thoracic breathers rather than diaphragmatic breathers.
- ○ 4. Clients with upper abdominal surgery usually have a nasogastric tube in place, which inhibits deep breathing.

122. Mrs. LaChance refuses to cough after surgery "because it hurts." Your action would be to:
- ○ 1. Administer an analgesic and wait a few minutes. **IMP** **6**
- ○ 2. Assist Mrs. LaChance to sit up on the side of the bed and splint her incision with a pillow during coughing. **SECE**
- ○ 3. Allow Mrs. LaChance to rest this time, but inform her she will be expected to cough the next time.
- ○ 4. Increase fluid intake so as to loosen secretions and ease expectoration.

123. Mrs. LaChance has a T-tube to dependent drainage. The nurse knows that the purpose of the T-tube is to:
- ○ 1. Maintain patency of the common bile duct. **AN**
- ○ 2. Reduce the occurrence of postoperative hemorrhage. **4** **PhI**
- ○ 3. Prevent infection.
- ○ 4. Reduce bile flow into the duodenum.

124. In observing the drainage from the T-tube during Mrs. LaChance's early postoperative period, you would notify the physician if:
- ○ 1. The drainage contained blood during the first 2–4 hours postsurgery. **AN** **6**
- ○ 2. The drainage was less than 500 mL on the first postoperative day. **PhI**
- ○ 3. The drainage turned greenish brown in color.
- ○ 4. The drainage was more than 500 mL on the fourth postoperative day.

125. On the fourth postoperative day, the surgeon orders Mrs. LaChance's T-tube clamped for 1 hour prior to her first solid meal. You explain to Mrs. LaChance that the purpose of clamping the T-tube is to:
- ○ 1. Inhibit excessive bile drainage during meals. **AN**
- ○ 2. Allow bile to flow into the duodenum and aid digestion. **4** **PhI**
- ○ 3. Relieve abdominal distention and promote normal peristalsis.
- ○ 4. Assess the patency of the common bile duct.

126. While the T-tube is clamped, the nurse should observe Mrs. LaChance for signs of:
- ○ 1. Abdominal discomfort or pain. **AS**
- ○ 2. Eructation. **3**
- ○ 3. Jaundice. **PhI**
- ○ 4. Increased respiratory rate.

127. While instructing Mrs. LaChance about her diet, you inform her that:
- ○ 1. She will not be able to include fatty food in her diet for at least 1 year. **IMP** **4**
- ○ 2. After approximately 3 months she will be able to begin to add polyunsaturated fats to her diet. **PhI**
- ○ 3. There are no specific dietary restrictions in the postoperative period, but she will be more comfortable if she avoids large, fatty meals.
- ○ 4. Her diet will be limited to 20 g of fat per day.

Mrs. Suzi Chan is a 44-year-old public health nurse admitted to the hospital with complaints of increasing fatigue, loss of appetite, and night sweats. She is tall, thin, and pale. She states she has recently returned from a Peace Corps assignment in India. Vital signs: BP 110/80, pulse 100, respirations 28. Temperature 102.2°F rectally. A skin test (Mantoux) is ordered, as well as sputum specimens for acid-fast bacilli and chest X ray.

128. In order to correctly administer the Mantoux test, you would inject 5 TU (tuberculin units) of PPD (purified protein derivative) of tuberculin:
- ○ 1. Intradermally. **IMP**
- ○ 2. Subcutaneously. **1**
- ○ 3. Intramuscularly. **SECE**
- ○ 4. Subdermally.

129. The nurse will plan to read the reaction to the Mantoux test in:
- ○ 1. 6–12 hours. **EV**
- ○ 2. 12–24 hours. **1**
- ○ 3. 24–48 hours. **SECE**
- ○ 4. 48–72 hours.

130. The nurse concludes that the Mantoux test is positive if the following is present:
- ○ 1. An induration of 10 mm or more. **EV**
- ○ 2. An induration of 10 cm or more. **1**
- ○ 3. An induration of 5–9 mm. **SECE**
- ○ 4. A hivelike vesicle.

131. Skin test and sputum culture are positive. The chest X ray demonstrated four small lesions and one of moderate density. Diagnosis: tuberculosis. Respiratory isolation was initiated by the nurse. This is defined as:
- ○ 1. Both client and attending nurse must wear masks at all times. **IMP** **1**
- ○ 2. Full isolation; that is, caps and gowns required during the period of contagion. **SECE**
- ○ 3. Nurse and visitors must wear masks until chemotherapy is begun. Client instructed in cough and tissue techniques.

○ 4. Gloves are worn when handling client's tissues, excretions, and linen.

132. Mrs. Chan is treated with INH (isoniazid) 300 mg PO, and RMP (rifampin). Which of the following vitamins would the nurse expect her to receive to prevent the peripheral neuritis that may occur with INH therapy?
○ 1. Ascorbic acid (vitamin C). **PL**
○ 2. Pyridoxine (vitamin B_6). **1**
○ 3. Vitamin E. **PhI**
○ 4. Vitamin B_{12}.

133. Although chemotherapy renders the client noninfectious within days to a few weeks, barring side effects, Mrs. Chan is instructed by the nurse to continue INH therapy for:
○ 1. Six months. **IMP**
○ 2. One year. **1**
○ 3. Two years. **PhI**
○ 4. The rest of her life.

Deanna Thomas, a 36-year-old operating room nurse, is admitted for a thyroid scan. Ms. Thomas, who is a part-time student working toward her baccalaureate degree in nursing, had discovered a nodule on her thyroid while practicing the neck exam for a physical-assessment class she was taking.

134. The most accurate description the nurse could give about a thyroid scan is that it:
○ 1. Assists in differentiating between primary and secondary hypothyroidism. **IMP** **3**
○ 2. Demonstrates increased uptake of radioactive iodine in areas of possible malignancy. **PhI**
○ 3. Demonstrates decreased uptake of radioactive iodine in areas of possible malignancy.
○ 4. Measures the effect of TSH on thyroid function.

135. Following a thyroid scan with ^{131}I, the nurse should plan for:
○ 1. No special radiation precautions. **PL**
○ 2. Full radiation precautions to be instituted, including segregating the client in a private room. **3** **SECE**
○ 3. Radiation precautions that are limited to urine and feces.
○ 4. Full radiation precautions to be instituted for 8 hours (the half-life of ^{131}I).

Ms. Thomas' thyroid scan revealed a positive cold nodule, and a total thyroidectomy was planned. Preoperative orders included:
- *Routine CBC and urinalysis.*
- *Type and cross-match for three units of blood.*
- *Electrocardiogram.*
- *200 mg Seconal hs.*
- *NPO after midnight.*

136. A total thyroidectomy is ordered following discovery of a cold nodule. In the case of hyperthyroidism versus malignancy, the nurse anticipates that the client will have:
○ 1. A complete thyroidectomy also. **AS**
○ 2. A partial thyroidectomy (approximately one-half of the thyroid is removed). **3** **SECE**
○ 3. A partial thyroidectomy (approximately five-sixths of the thyroid is removed).
○ 4. Administration of thyroid medication.

137. Preoperative teaching measures unique to the client having a thyroidectomy should encompass:
○ 1. Active flexion exercise of the neck, special coughing instructions, voice rest, and antithyroid medications postoperatively. **IMP** **3** **SECE**
○ 2. Active flexion and extension neck exercises, deep breathing and coughing, and thyroid replacement when necessary.
○ 3. Instruction on supporting the back of the neck when repositioning and/or ambulating; avoiding hyperextension and flexion of the neck when coughing.
○ 4. Instructions on supporting the back of the neck when ambulating and/or repositioning and active flexion exercises of the neck.

138. Which of the following is a complication of thyroidectomy?
○ 1. Hypercalcemia. **AN**
○ 2. Respiratory obstruction. **3**
○ 3. Elevated serum T4. **PhI**
○ 4. Paralytic ileus.

139. Muscular twitching and hyperirritability of the nervous system indicate tetany (hypocalcemia). The nurse can assess for this complication by:
○ 1. Checking the urine calcium. **AS**
○ 2. Palpating the calf muscle, with the ankle hyperflexed. **3** **PhI**
○ 3. Tapping the facial nerve just proximal to the ear.
○ 4. Checking for ankle clonus.

140. Nursing measures that should decrease the incidence of hemorrhage postthyroidectomy are:
○ 1. Frequent checking of dressing, semi-Fowler's position, and ice packs to neck. **IMP** **3**
○ 2. Frequent checking of dressing, supine position, and ice packs to neck. **SECE**
○ 3. Frequent checking of dressing, coughing every 2 hours, and moist packs to neck.
○ 4. Frequent checking of dressings and maintenance of neck flexion.

141. In anticipation of emergency complications post thyroidectomy, which of the following nursing measures is essential in the postoperative period?
○ 1. Having calcium gluconate available for possible tetany. **PL** **6**
○ 2. Having a thoracentesis tray available to reduce edema. **PhI**
○ 3. Having a tracheostomy tray available for possible airway obstruction.
○ 4. Having pressure dressings available for possible hemorrhage.

142. Signs and/or symptoms of respiratory obstruction vary with the degree of severity. Early warnings observed by the nurse might include:
○ 1. Hoarseness and weakness of the voice. **AS**
○ 2. Stridor and cyanosis. **6**
○ 3. Vague feeling of choking, difficulty swallowing, and fullness of the throat. **SECE**
○ 4. Pale nailbeds, disorientation, and combative behavior.

143. Upon returning from the recovery room, Ms. Thomas begins to complain of a choking sensation. The immediate nursing action should be to:
○ 1. Elevate the head to high Fowler's. **IMP**
○ 2. Suggest she suck on some ice chips. **6**
○ 3. Assess the wound and dressing for increased swelling, and loosen dressing if necessary. **PhI**
○ 4. Call the physician.

144. While assisting Ms. Thomas to dangle at the bedside on her first postoperative evening, the most appropriate nursing action would be to:
- ○ 1. Support her under the axilla while bringing her feet over the bedside. **IMP 3 SECE**
- ○ 2. Bring her feet to the side of the bed and support the back of her neck while assisting her to assume a sitting position.
- ○ 3. Allow her to assume the sitting position at her own pace, unassisted unless necessary.
- ○ 4. Bring her feet to the side of the bed, then pull her forward.

Mr. John Edwards, a 78-year-old retired engineer, is admitted to the short-stay unit for the removal of a cataract from his left eye. Nursing history and physical assessment reveal a wiry, well-nourished man who states he has always enjoyed good health.

145. The preoperative nursing care plan for Mr. Edwards includes:
- ○ 1. Keeping him flat in bed. **PL 2 PhI**
- ○ 2. Applying eye patches to both eyes.
- ○ 3. Orienting him to his environment and nursing personnel.
- ○ 4. Teaching him eye-drop instillation.

146. Mr. Edwards asks about the type of anesthesia he will be having. You tell him that cataract surgery is generally performed using a:
- ○ 1. Local. **IMP 2 SECE**
- ○ 2. General.
- ○ 3. Intravenous.
- ○ 4. Rectal.

147. During the procedure to remove the opacified lens, an iridectomy will also be performed. You tell the client that this procedure is done:
- ○ 1. To prevent secondary glaucoma from developing in the postoperative period. **IMP 2 SECE**
- ○ 2. To increase pupillary dilatation postoperatively.
- ○ 3. To facilitate circulation and postoperative healing.
- ○ 4. To prevent corneal scarring during the procedure.

148. Postoperatively Mr. Edwards should be positioned:
- ○ 1. In a semi-Fowler's position. **PL 2 SECE**
- ○ 2. In a prone position only.
- ○ 3. On his back or on the unoperated side.
- ○ 4. On his operative side.

149. Which of the following activities of daily living must a patient be instructed to avoid to prevent complications upon his return home following cataract removal?
- ○ 1. Self-feeding. **IMP 2 HPM**
- ○ 2. Self-dressing.
- ○ 3. Brushing his teeth.
- ○ 4. Ambulating.

150. One week after his surgery, Mr. Edwards was fitted with cataract glasses. Which of the following nursing statements would best prepare Mr. Edwards for adjusting to these glasses?
- ○ 1. "The cataract lenses magnify objects so that they will seem closer to you than they really are." **IMP 2 SECE**
- ○ 2. "While your central vision may be somewhat distorted, you will be able to see well peripherally."
- ○ 3. "These lenses will enable you to see as well as you did before the cataract formed."
- ○ 4. "The lenses on these glasses are quite narrow, and therefore you may have some double vision."

Mrs. Ryan, a 50-year-old history professor at the local university, is admitted to the hospital with complaints of postmenopausal bleeding. Following a D&C, a diagnosis of adenocarcinoma is made. Internal radiation therapy is initiated.

151. Mrs. Ryan has cobalt (^{60}Co) seeds implanted. On returning to the unit, she has a vaginal packing and a urinary catheter attached to continuous drainage. To prevent displacement of the radioactive substance, the nurse should position the client:
- ○ 1. With the foot of the bed elevated. **IMP 3 PhI**
- ○ 2. Flat in bed.
- ○ 3. With her head elevated 45° (semi-Fowler's).
- ○ 4. On her side only.

152. Which of the following are precautionary nursing measures to be used when caring for a client being treated with internal radioisotopes?
- ○ 1. Maintain strict client isolation, and limit professional contact with client. **IMP 3 SECE**
- ○ 2. Limit exposure, and maximize distance between client, professional, and family.
- ○ 3. Position the client in a prone position, and restrict turning to mealtimes only.
- ○ 4. Maintain the legs in a flexed position to decrease the likelihood of dislodgement.

153. Which of the following nursing problems should you expect following uterine isotope insertion?
- ○ 1. Bladder atony. **PL 3 SECE**
- ○ 2. Constipation.
- ○ 3. Foul-smelling vaginal discharge.
- ○ 4. Loss of sexual libido.

154. Mrs. Ryan is receiving internal radiation therapy for treatment of adenocarcinoma. She complains of nausea and a general feeling of weakness. Her stools are loose. The nurse might suspect:
- ○ 1. Extension of her cancer to the abdominal contents. **AN 3 PhI**
- ○ 2. Radiation syndrome.
- ○ 3. Electrolyte imbalances.
- ○ 4. Depression.

Juanita Gomez, a 33-year-old Spanish-speaking female, arrived in the labor room complaining of severe cramping and excessive bleeding. Juanita is presently 8 months (36 weeks) pregnant with her first child. She is gravida 1, para 0.

Juanita received adequate prenatal care as scheduled. She was very conscientious about restricting her intake of salt and alcohol. She had even stopped smoking after finding out that she was pregnant.

Juanita complained that cramping and bleeding started about a half hour before. The initial assessment showed that she was approximately 4 cm dilated with intact membranes, and contractions were coming about every 4–6 minutes. Her husband, Tyronne, was with her throughout the admission process and appeared to be very anxious and concerned.

After Juanita has been in labor for 4 hours in the hospital, her cervix is assessed to be 5 cm. Her vital signs are T:99–P:100–R:30. BP = 132/90. FHR = 180 and difficult to auscultate with the monitor and fetal scope. The fetus is now positioned in a transverse position. Juanita and Tyronne are quickly informed of the gravity of the situation.

PRE TEST

155. The *primary* priority of the nurse at this time would be:
- ○ 1. To obtain an operation permit. **PL**
- ○ 2. To attempt to alleviate Tyronne and Juanita's anxiety. **1** **PsI**
- ○ 3. To monitor maternal and fetal signs closely.
- ○ 4. To provide emotional and physiologic support.

156. Juanita is moved into the delivery room. Tyronne enters the delivery room and appears somewhat anxious. The nurse should ask Tyronne:
- ○ 1. "How are you feeling?" **IMP**
- ○ 2. "Are you feeling up to this?" **7**
- ○ 3. "Would you rather wait outside?" **PsI**
- ○ 4. "Can I get you anything?"

157. Juanita expresses some concern over feeling the incision and experiencing pain. The most appropriate response would be:
- ○ 1. "You will feel nothing at all." **IMP**
- ○ 2. "You may feel some pressure in the area during surgery." **7** **PsI**
- ○ 3. "You may feel slight pain when the incision is made."
- ○ 4. "If you feel any pain, it is only your imagination."

158. Juanita questions the nurse about the type of incision the physician will use in her operation. The nurse should realize that Juanita's *primary* concern involves the possibility of:
- ○ 1. Infection. **AN**
- ○ 2. Bleeding. **7**
- ○ 3. Scarring. **HPM**
- ○ 4. Rupture.

Juanita undergoes the operation without complications. However, the neonate's Apgar score at 1 minute is 1 and at 5 minutes is 4. Oxygen is administered to the neonate immediately. The pediatrician notes that the neonate has a cleft lip and palate that is obstructing adequate ventilation. The infant's birthweight is 2500 g (5.5 lb), and it is a boy.

159. An Apgar score of 4 at 5 minutes indicates that the neonate's condition is:
- ○ 1. Excellent. **EV**
- ○ 2. Good. **5**
- ○ 3. Fair. **HPM**
- ○ 4. Poor.

160. The nurse assisting with the care of this newborn should realize the *primary* goal is to:
- ○ 1. Establish an airway. **PL**
- ○ 2. Maintain an adequate temperature. **6**
- ○ 3. Reassure the parents. **HPM**
- ○ 4. Monitor the infant's vital signs.

161. While providing care for the newborn, the nurse must also be aware of the parents' feelings. Both Juanita and Tyronne appear stunned. However, they are still in touch with reality and are asking appropriate questions focused on the newborn's condition. The couple is functioning at what level of anxiety at this time?
- ○ 1. Mild. **AS**
- ○ 2. Moderate. **7**
- ○ 3. Severe. **PsI**
- ○ 4. Panic.

The neonate's respirations are established. He is placed in an incubator and transferred immediately to the high-risk neonatal nursery. The couple is informed that the baby's condition is serious but stable. Juanita is transferred to the recovery room.

162. Tyronne requests permission to see his wife and baby immediately. The most appropriate nursing response would be to:
- ○ 1. Take him to see Juanita. **IMP**
- ○ 2. Inform him that they both need their rest. **7**
- ○ 3. Refer him to Juanita's physician. **HPM**
- ○ 4. Allow him to go see the infant.

Part of the nurse's role is to provide psychologic and emotional support to the parents, especially after the birth of an abnormal or unhealthy infant. In this case the nurse realizes that Juanita and Tyronne will have many different feelings to work through in the future.

163. The nurse should expect Juanita and Tyronne's initial reactions to include:
- ○ 1. Depression. **EV**
- ○ 2. Apathy. **7**
- ○ 3. Withdrawal. **PsI**
- ○ 4. Anger.

164. In providing emotional support for the couple, the nurse should realize that at first they will probably:
- ○ 1. Wish to talk with other couples who have experienced the same circumstances. **EV** **7**
- ○ 2. Wish to be left alone, unless they seek out someone to talk to. **PsI**
- ○ 3. Need reassurance and emotional support.
- ○ 4. Avoid discussing the situation at this time.

165. Juanita and Tyronne ask to see their son. The most appropriate nursing action would encompass:
- ○ 1. Assessing and analyzing the couple's level of readiness. **PL** **7**
- ○ 2. Arranging for the couple to see and hold their son immediately. **PsI**
- ○ 3. Teaching the couple what to expect.
- ○ 4. Preparing the couple for what to expect while making the arrangements for visitation.

166. Juanita's initial reaction to seeing her son in the neonatal nursery is to cry and tremble slightly. The most appropriate nursing intervention would be to:
- ○ 1. Remove her from the area immediately. **IMP**
- ○ 2. Monitor her for vital signs. **7**
- ○ 3. Allow her to cry. **PsI**
- ○ 4. Ask her what she is feeling.

167. Initially Juanita is reluctant to touch or hold her son. She says, "I don't know what to do. He's so small, so helpless. He looks so awful." Crying, she turns into Tyronne's arms. Which of the following nursing diagnoses is the *least* accurate interpretation of her behavior?
- ○ 1. *Altered parenting.* **AN**
- ○ 2. *Ineffective family coping: compromised.* **7**
- ○ 3. *Impaired verbal communication.* **PsI**
- ○ 4. *Potential altered family processes.*

168. Juanita and Tyronne may use which of the following defense mechanisms in attempting to cope with their anxiety?
- ○ 1. Fixation. **AS**
- ○ 2. Displacement. **7**
- ○ 3. Conversion. **PsI**
- ○ 4. Sublimation.

169. Juanita and Tyronne are experiencing a reactive depression. The primary difference between a reactive depression and an endogenous depression is that in a reactive depression:
- ○ 1. There is substantial weight loss, usually over 10 lb. **AS** **7**

○ 2. The individual does not respond to environmental stimuli. **PsI**
○ 3. The individual generally feels worse as the day progresses.
○ 4. The precipitating event is usually difficult to identify.

The couple is now aware that their son has a unilateral cleft of the lip and palate. They are anxious to have surgery performed to repair the deformities.

170. The most appropriate response to the couple's request for surgery would be to:
○ 1. Reinforce what the physicians have told the parents. **PL** **5**
○ 2. Inform the couple that the lip may be repaired when their son is 2–3 months old and the palate repaired at 18 months. **HPM**
○ 3. Refer the couple to the surgeon.
○ 4. Tell the couple that surgery may be performed when their son weighs at least 10 lb.

171. When teaching Juanita and Tyronne about the cleft lip and palate, the nurse would need to be aware that:
○ 1. Cleft lip occurs most frequently in girls. **AS**
○ 2. Cleft palate occurs most frequently in boys. **5**
○ 3. Cleft lip and palate almost always occur simultaneously. **HPM**
○ 4. Cleft lip and palate are both influenced by hereditary factors.

172. Which of the following nursing actions is *least* likely to assist Juanita and Tyronne to adjust to the psychologic trauma of the birth of a deformed child?
○ 1. Encouraging verbalization of anxiety, fears, concerns. **PL** **7**
○ 2. Explaining all treatments and prognosis. **PsI**
○ 3. Interacting normally with the infant.
○ 4. Expressing sympathy.

173. When teaching the parents about the care of their son with a cleft lip and palate, the nurse should inform them that:
○ 1. It is important to use a nipple with large holes in order to make sucking easier. **IMP** **4**
○ 2. The infant will have difficulty feeding because he cannot create a vacuum in his mouth. **HPM**
○ 3. The infant should be given small amounts of formula while being maintained in a supine position to facilitate feeding.
○ 4. It is important to isolate the infant from others to prevent possible infection.

174. Juanita and Tyronne's son undergoes an operation for the repair of the cleft lip when he is 3 months old. In providing nursing care for the infant, the nurse should:
○ 1. Place the infant in a prone position to facilitate drainage. **PL** **1**
○ 2. Avoid moving the infant too much in order to keep from dislodging the Logan bar. **SECE**
○ 3. Cleanse the suture area frequently in order to prevent scarring.
○ 4. Encourage the infant to cry in order to promote adequate lung aeration.

175. The couple expresses concern about caring for the infant. Tyronne is especially worried about paying excessive hospital bills because his insurance has set limits. The most appropriate nursing action would be to:
○ 1. Refer the couple to a social worker. **PL**
○ 2. Validate the couple's perceived needs. **7**
○ 3. Discuss alternatives with the couple. **HPM**
○ 4. Implement health teaching regarding the physical care of the infant.

Mrs. Washington is a 42-year-old housewife admitted for right-breast biopsy and possible modified radical mastectomy. She had delayed seeking medical consultation until 18 days ago. Mrs. Washington answered questions in a rushed, breathless manner. She constantly straightened the bedclothes. Lungs were clear to auscultation. Apical heart sounds were rapid, regular, and accentuated. Vital signs were BP 186/110, pulse 90, respirations 22, temperature 98.4°F.

176. Breast self-examinations are best carried out:
○ 1. During the middle of the menstrual cycle. **AS**
○ 2. On the first day of each month. **2**
○ 3. One week after the onset of menses. **HPM**
○ 4. The week before the onset of menses.

177. Women who tend to delay seeking medical advice after discovering a lump in the breast are displaying what common defense mechanism?
○ 1. Suppression. **AN**
○ 2. Denial. **7**
○ 3. Repression. **PsI**
○ 4. Intellectualization.

178. A half-hour later you retake Mrs. Washington's vital signs. They are now BP 132/86, pulse 80, and respirations 16. Mrs. Washington's elevated blood pressure indicated:
○ 1. She may be an individual who is highly sensitive to sympathetic nervous system stimulation. **EV** **7** **PsI**
○ 2. She is emotionally labile and will need to be assessed closely in the postoperative period.
○ 3. She is psychologically unprepared for surgery and a psych consult is in order.
○ 4. She is denying the possible loss of her breast.

179. Mr. Washington has arrived early to be with his wife before surgery. After his wife leaves for the operating room, you would *initially:*
○ 1. Tell him to go on to work and come back in the early evening, when his wife is likely to be more responsive. **IMP** **7** **HPM**
○ 2. Explain that, following surgery, his wife will be taken to the recovery room, but the surgeon will contact him when the procedure is over.
○ 3. Get him a cup of coffee and tell him to make himself comfortable, as it will be some time before his wife returns to her room.
○ 4. Encourage him to express his feelings and concerns so as to plan for postoperative family teaching.

180. On the third postoperative day, Mrs. Washington voiced concern about her husband's reaction to her surgery. Of the following approaches by the nurse, which is most likely to minimize Mrs. Washington's concern?
○ 1. Emphasizing the life-saving aspects of her surgery. **IMP** **7**
○ 2. Explaining that depression and anxiety are common behaviors following radical surgery. **PsI**
○ 3. Interviewing Mr. Washington to ascertain his real reaction to his wife's surgery.
○ 4. Encouraging her to identify the strengths in her relationship with her husband.

Mrs. Arturri is a 55-year-old lawyer admitted to the hospital with a diagnosis of bacterial pneumonia. On admission she was pale to dusky in color. Her respiratory rate was 32, temperature 103°F, pulse 100. Oxygen per nasal cannula is administered at 7 L/minute. Mrs. Arturri's physician decides to perform a tracheostomy.

181. A preoperative *nursing priority* is:
- ○ 1. Establishing postoperative communication. **IMP**
- ○ 2. Drawing blood for serum electrolytes and blood gases. **7** **PsI**
- ○ 3. Inserting a Foley catheter and attaching it to dependent drainage.
- ○ 4. Doing a surgical prep of her neck and upper chest wall.

Ruth Fara has come to clinic for family planning counseling. She states, "I want to postpone getting pregnant again for at least a year." Her history notes two episodes of thrombophlebitis with her previous pregnancy, repeated Candida infections, and gestational diabetes.

182. Most accidental pregnancies in clients using "natural" family planning methods have been related to unprotected intercourse *prior* to ovulation. Which of the following factors explains why pregnancy may be achieved by unprotected intercourse during the preovulatory period?
- ○ 1. Spermatazoal viability. **EV**
- ○ 2. Ovum viability. **5**
- ○ 3. Tubal motility. **HPM**
- ○ 4. Secretory endometrium.

183. In order to use "natural" methods of family planning effectively to either avoid or achieve a pregnancy, the client must be able to identify the fertile period accurately. In analyzing the BBT record of a client who has a normal 30-day cycle, on which of the following days would the nurse expect to find evidence of ovulation?
- ○ 1. Day 5 or 6. **AS**
- ○ 2. Day 13 or 14. **5**
- ○ 3. Day 16 or 17. **HPM**
- ○ 4. Day 28 or 29.

184. The Billings method of natural family planning incorporates client examination of cervical mucus. Which of the following characteristics should the nurse teach are typical of the cervical mucus during the "fertile" period of the menstrual cycle?
- ○ 1. Thick, cloudy. **IMP**
- ○ 2. Thin, clear, spinnbarkeit. **5**
- ○ 3. Yellow, sticky. **HPM**
- ○ 4. Absence of ferning.

185. To assist clients in making an informed choice of an effective method of family planning that is consistent with individual needs, the nurse discusses available options and the comparative advantages and disadvantages. Which of the following methods acts by preventing implantation of the zygote?
- ○ 1. Tubal ligation. **IMP**
- ○ 2. Intrauterine device. **5**
- ○ 3. Oral contraceptives. **HPM**
- ○ 4. Diaphragm and spermicidal jelly.

186. Clients selecting oral contraceptives as their chosen method of family planning should be instructed to notify the clinic if they develop symptoms of potential problems. Which of the following symptoms require prompt evaluation?
- ○ 1. Mild to moderate nausea during the first few days on the medication. **IMP** **5**
- ○ 2. Chloasma. **HPM**
- ○ 3. Leg cramps and/or headaches.
- ○ 4. Breast tenderness and weight gain.

187. To evaluate a client's understanding of the use of a diaphragm for family planning, the nurse asks her to explain, in her own words, how she will use the appliance. Which of the following responses indicates a need for further health teaching?
- ○ 1. "I really need to use the diaphragm and jelly most during the middle of my menstrual cycle." **EV** **5** **HPM**
- ○ 2. "The diaphragm must be left in place for at least 6 hours after intercourse."
- ○ 3. "I may need a different size diaphragm if I gain or lose more than 10 pounds."
- ○ 4. "I should check the diaphragm carefully for holes everytime I use it."

188. After presenting a brief class on various methods of family planning to students in a health course, the nurse administers a post test. If teaching has been effective, which of the following statements should the students select as true?
- ○ 1. To be effective, rhythm requires avoiding intercourse during the last week of the menstrual cycle. **EV** **5** **HPM**
- ○ 2. Clients using coitus interruptus may become pregnant accidentally due to escape of pre-ejaculatory fluid containing spermatazoa.
- ○ 3. Spermicidal jellies are highly effective whether used alone or with a diaphragm.
- ○ 4. The intrauterine device is the most effective modern method of contraception.

Jana Wile is seen in clinic for the first time. Her last menstrual period (LMP) was over 2 months ago, and she thinks she may be pregnant. Jana is 19, unmarried, and works days as a waitress.

189. Which of the following assessment findings provides data to validate an 8-week gestation?
- ○ 1. Fundal height. **AS**
- ○ 2. Auscultation of fetal heart tones. **5**
- ○ 3. Positive radioimmunoassay (RIA) test. **HPM**
- ○ 4. Leopold maneuvers.

190. Jana develops preeclampsia. The physician orders a magnesium sulfate infusion. Which of the following assessments is most important when administering this drug?
- ○ 1. Monitoring the serum magnesium level every eight hours. **IMP** **1**
- ○ 2. Evaluating the apical heart rate every four hours. **PhI**
- ○ 3. Counting the respiratory rate every hour.
- ○ 4. Auscultating bowel sounds before meals.

Mrs. Kate Logan is a 41-year-old housewife and mother who works approximately 20 hours a week as a salesperson in a local boutique. She has had varicose veins in both legs since the birth of her first child 15 years ago. Currently she is experiencing increased muscle fatigue and ankle swelling, particularly after being on her feet for more than 2 or 3 hours.

191. A routine preoperative assessment would include the following laboratory studies:
- ○ 1. VDRL, NA, K, Cl. **AS**
- ○ 2. Prothrombin time, ALT[SGOT], VDRL. **6**
- ○ 3. UA, CBC, prothrombin time. **PhI**
- ○ 4. WBC, VDRL, serum glucose.

192. The Trendelenburg test is frequently used to evaluate the competence of venous valves. Prior to administering the test, you tell the client that this test will consist of:
- ○ 1. Her walking back and forth so you can observe venous changes during walking. **IMP 6**
- ○ 2. Injecting a contrast medium into the veins and taking multiple X rays as the dye flows in the veins. **SECE**
- ○ 3. Stripping a superficial vein, occluding flow, then releasing the vein and observing the direction of filling.
- ○ 4. Her elevating the involved leg to empty the veins, your applying a tourniquet to the upper thigh, her standing, and then your removing the tourniquet to observe the filling of the superficial veins.

193. The nurse concludes from the assessment and history that vein-stripping is indicated for this client because of:
- ○ 1. Advancing varicosities and cosmetic reasons. **AN**
- ○ 2. Stasis ulceration and thrombophlebitis. **6**
- ○ 3. Lymphedema and Reynaud's disease. **PhI**
- ○ 4. Advancing varicosities only.

194. Mrs. Logan asks what type of anesthesia is usually used during vein-stripping. You tell her to expect:
- ○ 1. Local. **IMP**
- ○ 2. Topical. **6**
- ○ 3. Regional. **SECE**
- ○ 4. General.

195. The postoperative nursing care plan following vein-stripping would include which of the following?
- ○ 1. Administration of anticoagulants to prevent clotting. **PL 1**
- ○ 2. Elastic stockings from toe to groin. **SECE**
- ○ 3. Sitting in a chair.
- ○ 4. Bedrest for 48 hours after surgery.

196. You would explain to the client that elevation of the foot of the bed after vein-stripping surgery is done to:
- ○ 1. Decrease pain. **IMP**
- ○ 2. Aid venous return. **6**
- ○ 3. Increase blood supply to feet. **PhI**
- ○ 4. Make the client more comfortable.

197. During a predischarge teaching session, you tell Mrs. Logan that elastic stockings are best applied:
- ○ 1. Before rising in the morning, to prevent pooling of blood in the lower extremities. **IMP 3**
- ○ 2. After showering and application of skin care to the legs, to prevent undue dermal irritation. **SECE**
- ○ 3. After 15 minutes of vigorous leg exercises designed to increase blood flow.
- ○ 4. Only when she plans to be on her feet for an extended period of time because undue constriction of the veins can cause a recurrence of varicosities.

Bart Gordon, 11 months old, is admitted to the hospital with intussusception.

198. In reviewing Bart's admission history, the nurse should know that intussusception most typically presents which two signs or symptoms?
- ○ 1. Currant-jelly stools and paroxysmal abdominal pain. **AS 8**
- ○ 2. Olive-shaped mass in the right upper quadrant and projectile vomiting. **PhI**
- ○ 3. Obstinate constipation and increasing abdominal girth.
- ○ 4. Excessive amounts of mucus and abdominal distention.

Betsy Sullivan, age 18 months, fractured her right femur in a car accident. She is placed in Bryant's traction and admitted to the hospital. During her first night in the hospital, Betsy lies still in her crib, sucks her thumb, and occasionally sobs quietly in a monotone voice.

199. The nurse should interpret these behaviors to mean that Betsy:
- ○ 1. Wants her mother. **AN**
- ○ 2. Might prefer to sleep in a bed. **5**
- ○ 3. Probably does not sleep through the night at home. **HPM**
- ○ 4. May be experiencing painful muscle spasms due to her fracture.

200. When Betsy's mother comes to visit the next morning, Betsy clings to the nurse, who is washing her, and refuses to look at her mother. How should the nurse explain this behavior to Betsy's mother?
- ○ 1. Betsy is upset because her mother left her at the hospital. **IMP 5**
- ○ 2. Betsy is spoiled and needs firm, consistent limits set for her. **HPM**
- ○ 3. Betsy has adjusted to the nurse and is doing fine.
- ○ 4. Betsy may be trying to make her mother jealous of the nurse.

■ ANSWERS/RATIONALE

1. (2) Many times, manipulative clients are not aware of any other mechanisms for fulfilling their needs. Teaching them to identify manipulative behaviors may help them to avoid being manipulative and to eventually adopt more appropriate means for meeting their needs. The clients should be involved in the decision-making process (No. 1). Limits must be realistically established (No. 3). Public confrontation (No. 4) may only exacerbate the power struggle.

2. (2) There is a physical tolerance, but the dependence is purely psychologic. Nos. 1 and 3 are imprecise; and No. 4 is incorrect because this drug is not physiologically addictive.

3. (3) This allows David some control over his care and makes him feel that the staff is interested in meeting his needs. No. 1 is inappropriate unless they have common interest. Frequent visits should initially be *dis*couraged (No. 2) to avoid the possibility of David's receiving drugs from the outside. No. 4 may be appropriate; however, it is not as important as allowing David some control over his own care.

4. (4) Provide activities David enjoys. No. 1 does not promote intellectual stimulation and may disturb his roommate. Furthermore, the nurse has not validated whether David enjoys watching television. No. 2 is not a recreational activity. The nurse does not yet know whether David enjoys board games (No. 3), and they also require a suitable partner.

5. (2) He is attempting to cope with his anxiety by denying reality. He may also be angry (No. 1), but his behavior and verbalization indicate denial. It is through the use of denial that he is displacing the blame (No. 3), so denial is the more appropriate answer. He is unable to think clearly enough to seek any type of intervention (No. 4); he is reacting rather than problem-solving.

respiratory rate and lack of other symptoms (lethargy, easy fatigue) tend to contradict the occurrence of respiratory acidosis.

29. (2) The primary purpose of the water-sealed drainage system is to remove excess fluid and air from the pleural space, thereby speeding reinflation of the lung, reestablishing normal negative intrapleural pressure, and preventing the development of pneumothorax in the unaffected lung. Secondarily, water-sealed drainage enables the nurse to monitor blood loss. Nos. 1 and 3 are incorrect because both effects are the opposite of those intended. No. 4 is incorrect because atelectasis is caused by insufficient removal of secretions from the bronchial tree.

30. (4) In a two-bottle, water-sealed drainage system, the first bottle, the one proximal to the client, collects the drainage from the chest tubes. The first bottle is attached to the second bottle by a short tube. In the second bottle there is also a long glass tube that is open to the atmospheric air at the top and submerged below the water on the bottom. It is the distance this tube is submerged below the water that determines the amount of pressure exerted on the intrapleural space. In some instances, the second bottle may have a third tube attached to suction. Nos. 1 and 2 are incorrect because the first bottle is the drainage bottle. No. 3 is incorrect because, with the exception of the Pleur-Evac system (which has a mechanism for removing specimens without interfering with the suction), the water-sealed drainage system is never opened.

31. (4) Your first nursing measure should be to mark the time and the amount of drainage in the collection bottle to assure a baseline measurement for further observations. The milking of chest tubes (No. 1) is a matter of debate at this time. Although the process of stripping or milking does assist in the removal of fibrin and clots from the chest tubes, compression of the tubes also increases intrapleural pressures by preventing the movement of air and fluid. Whether the chest tubes are milked or not will depend on institutional or individual physician's policies. No. 2 is incorrect because the drainage system is always kept in a dependent position to maintain gravity flow of air and fluids. Your next measure is to secure the tubes to the bed linen (No. 3) in order to prevent kinking or unnecessary looping of the drainage tubes, which would hinder the flow of air and fluid.

32. (1) Fluid in the long tube of the suction bottle will cease to fluctuate when the tubing is plugged by fibrin or a clot and/or when negative intrapleural pressures have been reestablished and the lung has reexpanded. The likelihood of lung reexpansion on the second postoperative day is quite small. Therefore it is necessary to check the tubing for fibrin, clots, or severe kinking. If the tubing is kinked, it needs to be repositioned. Milking of the tube may be ordered if fibrin or clots are suspected. No. 2 is incorrect because an air leak is indicated by bubbling in the water-sealed suction bottle. Pulmonary edema (No. 3) would be reflected in dyspnea, orthopnea, crackles, and pink, frothy sputum. No. 4 is not entirely incorrect since the client's position may be such that the chest tubes are unnecessarily looped or kinked and repositioning the client may facilitate flow; however, it is *not* the *best* answer.

33. (1) IPPB facilitates the flow of air deep into the lungs by exerting pressures greater than atmospheric pressure (positive pressure) on inspiration. The client needs to learn to take slow, controlled inspirations to prevent hyperventilation. Nos. 2, 3, and 4 are incorrect because negative inspiratory pressures are consistent with CPAP or PEEP ventilatory systems, and pressures normally become more negative as the client exhales.

34. (2) Arm exercises are initiated to prevent ankylosis of the shoulder. Most clients tend to splint incisional discomfort by limiting movement on the affected side. This protective mechanism may lead to "frozen shoulder," or ankylosis. Therefore, it is important to initiate movement early to maintain muscle tone and joint integrity. No. 1 is an example of wrist drop due to poor positioning of wrist joints. No. 3 is usually a normal finding, although it may occur with improper positioning with upper motor neuron lesions. Intercostal muscle spasticity (No. 4) is rare and is not due to positioning.

35. (4) Normal functioning of chest tubes is maintained, and the drainage system is transported below the level of the chest. Chest tubes are not removed (No. 1) to facilitate transportation of the client; they are removed only after the physician is satisfied with the degree of reexpansion. Removing the chest tubes from the suction drainage system (No. 2) will result in an equalization of intrapleural pressures with atmospheric pressures, thus also increasing the risk of pneumothorax. Current practice precludes the clamping of the chest tubes (No. 3). It is believed that clamping increases the risk of a tension pneumothorax because air may enter the intrapleural space during inspiration but cannot escape during expiration.

36. (1) When excessive quantities of fatty acids are oxidized, blood buffer systems may become exhausted. Ketoacidosis develops and acetone bodies are excreted in the urine. In an emergency room situation, diabetic acidosis can be recognized not only by the increased rate and depth of respirations (Kussmaul's respirations) but by the odor of acetone on the breath. Neither osmotic diuresis (No. 2) nor failure in the sodium-hydrogen ion exchange (No. 3) causes acetonuria. In the latter case, failure to excrete excess hydrogen ions would decrease urinary acids. Volatile hydrogen ions (CO_2) are excreted by the lungs; a decrease in nonvolatile hydrogen ions in the glomerular filtrate (No. 4) would move the pH of the urine toward the alkaline side.

37. (2) Ms. Phillips is demonstrating early signs of diabetic acidosis. Before notifying the physician (No. 1), it is necessary to collect the data, blood sugar and urine sugar and acetone, on which the physician will base the insulin order. The physician should also be notified of Ms. Phillips' vital signs and intake and output. Generally, urinary output is depressed for about 36 hours after surgery due to increased circulating levels of ADH. Given that Ms. Phillips has also had insensible water loss (respirations and perspiration), her assessment data strongly indicate dehydration or hypovolemia. An antiemetic (No. 3) may be administered if nausea persists *after* blood sugar and fluid balance are rectified. The physician may order an increase in the amount and rate of intravenous fluids (contrary to No. 4).

38. (2) Ms. Phillips' vital signs and urine output reflect a decrease in extracellular volume secondary to osmotic diuresis. Increased ADH release *decreases* urinary output (No. 1). A hypo-osmolar fluid imbalance is one in which there is more water than solute in the extracellular fluid compartment (No. 3). Like circulatory overload (No. 4), symptoms of a hypo-osmolar imbalance include widened pulse pressure, increased blood pressure, distended neck veins, and respiratory crackles.

39. (3) Glycogenolysis and therefore serum-glucose levels are increased due to the stresses of surgery. In order to control blood-glucose levels and prevent ketoacidosis, secondary to increased tissue metabolism (No. 1), regular insulin is given in doses adjusted according to the results of urine tests (rainbow or sliding scale). Regular insulin may be given alone until urine tests for glucosuria and ketonuria stabilize or as a supplement along with an intermediate-acting insulin such as NPH. No. 2, decreased insulin production, results from the extent of Ms. Phillips' dysfunction, not the stress of surgery. Insulin does facilitate the movement of potassium across the cellular membrane, thus preventing hyperkalemia (No. 4), but this is not the *best* answer.

40. (2) NPH is an intermediate-acting insulin with an onset time of 2 hours, peak action in 6–12 hours, and a duration of action of 24 hours. No. 1 is the peak action time for regular insulin. Nos. 3 and 4 are within the range for long-acting insulins.

41. (3) The client receiving NPH insulin is most likely to experience a hypoglycemic reaction in the late afternoon. Several factors may be involved, such as increased physical activity or inadequate dietary intake. Clients should be instructed to carry gumdrops or Lifesavers as a source of quickly absorbed carbohydrates should symptoms occur. Nos. 1, 2, and 4 are not as likely.

42. (3) Hypoglycemic or insulin reactions are the result of decreased circulatory serum glucose to the brain. This stimulates epinephrine release. Early symptoms include cold, clammy skin, nervousness, tremors, numbness of the hands or around the lips, and cardiac palpitations. Later symptoms may mimic alcoholic intoxication, such as staggering gait, slurring of words, combative behavior, or uncontrolled weeping. As hypoglycemia deepens, the client may develop convulsions and coma. Nos. 1, 2, and 4 are symptoms of ketoacidosis, which acts to depress the central nervous system.

43. (3) See rationale for question 42 above. No. 1 is incorrect, in that respirations in insulin shock, though shallow, are increased. No. 2 is incorrect because the breath of the client in insulin shock is noncontributory, not fetid. Fetid breath may occur with liver failure or poor dental hygiene. Behavioral responses in No. 4 are switched; that is, confusion and lethargy are common with ketoacidosis, and cold, clammy skin is consistent with insulin shock.

44. (1) Emergency surgery must be performed in order to save the life of the client, save the function of an organ or limb, remove a damaged organ or limb, or stop hemorrhage. Few emergency situations are so urgent as to require immediate response (No. 2), eliminating the necessary laboratory data to evaluate the client's physiologic response to the situation. Surgical preparation would be completed within 24 hours (No. 3), but this is not the *best* answer. True emergency situations cannot be postponed to the following surgical day (No. 4).

45. (4) An abdominal hysterectomy is generally the treatment of choice for uterine fibroids with excessive vaginal bleeding. If the ovaries are not pathologic, there is no reason for surgical removal. No. 1, panabdominal hysterectomy, involves the removal of the uterus, fallopian tubes, and ovaries and is usually performed for extensive endometriosis or carcinoma. A vaginal hysterectomy (No. 2) is the treatment of choice for a prolapsed uterus, and a D&C (No. 3) is primarily a diagnostic tool, not a measure to control excessive uterine bleeding.

46. (2) Few surgeries warrant immediate treatment (No. 1); however, the urgency of the situation does decrease client preparation time. Consequently, the client's physiologic stress will increase, not decrease (No. 3), placing greater demands on metabolic functions and increasing the risk of complications. Emergency surgery does not compromise the use of general anesthesia (No. 4). It is imperative to ascertain before an emergency surgery the time, type, and amount of the last oral intake, as gastric lavage or suctioning may be necessary to prevent aspiration during the surgery. Generally clients are NPO 12 hours before surgery.

47. (1) Anticoagulants increase bleeding time and tendency to hemorrhage. Antihypertensives such as reserpine, hydralazine, and methyldopa potentiate the hypotensive effects of anesthetic agents, thereby creating problems with maintenance of blood pressure. Thiazide diuretics may induce potassium depletion and lead to respiratory depression during anesthesia. Nos. 2, 3, and 4 are incorrect because neither insulin, digoxin, nor vitamins and minerals potentiate the central nervous system depression due to anesthesia.

48. (3) The initial response would be to notify the physician of the critical hemoglobin (oxygen-carrying protein) level. A hemoglobin of 10 is desirable for the client, decreasing the deleterious risks of general anesthetic and hypovolemic shock. The lab slip is then attached to the chart (No. 1). Most likely a blood transfusion will be ordered before surgery (No. 2), but there is no order yet. Your actions will be charted on the nurses' notes (No. 4), but charting is *not* the *first* priority.

49. (3) Manipulation of abdominal contents during surgery produces inhibition of peristalsis for 24–48 hours. Measures to avoid potential distention could include insertion of a nasogastric tube before surgery and continuous postsurgical suction until peristalsis returns; rectal tubes can be inserted to remove excess air in the lower colon; and early ambulation promotes return of gastrointestinal functioning. Auscultation of the abdomen for return of bowel sounds (No. 1) will be necessary in assessing the return and degree of peristalsis. Abdominal massage is not recommended (No. 2). When bowel sounds return, oral intake (No. 4) may be started.

50. (1) Sitting for long periods of time and wearing constrictive clothing tend to increase pelvic congestion. Daily bowel movements (No. 2) are not necessary as long as a normal pattern is achieved. It is important to reinforce the physician's instructions that sexual activity may be resumed within a specific period of time, usually 6–8 weeks. Six months (No. 3) is too long. Paced and gradual ambulation aids in increasing venous return and general strength. Complete avoidance of chores for 2 months (No. 4) is not necessary. Lifting of heavy objects, however, may injure the incision site and promote bleeding.

51. (3) Once the uterus is removed, the client is infertile and contraception is not necessary. Nos. 1, 2, and 4 *should* be included in the teaching plan. Following a hysterectomy, the vaginal flow is usually brownish in nature and will gradually diminish and cease. If the flow continues and is obviously red in nature, the physician must be notified. These signs could indicate a bleeding vessel. Menses will be absent following removal of the uterus.

52. (1) Liver functions are many and varied, including detoxification of chemicals (estrogen, adrenocorticoids, aldosterone, drugs, poisons, and heavy metals); synthesis of plasma proteins (albumin, fibrinogen, globulin) and several clotting factors (prothrombin, factor VII); storage of glycogen, iron, and vitamins (A, D, E, K, and B_{12}); gluconeogenesis (glucose from amino acids and fats); and deamination of amino acids. Fluid volume control and acid-base balance are functions of the *kidney* (No. 2). Most erythrocyte and leukocyte breakdown occurs in the *spleen* (No. 3). The *gallbladder* concentrates and stores bile (No. 4), and the liver is involved with synthesis and secretion of bile.

53. (2) Ecchymoses occur in cirrhosis due to decreased synthesis of clotting factors as well as decreased vitamin K storage. Dilatation and slow blood flow in veins causes the formation of spider angiomas (particularly on the upper chest), palmar redness, and varicosities (esophageal and rectal are common). Esophageal hemorrhage (No. 1) results in the vomiting of bright red blood. Vitamin K is fat-soluble, not water-soluble (No. 3). Venous pressures will increase, not decrease (No. 4), due to mechanical obstruction in the liver, which results in increased capillary fragility.

54. (1) The portal system becomes obstructed, causing a rise in portal venous pressure and portal hypertension, venous dilatation, and stasis. In cirrhosis, there is *decreased* hepatic synthesis of albumin, not increased (No. 2), and *increased* levels of aldosterone, not decreased (No. 3). Blood volumes are *decreased,* not increased (No. 4), while total body fluid is increased due to the physiologic effects of hypoproteinemia (decreased serum proteins). These factors, plus increasing obstruction of the portal vein, cause fluids, electrolytes, and serum proteins to move out of the vascular compartment and into the intestines. The abdomen provides a large potential space for the accumulation of these fluids.

55. (1) Anemia occurs in cirrhosis due to (a) erythrocyte destruction in the engorged spleen, (b) gastrointestinal blood losses, and (c) folic acid deficiencies from inadequate dietary intake. Kupffer cells (No. 2) line the venous sinusoids in the liver and are primarily macrophagic. Nos. 3 and 4 are incorrect because decreased amino acid breakdown and synthesis result in increasing serum-ammonia levels, which may further inhibit dietary intake.

56. (2) The diet of a cirrhotic client should provide ample protein for tissue repair, at least 0.5 g/lb. Some modification occurs if serum-ammonia levels are elevated (No. 1). Sufficient carbohydrate intake is needed to sustain weight and prevent proteins from being utilized for energy, not for the reason stated in No. 3. No. 4 is partially correct. Salt is restricted to assist in decreasing edema formation. However, the reason for high-carbohydrate foods is as discussed above. Fluids may also be restricted to 1000–1500 mL/day. Vitamin supplements, particularly fat-soluble vitamins (A, D, and K), are usually prescribed because of decreased bile production for their absorption and because of the inability of the liver to store them successfully. Initially, if the client has a very poor appetite, liquid protein supplements such as Sustagen may be given. Frequent, small feedings may also increase intake.

57. (4) Frequent, small meals do not visually overwhelm the client, and they require less energy for ingestion. Because clients with cirrhosis frequently have very poor appetites, the nurse may have to be very creative in approaches to assure adequate nutritional intake. Nos. 1, 2, and 3 take the responsibility away from the client and increase his dependency.

58. (2) After explaining the procedure to the client, the nurse should first instruct him to void. This prevents accidental nicking or perforation of the bladder during the procedure. The client is positioned in a chair or in high Fowler's position in bed (No. 1), after the vital signs have been taken to establish baseline information (No. 3) and the abdomen is prepared (No. 4).

59. (2) Hypotension and shock can occur during or after paracentesis. Fluid from the vascular compartment shifts into the abdomen to replace fluids that are withdrawn. This complication can be minimized if withdrawal of ascitic fluid is limited to 1000 mL and/or if lost fluid is replaced by administration of salt-poor albumin. To assess for this complication, vital signs are taken every 15 minutes during the procedure and afterward until stable, then every hour for 4 hours. Disequilibrium (No. 1) occurs with rapid removal of wastes during renal dialysis. Hypoalbuminuria (no protein in urine) is a normal physical finding; therefore No. 3 is incorrect. Paralytic ileus (No. 4) is rarely a complication of this procedure.

60. (2) See answer 59 above.

61. (1) The earliest clinical signs of bleeding include restlessness, pallor, tachycardia, and cooling of the skin. These symptoms occur as the result of vasoconstriction (increased sympathetic stimulation) in order to maintain venous return and cardiac output. No. 2 represents symptoms of ketoacidosis. When the vasoconstrictive mechanisms discussed above are no longer effective, the blood pressure begins to fall (No. 3). It is essential to identify bleeding early because liver cells are very susceptible to ischemia. No. 4 may occur with increases in intracranial pressure.

62. (3) The Sengstaken-Blakemore tube is a triple-lumen tube composed of a catheter that goes to the stomach for suctioning, a lumen that ends in a gastric balloon, and a lumen that ends in an esophageal balloon. The primary purpose of this tube is to stop bleeding by applying pressure to the cardiac portion of the stomach and against the esophageal varices. Thus, No. 1 is only partially correct. The secondary purposes of the tube are: (a) to prevent accumulation of blood in the gastrointestinal tract (No. 2), which could precipitate hepatic coma, and (b) to reduce blood transfusion requirements (No. 4).

63. (2) Symptoms of severe respiratory distress indicate that the tube has dislodged and is obstructing the airway. Reestablishing an airway is the first priority: deflate the balloons using a syringe. Following deflation, the doctor should be notified in order to assess Mr. Chuska's condition and determine ongoing medical therapy. A code blue (No. 1) would be called only after establishing the airway. Traction on the Sengstaken tube should be increased or decreased (No. 3) only by the attending physician. Iced saline (No. 4) is no longer used for irrigation during active bleeding, and this problem is respiratory, not hemorrhagic.

64. (2) Ammonia is formed in the intestines by the action of intestinal bacteria on proteins. Tap-water enemas may be given to remove protein-rich blood that has resulted from bleeding esophageal varices. Since ammonia is formed during muscle contraction, active range-of-motion exercises are contraindicated (No. 1). To prevent skin breakdown in a client who is jaundiced and edematous, passive exercises, turning, and frequent skin care are indicated. In an effort to reduce serum-ammonia levels, potassium levels need to be increased, not reduced (No. 3), because potassium is necessary for cerebral metabolism of ammonia. Antibiotics that are poorly absorbed by the intestines, such as neomycin, are given, rather than withheld (No. 4), to decrease the intestinal flora that manufacture ammonia.

65. (1) Prognosis is generally poor if hepatic coma lasts longer than 24 hours. Other measures that have been utilized to decrease serum ammonia and allow for regeneration of hepatocytes include hemodialysis, exchange blood transfusions, and administration of lactalose, which, when degraded in the large bowel, decreases the pH of the feces, thus preventing formation of ammonia and promoting its excretion. Nos. 2, 3, and 4 all exceed the 24-hour threshold.

66. (4) Both women are Rh-negative primiparas and are at some risk for Rh incompatibility; erythroblastosis fetalis results from hemolysis of fetal cells by maternal antibodies. No. 1 is wrong because Sue is at greater risk for spontaneous abortion due to her diabetes. No. 2 is wrong because the incidence of preeclampsia is higher in the pregnant diabetic. No. 3 is wrong because fetal macrosomia in infants of diabetic mothers may result in dystocia.

67. (2) Human placental lactogen (HPL) is an insulin antagonist and may complicate management of Sue's diabetes during pregnancy. No. 1 is incorrect because fatigue and varicosities are common complaints associated with decreased venous return from the lower extremities. No. 3 is wrong because increased cardiac output places additional work on the heart. No. 4 is wrong because relaxation of the cardiac sphincter is associated with heartburn and gastric reflux.

68. (3) Increased cardiac output has greater implications for Judi because her heart has been compromised by rheumatic fever. Judi should understand and be able to recognize signs of complications associated with her heart function. No. 1 is wrong because increased venous pressure in the lower extremities presents little more than an annoyance to either woman. No. 2 is wrong because placental production of HPL presents a greater problem for *Sue* (because of her diabetes). No. 4 is wrong because relaxation of the cardiac sphincter results in minor complaints for both women.

69. (4) Amniocentesis does not provide evidence as to whether or not the fetus is a potential diabetic, but it may be performed on diabetic women to test for fetal lung maturity or on Rh-negative women to monitor Rh-sensitized fetuses. No. 1 is incorrect because her statement indicates understanding of the interrelationship between her pregnancy and her diabetes. No. 2 is wrong because pregnant diabetics may be hospitalized for testing for placental function. No. 3 is wrong because nausea and vomiting in the pregnant diabetic may lead to acidosis.

70. (2) The most important single factor in maintaining good health for the pregnant cardiac client is adequate rest. The pregnant cardiac client should have approximately 8–10 hours rest each night and should lie down for one-half hour after each meal (Williams, 1980). No. 1 is incorrect because *reduced* activity reduces fatigue and supports preservation of cardiac reserve. No. 3 is wrong because moderate sodium intake (2000 mg) is allowable for the average class I cardiac; nutritional counseling focuses on increasing dietary intake of iron, protein, and essential nutrients to meet the increased demands of pregnancy. No. 4 is wrong because ferrous sulfate is prescribed to meet the increased demands for hemoglobin synthesis and to combat nutritional anemia.

71. (2) Activities of daily living will increase energy expenditures in the cardiac patient and may contribute to further decompensation. No. 1 is incorrect because dyspnea and shortness of breath will be exacerbated in the head-down position. No. 3 is incorrect because any activity that causes the patient to perform a Valsalva maneuver (coughing) will cause a sudden increase in blood return to the heart, which is contraindicated in cardiac disease. No. 4 is incorrect because the major goal of care is to reduce all energy expenditures.

72. (2) The woman who seems restless, with flushed face, rapid pulse, and rapid deep respirations, is exhibiting signs of hyperglycemia. No. 1 is incorrect because failure to react to a flash of light in the face is associated with an insulin reaction. No. 3 is wrong because diaphoresis during sleep is associated with insulin reactions. No. 4 is wrong because headaches are associated with insulin reactions.

73. (4) Hypoglycemia does inhibit the let-down reflex and interfere with successful breastfeeding. Further, maintaining a stable serum glucose is important to maternal health. No. 1 is incorrect because breastfeeding exerts a positive effect on diabetes, reducing blood-sugar levels by transfering glucose from serum to the breast for conversion to lactose; energy is expended in milk production. No. 2 is wrong because her caloric needs will increase with lactation; insulin dosage must be adjusted to maintain optimum serum-glucose levels. No. 3 is wrong because hypoglycemia jeopardizes both successful breastfeeding and maternal status.

74. (3) is correct because the primary goal is to prepare the new mother with diabetes to care for her infant while effectively managing her disease. No. 1 is incorrect because it will not ensure adequate home health maintenance of mother and infant. No. 2 is incorrect because potential problems will vary, depending on many factors such as maternal age, and does not address the primary health maintenance goal. No. 4 is incorrect because, although follow-up care is an important aspect of discharge teaching, it is subsumed under the broader goal of discussing coping strategies for managing diabetes.

75. (4) Bearing down is too strenuous for the pregnant cardiac. No. 1 is incorrect because relaxation in a semirecumbent position reduces the workload on the heart. No. 2 is wrong because increased pulse rate is an early sign of cardiac decompensation. No. 3 is wrong because regional anesthesia reduces pain and the physiologic response to pain, which may cause cardiac decompensation.

76. (3) Pelvic inflammatory disease is associated with adhesions and blockage of the fallopian tubes, preventing transport and joining of the ovum and sperm. No. 1 is incorrect because moderate alcohol intake is not implicated in infertility. No. 2 is incorrect because a normal menstrual cycle is not associated with infertility. No. 4 is incorrect because use of a diaphragm and spermicidal jelly is not implicated in infertility.

77. (2) Acute glomerulonephritis is an autoimmune response to an antigen produced by beta-hemolytic streptococci. Antibodies produced to fight the antigen also react against the glomerular tissue. This causes proliferation and swelling of endothelial cells in the glomerular capillary wall and results in passage of blood cells and protein into the glomerular filtrate. Acute glomerular nephritis is not the result of direct infection (Nos. 1 and 3) or of hypoxia (No. 4).

78. (1) The kidneys secrete the erythropoietin factor, which stimulates the bone marrow to produce red blood cells. In chronic kidney disease, secretion of this factor decreases as greater portions of the kidney are destroyed by the disease process. Hypertension does not suppress bone marrow centers (No. 2), because local blood flow regulators tend to compensate over the long run by supplying tissue with adequate blood flow for metabolic purposes. Unlike metabolic acidosis, metabolic alkalosis does not increase RBC fragility (No. 3). Frank bleeding into the urine is uncommon in chronic renal disease (No. 4).

79. (1) Hyperkalemia tends to develop in renal dysfunction for two reasons: in the kidneys, more hydrogen ions than potassium ions are selectively secreted in exchange for sodium ions, and decreasing glomerular filtration and urine output tend to decrease the excretion of all electrolytes and waste products of metabolism. Potassium does not move out of the cell to balance sodium shifts in edema (No. 2), nor does respiratory alkalosis affect potassium reabsorption in the kidneys (No. 3). Nausea and vomiting (No. 4) cause hypokalemia.

80. (3) Mr. Lawson's urine specific gravity indicates that his kidneys have lost their ability to concentrate his urine. Therefore he has a greater water loss than would normally be expected. ADH secretion (No. 1) would produce an elevated specific gravity. No. 2 is incorrect because water loss without concomitant electrolyte loss causes the extracellular fluids to become hyperosmolar (that is, the client is dehydrated). No. 4 is incorrect because hyperosmolarity of ECF causes the thirst receptors in the hypothalamus to shrink, which stimulates the thirst mechanism.

81. (2) The evening before an intravenous pyelogram, the client is administered oral cathartics or enemas to clean the bowel of fecal material and flatus, thereby improving visualization of the kidneys and ureters. The radiopaque dye used in this procedure is injected by a physician in the radiology department, not the night before (No. 1). No. 3 is *not* part of IVP preparation. If Mr. Lawson is having difficulty maintaining fluid volume balance, an intravenous infusion *may* be initiated to prevent dehydration, but it is not standard (No. 4).

82. (4) Lethargy, disorientation, and increased rate and depth of respirations are clinical manifestations of metabolic *acidosis*. As hydrogen ion concentration rises, the central nervous system is depressed, causing the client to become increasingly lethargic and slower in his responses. Likewise, the lungs endeavor to compensate for a metabolic acidosis by increasing both the rate and depth of respirations. Serum bicarbonates provide an estimate of metabolic components of acid-base balance. The level of these ions is controlled by the kidney's ability to secrete hydrogen ions and actively reabsorb bicarbonate ions. Decreased levels of bicarbonate indicate metabolic acidosis, and increased levels of serum bicarbonate indicate metabolic alkalosis. Nos. 1, 2, and 3 are symptoms of *alkalosis*.

83. (3) Methyldopa acts to decrease blood pressure by inhibiting the formation of dopamine, thus decreasing the amount of norepinephrine that is secreted in adrenergic synapses. Decreased adrenergic stimulation results in decreased vasoconstriction, which causes peripheral vascular resistance. No. 1 is an example of the effects of hydralazine; No. 2, of guanethidine SO_4; and No. 4, of diazepam.

84. (3) The single best measure for assessing Mr. Lawson's fluid volume status is daily weights. Significant water loss must occur before there are changes in skin turgor (No. 1). Similarly, blood pressure (No. 2) may not reflect changes in fluid volume status if the fluid is sequestered in the interstitial spaces (edema formation). Finally, intake and output measures are important (No. 4) but generally do not reflect insensible water losses (water lost per respiration and diaphoresis) and are not always as sensitive to decreases in urine output in chronic renal dysfunction as they are in more acute illnesses.

85. (2) Mr. Lawson's increasing symptomatology is due to a decrease in the number of functioning nephrons, with resultant decrease in glomerular filtration due to the extension of his disease process. No. 1 is incorrect because the cause of his renal failure was likely related to intrarenal damage from acute glomerulonephritis. Nos. 3 and 4 are incorrect because Mr. Lawson has moved from the second stage of chronic kidney disease (renal insufficiency, characterized by water diuresis and mild azotemia) to renal failure, which is characterized by acidosis, marked electrolyte imbalances, fluid retention, anemia, and increases in serum urea, uric acid, and creatinine.

86. (4) Increased circulating levels of uric acid, an end product of purine metabolism, are responsible for Mr. Lawson's goutlike joint discomfort. Thus his diet will exclude foods high in purines (e.g., high-protein foods, organ meats). Hyperphosphatemia does occur in the third stage of chronic kidney disease. Normally this would stimulate the parathyroid gland to increase parathormone, thus raising calcium levels and lowering phosphate (No. 1). However, in chronic renal failure the kidney fails to produce a metabolite of vitamin D, which effectively reduces parathormone activity, lowering serum-calcium levels. Amphogel (an aluminum hydroxide preparation) is given to bind the phosphate excreted in the bowel (No. 1). Dialysis is used to decrease the serum-creatinine level, which causes central nervous system depression (No. 2). Joint pain is usually related to inflammation or trauma rather than decreased activity level. Increasing his activity (No. 3) might aggravate his pain.

87. (1) Increased serum potassium (hyperkalemia) causes the T waves to lose their normal, rounded configuration and become more pointy or peaked (the difference in shape between a mountain and a mound); therefore No. 2 is incorrect. ST segments are not significantly affected by this electrolyte imbalance (Nos. 3 and 4).

88. (2) Mr. Lawson's blood gases indicate that he is mildly acidotic. pH is still within normal limits. No. 1 is incorrect because his remaining functional nephrons and his lungs have been able to compensate for the increase in circulating hydrogen ions. If respiratory alkalosis (No. 3) were the underlying pathology, the pH would demonstrate alkalosis (pH above 7.40). No. 4 is incorrect because Mr. Lawson does have respiratory alkalosis, but it represents respiratory compensation rather than the primary pathologic mechanism.

89. (2) Symptoms of circulatory overload result from varying degrees of cardiac decompensation, with blood backing up into the pulmonary (moist crackles) and systemic circuits (neck vein distention, dependent edema, periorbital edema, and hepatomegaly). Symptoms of circulatory failure or hypovolemia include apprehension, soft eyeballs, flattened neck veins, shock, decreased pulse pressure, and poor skin turgor (Nos. 1, 3, and 4).

90. (3) Before beginning the dialysis procedure, baseline information needs to be collected so that the therapy can be accurately evaluated. Baseline information will include vital signs, body temperature, weight, ECG, and electrolyte levels. If the client does not have a Foley catheter (often by this time they do because of the need to assess hourly outputs), then the client is asked to void. Following voiding, the client is positioned in a supine or low Fowler's position and the abdomen is prepared and draped. Nos. 1, 2, and 4 are actions subsequent to No. 3.

91. (2) The dialysate is warmed to body temperature before administration to minimize discomfort and optimize clearance of waste products. Warming the fluid tends to dilate the peritoneal vessels, increasing the amount of urea that passes through the membrane. It has little effect on the osmotic gradient (No. 1), does not prevent peritonitis, which is secondary to infection (No. 3), and does not speed infusion time (No. 4), although it does make it more comfortable.

92. (2) Generally, the dwell time of the dialysate is 20–30 minutes, occasionally longer. The dwell time as well as the instillation and outflow times are prescribed by the physician according to the client's needs. Ten to fifteen minutes (No. 1) is too short a time to allow for diffusion of waste products. Equilibrium between dialysate and body fluids occurs in 15–30 minutes. Longer times (Nos. 3 and 4) are not necessary.

93. (3) The cumulative inflow and outflow records should show an outflow equal to or in excess of the amount instilled. The amount of excess outflow allowed is also determined by the physician; this rarely exceeds 200 mL per cycle. Occasionally, drainage is less than expected. Nursing measures to enhance outflow include turning the client from side to side, elevating the head of the bed (increases intraabdominal pressures), and/or gently massaging the abdomen. If the problem continues, notify the physician before initiating another cycle; she or he may attempt to clear the catheter by rotation or by probing it for fibrin clots (No. 2). Nos. 1 and 4 will not improve flow.

94. (4) Flattened neck veins in a supine position are characteristic of hypovolemia. Inadequate drainage would result in fluid retention and hypervolemia. Indications of fluid retention include inadequate fluid drainage (greater intake than output), increased blood pressure, and signs of congestive heart failure, e.g., distended neck veins, increased dependent edema, crackles, and decreased mentation (Nos. 1, 2, and 3).

95. (3) A BUN of less than 20 mg% and serum creatinine less than 1.2 mg% would be optimal outcome measures for this client (that is, within normal range). Nos. 1, 2, and 4 are incorrect because: a serum K^+ of less than 3.5 mEq/L would be indicative of hypokalemia; a serum Na^+ above 148 mEq/L indicates hypernatremia (No. 1). Quantity of urine output should increase to over 500 mL/24 hours (No. 2); the abdomen should be soft and tympanic to percussion; so dullness to percussion in the abdomen is consistent with fluid excess (No. 4).

96. (1) To prevent contractures, the affected limb is kept straight (knee extension) and slightly abducted (to prevent pressure in hip joint), and the foot is supported (ankle flexion) to prevent footdrop. Nos. 2, 3, and 4 are incorrect because all or part of each response could produce a contracture.

97. (1) Quadriceps setting exercise is an appropriate activity to prevent complications of immobility. Range of motion exercises for joints not enclosed in the cast are encouraged. The primary purpose of the cast is to immobilize those joints above and below the fracture site; therefore (No. 2) extension and (No. 4) flexion of the knees are inappropriate. No. 3 is not correct because passive range of motion is *not as effective* as *active* range of motion in the prevention of complications of immobility.

98. (3) Before assessing and planning any rehabilitation program, the nurse must first assess the client's and the family's understanding of and attitudes toward myasthenia, as well as their emotional response and coping abilities. Before ascertaining any further information about job stresses (No. 1) and/or life-style (No. 2), any unusual fears, misconceptions, or problems relating to the client's condition need to be identified and dealt with (No. 4). It may be necessary to utilize the skills of a psychiatric nurse specialist, health psychologist, or psychiatrist to evaluate the situation and assist in planning interventions.

99. (2) Keeping the foot in the correct anatomical position is the *best* method of preventing footdrop, and a footboard is best when the client is in traction. A bed cradle (No. 1) is effective in keeping pressure off the legs and feet. Passive range of motion (No. 3) is most effective in preventing contractures. A trochanter roll (No. 4) is most effective in preventing external rotation of the hip.

100. (3) Coughing, vigorous exercise, and straining or lifting increase intraabdominal pressures, which tend to extrude the intestines through weakened areas of the abdominal wall. Mr. Kealey's history includes all of the above. Other causes of hernia include Nos. 1, 2, and 4.

101. (2) A truss should be applied before getting out of bed or after the hernia has been reduced, by lying down with the feet elevated in bed or in the bath. If the hernia cannot be reduced, the truss should not be applied (Nos. 1 and 3). Although the truss is not a cure for a hernia and its use is not as common as it once was, it is far more effective in keeping a hernia reduced than is an athletic supporter (No. 4).

102. (2) Mr. Kealey's smoking history and history of chronic cough necessitate directing preoperative nursing measures toward clearing his respiratory tract of excess secretions that might lead to postoperative complications. Besides oral hygiene, the following may be instituted or ordered before surgery: postural drainage, incentive spirometers, IPPB, and mucolytic agent. Since postoperative coughing is contraindicated with hernia repairs, removal of secretions is a priority, as is instruction in deep-breathing techniques. Nos. 1, 3, and 4, though not top priority, are correct and should also be included in your preoperative teaching plan.

103. (3) Since the client has a history of chronic cough, and since hernias can be repaired with spinal anesthesia, this approach may have the least amount of risk for postoperative complications. General anesthesia (No. 1) has the greatest risk for respiratory complications after surgery. Intravenous (No. 2) and local infiltration (No. 4) would not supply the depth of anesthesia needed to complete the repair.

104. (2) Timed forced expiratory volume measures the functional ability of an individual to remove air from his lungs. Reduction in FEV_1 is usually due to airway obstruction from excess mucus. Vital capacity measures the individual's ability to move a volume of air in and out of the lungs (No. 1). Though inadequate innervation of the intercostals (No. 3) would also reduce the FEV_1, there is nothing in this case study to indicate that Mr. Kealey has neuromuscular problems. Atelectasis (No. 4) is determined by X ray, clinical symptomatology, and blood gases.

105. (1) The skin preparation area for hernia repair includes the entire abdomen from just below the nipple line to the mid-thigh. It includes all pubic hair visible when the legs are together, and should extend to the bedline on each side. No. 2 is an example of an abdominal prep when the incision is above the umbilicus. No. 3 is a lower-extremities prep for surgeries such as a femoral arterial graft. No. 4 is a perineal prep used for vaginal or rectal surgeries.

106. (2) To avoid the complication of a painful spinal headache that can last for several days, the client is kept flat in a supine position for approximately 4–12 hours postoperatively. Headaches are believed due to the seepage of cerebral spinal fluid from the puncture site. By keeping the client flat, cerebral spinal fluid pressures are equalized, which avoid trauma to the neurons. No. 1 is the position for clients having general anesthesia. No. 3 is incorrect because knees are flexed. No. 4 is the position for clients with head traumas.

107. (2) Clients who have had spinal anesthesia have varying degrees of hypotension due to the vasodepressor effect of the anesthetic agent on the autonomic nervous system. Reflexes (No. 1) will be depressed in the lower extremities because of the anesthetic and should be checked *after* circulatory status. However, sensory impulses remain blocked longer than motor activity, so safety measures should be instituted to prevent injury from bedding, poor positioning, or sources of heat. Since the client is awake with a spinal anesthetic, level of consciousness (No. 3) and airway integrity (No. 4) are lower priorities than circulatory status.

108. (2) Postoperative inflammation and edema underlie the frequent occurrence of scrotal swelling after indirect hernia repair. This complication is very painful, and any movement by the client results in discomfort. Elevating the scrotum on rolled towels or providing support with a suspensory helps to reduce edema. Ice bags facilitate pain relief. No. 1 is inappropriate, as this is not an emergency side effect of surgery. Pain medication (No. 3) may also be administered, but vigorous coughing (No. 4) is contraindicated following herniorrhaphy.

109. (3) Although most clients are able to rest more comfortably and even sleep after administration of a narcotic, extreme or prolonged lethargy indicates that the medication dose may be too large. The physician should be consulted for both a change of dose and/or route of administration (Nos. 1 and 2). Alternate modes of pain relief can and should be instituted if Mr. Kealey's discomfort is not severe, but not as a delaying tactic (No. 4) when the issue is the appropriateness of a specific medication dose.

110. (4) If all the secondary measures have been tried and the client's bladder is distended, the physician should be notified if he or she has not left a catheterization order. Occasionally, drugs such as Prostigmin are ordered to stimulate bladder contractions before resorting to catheterization. No. 1 will only tire him more. Catheters should not be inserted without an order (No. 2), nor should the client be unduly fatigued by continuing to try other measures (No. 3) that most likely were unsuccessful prior to this point in time. The bladder should not be allowed to become overdistended.

111. (1) Urinary retention following spinal anesthesia is due to blockage of autonomic nervous system fibers, which innervate the bladder and sensory perception. No. 2, though correct, is not as complete as No. 1. All clients secrete ADH postoperatively because of the surgical insult. However, ADH reduces the volume of urine (No. 3), as does lowered blood pressure (No. 4), but neither causes urinary retention.

112. (2) Given Mr. Kealey's complaint and evidence of pink drainage, you should suspect dehiscence. Dehiscence is characterized by a gush of pink serous drainage and a parting of the wound edges. Dehiscence generally occurs in the fifth to seventh day following surgery, due to increased intraabdominal pressures from flatus, coughing, retching, or inadequate tissue support. Late hemorrhage (No. 1) would be accompanied by signs of shock such as decreased blood pressure, rapid pulse, and diaphoresis. Wound infection (No. 3) would be characterized by pain, redness, and fever. Evisceration (No. 4) occurs after dehiscence when loops of intestine escape through the opened incision.

113. (1) The client should remain quiet in a low Fowler's or horizontal position. He should be cautioned not to cough so as not to extrude any intestines by increasing intra-abdominal pressures. The physician should be notified next. Remain with the client, reassuring him, monitoring vital signs, and having others bring equipment such as an IV set-up, nasogastric tube, and suction equipment. The surgeon should also be notified that the client will be returning to the operating room. The client should be kept NPO (No. 2) in above position (No. 3) and the dressing left in place to prevent evisceration (No. 4).

114. (4) All straining and lifting should be avoided for at least 3 weeks to prevent undue stress on the sutures. Other less strenuous activities, such as Nos. 1, 2, and 3, are appropriate, though good body mechanics should be reviewed with the client.

115. (2) The functions of the gallbladder are to collect, concentrate, and store bile, which is produced by the liver, not by the gallbladder (No. 1). Bile reaches the gallbladder via the hepatic duct, which later joins the cystic duct emanating from the gallbladder to form the common bile duct. The common bile duct joins the pancreatic duct, which opens into the duodenum. Bile is not diluted (No. 3). No. 4 is incorrect because contraction of the gallbladder and therefore flow of bile are stimulated by the hormone cholecystokinin, which is secreted by the duodenal mucosa when food enters the duodenum.

116. (3) Fat-soluble vitamins, particularly vitamin K, are poorly absorbed in the absence of bile. Decreased absorption of vitamin K results in decreased levels of circulating prothrombin, thus reducing normal clotting levels. Peripheral neuritis (No. 1) occurs with vitamin B_6 deficiencies, and scurvy (No. 2) occurs with deficiency in vitamin C; these are water-soluble vitamins. Macrocytic anemia (No. 4) is consistent with a vitamin B_{12} deficiency, which may be due to lack of intrinsic factor in the stomach.

117. (3) Obstruction of the bile duct will cause elevated serum and urine bilirubin (dark urine) as well as a decreased amount of urobilinogen in the feces (clay-colored stools). Bilirubin is an end product of hemoglobin breakdown. Normally it is conjugated in the liver and secreted, in the bile, into the intestines, where it is converted into urobilinogen and excreted in the stools. No. 1 is incorrect because biliary obstruction itself does not directly affect blood pressure. However, if the obstruction is acute and accompanied by pain, changes in blood pressure in response to increased sympathetic tone can be expected. No. 2 is incorrect because between-meal eructation is a symptom of ulcer disease. Eructation in gallbladder disease occurs after eating, particularly if large amounts of fat have been ingested. No. 4 is also incorrect; longitudinal ridging of the fingernails is a sign seen frequently in anemia.

118. (2) The contrast medium utilized in IV cholangiograms, like that used in intravenous pyelogram, contains iodine. It is important to ascertain before the test whether the client is aware of any allergy to iodine. Saltwater fish generally leave a high iodine content, so it is helpful to ascertain if the client has an allergy to fish, and, if so, to what kind. No. 1 is helpful in planning client teaching and may also elicit No. 2. Nos. 3 and 4 are less specific responses that provide interesting, though not essential, data.

119. (3) Telepaque tablets are administered 1 hour after eating a fat-free meal (No. 1), one at a time and in 5-minute intervals (No. 2), with a minimal amount of water (usually 8 oz) in order to swallow *all* the tablets. Water is allowed until bedtime (No. 4), but food is withheld in order to allow as much dye as possible to concentrate in the gallbladder. The next morning an initial X ray is taken, after which the client is given a fatty meal, and several more pictures are taken to observe the functioning of the gallbladder.

120. (1) Fat-soluble vitamins, particularly vitamin K, are poorly absorbed in the absence of bile. This leads to decreased levels of circulating prothrombin, thus reducing normal clotting and increasing the tendency to bleed. Clients will have a T-tube postoperatively, not a Hemovac (No. 2). Heating pads (No. 3) are not used to relieve the abdominal discomfort of cholelithiasis and cholecystitis since they have little effect on reducing spasms of deeper organs. Instead, antispasmodics are used. A high-carbohydrate diet, rather than a low-carbohydrate (No. 4), would be given to build up glycogen stores in the liver.

121. (2) Clients with high-abdominal surgeries tend to breathe shallowly after surgery in order to splint incisional discomfort. Consequently, these clients need both assistance and encouragement to deep breathe and cough. Splinting of the incisional area by the nurse helps, as well as planning deep breathing and particularly coughing times to follow the administration of a pain reliever. Nos. 1 and 3 are correct statements but not the best answers. Clients with abdominal surgeries tend to guard against coughing as it increases intra-abdominal pressures and incisional discomfort. Women do tend to be thoracic breathers and need to be taught abdominal or diaphragmatic breathing in the preoperative period. No. 4 is incorrect, because NG tubes do not inhibit deep breathing; rather, they tend to increase oral respirations, which causes drying of the oral mucous membranes.

122. (2) Sitting the client up allows for deeper ventilation, and splinting of the incisional area reduces incisional discomfort. No. 1 is also correct but not specific enough. Generally 20–30 minutes should elapse before instituting coughing techniques following administration of an analgesic, to allow for the full effects of the drug. No. 3 is incorrect unless she is in a good deal of pain; if so, she should be medicated, then coughed. No. 4 is incorrect because oral intake is withheld until bowel activity is reestablished. Secretions can be kept mobilized by frequent turning and deep breathing.

123. (1) The purpose of the T-tube is to maintain the patency of the bile duct after surgery. Localized edema in the surgery area tends to obstruct the outflow of bile, which is continuously being synthesized by the liver. The T-tube does not directly prevent postoperative hemorrhage (No. 2) or postoperative wound infection (No. 3). A secondary effect of this procedure is that bile flow is directed away from the duodenum (No. 4).

124. (4) Normally drainage from the T-tube averages 300–500 mL during the first few days after surgery and then gradually decreases; the tube is generally removed in 7–10 days. By the fourth postoperative day, flow has usually begun to decrease. Excessive drainage at this time should be reported as it indicates possible re-obstruction of the duct. Nos. 1, 2, and 3 are normal postoperative findings.

125. (2) The T-tube is clamped prior to eating to increase bile flow into the duodenum and assist in the digestion of fats. No. 1 is incorrect because the act of eating normally stimulates bile secretion, and clamping of the T-tube will not inhibit its flow except to the dependent drainage bag. No. 3 is incorrect because bile does not affect peristalsis, although inadequate bile flow can result in abdominal distention. No. 4 is also correct, though it is not the best answer. If the client is able to tolerate clamping of the T-tube, then bile is flowing normally into the duodenum and the duct is patent.

126. (1) Following clamping of the T-tube, observe the client for signs of abdominal distress, pain, nausea, chills, or fever. These symptoms may be due to a localized reaction to the bile, edema, or obstructed flow. Severe abdominal pain may indicate leakage of bile into the peritoneal cavity. Eructation (No. 2) or burping may occur after eating if bile flow was insufficient. Jaundice (No. 3) is a late symptom of biliary obstruction. An increased respiratory rate (No. 4) may occur if the client has abdominal discomfort, pain, or nausea.

127. (3) There are no specific dietary restrictions following cholecystectomy. Clients are advised, however, to avoid foods high in fats. Most clients tend to avoid these foods anyway because they are more comfortable if they do so. Generally, after about 3 months, clients may begin to experiment with certain foods to ascertain their tolerance to them. No. 1 is incorrect because some fat is allowed in the diet at all times. No. 2 is incorrect because fats are not limited to those classified as polyunsaturates. No. 4 is incorrect because fats are allowed in the postcholecystectomy diet, to tolerance.

128. (1) The Mantoux test is injected intradermally on the polar aspect of the forearm. If correctly administered, a pale elevation similar to a mosquito bite should be apparent. Nos. 2, 3, and 4 are not used for this test.

129. (4) The Mantoux test is read in 48–72 hours. Color is observed, and the injection site is palpated for induration. Reading the test in less than 48 hours may lead to inaccurate interpretation (Nos. 1, 2, and 3).

130. (1) An induration of 10 mm or more (not cm, as in No. 2) is considered a positive reaction. The skin is generally reddened. Indurations of 5–9 mm (No. 3) are considered doubtful reactions. Individuals with doubtful reactions should be retested, unless they have had a known contact with persons with tuberculosis. Indurations of less than 5 mm are considered negative reactions. The reaction is not hivelike (No. 4).

131. (3) Proper handling of sputum is essential to allay droplet transference of bacilli in the air. Clients need to be taught to cover their nose and mouth with tissues when sneezing or coughing. Chemotherapy generally renders the client noninfectious within days to a few weeks, usually before cultures for tubercle bacilli are negative. Until chemical isolation is established, many institutions require the client to wear a mask when visitors are in the room or when the nurse is in attendance. Clients should be in a well-ventilated room, without air recirculation, to prevent air contamination. Nos. 1, 2, and 4 are unnecessary precautions.

132. (2) Pyridoxine (vitamin B_6) 25–50 mg a day is ordered prophylactically to prevent symptoms of peripheral neuritis. Serious side effects of INH therapy are rare. Nos. 1, 3, and 4 have no effect on peripheral neuritis.

133. (3) Since tubercle bacilli multiply very slowly, and since antitubercular drugs are bacteriostatic, not bacteriocidal, the client must continue therapy for at least 2 years to allow time for the body's defenses to contain the organisms. Six months (No. 1) would be insufficient treatment. Individuals who have been inspected for tuberculosis but who do not have evidence of active disease are treated prophylactically with INH for a 1-year period (No. 2). No. 4 is an excessive length of time.

134. (3) A thyroid scan utilizes the uptake of ^{131}I by the thyroid gland to determine the size, shape, and function of the gland. Also identified are areas of increased uptake (hot areas), indicating increased metabolic function, as in hyperthyroidism, not malignancy (No. 2), and areas of decreased or no uptake (cold areas), which are associated with malignancy. Nos. 1 and 4 both describe the TSH stimulation test.

135. (1) Following an injection of the small dose of ^{131}I used in a thyroid scan, no radiation precautions are necessary. Full radiation precaution (No. 2) is utilized for radium implants. No. 3 may be employed when ^{131}I therapy is utilized to control and reduce hypersecretion by the thyroid (hyperthyroidism). No. 4 is not an example of normal radiation therapy policy.

136. (3) Surgical treatment of hyperthyroidism involves a subtotal thyroidectomy in which approximately five-sixths of the thyroid tissue is removed. While this procedure does not cure hyperthyroidism, it reduces the amount of circulating thyroid hormone by reducing the amount of functioning tissue. No. 1, complete or total thyroidectomy, is rarely done for hyperthyroidism today but is indicated for thyroid malignancy. No. 2, removal of half of the thyroid, would leave enough functioning hyperactive tissue to prevent diminution of symptoms in the client. No. 4 is incorrect because the client with hyperthyroidism needs no additional thyroid hormone; he or she receives antithyroid medications such as propylthiouracil (PRU) or methimazole (Tapizole) to reduce both circulating and stored thyroid hormone.

137. (3) To prevent undue stress on the suture line and underlying surgical repair, the client is taught to support the back of the neck when repositioning and to avoid both hyperextension and flexion of the neck. No. 1 is incorrect because active flexion of the neck is avoided and because after a total thyroidectomy the client will receive thyroid medications to prevent hypothyroidism and to maintain a euthyroid state. No. 2 is also incorrect due to the focus on active flexion and extension neck exercises, which would put undue stress on the suture line. No. 4 is partially correct; however, again active flexion exercises are contraindicated.

138. (2) Respiratory obstruction, hemorrhage, tetany, and laryngeal nerve injury are the major complications following thyroid surgery. *Hypocalcemia,* not hypercalcemia (No. 1) is a complication resulting from damage to the parathyroid glands during surgery. Serum T4 will be *decreased* or absent, *not* elevated (No. 3), and the client will need replacement therapy because no thyroid hormone is secreted once the total thyroid gland is removed. No. 4 is not a good answer. Since the integrity of the gastrointestinal tract is not interrupted during thyroid surgery, paralytic ileus is a *rare* complication.

139. (3) Tetany caused by hypocalcemia can be assessed for by briskly tapping the facial nerve, which is located near the middle of the masseter muscle just proximal to the ear lobe (Chvostek's sign). A positive reaction occurs when there is facial-muscle contraction, which includes a twitch of the upper lip on that side. Checking urine-calcium levels (No. 1) is not helpful in assessing for early signs of hypocalcemia because urine-calcium levels are dependent not only on parathormone excretion but also on oral intake. No. 2 describes Homans' sign, which is used to determine the presence of deep-vein thrombosis. No. 4 is a late sign of hypocalcemia.

140. (1) Nursing measures designed to reduce the occurrence of postthyroidectomy hemorrhage include frequent checks of the dressings and bedclothes under the client, semi-Fowler's to prevent hyperextension of the neck, and ice packs to reduce hematoma formation and edema. No. 2 is partially correct; however, the supine position would increase edema because it prevents gravity drainage of the wound site. No. 3 is incorrect because coughing will increase stress on the sutures unless the head and neck are well supported, and moist packs tend to increase local blood flow, which in turn tends to increase edema formation in this client. No. 4 is incorrect because flexionlike hyperextension puts increased stress on the suture line.

141. (3) Maintenance of an adequate airway is always the primary goal of nursing care. Respiratory obstruction is a very serious complication; therefore it is wise to have both an emergency tracheostomy set and suctioning apparatus available at the bedside of the client who has had a thyroidectomy. No. 1 is also correct, but it is not the best answer since the onset of this complication is more gradual. With adequate nursing observation, it can be handled before it becomes life-threatening. No. 2 is incorrect because thoracentesis is utilized to remove excess fluid from the pleural space. The correct nursing strategy for postoperative bleeding (No. 4) is to notify the physician immediately.

142. (3) In early respiratory obstruction, the client generally complains of a feeling of fullness or a choking sensation. Swallowing difficulties are fairly common due to tracheal irritation; however, difficulty in swallowing in conjunction with a choking sensation is indicative of airway obstruction. No. 1, hoarseness and weakness of the voice, is common and is secondary to edema of the larynx. No. 2, stridor and cyanosis, is a late sign of airway obstruction. No. 4, disorientation and combative behaviors, is indicative of severe anoxia.

143. (3) An immediate response to the choking sensation is assessment of the surgical site by examining under the dressing. If it appears edematous, loosen the dressing and have someone remain with the client. Elevating the head to a high Fowler's position (No. 1), though the preferred position for improving ventilation of the lung, will not reduce upper-airway obstruction. No. 2 is inappropriate for this situation and may actually increase the client's distress. Notify the physician (No. 4), who might order the sutures or clips to be removed, *after* assessing the surgical site.

144. (2) The client who has had thyroid surgery should be assisted in supporting the head and neck whenever the position is changed during the first three postoperative days. Supporting the head is particularly important during early ambulation procedures, when sudden movement may result in hyperextension of the neck. Nos. 1, 3, and 4 are incorrect because none of these responses takes into account the need to prevent hyperextension of the neck.

145. (3) Even though Mr. Edwards will have only one eye patched after surgery, familiarization with the physical arrangement of his room and with nursing personnel will decrease the occurrence of disorientation, which affects many elderly clients. It is not necessary to keep Mr. Edwards flat in bed before or after surgery (No. 1). Patches (No. 2) are not generally applied to both eyes. Eye-drop instillations (No. 4) are part of the postoperative or predischarge teaching plan.

146. (1) Local anesthesia is used in cataract surgery, not only because this surgery is a short procedure but also because most clients are elderly, with one or more chronic disease, which may be exacerbated by general anesthesia (No. 2). Intravenous anesthesia (No. 3) with sodium pentothal is most frequently used when unconsciousness is desirable for short procedures or when an anesthetic induction is desired for general anesthesia. Rectal anesthesia (No. 4), though rarely used today, has been employed to induce short-term anesthesia in children.

147. (1) An iridectomy, or removal of a wedge from the iris, is performed with cataract removal to prevent the forward push of the aqueous humor from blocking the canal of Schlemm, which would produce a secondary glaucoma. Iridectomy does not affect pupillary dilatation (No. 2), facilitate retinal circulation (No. 3), or prevent corneal scarring (No. 4).

148. (3) Postoperatively the cataract client may be placed in a flat or low Fowler's position on his back or turned to the unoperated side. Turning the client to the operated side (No. 4) or raising the head of the bed (No. 1) increases the stress on the sutures and may lead to hemorrhage. The client may assume a prone position with the head turned to the unoperated side (No. 2), though most clients find a side-lying position more comfortable.

149. (3) Coughing, brushing the teeth, and shaving are activities that tend to increase intraocular pressures and are therefore restricted during the early postoperative period. Other activities to avoid include vomiting, bending, and stooping. Self-feeding (No. 1) is encouraged to help reduce the client's perception of helplessness, though food may need to be cut up for the client, to reduce exertion. Self-dressing (No. 2) and ambulation (No. 4) are permitted. The ambulating client should wear slip-on slippers or shoes to avoid bending or stooping.

150. (1) Clients should be informed that the cataract glasses will magnify objects; this not only causes distortions in the shape of an object but may also result in color distortions. The spatial changes that result from these lenses may cause the client to underreach for an object or have difficulty walking and climbing stairs. Peripheral vision is decreased (No. 2), so the client needs to be taught to turn his head and utilize the central vision provided by the lenses. Nos. 3 and 4 are incorrect because the magnification created by these lenses (up to 35%) is not similar to the size perception before the cataract formed, nor do they cause double vision.

151. (2) Clients with radioactive implants should be positioned flat in bed to prevent dislodgement of the vaginal packing. The client may roll to the side for meals, but the upper body should not be raised more than 20°. Nos. 1, 3, and 4 are incorrect because these positions are more likely to change the position of the cobalt seeds.

152. (2) It is not necessary to isolate the client with radioactive implants (No. 1); but to prevent undue exposure to radiation contacts, contact time should be brief and distance between the client and others maximized. Specific instructions as to the amount of time permitted with the client and the safe distance should be posted. Nos. 3 and 4 are incorrect because the best position for the client is supine.

153. (3) During treatment (total insertion time varies from 48–144 hours), vaginal discharge may become foul-smelling due to tissue destruction; however, perineal care is generally not allowed due to the danger of dislodging the needles. Frequently, clients find this quite distressing. A douche given under low pressure following removal of the applicator helps to reduce this side effect of therapy. Bladder atony (No. 1) is a rare complication; diarrhea, rather than constipation (No. 2), is more likely to occur. Sexual libido (No. 4) following this therapy seems more dependent on the relationship of the partners before therapy than on the therapy itself.

154. (2) Local radiation is generally used under four conditions: the tumor is relatively well defined; a larger dose of radiation can be delivered than by an external source; there is a critical need to reduce involvement of other tissue; and the site is accessible for introduction of seeds or implants. As a result of cobalt implantation, diarrhea may occur due to radiation-induced toxicosis of the mucous membranes of the large bowel. Diarrhea may be painful as well as profuse and bloody. No. 1 is incorrect because the rationale for doing an implant is that the tumor is generally well defined. The effects of severe diarrhea may indeed be electrolyte imbalance (No. 3), but this is not the cause in this situation. No. 4 may indeed be occurring, but is not the basis for Mrs. Ryan's present symptoms.

155. (4) This is the most appropriate response because it attempts to provide total intervention for all parties involved. No. 1 is essentially the physician's role. It would be almost impossible to alleviate the couple's anxiety at this time (No. 2). The most appropriate intervention is to assist the couple to cope with their anxiety as effectively as possible. No. 3 is essential, but it neglects the psychologic needs of the clients.

156. (1) This is an open-ended question that allows Tyronne to identify what his needs are at this time. No. 2 is too threatening. No. 3 assumes he cannot tolerate the situation, which is unfair. No. 4 is unrealistic because the nurse has many responsibilities at this time. In addition, Tyronne would have to leave the room anyway to drink or take anything.

157. (2) The effect of the anesthesia will be closely checked prior to making the incision, and the level of anesthesia will be monitored throughout the procedure. Many times the woman complains of tightness or pressure in the area where the physician is working (No. 1). No significant pain should be felt as long as the anesthesia is closely monitored and maintained (No. 3). No. 4 is inappropriate because it makes her feel that she should not complain about pain even if she actually does feel it.

158. (3) Usually with a transverse lie the classical or longitudinal incision is used, and the woman is concerned about her body image. Nos. 1, 2, and 4 may be concerns, but they are not usually primary in the client's mind.

159. (3) An Apgar score of 4–6 indicates the infant is in fair condition. "Excellent" (No. 1) is not a category in the Apgar score. "Good" (No. 2) is a score of 7–10. "Poor" (No. 4) is a score of 0–3.

160. (1) Ensuring adequate oxygenation of the infant's system is the number one priority in order to sustain life. Nos. 2, 3, and 4 are all appropriate *secondary* goals.

161. (2) The couple is able to perceive events and communicate their concerns, although there is overt tension present. No. 1 is usually indicated by restlessness and increased alertness. No. 3 is indicated by an increase in physical symptoms (headaches, nausea, dizziness, etc.) and perceiving only details. No. 4 is indicated by an inability to communicate or function.

162. (1) It is important for the couple to be able to rely on each other at this time. They need time to communicate and to begin to cope with their feelings. As long as Juanita's vital signs are stable, it may be most therapeutic to allow Tyronne into the recovery room. No. 2 isolates the husband from all significant others. No. 3 evades the problem and does not alleviate any anxiety. No. 4 is a physician's decision, and the infant is probably still being worked up and treated at this time.

163. (4) This couple is experiencing an actual loss and will probably exhibit many of the same symptoms as a person who has lost someone to death. Nos. 1, 2, and 3 will most likely occur at some later time.

164. (3) Initially this couple will be unable to make appropriate decisions regarding their own needs. They need tender support, empathy, and reassurance in order to assist them in coping with this stress. No. 1 may be appropriate at a later time. No. 2 is incorrect because this couple is probably incapable of seeking out someone to talk to or to listen. They need guidance. If left alone, they may isolate themselves, withdraw, and become depressed. Avoidance (No. 4) is nontherapeutic; the problems must be faced eventually.

165. (4) It is essential that the couple be prepared for what they will see. However, it is equally as important for them to be able to see, touch, and hold their son as soon as possible, to begin the attachment process. No. 1 merely delays the couple's seeing their son. The nurse continually assesses the parents' readiness while caring for the infant. Juanita and Tyronne *do* need some preparation prior to seeing their son (No. 2). Teaching without immediate parent–child contact can increase the parents' anxiety (No. 3).

166. (3) Crying is an appropriate, expected, and natural response. Nos. 1, 2, and 4 all invade the woman's need for privacy at this time.

167. (3) Juanita is communicating her feelings of distress at seeing her physiologically compromised son. No. 1 is wrong because interference with the bonding process may affect later parenting. No. 2 is wrong because the mother is demonstrating her inability to cope with the situation at present. No. 4 is wrong because the family system is unable to meet the neonate's emotional needs at present due to being overwhelmed by their own reactions to the baby.

168. (2) Both Juanita and Tyronne will probably attempt to place the blame for their son's deformities on someone or something else, such as "inadequate prenatal care," "bad counseling," or "God's wish." No. 1 involves a state in which personality development is arrested in one or more aspects at a level short of maturity. No. 3 involves unconsciously translating psychic problems into physical symptoms. No. 4 involves channeling a destructive or instinctual impulse that is socially unacceptable into a socially acceptable behavior, such as coping with anger by participating in sports that require the release of a lot of energy.

169. (3) This is characteristic of a reactive depression. The individual experiencing an endogenous depression usually feels worse in the morning but better as the day progresses. There is usually a weight loss of less than 10 lb (No. 1). The individual usually responds to environmental stimuli (No. 2). The precipitating event is usually an identifiable stressor, such as the birth of an unhealthy baby (No. 4).

170. (1) This is the most appropriate response congruent with the nurse's role. No. 2 is the physician's role. The nurse should accurately reinforce the information the physician gives the couple. In addition, the information is incomplete, in that the initial repair of the palate may begin as early as 6 months or as late as 2 years, depending on the condition of the infant. No. 3 avoids answering the couple's question and may stimulate an increase in anxiety. No. 4 is the physician's role.

171. (4) The exact cause of the failure of the embryonic structures of the face to form a union is unclear. However, there is a significant familial pattern, and a hereditary factor is involved. Cleft palate is seen more frequently in girls, whereas cleft lip is seen more frequently in boys (Nos. 1 and 2). Although cleft lip and palate sometimes do occur together (No. 3), in many cases they occur independently.

172. (4) Empathy and understanding, rather than sympathy, are more effective in providing emotional support to families in crisis. No. 1 is wrong because the family may need to openly communicate their anxiety, fears, and concerns about the baby in order to begin positive coping. No. 2 is wrong because understanding the treatment being given and the potential for a successful surgical repair may aid them in coping with their fears. No. 3 is wrong because staff attitudes in working with compromised infants affects parental perceptions of the infant.

173. (2) The nurse must meet the parents at their level of readiness while at the same time providing them with enough information to allow them to care adequately for the infant. Sucking needs to be avoided in an infant with a cleft palate because of the possibility of aspiration and because he will not be allowed to suck postoperatively (No. 1). A special nipple or feeder is helpful, such as Lamb's nipple or Brecht feeder. The infant should be fed in an upright position to decrease the likelihood of aspiration (No. 3). The infant needs to be isolated only from those individuals with infectious diseases such as colds or chickenpox (No. 4). The infant should be treated as normally as possible in order to stimulate growth and development.

174. (3) The prevention of scarring is essential. All crusts should be cleaned away as gently as possible, and the area should be cleansed frequently in order to prevent infection. The infant should be placed on his back or side and minimally restrained to prevent him from turning onto his face. The side position is preferred in order to prevent the aspiration of mucus or the regurgitation of milk (No. 1). The infant needs to be repositioned frequently to lessen the danger of hypostatic pneumonia (No. 2). Crying should be minimized as much as possible to avoid unnecessary strain on the suture line (No. 4).

175. (2) It is important to assess and validate the couple's perceived needs in order to plan care effectively. The couple may need a social worker as well as a public health nurse, speech pathologist, audiologist, etc. Therefore it is essential to make an accurate and continual assessment of the family's needs (No. 1). Alternatives (No. 3) may be more appropriately identified after performing a total assessment. Health teaching (No. 4) is necessary, but it must be based on an assessment and validation of the family's needs as well as of their level of readiness.

176. (3) Breast self-examinations are best done the week following onset of menses. The breasts are then the softest, and any lumps not associated with hormonal changes are more evident. No. 1 is incorrect because breast changes due to hormonal changes, such as fullness or tenderness, may occur at this time, obscuring possible pathology. No. 2 is a good idea (that is, having a regular time or pattern for examination), but does not take into account the normal breast-tissue changes during the menstrual cycle. No. 4 is incorrect for the same reason as No. 1.

177. (2) Denial is a very strong defense mechanism used to allay the emotional effects of discovering a potential threat. Although denial has been found to be an effective mechanism for survival in some instances, such as during natural disasters, it may result in greater pathology in a woman with potential breast carcinoma. Suppression (No. 1) occurs when the individual recognizes the threat but consciously refuses to think about it. Repression (No. 3) is an unconscious mechanism that keeps the knowledge of the threat from coming to one's conscious awareness. Intellectualization (No. 4) occurs when the individual attempts to consciously allay anxiety by attributing symptoms to other possible causes, such as cystic breast disease. However, the client who intellectualizes does not attempt to deny the possibility that a more serious pathology may be present.

178. (1) Anxiety, like pain, glucose imbalance, or changes in blood pressure, stimulates discharge of the sympathetic nervous system. In some clients this increased adrenergic discharge results in moderate to severe increases in systolic and diastolic pressures that decrease to normal levels when emotional equilibrium is restored. Mrs. Washington may be emotionally labile (No. 2), but at this time there are insufficient data to make this judgment. Mrs. Washington is fearful, but that does not mean she is unprepared for this surgery (No. 3). Should her anxiety remain high, however, the attending physician should be notified. Though Mrs. Washington may be attempting to employ denial ("I only have a cyst"), her emotional response (restlessness and increased blood pressure) indicates this defense mechanism is ineffective in allaying her present anxieties (No. 4).

179. (2) After the client has left for surgery, family members should be told the approximate time the client will be in surgery and that from there the client will go to the recovery room until awake and all vital signs are stable. Clarify that delays may occur and that the induction of, as well as the emergence from, anesthesia take time. Nos. 1 and 3 are incorrect because family members should be allowed to decide whether they will stay or go and come back later. If family members decide to wait, direct them to a waiting area where they can be comfortable. Assure them that you will direct the surgeon to them after the surgery is finished. No. 4 is not an initial action. The nurse does answer any questions and/or concerns the family members may have, being as supportive as possible.

180. (4) Initial intervention when clients are reacting to the loss of a significant body part is to encourage verbalization of their fears and to assist them in identifying how they see the change in their body image as well as how it may affect their marriage relationship. One of the most important factors in the mastectomy client's response to surgery is the reaction of her husband or the person with whom she is intimately involved. Nos. 1 and 2 tend to cut off communication in this instance. Many partners are very supportive, others are not. It is therefore also important to assist the partners to acknowledge their feelings and concerns (No. 3). The client needs the reassurance of the partner's love and support to work through her own emotional reaction and begin the work of recovery.

181. (1) Since tracheostomy inhibits the client from talking, it is essential to establish a mode of postoperative communication so that the client can express her needs. The mode chosen should be communicated to the rest of the staff so that the approach to the client is consistent. Blood work (No. 2) may or may not be ordered before tracheostomy, though blood gases are frequently ordered to establish baseline data in order to evaluate the effectiveness of the intervention. Inserting a Foley catheter (No. 3) is not a priority unless urinary output has decreased. A standard surgical prep (No. 4), cleansing and shaving the operative area, is not done before tracheostomy. However, the physician does cleanse the area with an antiseptic before performing the tracheostomy.

182. (1) Sperm deposited during intercourse may remain viable for about 3 days. If ovulation occurs during this period, conception may result. No. 2 is incorrect because the ovum is present only *after* ovulation. No. 3 is wrong because tubal motility is important in the union of ovum and sperm (and transport of the zygote) *after ovulation*. No. 4 is wrong because the uterine endometrium becomes secretory postovulation.

183. (3) Ovulation occurs most commonly 14 days prior to the next menstrual period. In a 30-day cycle, this would be day 16 or 17. Answers 1 and 2 are incorrect because they describe a time *prior* to normal ovulation; No. 4 is wrong because ovulation occurs *prior to* the last week of the menstrual cycle.

184. (2) Under high estrogen levels, during the period surrounding ovulation, the cervical mucus becomes thin, clear, and elastic (spinnbarkeit), facilitating sperm passage. No. 1 is incorrect because cervical mucus becomes thicker and opaque under progesterone stimulation after ovulation. No. 3 is wrong because cervical mucus is essentially colorless, and postovulation, under progesterone stimulation, it becomes thick and sticky. No. 4 is wrong because ferning is absent during the postovulatory period.

185. (2) Intrauterine devices are believed to prevent implantation of the fertilized ovum by producing a sterile local inflammation. No. 1 is incorrect because tubal ligation prevents union of sperm and egg by closing the passage. No. 3 is wrong because oral contraceptives prevent maturation of the graafian follicle and expulsion of the egg. No. 4 is wrong because the diaphragm and spermicidal jelly serve as mechanical and chemical barriers to prevent viable sperm from gaining access to the egg.

186. (3) Clients should be instructed to contact the clinic doctor or nurse if they have leg cramps or headaches (signs of possible thrombophlebitis caused by the hypercoagulability that occurs under estrogen/progesterone stimulation). No. 1 is incorrect because mild to moderate nonpathologic nausea may occur during the first few days on oral contraceptives as the body adjusts to the elevated hormone levels. No. 2 is wrong because chloasma, the "mask of pregnancy," is merely hyperpigmentation related to the high hormone levels. No. 4 is wrong because breast tenderness and weight gain are nonpathologic and are associated with an increased tendency to retain fluid in the interstitial spaces.

187. (1) The client must understand that, although the "fertile" period is approximately mid-cycle, hormonal variations do occur that result in early or late ovulations. To be effective, the diaphragm should be inserted prior to every intercourse. No. 2 is incorrect because the diaphragm must be left in place for a minimum of 6 hours after intercourse. Premature removal may permit passage of viable sperm. No. 3 is incorrect because marked variations in weight may result in the need for a larger or smaller appliance. No. 4 is wrong because pin holes in the diaphragm may permit viable sperm to pass the barrier.

188. (2) Withdrawal of the penis prior to orgasm is not reliable as a method of birth control because fluid containing semen, stored in the prostate or Cowper's glands, may release viable sperm into the vaginal canal preejaculation. No. 1 is incorrect because the rhythm method of birth control requires avoiding intercourse around the time of ovulation (approximately 16 days prior to next menses). No. 3 is incorrect because spermicidal jellies are most effective when used in conjunction with the barrier diaphragm. No. 4 is wrong because oral contraceptives provide the most effective modern method of contraception when used appropriately.

189. (3) Serum radioimmunoassay (RIA) is accurate within 7 days of conception. This test is specific for HCG, and accuracy is not compromised by confusion with LH levels. No. 1 is incorrect because the pregnant uterus is not palpable at or above the pubic symphysis before 12-weeks gestation. No. 2 is incorrect because fetal heart tones are not audible by present methods before 9–12 weeks (Doppler) or 20 weeks (fetoscope). No. 4 is wrong because Leopold maneuvers are neither possible nor applicable until much later in pregnancy.

190. (3) Respiratory depression is a cardinal sign of magnesium toxicity. No. 1 is incorrect because individual variations in respiratory depression are observed at the same serum magnesium level. No. 2 is incorrect because respiratory compromise normally precedes depressed cardiac function and is a late sign of magnesium toxicity. No. 4 is incorrect because, although decreased peristalsis can occur with a magnesium infusion, it is not the most important assessment to make.

191. (3) For clients having elective surgery, routine preoperative laboratory studies generally include a complete blood count, urinalysis, and prothrombin time. Some institutions also require a VDRL. The urinalysis provides information about specific gravity (indicating the ability of the kidney to concentrate and dilute urine); the presence of albumin or pus, indicating renal infection; and the presence of sugar and acetone. The CBC detects the presence of anemia, infection, allergy, and leukemia. Prothrombin time (increased) may indicate a need for preoperative vitamin K therapy. Electrolytes (No. 1), enzymes such as ALT[SGOT] (No. 2), and serum glucose (No. 4) are ordered only if the client's history or physical condition warrants a more complete workup.

192. (4) The Trendelenburg test evaluates the competency of the superficial veins. The client is asked to elevate the involved leg to empty the veins. A tourniquet is then applied lightly to occlude the superficial veins. The client is then asked to stand, the tourniquet is removed, and the direction and degree of vein-filling is observed. No. 1 is also a test of venous competence: ordinarily, distended veins decrease markedly during walking because muscular contractions facilitate venous flow in deeper veins. No. 2 describes a phlebography, and No. 3 is a test generally used on the jugular vein when pump failure is suspected.

193. (1) Vein-stripping is done not only for advancing varicosities but also for cosmetic reasons. Vein-stripping is *not* done for thrombophlebitis (No. 2), though it is done for stasis ulcerations following successful healing of the ulcer. No. 3 is incorrect because lymphedema is due to blockage of lymph channels and Reynaud's disease is a syndrome that affects the arterial vasculature. No. 4 is incomplete.

194. (4) Vein-stripping is a painful and tiresome procedure and, for the client's comfort, is almost always done under general anesthesia. No. 1 is incorrect because local anesthesia is limited to small areas such as with laceration repair. Topical anesthesia (No. 2) only decreases pain sensation in mucous membranes. And, since the incisions for vein-stripping are made in the groin as well as the ankle, regional anesthesia (No. 3) would be impractical. Vein-stripping could be done using spinal anesthesia.

195. (2) The legs of the client undergoing vein-stripping are wrapped from foot to groin with elastic bandages. Anticoagulants (No. 1) are not routinely ordered following surgery, although analgesics will be ordered for pain. Sitting in a chair (No. 3) is contraindicated because the pressure this position exerts behind the knees and at the hips impedes venous return and increases dependent venous pressures. No. 4 is incorrect because the client is usually ambulated the day of vein-stripping surgery to enhance venous return by way of muscle contraction.

196. (2) Elevation of the foot of the bed enhances venous return and reduces edema by utilizing the force of gravity. Pain is decreased (No. 1) as the edema is reduced. No. 3 is incorrect because raising the foot of the bed should not greatly affect arterial blood flow. Reducing edema is what makes the client more comfortable (No. 4).

197. (1) Elastic stockings are applied before standing up in order to prevent stagnation of blood in the lower extremities. If the client has been standing or exercising (No. 3), he or she should sit in a chair, with legs elevated, for at least 15 minutes before applying the stockings. Elastic stockings should be removed regularly, both to inspect the skin and to provide skin care (No. 2). The client should be cautioned not to sit or stand in any one position for a prolonged period of time. Stockings should fit properly and be kept wrinkle-free because when improperly used they can cause venous stasis, the condition they are designed to prevent (No. 4).

198. (1) Severe, crampy, intermittent pain accompanies the progressive telescoping of the bowel wall found in intussusception; as this progresses, the stools become bloody and full of mucus ("currant jelly"). An olive-shaped mass in the right upper quadrant and projectile vomiting (No. 2) are found in pyloric stenosis. Obstinate constipation and increasing abdominal girth (No. 3) are found in Hirschsprung's disease. Excess mucus and abdominal distention (No. 4) are found in tracheoesophageal fistula.

199. (1) As a toddler, Betsy will most likely experience separation anxiety when separated from her parents, especially her mother. In the "despair" phase, the child appears to be mourning the apparent loss of the parent, as evidenced by nonverbal behavior cues such as monotone crying, regressive behavior (thumb sucking), and sleep disturbances. If Betsy were experiencing muscle spasms due to her fracture (No. 4), she would most likely scream out in severe pain intermittently. The other explanations for Betsy's behavior (Nos. 2 and 3) do not take her developmental level into account.

200. (1) After a settling-in period, the child experiencing separation anxiety may enter the phase of "denial," covering up painful feelings toward parents and seeming to turn instead to others, such as the nurse. Although it may seem like the child is doing fine (No. 3), she is actually denying feelings that are too painful to deal with just now. At her age, Betsy is not trying to make her mother jealous (No. 4); neither does she need discipline (No. 2).

Post Test

INTRODUCTION

The **Post Test** is a *follow-up assessment* tool designed to assess areas of improvement from your initial self-assessment using the **Pre Test**. Take the **Post Test** immediately after reading the specific content areas related to your specific problem areas as identified by the **Pre Test**. Determine that you are now able to meet the goal of 75% correct answers in this integrated exam.

Note that many of the case studies in the **Post Test** are the same case studies that are in the **Pre Test**, but the questions are entirely new.

After taking the **Post Test**, compare your results with the nationwide results of a normative group of test subjects by taking the **Prep Test**. Fill out the answer sheet inside the front cover of this book, and send away for the computerized evaluation of your answers. Specific diagnostic information concerning your performance will be mailed to you. It should prove beneficial in preparing you for the licensure examination since it parallels the NCLEX-RN test plan in its distribution of questions concerning client needs and phases of the nursing process.

QUESTIONS

Charlie, a 14-year-old male, lives in the inner city with his mother (age 32), his father (age 35), his sister (age 12), and his brother (age 15). Charlie's mother is white and his father is black. His father is a mechanical engineer, and his mother is a real estate agent.

Three weeks ago a janitor discovered Charlie setting fires in the locker room of his school. This was the fifth such incident in the past 8 months. The school counselor suggested that Charlie's family seek professional counseling. Charlie was placed in a private inpatient mental hospital on a coed adolescent unit with 16 other clients.

1. As an adolescent, Charlie's main life-stage task is:
- ○ 1. Developing a sense of trust in others and in his environment. **EV 5**
- ○ 2. Finalizing his goals and plans for the future. **HPM**
- ○ 3. Striving to attain independence and identity.
- ○ 4. Resolving inner conflicts and turmoil.

2. During the adolescent period, the *least* important task for Charlie to complete is:
- ○ 1. Developing an individualized personality. **PL**
- ○ 2. Attaining adequate defense mechanisms. **5**
- ○ 3. Establishing an ego identity. **HPM**
- ○ 4. Refining and stabilizing the superego.

3. To establish a relationship with Charlie, which of the following would be inappropriate for the nurse to consider?
- ○ 1. Boys in early adolescence feel threatened by female authority figures. **AN 7**
- ○ 2. Enforced inactivity will deprive the adolescent of a major avenue for relieving frustration. **PsI**
- ○ 3. Impulse control is a major problem for males.
- ○ 4. Fear and ambivalence will usually dissipate with the passage of time.

4. Charlie is experiencing several biologic and psychosocial changes at this time. Which of the following behaviors would you expect to see?
- ○ 1. An increase in imaginative thinking. **EV**
- ○ 2. An increased ability to learn by rote. **7**
- ○ 3. An increase in academic achievement. **HPM**
- ○ 4. An increased ability to cope with frustration.

POST TEST

5. During adolescence, Charlie *least* needs which of the following?
- ○ 1. External control on his behavior by adults. **PL**
- ○ 2. Limit-setting based on fear and reprimands. **5**
- ○ 3. Adult role models for identification. **HPM**
- ○ 4. Stable relationships and interactions.

6. Charlie's arson attempts may exhibit which of the following behaviors?
- ○ 1. Acting out. **AS**
- ○ 2. Depression. **7**
- ○ 3. Paranoia. **PsI**
- ○ 4. Mania.

7. Charlie may exhibit his depression differently from an adult. An adolescent who is depressed is most likely to exhibit which of the following behaviors?
- ○ 1. Withdrawal. **AS**
- ○ 2. Apathy. **7**
- ○ 3. Violence. **PsI**
- ○ 4. Regression.

Charlie's stay in the psychiatric hospital is punctuated by frequent outbursts of maladaptive behavior.

8. After his admission to the hospital, Charlie started hitting other clients and even struck a nurse. In assessing Charlie's behavior, the nurse should consider which of the following facts to be *most* relevant?
- ○ 1. Hitting others makes Charlie feel satisfied because he is in control of the situation. **AN** **7**
- ○ 2. Hitting others provides Charlie with an escape from his feelings of hopelessness. **PsI**
- ○ 3. Hitting others is Charlie's mechanism for alleviating anxiety.
- ○ 4. Hitting others allows Charlie to instill fear in others.

9. After Charlie has been hospitalized in the psychiatric institution for several days, he is introduced to the other adolescents in group therapy. The *most* significant factor the nurse should consider in initiating group therapy is that:
- ○ 1. Confrontation could lead to elopement. **AN**
- ○ 2. Charlie may refuse to verbalize. **7**
- ○ 3. Group members may ignore Charlie. **PsI**
- ○ 4. Charlie may act out during group therapy.

10. Charlie has been attending group therapy twice a week for 3 weeks. He is still fairly quiet during group therapy and speaks only when questioned. The nurse should assume that:
- ○ 1. Charlie feels comfortable within the group. **EV**
- ○ 2. Charlie is threatened by the group. **7**
- ○ 3. Charlie does not feel the need to verbalize. **PsI**
- ○ 4. Charlie is progressing as expected.

11. Charlie is becoming increasingly combative. He hits other clients as well as the nursing staff at least once or twice each day. Which of the following is an inappropriate nursing goal?
- ○ 1. Helping Charlie develop impulse control. **PL**
- ○ 2. Helping Charlie manage his feelings appropriately. **7** **PsI**
- ○ 3. Helping Charlie learn socially acceptable behavior.
- ○ 4. Helping Charlie internalize his feelings.

12. By the time Charlie has been hospitalized 3 months, he has become apathetic and withdrawn. He sits in his room at least 3–4 hours each day. When he is requested to sit in the recreation room, he generally sits alone and stares into space. The most appropriate nursing intervention would include:
- ○ 1. Selecting a group activity for Charlie to participate in. **PL** **7**
- ○ 2. Stimulating self-growth by providing challenging activities for Charlie. **PsI**
- ○ 3. Allowing Charlie to spend at least 3 hours a day in his room, for inner reflection.
- ○ 4. Encouraging staff members to sit with Charlie during group activities until he socializes voluntarily.

13. During the fourth month of hospitalization, Charlie begins mutilating his forearms with lighted cigarettes and scratching his wrists with thumbtacks and staples he finds on the unit. Which of the following is the *least* appropriate nursing goal?
- ○ 1. Supervising Charlie closely. **PL**
- ○ 2. Avoiding confrontations with Charlie regarding his behavior. **7** **PsI**
- ○ 3. Removing all items that could be used for destructive purposes.
- ○ 4. Assisting Charlie to increase his self-esteem.

14. Charlie has developed a homosexual relationship with a 16-year-old named Rich. In planning care, the nurse should *primarily:*
- ○ 1. Avoid confronting Charlie about his attention-getting behavior. **PL** **7**
- ○ 2. Validate Charlie's rationale for establishing the relationship. **PsI**
- ○ 3. Explore Charlie's thoughts, feelings, and attitudes.
- ○ 4. Enforce limits on interactions between Rich and Charlie.

During Charlie's hospitalization, his father continues to work 8–10 hours a day; his mother, however, is extremely upset. She has increased her consumption of alcoholic beverages to 24 oz of 80-proof drinks per day. She gets angry with the other children very quickly, cries spontaneously several times every day, and complains of headaches constantly.

15. In planning care for Charlie's mother, what would be considered the *least* appropriate nursing intervention?
- ○ 1. Stimulating her to work at a concrete task. **PL**
- ○ 2. Encouraging her to cry. **7**
- ○ 3. Providing her with someone to talk to. **PsI**
- ○ 4. Isolating her from stimuli.

16. The most important nursing intervention in planning care for Charlie's mother would include:
- ○ 1. Referring her to an alcohol rehabilitation program. **IMP** **7**
- ○ 2. Identifying how she has coped with anxiety in the past. **PsI**

Key to codes following questions Nursing process: **AS**, Assessment; **AN**, Analysis; **PL**, Plan; **IMP**, Implementation; **EV**, Evaluation. Category of human function: **1**, Protective; **2**, Sensory-perceptual; **3**, Comfort, Rest, Activity, and Mobility; **4**, Nutrition; **5**, Growth and Development; **6**, Fluid-Gas Transport; **7**, Psycho-Social-Cultural; **8**, Elimination. Client need: **SECE**, Safe, Effective Care Environment; **PhI**, Physiological Integrity; **PsI**, Psychosocial Integrity; **HPM**, Health Promotion/Maintenance. See frontmatter for full explanation.

○ 3. Arranging for inpatient hospitalization.
○ 4. Requesting a prescription for an antidepressant.

After Charlie has been in the hospital about 5 months, his mother takes an overdose of sleeping pills and alcohol. She is brought to the emergency room in an ambulance called by a neighbor, who discovered her unconscious on the living room sofa. Upon admission, she is unconscious. Her vital signs are TPR 98–60–10, BP 90/50. Her reflexes are dull.

17. The emergency room nurse's initial response should include which of the following?
○ 1. Administering a central nervous system stimulant. **IMP**
○ 2. Paging the resident on call. **6**
○ 3. Maintaining a patent airway. **PhI**
○ 4. Assessing her neurologic signs.

18. Charlie's mother is hospitalized. In planning nursing care for a suicidal client, which of the following is the *least* appropriate nursing action?
○ 1. Searching personal effects for toxic agents. **IMP**
○ 2. Removing straps from clothing. **7**
○ 3. Placing the client in small groups for observation. **PsI**
○ 4. Removing sharp objects from the environment.

19. Since Charlie's mother has a history of alcohol abuse, the nurse should be aware that she is most likely to exhibit which of the following in the first 72 hours following admission to the hospital?
○ 1. Withdrawal delirium. **AS**
○ 2. Suspiciousness. **7**
○ 3. Mood swings. **PsI**
○ 4. The use of coping mechanisms such as reaction formation.

20. The *least* appropriate nursing intervention for a client experiencing withdrawal delirium would be:
○ 1. Reinforcing time, place, and person. **IMP**
○ 2. Providing consistent and concrete answers to questions. **7** **PsI**
○ 3. Administering ordered vitamins and glucose.
○ 4. Applying and maintaining physical restraints.

21. During Charlie's mother's twenty-first day of hospitalization, she begins to verbalize more and has interacted with one other client on the inpatient psychiatric unit. The nurse should realize that this increase in her energy level may indicate that:
○ 1. She needs less individual attention. **EV**
○ 2. She needs more individual attention. **7**
○ 3. She needs a decrease in her antidepressant medications. **PsI**
○ 4. She is presently motivated to get well.

After Charlie's mother's release from the hospital, the entire family resumes attending family therapy once a week, and the parents begin individual and marital counseling.

22. One of the primary goals of therapy with this family system is to provide:
○ 1. A forum in which familial conflicts can be verbalized. **PL** **7**
○ 2. Individual therapy for each family member. **PsI**
○ 3. Treatment for the identified problem child.
○ 4. Crisis intervention for the family system.

23. Charlie's parents are a biracial couple. They are very reluctant to discuss this issue during family therapy sessions or even during marital counseling sessions. The nurse therapist's best response to this hesitancy would be to:
○ 1. Confront the couple's resistance to discussing the issue. **PL** **7**
○ 2. Avoid the issue unless the couple raises it. **PsI**
○ 3. Encourage a trusting relationship between the therapist and the couple.
○ 4. Refer the couple to individual psychotherapy.

24. Charlie's father is assessed as having an obsessive-compulsive personality. Which of the following behaviors would you *least* expect him to exhibit?
○ 1. Working 50- to 60-hour weeks. **AS**
○ 2. Smoking two packs of cigarettes a day. **7**
○ 3. Showing flexibility in decision making. **PsI**
○ 4. Exhibiting a low level of concentration.

25. Charlie's father does not remember ever seeing his wife take an alcoholic drink. He also states that he has never seen his wife drunk or tipsy. Given the fact that his wife has admitted to drinking several drinks each day, what coping mechanism is Charlie's father using?
○ 1. Projection. **AN**
○ 2. Denial. **7**
○ 3. Repression. **PsI**
○ 4. Sublimation.

26. Charlie's mother is diagnosed as having an affective disorder. What drug is usually administered in treating such disorders?
○ 1. Lithium (lithium carbonate). **IMP**
○ 2. Librium (chlordiazepoxide HCl). **7**
○ 3. Prolixin (fluophenazine hydrochloride). **PsI**
○ 4. Mellaril (thioridazine).

27. When administering lithium to a client with an affective disorder, which of the following is the least relevant consideration?
○ 1. If the client's urinary output decreases significantly, diuretics should be ordered. **EV** **7**
○ 2. The client needs to be given a complete physical examination prior to administering the drug. **PsI**
○ 3. If the client experiences nausea, vomiting, and muscle weakness, the dosage may need regulating.
○ 4. If the client exhibits symptoms of mania during the first 10 days of receiving the drug, Haldol may also be administered.

Charlie has now been hospitalized 8 months. Two days ago he was granted permission to walk across the hospital grounds to various activities, without a staff escort. This afternoon he argued with the recreational therapist and disappeared from the hospital. The hospital security staff found him walking about a mile from the hospital grounds.

28. In planning care for Charlie after this incident, the nurse would consider which of the following factors most significant?
○ 1. Charlie's need to be reprimanded for his deviant behavior. **AN** **7**
○ 2. Charlie's need to be medicated to calm him down. **Psi**
○ 3. Charlie's need to be listened to in order to identify his feelings.
○ 4. Charlie's need to understand the consequences of his actions.

After Charlie has been in the hospital a year and a half, the professional staff at the psychiatric hospital considers discharging him.

29. Charlie asks the nurse whether he must tell other people that he has been in a mental hospital. The most appropriate response the nurse could make would be:
- ○ 1. "Yes, especially to all future school officials." **IMP**
- ○ 2. "Yes, especially to all prospective employers." **7**
- ○ 3. "No, this is an individual decision." **PsI**
- ○ 4. "No, there is no specific requirement."

30. Charlie's parents have decided that they would rather have Charlie placed outside of the home when he is discharged from the hospital. The most appropriate response the nurse could make would include:
- ○ 1. Asking Charlie's parents to reassess their feelings about this decision. **IMP** **7**
- ○ 2. Suggesting that Charlie's parents discuss this decision with the entire family. **PsI**
- ○ 3. Referring Charlie's parents to a social worker to assist in finding an alternative placement.
- ○ 4. Assisting Charlie's parents in finding an appropriate discharge placement.

31. Charlie has been living in a group home for the past 2 months. He has asked permission to visit a friend in the psychiatric hospital. The nurse should:
- ○ 1. Allow him to visit. **IMP**
- ○ 2. Assess his motives. **7**
- ○ 3. Ask his parents' permission. **PsI**
- ○ 4. Consult with the hospital staff.

Sue Way is admitted in active labor. She has dilated to 5 cm and is having moderate to strong contractions every 3 minutes, lasting 50 seconds. Her membranes ruptured spontaneously 2 hours ago. Sue states that she is prepared for natural childbirth and that she is very excited about having her first baby. Her EDD is tomorrow.

32. While auscultating for the point of maximum clarity of the fetal heart tones before applying an external fetal monitor, the nurse counts 100 beats per minute. Which of the following actions should she take *immediately?*
- ○ 1. Examine Sue for signs of a prolapsed cord. **IMP**
- ○ 2. Turn Sue on her left side to increase placental perfusion. **6** **HPM**
- ○ 3. Take Sue's radial pulse while still auscultating her abdomen.
- ○ 4. Start oxygen by mask to reduce fetal distress.

33. Later, external fetal monitor tracings show consistent fetal decelerations of uniform shape, which begin with the contraction and return to baseline as the contraction subsides. Which of the following is the correct interpretation of these data?
- ○ 1. Acute fetal distress. **AN**
- ○ 2. Uteroplacental insufficiency. **6**
- ○ 3. Umbilical cord compression. **PhI**
- ○ 4. Physiologic fetal bradycardia.

34. Sue expresses concern about her baby's status. If the nurse identifies the presence of early decelerations, which of these interventions should be instituted?
- ○ 1. Elevate Sue's hips, and start oxygen by mask. **IMP**
- ○ 2. Lower the head of the bed, and place Sue in supine position. **5** **SECE**
- ○ 3. Mark the tracing in red, and check for dislodged electrode.
- ○ 4. Reassure Sue that this represents a normal tracing.

35. Sue appears tired, tense, and uncomfortable. She complains that her back aches, the monitor "bothers" her, and she wants people to leave her alone and let her rest. Which of the following nursing interventions, implemented by the nurse, demonstrates *proper* nursing judgment?
- ○ 1. Offer to get an order for some pain medication. **IMP** **3**
- ○ 2. Reposition Sue and apply sacral pressure. **SECE**
- ○ 3. Turn monitor off audible reading.
- ○ 4. Darken room and leave her alone for 5 minutes.

36. Sue says, "I can't stand it any longer. I have to push." On vaginal exam, she has dilated to 8 cm and the head is at station 0. For which of the following reasons should the nurse encourage Sue to pant, or breathe naturally, with her contractions?
- ○ 1. Pushing now could cause the cord to prolapse. **AN** **5**
- ○ 2. She should increase her oxygen level before completion of the first stage. **HPM**
- ○ 3. Pushing before complete dilatation may cause cervical edema and may prolong labor.
- ○ 4. Panting will speed cervical dilatation.

Milly Rust is seen in clinic complaining of amenorrhea, fatigue, urinary frequency, and morning nausea. She states that her LMP was 7 weeks ago and that her menses have been normal except for one episode following a spontaneous abortion at 8 weeks gestation. She states she has a 5-year-old boy and 3-year-old twin girls at home.

37. Which of the following would accurately describe Milly if she is pregnant now?
- ○ 1. Gravida 4 Para 2. **AS**
- ○ 2. Gravida 5 Para 3. **5**
- ○ 3. Gravida 4 Para 3. **HPM**
- ○ 4. Gravida 3 Para 2.

38. Milly's last menstrual period began on April 3. Which of the following is an accurate estimate of her EDD?
- ○ 1. January 3. **AN**
- ○ 2. January 10. **5**
- ○ 3. January 27. **HPM**
- ○ 4. December 10.

39. Milly complains her nausea is very "bothersome" in the morning, when she must prepare breakfast for her family. Which of the following actions should the nurse recommend?
- ○ 1. Avoid eating before retiring. **IMP**
- ○ 2. Drink a glass of fruit juice immediately on rising. **4** **HPM**
- ○ 3. Eat one or two soda crackers before rising.
- ○ 4. Make and eat her breakfast first.

40. Milly returns for a routine visit 5 weeks later. Which of the following nursing assessments could the nurse use to verify the EDD and estimate uterine/fetal growth?
- ○ 1. Leopold's maneuvers. **AS**
- ○ 2. Weight-gain pattern. **5**
- ○ 3. Vital signs and fetal heart tones. **SECE**
- ○ 4. Height of the fundus.

41. Milly complains of constipation. Which of the following should the nurse recommend to relieve her symptoms of constipation?
- ○ 1. Regular bedtime use of mild laxatives like mineral oil. **PL** **8**
- ○ 2. Limit fluid intake to 1000 mL daily. **HPM**

POST TEST

○ 3. Increase dietary intake of fresh fruit and salads.
○ 4. Begin Kegel exercises to increase tone.

Amy Dohn, age 23, Gravida 1 Para 0, has returned for a routine prenatal visit in her eighteenth week of pregnancy. Pregnancy has been progressing normally. Amy and her husband Jim have registered to take Lamaze classes and are apartment hunting in anticipation of the new baby.

42. Amy complains of severe "charley horses" during the night. Which of the following actions should the nurse recommend to provide symptomatic relief?
○ 1. Drink a glass of milk at bedtime. **PL**
○ 2. Extend affected leg, and dorsiflex the foot. **4**
○ 3. Increase dietary intake of vitamin C. **HPM**
○ 4. Mild exercise every evening, such as walking.

43. Which of the following assessment findings indicates a need for further assessment of Amy's general health status at this point in the pregnancy?
○ 1. Rheumatic fever at age 12. **AS**
○ 2. Rubella titer negative. **1**
○ 3. Family history of multiple births. **PhI**
○ 4. Treatment for chlamydial infection prior to pregnancy validation.

44. Anticipatory guidance may be indicated to assist Amy and Jim achieve the normal developmental tasks of the beginning family. Which of the following is *least likely* to cause anxiety and stress at this point in the pregnancy?
○ 1. Economic demands of having a child. **AN**
○ 2. Change in intrafamily relationships. **7**
○ 3. Increasing awareness of the need to be responsible for another individual (the baby). **PsI**
○ 4. Feelings of having to "compete" for attention.

Amy states, "I don't feel like myself lately." Further assessment identifies feelings of discomfort due to mood swings, fluctuating sexual desire, and worries over a changing life-style.

45. Which of the following nursing diagnoses is *most* appropriate?
○ 1. *Body image disturbance* related to second trimester physiologic and psychologic adaptations. **AN** **7** **PsI**
○ 2. *Altered nutrition, less than body requirements,* related to increased need for vitamin B_6 during pregnancy.
○ 3. *Ineffective individual coping* related to perceived need to alter life-style, role-change.
○ 4. *Personal identity disturbance* related to introspection and self-focusing.

46. Which of the following nursing interventions should be implemented to reduce Amy's stress regarding her feelings?
○ 1. Validate normalcy of emotional lability. **PL**
○ 2. Recommend high-protein, high-vitamin diet. **7**
○ 3. Refer Amy to a psychologist for counseling. **PsI**
○ 4. Reinforce positive feelings about the pregnancy.

Tara Ode, age 15, is seen in clinic with complaints of severe vulvovaginal itching, burning on urination, and thin, watery vaginal discharge for the past 4 days. During the history and physical exam, she appears very embarrassed and upset. Looking at the floor, she admits to being sexually active. She says, "Do you think I'm pregnant, or have something awful? How can I tell my mother?"

47. Which of the following nursing diagnoses is *least likely* to apply in this situation?
○ 1. *Anxiety/fear* related to the perceived possibility of diagnosis of pregnancy or venereal disease. **AN** **7** **PsI**
○ 2. *Ineffective individual coping* related to situational crisis.
○ 3. *Self-esteem disturbance* related to inability to reconcile expectations of peers and family; situational crisis.
○ 4. *Powerlessness* related to life-style of helplessness.

48. The vaginal examination disclosed several painful red papules on the inner surfaces of the labia minora and in the vagina. Lesions were extremely painful on gentle touch with an applicator. Discharge had a very foul odor. Inflammatory regional lymph nodes were easily palpated. With which of the following infectious organisms are these assessment findings associated?
○ 1. *Trichomonas vaginalis.* **AS**
○ 2. *Candida albicans.* **1**
○ 3. Herpesvirus type 2. **PhI**
○ 4. *Neisseria gonorrhea.*

49. Health teaching for Tara should include which of the following?
○ 1. "Abstain from intercourse until lesions heal." **IMP**
○ 2. "Penicillin is the drug of choice for treatment." **1**
○ 3. "Therapy is curative." **HPM**
○ 4. "Organism is associated with later development of hydatidiform mole."

Lupe Lopez is admitted via the emergency room. No prenatal information is available because Lupe is not a local resident, speaks little English, and appears very apprehensive. Her husband, José, says this is their first baby and "it was not supposed to come for 2 weeks." She is 4 cm dilated; cervix is 60% effaced.

50. Which of the following nursing diagnoses is least likely to prove a problem during Lupe's labor and delivery?
○ 1. *Pain* related to uterine contractions and fear. **AN**
○ 2. *Impaired verbal communication* related to language barrier. **5** **HPM**
○ 3. *Anxiety/fear* related to poor communication and labor.
○ 4. *Altered nutrition, less than body requirements.*

51. Lupe is in active labor, with moderate to strong contractions every 2–3 minutes, lasting 45 seconds. She appears very frightened. By which of the following modalities can the nurse convey caring and allay anxiety?
○ 1. Asking José to translate all interactions. **PL**
○ 2. Touching, smiling, and speaking in a calm, assured voice. **7** **PsI**
○ 3. Speaking slowly, loudly, and clearly, to facilitate Lupe's understanding.
○ 4. Offering to notify the doctor on call.

52. Suddenly, Lupe screams and shouts in Spanish. José translates that she has a "terrible pain in her calf," a charley horse. Which of the following should the nurse do *immediately?*
○ 1. Inform the doctor that Lupe has signs of thrombophlebitis. **IMP** **3**
○ 2. Administer oxygen by mask to expedite conversion of muscle lactic acid. **PhI**
○ 3. Straighten Lupe's knee and dorsiflex her foot.
○ 4. Turn Lupe on her left side to increase placental perfusion.

53. Suddenly, during a contraction, Lupe's water breaks. If present, which of the following assessment findings indicates a deviation from normal labor patterns?
○ 1. Issue of colored amniotic fluid. **AS**
○ 2. Lupe complains of nausea, and she vomits. **5**
○ 3. Fetal bradycardia with contractions. **PhI**
○ 4. Lupe becomes diaphoretic and irritable.

54. Lupe begins to push. Vaginal examination reveals she is 8 cm dilated. For which of the following reasons does the nurse ask José to tell Lupe to pant with her "pains"?
○ 1. To increase oxygenation of the fetus during transitional phase. **PL** **6**
○ 2. Pushing on an incompletely dilated cervix may cause cervical edema and may prolong labor. **PhI**
○ 3. Hyperventilating will make her dizzy, reduce pain, and encourage complete dilatation.
○ 4. To reduce stress on the fetal head during internal rotation.

55. Lupe delivers a viable 7-lb 12-oz. boy. Apgar scores are 7 and 9. In assessing the baby, the nurse notes he appears slightly cyanotic. Which of the following should the nurse perform *first?*
○ 1. Wrap him in another blanket, to reduce heat loss. **IMP** **6**
○ 2. Stimulate him to cry, to increase oxygenation. **SECE**
○ 3. Aspirate his nose and mouth with bulb syringe.
○ 4. Elevate his head to promote gravity drainage of secretions.

56. Lupe wants to breastfeed her baby. Which of the following hormones, normally secreted during the postpartum period, influences both the milk ejection reflex and uterine involution?
○ 1. Estrogen. **AN**
○ 2. Progesterone. **5**
○ 3. Relaxin. **PhI**
○ 4. Oxytocin.

57. When Juan is nearly 24 hours old, a nursing assessment notes that his skin is dry and flaking and that there are several areas of an apparent macular rash. The nurse charts this as which of the following?
○ 1. Erythema toxicum. **IMP**
○ 2. Milia. **5**
○ 3. Icterus neonatorum. **HPM**
○ 4. Multiple hemangiomas.

58. Lupe is leaving in the morning and will be returning immediately to San Juan. Anticipatory guidance and health teaching should be directed toward the goals of Lupe's demonstrating confidence and competence in caring for Juan. Which of the following modalities will be most effective in facilitating and evaluating Lupe's achievement of the nursing goals?
○ 1. Giving Lupe a Spanish-language booklet describing basic techniques of baby care. **PL** **7**
○ 2. Discussing the pattern and procedures of basic newborn care with Lupe. **HPM**
○ 3. Demonstrating basic baby care procedures and having Lupe perform them with Juan.
○ 4. Referring Lupe to the San Juan Public Health Department nurses.

Frank Henry, a 65-year-old retired merchant seaman, has been hospitalized for 2 weeks for severe vascular insufficiency and gangrene of the left foot. He has been an insulin-dependent diabetic for 20 years. Frank is scheduled for an above-the-knee amputation in 4 days.

59. Mr. Henry verbalizes feelings of decreased self-worth and of being less of a man. His acceptance of the surgery is largely dependent on:
○ 1. What his doctor says. **AN**
○ 2. How his family is reacting. **7**
○ 3. How the nursing staff reacts and responds to his behavior. **PsI**
○ 4. His ability to grieve.

60. Two days before surgery, Frank expresses a desire to learn more about the surgery and outcome. Preoperative teaching is directed toward:
○ 1. Discussing the possibility of another vocation. **PL**
○ 2. Learning crutch-walking. **1**
○ 3. Instruction in postoperative exercises. **HPM**
○ 4. Encouraging the client to verbalize fears and concerns.

As Mr. Leonard begins to regain consciousness following surgery, it is noted that he is not moving his left extremities. Further neurologic examination reveals he has suffered a cerebral vascular accident in the right hemisphere. He seems to be trying to talk, but you are unable to understand him.

61. The appropriate nursing action with a client experiencing expressive aphasia following a CVA would be:
○ 1. Help the client and family accept this permanent disability. **IMP** **2**
○ 2. Associate words with physical objects. **HPM**
○ 3. Wait indefinitely for the client to verbalize.
○ 4. Tell the family that the client cannot communicate.

Amy Black, 5 years old, is admitted for cardiac catheterization to evaluate the status of her ventricular septal defect (VSD). Amy also has Down syndrome.

62. Amy's cardiac catheterization is scheduled for the next morning. Which action by the nurse would be most helpful in preparing Amy for this procedure?
○ 1. Describe the procedure to Amy in very simple terms. **IMP** **5**
○ 2. Take Amy to the lab to allow her to observe such a procedure. **PsI**
○ 3. Answer only those questions Amy herself asks.
○ 4. Use puppets to dramatize the procedure for Amy.

63. While Amy is in the hospital, she is found to have lice. Mrs. Black asks the nurse how Amy got lice. Which one factor should the nurse identify as the most probable cause of Amy's lice?
○ 1. Amy washes her hair only once a week. **AS**
○ 2. Amy shares her comb and brush with her friend. **1** **HPM**
○ 3. Amy wears a hat to school every day.
○ 4. Amy's hair is long, thick, and curly.

64. The nurse should also teach Mrs. Black that, to prevent other members of the Black family from getting lice:
○ 1. Amy should sleep alone and in her own bed. **IMP**
○ 2. All family members should get a very short haircut. **1** **HPM**
○ 3. Amy should wear a hair net for a few days.
○ 4. All family members should comb their hair with a fine-toothed comb after regular shampooing.

Trevor Roberts, 14 years old, is admitted to the adolescent unit following surgery for a ruptured appendix. Admitting orders include:

- *Salem sump to suction*
- *IV Ringer's Lactate at 110 cc/hour*
- *NPO*

65. If Trevor's Salem sump tube is functioning properly, the nurse should expect to make which of these observations?
- ○ 1. There is no drainage on Trevor's surgical dressing. **EV**
- ○ 2. Trevor's abdomen is soft. **8**
- ○ 3. Trevor is able to swallow his saliva. **PhI**
- ○ 4. There are bowel sounds in all four quadrants.

66. In monitoring Trevor's postop course, the nurse would be most correct in expecting that Trevor will:
- ○ 1. Have moderate to severe pain for 24 hours. **EV**
- ○ 2. Be discharged within 48 hours. **8**
- ○ 3. Make a slow, steady recovery. **PhI**
- ○ 4. Make a fairly rapid and complete recovery.

67. Trevor complains of having nothing to do while he is recovering. The nurse should:
- ○ 1. Ask Trevor to place routine lab slips in the charts. **IMP**
- ○ 2. Refer Trevor to the tutor and arrange for him to get his school books and homework. **5** **PsI**
- ○ 3. Bring in several board games, and encourage Trevor and his 13-year-old roommate to start playing with one of them.
- ○ 4. Introduce Trevor to the two 13-year-old girls in the room next door.

Following a fire in her family's apartment, 7-year-old Amber Larson is admitted to the burn unit in serious condition with second-degree burns over her head, face, neck, and anterior chest.

68. As Amber is lying on the stretcher during her admission, she suddenly complains of nausea and begins to vomit. The nurse should immediately:
- ○ 1. Turn Amber's head to the side. **IMP**
- ○ 2. Suction her oropharynx. **1**
- ○ 3. Raise the head of the stretcher. **SECE**
- ○ 4. Insert an NG tube.

69. On Amber's first night in the hospital, the nurse enters her room and finds her crying softly and moaning in pain. Recognizing the extent of Amber's injuries, the nurse should:
- ○ 1. Do nothing at this time. **IMP**
- ○ 2. Offer Amber 2 Tylenol as ordered and a glass of warm milk. **3** **PhI**
- ○ 3. Give Amber an IM injection of 40 mg of demerol as ordered.
- ○ 4. Inject 25 mg of demerol as ordered via Amber's central IV line.

70. In positioning Amber during her recovery, the nurse should:
- ○ 1. Avoid head flexion. **IMP**
- ○ 2. Keep Amber as still as possible. **3**
- ○ 3. Avoid sitting her up in a chair. **PhI**
- ○ 4. Place 2 firm pillows under Amber's head.

71. Amber is to have daily debridement and whirlpool therapy for her burns. In cleansing Amber's burns, the nurse should use sterile:
- ○ 1. 4x4 gauze pads. **IMP**
- ○ 2. Cotton balls. **1**
- ○ 3. Washcloths. **SECE**
- ○ 4. Telfa pads.

72. Amber is fitted for a pressure stockinette to cover her head, face, and neck to minimize scarring as her burns are healing. In order to help Amber cope with her injuries, treatment, and recuperation, the nurse should ask Amber's parents to bring:
- ○ 1. Amber's favorite toys and stuffed animals. **IMP**
- ○ 2. Some of Amber's friends for a short visit. **5**
- ○ 3. Amber's favorite foods, including pizza and ice cream. **PsI**
- ○ 4. Colorful scarves and hats.

Mr. Sam Gold is a 68-year-old retired engineer who has been in consistent good health since childhood. Lately he has been having problems with intermittent diarrhea and constipation. Two weeks ago he noted blood in the stool. Manual examination of the rectum and anal canal by the physician revealed no abnormalities. A lower GI series was set on an outpatient basis. Three days later, Mr. Gold's physician called to schedule a sigmoidoscopy for the morning.

73. The nurse explains that a sigmoidoscopy involves:
- ○ 1. Instillation of a radiopaque dye into the lower gastrointestinal tract. **IMP** **8**
- ○ 2. Insertion of a rigid instrument that allows for direct visual examination of the anal canal, rectum, and sigmoid colon. **PhI**
- ○ 3. Insertion of a fiber-optic scope that allows for direct visualization of the sigmoid colon, transverse colon, and ileocecal valve.
- ○ 4. Surgical removal of polyps and biopsy of suspicious gastrointestinal mucosa.

Proctoscopy reveals severe diverticulitis of the upper sigmoid colon. The physician decides to do a temporary colostomy to prevent perforation of the bowel.

74. Preoperative preparation of Mr. Gold included administration of neomycin SO_4. The nurse expects that this antibiotic will:
- ○ 1. Combat postoperative wound infection. **EV**
- ○ 2. Decrease bacterial count of the colon. **8**
- ○ 3. Reduce the size of the suspected tumor before surgery. **PhI**
- ○ 4. Stimulate peristalsis and facilitate action of cleansing enemas.

Postoperatively Mr. Gold had a double-barrel transverse colostomy. Postoperative orders were:

- *1000 cc 5% D/Ringer's every 8 hours.*
- *Meperidine 100 mg IM every 4 hours p.r.n. for pain.*
- *IPPB with normal saline 15 min tid.*
- *Attach nasogastric tube to low intermittent suction.*
- *Out of bed tonight × 1.*

75. Which of the following statements by the nurse correctly describes a double-barrel colostomy?
- ○ 1. It is the least common type of colostomy, and it discharges liquid or unformed stool. **PL** **8**
- ○ 2. A single loop of the transverse colon is exteriorized and supported by a glass rod. There are two openings, a proximal loop and a distal loop. **PhI**
- ○ 3. It has two stomas. A proximal loop discharges feces, and a distal loop discharges mucus.
- ○ 4. It is most often permanent and is done to treat disorders of the sigmoid colon.

76. The nurse knows that a colostomy begins functioning:
- ○ 1. Immediately. **PL**
- ○ 2. Two to three days postoperatively. **8**
- ○ 3. One week postoperatively. **SECE**
- ○ 4. Two weeks postoperatively.

77. You explain to Mr. Gold that the colostomy appliance should be changed:
- ○ 1. Every day. **PL**
- ○ 2. When drainage leaks through seal. **8**
- ○ 3. Once a week. **PhI**
- ○ 4. At a time selected by the visiting nurse.

78. You are teaching methods to reduce flatus and odor. What would be the *least* effective method to achieve this?
- ○ 1. Avoid eating broccoli and cabbage. **PL**
- ○ 2. Utilize *Banish* deodorant drops in bottom of appliance. **8** **PhI**
- ○ 3. Put pinhole in appliance to let flatus escape.
- ○ 4. Empty feces and gas from appliance as necessary.

John Garcia is a 56-year-old man admitted to the hospital with increasing breathlessness for the past 5 days. Past history included frequent bronchitis. He has smoked 2 packs of cigarettes a day since age 25 and has had a productive cough on rising for the past 15 years. Physical examination reveals a short, stocky, barrel-chested male, blood pressure 150/96, pulse 88, respirations 16, temperature 98°F. Percussion note hyperresonant, breath sounds soft and flat, medium-pitched rhonchi and wheezes heard in right upper lobe and both lower lung lobes.

79. The nurse explains to Mr. Garcia that bronchitis is characterized by:
- ○ 1. Hypertrophy of the bronchial mucous glands and the production of mucoid sputum sometimes difficult to expectorate. **AS** **6** **SECE**
- ○ 2. Bronchoconstriction and edema of the wall of the bronchioles.
- ○ 3. Exudate in the alveoli.
- ○ 4. Increasing lung stiffness.

80. Which statement by the nurse correctly describes a wheeze?
- ○ 1. A high-pitched musical sound produced by airflow in narrowed bronchioles. **AS** **6**
- ○ 2. Rarely considered pathological. **PhI**
- ○ 3. A medium-pitched sonorous sound produced by airflow in obstructed bronchi.
- ○ 4. A high-pitched crowing sound produced by edema in the trachea.

Mr. Garcia's laboratory work reveals: Hct 50%, Hgb 17, Na^+ 144, K^+ 4.2, Cl^- 92, HCO^{3-} 32. Arterial blood gases: pH 7.38, Po_2 65, Pco_2 55.

81. The nurse's interpretation of Mr. Garcia's blood gases is that he has:
- ○ 1. Uncompensated respiratory acidosis. **AN**
- ○ 2. Compensated respiratory acidosis. **6**
- ○ 3. Uncompensated metabolic alkalosis. **PhI**
- ○ 4. Compensated metabolic alkalosis.

82. The nurse observes that Mr. Garcia demonstrates the "increased work of breathing" during this acute period by:
- ○ 1. Increasing the rate and depth of his respirations. **AS** **6**
- ○ 2. Increasing diaphragmatic excursion. **PhI**
- ○ 3. Using pursed-lip exhalations.
- ○ 4. Using accessory muscles for ventilation.

83. Pulmonary function data were also collected on Mr. Garcia. The results were:

	TLC	FRC	RV	VC	FEV_1
Predicted	6000	3000	2000	4000	3000
Observed	7000	5000	4200	2800	2000

The nurse's analysis of these data reveals:
- ○ 1. Hyperinflation. **AN**
- ○ 2. Hyperventilation. **6**
- ○ 3. Hyperpnea. **SECE**
- ○ 4. Hypercapnia.

84. The nurse recognizes that the pattern of pulmonary dysfunction reflected by these lung volumes is characteristic of:
- ○ 1. Restrictive lung disease. **AN**
- ○ 2. Obstructive lung disease. **6**
- ○ 3. Vascular lung disease. **PhI**
- ○ 4. A combination of restrictive and obstructive lung disease.

85. After a nebulizer treatment with isoproterenol (Isuprel), the following measurements were obtained:

	TLC	FRC	RV	VC	FEV_1
Observed	7000	4000	3000	3800	2500

The nurse would conclude that the change in lung volumes indicates:
- ○ 1. Improvement. **EV**
- ○ 2. Deterioration. **6**
- ○ 3. No change. **PhI**
- ○ 4. Data inadequate to decide.

Physician orders for Mr. Garcia included:
- *IPPB tid with Mucomyst (acetylcysteine).*
- *Postural drainage with percussion and vibration for 30 min bid.*
- *Theophylline elixir 1 tbsp every 6 hours.*
- *Sputum for culture and sensitivity.*

86. Nursing actions that will facilitate Mr. Garcia's medical therapy include:
- ○ 1. Limiting fluid intake to prevent volume overload and right-sided heart failure. **IMP** **6**
- ○ 2. Oral and endotracheal suctioning as necessary. **PhI**
- ○ 3. Instructing the client in deep breathing and coughing techniques as well as pursed-lip exhalations.
- ○ 4. Maintenance of bedrest and activity restrictions to reduce acidosis.

87. The nurse can also increase Mr. Garcia's ventilatory efficiency by positioning him as follows:
- ○ 1. High Fowler's. **IMP**
- ○ 2. Prone. **6**
- ○ 3. Sitting up and leaning slightly forward. **SECE**
- ○ 4. Trendelenburg.

88. Mr. Garcia's teaching plan should emphasize:
- ○ 1. Smoking and alcohol restrictions. **IMP**
- ○ 2. Nutrition, fluid balance, and ways to stop smoking. **6** **SECE**
- ○ 3. Vocational rehabilitation programs available in the community.
- ○ 4. Activity restrictions and pulmonary physiology.

89. Chronic obstructive pulmonary disease can progress to respiratory failure. A client with emphysema becomes increasingly drowsy, tachypneic, and tachycardic. The nurse should first:
- ○ 1. Prepare IV aminophylline. **IMP**
- ○ 2. Position the client in high Fowler's. **6**
- ○ 3. Give 2 L of O_2 per nasal cannula. **PhI**
- ○ 4. Administer 60% O_2 via mask.

90. Another complication of chronic obstructive pulmonary disease is the possible rupture of an emphysematous bleb. You suspect that the client has a right tension pneumothorax. What signs would you expect to see?
- ○ 1. Flushed appearance from elevated blood pressure. **AS 6 PhI**
- ○ 2. Tracheal deviation to the unaffected side.
- ○ 3. Hyporesonance on the affected side.
- ○ 4. Medial shift of the heart.

Mrs. Rhonda Sanches is a 32-year-old flight attendant admitted to the hospital with acute rheumatoid arthritis. Vital signs are: temperature 101°F orally, BP 102/68, pulse 96, respirations 22. Her hands are painful and edematous with severe (L) hip pain. Medical orders: bed rest, ASA gr$\bar{x}$ q.i.d.; passive range of motion b.i.d.

91. The nurse can expect Mrs. Sanches' temperature and pulse to be elevated because of:
- ○ 1. Increased fluid losses. **AN 3 PhI**
- ○ 2. Inflammation of her hand and hip joints.
- ○ 3. Stress response.
- ○ 4. Side effect of salicylate therapy.

92. The primary purpose of the nurse's performing passive range-of-motion exercises to Mrs. Sanches' affected limbs is to:
- ○ 1. Prevent contractures and limited range of motion. **IMP 3 SECE**
- ○ 2. Continually evaluate her functional abilities.
- ○ 3. Assess her pain tolerance.
- ○ 4. Evaluate the effectiveness of drug therapy.

93. Which of the following laboratory tests would be increased on assessment for acute rheumatoid arthritis?
- ○ 1. Hemoglobin and hematocrit. **AN 3 PhI**
- ○ 2. Sedimentation rate and C-reactive protein.
- ○ 3. Wasserman test.
- ○ 4. Platelet count.

94. To reduce symptoms of early morning stiffness, the nurse can encourage the client to:
- ○ 1. Take a hot tub bath or shower in the morning. **PL 3 PhI**
- ○ 2. Put joints through passive ROM before trying to move them actively.
- ○ 3. Sleep with a hot pad.
- ○ 4. Take two aspirins before arising, and wait 15 minutes before attempting locomotion.

95. The physician orders prednisone 10 mg every morning for Mrs. Sanches. Which of the following precautions should the nurse advise the client of during predischarge teaching?
- ○ 1. Take oral preparations of prednisone before meals. **IMP 3 SECE**
- ○ 2. Never stop or change the amount of the medication without medical advice.
- ○ 3. Have periodic complete blood counts while on the medication.
- ○ 4. Wear sunglasses if exposed to bright light for an extended period of time.

96. Which of the following is a reliable index of Mrs. Sanches' exercise tolerance?
- ○ 1. Pulse and respiratory rate. **EV 3 PhI**
- ○ 2. Occurrence and duration of pain in the affected joint.
- ○ 3. Mobility of joints.
- ○ 4. Decreased redness and swelling of joints.

The following are individual items.

97. Julie Cross, age 25, has been scheduled for surgery to remove the lesions at the footplate of the stapes, associated with *otosclerosis*. A client who is scheduled for a *stapedectomy* should be told to expect which of the following?
- ○ 1. Tinnitus for several weeks after surgery. **IMP 2 SECE**
- ○ 2. Rhinitis as the edema from surgery resolves.
- ○ 3. The hearing loss will continue for a while.
- ○ 4. Showering and swimming will no longer be permitted.

98. The nurse would know that the appropriate positioning for a client with *ruptured appendix* is:
- ○ 1. Semi-Fowler's. **PL 8 SECE**
- ○ 2. Trendelenburg.
- ○ 3. Left Sims'.
- ○ 4. Dorsal recumbent.

99. A peripheral iridectomy is the surgical procedure of choice following an acute episode of closed-angle glaucoma. Which of the following nursing measures is *inappropriate* for the client who has had an *iridectomy*?
- ○ 1. Instill eye drops to mobilize the affected pupil by alternate dilatation and constriction. **IMP 2 SECE**
- ○ 2. Ambulate the client as soon as possible after the surgery.
- ○ 3. Reinforce the surgical dressing as needed to prevent infection.
- ○ 4. If ordered, instruct the client to massage the affected eye.

100. Which of the following should the nurse recognize as an *inappropriate* method of treating *hyperthyroidism*?
- ○ 1. Subtotal thyroidectomy. **IMP 3 SECE**
- ○ 2. Administration of propylthiouracil.
- ○ 3. Radioiodine therapy.
- ○ 4. Administration of thyroglobulin.

■ ANSWERS/RATIONALE

1. (3) The adolescent is striving to attain a sense of independence and identity. Trust (No. 1) is usually developed during infancy and matures as the individual develops. Goals and plans (No. 2) are made during the adolescent period, but they are rarely finalized realistically until late adulthood. During this period, inner conflicts (No. 4) are rarely resolved and are usually heightened.

2. (4) The superego may never be completely refined or stabilized. Some individuals may achieve an optimal level of functioning some time in late adulthood; however, rarely will the superego become stabilized during adolescence. As stated in No. 1, the individual does strive to develop an independent and unique personality during adolescence. In order to maintain a steady state of functioning, the adolescent must learn to use defense mechanisms (No. 2) in an appropriate manner. Developing a positive ego identity (No. 3) is one of the major goals of adolescence.

3. (4) The passage of time will *not* help Charlie cope effectively with his feelings of fear and ambivalence. These feeling are a normal part of the maturation process, and *only* with effective limit-setting and psychologic support will the adolescent's ability to cope be strengthened. In early adolescence boys generally are intolerant of female authority figures (No. 1). They perceive these females as a threat to their emerging masculine identity. Adolescents need physical activity to alleviate tension (No. 2). Males in general have problems dealing with impulse control (No. 3) and need consistent limits set on their behaviors.

4. (1) Adolescents are preoccupied with their changing bodies, their relationships, and their fantasies. Although they have difficulty with rote learning (No. 2), they have an increased potential for imaginative thinking. During this period they are less able to concentrate on their academic work (No. 3), which leads to increased feelings of frustration that are usually *not* accompanied by an increased ability to cope (No. 4).

5. (2) Limits *do* need to be set, but they should be based on *mutual respect* rather than fear. Adult (or external) controls on behavior (No. 1) are essential and must be consistent. Role models serve to stimulate the identification process (No. 3) both consciously and unconsciously. Stable relationships (No. 4) are essential if the adolescent is to mature and develop a sense of trust.

6. (1) Acting out is the expression through behavior (rather than through words) of emotions that occur when the client relives or reproduces the feelings, wishes, or conflicts that are operating unconsciously. Charlie may be feeling frustrated, angry, ambivalent, etc., for numerous reasons, such as conflict between himself and his parents, a reaction to his parents' intramarital conflicts, sibling rivalry, or frustration due to poor self-esteem.

7. (3) Hostility and aggression are considered the underlying factors in the psychogenesis and psychodynamics of depression. The adolescent is in a stage of development where he experiences extensive anger due to frustration. The adolescent has a greater energy level because of the increased libidinal energy available in his system. In order to expend this energy, many adolescents act out their feelings of depression in violent ways rather than become withdrawn, apathetic, or regressive (Nos. 1, 2, and 4).

8. (2) Hitting others provides Charlie with an outlet for his feelings of hopelessness and despair. Although this behavior may not make him feel happy or satisfied, it does provide a defense against feeling unhappy. Nos. 1, 3, and 4 are not primary motivations of this behavior.

9. (1) If a confrontation develops too soon, Charlie may feel threatened and run away from the hospital. Although the other answers are all true, they have less significant consequences. Charlie's refusal to verbalize (No. 2) is expected only initially, because he probably will not trust the group members at first. The other group members may also feel threatened by a new member and may not trust him (No. 3). Acting out (No. 4) is a coping mechanism that Charlie uses to mask his fear of a new situation or his sense of being threatened.

10. (4) Since Charlie has only attended six sessions of group therapy, it is expected that he would only speak when questioned. He is probably still unsure of his own feelings and is in the preinteraction phase of trusting other group members. Nos. 1, 2, and 3 are probably not true at this point.

11. (4) It is important for the angry client to express his feelings overtly. Internalizing them would cause increased feelings of frustration and anxiety and would therefore be counterproductive. Nos. 1, 2, and 3 are all appropriate goals.

12. (4) Charlie *initially* needs staff's help in one-to-one socialization. He *next* must be stimulated by the staff to participate in minimally demanding group acitivites (No. 1). Allowing him a minimum of 3 hours in his room (No. 3) will probably increase his isolation and his withdrawal. Perhaps the nurse could establish a behavior-modification program involving a trade-off of 15 minutes in his room for every 45 minutes spent socializing and interacting with others. If activities are too challenging (No. 2), Charlie may become frustrated and feel incompetent, which would lead to a decrease in self-esteem.

13. (2) Confrontation *could* help Charlie identify the inappropriateness of mutilation and other destructive behaviors as attention-getting devices. Nos. 1, 3, and 4 are all appropriate interventions.

14. (3) Charlie's thoughts, feelings, and attitudes toward sexual relationships need to be explored in order to assess his level of maturity in deciding his sexual preference. Confrontation (No. 1) could help Charlie identify his use of homosexual behavior as an attention-seeking device. Validation of his rationale for seeking homosexual relationships (No. 2) may be identified more appropriately through exploring his thoughts, feelings, and attitudes regarding his sexual orientation. Enforcing limits on his relationships (No. 4) will only make him angry and is in any case an invasion of his right to privacy and freedom of choice. As long as neither Charlie nor Rich is forcing himself on the other, their relationship should not be interfered with. However, if it is determined that for some appropriate reason this relationship is detrimental to either individual's optimal level of functioning, then limits should be set.

15. (4) Isolation may lead to withdrawal and depression. Charlie's mother needs positive reinforcement and reassurance to increase her self-esteem. Isolation may also lead to an increase in her drinking and depression. Based on the symptoms Charlie's mother is exhibiting, involving her in simple, concrete tasks (No. 1) may help her feel useful. Crying (No. 2) helps her alleviate anxiety through the physical expression of her feelings. Encouraging the verbalization of her feelings (No. 3) will demonstrate that someone cares for her enough to listen, and may decrease her anxiety level.

16. (2) Past coping mechanisms are important in assessing the client's ability to return to a steady state of functioning. Strengths and weaknesses in the client's ability to rationally assess and cope with her feelings need to be explored. Referrals may need to be made (No. 1), but an initial assessment of the client needs to be completed first. Inpatient hospitalization may be needed (No. 3); however, the assessment of her ability to cope with the situation may assist in identifying whether hospitalization is needed. Obtaining a prescription for an antidepressant at this time (No. 4) may prove to be detrimental. Even if she does not decide to overdose, medication without psychologic support is generally ineffective.

17. (3) The first priority with any unconscious client is to maintain a patent airway. The nurse would need a physician's order to administer any medication or stimulant (No. 1), which may not be appropriate in this situation. The emergency room nurse would see that the attending resident was paged (No. 2), but this task could be delegated while the nurse administered primary care. Monitoring neurologic signs (No. 4) is also essential but can be done after ensuring that the client can breathe.

18. (3) The client should be placed under one-to-one, not group, observation to ensure effective protection against suicidal behaviors. Nos. 1, 2, and 4 are all appropriate actions.

19. (1) Individuals who have used alcohol habitually over an extended time period usually exhibit symptoms of withdrawal delirium when the alcohol intake is severely decreased or curtailed. Nos. 2, 3, and 4 are less likely reactions.

20. (4) The psychologic effect of being restrained can be severe. Therefore any form of restraint should be applied as a last resort. Isolating the client from other clients during the initial adjustment period would serve to decrease stimuli and possibly prevent the need for restraints. Nos. 1, 2, and 3 are all more appropriate interventions.

21. (2) An increase in Charlie's mother's energy level may provide her with enough motivation to make another suicide attempt. Generally, depressed clients do not kill themselves because their energy level is very low. Therefore the one-to-one relationship needs to be maintained and stressed at this time. Nos. 1, 3, and 4 are dangerous assumptions at this time.

22. (1) Family therapy should promote the expression of feelings. Intragroup dynamics of the family system should be assessed, and appropriate coping strategies identified. The objectives of family therapy are not primarily to provide individual therapy for each family member (No. 2). If a family member needs one-to-one therapy, individual therapy is usually provided in conjunction with, but at a separate time from, family therapy sessions. The identified client is treated in individual and family therapy sessions (No. 3). However, the primary focus of family therapy is not just treatment of this particular individual. Crisis intervention may be one aspect of family therapy (No. 4), but it is not necessarily the primary goal in this case. Crisis intervention may be used initially to assist in returning the family system to a steady state of functioning.

23. (3) Establishing trust between the therapist and the couple is essential to facilitate effective therapy and possible resolution of the marital and familial conflicts. Confrontation (No. 1) may prove very theatening in this situation, and the couple may leave therapy to avoid feelings of anxiety. Avoidance (No. 2) is nontherapeutic in this situation because it does not help resolve the conflict. A referral (No. 4) may be appropriate; however, the nurse should initially use all her therapeutic techniques in assisting the couple to identify relevant issues and possibly to resolve conflicts before making a referral.

24. (3) Most obsessive-compulsive individuals are highly inflexible and resist change because change stimulates anxiety and they are unable to cope with stress. Nos. 1, 2, and 4 are all likely behaviors.

25. (2) Denial is the failure to acknowledge the existence of an affect, experience, idea, or memory. The person blocks from conscious awareness that which is painful, anxiety provoking, or threatening. Charlie's father may perceive that his behavior contributes to his wife's use of alcohol, and he may use denial to avoid facing feelings of guilt. Projection (No. 1) is the attribution of one's feelings, impulses, thoughts, and wishes to others or to the environment. Repression (No. 3) is an unconscious mechanism used to avoid painful experiences, unacceptable thoughts and impulses, and disagreeable memories by "forgetting." Sublimation (No. 4) is the transformation of psychic energy associated with unacceptable sexual or aggressive behaviors into socially acceptable outlets.

26. (1) Lithium is used to treat affective disorders. Mellaril (No. 4) is a major tranquilizer used to treat schizophrenia. Mellaril has been used to treat the manic phase of bipolar affective disorders, but it is not the primary drug. Librium (No. 2) is a minor tranquilizer used to relieve the mild or moderate anxiety usually associated with affective and somatoform disorders. Prolixin (No. 3) is a long-acting psychotropic used primarily to treat schizophrenia. It can be administered biweekly in an injection for a long-term effect.

27. (1) Lithium is excreted through the kidneys. Consequently, the kidneys must function adequately to avoid lithium toxicity. Diuretics should *not* be given concurrently with lithium because they may potentiate sodium and fluid depletion, which may lead to lithium toxicity. Haldol (No. 4) is a major tranquilizer that is sometimes administered simultaneously with lithium during the first week to 10 days to control manic symptoms. Nausea, vomiting, and muscle weakness (No. 3) are all possible side effects of lithium. They indicate a need for close observation and regulation of the drug if they disrupt the person's level of functioning. Every client should be screened prior to the administration of any medication (No. 2). However, since lithium is a drug that is taken over a long period of time, blood levels must be consistently regulated and physical examinations routinely scheduled (i.e., every 3 months initially, then every 6 months once the client appears to be regulated).

28. (3) Charlie is probably very frightened and angry. He needs to feel that his side will be considered if he is to cope effectively with these feelings and with his behavior. Nos. 1, 2, and 4 are all staff-oriented and provide little psychologic support for Charlie as an individual striving for independence.

29. (3) Although there are several forms that elicit disclosure of this information, there is no law that mandates disclosure (No. 4). Charlie has to make this decision independently. The nurse should provide therapeutic support for whatever he decides. Nos. 1 and 2 are untrue statements.

30. (2) Although Charlie's parents may perceive this as a parental decision, it is important for Charlie's sister and brother to be included in the decision-making process because the entire family system will be affected by this change. Asking the parents to reassess their feelings (No. 1) may help them evaluate the situation, but it avoids facing the issue as a family decision. A referral may be appropriate (Nos. 3 and 4); however, all parties involved in the decision must be listened to before making a referral or searching for an alternative placement.

31. (2) Charlie may have valid reasons for wanting to visit his friend, but allowing him to visit without assessing his motives (No. 1) may prove detrimental to Charlie, his friend, and the staff. Charlie's parents (No. 3) essentially relinquished their decision-making authority by allowing Charlie to become a ward of the state. The hospital staff would have to be consulted prior to Charlie's visit, regardless of his motive. However, No. 4 is too vague, in that it does not specify what issues would be covered in the consultation.

32. (3) Taking Sue's pulse while listening to the abdominal beat will differentiate between the maternal and fetal heart rates and rule out fetal bradycardia. No. 1 is wrong because, although the cord may prolapse at any time before the oncoming head occludes the cervix, the most common time of occurrence is when the membranes rupture. No. 2 is wrong because she shows no signs of supine hypotensive syndrome, and, in the absence of fetal bradycardia, she may assume any position of comfort; No. 4 is wrong because, if the FHR is normal, there is no need for supplemental oxygen therapy.

33. (4) Early decelerations represent the normal fetal response to head compressions during contractions. No. 1 is wrong because head compression does not cause fetal distress. Nos. 2 and 3 are wrong because there are no signs of late or variable decelerations.

34. (4) Early decelerations represent the normal fetal response to contractions. No. 1 is wrong because this action would be taken to relieve possible cord compression. No. 2 is wrong because use of Trendelenburg position is not necessary. No. 3 is an inaccurate interpretation of the assessment data.

35. (2) Sue is demonstrating signs of beginning transition. Sacral pressure and backrubs assist in reducing her discomfort at this time. No. 1 is wrong because assessment indicates irritability, not pain. Further, she has expressed a desire to use Lamaze for labor and delivery. No. 3 is wrong because it is important to maintain continual assessment of fetal status during the transitional stage. No. 4 is wrong because the client should be attended continually during transition.

36. (3) Pushing on an incompletely dilated cervix may contribute to development of cervical edema and/or lacerations. No. 1 is wrong because an engaged head occludes the cervix. Neither panting nor normal breathing increase oxygen level (No. 2). No. 4 is wrong because breathing patterns do not affect cervical dilatation.

37. (1) History of three pregnancies plus current pregnancy (Gravida 4). Parity refers to the number of pregnancies carried to viability, *not* the number of babies. Two pregnancies have ended with viable children (Para 2). Nos. 2, 3, and 4 are wrong based on the definitions of gravida and parity.

38. (2) By calculation of EDD using Naegele's rule of counting back 3 months and adding 7 days to the date of LMP: 4th month – 3 months = 1st month (January); third day plus 7 days = tenth day; January 10 is her EDD. No. 1 is wrong because of failure to add 7 days to LMP. No. 3 is wrong because 7 days were subtracted from date of LMP. No. 4 is wrong because of counting back 4 months instead of 3.

39. (3) Dry soda crackers will absorb gastric juices and increase blood sugar, thereby reducing nausea. No. 1 is wrong because eating before retiring has no effect on morning nausea. No. 2 is wrong because drinking fruit juice on an empty stomach may increase nausea. No. 4 is wrong because demands of physical activity may increase nausea.

40. (4) At 12 weeks gestation, fundus should be palpable at the pubic symphysis. No. 1 is wrong because of inability to palpate due to current uterine size and position. No. 2 is wrong because weight-gain patterns provide no information regarding uterine or fetal growth. No. 3 is wrong because maternal vital signs are not diagnostic of gestational age or uterine growth, and fetal heart tones may be heard with a Doppler as early as 9–10 weeks.

41. (3) Increased dietary bulk and adequate fluids relieve symptoms of constipation naturally, by stimulating peritalsis. No. 1 is wrong because regular use of laxatives reduces normal bowel functions; mineral oil contributes to loss of fat-soluble vitamins A, D, and E. No. 2 is wrong because adequate fluid intake is needed to avoid dry, packed stools associated with constipation. No. 4 is wrong because Kegel exercises increase sphincter control and do not encourage defecation.

42. (2) "Charley horse" pain is due to sudden spasm and acute flexion of leg muscles; it is relieved by dorsiflexing the foot, which reduces the muscle spasm. No. 1 is wrong because such action will not eliminate the possibility of muscle spasm during pregnancy. No. 3 is wrong because the actions of vitamin C do not affect muscle spasms. No. 4 is wrong because exercise does not prevent muscle spasm.

43. (1) Definitive (30%) increase in blood volume occurs at this point in pregnancy; rising cardiac load imposes stress on the heart valves affected during the episode of rheumatic fever. No. 2 is wrong because first trimester rubella infection presents the greatest hazard to the fetus, and immunization should be planned for the immediate postpartum. No. 3 is wrong because diagnosis of multiple pregnancy would be based not on discussions of general health status but on physical evidence (fundal height, ultrasound). No. 4 is wrong because once treatment is ended, infection is gone.

44. (4) During pregnancy, attention is focused on the expectant parents; feelings of competition for attention with the baby arise during the postpartum. No. 1 is wrong because pressures of present and anticipated expenses associated with childbearing impose stress on the family. No. 2 is wrong because both expectant parents must adjust to changing relationships between themselves and their extended families. No. 3 is wrong because both parents may experience stress on recognizing the need to be totally responsible for the health and development of a baby and the concomitant need to change their life-styles to meet those obligations.

45. (1) Amy's behavior typifies patterns expressed during the second trimester. No. 2 is wrong because her symptoms are related both to fluctuating hormone levels and to psychologic reevaluation of self and marriage. Nos. 3 and 4 are wrong because of the physiologic component of her symptoms.

46. (1) Understanding the reasons for disconcerting symptoms, and receiving assurance of their normalcy, assists in coping. No. 2 is wrong because, although diet may improve the general sense of well-being, diet will not affect feelings generated by the developmental tasks of pregnancy. No. 3 is wrong because Amy is demonstrating normal behavioral changes associated with second trimester pregnancy. No. 4 is wrong because it does not address the problem.

47. (4) Adolescents rarely demonstrate a life-style characterized by helplessness; rather, they are striving to gain control over their own lives. No. 1 is wrong because Amy has verbalized anxiety and fear over possible diagnoses. No. 2 is wrong because the threat of adolescent pregnancy evidently presents a situational crisis for her. No. 3 is wrong because either diagnosis will provide her with evidence that she failed to meet family expectations, and precipitates situational crisis.

48. (3) Painful, red, papular lesions associated with foul-smelling vaginal discharge are characteristic of herpesvirus type 2 infection. No. 1 is wrong because discrete lesions do not accompany trichomonal infections; discharge usually is thin, frothy, and grayish and has no odor. No. 2 is wrong because monilial vaginal infections produce a characteristic white, cheesy discharge. No. 4 is wrong because gonorrhea in women is often totally asymptomatic or may produce a purulent vaginal discharge.

49. (1) Abstinence will eliminate any unnecessary pain due to intercourse and will reduce the possibility of transmitting infection to one's sexual partner. No. 2 is wrong because the current drug of choice is acyclovir (Zovirax). No. 3 is wrong because currently available therapy is only palliative; the virus remains in the body after symptoms subside. No. 4 is wrong because hydatidiform mole is associated with benign degeneration of the chorionic villi of pregnancy.

50. (4) Although hydration may be affected by the physiologic stress of labor, the duration is insufficient to significantly affect nutritional status. No. 1 is wrong because discomfort generally accompanies labor. No. 2 is wrong because the inability to communicate clearly affects nurse–client relationships and may induce or augment anxiety. No. 3 is wrong because labor is commonly accompanied by anxiety, and Lupe was already demonstrating apprehension at admission.

51. (2) Touch, facial expression, and tone of voice may be used effectively to reduce anxiety, apprehensions, and fear in situations where verbal communication is inhibited by language barriers. No. 1 is wrong because the continual use of an intermediary (José) may impede establishing the rapport necessary for a successful labor experience. No. 3 is wrong because incomprehensible words become no more understandable spoken slowly or distinctly; loud voices are disconcerting during labor. No. 4 is inappropriate because the *nurse,* not the MD, is there to provide ongoing care and allay anxiety.

52. (3) Sudden spasm and extreme flexion of the calf muscles is relieved by forcibly extending the muscle by dorsiflexion of the foot. No. 1 is wrong because Lupe's complaint is due to muscle spasm. No. 2 is wrong because relief is accomplished by stretching the muscle; the pain is not due to lowered levels of oxygen in the muscle. No. 4 is wrong because increasing placental perfusion will be ineffective in relieving the muscle spasm.

53. (1) Normal amniotic fluid is essentially colorless; any color may signify fetal or maternal problems. For example, green amniotic fluid indicates meconium released due to fetal hypoxia; bloody amniotic fluid may indicate abruptio placentae. No. 2 is wrong because nausea with or without emesis is common in labor, due to physiologic stress. No. 3 is wrong because fetal bradycardia commonly manifests at contraction acme, due to head compression. No. 4 is wrong because diaphoresis and irritability are signs of transitional phase of labor.

54. (2) Pushing before complete dilatation may result in edema of the cervix and increase the resistance to be overcome by the oncoming head. No. 1 is wrong because panting is recommended to reduce the urge and ability to push. No. 3 is wrong because hyperventilating has no effect on cervical dilatation. No. 4 is wrong because the open fontanelles and flexibility of the sutures of the fetal head reduce pressure imposed by the force of uterine contractions.

55. (3) Gentle aspiration of mucus helps maintain a patent airway, required for effective gas exchange. No. 1 is wrong because the first priority is a patent airway. No. 2 is wrong because the baby may aspirate mucus, which would occlude the airway. No. 4 is wrong because gravity drainage is accomplished in head-dependent position.

56. (4) Contraction of the milk ducts and the let-down reflex occur under the stimulation of oxytocin released by the posterior pituitary gland. Nos. 1, 2, and 3 are wrong because these hormones have no effect on the let-down reflex or uterine involution.

57. (1) Erythema toxicum is the normal, nonpathologic macular newborn rash. No. 2 is wrong because milia are small white nodules due to clogged sebaceous glands. No. 3 is wrong because *icterus neonatorum* is the term for normal physiologic jaundice of the newborn, which occurs 48–72 hours after birth. No. 4 is wrong because hemangiomas are small elevated clusters of capillaries ("stork bites").

58. (3) Assisting the mother to develop basic skills in infant care under comfortable professional supervision is the most effective way of increasing Lupe's confidence and competence in caring for Juan. No. 1 is wrong because, although the booklet is a helpful adjunct to teaching, skills are most effectively gained by actual experience. No. 2 is wrong because clear, meaningful communication is inhibited by the language barrier, and actual experience in providing care will be of most assistance to Lupe. No. 4 is wrong because basic infant care techniques should be mastered before the mother leaves the hospital with her newborn.

59. (4) The loss of a limb is significant. The client facing the amputation must deal with his perception of himself, incorporate the changes in body image, and be allowed to grieve. The nurse must be sensitive to the client's stage of grieving and provide information as he asks, at a level consistent with his ability to comprehend. Although the attending physician (No. 1), his family (No. 2), and the nursing staff (No. 3) may affect the client's perception of a situation, the work of grieving is primarily personal, with movement both forward and backward as the client progresses through the stages.

60. (3) Although Mr. Henry expresses a willingness to learn, his apprehension will limit his ability to assimilate much. He must be taught specific arm and leg exercises, including frequent repositioning onto the abdomen to prevent contracture. Prior to discharge, alternate vocational pursuits (No. 1) may be discussed, as indicated. In the postoperative period the focus changes to crutch-walking (No. 2). Encouraging the client to verbalize fears and concerns (No. 4) is not a specific teaching strategy but rather an intervention designed to give support as well as identify potential problems.

61. (2) The client needs an opportunity to receive word images. Point to the object and clearly enunciate its name, e.g., "spoon." Also, the expressive aphasia client needs the chance to practice repeating words. Begin with sample words, such as *yes* and *no,* and then progress to complete phrases. Recovery from aphasia depends on the area of the brain involved and the extent of damage. There may be spontaneous recovery or improvement with speech therapy 2 years after the stroke. To consider the impairment permanent (No. 1) would be premature. No. 3 is incorrect because waiting may increase the client's frustration. Try to anticipate client needs to reduce feelings of helplessness. The nurse plays an important part in showing the family members how to communicate and in not discouraging communication (No. 4).

62. (4) As a preschooler, Amy would probably respond best to the use of puppets to dramatize the procedure. Any description of the procedure alone (No. 1), no matter how simple, would probably not be enough to enable most preschoolers to understand what will happen to them. Taking a client to the operating room or the catheterization lab (No. 2) would probably be unnecessarily frightening for any client, especially a child. Amy may not ask any questions herself (No. 3); and if she does not, then the nurse would be unable to do any teaching.

63. (2) Lice are spread by direct or indirect contact: sharing combs and brushes, sharing hats, sleeping together, etc. It is generally unrelated to frequency of hair washing (No. 1), wearing a hat (No. 3), or having long hair (No. 4).

64. (1) Lice are spread by direct or indirect contact; Amy should sleep alone to prevent other family members from also getting lice. In addition, Amy's mother should be taught to wash the linens in hot soapy water to kill any lice that are on them. Having the family all get short haircuts (No. 2), or use a fine-toothed comb (No. 4), or having Amy wear a hair net (No. 3) would not necessarily prevent the other family members from getting lice.

65. (2) The main purpose of a Salem sump tube is to drain fluid and gas from the stomach; if it is functioning properly, Trevor's abdomen should be soft, and the tube should drain stomach contents, including bile. The Salem sump tube will not affect the drainage on his dressing (No. 1) or his bowel sounds (No. 4). Trevor may complain of a sore throat from this tube, but it should not affect his ability to swallow saliva (No. 3).

66. (4) Children who have had an appendectomy are expected to make a complete, rapid recovery; they should have *minimal,* not moderate or severe, pain during the first 24 hours (No. 1). Discharge is expected with 5 days, not within 48 hours or after a *slow* recovery (Nos. 2 and 3).

67. (3) As a young adolescent, Trevor will most likely prefer the companionship of another boy close to his age. Although he may be interested in girls (No. 4), being introduced to them would not necessarily prove helpful for Trevor. Children, even 14-year-olds, cannot be relied on to place materials into hospital charts (No. 1). Because Trevor's recovery is expected to be quite rapid and complete, he will miss little school, and there is no need to get him involved with in-hospital tutoring (No. 2); he can easily catch up with his school work when he gets home.

68. (1) To prevent aspiration, the first and immediate action the nurse should take is to turn Amber's head to the side. All of the other actions (Nos. 2, 3, and 4) may also prevent aspiration but will take considerably longer and are not effective immediately.

69. (4) The nurse should know that second-degree burns cause severe pain. The nurse should also know that, during the first 48–72 hours following a serious burn, there is a very poor peripheral circulation due to hypovolemia; therefore, medications should be given via the IV route. PO (No. 2) and IM (No. 3) medications are generally contraindicated during this time. To do nothing (No. 1) would be inappropriate, given the nature and extent of Amber's injuries.

70. (1) In positioning Amber during her recovery, the nurse should avoid those positions where contractures and flexion deformities may occur. With burns on Amber's neck, the nurse should keep Amber's neck extended and help her avoid flexing her neck (No. 4). Keeping Amber still (No. 2) will predispose her to complications of immobility. There is no reason Amber cannot sit in a chair (with help as needed) during her recovery (No. 3).

71. (1) The best topical cleansing material to use in debriding burns are sterile 4x4 gauze pads. Cotton balls (No. 2) may pull and stick to burned tissue. Washcloths (No. 3) are too harsh and may damage new healing tissue. Telfa pads (No. 4) are too smooth and will not cleanse the area as well as gauze pads.

72. (4) To help Amber cope with body image changes associated with her burns, the nurse should work with Amber's parents to help Amber with her physical appearance. Colorful scarves and hats will cover her hairless scalp and pressure stocking, making her look more like other school-age children. It may also boost her morale. Stuffed animals (No. 1) may harbor bacteria and be a possible source of infection. Amber's friends (No. 2) will probably not be allowed to visit in the hospital, especially in the burn unit, which is a frightening place for most children. They can call her or send cards and pictures instead; they can visit her when she returns home. Favorite foods (No. 3) won't specifically help Amber cope with her injuries and treatment; thus, this is not a good choice.

73. (2) Sigmoidoscopy involves the insertion of a rigid instrument into the anus that allows direct visualization of the anal canal, rectum, and sigmoid colon. The client is usually prepared for this procedure with enemas or rectal suppositories. No. 1 is an example of a lower GI. No. 3 describes a colonoscopy, and No. 4 describes two of the procedures that can be accomplished with a colonoscope.

74. (2) Neomycin sulfate is used preoperatively because it is poorly absorbed in the intestinal tract and acts to decrease the bacteria count in the colon. As the result of this action, postoperative infection is reduced (No. 1). Neomycin does not reduce tumor size (No. 3) or directly affect peristalsis (No. 4).

75. (3) A double-barrel colostomy has two stomas that may or may not be separated by skin. The proximal loop discharges feces, and the distal loop discharges mucus. The closure of this temporary colostomy usually occurs in approximately 6 months. No. 1 is an example of an ascending colostomy, No. 2 describes a transverse loop colostomy, and No. 4 describes a descending colostomy.

76. (2) The stomas will begin to secrete mucus within 48 hours, and the proximal loop should begin to drain fecal material within 72 hours. Ileostomies (No. 1) begin to drain immediately. Nos. 3 and 4 are incorrect because peristalsis generally returns within 48–72 hours postoperatively.

77. (2) Appliance should be changed every 2–3 days or as soon as there is leakage. Drainage can excoriate the skin; therefore a new appliance needs to be applied as soon as leakage appears. No. 1 is wrong because every day is too often; there will be damage to the skin from pulling the appliance off so often. No. 3 is wrong because one week is too long for the skin to go without being examined and cleansed. No. 4 is incorrect; the visiting nurse does not determine when the appliance should be changed.

78. (3) Putting a pinhole in the appliance is the least effective method because it allows flatus to escape immediately and the client has no control. No. 1 is incorrect because foods that cause increased flatus, such as cabbage and brussel sprouts, *should* be avoided. No. 2 is incorrect because any deodorant that is safe for mucous membranes *can* be utilized; or the client can purchase appliances that have an odor barrier. No. 4 is incorrect because emptying the appliance *does* protect the seal since extra weight from a full pouch will pull at a seal; once the seal is broken, odor can escape.

79. (1) The basic pathophysiologic changes associated with chronic bronchitis are hypertrophy of the mucous glands lining the bronchi and the production of increased amounts of mucus (sometimes thick and difficult to expectorate) that tend to narrow the airway and trap air distal to the mucus. Bronchoconstriction and edema of the bronchial walls (No. 2) is characteristic of asthma. Exudate in the alveoli (No. 3) and increasing lung stiffness (No. 4) are consistent with pneumonia.

80. (1) A wheeze is a high-pitched, musical chest sound produced by airflow in narrowed bronchioles. It is primarily an expiratory sound and is always, not rarely (No. 2), considered pathologic. Rhonchi are medium-pitched sonorous sounds (No. 3) produced by airflow obstruction in larger airways. Stridor is a high-pitched crowing sound (No. 4) on inspiration and is due to an upper-airway obstruction, such as edema, adhesions, or tracheal hypertrophy.

81. (2) To read blood gases, first note the pH. In this case, pH is 7.38, which is within the normal range (7.35–7.45) but is on the acidotic side. Next you need to look at the Pco_2 and HCO_3^- to see which one is causing the shift to acidosis. In this case the Pco_2 is 55 (acidosis) and the HCO_3^- is 32 (alkalosis). Therefore, Mr. Garcia has compensated respiratory acidosis because his kidneys have been able to conserve enough bicarbonate to keep pH within normal range. In this case a pH below 7.35 would indicate uncompensated respiratory acidosis (No. 1). If Mr. Garcia had uncompensated metabolic alkalosis (No. 3), then pH would be above 7.45. If he had compensated metabolic alkalosis (No. 4), pH would be between 7.41 and 7.45.

82. (4) Indications of respiratory distress and the increased work of breathing in this client are characterized by the use of the accessory muscles of respiration, the sternocleidomastoid and trapezius muscles. Using these muscles enables the client to increase the size of his thorax, thus allowing air to move in. Clients with chronic bronchitis and air-trapping generally are not able to increase the depth of breathing (No. 1) by increasing diaphragmatic excursion (No. 2). Some clients may be using pursed-lip exhalations (No. 3), but these help maintain open airways for the expulsion of gases.

83. (1) The observed total lung capacity (TLC), functional residual capacity (FRC), and residual volume (RV) are all increased over expected values. These values indicate that Mr. Garcia is hyperinflated, a common phenomenon with air obstruction and air-trapping. Hyperventilation is characterized by an increase in Po_2 and pH (No. 2). Hyperpnea is simply an increase in respiratory rate (No. 3). Hypercapnia is identified when Pco_2 is elevated (No. 4).

84. (2) Increased lung volumes (TLC, FRC, RV) and decreased airflow—vital capacity (VC) and forced expiratory volume in 1 second (FEV_1)—are functional problems consistent with obstructive lung disease. In restrictive lung disease (No. 1), volumes generally are decreased. Vascular lung disease (No. 3) has no effect on ventilatory capacity but directly affects diffusion of gases; that is, pulmonary infarction decreases blood flow to the lungs, so some alveoli that are ventilated are no longer perfused. Restrictive lung disease is incorrect in No. 4.

85. (1) Treatment with bronchodilators such as isoproterenol will decrease bronchoconstriction, improving the movement of air in and out of the lungs. Nos. 2, 3, and 4 are incorrect because these pulmonary function studies indicate that Mr. Garcia has been able to increase his inspiratory capacity by 1000 mL (VC 2800–3800) and his expiratory capacity (RV decreased, FRC decreased, and FEV_1 increased).

86. (3) Deep breathing, coughing, and pursed-lip exhalations are all techniques that the nurse can teach the client to improve ventilation. Adequate fluid intake (No. 1) is essential for keeping sputum liquified; however, very hot and very cold drinks should be avoided since they may cause bronchospasm. Clients with COPD also need to be taught to avoid exposure to infections, early signs of infection, and the need to seek medical intervention promptly should symptoms occur. Nos. 2 and 4 are not indicated in this client's therapy.

87. (3) The position that allows for the greatest amount of lung expansion is sitting up and leaning slightly forward. This position can be facilitated by allowing the client to rest his arms on a bedside table. The position that also facilitates lung expansion, but not to the same degree, is high Fowler's (No. 1). Both the prone position (No. 2) and the Trendelenburg position (No. 4) tend to decrease full lung expansion due to increased pressure of abdominal contents on the diaphragm.

88. (2) Although it is not possible to make a client stop smoking, the client should be presented with information about methods used by other people who were successful in stopping. Although most people are aware of the deleterious effects of smoking, clients need to be reminded of the relationship between smoking and their present condition. Fluid intake and nutrition need to be discussed and adapted to individual needs. Clients should be able to identify drugs, giving the name, correct dosage, timing, and potential side effects. Alcohol in moderation is not restricted (No. 1). Vocational rehabilitation should be present as an option but not emphasized (No. 3). Activities should be encouraged to tolerance (No. 4).

89. (2) Position the conscious client sitting upright in a supported, forward-leaning position (high Fowler's, orthopneic) to improve ventilation and oxygenation. A calm and reassuring approach will decrease hyperactivity of the client and oxygen need. Acute respiratory failure is a medical emergency. Aminophylline (No. 1) is indicated to combat bronchospasm, but it is not an independent nursing action. Low-flow oxygen (2 L) is also administered to the client in respiratory failure; however, nasal cannulas (No. 3) do not provide predictable O_2 concentrations. A Venturi mask would be more appropriate. No. 4 is incorrect because the higher concentration of O_2 (60%) may lead to respiratory depression unless the client is maintained on controlled mechanical ventilation.

90. (2) Indications of mediastinal shift and tension pneumothorax include cyanosis, severe dyspnea, and deviation of the trachea and larynx from the normal midline position toward the side of the chest *opposite* the pneumothorax (the unaffected side). Because no blood is available for cardiac output, the blood pressure is absent, not elevated (No. 1). No. 3 is incorrect because the lung has collapsed on the affected side, resulting in tympany on percussion, reduced or absent breath sounds, and hyperresonance. With a right tension pneumothorax, the heart will shift laterally from the normal midclavicular line. If the *left* lung were involved, the heart would shift medially (No. 4).

91. (2) Fever and increased pulse rates occur in rheumatoid arthritis due to the systemic inflammatory process of this dysfunction. If the fever is high or prolonged, increased fluid losses could occur due to insensible water loss (No. 1); however, the effects on body temperature would be secondary to the primary inflammatory response. Though the stress response (No. 3) does increase pulse rate, normally it does not significantly affect body temperature. No. 4 is incorrect because salicylates have an antipyretic effect.

92. (1) The primary purpose of passive range-of-motion exercises is to prevent contractures and decreased range of motion. Secondarily, passive range-of-motion exercises assist the nurse in evaluating functional abilities (No. 2), pain tolerance (No. 3), and the effectiveness of drug therapy (No. 4).

93. (2) In rheumatoid arthritis both the erythrocyte sedimentation rate and C-reactive protein levels are increased. Anemia is common, so hemoglobin and hematocrit are usually decreased, not increased (No. 1). The Wasserman (No. 3) is normally negative. The platelet count (No. 4) is not affected either.

94. (1) A hot tub bath or shower in the morning helps many clients limber up and reduces the symptoms of early morning stiffness. Cold and ice packs are used to a lesser degree, though some clients state that cold decreases localized pain, particularly during acute attacks. Passive ROM exercises (No. 2) may be helpful, but this is not the response of choice. Sleeping with a hot pad (No. 3) may cause localized injury. Some clients, however, have found electric blankets helpful in reducing early morning stiffness. Taking salicylates on an empty stomach (No. 4) may increase gastric irritation and distress.

95. (2) In preparing the client for discharge on prednisone therapy, you should caution him or her to: (a) take oral preparations after meals; (b) remember that routine checks of vital signs, weight, and lab studies are critical; (c) never stop or change the amount of medication without medical advice; and (d) store the medication in a light-resistant container. No. 1 is incorrect because prednisone, as well as other medications given in rheumatoid arthritis therapy, is irritating to the GI tract and should be taken after meals. No. 3 is incorrect because, although fluid, electrolyte, and serum-glucose levels need frequent evaluation during prednisone therapy, CBCs need regular checking if the client is on phenylbutazone (Butazolidin), oxyphenbutazone (Tandearil), or ibuprofen (Motrin) therapy. No. 4 is a precaution given to clients on hydroxychloroquine SO_4 (Plaquenil) or chloroquine (Aralen) therapy.

96. (2) Clients should not be encouraged to do exercises to the point of unusual pain, and pain should not last longer than one-half hour after exercise. If pain lasts longer than this, the exercises are too strenuous. No. 1 is incorrect because pulse and respiratory rates are affected not only by physical stress but by emotional or psychologic stress as well. Nos. 3 and 4 indicate that therapy has been effective.

97. (3) Stapedectomy is the surgical procedure for the treatment of otosclerosis. Its success cannot be determined in the immediate postoperative period. The client must be told that hearing is affected for a while after surgery because of edema. Tinnitus (No. 1) is a postoperative complication that must be reported, but is not expected. The resolution of postoperative edema (No. 2) does not result in rhinitis. Once the ear has healed, normal activities are permitted, including showering and swimming (No. 4). With an upper respiratory infection, deep-sea diving and flying are usually restricted.

98. (1) The client is placed in a semi-Fowler's position to promote the flow of drainage to the pelvic region, where a localized abscess can be drained or be resolved by the body's normal defenses. The elevated position also keeps the infection from spreading upward in the peritoneal cavity. Nos. 2, 3, and 4 are incorrect because none of them elevates the trunk of the body.

99. (3) An iridectomy is performed in the upper segment of the iris and is covered by the upper eyelid, as normally. The excision in the iris is occluded, which decreases discomfort. Infection is less likely since bacteria are carried in the tears, by gravity, to the lower cul-de-sac. The need for a dressing is usually indicated, to decrease infection or eye movement. Since infection is not likely and mobilization of the eye (No. 1) is desirable in order to prevent posterior synechiae (adhesion of iris to cornea or lens), no dressing is needed. Nos. 2 and 4 are appropriate actions. Massage of the eye, if ordered, encourages continuous flow of fluids through the surgical opening.

100. (4) Thyroglobulin (Proloid) is a purified extract of pig thyroid and is utilized in the treatment of hypothyroidism. Nos. 1, 2, and 3 are current methods for treating Graves' disease, or hyperthyroidism.

Prep Test

WHAT IS THE PREP TEST?

The **Prep Test** is a computer-scored and analyzed multiple-choice exam designed to assess your baseline nursing knowledge and evaluate your ability to apply that knowledge to various clinical situations and to items presented in a simulated NCLEX-RN exam. Individual analysis of your scores will be provided to help you prioritize what to study by identifying your individual problem areas.

Written to reflect the content framework and the purpose of the NCLEX-RN Test Plan, ". . . to measure a candidate's ability to practice safely and effectively as a Registered Nurse in an entry-level position," the **Prep Test** can be used as preparation and review for the licensure examination. It can also be used for review by *nurses returning to active practice* as well as by *graduates of foreign nursing schools* who are preparing for qualifying examinations.

Each question on the **Prep Test** was field tested in a pilot test given to NCLEX-RN candidates in order to develop national norms. The norm sample represented examinees who are geographically distributed as well as from various types of nursing programs. When you send in your answer sheet for scoring, your individual performance will be compared with the performance of other candidates in the norm sample.

SELECTION OF CONTENT AND DISTRIBUTION OF THE QUESTIONS

The **Prep Test** is comprised of 200 content-integrated, multiple-choice questions, with 4 options. *One* of the answers is most complete and therefore the best choice. The other 3 answers (distractors) are not always wrong but are usually not as complete or as important as the best answer.

Using a nursing process framework, the questions on the **Prep Test** reflect nursing situations that involve different clinical areas and diagnoses. As on the NCLEX-RN, the number of questions for each content area varies. The percentage distribution of items in this test related to client needs follows the NCLEX-RN blueprint (see Appendix I).

Based on the blueprint for the *Test Plan for The National Council Licensure Examination* (NCLEX-RN) published by the National Council of State Boards of Nursing, Inc., the **Prep Test** assesses your knowledge, skills, and abilities in the 5 phases of the *nursing process:* Assessment (AS), Analysis (AN), Plan (PL), Implementation (IMP), Evaluation (EV), and 4 areas of *client needs:* Safe, Effective Care Environment (SECE), Physiologic Integrity (PhI), Psychosocial Integrity (PsI), and Health Promotion and Maintenance (HPM). Each question in the **Prep Test** has also been classified according to the categories of human functions listed in Appendix B.

INSTRUCTIONS FOR TAKING THE PREP TEST

Have on hand the following items:

1. Test questions beginning on p. 605.
2. Answer sheet (included inside the envelope inside the front cover of this textbook).
3. Several sharpened #2 (soft, black lead) pencils with clean eraser tips. *Do not use* ballpoint pens or colored pencils.
4. Preaddressed envelope (inside the front cover) to return answer sheet.

Addison-Wesley's Nursing Examination Review Prep Test

Page No. 1

Performance Profile for: SMITH MARY J
Social Security No: 123456789
Date of Birth: 05/14/58
Test Date/Number: 05/22/90-10000001
Report Date: 10/11/90

PERFORMANCE SUMMARY

Category	# of Questions You Answered Correctly		Percentile Ranking
I. NURSING PROCESS:			
Assessment (AS)	18 of 19	(95%)	72
Analysis (AN)	14 of 26	(54%)	99
Planning (PL)	21 of 32	(66%)	72
Implementation (IMP)	62 of 89	(70%)	67
Evaluation (EV)	21 of 34	(62%)	39
Total	136 of 200	(68%)	
II. CLIENT NEEDS:			
Safe, Effective Care Environment (SECE)	36 of 54	(67%)	39
Physiological Integrity (PhI)	63 of 89	(71%)	90
Psychosocial Integrity (PsI)	18 of 27	(67%)	44
Health Promotion and Maintenance (HPM)	19 of 30	(63%)	34
Total	136 of 200	(68%)	
III. HUMAN FUNCTIONS:			
Protective (1)	19 of 33	(58%)	44
Sensory-Perceptual (2)	7 of 10	(70%)	49
Comfort, Rest, Activity and Mobility (3)	6 of 14	(43%)	6
Nutrition (4)	8 of 10	(80%)	58
Growth and Development (5)	18 of 24	(75%)	67
Fluid-Gas Transport (6)	54 of 75	(72%)	90
Psycho-Social-Cultural (7)	21 of 30	(70%)	63
Elimination (8)	3 of 4	(75%)	34
Total	136 of 200	(68%)	
OVERALL PERFORMANCE	136 of 200	(68%)	85

PERFORMANCE PROFILE

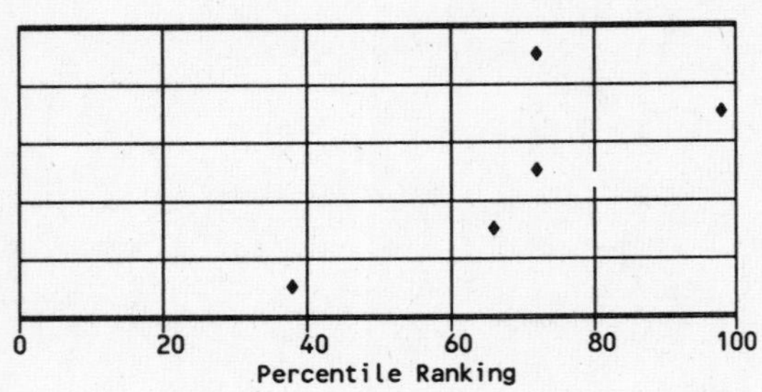

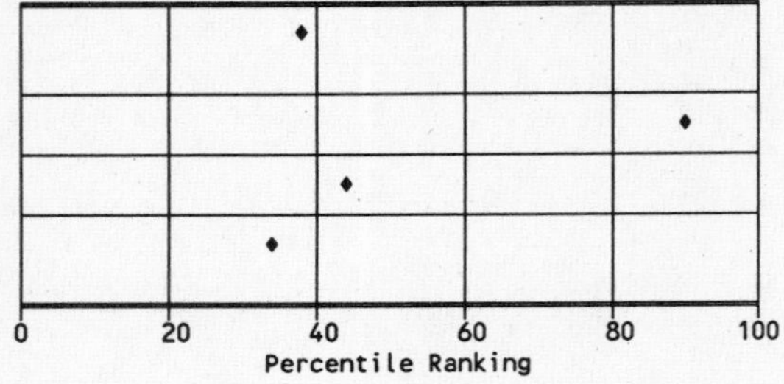

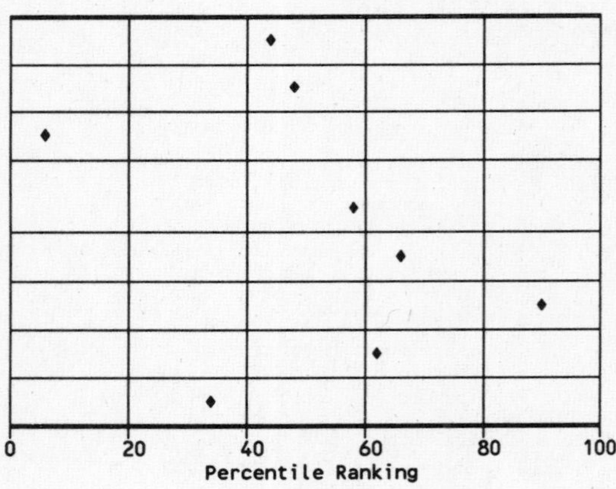

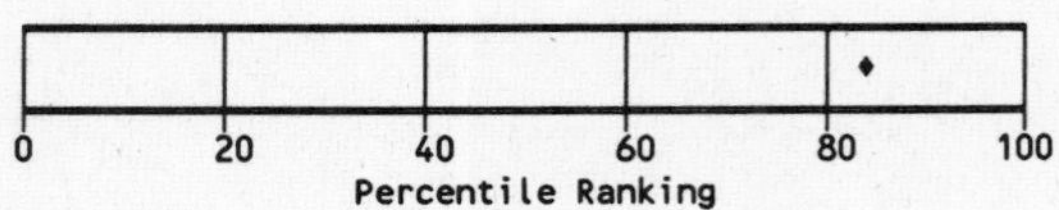

Continued...

■ Sample Prep Test Computer-Scored Performance Profile. (Courtesy of ACT Data Services, ©1990.)

Addison-Wesley's Nursing Examination Review Prep Test

Page No. 2

Performance Profile for: SMITH MARY J
Social Security No: 123456789
Date of Birth: 05/14/58
Test Date/Number: 05/22/90-10000001
Report Date: 10/11/90

RESPONSE ANALYSIS FOR INCORRECT ANSWERS

Ques #	Correct Answer	Your Answ	Rationale For Correct Answer	Reason Your Answer Is Incorrect
1	2	1	Category Codes: AS, PhI, 6 Hypertension is considerably more severe in men than women and tends to occur more frequently at an earlier age.	No. 1 is incorrect because currently it is estimated that 20-25 million Americans (about 10% of the population) have hypertension. This is due largely to the slow onset and lack of specific symptoms in its early stages.
4	3	2	Category Codes: EV, HPM, 6 Both systolic and diastolic pressures should decrease as the result of the pharmacologic interventions.	No. 2 is incorrect because vasodilation and decreases in fluid volume decrease peripheral resistance, thereby lowering the diastolic pressure. A concomitant drop in systolic pressure occurs because the left ventricle is delivering its stroke volume at considerably less resistance.
11	1	3	Category Codes: IMP, PhI, 6 An early indication of cardiac decompensation is tachycardia. Therefore, Mr. Smith's vital signs, mentation, and pulmonary status should be assessed to rule out this complication of myocardial infarction. Other causes of tachycardia are hypovolemia, anxiety and pain. Assessment of pain and emotional status can be determined during cognitive assessment.	No. 3 is incorrect because actions such as administering oxygen will be determined by your assessment of vital signs.
14	2	4	Category Codes: IMP, PhI, 6 While summoning the physician, you should ensure that the client's head is elevated. A sitting position bent slightly forward is best (a bedside table with pillows can be used for the client to rest on), as it allows for the greatest lung expansion and gravity aids in shifting fluids toward the bases of the lungs. Lowering the legs tends to decrease venous return by pooling blood in the periphery.	No. 4 is incorrect because supplemental O2 may be given while awaiting medical orders, but initial nursing actions should be directed toward decreasing venous return and improving ventilation.
19	2	1	Category Codes: AS, HPM, 5 The date of Lauren's last period is the most relevant question to ask in performing the initial assessment, because it will assist the nurse in making a preliminary determination of possible pregnancy.	No. 1 is incorrect because, whether Lauren is presently taking oral contraceptives may be relevant, but it would be more pertinent to assess what general type of birth control the couple may be using and if they have been using it effectively.
22	3	2	Category Codes: AS, HPM, 5 This is a common indicator of pregnancy. Eighty percent experience breast tingling sensation during the first few weeks of gestation.	No. 2 is incorrect because not all women have amenorrhea, especially during the first trimester.
32	4	1	Category Codes: IMP, PsI, 7 An effective assessment of the couple's needs is obtained through discussing the couple's own perceptions of those needs.	No. 1 is incorrect because, although referral to social services may be an appropriate action once a thorough assessment is complete, it should never precede discussion with the couple.
34	4	2	Category Codes: IMP, HPM, 5 In this case the nurse's calm, assured manner would be most therapeutic. It would serve to decrease the couple's anxiety and to facilitate an effective admission and delivery.	No. 2 is incorrect because although Lauren is in active labor, she is not ready to deliver at this time.
39	2	1	Category Codes: IMP, HPM, 5 All physicians and/or institutions have their own guidelines. However, 3 weeks is generally appropriate if the lochia has decreased and becomes fairly clear in color, and if there are not other problems.	No. 1 is incorrect because six weeks is longer than is usually necessary.

■ Sample Prep Test Computer-Scored Performance Profile. (Courtesy of ACT Data Services, ©1990.)

5. Note paper on which to make calculations (in the actual NCLEX-RN exam, space will be provided in the exam booklet).

Timing

Allow about one minute per question. Time yourself and plan to complete the 200-question test in no more than 3½ hours. Simulate test-taking conditions as closely as possible by having uninterrupted time of 3½ hours, or divide the exam into 2 sessions of 100 questions for 1 hour and 45 minutes each session.

Directions for Taking the Test

1. Answer *all* the questions by completely darkening the correct circle. Avoid stray marks. Erase completely if you change an answer.
2. First, answer the ones you think are correct.
3. Then, go back and guess on the remaining questions. There is no penalty for guessing. Because the NCLEX-RN is based on the number of items you answered correctly, the **Prep Test** will also determine your raw score (number correct) by subtracting the number of questions missed from the *total* number of questions (200).
4. Since the computer printout will track and give you feedback only on the questions you answered *incorrectly,* you may want to track *all* of your responses by marking your answers directly on the following book pages as well as on the special answer sheet bound inside the back cover.

Completing the Answer Sheet

1. Fill in your personal data section. Print clearly where indicated. Do *not* make dots ⦿, crosses ⊗, or lines ⊖; only fill in single circles ●. Be sure to answer all the exam questions and supply the information requested. This information will be used for statistical purposes and will not affect your scores.
2. Start the test by marking the answer sheet, selecting the *one* best answer from the 4 choices given for each question. This differs from NCLEX-RN, where you will mark directly in the exam booklet and return the entire booklet for scoring. We want you to keep the questions in this book to allow further review and study.

Returning the Answer Sheet for Scoring

1. Complete the **Prep Test**, answering all 200 questions and the information requested on the answer sheet.
2. Mail in the answer sheet and a certified check or postal money order for $25 (U.S. currency only), payable to ACT Data Services, Inc., using the preaddressed envelope. Your answer sheet will not be processed if the correct fee is not enclosed.
3. Remember to *print* your name and return address and add sufficient postage on the envelope, to avoid delays in processing your results.
4. An individualized computer evaluation of your performance will be returned to you about 2 weeks after your answer sheet is received.

HOW TO INTERPRET YOUR PREP TEST RESULTS

Approximately two weeks after you mail in your answer sheet, you will receive a computerized analysis of your performance. The *Performance Profile* will provide analysis of your results in each of the 3 categories measured by the **Prep Test** (nursing process, client needs, and human functions) as well as a ranking of your overall performance. The analysis will include 3 parts: *Overall Performance, Performance Summary and Profile*, and *Response Analysis for Incorrect Answers*.

Interpreting Your Overall Performance

Refer to the bottom of page 1 of the Performance Profile on page 602, to the box labeled *Overall Performance*. To get a general idea of how you scored in comparison to the normative group, first note the number and percentage of the 200 questions that you answered correctly. Next, note your percentile ranking. If you scored higher than 50% of the normative group (the percentile ranking), your score is higher than the average score. (Note: The average score for all students taking the **Prep Test** may be higher than the passing score for NCLEX-RN.)

Interpreting the Performance Summary and Profile

The *Performance Summary* gives you a detailed breakdown of your results according to the categories tested by each question. It also shows how you compared with the normative group in each category. Your response to each question is evaluated in 3 categories:

1. *Nursing process*—measures your problem-solving ability in terms of assessment, analysis, planning, implementation, or evaluation.
2. *Client needs*—measures your ability to apply knowledge in the areas of safe, effective care, physiological integrity, psychosocial integrity, and health promotion and maintenance (see Appendix H for definitions of these terms).
3. *Human functions*—measures your ability to apply knowledge to more specific situations related to client needs (see Appendix B for a list of categories and definitions).

Look at the number and percentage of questions you answered correctly. For example, under Nursing Process, Assessment, the sample profile states that there were 19 assessment questions on the **Prep Test** and that Mary Smith correctly answered 18 of them, or 95% of the total number of assessment questions.

Compare your percentage answered correctly in all the various categories. For example, in the sample summary, Mary Smith scored *highest* in assessment (95%), knowledge of nutrition (80%), related to physiological integrity (71%). Mary Smith scored *lowest* in ability to analyze (44%), knowledge of comfort and mobility conditions (43%), related to health promotion and maintenance (63%).

The *Percentile Ranking* column shows what percent of the normative group scored lower than you did in each category. For example, on the sample summary, Mary Smith scored *higher* than 72% of the normative group and *lower* than 28% of the group in assessment questions. Note your percentile ranking in each category to compare your results with the normative group.

The *Performance Profile* is a *graphic* summary of your results (percentile ranking in each category) so that you may easily see how you compare with the normative group in your individual areas of strength and weakness. Check for patterns; where do the scores cluster? If your scores cluster around the 60th percentile or higher, you are relatively strong in these areas. You need to concentrate further on areas where your performance is below the 60th percentile.

Interpreting the Response Analysis

This part of the computerized evaluation is especially valuable in providing you with in-depth analysis of your problem areas. It lists all the questions that you answered *incorrectly*, provides the *correct* answer with the reason *why* it was correct, and gives your answer and the reason why it was *not correct*. Codes are also included for each question that you missed, describing the type of ability and knowledge tested by that question.

SUGGESTIONS FOR FURTHER STUDY

Your results in the category of *nursing process* will provide you with an assessment of how you process information (your ability to assess or analyze a situation). For further practice in answering test questions in identified areas of weakness (scores lower than 60th percentile ranking) in nursing process, refer to Appendix J, Index to Nursing Process Questions, for specific practice questions that are examples of a particular step of the nursing process. These practice questions are found at the end of each content unit in this book.

Your results in the categories of *client needs* and *human functions* will give you an evaluation of your knowledge of subject matter. For additional review of specific problem content areas, refer to Appendix C (Index to Categories of Human Functions) and Appendix I (Detailed NCLEX-RN Test Plan: Knowledge, Skills, and Abilities) for specific page references of particular subject matter to study in this book to improve your scores in these problem areas.

With the *Prep Test Performance Profile*, you will now have an individualized evaluation with which to develop your plan for *what* you need to study and *where* to find the material for further study. Our good wishes for your success!

■ QUESTIONS

Mr. Smith, a 50-year-old Caucasian man, complained of increasing shortness of breath on exertion. Physical exam revealed a moderately overweight (20 lb) male, fine basilar crackles in both lung fields, PMI (point of maximal impulse) shifted to the left and down by 1.5 cm, heart rate regular, BP 152/105, heart rate 81, respirations 16.

1. Which of the following statements by the nurse would correctly characterize essential hypertension?
- ○ 1. Forty percent of the American adult population is affected by hypertension.
- ○ 2. Essential hypertension is more severe in men than women.
- ○ 3. American blacks develop hypertension at an earlier age than Caucasians but have a lower mortality rate.
- ○ 4. Given newer screening devices, most hypertensive persons are now being detected.

2. The best explanation the nurse could offer Mr. Smith is that his increasing shortness of breath with exercise is most likely related to:
- ○ 1. Inadequate functioning of the left ventricle.
- ○ 2. Insufficient blood return to the right side of the heart.
- ○ 3. Asynergistic pumping of the left ventricle.
- ○ 4. Obesity and sedentary life-style.

Initial medical therapy for Mr. Smith included:
- *Hydrochlorothiazide (HydroDiuril) 50 mg bid.*
- *Reserpine (Serpasil) 0.25 mg daily*
- *1500-cal reducing diet*

3. Mr. Smith is to be discharged on the antihypertensive drug reserpine. Your instructions to avoid intermittent hypotension would include:
- ○ 1. "Rise slowly from sitting or lying."
- ○ 2. "Ingest alcohol to prevent hypotension."
- ○ 3. "Avoid cold weather, which precipitates attacks."
- ○ 4. "Exercise to decrease sudden vasodilation."

4. If Mr. Smith's therapy is effective, you would expect:
- ○ 1. A greater decrease in systolic than diastolic pressure.
- ○ 2. A greater decrease in diastolic than systolic pressure.
- ○ 3. An approximately equal decrease in both systolic and diastolic pressures.
- ○ 4. Little change in blood pressure initially, but pulse will slow.

Three months later, Mr. Smith is admitted to CCU with an anterior MI. He had been experiencing occasional substernal chest pains lasting approximately 15 minutes that were relieved by rest. Mr. Smith explained he believed that the pains were related to indigestion since they generally occurred after a heavy meal.

5. The nurse knows that angina pectoris, which occurs after eating, may be due to:
- ○ 1. Incomplete digestion of fats due to a decrease in pancreatic enzyme, thereby increasing reflux.
- ○ 2. Local blood flow regulators that shunt blood to gut during digestion, thereby decreasing coronary artery perfusion pressures.
- ○ 3. Abdominal distention from air-swallowing during eating, thereby decreasing diaphragmatic excursion and arterial Po_2.
- ○ 4. Decreased heart rate and blood pressure resulting in increased myocardial oxygen consumption.

The nursing notes on admission gave the following assessment date: BP 124/84, apical pulse 100 and regular, respirations 24, skin cool, pale, and slightly diaphoretic. Blood gases: Po_2 *85,* Pco_2 *37, pH 7.35,* HCO_3 *19.*

6. Given that Mr. Smith's normal BP is 144/96 and his average pulse is 80, you conclude that his present vital signs are related to:
- ○ 1. Increased vagal stimulation of SA node.
- ○ 2. Arrhythmias.
- ○ 3. Cardiogenic shock.
- ○ 4. Sympathetic nervous system response.

7. Your analysis of Mr. Smith's blood gases indicate:
- ○ 1. Compensated metabolic acidosis.
- ○ 2. Hyperventilation.
- ○ 3. Uncompensated metabolic acidosis.
- ○ 4. Alveolar hypoventilation.

8. Morphine sulfate 0.6 mg has been ordered to relieve Mr. Smith's chest pain. You would give this narcotic to:
- ○ 1. Increase the threshold for pain tolerance and decrease arterial resistance.
- ○ 2. Increase arterial resistance and reduce apprehension and anxiety as well as pain.
- ○ 3. Relieve apprehension, anxiety, and pain and stimulate medullary respiratory centers.
- ○ 4. Reduce venous capacitance and reduce pain threshold.

9. Three hours after admission to the CCU, Mr. Smith develops increasing ventricular ectopy, followed by a short burst of ventricular tachycardia. Your first nursing action is to:
- ○ 1. Notify the attending physician.
- ○ 2. Increase the flow of O_2 from 4 L to 8 L.
- ○ 3. Administer a bolus of lidocaine, per order.
- ○ 4. Repeat the morphine sulfate, per order.

10. An assessment finding that would be an early indicator of the extent of tissue necrosis in Mr. Smith's heart is:
- ○ 1. The duration of sinus tachycardia.
- ○ 2. CPK and ALT[SGOT] enzyme measures.
- ○ 3. The duration of his chest pain.
- ○ 4. The occurrence of primary ventricular fibrillation.

On the third day of hospitalization, Mr. Smith becomes increasingly restless. Pulse rate has increased to 126 beats per minute.

11. Your first nursing action is to:
- ○ 1. Do a partial physical assessment, which includes vital signs, pulmonary auscultation, and cognitive functions.
- ○ 2. Ask Mr. Smith if he is upset, since depression is common on the third day of hospitalization.
- ○ 3. Readminister oxygen per nasal catheter (prongs or tongs) at 6 L as restlessness is an early sign of cerebral hypoxia.
- ○ 4. Decrease the rate of Mr. Smith's intravenous infusion to prevent fluid volume overload.

12. Increased restlessness with tachycardia can be expected because:
- ○ 1. Decreased ventricular filling time results in decreased venous return and cerebral edema.
- ○ 2. Palpitations result in anxiety.
- ○ 3. Decreased ventricular filling time always results in decreased cardiac output and tissue perfusion.
- ○ 4. A significant decrease in stroke volume may occur, causing a decrease in cardiac output.

13. Your assessment of the client in pulmonary edema would reveal:
- ○ 1. Rapid respiration, frequent cough, flushed face.
- ○ 2. Persistent cough, rapid respiration, hemoptysis.
- ○ 3. Dyspnea, hacking cough, purulent sputum.
- ○ 4. Air hunger, orthopnea, elevated temperature.

14. Mr. Smith states that he can hardly get his breath. His vital signs are BP 100/70, apical pulse 126, respirations 26. Pulmonary rales and rhonchi are heard halfway up his chest. Your first nursing action is to:
- ○ 1. Administer morphine sulfate to allay Mr. Smith's apprehension.
- ○ 2. Assist Mr. Smith to a sitting position and lower his legs.
- ○ 3. Remove excess pulmonary secretions with suction.
- ○ 4. Administer oxygen at 10 L, per mask instead of nasal catheter.

15. Given his diagnosis, you know that Mr. Smith's dyspnea is the result of:
- ○ 1. Increased lung compliance due to mechanical congestion.
- ○ 2. Decreased CO_2 retention.
- ○ 3. Decreased venous return.
- ○ 4. Fluid shift from systemic circulation to lungs.

16. In order to monitor Mr. Smith's fluid volumes more closely, a CVP line has been inserted via the right subclavian vein. CVP assesses the pressure in:
- ○ 1. The left atrium.
- ○ 2. The right atrium.
- ○ 3. The left ventricle.
- ○ 4. The right ventricle.

17. You would interpret Mr. Smith's CVP as normal if the pressure were between:
- ○ 1. 4–10 cm H_2O.
- ○ 2. 20–30 mm Hg.
- ○ 3. 10–20 cm H_2O.
- ○ 4. 7–14 mm Hg.

18. While you are changing Mr. Smith's CVP dressing, the client becomes tachypneic and complains of chest pain. You suspect the symptoms are related to an air embolism. Your first priority would be to position the client:
- ○ 1. In Trendelenburg.
- ○ 2. On the left side, head down.
- ○ 3. On the right side, head up.
- ○ 4. Supine, in high Fowler's.

Lauren is a 28-year-old female who suspects that she is 3 months pregnant. She has scheduled an appointment next week to see her physician. Lauren is married and works full time as an administrative assistant for the bus company. Lauren's pregnancy was unexpected and unplanned, and the couple has not yet decided whether they really want to have any children at all.

Lauren is the eldest of three children; her two younger siblings both have Down syndrome. Her parents are both alive and healthy. Justin, her husband, is an only child. His father died of a myocardial infarction at age 35, when Justin was 15. His mother was recently diagnosed as extremely hypertensive, with a blood pressure of 180/90–100. Lauren appears to have adequate understanding of healthy nutrition but does admit to infrequent alcoholic beverages and occasional smoking.

19. In assessing Lauren's reasons for suspecting she may be 3 months pregnant, the most relevant question for the nurse to ask would be:
- ○ 1. "Are you currently taking oral contraceptives?"
- ○ 2. "When was your last menstrual period?"
- ○ 3. "How much weight have you gained?"
- ○ 4. "Have you ever been pregnant before?"

20. If the first day of Lauren's LMP was July 10, what is her EDD?
- ○ 1. April 17.
- ○ 2. May 30.
- ○ 3. March 14.
- ○ 4. June 1.

21. If this is Lauren's second pregnancy but the first did not reach viability, what would be her parity?
○ 1. 1001.
○ 2. 0010.
○ 3. 0100.
○ 4. 0101.

22. Given that Lauren is 3 months pregnant, what symptoms would the nurse's assessment most likely discover?
○ 1. Quickening.
○ 2. Amenorrhea.
○ 3. Positive HCG test.
○ 4. Nausea and vomiting.

23. In providing health teaching for Lauren and Justin, which of the following should the nurse tell them is a *probable* sign of pregnancy?
○ 1. Fetal heart sounds.
○ 2. Positive pregnancy test.
○ 3. Fetal movements felt by examiner.
○ 4. Outline of fetal skeleton on sonogram.

Lauren has expressed anxiety over the fact that her brother and sister have Down syndrome, and she asks the nurse what this involves. In her health teaching, the nurse discusses Down syndrome with Lauren.

24. To evaluate Lauren's understanding of the discussion, the nurse would ask her to explain Down syndrome in her own words. Which of the following responses indicates a need for further health teaching?
○ 1. "Down syndrome is an abnormality that can result from an extra chromosome."
○ 2. "Only children born to older women have Down syndrome."
○ 3. "A test can be done to diagnose Down while the fetus is still in utero."
○ 4. "Down syndrome is a form of mental retardation."

25. An amniocentesis is ordered for Lauren. Which of the following actions is *least* likely to be within the role and legal responsibilities of the nurse who is assisting with the amniocentesis?
○ 1. Informing Lauren about the risks involved in amniocentesis.
○ 2. Explaining/reinforcing how the procedure will be done.
○ 3. Monitoring the fetal heart rate.
○ 4. Observing Lauren for signs of bleeding or contractions after the procedure is completed.

Lauren is discharged, and her pregnancy continues to progress.

26. Lauren is concerned about her weight gain of 15 pounds in week 29 of pregnancy. The nurse assessing Lauren should identify that Lauren is primarily concerned about:
○ 1. The baby's nutrition status.
○ 2. Her own body image.
○ 3. Her need to diet.
○ 4. Her need to gain more weight.

27. Because Lauren remains essentially healthy, the nurse's health teaching about safeguards to maintain throughout pregnancy should advise Lauren to:
○ 1. Stop working by week 32 of gestation.
○ 2. Avoid intercourse.
○ 3. Avoid alcohol and smoking.
○ 4. Eat a minimum of three full meals each day.

Lauren and Justin ask the nurse about the possibility of participating in natural childbirth classes.

28. In teaching the couple about natural childbirth, the nurst should *first:*
○ 1. Evaluate the couple's knowledge base of childbirth techniques.
○ 2. Assess the couple's level of readiness to learn.
○ 3. Consult a childbirth nurse practitioner regarding what to tell the couple.
○ 4. Refer the couple to a Lamaze childbirth class.

During Lauren's thirty-second week of pregnancy, she is diagnosed with mild PIH. She is admitted to the hospital.

29. In planning Lauren's care during this hospitalization, which of the following nursing orders is *least* likely to be implemented?
○ 1. Vital signs and FHTs q4h while awake.
○ 2. Daily weight.
○ 3. Deep tendon reflexes once per shift.
○ 4. Absolute bedrest.

30. At 36 weeks, Lauren's status changes: hyperreflexia, generalized edema, and ataxia. If she begins to have a convulsion, the nurse's *primary* action should be:
○ 1. Maintain patent airway.
○ 2. Observe for bowel or bladder evacuation.
○ 3. Administer cardiac pulmonary resuscitation.
○ 4. Maintain a safe environment.

31. Lauren verbalizes concern about the possibility of having to remain hospitalized for the next 8 weeks because of her preeclampsia. The *most* therapeutic response the nurse could make would be:
○ 1. "It may not be that bad if you keep busy."
○ 2. "Tell me how you are feeling."
○ 3. "I'll sit with you a while."
○ 4. "Maybe you should tell your doctor how you are feeling."

32. Lauren and Justin express anxiety about having limited insurance coverage. The *most* appropriate nursing intervention would be to:
○ 1. Refer the couple to social services for possible assistance.
○ 2. Initiate a family-counseling referral.
○ 3. Provide supportive counseling.
○ 4. Assess the couple's needs through discussion.

33. Lauren and Justin are concerned about what effect preeclampsia may have on the fetus. Which of the following indicators of fetal well-being should the nurse teach Lauren and Justin to expect most commonly during the rest of the prenatal period?
○ 1. Nonstress test.
○ 2. Amniocentesis.
○ 3. Urinary estriols.
○ 4. Fetal blood gases.

In week 38 of Lauren's pregnancy, active labor starts (i.e., contractions are every 10 minutes). Her membranes ruptured approximately 45 minutes ago.

34. The nurse's primary intervention would be to:
○ 1. Teach the couple about the stages of labor.
○ 2. Prepare Lauren for delivery.
○ 3. Assess the couple's level of preparation.
○ 4. Reassure the couple and answer any questions.

35. Lauren is in the transitional phase of the first stage of labor. During this time the nurse would expect Lauren to be:

○ 1. Irritable.
○ 2. Excited.
○ 3. Euphoric.
○ 4. Serious.

36. Immediately before Lauren goes into the delivery room, Justin expresses anxiety about going in with her. The *most* appropriate response the nurse could make would be:
○ 1. "Many people feel frightened at this time."
○ 2. "You'll do fine, don't worry."
○ 3. "Think of Lauren. How will she feel if you don't go in?"
○ 4. "Once you get in there, you'll forget about being afraid."

37. After Lauren delivers, the infant's condition is assessed. His respirations do not establish readily, he is slightly cyanotic, and there is some muscle flaccidity. The most appropriate nursing action would be to:
○ 1. Initiate CPR immediately.
○ 2. Clear airway and administer oxygen.
○ 3. Reassure the parents.
○ 4. Check Lauren's chart for her last medication (drug, time, and amount).

38. Lauren has decided to breastfeed. The nurse has discussed important aspects of breastfeeding with her. To evaluate the effects of her teaching, she asks Lauren to put it in her own words. Which of the following responses indicates a need for further teaching?
○ 1. "Rest and relaxation are essential."
○ 2. "An adequate diet is important."
○ 3. "Large breasts produce more milk."
○ 4. "Birth control is necessary throughout breastfeeding if I don't want to become pregnant."

39. Lauren and Justin express concern about when they can resume intercourse. After validating the information with Lauren's physician, the nurse would inform the couple that:
○ 1. Generally it's a good idea to wait until after the sixth-week postpartum check-up.
○ 2. If there are no unforeseen problems, 3 weeks is usually the recommended waiting time.
○ 3. The couple may have sex as soon as they arrive home from the hospital, as long as Lauren feels up to it.
○ 4. The couple should wait until Lauren ceases to breastfeed.

40. Ten days after delivery, Justin comes in with Lauren and their new son because he is concerned about Lauren's mood. He states that she is tearful and apathetic and doesn't eat much. What would be the nurse's most appropriate response?
○ 1. "Many women experience some degree of depression after the birth of a baby."
○ 2. "I will suggest a psychiatric referral to assist Lauren in coping with this crisis."
○ 3. "I will notify the physician of your concern and ask the physician to prescribe an antidepressant for Lauren."
○ 4. "You need to be patient since these symptoms will dissipate."

41. After the baby is 6 months old, Justin and Lauren bring him in for a physical examination. As all his immunizations are up to date, what should he receive at this visit?
○ 1. DTP and TOPV.
○ 2. TOPV.
○ 3. DTP.
○ 4. MMR.

42. At the 6-month physical exam for the baby, Lauren mentions that she has been experiencing a heavy vaginal discharge and severe itching for the past 3 days. She is diagnosed as having *Trichomonas vaginalis*. Health teaching for Lauren should include dosage, administration, and signs and symptoms of side effects of which of the following medications as treatment for this condition?
○ 1. Tetracycline.
○ 2. Erythromycin.
○ 3. Nystatin.
○ 4. Metronidazole.

43. Justin is diagnosed as being mildly hypertensive. In assessing Justin's BP, the nurse most likely finds that his resting diastolic pressure is:
○ 1. Between 110 and 120 mm Hg.
○ 2. Between 90 and 100 mm Hg.
○ 3. Between 120 and 140 mm Hg.
○ 4. Between 100 and 115 mm Hg.

44. Justin is eventually hospitalized with a BP of 170/100, difficulty breathing, dizziness, and weakness. The nurse establishing his care should consider which one of the following?
○ 1. Ensuring that a different nurse takes care of Justin each day to prevent hospital fatigue.
○ 2. Planning care to allow for periods of activity.
○ 3. Identifying any misconceptions Justin may have regarding hypertension.
○ 4. Instructing the client to report only major symptoms to the physician.

45. In planning discharge care for Justin after his treatment for hypertension, the nurse should consider which one of the following?
○ 1. Medication scheduling and side effects.
○ 2. Need to change jobs.
○ 3. Importance of smoking less.
○ 4. Sexual activity restrictions.

Laura, a three-year-old black female, was playing in the family garage when she found a glass container and drank the liquid. She immediately began to scream in pain, vomiting the liquid and some gastric juices. She was brought by ambulance to the emergency room. The nurse identified that Laura had swallowed approximately 1 oz of liquid lye, which caused inflammatory first- and second-degree burns over the entire oral cavity and outer and inner lips and possible burning of the pharynx, esophagus, and larynx.

46. Since Laura has experienced severe burning of the oral cavity and possibly of the esophagus, pharynx, and larynx, the primary nursing intervention should be:
○ 1. Observe for symptoms of shock.
○ 2. Check airway for signs of obstruction.
○ 3. Maintain adequate hydration by offering Laura small amounts of clear liquid.
○ 4. Initiate intravenous therapy immediately.

47. Laura is scheduled to undergo dilation of the pharynx the first morning following her admission to the hospital. When teaching Laura about the procedure, the nurse should realize that the *most* important factor influencing Laura's ability to learn is her:
○ 1. Chronological age.
○ 2. Developmental level.
○ 3. Present state of anxiety.
○ 4. Previous experience with illness and hospitalization.

48. In preparing Laura's preop injections, which size needle would the nurse be most correct in selecting to administer her IM?

○ 1. 25 G, ⅝ in.
○ 2. 21 G, 1 in.
○ 3. 18 G, 1 in.
○ 4. 18 G, 1½ in.

49. The best approach for Laura's nurse to take in administering Laura's preop injection would be to:
○ 1. Ask Laura's mother to explain the injection to her.
○ 2. Simply give the injection as quickly as possible without telling Laura anything, as it may scare her.
○ 3. Give Laura a short and simple explanation immediately before giving the injection.
○ 4. Tell Laura you have to give her the injection and then her father can read her a story.

50. After being dilated, Laura begins to hemorrhage internally, and she is returned to surgery. When she comes back to the floor, whole blood is ordered for her. The nurse planning to administer the blood should know that, after removing it from the refrigerator, the blood should be transfused within:
○ 1. Six hours.
○ 2. Two hours.
○ 3. Four hours.
○ 4. One hour.

51. While observing Laura throughout the blood transfusion, the nurse should be alert to which of the following as possible signs of a transfusion reaction?
○ 1. Hypothermia.
○ 2. Low back pain.
○ 3. Polyuria.
○ 4. Anemia.

52. Laura has been in the hospital one week. She has failed to talk with anyone, including her family. She sits in the corner of her crib crying and rocking back and forth. The most important nursing intervention at this time should be:
○ 1. Establish a one-to-one relationship with Laura to develop trust.
○ 2. Assign different staff to work with Laura each day to promote socialization.
○ 3. Ignore Laura's behavior because it probably indicates normal regression.
○ 4. Refer Laura to the Pediatric Clinical Nurse Specialist for further evaluation.

Four-year-old Juan Nuncio was screened for lead poisoning in the child health clinic and was found to be toxic. He is admitted to the pediatric unit for chelating therapy.

53. In doing Juan's admission assessment, the nurse should be alert to note which of the following signs and symptoms of chronic lead poisoning?
○ 1. Irritability and seizures.
○ 2. Dehydration and diarrhea.
○ 3. Bradycardia and hypotension.
○ 4. Petechiae and hematuria.

54. Juan is being treated with EDTA. Which system should the nurse monitor carefully for possible toxic effects of EDTA?
○ 1. Neurological.
○ 2. Renal.
○ 3. Cardiovascular.
○ 4. Hematological.

55. To help Juan cope most effectively with repeated painful injections of EDTA, the nurse should:
○ 1. Teach his mother the importance of bringing him his favorite toys.
○ 2. Encourage him to spend most of the day in the play room, engaged in free play.
○ 3. Offer him the opportunity for therapeutic play.
○ 4. Allow him to play with other preschool children as much as he wants.

56. Prior to entering Juan's room, the nurse should wash her hands for a minimum of:
○ 1. 10 seconds.
○ 2. 30 seconds.
○ 3. 45 seconds.
○ 4. 60 seconds.

57. The best cleansing agent for the nurse to use in handwashing is:
○ 1. Soap and water.
○ 2. Isopropyl alcohol.
○ 3. Hexachlorophene (Phisohex).
○ 4. Chlorhexidane gluconate (CHG)(Hibiclens).

58. Juan is diagnosed as having iron deficiency anemia. In addition to teaching Mrs. Nuncio to give Juan his Fer-In-Sol between meals, the nurse should also instruct her to give this medication with:
○ 1. Citrus juice.
○ 2. Milk.
○ 3. Apple juice.
○ 4. Bananas.

Luke Bronson, age 15, is admitted to the hospital with a compound fracture of his left tibia and patella following a minibike accident. Luke's fractures are repaired surgically, and a long leg cast is applied.

59. Postop orders include "IV of D5 1/4 NS at 75 cc/per hour." At 7:00 P.M., a new 1000 cc bag of fluid is hung. If the IV infuses at the prescribed rate, how much fluid should be left in the bag at 7:00 A.M.?
○ 1. 100 cc.
○ 2. 900 cc.
○ 3. Nothing should be left; bag should be empty.
○ 4. Not enough information given to determine this.

60. During his first night in the hospital, Luke complains of severe pain in his left leg. At this time, it would be most appropriate for the nurse to:
○ 1. Obtain more information about the characteristics of Luke's pain.
○ 2. Give Luke a dose of "Demerol 50 mg IM p.r.n. q4–6h" as ordered.
○ 3. Reassure Luke that the pain will diminish in a few days.
○ 4. Distract Luke by turning on the television.

61. Luke's cast is damp. To facilitate the proper drying of Luke's cast, the nurse should include which of these measures in Luke's plan of care?
○ 1. Leave Luke's cast exposed to the air.
○ 2. Encourage Luke to remain in one position.
○ 3. Place Luke on a bedboard.
○ 4. Use only tips of her fingers to handle Luke's cast.

62. Luke is to be taught the three-point gait prior to discharge. Luke should be given which of these instructions by his nurse?
○ 1. "Advance your right crutch, swing the left foot forward, advance the left crutch, and then bring the right foot forward."
○ 2. "Move your right crutch and left foot forward together, and then swing the right foot and left crutch in one movement."

○ 3. "While partially bearing weight on your left leg, advance both crutches and then bring your right leg forward."
○ 4. "Using one movement, advance your right foot and both crutches and then bring your left leg forward."

63. When Luke returns to the clinic 2 weeks later, a foul odor is detected at the lower end of his cast. A window is made in the cast over the infected area and an antibiotic is prescribed. After three days on antibiotic therapy, which of these effects would be most indicative of a therapeutic response?
○ 1. Luke's white blood cell count is 7,900 per mm^3.
○ 2. Luke's temperature is 99.4 °F.
○ 3. Luke has no complaints of pain.
○ 4. Luke says that his appetite is fairly good.

64. Luke is also screened for possible scoliosis during his final clinic visit. The nurse should know that the best position to check Luke for scoliosis is:
○ 1. Standing up straight.
○ 2. Lying flat on his stomach.
○ 3. Standing and bending 90 degrees at the waist.
○ 4. Sitting in a straight-back chair.

Fred Stark, 2 ½ years old, is admitted to the hospital with severe eczema, with lesions on his face, scalp, neck, and arms.

65. Ms. Stark states that the pediatrician told her Fred has numerous allergies, including milk allergies. The nurse should offer Fred which of the following formulas?
○ 1. Lofenalac.
○ 2. Lonalac.
○ 3. Similac with iron.
○ 4. Isomil.

66. The best nursing intervention to prevent Fred from scratching the affected areas would be to apply:
○ 1. Clove-hitch restraints to Fred's hands.
○ 2. Elbow restraints to Fred's arms.
○ 3. Mittens to Fred's hands.
○ 4. Posey jacket to Fred's torso.

67. In discussing what clothes Fred should wear, both in the hospital and at home, the nurse would be most correct in teaching Ms. Stark that Fred should wear only:
○ 1. Cotton.
○ 2. Linen.
○ 3. Natural wool.
○ 4. Polyester blend.

68. The doctor orders Burow's solution soaks for Fred. In order to gain Fred's cooperation with this treatment, the nurse should tell him:
○ 1. "Let's do this real fast and then you can see mommy and daddy."
○ 2. "You don't want to have to stay here forever, do you? Let's make you all better now!"
○ 3. "This medicine will help you get better so you can go home. Will you help me pour some on your arms?"
○ 4. "This is magic medicine that will make all your boo-boos go away. Don't you want to chase away those boo-boos?"

69. In preparation for discharge, Ms. Stark asks the nurse if she can bathe Fred in the bathtub at home. The best response by the nurse would be:
○ 1. "It would probably be a good idea to check with your doctor first."
○ 2. "Perhaps in a week to ten days you can begin tub baths; until then, a sponge bath will be adequate."
○ 3. "No, baths are not generally permitted for children with eczema."
○ 4. "Yes, frequent baths will help dry his lesions."

David, a 16-year-old white Jewish male, attends a private school and was doing exceptionally well until 6 months ago, when he was arrested for drunk driving and his license was temporarily suspended. His parents placed him on house restriction for several months. When David's mother was cleaning his room she found some pills and some things that looked like cigarettes. David accused his mother of being "nosy" and of "invading his privacy," and he stormed out of the house. David's mother received a call from University Hospital's emergency room informing her that her son had just been brought there by the police after he was found on school property running around in the nude with several other students. He appeared to be hallucinating. He was admitted and sent to the adult medical/surgical unit because the adolescent unit was full.

70. The nurse who admits David to the unit should be primarily concerned with:
○ 1. Providing a general orientation to the unit.
○ 2. Maintaining a quiet environment.
○ 3. Taking precautions against seizures.
○ 4. Taking vital signs every 4 hours.

71. Since David is not in touch with reality, the most appropriate nursing intervention would be to:
○ 1. Maintain a safe environment.
○ 2. Establish a trusting relationship.
○ 3. Orient David to time, place, and person.
○ 4. Isolate David from other clients.

72. David tells the nurse that he sees big white ants crawling all over the wall. The most appropriate nursing response would be:
○ 1. "Where are they? I'll kill them for you."
○ 2. "You must be seeing things."
○ 3. Silence.
○ 4. "I don't see any ants; but you seem afraid."

73. David constantly asks the nurse to bring him french fries and a piece of apple pie. The nurse should realize that David is probably:
○ 1. Starving.
○ 2. Hallucinating.
○ 3. Disoriented.
○ 4. Playing a game.

74. The nurse assessing a drug abuser would expect to find which of the following characteristics?
○ 1. A very assertive individual.
○ 2. A very dependent individual.
○ 3. A very mature individual.
○ 4. A very aggressive individual.

75. The nurse would expect to find drug abuse *least* prevalent in:
○ 1. An upper socioeconomic family.
○ 2. An elderly individual.
○ 3. A lower socioeconomic family.
○ 4. An adolescent.

76. David's mother is very upset. She is in the waiting room crying uncontrollably. The most appropriate nursing action would be to:
○ 1. Provide privacy for her.
○ 2. Ask the physician to order Valium for her.
○ 3. Contact her husband.
○ 4. Offer to sit with her.

77. The nurse assessing David's mother would expect her initial reaction to David's illness and hospitalization to be:
- ○ 1. Anger.
- ○ 2. Denial.
- ○ 3. Acceptance.
- ○ 4. Shock.

78. David's mother asks the nurse what caused her son to take drugs. The most therapeutic response would be:
- ○ 1. "David probably wanted to be like his peers."
- ○ 2. "Inappropriate limits were probably set on David's behavior."
- ○ 3. "It involves many factors."
- ○ 4. "David felt isolated and unloved."

79. The most important aspect of David's treatment is:
- ○ 1. Teaching him about the hazards of taking drugs.
- ○ 2. Informing him that using drugs is illegal.
- ○ 3. Encouraging him to want to change his behavior.
- ○ 4. Assisting him to develop alternative coping mechanisms.

80. In planning David's initial care, the nurse should:
- ○ 1. Be very direct with him.
- ○ 2. Allow him to make all the decisions about his care.
- ○ 3. Help him to feel very secure to prevent anxiety.
- ○ 4. Encourage him to begin to depend on others.

David's father returns home the afternoon after David's admission to the hospital. His initial response to his wife is, "I always knew you were too easy on him. You see what giving him his way has done!"

81. In analyzing David's father's response, the nurse should realize that his behavior indicates a nursing diagnosis of defensive coping as evidenced by:
- ○ 1. Guilt.
- ○ 2. Sublimation.
- ○ 3. Projection.
- ○ 4. Displacement.

82. David's mother asks the nurse if she would talk with David's father when he arrives at the hospital. She says that she is afraid of what he might say to David. The most appropriate nursing intervention would be to:
- ○ 1. Inform David's mother that you think she and her husband can work through this problem themselves.
- ○ 2. Refer David's mother to the hospital social worker.
- ○ 3. Agree to talk with David's mother and father together.
- ○ 4. Suggest that father and son works things out.

83. As David's hospitalization continues, the nurse must be able to handle a variety of behavior problems. In implementing care for David, which of the following actions would be the *least* appropriate?
- ○ 1. Allowing David to select some of the food he wants to eat.
- ○ 2. Restricting his activity level.
- ○ 3. Encouraging friends to visit.
- ○ 4. Closely monitoring his behavior.

84. David asks the nurse, "Have you ever used drugs?" The most appropriate nursing response would be:
- ○ 1. "Yes, once I tried grass."
- ○ 2. "Why do you want to know?"
- ○ 3. "How will my answer help you?"
- ○ 4. "No, I don't think so."

85. David's girlfriend comes to visit him in the hospital. The nurse suspects that they may become intimate. What is the most appropriate nursing intervention?
- ○ 1. Don't allow his girlfriend to visit.
- ○ 2. Inform the couple that "necking" is prohibited.
- ○ 3. Provide privacy from staff and other clients.
- ○ 4. Allow visitation with supervision.

86. David's friend John brings him a marijuana cigarette. The nurse finds the cigarette under David's pillow. The most appropriate nursing action would be to:
- ○ 1. Ignore the situation.
- ○ 2. Inform the police.
- ○ 3. Discuss the incident with his parents.
- ○ 4. Confront David.

87. David asks the nurse not to tell anyone that he was smoking a marijuana joint in his room, and he promises that he'll never do it again. The nurse should realize that David is *mostly:*
- ○ 1. Being sincere and wanting to change.
- ○ 2. Seeking attention.
- ○ 3. Being manipulative.
- ○ 4. Trying to avoid punishment.

88. When assessing the client who has been abusing amphetamines, the nurse would expect to see which of the following symptoms?
- ○ 1. Bradycardia.
- ○ 2. Increased irritability.
- ○ 3. Hypotension.
- ○ 4. Constipation.

89. When planning to teach a client about the side effects of amphetamines, the nurse should emphasize that:
- ○ 1. Withdrawal from these drugs usually causes death.
- ○ 2. The body develops a tolerance to these drugs.
- ○ 3. An overdose of these drugs induces sleepiness.
- ○ 4. Physiologic dependence may develop.

90. David has a friend who takes Seconal whenever he feels "too stressed," such as whenever he has an exam or feels too pressured, which happens at least four or five times a week. The nurse should be aware that large doses of Seconal can cause which of the following?
- ○ 1. Tachycardia.
- ○ 2. Hypertension.
- ○ 3. Assaultive behavior.
- ○ 4. Increased respirations.

Later in the evening following the discussion with David's physician, David's father begins experiencing severe abdominal cramping and vomits a moderate amount of blood. His wife immediately drives him to the emergency room.

91. On David's father's arrival at the emergency room, the nurse's *primary* concern should be:
- ○ 1. Observing for signs and symptoms of shock.
- ○ 2. Immediately paging the physician on call.
- ○ 3. Filling out the appropriate assessment tool.
- ○ 4. Immediately administering CPR.

92. During the first 24–48 hours after admission, the most appropriate diet for David's father is likely to be:
- ○ 1. NPO.
- ○ 2. Clear liquids.
- ○ 3. A soft, bland diet.
- ○ 4. Skim or regular milk.

93. The physician suspects that David's father has a peptic ulcer. The nurse should expect the physician to order which of the following diets after the first 48–72 hours?
- ○ 1. Small feedings of bland food.
- ○ 2. Frequent feedings of clear liquids.
- ○ 3. A regular diet given frequently in small amounts.
- ○ 4. NPO.

94. The nurse knows that a person with a peptic ulcer who is on a bland diet may *lack* which of the following essential nutrients?
○ 1. Vitamin C.
○ 2. Carbohydrates.
○ 3. Protein.
○ 4. Vitamin A.

95. The nurse caring for David's father at this time should:
○ 1. Plan care so he can receive at least 8 hours of uninterrupted sleep each night.
○ 2. Monitor his vital signs every 2 hours.
○ 3. Make sure that he takes his food and medications at prescribed intervals.
○ 4. Provide milk for him every 2–3 hours.

Mr. and Mrs. Franco arrive in the emergency room at 4:00 A.M. with their son José, a 3-month-old born at 8-months gestation. Mrs. Franco tells the nurse that she had just finished nursing Carlos, the twin brother, when she noticed José was not moving and not breathing. Mr. Franco grabbed José and shook him to try to make him breathe. José did not respond. He never regained consciousness and was pronounced dead at 5:00 A.M.

96. The nurse needs to know that SIDS usually occurs:
○ 1. Between 2 and 4 months after birth.
○ 2. Within 3 weeks of birth.
○ 3. More than 6 months after birth.
○ 4. Between 6 and 9 months after birth.

97. Sudden infant death occurs *most* frequently when which of the following factors is involved?
○ 1. Low birthweight.
○ 2. Multiple births.
○ 3. Middle-class family.
○ 4. Familial history of the syndrome.

98. Mrs. Franco insists on seeing José before leaving the hospital. The most therapeutic nursing action includes:
○ 1. Arranging for her to see her son.
○ 2. Discussing this with the family's priest.
○ 3. Informing Mr. Franco that seeing José would be detrimental to his wife's health.
○ 4. Telling the Francos that hospital policy forbids her seeing José.

99. Several weeks after the funeral, Mrs. Franco tells the public health nurse that she is experiencing difficulty producing enough breast milk to satisfy Carlos. The most appropriate response for the nurse to make would be:
○ 1. "You probably have a virus and should see a doctor right away."
○ 2. "Carlos is probably reacting to the loss of his brother and not sucking long enough to stimulate an adequate supply."
○ 3. "Milk production may decrease with an increase in stress."
○ 4. "The lactation ducts may be occluded."

100. When teaching Mrs. Franco about a decrease in milk production, the nurse should:
○ 1. Recommend weaning the baby onto formula.
○ 2. Assess Mrs. Franco's feelings about nursing.
○ 3. Refer Mrs. Franco to La Leche League.
○ 4. Suggest supplemental feedings of glucose water.

Henry Miller, 8 weeks old, is diagnosed as being susceptible to extended periods of apnea. The physician suggests placing Henry on an apnea monitor at home.

101. The Millers ask the nurse what the monitor will do. The nurse's most appropriate response would be:
○ 1. "It will stimulate his breathing."
○ 2. "It will monitor his vital signs."
○ 3. "It will sound an alarm if his breathing stops."
○ 4. "It will maintain his respirations."

102. The Millers agree to place Henry on the monitor. When teaching the parents about the monitor, the nurse should stress which of the following?
○ 1. "Always respond to the monitor alarm immediately."
○ 2. "Initiate CPR whenever the alarm sounds."
○ 3. "A responsible adult must remain in the room with the infant at all times."
○ 4. "Call the emergency room during any episodes of apnea."

103. When teaching the Millers to provide CPR for Henry, it is important to stress:
○ 1. Applying systematic pressure to the chest with the heel of the hand.
○ 2. Compressing the chest at a rate of 100–120 compressions per minute.
○ 3. Placing the resuscitator's mouth over the infant's mouth to ensure an adequate seal.
○ 4. Blowing forcefully into the infant's air passages to fully inflate the lungs.

104. The nurse working with a family that is using an apnea monitor should know that the monitor's most problematic side effect is:
○ 1. Sounding the alarm whenever the infant moves around the crib.
○ 2. Overprotectiveness by the parents.
○ 3. Developmental lag in the infant.
○ 4. Unreliability of the monitor.

Ten days after admission of Mr. Smith for a myocardial infarction, his physician decides that he has stabilized sufficiently to be transferred to floor care. Mrs. Smith has stopped by the nurses' station on her way out after visiting hours. She states, "Keep an eye on Mr. Smith, will you? He doesn't seem himself tonight." You decide to check Mr. Smith immediately, and you find him slumped on the siderails of his bed. He does not respond when you shake his shoulder or loudly call his name.

105. In an unmonitored arrest in the hospital, when you are the only person present, your *first* action is to:
○ 1. Call for help and note the time.
○ 2. Clear the airway.
○ 3. Give two sharp thumps to precordium.
○ 4. Administer two quick breaths.

106. Your *second* nursing action is to:
○ 1. Clear the airway.
○ 2. Position the client for possible resuscitation—roll on back, remove pillows.
○ 3. Administer two sharp thumps to precordium.
○ 4. Call for help and note the time.

107. Your next nursing action in the arrest procedure is to:
○ 1. Open airway.
○ 2. Check for breathing by placing your ear within an inch of the client's mouth.
○ 3. Check the carotid pulse for 5–10 seconds.
○ 4. Summon help.

108. Following the above actions, you would next:
○ 1. Bag the client.
○ 2. Deliver two sharp blows to the precordium.

○ 3. Check for breathing and ventilate with ambu-bag if the client is not breathing.
○ 4. Palpate the carotid pulse for 5–10 seconds and, if absent, initiate closed-chest massage.

109. To complete this arrest procedure sequence you would:
○ 1. Monitor vital signs.
○ 2. Palpate the carotid pulse and, if absent, give closed-chest cardiac massage.
○ 3. Increase IV infusion rate to prevent hypovolemia.
○ 4. Continue ventilating until arrest team arrives.

On getting Mr. Smith up to the commode, you observed that he suddenly became dizzy, turning ashen and diaphoretic. On returning Mr. Smith to bed, you note his vital signs are now BP 128/60, HR 42, RR 24. Continuous EKG monitoring reveals a pattern of complete heart block.

110. The nurse knows that Mr. Smith's signs and symptoms are related to:
○ 1. Inability of heart to increase its rate during exertion.
○ 2. Insufficient blood flow to the coronary arteries.
○ 3. Increased stroke volume.
○ 4. Inability of the circulatory reflexes to increase venous return.

111. Mr. Smith's physician orders the insertion of a permanent pacemaker. In preparing a preoperative teaching plan for Mr. Smith, the nurse would initially:
○ 1. Assess Mr. Smith's interest in learning about the procedure and his current understanding.
○ 2. Invite Mrs. Smith to join the preoperative teaching session.
○ 3. Ascertain from the physician the amount of information she or he has given the client.
○ 4. Have the operative permit signed, then institute the teaching plan.

112. Which of the following nursing care procedures is *least* important during the period prior to insertion of the pacemaker?
○ 1. Providing sedation to relieve anxiety and promote relaxation as needed.
○ 2. Instituting arm and leg range-of-motion exercises to prevent postinsertion complications.
○ 3. Establishing an intravenous line and having emergency equipment and medications available.
○ 4. Weighing the client and instituting strict intake and output records.

113. Which of the following medications should the nurse have available during Mr. Smith's preoperative period?
○ 1. Lidocaine xylocaine.
○ 2. Atropine sulfate.
○ 3. Digoxin.
○ 4. Propranolol hydrochloride (Inderal).

114. The nurse knows that Isuprel is also used because of which of the following drug effects?
○ 1. Beta mimetic.
○ 2. Cardiac glycoside.
○ 3. Anticholinergic.
○ 4. Beta blocker.

115. Besides enhancing pacemaker automaticity and facilitating AV conduction during heart block, what other effect of Isuprel would the nurse look for?
○ 1. Increased peripheral vascular resistance.
○ 2. Decreased automaticity of Purkinje fibers.
○ 3. Decreased broncoconstriction.
○ 4. Decreased oral secretion.

116. The physician orders an IV started, for easy administration of medications. The IV rate is to be regulated to keep vein open (KVO). You know that the longest possible time that a single 1000-cc bottle can infuse safely is:
○ 1. 24 hours.
○ 2. 5 hours.
○ 3. 18 hours.
○ 4. 12 hours.

Mr. Smith's demand pacemaker was inserted under fluoroscopy and local anesthesia in the cardiac catheterization laboratory. The pacing catheter was inserted into the right external jugular vein and positioned in the right ventricle. The pulse generator was implanted in the right anterior chest below the clavicle.

117. Which of the following nursing care activities is your *first* priority in the *early* postimplantation period?
○ 1. Restricting activity to prevent pacing catheter displacement.
○ 2. Monitoring the ECG continually, noting rhythm, rate, appearance, and amplitude of pacing spike.
○ 3. Implementing passive range-of-motion exercise to the right arm to prevent "frozen shoulder."
○ 4. Maintaining sterile dressings over the operative site to prevent infection.

118. Which of the following would receive the *least* emphasis in your predischarge education plan?
○ 1. Rationale for pacemaker implantation.
○ 2. Pacemaker function and signs indicating malfunction.
○ 3. Therapeutic program, including medication, diet, activity schedule, and safety precautions.
○ 4. Necessity for periodic follow-up visits to physician.

119. Which of Mr. Smith's hobbies will most likely be restricted following recovery from pacemaker insertion?
○ 1. Swimming.
○ 2. Fashioning lamps from driftwood and metal.
○ 3. Operating ham radio.
○ 4. Playing golf.

120. Mr. Smith and his wife should be able to describe signs of pacemaker malfunction. Which of the following behaviors would indicate that his goal has been met?
○ 1. Counts pulse correctly and identifies need to monitor rate daily.
○ 2. Counts pulse correctly and identifies the significance of drainage or discoloration around the battery insertion site.
○ 3. Counts pulse correctly, states the estimated life of the battery, and understands need of prophylactic replacement.
○ 4. Counts pulse correctly and identifies need to report rate changes and symptoms such as dizziness, palpitations, and hiccoughs.

121. During a predischarge teaching session, Mrs. Smith states, "Don't worry, I'll be sure that he obeys the doctor's orders to the letter." Your best response would be:
○ 1. "Mrs. Smith, I can see that with your help, Mr. Smith should do just fine."
○ 2. "Are you worried?"
○ 3. "I'm not worried. You both have a lot of common sense."
○ 4. "This has been a difficult period for both of you. Can you foresee any problems with these instructions?"

122. Mr. Smith is taking nitroglycerine to control his angina. Client teaching regarding administration of nitroglycerine includes the importance of notifying the physician if repeated doses do not relieve chest pain. Additional information would include:
- ○ 1. Notifying the physician if headaches occur.
- ○ 2. Storing the medication in the refrigerator.
- ○ 3. Taking nitroglycerine prophylactically before exercise.
- ○ 4. Ingesting the tablets with liquid.

123. The nurse knows that following administration of nitroglycerine the client's angina will be relieved because the drug:
- ○ 1. Constricts cardiac chambers in order to reduce workload.
- ○ 2. Stimulates the heart rate to increase blood supply to the myocardium.
- ○ 3. Increases myocardial contractility.
- ○ 4. Decreases workload of the heart through lowering the systemic blood pressure.

124. Mr. Smith is to be discharged on a 2-g sodium diet. You would know that he understands his dietary limitations if he selected which of the following?
- ○ 1. Filet of sole, tossed salad with lemon juice, coffee.
- ○ 2. Chow mein, fried rice, tea.
- ○ 3. Canned tomato soup, unsalted crackers, skim milk.
- ○ 4. Two hot dogs with mustard, macaroni salad, ginger ale.

Juanita Perez, a 33-year-old Spanish-speaking female, arrived in the labor room complaining of severe cramping and excessive bleeding. Juanita is presently 8 months (36 weeks) pregnant with her first child. She is Gravida 1, Para 0.

Juanita received adequate prenatal care as scheduled. She was very conscientious about restricting her intake of salt and alcohol. She had even stopped smoking cigarettes and marijuana after finding out that she was pregnant.

Juanita complained that cramping and bleeding started about a half hour before her arrival at the hospital. The initial assessment showed that she was approximately 4 cm dilated, with intact membranes; contractions were coming about every 4–6 minutes. Her husband, Tyronne, was with her throughout the admission process and appeared to be very anxious and concerned.

125. The nurse considers information regarding smoking cigarettes and marijuana essential because it is well established that these activities may lead to:
- ○ 1. Retarded infants.
- ○ 2. Low-birthweight infants.
- ○ 3. Deformed infants.
- ○ 4. Malnourished infants.

126. Tyronne expresses some concern over Juanita's previous smoking habits. The nurse should inform Tyronne that:
- ○ 1. Although Juanita no longer smokes, she was exposed to cigarette and marijuana smoke, which could affect her pregnancy.
- ○ 2. Juanita is assured of a healthy infant because she stopped smoking as soon as she knew she was pregnant.
- ○ 3. The early labor is probably due to Juanita's smoking marijuana.
- ○ 4. Alcohol is considered much safer than marijuana.

127. The nurse in assessing Juanita should identify that she is in what stage of active labor at this time?
- ○ 1. First.
- ○ 2. Second.
- ○ 3. Third.
- ○ 4. Fourth.

128. In observing women in the latent phase of the first stage, the nurse would expect to see which of the following behaviors?
- ○ 1. Tendency to hyperventilate.
- ○ 2. Euphoria, excitement, and talkativeness.
- ○ 3. Fairly quiet and introverted behavior.
- ○ 4. Irritability and crying.

129. The nurse should recognize that which of the following procedures may be *contraindicated* on Juanita's arrival in the labor room?
- ○ 1. Initiating intravenous therapy.
- ○ 2. Taking her blood pressure.
- ○ 3. Examining her vaginal canal.
- ○ 4. Monitoring FHR.

130. Juanita's membranes are ruptured by the attending physician. The nurse should expect the amniotic fluid to:
- ○ 1. Be clear in color.
- ○ 2. Have a slightly pungent odor.
- ○ 3. Have a thick consistency.
- ○ 4. Turn litmus paper blue.

131. During the first stage of labor, maternal and fetal vital signs need to be closely monitored. The best time to observe maternal vital signs is:
- ○ 1. Immediately before a contraction.
- ○ 2. Between contractions.
- ○ 3. Immediately after a contraction.
- ○ 4. Any time the mother feels totally comfortable.

132. Juanita's physician orders a soapsuds enema. The most appropriate nursing action would be to:
- ○ 1. Administer the enema as soon as possible.
- ○ 2. Recheck the order for the type of enema.
- ○ 3. Refuse to administer the enema because this is a premature labor and membranes have ruptured.
- ○ 4. Ask the physician to check the fetal position prior to giving the enema.

133. When Juanita is in labor, which of the following actions requested by the nurse could cause problems?
- ○ 1. Empty her bladder.
- ○ 2. Lie on her back to facilitate adequate ventilation.
- ○ 3. Not bear down until she enters the second stage.
- ○ 4. Breathe slowly and evenly.

134. If the nurse observes the discharge of green amniotic fluid, she should realize this may indicate:
- ○ 1. Rh or ABO incompatibility.
- ○ 2. Fetal distress occurred approximately 36 hours ago.
- ○ 3. Recent or current hypoxia.
- ○ 4. Abruptio placentae has occurred.

135. Juanita requests a sip of water after being in labor for 2 hours in the hospital. The most appropriate nursing action would be:
- ○ 1. Checking the physician's orders.
- ○ 2. Giving her a small sip of water.
- ○ 3. Offering her ice chips.
- ○ 4. Telling her she cannot have fluids at this time.

After Juanita has been in labor for 4 hours in the hospital, her cervix is assessed to be 5 cm. Her vital signs are T:99-P:100-R:30, BP 132/90, FHR 180 and difficult to auscultate with the monitor and fetal scope. The fetus is now positioned in a transverse position. Juanita and Tyronne are quickly informed of the gravity of the situation.

136. Tyronne tells the nurse that he and Juanita had counted on his being in the delivery room throughout their baby's birth. The most therapeutic response would be to:
- ○ 1. Refer him to the attending physician for permission to attend the birth.
- ○ 2. Assess whether he has attended childbirth education classes.
- ○ 3. Check with the attending physician and relay the response to Tyronne.
- ○ 4. Tell Tyronne to dress and meet you in the delivery room.

137. Juanita and Tyronne are informed that a cesarean delivery will be performed immediately. The couple inquire whether Juanita must be put to sleep. The most appropriate nursing response would be to:
- ○ 1. Refer the couple to the anesthesiologist.
- ○ 2. Ask the attending physician to explain the procedure to the couple.
- ○ 3. Tell the couple that she probably will receive general anesthesia.
- ○ 4. Inform the couple that most women who have a cesarean delivery receive spinal anesthesia.

138. The attending physician and anesthesiologist decide to administer spinal anesthesia. However, the amount of anesthesia used will be as minimal as possible because spinal anesthesia:
- ○ 1. Produces severe fetal depression.
- ○ 2. Causes maternal hypotension.
- ○ 3. Rapidly crosses the placenta.
- ○ 4. Depresses maternal respirations.

139. In assessing Juanita following the administration of the spinal anesthesia, the nurse should realize that if she can wiggle her toes:
- ○ 1. The effect of the spinal anesthesia has dissipated.
- ○ 2. She may still become hypotensive.
- ○ 3. This behavior is essentially meaningless.
- ○ 4. She is prone to hypertension.

140. Tyronne asks the nurse whether he will see any gore or blood during the operation. The most realistic response would be:
- ○ 1. "I'm not sure."
- ○ 2. "It depends on the technique the physician uses."
- ○ 3. "Probably not, because a drape keeps the operation from view by both you and Juanita, if you sit by her head."
- ○ 4. "Yes, blood and tissue will be all over the table."

Mrs. Washington is a 42-year-old housewife admitted for right-breast biopsy and possible modified radical mastectomy. She had delayed seeking medical consultation until 18 days ago. Mrs. Washington answered questions in a rushed, breathless manner. She constantly straightened the bedclothes. Lungs were clear to auscultation. Apical heart sounds were rapid, regular, and accentuated. Vital signs were BP 186/110, pulse 90, respirations 22, temperature 98.4°F.

141. Preoperative teaching for Mrs. Washington included deep breathing and coughing. Which of the following is the *least* desired outcome of the teaching plan? Mrs. Washington:
- ○ 1. States the rationale for repeating these exercises every 1–2 hours postoperatively.
- ○ 2. Demonstrates coughing technique.
- ○ 3. Inhales through both nose and mouth and raises abdomen with each respiration.
- ○ 4. States she recognizes the need to repeat exercises until she is feeling lightheaded.

142. In preparation for surgery, Mrs. Washington's right upper chest, right upper arm, and axilla were cleansed with Betadine and shaved. The nurse explains that the *primary* objective of a skin prep is:
- ○ 1. To clean the skin of excess oils and hair.
- ○ 2. To prevent postoperative infection by sterilizing the skin.
- ○ 3. To prevent postoperative infection by reducing the number of microorganisms on the skin.
- ○ 4. To provide a clear field for the incision.

143. On the morning of surgery, you are assigned to assist Mrs. Washington in the final preparations before going to surgery. Before going to see Mrs. Washington, your first action is to:
- ○ 1. Prepare her preoperative medication.
- ○ 2. Check to be sure the operative permit has been signed.
- ○ 3. Check to see if the preoperative laboratory reports have been placed in the chart.
- ○ 4. Check the diet orders to be sure she has been placed on the NPO list.

144. In assisting Mrs. Washington to prepare herself for surgery, which of the following would you do?
- ○ 1. Remove her wedding band.
- ○ 2. Begin exploring her fears and anxieties about surgery.
- ○ 3. Assist in removing hairpins and nail polish.
- ○ 4. Remind her to void following preoperative medication.

145. The preoperative medications ordered for Mrs. Washington by the anesthesiologist are morphine sulfate 15 mg and atropine SO_4 0.4 mg, subcutaneously. You can expect to give these drugs:
- ○ 1. Right before the client leaves for surgery.
- ○ 2. 45–60 minutes before anesthetic induction.
- ○ 3. 20–30 minutes before anesthetic induction.
- ○ 4. 10–15 minutes before anesthetic induction.

146. While preparing Mrs. Washington's preoperative medication, you note that the atropine SO_4 you have on hand is in a strength of 0.6 mg per mL. The correct amount of atropine to administer is:
- ○ 1. 1.5 milliliters.
- ○ 2. 1 milliliter.
- ○ 3. 10 minims.
- ○ 4. 8 minims.

147. The nurse knows that the desired effects of morphine SO_4 and atropine SO_4 have been achieved when:
- ○ 1. Pain is relieved and anxiety is reduced.
- ○ 2. Secretions are decreased and sensitivity to stimuli reduced.
- ○ 3. Sleep occurs and oral secretions are reduced.
- ○ 4. Sensitivity to pain is reduced and muscular relaxation occurs.

148. The nurse must recognize the side effects of morphine and atropine administration, which include:
- ○ 1. Bradycardia, anorexia, and decreased urine output.
- ○ 2. Hypertension, nausea, vomiting, tachycardia.
- ○ 3. Hypotension, cotton-mouth, nausea, and vomiting.
- ○ 4. Dryness, cotton-mouth, constricted pupils, and bradycardia.

149. Following administration of Mrs. Washington's preoperative medication, it is important to:
- ○ 1. Position her in high Fowler's position to improve ventilation.
- ○ 2. Let her know she will be asleep when she leaves the unit.

○ 3. Tell her that you or another nurse will be there when she returns.
○ 4. Get her up to the bathroom when she complains of bladder fullness.

150. Mrs. Washington's frozen section is positive for carcinoma, and the surgeon performs a modified radical mastectomy. The nurse knows that this procedure involves removal of:
○ 1. The right breast only.
○ 2. The right breast and axillary nodes.
○ 3. The right breast, pectoralis major muscle, and axillary lymph nodes.
○ 4. The right breast, underlying chest muscle, axillary lymph nodes, and internal mammary lymph nodes.

151. On admission to the recovery room, Mrs. Washington is very restless. Her respirations are deep and somewhat irregular; she startles easily and moans when you touch her. The best nursing action is:
○ 1. Continue to stimulate her by telling her the operation is over.
○ 2. Raise the siderails and remain quietly in attendance.
○ 3. Administer meperidine (Demerol) HCl 100 mg IM.
○ 4. Check her nailbeds for cyanosis.

152. Mrs. Washington has an airway in place and is in a supine position. To prevent airway obstruction, the nurse should:
○ 1. Leave the airway in and turn her head to the side.
○ 2. Maintain her present position.
○ 3. Remove the airway and turn her head to the side.
○ 4. Remove the airway and maintain a prone position.

153. You are monitoring Mrs. Washington's vital signs every 15 minutes. Which of the following changes should be reported immediately to the surgeon?
○ 1. Dry, cool skin.
○ 2. A systolic blood pressure that drops 20 mm Hg or more.
○ 3. A diastolic pressure below 70.
○ 4. A pulse rate that increases and decreases with respirations.

154. A unit of blood is ordered for Mrs. Washington when her BP drops to 90/60. Which of the following is the most important safeguard prior to administering blood?
○ 1. Refrigerate unit of blood until immediately before giving.
○ 2. Agitate the blood so it is well mixed.
○ 3. Carefully check labeled blood against client's wrist band.
○ 4. Infuse the blood through a blood warmer.

155. Mrs. Washington has a unit of whole blood transfusing in her left arm. The earliest signs of transfusion reaction are:
○ 1. Headache and elevated temperature.
○ 2. Hypertension and flushing.
○ 3. Urticaria and wheezing.
○ 4. Oliguria and jaundice.

156. Mrs. Washington's incision is covered with a pressure dressing, and she has two drains attached to a Hemovac pump. Which nursing intervention for the client with a Hemovac is *inappropriate?*
○ 1. Observing and recording the amount and color of the drainage.
○ 2. Maintaining suction by emptying and recompressing the apparatus regularly.
○ 3. Increasing suction by attaching the Hemovac to wall suction as the drainage increases.
○ 4. Preventing traction on the drainage tubes by repositioning the Hemovac each time the client is repositioned.

157. The nurse knows that the *primary* advantage of Hemovac wound suction is that it:
○ 1. Exerts high, even suction.
○ 2. Allows easy mobility because it is lightweight.
○ 3. Speeds wound-healing by removing excess fluids.
○ 4. Reduces the occurrence of postoperative infection.

158. The pressure dressing encircles Mrs. Washington's chest and fits very snugly. The nurse should anticipate difficulty in which of the following postoperative nursing functions?
○ 1. Maintaining good body alignment.
○ 2. Initiating arm exercises.
○ 3. Promoting deep breathing and coughing.
○ 4. Taking vital signs.

159. On turning Mrs. Washington to her left side, you note a moderately large amount of serosanguineous drainage on the bedsheets. You should:
○ 1. Remove the dressing to ascertain the origin of the bleeding.
○ 2. Milk the Hemovac tubing, using a downward motion.
○ 3. Note vital signs, reinforce the dressing, and notify the surgeon immediately.
○ 4. Recognize that this is a frequent occurrence with this type of surgery.

160. If Mrs. Washington begins to demonstrate some early signs of shock, such as increased pulse, cool, clammy skin, and restlessness, you could enhance venous return by:
○ 1. Administering oxygen via mask to reduce restlessness.
○ 2. Keeping trunk flat and raising foot of bed.
○ 3. Placing her in Trendelenburg position.
○ 4. Wrapping her entire body in warmed blankets.

161. Which of the following arm positions will best facilitate venous return on the operative side and reduce the occurrence of lymphedema?
○ 1. Semi-Fowler's position with the elbow flexed and the arm across the chest.
○ 2. Low Fowler's position with the arm elevated so that the hand and elbow are slightly higher than the shoulder.
○ 3. High Fowler's position with the elbow flexed and the right hand positioned next to the head.
○ 4. Adduction of the shoulder, extension of the elbow, and flexion of the wrist.

162. Depending on the extent of surgery and the physician's orders, it is possible to initiate arm exercises as early as 24 hours after surgery. Which of the following will the nurse encourage Mrs. Washington to do as appropriate *initial* therapy?
○ 1. Self-feeding and hair-combing.
○ 2. Passive/active flexion and extension of the elbow and pronation and supination of the wrist.
○ 3. Abduction and external rotation of the right shoulder.
○ 4. Early ambulation and active extension and flexion of the elbow.

163. To which of the following postoperative complications is Mrs. Washington predisposed because of the nature of her surgery?
- ○ 1. Peripheral thrombophlebitis.
- ○ 2. Wound dehiscence.
- ○ 3. Atelectasis.
- ○ 4. Paralytic ileus.

164. In your planning for discharge, Mrs. Washington should be informed of actions that may increase lymphedema. Which of the following activities is *most likely* to increase symptoms?
- ○ 1. Wearing gloves for household tasks or gardening.
- ○ 2. Carrying heavy groceries in her right arm.
- ○ 3. Wearing dresses with elasticized sleeves.
- ○ 4. Driving to and from work.

Mrs. Arturri is a 55-year-old lawyer admitted to the hospital with a diagnosis of bacterial pneumonia. On admission she was pale to dusky in color. Her respiratory rate was 32, temperature 103°F, pulse 100. Oxygen per nasal cannula was administered at 7 L/minute.

165. Mrs. Arturri's physician decides to perform a tracheostomy. The purpose of a tracheostomy is to:
- ○ 1. Decrease client anxiety by increasing the size of the airway.
- ○ 2. Provide more controlled ventilation and ease removal of secretions the client is unable to handle.
- ○ 3. Provide increased cerebral oxygenation, thereby preventing further respiratory depression.
- ○ 4. Facilitate nursing care, since tracheal tubes have fewer side effects than nasotracheal tubes.

Following insertion of the tracheostomy tube, Mrs. Arturri appeared less distressed. Oxygen therapy was reinstituted with nebulization. The tracheostomy was to be suctioned every hour and p.r.n.

166. Which of the following nursing actions is essential to prevent hypoxemia during tracheal suctioning?
- ○ 1. Removal of oral and nasal secretions.
- ○ 2. Encouraging the client to deep breathe and cough to facilitate removal of upper-airway secretions.
- ○ 3. Administer 100% oxygen to reduce the effects of airway obstruction during suctioning.
- ○ 4. Auscultate the lungs to determine the baseline data to assess the effectiveness of suctioning.

167. The proper method of suctioning includes:
- ○ 1. Suctioning only while inserting the catheter.
- ○ 2. Suctioning only while withdrawing the catheter.
- ○ 3. Suctioning during both insertion and withdrawal of the catheter.
- ○ 4. Suctioning on insertion only if secretions are copious.

168. If a double-lumen tracheostomy tube is used, the inner cannula should be removed and cleansed with hydrogen peroxide and normal saline:
- ○ 1. Only as necessary.
- ○ 2. Every 2–4 hours.
- ○ 3. Once a day.
- ○ 4. Never—do not remove the inner cannula for any reason.

169. The rationale for using humidified oxygen with tracheal tubes is:
- ○ 1. It is a traditional procedure.
- ○ 2. It is a means of providing fluid intake.
- ○ 3. It decreases insensible water loss.
- ○ 4. The natural humidifying pathway has been bypassed.

170. Crepitus in Mrs. Arturri's neck and upper chest is caused by:
- ○ 1. Air from displaced tracheal tube.
- ○ 2. An inadequately inflated tracheostomy cuff.
- ○ 3. An overinflated tracheostomy cuff.
- ○ 4. Edema from the trauma of surgery.

Zariel Anakutty, a 7-week-old boy, is admitted to the hospital with a diagnosis of pyloric stenosis and a 2-week history of vomiting and weight loss.

171. Zariel's parents ask how their baby might have gotten pyloric stenosis. The nurse should tell them that:
- ○ 1. Zariel was born with this condition.
- ○ 2. Zariel acquired it due to a formula allergy.
- ○ 3. Zariel was normal at birth and it developed spontaneously.
- ○ 4. There is no way to determine this preoperatively.

172. Zariel vomits soon after his feeding. What should the nurse see in the vomitus that is characteristic of infants with pyloric stenosis?
- ○ 1. Stomach contents only.
- ○ 2. Stomach contents plus bile.
- ○ 3. Stomach contents streaked with blood.
- ○ 4. Stomach contents with flecks of feces.

173. Zariel is scheduled for a Fredet-Ramstedt procedure. The nurse administers Zariel's preop medication, atropine (0.15 mg) IM. Fifteen minutes later, his mother tells the nurse that Zariel is breathing rapidly and has a flushed, red face. The nurse should:
- ○ 1. Administer the atropine antidote stat.
- ○ 2. Give Zariel a cool sponge bath.
- ○ 3. Tell the mother these are normal side effects of atropine.
- ○ 4. Page the surgeon and advise him of Zariel's condition prior to transporting him to the operating room.

174. Upon his return from the OR at 11:30 A.M., Zariel has 425 cc left in his IV bag of 5% Dextrose and 1/2 NS. The postop MD orders include "IV to infuse at 320 cc every 8 hours." When should Zariel's nurse anticipate having to change his IV bag?
- ○ 1. 3:00 P.M.
- ○ 2. 6:00 P.M.
- ○ 3. 9:00 P.M.
- ○ 4. 12:00 midnight.

175. Potassium chloride is to be added to Zariel's intravenous fluids. Before adding this electrolyte, the nurse should determine that:
- ○ 1. Zariel is voiding.
- ○ 2. Zariel's Moro reflex is present.
- ○ 3. Zariel's respiratory rate is between 25 and 40.
- ○ 4. Zariel's mucous membranes are moist.

Bart Gordon, 17 months old, is admitted to the hospital with intussusception.

176. In reviewing Bart's admission history, the nurse should know that intussusception most typically presents with which two signs or symptoms?
- ○ 1. Currant-jelly stools and paroxysmal abdominal pain.
- ○ 2. Olive-shaped mass in the right upper quadrant and projectile vomiting.
- ○ 3. Obstinate constipation and increasing abdominal girth.
- ○ 4. Excessive amounts of mucus and abdominal distention.

177. Bart's MD orders an IV of D5W at 40 cc/hour. A 500 cc bag, with a pediatric microdrip chamber, is hung at 11:00 A.M. At 3:15 P.M., the nurse notes that the bag has 100 cc left. After slowing the IV initially, which action would be *most appropriate* for the nurse to take next?
- ○ 1. Readjust the flow rate to 40 microdrops per minute and check it frequently.
- ○ 2. Hang a new 500 cc bag of fluid.
- ○ 3. Maintain the flow rate at 20 microdrops per minute until his IV is back on schedule.
- ○ 4. Notify the physician.

178. Bart is scheduled for a barium enema. The nurse should teach Bart's parents that the major purpose of this procedure is to:
- ○ 1. Confirm the diagnosis.
- ○ 2. Reduce the telescoping.
- ○ 3. Ease the passage of stool.
- ○ 4. Provide symptomatic relief.

Betsy Sullivan, age 18 months, fractured her right femur in a car accident. She is admitted and placed in Bryant's traction.

179. In considering the equipment for Bryant's traction, the nurse should expect to see that Betsy has:
- ○ 1. A Kirschner wire in the fractured femur.
- ○ 2. A Steinman pin in the fractured femur.
- ○ 3. Adhesive material taped to the skin of both legs.
- ○ 4. Adhesive material taped to the skin of the right leg only.

180. At 7:00 A.M., the night nurse hangs a new 500 cc bag of D5 1/2 NS and adjusts the flow rate to 35 cc/hour per MD order. If the IV infuses at the proper rate, how much fluid should be left in the bag when the day nurse makes her rounds at 11:30 A.M., halfway through her shift?
- ○ 1. 160 cc.
- ○ 2. 250 cc.
- ○ 3. 340 cc.
- ○ 4. Unable to determine.

181. The nurse's aide reports that Betsy's buttocks are resting on the mattress. The nurse would be most correct in telling the aide that:
- ○ 1. This is where her buttocks should be.
- ○ 2. Betsy's buttocks should be slightly off the mattress.
- ○ 3. This is the responsibility of the nurse.
- ○ 4. Betsy will need special skin care to avoid pressure areas or breakdown.

Frank Henry, a 65-year-old retired merchant seaman, has been hospitalized for 2 weeks for severe vascular insufficiency and gangrene of the left foot. He has been an insulin-dependent diabetic for 20 years. Frank is scheduled for an above-the-knee amputation in 4 days.

182. The nurse should know that the majority of amputatiaons are attributed to:
- ○ 1. Chemical burns.
- ○ 2. Diabetic ulcers.
- ○ 3. Arteriosclerosis obliterans.
- ○ 4. Bone tumors.

183. Which type of anesthesia should the nurse anticipate being used generally for an amputation?
- ○ 1. IV regional.
- ○ 2. Spinal.
- ○ 3. General intravenous and inhalation anesthesia.
- ○ 4. Muscle relaxant.

184. The best explanation by the nurse for why Mr. Henry is having an above-the-knee (AK) amputation would be:
- ○ 1. The degree of vascular insufficiency is extensive.
- ○ 2. AK amputations are better suited for a prosthesis.
- ○ 3. The higher the amputation, the less energy required for rehabilitation of balance and walking.
- ○ 4. Below-the-knee amputation heals less successfully.

185. Because Mr. Henry is NPO prior to surgery, an appropriate nursing measure on the day of surgery is:
- ○ 1. To withhold the daily insulin dose.
- ○ 2. To administer the daily insulin dose.
- ○ 3. To administer the insulin and request that Frank drink a glass of juice.
- ○ 4. To request specific orders regarding insulin administration.

186. Despite the occurrence of gangrene, Mr. Henry's physician chooses to do a flap amputation in order to avoid the necessity of another surgery. Immediately on returning to the recovery room, Mr. Henry's stump should be:
- ○ 1. Elevated on a pillow to reduce occurrence of edema and hemorrhage.
- ○ 2. Placed in Buck's traction to prevent skin and muscle retraction.
- ○ 3. Firmly bandaged to a padded board to prevent contractures.
- ○ 4. Wrapped in an ace bandage to reduce edema formation.

187. Among the elderly, which of the following is the most common postoperative complication after amputation?
- ○ 1. Hemorrhage and shock.
- ○ 2. Pulmonary embolus.
- ○ 3. Disseminated intravascular clotting.
- ○ 4. Thrombophlebitis.

188. On the first postoperative day, Frank's vital signs are stable, his IV is discontinued, and he is getting solid foods. The surgeon has ordered rehabilitation exercises to begin. Which is most important for the nurse to initiate *first?*
- ○ 1. External rotation of the stump.
- ○ 2. Hyperextension of the thigh and stump.
- ○ 3. Lifting the buttock and stump off the bed while Frank is lying flat on his back.
- ○ 4. Arm exercises to prepare for crutch-walking.

189. While being repositioned onto his abdomen, Frank states that he can't turn because his "left foot is causing him too much pain." The first response by the nurse should be:
- ○ 1. To insist he lie on his abdomen.
- ○ 2. To ignore his comment and state that he or she will return later.
- ○ 3. To discuss the principle of phantom pain postamputation.
- ○ 4. To offer some form of pain control.

190. A nursing measure to help reduce the size of the stump once the surgical wound is healed is:
- ○ 1. Elevation of the stump on a pillow when reclining.
- ○ 2. Pushing the stump against hard surface.
- ○ 3. Wrapping moist, warm soaks on the thigh.
- ○ 4. Applying an elastic bandage.

Mr. David Leonard, age 60, had been cleaning the gutters of his roof when the ladder gave way and he fell to the ground, hitting his head on the driveway. He arrived unconscious at the emergency room by ambulance. A diagnosis of right subdural hematoma was made, and he was scheduled for a craniotomy and evacuation of the hematoma.

191. After Mr. Leonard returns from surgery following the craniotomy, the nurse knows that the optimum positioning of a neurosurgery client, unless otherwise indicated, would be:
- ○ 1. Flat on back.
- ○ 2. Head elevated 30°.
- ○ 3. Head elevated 45°.
- ○ 4. Head elevated 90°.

192. On completion of your nursing assessment, you conclude that the client is showing signs of increased intracranial pressure. Data to support this conclusion would include:
- ○ 1. Decreased blood pressure, tachycardia, tachypnea.
- ○ 2. Increase in level of consciousness.
- ○ 3. Dilation of the pupil on the side opposite the hematoma.
- ○ 4. Bradycardia, increased pulse pressure, and Biot's breathing.

Amy Black, 5 years old, is admitted for cardiac catheterization to evaluate the status of her ventricular septal defect (VSD). Amy also has Down syndrome.

193. Because Amy receives Valium "IV push" × 2 during the procedure, which one vital sign should the nurse evaluate *first*?
- ○ 1. Temperature.
- ○ 2. Pulse.
- ○ 3. Respirations.
- ○ 4. Blood pressure.

194. In the first few hours after Amy's catheterization, which of the following nursing measures would be most essential in caring for Amy?
- ○ 1. Checking Amy's pulse in the extremity used for the cut-down.
- ○ 2. Encouraging Amy to cough and deep breathe hourly.
- ○ 3. Keeping Amy sedated to maintain the pressure dressing.
- ○ 4. Monitoring Amy's urine output.

195. Two hours after Amy returns to the unit, her dressing is soaked with bright red blood. The nurse first reinforces the dressing. What should the nurse do next?
- ○ 1. Check Amy's vital signs.
- ○ 2. Increase the flow rate of Amy's IV.
- ○ 3. Place Amy in reverse Trendelenburg position.
- ○ 4. Notify Amy's cardiologist.

Trevor Roberts, 14 years old, is admitted to the adolescent unit following surgery for a ruptured appendix. Admitting orders include: Salem sump to suction, IV Ringer's Lactate at 110 cc/hour, NPO.

196. When admitting Trevor, the *first* action the nurse should take is to:
- ○ 1. Attach Salem sump tube to suction.
- ○ 2. Calculate the IV flow rate and adjust the drip.
- ○ 3. Take Trevor's blood pressure.
- ○ 4. Check Trevor's ID band.

197. Once Trevor is back in his room, the nurse should place Trevor in a semi-Fowler's position primarily to:
- ○ 1. Fully aerate the lungs.
- ○ 2. Promote drainage and prevent subdiaphragmatic abscesses.
- ○ 3. Splint the wound.
- ○ 4. Facilitate movement and reduce complications from immobility.

198. At 2:30 A.M., the nurse hangs a 1000 cc bottle of IV fluid. If the IV infuses at the proper rate, how much fluid should infuse by 6:00 A.M.?
- ○ 1. 385 cc.
- ○ 2. 500 cc.
- ○ 3. 615 cc.
- ○ 4. 740 cc.

199. At 7:00 A.M., Trevor's IV site appears red and swollen. The nurse should:
- ○ 1. Apply warm soaks.
- ○ 2. Decrease the flow rate.
- ○ 3. Elevate the IV site.
- ○ 4. Remove the IV.

200. After Trevor's appendectomy, the nurses' notes in his chart should include documentation of:
- ○ 1. Teaching to prevent dumping syndrome and to promote early ambulation.
- ○ 2. Frequent mouth care and dressing changes, including drainage.
- ○ 3. Bowel sounds, intake and output, and the need for a low-residue diet.
- ○ 4. Dressing changes, intake and output, and bowel sounds.

A
Directory of State Boards of Nursing

Board of Nursing
770 Washington Ave.
Montgomery, AL 36131

Health Services Regulatory Board
LBJ Tropical Medical Center
Pago Pago, American Samoa 96799

Board of Nursing
Dept of Commerce and Economic Development
Division of Occupational Licensing
3601 C St., Suite 722
Anchorage, AK 99503

State Board of Nursing
1123 S University Avenue
Univ. Tower Bldg.
Suite 800
Little Rock, AR 72204

State Board of Nursing
2001 W. Camelback Road
Suite 350
Phoenix, AZ 85015

Board of Registered Nursing
PO Box 944210
Sacramento, CA 95814-2100

State Board of Nursing
1560 Broadway, Suite 670
Denver, CO 80202

Department of Health Services, Nurse Licensure
150 Washington St
Hartford, CT 06106

Board of Nursing
Margaret O'Neill Bldg
PO Box 1401
Federal & Court Sts
Dover, DE 19901

District of Columbia
Board of Nursing
614 H Street NW
Rm 904
Washington, DC 20013

Board of Nursing
111 E Coastline Drive
Suite 504
Jacksonville, FL 32202

Board of Nursing
166 Pryor St SW
Suite 400
Atlanta, GA 30334

Board of Nurse Examiners
PO Box 2816
Agana, Guam 96910

Board of Nursing
PO Box 3469
Honolulu, HI 99503

State Board of Nursing
280 N. 8th St, Suite 210
Boise, ID 83720

Nursing Coordinator
Dept. of Professional Regulations
320 W Washington St
Springfield, IL 62786

State Board of Nursing
One American Sq Suite 1021
Box 82067
Indianapolis, IN 46282-0001

Board of Nursing
State Office Bldg
1223 E Court Ave
Des Moines, IA 50319

State Board of Nursing
900 SW Jackson St
Suite 551-S
Topeka, KS 66612-1256

Board of Nursing
4010 Dupont Circle
Suite 430
Louisville, KY 40207

State Board of Nursing
907 Pere Marquette Bldg
New Orleans, LA 70112

State Board of Nursing
35 Anthony Ave
State House Station 158
Augusta, ME 04333-2240

Board of Nursing
4201 Patterson Ave
Baltimore, MD 21215-2299

Board of Registration in Nursing
100 Cambridge St
Rm 150
Boston, MA 02202

Board of Nursing
611 W Ottawa
PO Box 30018
Lansing, MI 48909

Board of Nursing
2700 University Ave W
Suite 108
St. Paul, MN 55114

Board of Nursing
239 N. Lamar St, Suite 401
Jackson, MS 39201

Board of Nursing
3523 N Ten Mile Drive
PO Box 656
Jefferson City, MO 65102

State Board of Nursing
Arcade Bldg—Lower Level
111 N Jackson
Helena, MT 59620-0407

Board of Nursing
Dept of Health
Bureau of Examining Boards
PO Box 95007
Lincoln, NE 68509

State Board of Nursing
1281 Terminal Way
Suite 116
Reno, NV 89502

State Board of Nursing
Div of Public Health
6 Hazen Drive
Concord, NH 03301

Board of Nursing
PO Box 45010
Newark, NJ 07101

Board of Nursing
4253 Montgomery NE, Suite 130
Albuquerque, NM 87109

State Board of Nursing
State Education Department
Cultural Education Center
Rm 3013
Albany, NY 12230

Board of Nursing
PO Box 2129
Raleigh, NC 27602

Board of Nursing
Kirkwood Office Tower
919 S 7th St
Suite 504
Bismarck, ND 58504-5881

Board of Nursing
Education & Registration
77 S High St, 17th Floor
Columbus, OH 43266-0316

Board of Nursing
Registration & Nursing Education
2915 N Classen Blvd
Suite 524
Oklahoma City, OK 73106

State Board of Nursing
800 NE Oregon St #25
Portland, OR 97232

State Board of Nursing
PO Box 2649
Harrisburg, PA 17105-2649

Board of Nurse Examiners
Council on Higher Educ. of PR
Rio Piedras, Puerto Rico 00933

Board of Registration in Nursing
3 Capitol Hill
Suite 104
Providence, RI 02908-5097

State Board of Nursing for South Carolina
220 Executive Dr, Suite 220
Columbia, SC 29210

Board of Nursing
3307 South Lincoln
Sioux Falls, SD 57105

Board of Nursing
283 Plus Park Blvd
Nashville, TN 37217

Board of Nurse Examiners
9101 Burnet Rd
Suite 104
Austin, TX 78758

State Board of Nursing
Division of Professional Licensure
160 E 300 South
PO Box 45802
Salt Lake City, UT 84145

Board of Nursing
109 State St
Montpelier, VT 05602

State Board of Nursing
1601 Rolling Hills Drive
Richmond, VA 23229

Board of Nursing Licensure
PO Box 7309
Charlotte Amalie
St. Thomas
Virgin Islands 00801

State Board of Nursing
Division of Professional Licensing
1300 Quince EY-27
Olympia, WA 98504

Board of Examiners for Registered Nurses
Embleton Bldg
Suite 309
922 Quarrier St
Charleston, WV 25301

Board of Nursing
State Bureau of Health Service Prof.
PO Box 8935
Rm 174
Madison, WI 53708-8935

Board of Nursing
Barrett Bldg 3rd Floor
2301 Central Ave
Cheyenne, WY 82002

APPENDIX

B

Categories of Human Functions

Protective Functions

Client's ability to maintain defenses and prevent physical and chemical trauma, injury, infection, and threats to health status. Examples: communicable diseases (including sexually transmitted diseases), immunity, physical trauma and abuse, asepsis, safety hazards, poisoning, skin disorders, and preoperative care and postoperative complications.

Sensory-Perceptual Functions

Client's ability to perceive, interpret, and respond to sensory and cognitive stimuli. Examples: auditory, visual, and verbal impairments, sensory deprivation, sensory overload, aphasia, brain tumors, laryngectomy, organic brain syndrome, body image, reality orientation, learning disabilities, and seizure disorders.

Comfort, Rest, Activity, and Mobility Functions

Client's ability to maintain mobility, desirable level of activity, and adequate sleep, rest, and comfort. Examples: joint impairment, body alignment, pain, sleep disturbances, activities of daily living, neuromuscular impairment, musculoskeletal impairment, and endocrine disorders that affect activity.

Nutrition

Client's ability to maintain the intake and processing of essential nutrients. Examples: normal nutrition, diet in pregnancy and lactation, obesity, conditions such as diabetes, gastric disorders, and metabolic disorders that affect primarily the nutritional status.

Growth and Development

Client's ability to maintain maturational processes throughout the life span. Examples: child-bearing, child-rearing, conditions that interfere with the maturation process, maturational crises, changes in aging, psychosocial development, sterility, and conditions of the reproductive system.

Fluid-Gas Transport Functions

Client's ability to maintain fluid/gas transport. Examples: fluid volume deficit and overload, cardiopulmonary diseases, acid–base balance, cardiopulmonary resuscitation, anemias, hemorrhagic disorders, leukemias, and infectious pulmonary diseases.

Psycho-Social-Cultural Functions

Client's ability to function in intrapersonal, interpersonal, intergroup, and sociocultural relationships. Examples: grieving, death and dying, psychotic and neurotic behaviors, self-concept, therapeutic communication, group dynamics, ethical-legal aspects, community resources, spiritual needs, situational crises, and substance abuse.

Elimination Functions

Client's ability to maintain functions related to relieving the body of waste products. Examples: conditions of the gastrointestinal system, such as vomiting, diarrhea, constipation, ulcers, neoplasms, colostomy, and hernia; conditions of the urinary system, such as kidney stones, transplants, renal failure, and prostatic hypertrophy.

■ APPENDIX

C

Index to Content Related to Categories of Human Functions

APPENDIX

■ APPENDIX

D
Community Resources

AIDS Project Los Angeles, Inc.
7362 Santa Monica Boulevard
West Hollywood, CA 90046
Phone: (213) 876-8951

An organization that provides support groups, information, and referral services for persons with AIDS. Publishes *Living with AIDS: A Self Care Manual.*

Al-Anon Family Group Headquarters
PO Box 862
Midtown Station
New York, NY 10018-0862
Phone: (212) 302-7240

For relatives and friends of alcoholics. Includes Alateen for children of alcoholics. Functions separately from Alcoholics Anonymous.

Alcoholics Anonymous World Services, Inc.
PO Box 459
Grand Central Station
New York, NY 10163
Phone: (212) 686-1100

A self-help organization of people who share experiences with alcoholism and provide support for each other in overcoming alcoholism.

Alzheimer's Disease and Related Disorders Association (ADRDA)
70 E Lake Street
Chicago, IL 60601
Phone: (800) 621-0379; in Illinois (800) 572-6037 or (312) 853-3060

Provides information to the public and to health professionals, advocates and aids research, provides emotional support to family and friends, and makes referrals to other appropriate services.

American Alliance for Health, Physical Education, Recreation, and Dance
1900 Association Drive
Reston, VA 22091
Phone: (703) 476-3400

Provides information about recreation and fitness opportunities for the handicapped.

American Anorexia/Bulimia Association, Inc.
133 Cedar Lane
Teaneck, NJ 07666
Phone: (201) 836-1800

A self-help group that provides information and help as well as referrals to physicians and therapists. On Wednesdays from 10 AM to 2 PM, a recovered person takes calls.

---

* *Source:* Adapted with permission from Wilson HS, Kneisl CR: *Psychiatric Nursing*, 3rd ed., Redwood City, CA: Addison-Wesley, 1988, pp. 1155–61.

American Association of Retired Persons
1909 K Street, NW
Washington, DC 20049
Phone: (202) 872-4700

An association that provides informational material related to retirement and aging, a monthly newsletter, educational seminars, discounts on purchases and health insurance, etc.

Association for Voluntary Surgical Contraception
122 E 42d Street
New York, NY 10168
Phone: (212) 351-2500; for information call (212) 351-2555

Refers clients considering tubal ligation or vasectomy to specialists and treatment centers for consultation. Offers information and sponsors educational programs.

Autism Society of America
1234 Massachusetts Avenue, NW
Suite 1017
Washington, DC 20005
Phone: (202) 783-0125

A self-help organization for professionals, caregivers, and educators as well as for parents of children and adults with autism.

Biofeedback Society of America
10200 W 44th Avenue, Suite 304
Wheat Ridge, CO 80033
Phone: (303) 422-8436

Provides referrals and information on biofeedback.

Children of Alcoholics Foundation
540 Madison Avenue
New York, NY 10022

Provides information and free materials.

Committee on Pain Therapy
American Society of Anesthesiologists
515 Busse Highway
Park Ridge, IL 60068
Phone: (312) 825-5586

Distributes literature and provides information on chronic pain and its treatment.

Concern for Dying
250 W 57th Street, Room 831
New York, NY 10107
Phone: (212) 246-6962

Distributes literature, promotes research on death and dying, and works for the right of dying individuals to refuse extraordinary life-prolonging measures. Formerly called the Euthanasia Educational Council.

Gerontological Society of America
1411 K Street NW, Suite 300
Washington, DC 20005
Phone: (202) 393-1411

Provides information on aging and advocacy for the elderly.

The Hemlock Society
PO Box 66218
Los Angeles, CA 90066
Phone: (213) 391-1871

Promotes tolerance of the right of terminally ill persons to end their lives in a planned manner. Publishes the *Hemlock Quarterly* newsletter, various legal declarations and documents such as a "living will" and a durable power of attorney for health care, and the only guide to self-deliverance ("Let Me Die Before I Wake") for the dying in the United States.

Huntington's Disease Society of America, Inc.
140 W 22d Street, 6th floor
New York, NY 10011
Phone: (800) 345-HDSA (345-4372); in New York (212) 242-1968

Sponsors educational programs, raises funds for research, and maintains a comprehensive listing of specialists.

National Committee for Prevention of Child Abuse
332 S Michigan Avenue
Suite 950
Chicago, IL 60604
Phone: (312) 663-3520

An organization concerned with physically and emotionally abused and neglected children.

National Committee on the Treatment of Intractable Pain
9300 River Road
Potomac, MD 20854
Phone: (202) 944-8140

Promotes education and research on more effective management of intractable pain. Information on the latest methods of pain management and current research can be obtained by contacting their Pain Control Information Clearinghouse. Referrals to other agencies for pain control information or treatment are available upon request.

National Council on the Aging, Inc.
600 Maryland Avenue, SW
West Wing 100
Washington, DC 20024
Phone: (202) 479-1200

Provides information on aging to the public and to the health professionals.

National Council on Alcoholism, Inc.
12 W 21st Street, 7th floor
New York, NY 10010
Phone: (800) NCA-CALL (622-2255); in New York (212) 206-6770

Consists of state and local affiliates. Supports and cooperates with self-help groups. The NCA Publications Office invites questions by telephone or letter.

National Health Information Center
PO Box 1133
Washington, DC 20013-1133
Phone: (800) 336-4797; in Washington, DC area (202) 429-9091

A service of the Office of Disease Prevention and Health Promotion (ODPHP), US Department of Health and Human

Services. Provides health and medical information, lists of other toll-free numbers and referrals to appropriate organizations and researches answers to health questions. Also provides government-produced pamphlets such as "Healthstyle: A Self Test."

National Hospice Organization
1901 N Fort Myer Drive, Suite 307
Arlington, VA 22209
Phone: (703) 243-5900

An organization of hospices and individuals that encourages public and professional education on caring for the terminally ill, monitors legislation affecting the hospice movement, and publishes a quarterly newsletter.

National Institute of Mental Health
Public Inquiries Branch
Room 15C05
5600 Fishers Lane
Rockville, MD 20857
Phone: (301) 443-4517

This division of the federal government provides information on mental health, mental disorders, and programs and resources throughout the country.

National Nurses Society on Addictions (NNSA)
2506 Grosse Pointe Road
Evanston, IL 60201
Phone: (312) 475-7300

Publishes a newsletter four times a year for nurses working in the addiction field. Provides information on treatment and research in addiction, certification for nurses working in the field, and a network for nurses working with chemically dependent clients.

National Self-Help Clearinghouse
Graduate School University Center
City University of New York
33 W 42d Street
New York, NY 10036
(Letters only, please)

Monitors hundreds of self-help organizations throughout the United States and Canada.

Nightingale
77 Warren Street
Brighton, MA 02135
Phone: (617) 783-3522

A back-to-practice 18-bed in-patient recovery program for the licensed health care professional having trouble with alcohol and other chemical dependencies.

Overeaters Anonymous (OA)
PO Box 92870
Los Angeles, CA 90009
Phone: (213) 542-8363

Patterned after the philosophy of Alcoholics Anonymous, this self-help organization views compulsive eating as a disease that can be arrested but not cured. Literature available on request.

Parents Anonymous
7120 Franklin Avenue
Los Angeles, CA 90046
Phone: (800) 421-0353; in California (800) 352-0386

Provides confidential assistance about possible child abuse cases. Offers referrals to local chapters for help or information.

Parents Without Partners, Inc.
8807 Colesville Road
Silver Spring, MD 20910
Phone: (301) 588-9354

A self-help organization concerned with single, widowed, or divorced parents and their children. Provides referrals to local chapters throughout the United States.

Parkinson's Disease Foundation
Columbia University Medical Center
640–650 W 168th Street
New York, NY 10032
Phone: (212) 923-4700

Provides information and referral for people with Parkinson's disease and other diseases of the basal ganglia. Serves as a clearinghouse for clients, families, and health professionals.

Phobia Society of America
133 Rollins Avenue, Suite 4B
Rockville, MD 20852-4004
Phone: (301) 231-9350

Provides information on phobias and referrals to therapists and support groups.

Recovery, Inc.: The Association of Nervous and Former Mental Patients
802 Dearborn Street
Chicago, IL 60610
Phone: (312) 337-5661

A self-help organization for people with mental problems and former mental patients.

Resolve, Inc.
5 Water Street
Arlington, MA 02174
Phone: (617) 643-2424

Assists people who face problems of infertility. Offers counseling, information, and support concerning issues such as treatment and options for becoming parents (e.g., adoption). Branch offices available in many areas.

Sex Information and Education Council of the United States (SIECUS)
New York University
32 Washington Place, Room 52
New York, NY 10003
Phone: (212) 673-3850

Maintains an information clearinghouse on all aspects of human sexuality and will help clients locate information.

Stepfamily Foundation, Inc.
333 West End Avenue
New York, NY 10023
Phone: (212) 877-3244

Offers a newsletter, awareness workshops, telephone counseling, and private and group counseling for step-parents and complex households with children of both spouses.

Toughlove
PO Box 1069
Doylestown, PA 18901
Phone: (215) 348-7090

A parent support group for parents whose children are in trouble.

Women for Sobriety, Inc.
PO Box 618
Quakertown, PA 18951
Phone: (215) 536-8026

A network of over 200 self-help groups for women alcoholics only.

Youth Suicide National Center
1811 Trousdale Dr.
Burlingame, CA 94010
Phone: (415) 877-5604

Provides resource material on youth suicide.

In Canada

Alcoholism and Drug Addiction Research Foundation
33 Russell Street
Toronto, Ontario M5S 2S1
Phone: (416) 595-6000

Canadian Association on Gerontology
Suite 1080
167 Lombard Avenue
Winnipeg, Manitoba R3B OV3
Phone: (204) 944-9158

Canadian Rehabilitation Council for the Disabled (CRCD)
One Yonge Street, Suite 2110
Toronto, Ontario M5E 1E5
Phone: (416) 862-0340
(A chapter is also located in Fredericton, New Brunswick)

Dying With Dignity
175 St. Clair Avenue, West
Toronto, Ontario M4V 1P7
Phone: (416) 921-2329

Chapters are also located in Vancouver, British Columbia, and Ottawa, Ontario. Several others will be forming in the near future.

National Alliance for the Mentally Ill
(Check local telephone book.)

Overeaters Anonymous
Central Ontario Intergroup
175 St. Clair Avenue, West, Suite 25
Toronto, Ontario M4V 1P7
Phone: (416) 929-5361

The Parkinson Foundation of Canada
55 Bloor Street, West, Suite 232
Toronto, Ontario M4W 1A6
Phone: (416) 964-1155

Patients' Rights Association
40 Homewood Avenue, Suite 315
Toronto, Ontario M4Y 2K2
Phone: (416) 923-9629

Hot Lines

AIDS Hot Line
Phone: (800) 342-AIDS [342-2437] [8:30 AM to 5:30 PM EST]

Sponsored by the US Public Health Service and operated by the American Social Health Association. Gives a recorded informational message on AIDS. If the caller stays on the line, someone will be available to answer questions or respond to concerns.

Alcohol Hotline
Phone: (800) ALCOHOL [252-6465]

Operated by the Ad Care Hospital in Worcester, Massachusetts. Provides information on alcohol- and drug-related problems.

Alcoholics Anonymous
Local phone books in the United States and Canada list the number of the closest 24-hour answering service.

Alzheimer's Disease and Related Disorders Association
Phone: (800) 621-0379; in Illinois (800) 572-6037

Counseling for families and friends of those with Alzheimer's disease and related disorders.

National Cocaine Helpline
Phone: (800) COCAINE [262-2463]

A 24-hour nationwide referral and information service for cocaine users, nonuser victims, and health care professionals. Based at Fair Oaks Hospital in Summit, New Jersey.

National Gay Task Force Crisis Line
Phone: (800) 221-7044; in New York (212) 807-6016 [5–10 PM EST]; in San Francisco (800-FOR-AIDS); in Los Angeles (800-922-AIDS)

Provides up-to-date information on AIDS.

National Institute on Drug Abuse—Cocaine Hotline
Phone: (800) 662-HELP [662-4357]

National Runaway Switchboard—Adolescent Suicide Hotline
Phone: (800) 621-4000

Parents Anonymous
Phone: (800) 421-0353; in California (800) 352-0386 [24 hours]

Provides confidential assistance with possible child abuse cases. Offers referrals to local chapters for help or information.

Sleep Helpline
Sleep Disorder Center
Thomas Jefferson University Hospital
Philadelphia, PA
Phone: (215) 928-8019

APPENDIX

E

Communicating With Clients From Other Cultures

If you don't speak the language of your client, try the following:

1. Enlist the aid of a family member or friend of the client. Being able to help will increase the helper's self-esteem. Knowing that a concerned person is directly participating may help the client feel less anxious.
2. Seek out a bilingual staff member in the setting. Larger institutions often have bilingual employees on their staffs. Smaller agencies often employ indigenous staff.
3. Ask another client to translate. Another client can be helpful in translating cultural beliefs as well as language. Being able to help boosts self-esteem.
4. Use other agencies as resources. Health and social services departments, international institutes, college language departments, neighborhood houses, or cultural centers will often know of people who are willing to volunteer as translators.
5. Select the words you use carefully, avoiding buzz words and jargon. Speak clearly, pacing yourself to be neither too fast nor too slow. Words that are slurred, have many syllables in them, or are too technical make communication more difficult. Speaking too fast may overload the client and make it difficult for the client to follow. Speaking too slowly may lose the client's attention.
6. Select the gestures you use with care, using your nonverbal behavior to underscore your words and your actions. The proper use of gestures can clarify a message, and drawings can sometimes be helpful. Be careful, however; not all gestures mean the same thing in all cultures.
7. Listen to your client's words and watch your client's gestures carefully. Do your best to understand and validate the meaning they have for you. Listening carefully to the client will help you avoid focusing on what you will say or do next and will demonstrate your genuine concern for the client's distress.

Source: Reprinted with permission from Wilson HS, Kneisl CR: *Psychiatric Nursing*, 3rd ed., Redwood City, CA: Addison-Wesley, 1988.

F

Family Assessment: Cultural Profile

Communication Style

1. Language and dialect preference (understand concept, meaning of pain, fever, nausea).
2. Nonverbal behaviors (meaning of bowing, touching, speaking softly, smiling).
3. Social customs (acting agreeable or pleasant to avoid the unpleasant, embarrassing).

Orientation

1. Ethnic identity and adherence to traditional habits and values.
2. Acculturation: extent.
3. Value orientations:
   a. *Human nature:* evil, good, both.
   b. *Relationship between humans and nature:* subjugated, harmony, mastery.
   c. *Time:* past, present, future.
   d. *Purpose of life:* being, becoming, doing.
   e. *Relationship to one another:* lineal, collateral, individualistic.

Nutrition

1. Symbolism of food.
2. Preferences, taboos.

Family Relationships

1. Role and position of women, men, aged, boys, girls.
2. Decision-making styles/areas: finances, childrearing, health care.
3. Family: nuclear, extended, or tribal.
4. Matriarchal or patriarchal.
5. Life-style, living arrangements (crowded; urban/rural; ethnic neighborhood or mixed).

Health Beliefs

1. Alternative health care: self-care, folk medicine; cultural healer: herbalist, medicine man, curandero.
2. Health crisis and illness beliefs concerning causation: germ theory, maladaptation, stress, evil spirits, yin/yang imbalance, envy and hate.
3. Response to pain, hospitalization: stoic endurance, loud cries, quiet withdrawal.
4. Disease predisposition:
   a. *Blacks:* sickle cell anemia, CVD/CVA and hypertension; high infant mortality, diabetes.
   b. *Asians:* lactose intolerance, myopia.
   c. *Hispanics:* cardiovascular, diabetes, cancer, obesity, substance abuse, TB, AIDS, suicide, homicide.
   d. *Native Americans:* high infant and maternal mortality, cirrhosis, fetal alcohol abnormalities, pancreatitis, malnutrition, TB, alcoholism.
   e. *Jews:* Tay-Sachs.

Source: Adapted from *Topics in Clinical Nursing,* Vol. 7, No. 3, p. 4, with permission of Aspen Publishers, Inc., © 1985.

5. Disease resistance:
   a. *Jews:* cervical cancer.
   b. *Blacks:* skin cancer.

Education

1. Learning style (prefers printed word or audio-visual tools; learns by trial and error or didactic methods).
2. Informal/formal education.
3. Occupation and socioeconomic level (who works, health insurance).

Religion

1. Preferences.
2. Beliefs, rituals, taboos.

APPENDIX

G

Laboratory Values

Test	Normal Values	Possible Significance: Increases	Possible Significance: Decreases
HEMATOLOGY			
Bleeding time—indication of hemostatic efficiency	1–7 minutes	Hemorrhagic purpura, acute leukemia, aplastic anemia, DIC, oral anticoagulant therapy.	
Hematocrit—volume of packed red blood cells per 100 mL of blood	*Men:* 45% (38–54%) *Women:* 40% (36–47%)	Dehydration, polycythemia.	Anemia, hemorrhage, leukemia.
Hemoglobin-oxygen-combining protein	*Men:* 14–18 g/100 mL *Women:* 12–16 g/100 mL	Same as for Hematocrit.	Same as for Hematocrit.
Partial thromboplastin time—tests coagulation mechanism; stage I deficiencies	*Activated:* 30–46 seconds *Nonactivated:* 40–100 seconds	Deficiency of Factors VIII, IX, X, XI, XII; anticoagulant therapy.	Extensive cancer.
Platelets—thrombocytes	150,000–400,000/mm³	Polycythemia, postsplenectomy, anemia.	Leukemia, aplastic anemia, cirrhosis, multiple myeloma.
Prothrombin time—tests extrinsic clotting; stages II and III	11–15 seconds	Anticoagulant therapy, DIC, hepatic disease, malabsorption.	Digitalis therapy, diuretic reaction, vitamin K therapy.
Red blood cell count—number of circulating erythrocytes in 1 μL of whole blood	*Men:* 4.5–6.2 million/μL *Women:* 4.0–5.5 million/μL	Polycythemia vera, anoxia, dehydration.	Leukemia, hemorrhage, lupus erythematosus.
Sedimentation rate—speed at which red blood cells settle in uncoagulated blood	*Men:* 0–9 mm/hour *Women:* 0–20 mm/hour	Acute bacterial infection, cancer, infectious disease, numerous inflammatory states.	Polycythemia vera, sickle cell anemia.
White blood cell count—number of leukocytes in 1 mL³	4500–11,000/μL	Leukemia, bacterial infection, severe sepsis.	Viral infection, overwhelming bacterial infection, lupus erythematosus.
White blood cell differential—enumeration of individual leukocyte distribution:			
Neutrophils	3000–7500 μL, or 54–75%	Bacterial infection, tumor, inflammation, stress, drug reaction.	Acute viral infection, anorexia nervosa, splenic neutropenia, drug-induced, alcoholic ingestion.
Eosinophils	50–400 μL, or 1–4%	Allergic disorder, parasitic infestation, eosinophilic leukemia.	Acute or chronic stress; excess ACTH, cortisone, or epinephrine; endocrine disorder.
Basophils	25–100 μL, or 0–1%	Myeloproliferative disease.	Anaphylactic reaction, hyperthyroidism, radiation therapy, infections, ovulation, pregnancy, aging.

continued

Test	Normal Values	Possible Significance: Increases	Possible Significance: Decreases
HEMATOLOGY (cont.)			
White blood cell differential (cont.)			
Lymphocytes	1500–4500 μL, or 25–40%	Chronic lymphocytic leukemia, infectious mononucleosis, chronic bacterial infection, viral infection.	Leukemia, systemic lupus erythematosus.
BLOOD CHEMISTRY			
Alkaline phosphatase, total serum	1.4–4.1 U/100 mL (Bodansky method) 4–13 U/100 mL (King-Armstrong method) 20–48 IU/mL	Hyperparathyroidism, Paget's disease, cancer with bone metastasis, obstructive jaundice, cirrhosis, infectious hepatitis, rickets.	Malnutrition, scurvy, celiac disease, chronic nephritis.
Amylase	60–160 U/mL	Acute pancreatitis, mumps, duodenal ulcer, pancreatic cancer.	Chronic pancreatitis, cirrhosis, acute alcoholism, toxemia of pregnancy.
Bilirubin, serum	*Direct:* 0–0.3 mg/100 mL *Indirect:* 0.1–1.0 mg/100 mL *Total:* 0.1–1.2 mg/100 mL	Massive hemolysis, low-grade hemolytic disease, cirrhosis, obstructive liver disease, hepatitis, biliary obstruction	
Bromsulphalein (BSP)	Less than 5% of dye after 45 minutes	Acute hepatic disease, cholelithiasis, cholecystitis.	
Calcium, serum	9–11.5 mg/100 mL, or 4.5–5.7 mEq/L	Hyperparathyroidism, multiple myeloma, bone metastasis, bone fracture, thiazide-diuretic reaction.	Hypoparathyroidism, renal failure, pregnancy, massive transfusion.
Carbon-dioxide combining power	50–65% vol, or 24–30 mEq/L	Serum alkalosis, vomiting, hypoventilation.	Uremia, diabetic ketoacidosis, diarrhea, hyperventilation.
Chloride, serum	95–106 mEq/L, or 355–376 mg/100 mL	Hyperventilation, diabetes insipidus, uremia.	Congestive heart failure, pyloric obstruction, hypoventilation, vomiting.
Cholesterol (total serum)	100–300 mg/100 mL	Liver disease with biliary obstruction, nephrotic stage of glomerulonephritis, runs in family.	Malnutrition, extensive liver disease, hyperthyroidism.
Creatinine, serum	0.6–1.2 mg/100mL	Chronic glomerulonephritis, nephritis, congestive heart failure, muscle disease.	
Creatine phosphokinase (CPK)	*Men:* 55–170 U/L *Women:* 30–135 U/L	Acute myocardial infarction, reaction to exercise, surgery, CVA, head injury, salicylate intoxication, muscular dystrophy.	
Fatty acids, serum	250–390 mg/100 mL	Diabetes mellitus, anemia, nephrosis, hypothyroidism.	Hyperthyroidism.
Fibrinogen, serum	0.2–0.4 g/100 mL	Pneumonia, acute infection, nephrosis.	Cirrhosis, toxic liver necrosis, anemia, obstetric complications, DIC.
Glucose (fasting)	80–120 mg/100 mL	Acute stress, Cushing's syndrome, hyperthyroidism, acute or chronic pancreatitis, diabetes mellitus, ketoacidosis.	Addison's disease, liver disease, reactive hypoglycemia, pituitary hypofunction.
Iodine, protein-bound, serum (PBI)	4–8 μg/100 mL	Hyperthyroidism.	Hypothyroidism.
Iron-binding capacity	250–450 μg/100 mL	Iron-deficiency anemia.	Chronic infection.
Lactic dehydrogenase (LDH)	80–120 Wacker units 150–450 Wroblewski units 71–207 IU/L	Myocardial infarction, pernicious anemia, chronic viral hepatitis, pneumonia, pulmonary emboli, CVA, renal tissue destruction.	
Lipids (total serum)	400–1000 mg/100 mL	Hypothyroidism, diabetes, nephrosis, glomerulonephritis.	Hyperthyroidism.
Phosphorus, inorganic, serum	1.8–2.6 mEq/L, or 3.0–4.5 mg/100 mL	Chronic glomerular disease, hypoparathyroidism, milk-alkali syndrome, sarcoidosis.	Hyperparathyroidism, rickets, osteomalacia, renal tubular necrosis, malabsorption syndrome.

continued

Test	Normal Values	Possible Significance: Increases	Possible Significance: Decreases
BLOOD CHEMISTRY (cont.)			
Potassium, serum	3.5–5.0 mEq/L	Diabetic ketosis, renal failure, Addison's disease.	Thiazide diuretics, Cushing's syndrome, cirrhosis with ascites, hyperaldosteronism, steroid therapy, malignant hypertension, poor dietary habits, chronic diarrhea, diaphoresis, renal tubular necrosis, malabsorption syndrome, vomiting.
Protein, serum (albumin/globulin)	*Total:* 6.0–7.8 g/100 mL; *Albumin:* 3.2–4.5 g/100 mL; *Globulin:* 2.3–3.5 g/100 mL	Dehydration, multiple myeloma.	Chronic liver disease, myeloproliferative disease.
Sodium, serum	138–144 mEq/L	Increased intake, either orally or IV; CNS disease or damage.	Addison's disease, sodium-losing nephropathy, vomiting, diarrhea, fistulas, tube drainage, burns, renal insufficiency with acidosis, starvation with acidosis, paracentesis, thoracentesis, ascites, congestive heart failure, hypothermia, diabetic hyperglycemia.
T_3 uptake	25–38%	Hyperthyroidism, thyroxine-binding globulin (TBG) deficiency.	Hypothyroidism, pregnancy, TBG excess.
Thyroxine	5–11 μg/100 mL	Hyperthyroidism, pregnancy, TBG excess.	Hypothyroidism, TBG deficiency.
Serum glutamic oxaloacetic transaminase (SGOT)	Up to 40 U/100 mL	Hepatitis, severe liver necrosis, myocardial infarction, cirrhosis, skeletal muscle disease, pulmonary infarction, shock, thyrotoxicosis, burns, infection, GI hemorrhage, excessive protein catabolism.	Increased fluid intake, hepatic failure.
Urea nitrogen, serum (BUN)	10–18 mg/100 mL	Acute or chronic renal failure, congestive heart failure; obstructive uropathy, dehydration.	Cirrhosis, malnutrition, nephrosis.
Uric acid, serum	*Men:* 2.1–7.8 mg/100 mL *Women:* 2.0–6.4 mg/100 mL	Gout, chronic renal failure, starvation, diuretic therapy.	
Vitamin B_{12}	300–1000 pg/mL	Hepatic cellular damage, myeloproliferative disorder.	Alcoholism, vegetarianism, total or partial gastrectomy, sprue and celiac disease, fish tapeworm infestation.
Zinc	55–150 μg/100 mL	Hyperthermia.	Alcoholic cirrhosis, leukemia, pernicious anemia.
BLOOD GASES			
pH, serum	7.35–7.45	Metabolic alkalosis-alkali ingestion, respiratory alkalosis-hyperventilation.	Metabolic acidosis-ketoacidosis, shock, respiratory acidosis-alveolar hypoventilation.
Oxygen pressure (Po_2), whole blood, arterial	95–100 mm Hg	Oxygen administration in the absence of severe lung disease.	Chronic obstructive lung disease, severe pneumonia, pulmonary embolism, pulmonary edema, respiratory muscle disease.
Carbon dioxide pressure (Pco_2), whole blood, arterial	35–45 mm Hg	Alveolar hypoventilation, loss of H^+ through nasogastric suctioning or vomiting.	Hyperventilation.
IMMUNODIAGNOSTIC STUDIES			
Carcinoembryonic antigen	0–2.5 ng/mL	Cancer of colon, lung, metastatic breast, pancreas, stomach, prostate, ovary, bladder, limbs; also neuroblastoma, leukemias, osteogenic carcinoma. Elevated in noncancer conditions, such as hepatic cirrhosis, uremia, pancreatitis, colorectal, polypoidosis, or peptic ulcer disease, ulcerative colitis, and regional enteritis.	

continued

Test	Normal Values	Possible Significance: Increases	Possible Significance: Decreases
URINALYSIS			
pH	4.8–8.0	Metabolic alkalosis.	Intracellular acidosis due to potassium depletion.
Specific gravity	1.015–1.025	Dehydration.	Distal renal tubular disease, polycystic kidney disease, diabetes insipidus.
Glucose	Negative	Diabetes mellitus.	
Protein	Negative	Nephrosis, glomerulonephritis, lupus erythematosis.	
Casts	Negative	Nephrosis, glomerulonephritis, lupus erythematosus.	
Red blood cells	Negative	Renal calculi, hemorrhagic cystitis, tumors of the kidney.	
White blood cells	Negative	Inflammation of the kidneys, ureters, or bladder.	
Color	Normal yellow	*Abnormal:* red to reddish brown—hematuria; brown to brownish gray—bilirubinuria or urobilinuria; tea-colored—possible obstructive jaundice.	*Almost colorless:* chronic kidney disease, diabetes insipidus, diabetes mellitus, effect of alcohol ingestion.
Sodium	80–180 mEq/24 hours	Salt-wasting renal disease.	Congestive heart failure, primary aldosteronism.
Chloride	110–250 mEq/24 hours	Chronic obstructive lung disease.	Metabolic alkalosis.
Potassium	40–80 mEq/24 hours	Osmotic diuresis.	Renal failure.
Creatinine clearance	1.0–1.6 g/24 hours		Renal disease.
Hydroxycorticosteroids	2–10 mg/24 hours	Cushing's disease.	Addison's disease.
Ketosteroids	*Male:* 1–22 mg/24 hours *Female:* 6–16 mg/24 hours	Hirsutism, adrenal hyperplasia.	Thyrotoxicosis, Addison's disease, myxedema.
Catecholamines (VMA)	*Epinephrine:* 10 mg/24 hours *Norepinephrine:* 100 mg/24 hours	Pheochromocytoma, myasthenia gravis, severe anxiety, numerous medications.	Malnutrition, cervical spine transection.
URINE TESTS			
Schilling test	Excretion of 8% or more of test dose should appear in urine.		Gastrointestinal malabsorption, pernicious anemia.

■ APPENDIX

H

NCLEX-RN Test Plan: Categories of Client Needs

The latest NCLEX-RN test plan follows the categories of client needs, described below. See Appendix I for page references to specific topics for review.

■ Safe, Effective Care Environment

See Appendix B, Categories of Human Functions: Protective Functions.

The nurse meets client needs for a safe and effective environment by providing and directing nursing care that promotes achievement of the following client needs:

1. Coordinated care
2. Quality assurance
3. Goal-oriented care
4. Environmental safety
5. Preparation for treatments and procedures
6. Safe and effective treatments and procedures

Knowledge, Skills, and Abilities

In order to meet client needs for a safe, effective environment, the nurse should possess knowledge, skills, and the abilities in areas that include but are not limited to the following examples:

> knowledge of bio/psycho/social principles, teaching/learning principles, basic principles of management, principles of group dynamics and interpersonal communication, expected outcomes of various treatment modalities, general and specific protective measures, environmental and personal safety, client rights, confidentiality, cultural and religious influences on health, continuity of care, and spread and control of infectious agents.

■ Physiological Integrity

See Appendix B, Categories of Human Functions: Sensory-Perceptual, Comfort, Rest, Activity, and Mobility, Nutrition, Fluid-Gas Transport, Elimination.

The nurse meets the physiological integrity needs of clients with potentially life-threatening and/or chronically recurring physiological conditions, and of clients at risk for the development of complications or untoward effects of treatments or management modalities, by providing and directing nursing care that promotes achievement of the following client needs:

1. Physiological adaptation
2. Reduction of risk potential
3. Mobility
4. Comfort
5. Provision of basic care

Knowledge, Skills, and Abilities

In order to meet client needs for physiological integrity, the nurse should possess knowledge, skills, and abilities in areas that include but are not limited to the following examples:

Source: NCLEX-RN Test Plan for the National Council Licensure Examination for Registered Nurses, August 1987.

normal body structure and function, pathophysiology, drug administration and pharmacological actions, intrusive procedures, routine nursing measures, documentation, nutritional therapies, managing emergencies, expected and unexpected response to therapies, body mechanics, effects of immobility, activities of daily living, comfort measures, and use of special equipment.

■ Psychosocial Integrity

See Appendix B, Categories of Human Functions: Psycho-Social-Cultural Functions.

The nurse meets client needs for psychosocial integrity in stress and crisis-related situations throughout the life cycle by providing and directing nursing care that promotes achievement of the following client needs:

1. Psychosocial adaptation
2. Coping/Adaptation

Knowledge, Skills, and Abilities

In order to meet client needs for psychosocial integrity, the nurse should possess knowledge, skills, and abilities in areas that include but are not limited to the following examples:

communication skills, mental health concepts, behavioral norms, psychodynamics of behavior, psychopathology, treatment modalities, psychopharmacology, documentation, accountability, principles of teaching and learning, and appropriate community resources.

■ Health Promotion/Maintenance

See Appendix B, Categories of Human Functions: Growth and Development, Nutrition.

The nurse meets client needs for health promotion/maintenance throughout the life cycle by providing and directing nursing care that promotes achievement, within clients and their significant others, of the following needs:

1. Continued growth and development
2. Self-care
3. Integrity of support systems
4. Prevention and early treatment of disease

Knowledge, Skills, and Abilities

In order to meet client needs for health promotion/maintenance, the nurse should possess knowledge, skills, and abilities in areas that include but are not limited to the following examples:

communication skills, principles of teaching and learning, documentation, community resources, family systems, concepts of wellness, adaptation to altered health states, reproduction and human sexuality, birthing and parenting, growth and development including dying and death, pathophysiology, body structure and function, and principles of immunity.

APPENDIX I

Index to Detailed NCLEX-RN Test Plan: Knowledge, Skills, and Abilities

The following outline of nursing knowledge, skills, and abilities is organized in terms of four categories of client need: *Safe, Effective Care Environment* (SECE), *Physiological Integrity* (PhI), *Psychosocial Integrity* (PsI), and *Health Promotion/Maintenance* (HPM). Included in the outline of topics are 17 numbered subcategories and corresponding task statements. These items are derived from study of nursing tasks and are used in the development of the NCLEX-RN test plan.

Students who have taken and evaluated their performance on the **Pre Test**, **Post Test**, or **Prep Test** in this book will find this outline a useful guide for a concentrated review of specific problem topics. **Repeat NCLEX-RN test-takers** will also find this outline to be a useful guide for review of their areas of weakness. Refer to the pages listed in the right column for review of a particular topic.

APPENDIX

	Pages
h. Fear/phobia: effectiveness of desensitization techniques	75
i. Behavior modification program: teach family techniques to manage emotionally disturbed	42, 87
j. Disruptive behavior: measures to control (anger, demanding, hostility, manipulation)	38, 41–45
k. Noncompliance	45
l. Sleep pattern disturbance	53
m. Disturbance in self-concept; self-esteem: how to emphasize strength	69–70
n. Anxiety: reduce symptoms	46, 71–75
o. Posttrauma response	75
p. Rape trauma syndrome	51–53
q. Development of trusting, therapeutic nurse/client relationship	61, 64–66
r. Reality orientation; milieu, group, resocialization	87–90

13. *Coping Adaptation (CA)*

	Pages
a. Coping behaviors (dependence, denial, dissociative, somatoform disorders)	41–42, 72–73, 76–77
b. Relaxation techniques	9–10
c. Altered body image	16–19
(1) Adjustment to changes (phases of body image development)	16, 18
(2) Adjustment to physical or emotional impairment	19–21
d. Sensory disturbance: confusion, disorientation related to need for increase or decrease in stimulation	40–41, 54
e. Impaired verbal communication (nontherapeutic, noneffective)	67–69
f. Open communication: accepting, nonjudgmental, acknowledges feelings, etc.	66–67
g. Making referrals	626–629

D. Health Promotion/Maintenance (HPM)

Assessment: Physiological, Psychosocial, Developmental, Environmental

Period: Antepartal, Labor, Delivery, Postpartal, Newborn

14. (Part I) *Continued Growth and Development (CGD)*

	Pages
a. Risk factors: identify maternal, fetal, newborn	130, 135–137, 191, 193–196
b. Complications (pregnancy and labor)	130–135, 139–149, 167–174
c. Prevention of maternal, fetal, and newborn complications	130, 180–186, 191–202
d. Emergencies: measures to deal with maternal, fetal, and newborn	138–139, 156–157, 173, 175
e. Antepartal	120–150
(1) Nursing history (reproduction, sexual)	128–129
(2) Assessment of maternal physical status (e.g., breast, abdomen, pelvis)	120–125
(3) Maternal psychosocial profile (perception of pregnancy, coping mechanism)	127
(4) Routine care (nutrition, methods of childbirth)	129–130, 134, 157
(5) Maternal, fetal diagnostic tests	149–150
■ Chorionic villii sampling	150
■ Ultrasound	150
■ Amniocentesis	150
■ Non-stress test	150
■ Contraction stress test, etc.	150
(6) Common discomfort and complications	126
f. Labor	151–160, 163–164
(1) Assess maternal and fetal status (fetal heart rate, electronic fetal monitoring, descent of parts, etc.)	157–159
(2) Teach relaxation techniques	157, 165–167
g. Delivery	159–160
(1) Immediate care	160–161
(2) Promote adaptation to extrauterine life	186
(3) Emergency delivery	162–163
h. Newborn	186–202
(1) Newborn care (airway, cord, Apgar, eyes, weight and measuring, heat support, identification)	161–162, 169, 189
(2) Assist with infant feeding: assess skills of new parents at infant feeding	179

J

Index to Nursing Process Questions

Unit	Assessment Question #	Analysis Question #	Plan Question #	Implementation Question #	Evaluation Question #
Unit 1 Behavioral and Emotional Problems (Mental Health Nursing)	7, 22, 29, 51, 66, 74, 99, 130, 133, 148, 162	5, 12, 14, 18, 19, 20, 21, 23, 24, 28, 30, 31, 32, 44, 46, 47, 52, 53, 55, 58, 61, 62, 63, 65, 68, 72, 77, 79, 80, 97, 98, 100, 102, 105, 106, 108, 109, 114, 117, 131, 132, 134, 136, 137, 138, 139, 140, 141, 142, 143, 144, 145, 146, 155, 166	3, 8, 10, 15, 34, 37, 40, 41, 42, 43, 45, 48, 54, 60, 73, 75, 76, 78 82, 83, 86, 87, 89, 90, 96, 120, 125, 128, 135, 149, 152, 153, 154, 157, 158, 160	1, 2, 4, 6, 9, 11, 13, 16, 17, 26, 35, 36, 38, 39, 49, 50, 56, 57, 59, 69, 71, 81, 84, 85, 88, 91, 92, 93, 94, 101, 103, 104, 107, 110, 111, 112, 113, 115, 118, 119, 121, 122, 123, 124, 126, 127, 129, 147, 150, 151, 156, 159, 161, 164, 165	25, 27, 33, 64, 67, 70, 95, 116, 163
Unit 2 Childbearing Family (Maternal-Infant Nursing)	4, 7, 9, 10, 11, 13, 15, 18, 23, 25, 26, 27, 28, 29, 30, 34, 35, 36, 37, 38, 39, 40, 42, 45, 46, 48, 61, 66, 71, 72, 73, 80	49, 50, 64, 67, 68, 69, 70, 76, 78, 84		1, 2, 3, 5, 6, 8, 12, 14, 16, 17, 19, 20, 21, 22, 24, 31, 32, 33, 41, 43, 44, 47, 51, 52, 54, 55, 56, 57, 58, 59, 60, 62, 63, 65, 74, 75, 77, 80, 81, 82, 83	53, 79
Unit 3 Children and Families (Pediatric Nursing)	10, 16, 20, 43, 72, 85, 120	2, 4, 5, 8, 9, 19, 21, 22, 23, 26, 27, 28, 38, 44, 45, 48, 50, 51, 52, 58, 64, 78, 86, 91, 95, 97, 101, 109, 116, 117, 118, 119	11, 30, 54, 67, 74, 81, 87, 103	1, 6, 7, 12, 13, 15, 17, 24, 25, 29, 31, 32, 33, 34, 35, 37, 39, 40, 41, 42, 46, 47, 49, 53, 55, 57, 60, 62, 63, 65, 68, 70, 75, 76, 77, 79, 80, 82, 83, 84, 88, 89, 90, 92, 93, 94, 96, 98, 100, 102, 104, 105, 106, 107, 111, 112, 113, 115	3, 14, 18, 36, 56, 59, 61, 66, 69, 71, 73, 99, 108, 110, 114
Unit 4 Acutely Ill and Chronically Ill Adult (Adult Nursing)	4, 6, 20, 38, 42, 43, 45, 51, 57, 62, 63, 76, 79, 80, 82, 84, 85, 87, 90, 94	5, 7, 8, 9, 10, 12, 16, 17, 21, 22, 25, 28, 30, 35, 56, 61, 64, 69, 73, 78, 83, 91, 95	1, 11, 13, 19, 26, 27, 31, 33, 34, 36, 37, 40, 41, 47, 54, 59, 70, 72, 75, 77, 93	2, 3, 14, 18, 23, 24, 29, 39, 44, 46, 48, 49, 52, 53, 55, 58, 60, 65, 66, 67, 74, 89, 92	15, 32, 50, 68, 71, 81, 86, 88

Unit	Assessment Question #	Analysis Question #	Plan Question #	Implementation Question #	Evaluation Question #
Unit 5 Nutrition	8		2, 4, 5, 7, 9	1, 3, 6	
Unit 6 Pharmacology	1, 11, 20, 29	14, 19, 23, 35, 36, 37, 41, 44, 47, 50	2, 4, 9, 13, 27, 31, 33, 39, 40, 45, 49	3, 6, 8, 12, 16, 21, 22, 24, 25, 26, 30, 32, 38, 46, 48, 51, 52, 53, 54, 55	5, 7, 10, 15, 17, 18, 28, 34, 42, 43
Unit 7 Nursing Treatments	9	1, 2, 3, 5, 6	8, 12	4, 10, 11	7, 13
Unit 8 Ethical and Legal Aspects		15, 16, 18, 22, 23, 24	5	1, 2, 3, 4, 7, 11, 12, 17, 19	6, 8, 9, 10, 13, 14, 20, 21, 25, 27, 33

Bibliography

ORIENTATION

Alexander AB: Relaxation training script, modified Jacobsonian method, 1972. Denver: Children's Asthma Research Hospital.

Benson H: *The Relaxation Response*, 1975. New York: William Morrow.

Bernstein DA, Borkovec TD: *Progressive Relaxation Training*, 1973. Champaign, Illinois: Research Press.

Fuller G: *Relaxation Approaches for Nurses*, Audiocassette tape available from Review for Nurses Tapes Co., PO Box 16347, San Francisco, CA 94116.

Helm P: *Strategies for Success on Nursing Exams*. Audiocassette tape with booklet available from Review for Nurses Tapes Co., PO Box 16347, San Francisco, CA 94116.

Jacobson E: *Progressive Relaxation*, 3rd ed., 1974. Chicago: University of Chicago Press.

Jacobson E: *You Must Relax*, 4th ed., 1957. New York: McGraw-Hill.

Lagerquist S: *Effective Test-Taking Techniques*. Audiocassette tape available from Review for Nurses Tapes Co., PO Box 16347, San Francisco, CA 94116.

Lagerquist S: *How To Pass Nursing Exams*, 1992. San Francisco: Review Press.

Lagerquist S et al., *N.S.A.T. (Nursing Student Assessment Test)*. Computer software available from Review for Nurses Tapes Co., PO Box 16347, San Francisco, CA 94116.

Lagerquist S: *Stress Management While Studying*. Videocassette tape available from Review for Nurses Tapes Co., PO Box 16347, San Francisco, CA 94116.

Lagerquist S: *Successful Test-Taking Techniques*. Videocassette tape available from Review for Nurses Tapes Co., PO Box 16347, San Francisco, CA 94116.

Lagerquist S: *What To Study for the NCLEX-RN*. Videocassette tape available from Review for Nurses Tapes Co., PO Box 16347, San Francisco, CA 94116.

Lagerquist S: *What You Need To Know About NCLEX-RN*. Audiocassette (also videocassette) tape available from Review for Nurses Tapes Co., PO Box 16347, San Francisco, CA 94116.

Trygstad LS: "Simple New Way To Help Anxious Patients," *R.N.* 43 (12):28, 1980.

Von Bozzay G: *Stress Management for Nurses*. Audiocassette tape available from Review for Nurses Tapes Co., PO Box 16347, San Francisco, CA 94116.

UNIT 1

American Psychiatric Association: *Diagnostic and Statistical Manual of Mental Disorders* (DSM–III-R), 3rd ed., 1987. Washington, D.C. A systematic descriptive approach to the classification of mental disorders. Provides specific diagnostic criteria. Each disorder is described in the following areas: essential features, associated features, age at onset, course, impairment, complications, predisposing factors, prevalence, and differential diagnosis.

Beck C, Rawlins R, and Williams S: *Mental Health—Psychiatric Nursing—A Holistic Life-Cycle Approach*, 2nd ed., 1988. St. Louis: C.V. Mosby. This comprehensive textbook is unique in its use of *drugs* and *nursing process* applied to *psychotropic behavioral concepts* (such as anxiety, anger, guilt, hope-despair, flexibility-rigidity, dependence-independence, trust-mistrust). Additional valuable content is included: *cultural diversity*, therapy with vic-

content is included: *cultural diversity*, therapy with victims of *abuse*, legal and ethical issues, and coverage of *life-cycle phases* (infant, child, adolescent, young adult, middle-aged adult, aged adult). DSM–III-R classifications are discussed in relation to client behaviors. Numerous charts and case examples boxed-in and in bold print add to the readability of this mammoth textbook.

Burgess A, Lazare A: *Psychiatric Nursing in the Hospital and the Community*, 5th ed., 1989. Englewood Cliffs, NJ: Prentice-Hall. The most valuable feature of this book is the simple format and writing style. It is not as comprehensive in scope or theory as Kyes and Hofling. However, the intent is to devote a major part of the book to the application of basic concepts to nursing management of clinical syndromes. The art work is effective, key points are enumerated in outline form, key phrases are placed in the margins, and end-of-chapter summaries serve to promote this as a useful book for initial learning and review of major psychiatric conditions.

Cook SJ, Fontaine KL: *Essentials of Mental Health Nursing*, 2nd ed., 1991. Redwood City, California: Addison-Wesley. This new text focuses on core topics and is organized in a nursing process format. It contains objectives, case examples, numerous nursing care plans, and chapter summaries. It focuses specifically on assessment tools unique to the psychiatric setting. Also includes such timely issues as AIDS, homelessness, aging, and new research regarding organic brain disorders.

Haber J, Leach A, Schudy S, and Sideleau BF: *Comprehensive Psychiatric Nursing*, 3rd ed., 1987. New York: McGraw-Hill. This excellent book uses an integrated approach throughout the life span in a variety of settings. The focus is on nursing management of clients with a variety of behavioral difficulties, for example, anxiety, fear, frustration, anger, depression, and guilt. The nursing process is continually stressed, with sections labeled "Nursing Assessment," "Planning and Implementation," "Nursing Intervention," and "Evaluation."

Sundeen S, Stuart G: *Principles and Practice of Psychiatric Nursing*, 3rd ed., 1987. St. Louis: C.V. Mosby. This comprehensive overview of the field of psychiatric nursing reflects the changing emphasis in psychiatric nursing practice through its use of the nursing process model as a framework. The nursing role is viewed as one that influences health promotion, treatment of disturbances, and rehabilitation. There is an excellent section of the various models of psychiatric care, as well as current treatment modalities. Patient disturbances are seen as adaptive or maladaptive; terminology emphasizes the concepts of stress and stressors, with levels of primary, secondary, and tertiary prevention. A valuable feature is the summary of important points at the end of each chapter.

Taylor, CM: *Mereness' Essentials of Psychiatric Nursing*, 13th ed. St. Louis: C.V. Mosby. A classic textbook featuring a holistic conceptual approach with an informal narrative style.

Varcarolis EM: *Foundations of Psychiatric Mental Health Nursing*, 1990. Philadelphia: W. B. Saunders. A concise yet comprehensive textbook with a variety of visual learning tools. Focuses on teaching skills to attend to psychosocial needs in a variety of settings. Features issues of mental health needs regarding violence, substance abuse, and other contemporary issues.

Wilson H, Kneisl C: *Psychiatric Nursing*, 3rd ed., 1988. Redwood City, California: Addison-Wesley. This is the most inclusive book available in the field of psychiatric nursing. It can be used as an overall reference. An award-winning book, it is considered by many to be "the" classic (it is the only text cited in the bibliography of ANA Standards). It contains the most thorough information, concepts, theories, and ideas relevant to the field of psychiatric nursing. A unique feature is its extensive use of charts and tables. It includes unique chapters on human sexuality, parenting, group dynamics, psychiatric nursing ethics, and alternative therapies.

CLASSIC SUGGESTED READINGS

Psychiatric Emergencies

Rogerson K: "Psychiatric Emergencies," *Nursing Clinics of North America*, 8(3):457–466, September 1973.

Psychosocial Assessment

Snyder J, Wilson M: "Elements of a Psychological Assessment," *American Journal of Nursing*, 77(2):235–239, 1977.

Vincent P, Broad J, and Dylworth L: "Developing a Mental Health Assessment Form," *Journal of Nursing Administration*, 6(1):25–28, 1976.

Psychosocial Development

Duvall EM: *Marriage and Family Development*, 1977. Philadelphia: J. B. Lippincott.

Erikson E: *Childhood and Society*, 1963. New York: W.W. Norton.

Kalish R: *The Psychology of Human Behavior*, 1973. Monterey, California: Wadsworth.

Maslow A: *Motivation and Personality*, 1970. New York: Harper & Row.

Piaget J: *Origins of Intelligence in Children*, 1963. New York: W. W. Norton.

Stress and Crisis

Aguilera D, Messick J: *Crisis Intervention*, 5th ed., 1986. St. Louis: C.V. Mosby.

Sedgwick R: "Psychological Response to Stress," *Journal of Psychiatric Nursing and Mental Health Services*, 13(5): 20–23, September–October 1975.

Selye H: *Stress Without Distress*, 1974. Ontario: New American Library of Canada.

General Behavioral Problems

Disturbance in body image

Blaesing S et al.: "The Development of Body Image in the Child, the Adolescent, and Adulthood," *Nursing Clinics of North America*, 7(4):597–630, December 1972.

Corbeil M: "The Nursing Process for a Patient with a Body Image Disturbance," *Nursing Clinics of North America*, 6(1):155–163, March 1971.

Immobility

Carnevali D, Brueckner S: "Immobilization—Reassessment of a Concept," *American Journal of Nursing*, 70(7):1502–1507, July 1970.

Sensory disturbance

Bolin R: "Sensory Deprivation: an Overview," *Nursing Forum*, 13(3):240–258, Summer 1974.

Chodil J et al.: "The Concept of Sensory Deprivation," *Nursing Clinics of North America*, 5(3):544–548, September 1970.

Health Teaching

Murray R, Zentner J: "Guidelines for More Effective Health Teaching," *Nursing '76*, 6(2):44–53, February 1976.

Redman B: *The Process of Patient Teaching in Nursing*, 1976. St. Louis: C.V. Mosby.

UNIT 2

Benoit J: "Sexually Transmitted Disease During Pregnancy." *Nursing Clinics of North America*, 23(4), 937–943, 1988. A succinct review of the range of sexually transmitted diseases found in pregnancy. Discusses pharmacologic therapy safe during pregnancy and reviews appropriate patient teaching.

Bobak I, Jensen M: *Essentials of Maternity Care: The Nurse and the Childbearing Family*, 2nd ed., 1987. St. Louis: C.V. Mosby. A comprehensive maternal–newborn nursing text emphasizing nursing process and nursing diagnosis. Concepts, principles, and approaches to care are easily retrievable; definitions of terms are included in context. Comprehensive chapter outlines facilitate rapid identification and review of contents.

Brunner L, Suddarth D: *Textbook of Medical-Surgical Nursing*, 6th ed., 1988. Philadelphia: J.B. Lippincott. Popular medical-surgical nursing text; emphasizes nursing process approach to basic concepts of nursing care.

Galvan BJ, Van Mullem C, and Broekhuizen F: "Using Amnioinfusion for the Relief of Repetitive Variable Decelerations During Labor." *JOGNN*, 18(6), 222–229, 1989. Describes the process of amnioinfusion to relieve umbilical cord compression during labor and outlines the appropriate nursing observations and care during this procedure.

George D, Stephen S, Fellow R, and Bremer D: "The Latest on Retinopathy of Prematurity." *JOGNN*, 13(4), 254–258, 1988. Describes updated information on this major complication of oxygen therapy in the preterm infant. Reviews pathophysiology of disease and essential nursing care to prevent this complication.

Hatcher R et al.: *Contraceptive Technology, 1986–87*, 13th ed., 1986. Philadelphia: Irvington. Definitive discussion of modern contraceptive modalities. Incorporates relevant physiology and important concepts and principles needed for effective health teaching. Excellent reference for family planning.

Ippolito C, Gibes R: "AIDS and the Newborn." *Journal of Perinatal and Neonatal Nursing*, 1(4), 78–86, 1988. Reviews current knowledge regarding AIDS in the newborn and outlines appropriate nursing interventions for the infant.

Kennard M: "Cocaine Use During Pregnancy: Fetal and Neonatal Effects." *Journal of Perinatal and Neonatal Nursing*, 3(4), 53–63, 1990. Reviews major teratogenic effects of cocaine use during pregnancy and the physical and neurobehavioral sequelae of drug use in the neonatal period. Discusses major aspects of nursing management, including legal considerations of toxicology testing.

Mackey M, Lock S: "Women's Expectations of the Labor and Delivery Nurse." *JOGNN*, 18(6), 505–512, 1989. Nursing study describes the expectations of multiparous patients for nursing support and care during labor and delivery. Describes a wide range of anticipated nursing behaviors desired by the subjects.

May K, Mahlmeister L: *Comprehensive Maternity Nursing*, 1990. Philadelphia: J.B. Lippincott. A comprehensive maternal–newborn nursing text that emphasizes the cultural aspects of maternity care. Uses nursing diagnosis to delineate care for the childbearing family. Describes legal and ethical concerns of perinatal nursing in each chapter.

NAACOG: *Fetal Heart Rate Auscultation*, 1990. Washington, D.C.: NAACOG. This OGN Nursing Practice Resource from the Organization for Obstetric, Gynecologic and Neonatal Nurses delineates the current standards for intermittent auscultation of the fetal heart rate during labor. Discusses indications for use of method over electronic monitoring during labor.

NAACOG: *Mother-Baby Care*, 1989. Washington, DC: NAACOG. This OGN Nursing Practice Resource from the Organization for Obstetric, Gynecologic and Neonatal Nurses delineates the current standards for combined mother-baby care during the postpartum period. Excellent review of physical and emotional needs of new dyad.

NAACOG: *The Nurse's Role in the Induction and Augmentation of Labor*, 1988. Washington, DC: NAACOG. This OGN Nursing Practice Resource from the Organization for Obstetric, Gynecologic and Neonatal nurses delineates the current standards for the nurse administering oxytocin to initiate contractions during labor. Describes risks and benefits of drug and contraindications to its use during labor.

Norr K, Nacion K, and Abramson R: "Early Discharge With Home Follow-Up: Impacts on Low-Income Mothers and Infants." *JOGNN*, 18(2), 133–141, 1989. This study describes positive outcomes in high-risk women when early discharge is coupled with intensive follow-up care by nurses. Discusses specific interventions to improve outcomes for this group of women.

Sala J, Moise K: "The Treatment of Preterm Labor Using a Portable Subcutaneous Terbutaline Pump." *NAACOG*, 19(2), 108–115, 1990. An in-depth discussion of the most current treatment of preterm labor, including indications, risks, benefits and appropriate nursing care of the woman using this new device. Photographs of the pump and its use enhance discussion.

Sleutel M: "An Overview of Vibroacoustic Stimulation." *JOGNN*, 18(6), 447–452, 1989. Provides an in-depth overview of this new fetal assessment tool and delineates appropriate patient teaching and nursing care during the procedure.

Stringer M: "Chorionic Villi Sampling: A Nursing Perspective." *JOGNN*, 17(1), 19–22, 1988. This review article describes the new diagnostic procedure, its risks, advantages, and nursing implications.

Sullivan K: "Maternal Implications of Cocaine Use During Pregnancy." *Journal of Perinatal and Neonatal Nursing*, 3(4), 12–25, 1990. Describes pharmacology of cocaine and the physiologic, psychologic, and social consequences of its use during pregnancy. Also delineates major complications of use and appropriate nursing care of the woman.

Tighe D, Sweezy: "The Perioperative Experience of Cesarean Birth." *Journal of Perinatal and Neonatal Nursing*, 3(3), 14–30, 1990. Covers preparation, considerations, and complications of cesarean birth. Includes case studies to illustrate major points.

Tribotti S, Lyons N, Blackburn S, Stein M, and Withers J: "Nursing Diagnoses for the Postpartum Woman." *JOGNN*, 17(6), 410–416, 1988. This study lists the most common nursing diagnoses identified by postpartum nurses. Excellent review of common NANDA-approved diagnoses for the postpartum nurse.

Wiley K, Grohar J: "Human Immunodeficiency Virus and Precautions for Obstetric, Gynecologic, and Neonatal Nurses." *JOGNN*, 17(3), 165–168, 1988. Describes the recommendations for universal body substance precautions developed by the Centers for Disease Control. Addresses specific guidelines for perinatal nurses.

UNIT 3

Betz CL, Poster EC: *Pediatric Nursing Reference*, 1989. St. Louis: C.V. Mosby. The concise format of this handbook offers the nurse an easily accessible reference on 72 frequently encountered medical-surgical conditions in the pediatric population and major diagnostic tests and procedures. Appendices cover growth and development, immunization schedules, commonly used antibiotics, laboratory values, and guidelines for taking blood pressures. All material is tabbed for immediate access.

Clarke PH, Deeds NC: "The Child in a Mist Tent." *Pediatric Nursing*, 14(6):446–450, 1988. This recent article offers pictures of a mist tent as well as nursing care plan guidelines. It provides an excellent, detailed review of nursing care of the child in a mist tent.

Engel J: *Pocket Guide to Pediatric Assessment*, 1989. St. Louis: C.V. Mosby. This pocket guide is specifically designed to provide comprehensive information for health assessment of infants, children, and adolescents. It contains clinically relevant material in a quick reference outline format. Appendices cover developmental assessment, growth charts, lab values, and immunization schedules.

Foster RL, Hunsberger MM, and Anderson JT: *Family-Centered Nursing Care of Children*, 1989. Philadelphia: W.B. Saunders. This state-of-the-art textbook, with over 2,000 pages, details both the theoretical concepts and specific nursing strategies necessary to today's nursing practice with children and their families. The framework for this text includes the nursing process, a conceptual approach, development, nursing care across health care settings, and research-based intervention strategies. Appendices cover NANDA diagnoses, growth and development, laboratory values, resources for families, and nutrition.

James SR, Mott SR: *Child Health Nursing: Essential Care of Children and Families*, 1988. Menlo Park, California: Addison-Wesley. This text, specifically redesigned to be more manageable for students, covers both the ill child and the well child, including health maintenance and prevention of illness and disability. It consistently addresses the emotional, social, cultural, and psychologic needs of children and families. Home care, patient and family teaching, and discharge planning are emphasized throughout. The clarity and consistency of this text are enhanced through the use of numerous tables and charts, a focus on essential principles of nursing care, and preparations for and interpretation of diagnostic tests.

Lederer JR et al.: *Care Planning Pocket Guide*, 3rd ed., 1990. Redwood City, California: Addison-Wesley. This quick, complete pocket guide to writing individualized care plans includes 83 NANDA diagnoses. It details complete plans of care with specific nursing diagnoses across the life span and including pediatric conditions. Easy cross references to related diagnoses are included.

Marlow DR, Redding BA: *Textbook of Pediatric Nursing*, 6th ed., 1988. Philadelphia: W.B. Saunders. A basic text for beginning students, this text provides a complete guide to nursing care of children and their families. This classical pediatric nursing text contains new photos, drawings, tables, and graphs in order to clarify content for students. The nursing process is integrated in the knowledge base through the identification of relevant NANDA diagnoses for various pathologic conditions. Developmental needs are also included throughout. Appendices cover pediatric nursing history and family assessment, growth charts, vital signs, lab values, and nutrition.

Nelson NP, Beckel J: *Nursing Care Plans for the Pediatric Patient*, 1987. St. Louis: C.V. Mosby. This book provides an overview of well over 100 medical-surgical conditions in the pediatric population and their respective "standard" nursing care plans. Organized by systems, this book includes nursing diagnoses, defining characteristics, nursing orders, and expected outcomes for each condition. Appendices cover developmental assessment, lab values, and therapeutic drug levels.

Newman, JT, Scott GR: *Pediatric Nursing*, 1990. Springhouse, Pennsylvania: Springhouse Corporation. This clinical rotation guide is concise, easy to read, and small enough to carry to the clinical unit for fast reference. It identifies and explains pediatric clinical terminology as well as NANDA diagnoses and accompanying care plan guidelines. It includes diagrams to demonstrate common procedures and a separate section on pediatric medications. Appendices cover pediatric-related abbreviations, terminology, fluid and electrolyte imbalances, and clinical signs of dehydration.

Whaley, LF, Wong DL: *Essentials of Pediatric Nursing*, 1989. St. Louis: C.V. Mosby. This third edition maintains the emphasis on basic information essential to the delivery of safe, comprehensive, and holistic nursing care to children and families. A major new feature is the use of nursing process as the framework for presenting nursing care, including both observational guidelines and expected outcomes. Special features include numerous tables and boxes, particularly "Nursing Guidelines," to assist the reader to consolidate content. Content on emergency treatment of life-threatening conditions is clearly outlined and designated by a colored tab. Vignettes, or "therapeutic dialogues," as well as study questions and activities are also included.

UNIT 4

Beare PG, Myers JL: *Principles and Practices of Adult Health Nursing*, 1990. St. Louis: C.V. Mosby. Focuses on all settings where nursing has a role in health care delivery—acute care, outpatient, rehabilitation, longterm, and home care. The nursing science content is reinforced with information from the related sciences and humanities. All dimensions of the nurse's role are addressed as well as recent trends in health care, prevention, technological advances, family involvement in patient education, therapeutic communication, and the needs of the aging population.

Bullock B, Rosendahl P: *Pathophysiology, Adaptations and Alterations in Function*, 1988. Glenview, Illinois: Scott, Foresman. Comprehensive pathophysiology text that describes how alterations in structure and function can disrupt the whole body. Each chapter has learning objectives and excellent diagrams.

Holloway N: *Nursing the Critically Ill Adult*, 3rd ed., 1989. Redwood City, California: Addison-Wesley. Presents practical information basic to critical care nursing. Provides an approach to care in acute settings that has been tested, is pragmatic, and gives a framework for nursing practice.

Kozier B, Erb G: *Techniques in Clinical Nursing*, 1989. Redwood City, California: Addison-Wesley. Describes nursing actions pre, during, and post procedures. Identifies critical elements for procedures. Discusses home care adaptations. Many pictures and diagrams.

Luckman J, Sorenson K: *Medical-Surgical Nursing: A Psychophysiologic Approach*, 3rd ed., 1987. Philadelphia:

Saunders. This text offers an in-depth presentation of current medical-surgical nursing practice as well as a discussion of basic behavioral and physiologic concepts. A wide range of specific health problems are presented, and the components of the nursing process are consistently related to underlying psychophysiologic principles. The authors have included unit objectives and varied learning activities to facilitate mastery of the material and to enhance learning. References are extensive.

Olson E: "The Hazards of Immobility." *American Journal of Nursing*, April, 1967. *Classic* work describing the effects of immobility on physiological and psychological functioning.

Patrick M et al.: *Medical-Surgical Nursing: Pathophysiological Concepts*, 1986. Philadelphia: J.B. Lippincott. Comprehensive nursing text utilizing a strong nursing process framework. Sample nursing care plans offered throughout the book.

Phipps W, Long B, Woods N: *Medical-Surgical Nursing, Concepts and Clinical Practice*, 3rd ed., 1987. St. Louis: C.V. Mosby. The text begins with an examination of the social, cultural, and environmental factors that influence nursing. The nursing process is utilized with outcome criteria clearly identified for interventions described. Concepts necessary to understand the process of stress and adaptation are presented. Common problems resulting from pathophysiological changes are presented using a systems approach.

Thompson J et al.: *Clinical Nursing*, 1986. St. Louis: C.V. Mosby. The framework for this text is based on the Social Policy Statement of the ANA. Using this definition, the text focuses on applying nursing theory to observable phenomena and identifying appropriate nursing actions.

UNIT 5

Dudek SG: *Nutrition Handbook for Nursing Practice*, 1987. Philadelphia: J.B. Lippincott. A comprehensive handbook that uses the nursing process to integrate nutrition into nursing care plans. Where applicable, possible adverse nutritional side effects of commonly used medications and appropriate interventions have been included. Many useful reference tables are also provided.

Whitney E, Cataldo C, Rolfes S: *Understanding Normal and Clinical Nutrition*, 1987. St. Paul: West. Considers nutritional issues from a developmental and systems approach. Informative pictures and charts. Drawings assist in the learning of difficult concepts.

Williams SR: *Essentials of Nutrition and Diet Therapy*, 6th ed., 1989. St. Louis: C.V. Mosby. This in-depth nutrition text presents material concerning the foundation of nutrition in great detail. The second section of the book deals with applied nutrition in the community, focusing on personal beliefs, cultural influences, nutrition counseling, and education. Nutritional influences throughout the life cycle include physical fitness, weight management, and clinical care. The appendices and glossary are extremely helpful.

UNIT 6

Clark J, Queener S, and Karb V: *Pharmacological Basis of Nursing Practice*, 2nd ed., 1986. St. Louis: C.V. Mosby. Revised text presents the concepts of pharmacology, information on drug classifications, and client care implications of drug groups.

Govoni L, Hayes J: *Drugs and Nursing Implications*, 5th ed., 1988. Norwalk, Conn.: Appleton & Lange. Text presents precise information to assist the professional nurse in the important responsibility related to medication administration and education. Nursing implications are clearly identified.

Hahn A, Barkin S: *Pharmacology in Nursing*, 17th ed., 1988. St. Louis: C.V. Mosby. Excellent comprehensive text featuring principles of pharmacology and a unit on the nursing process and pharmacology. The second section of the book focuses on clinical aspects of pharmacology. Nursing considerations are clearly identified.

Shlafer M, Marieb E: *The Nurse, Pharmacology and Drug Therapy*, 1989. Redwood City, California: Addison-Wesley. To make it feasible to learn so many drugs, this text focuses on prototype drugs as representative of their class or the drug most commonly used. Integrated throughout each chapter are nursing implications, including special sections on the elderly, children, and drug therapy during pregnancy and lactation. Each chapter ends with a nursing process summary.

UNIT 7

Brunner L, Suddarth D: *The Lippincott Manual of Nursing Practice*, 4th ed., 1986. Philadelphia: J.B. Lippincott. Comprehensive manual dealing with nursing interventions of adults, new families and children. The text utilizes the nursing process to present information. It includes a brief description of the health problem, diagnostic tests used to confirm the problem, and excellent rationales for care.

Kozier B, Erb G: *Fundamentals of Nursing Concepts and Procedures*, 4th ed., 1991. Redwood City, California: Addison-Wesley. Excellent text featuring the nursing process, information about nursing as a profession, and indepth material regarding procedures. Rationales for specific intervention provide the student with understanding of the basic principles utilized. The classic introductory text.

Kozier B, Erb G: *Techniques in Clinical Nursing*, 1989. Redwood City, California: Addison-Wesley. Describes nursing actions pre, during, and post procedures. Identifies critical elements for procedures. Discusses home care adaptations. Many pictures and diagrams.

Perry A, Potter P: *Clinical Nursing Skills and Techniques*, 1986. St. Louis: C.V. Mosby. Text contains many chapters organized by broad subject material and the skills necessary to accomplish the intervention planned.

Potter P, Perry A: *Fundamentals of Nursing Concepts, Process and Practice*, 2nd ed., 1988. St. Louis: C.V. Mosby. A basic textbook for the beginning nursing student. A major portion of the text is devoted to skills essential to nursing practice.

UNIT 8

American Nurses Association: *Code for Nurses,* 1985. Kansas City, Missouri.

American Nurses Association: *Standards of Nursing Practice,* 1973, Kansas City, Missouri.

Creighton, H.: *Law Every Nurse Should Know,* 1986. Philadelphia: W. B. Saunders.

International Council of Nurses: *ICN Code for Nurses: Ethical Concepts Applied to Nursing,* 1973, Geneva.

National Commission for the Study of Nursing and Nursing Education: "Summary Report and Recommendations," in Jerome Lysaught: *Action in Nursing: Progress in Professional Purpose,* 1974. New York: McGraw-Hill.

Index